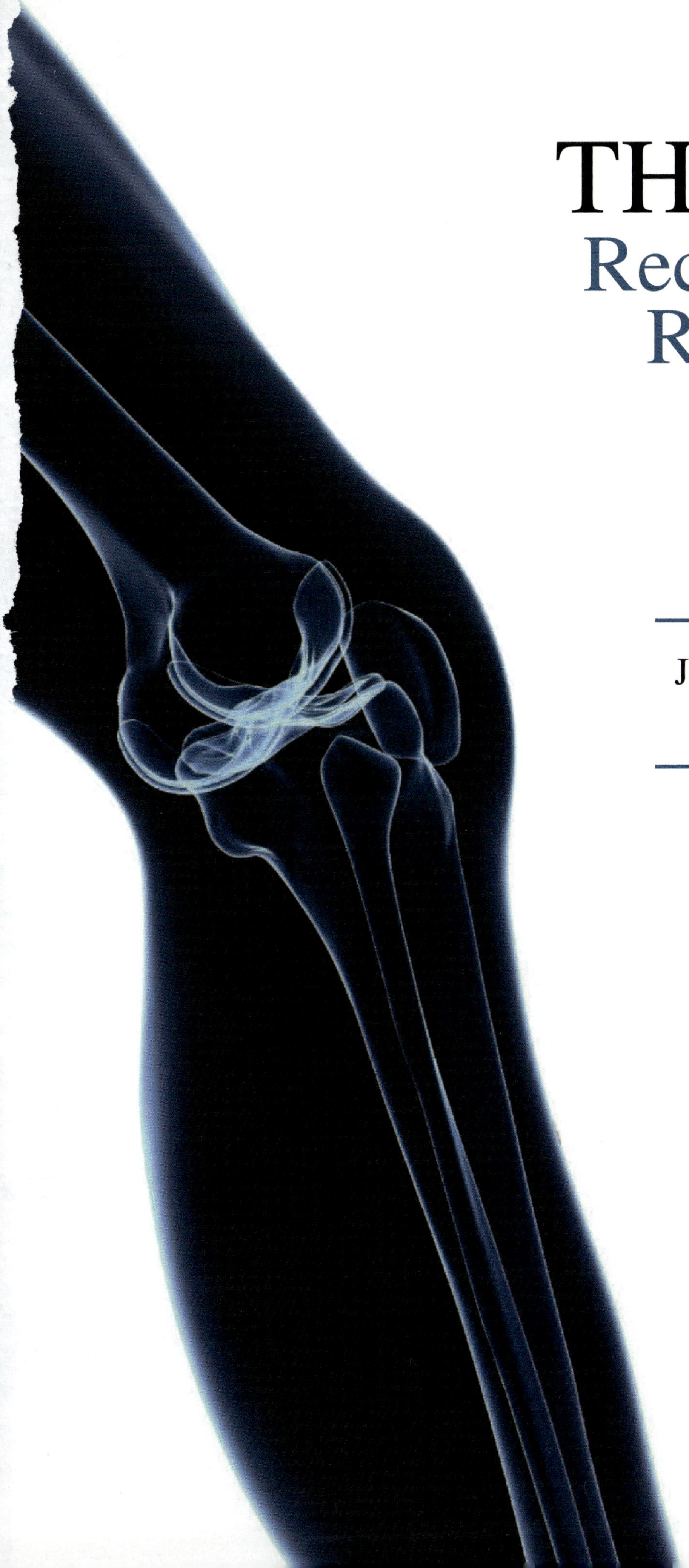

THE KNEE
Reconstruction Replacement and Revision

Volume 1

Javad Parvizi, MD, FRCS
Editor

Section Editors:

James Cashman, MD
Nitin Goyal, MD
Matthew Morrey, MD
Camilo Restrepo, MD

dtp data trace
PUBLISHING COMPANY

Printed in the United States of America

Published by
Data Trace Publishing Company
P.O. Box 1239
Brooklandville, Maryland 21022-9978
410-494-4994 Fax: 410-494-0515

ISBN 978-1-57400-139-6

Care has been taken to confirm the accuracy of the information presented and to describe generally accepted practices. However, the authors, editors, and publisher are not responsible for errors or omissions or for any consequences from application of the information in this book and make no warranty, expressed or implied, with respect to the currency, completeness, or accuracy of the contents of the publication.

Application of this information in a particular situation remains the professional responsibility of the practitioner. The authors, editors, and publisher have exerted every effort to ensure that procedures set forth in this text are in accordance with current recommendations and practice at the time of publication. However, in view of ongoing research, changes in government regulations, and the constant flow of information relating to medical advances, the reader is urged to check device manufacturers' instructions for use for any device and keep abreast of new research regarding the orthopaedic treatment of the knee.

Library of Congress Cataloging-in-Publication Data

The knee : reconstruction, replacement, and revision / Javad Parvizi, editor.
p. ; cm.
Includes bibliographical references and index.
ISBN 978-1-57400-139-6
I. Parvizi, Javad.
[DNLM: 1. Knee--surgery. 2. Anterior Cruciate Ligament Reconstruction. 3. Arthroplasty, Replacement, Knee. 4. Knee Prosthesis. 5. Osteoarthritis, Knee. 6. Reoperation--methods. WE 870]

617.5'84--dc23

2012022975

THE KNEE
Reconstruction Replacement and Revision

Volume 1

Javad Parvizi, MD, FRCS
Editor

Section Editors

James Cashman, MD
Nitin Goyal, MD
Matthew Morrey, MD
Camilo Restrepo, MD

Editor

Javad Parvizi, MD, FRCS
Professor of Orthopaedic Surgery
Rothman Institute
Thomas Jefferson University Hospital
Philadelphia, Pennsylvania

Section Editors

James P. Cashman, MD
Arthroplasty Fellow
Rothman Institute
Philadelphia, Pennsylvania

Nitin Goyal, MD
Arthroplasty Surgeon
Anderson Orthopaedic Clinic
Alexandria, Virginia

Matthew C. Morrey, MD, MS
Assistant Professor of Orthopedic Surgery
Department of Orthopedic Surgery
University of Texas Health Science Center
San Antonio, Texas

Camilo Restrepo, MD
Joint Research Fellow
Rothman Institute
Philadelphia, Pennsylvania

Contributors

Matthew P. Abdel, MD, MS
Assistant Professor of Orthopedic Surgery
Department of Orthopedic Surgery
Mayo Clinic
Rochester, Minnesota

Kelsey Adair, BS
Research Associate
Joint Preservation Institute
Sacramento, California

Vinay Aggarwal, BS
Joint Reconstruction Research Fellow
Rothman Institute of Orthopaedics
Philadelphia, Pennsylvania

Joseph F. Alderete, Jr., MD
Major, Medical Corps
Chief, Orthopaedic Oncology Service
Consultant, Center for the Intrepid Amputee Care
Associate Program Director, Orthopaedic Surgery Residency
San Antonio Military Medical Center
San Antonio, Texas

Ahmed Alghamdi, MD, FRCSC
Clinical Fellow, Adult Reconstruction
MSc Candidate
Biomedical Science and Clinical Research
Department of Orthopaedic Surgery
Université de Montréal
Montreal, Quebec, Canada

Carles Amat, MD
Septic and Reconstructive Surgery Unit
Department of Orthopaedic Surgery
Hospital Universitario Vall d´Hebron
Barcelona, Spain

Paweł Ambroziak, MD
Clinic of Orthopedic Surgery and Traumatology
Central Clinical Hospital of the Ministry of the Interior and Administration
Warsaw, Poland

Jean-Noel Argenson, MD, PhD
Aix-Marseille University
Department of Orthopedic Surgery
Institute for Locomotion
Hospital Sainte-Marguerite
Marseille, France

Matt Austin, MD
Associate Professor of Orthopaedic Surgery
Rothman Institute
Thomas Jefferson University Hospital
Philadelphia, Pennsylvania

David Backstein, MD, MEd, FRCSC
Associate Professor, Surgery
Division Head Orthopaedic Surgery
Mount Sinai Hospital
Toronto, Ontario, Canada
Medical Director
Mount Sinai MSK Centre of Excellence
Toronto, Ontario, Canada

Dae-Kyung Bae, MD, PhD
Professor
Department of Orthopaedic Surgery
Kyung Hee University Hospital
Seoul, South Korea

Jean Bahebeck, MD
Consultant Orthopaedic Surgeon
University Hospitals of Yaounde
Cameroon
Associated Professor of Orthopaedics
Faculty of Medicine
University of Yaounde
Cameroon

Yaron Bar Ziv, MD
Division of Arthroplasty
Orthopedic Department
Assaf Harofeh Medical Centre
Zerrifin, Israel

Jaime L. Baratta, MD
Clinical Assistant Professor
Department of Anesthesiology
Jefferson Medical College
Philadelphia, Pennsylvania

Robert L. Barrack, MD
Charles F. and Joanne Knight Distinguished Professor
Chief of Service
Department of Orthopaedic Surgery
Washington University School of Medicine
Saint Louis, Missouri

Thomas W. Bauer, MD, PhD
Departments of Pathology
Orthopedic Surgery and The Spine Center
The Cleveland Clinic Foundation
Cleveland, Ohio

Peter M. Bonutti, MD
Bonutti Clinic
Effingham, Illinois
Associate Clinical Professor
University of Arkansas
Little Rock, Arkansas

Robert E. Booth, Jr., MD
Chief of Orthopaedic Surgery
University of Pennsylvania Health System
Pennsylvania Hospital
Philadelphia, Pennsylvania

Kevin J. Bozic, MD, MBA
Associate Professor and Vice Chair
University of California
San Francisco, California
Department of Orthopaedic Surgery
Core Faculty
Philip R. Lee Institute for Health Policy Studies
San Francisco, California

Elena M. Brach del Prever, MD
Department of Traumatology
Orthopaedics and Health Medicine
University of Turin
Turin, Italy

R. Stephen J. Burnett, MD, FRCS(C), Dipl ABOS
Division of Orthopaedic Surgery
Adult Reconstructive Surgery of the Hip & Knee
Vancouver Island Health
South Island University of British Columbia
Island Medical School Royal Jubilee Hospital
Victoria, British Columbia, Canada

Cathy Buyea, MD
State University of New York at Buffalo
Department of Orthopaedic Surgery
Buffalo, New York

Tyler Cannon, MD
Resident Physician
Campbell Clinic Orthopaedics
University of Tennessee
Memphis, Tennessee

Antonia F. Chen, MD, MBA
University of Pittsburgh
Pittsburgh, Pennsylvania

Jiying Chen, MD
Professor in Orthopedics
Chief, Division of Arthroplasty
Vice Chair, Orthopedic Hospital
PLA General Hospital
Beijing, China

Naga Suresh Prasad Reddy Cheppalli, MD
Fellow
Adult Reconstruction
Virginia Commonwealth University
Richmond, Virginia

Kye-Youl Cho, MD
Clinical Instructor
Department of Orthopaedic Surgery
Center for Joint Diseases & Rheumatism
Kyung Hee University Hospital at Gangdong
Seoul, South Korea

Michael G. Ciccotti, MD
Professor of Orthopaedic Surgery
Chief, Division of Sports Medicine
Director, Orthopaedic Sports Medicine Fellowship
Rothman Institute
Thomas Jefferson University Hospital
Philadelphia, Pennsylvania
Head Team Physician
Philadelphia Phillies Baseball
Philadelphia, Pennsylvania

Janet D. Conway, MD
Head of Bone and Joint Infection
International Center for Limb Lengthening
Rubin Institute for Advanced Orthopedics
Sinai Hospital of Baltimore
Baltimore, Maryland

Pablo Corona, MD
Septic and Reconstructive Surgery Unit
Department of Orthopaedic Surgery
Hospital Universitario Vall d'Hebron
Barcelona, Spain

Luigi Costa, PhD
Chemistry Department
Torino University
Torino, Italy

Michael B. Cross, MD
Hospital for Special Surgery
Department of Adult Reconstruction and Joint Replacement
New York, New York

Emmet Cullen, MD
Orthopaedic Specialist Registrar
Department of Trauma and Orthopaedics
Midland Regional Hospital Tullamore
County Offaly, Ireland

Carl Deirmengian, MD
Assistant Professor of Surgery
Department of Orthopaedic Surgery
Jefferson Medical College
Lankenau Institute for Medical Research
Wynnewood, Pennsylvania

Gregory K. Deirmengian, MD
Assistant Professor of Orthopaedic Surgery
Rothman Institute of Orthopaedics
Thomas Jefferson University Medical School
Philadelphia, Pennsylvania

Craig J. Della Valle, MD
Associate Professor of Orthopaedic Surgery
Rush University Medical Center
Chicago, Illinois

Douglas A. Dennis, MD
Colorado Joint Replacement
Adjunct Associate Professor of Bioengineering
Department of Mechanical and Materials Engineering,
University of Denver
Clinical Co-Director
Rocky Mountain Musculoskeletal Research Laboratory
Denver, Colorado
Adjunct Professor, Department of Biomedical Engineering
University of Tennessee
Knoxville, Tennessee
Assistant Clinical Professor
University of Colorado Health Sciences Center
Denver, Colorado

Claudio Diaz, MD
Joint Reconstruction Research Fellow
Rothman Institute of Orthopaedics
Philadelphia, Pennsylvania

Florian F. Dibra, MD
Thomas Jefferson University Hospital
PGY-1, Internal Medicine
Philadelphia, Pennsylvania

Paul DiMuzio, MD
William M. Measey Professor of Surgery
Director, Division of Vascular and Endovascular Surgery
Thomas Jefferson University Hospital
Philadelphia, Pennsylvania

Christopher C. Dodson, MD
Assistant Professor of Orthopaedic Surgery
Thomas Jefferson Medical College
Attending Surgeon, Sports Medicine Division
Rothman Institute
Philadelphia, Pennsylvania

Christina Dorey, BS
Universal Research Solutions, LLC
Columbia, Missouri

Michael Dragone
Pre-Med
Franklin and Marshall University
Lancaster, Pennsylvania

Michael J. Dunbar, MD, FRCSC, PhD
Division of Orthopaedics
Dalhousie University
Halifax, Nova Scotia, Canada

Kenneth A. Egol, MD
Professor and Vice Chairman
Department of Orthopaedic Surgery
NYU Hospital for Joint Diseases
New York, New York

Joshua Eisenberg, MD
Assistant Professor of Surgery
Division of Vascular and Endovascular Surgery
Thomas Jefferson University Hospital
Philadelphia, Pennsylvania

Gerard A. Engh, MD
Anderson Orthopaedic Clinic
Alexandria, Virginia

Aidin Eslam Pour, MD
Orthopaedic Surgeon
Adult Reconstruction Fellow
Department of Orthopaedic Surgery
Emory University
Atlanta, Georgia

Chris S. Estes, DO
Banner Good Samaritan Orthopaedic Residency
Banner Good Samaritan Medical Center
Phoenix, Arizona

Nicholas J. Farber, BS
University of Pittsburgh Medical School
Pittsburgh, Pennsylvania

Sarah Fernandez, MD
Chief Resident
General Surgery
Thomas Jefferson University Hospital
Philadelphia, Pennsylvania

Steven J. Fitzgerald, MD
Assistant Professor
Adult Reconstruction and Joint Replacement
Department of Orthopaedic Surgery
University Hospitals
Case Medical Center
Case Western Reserve University
Cleveland, Ohio

Xavier Flores, MD
Chief of Septic and Reconstructive Surgery Unit
Department of Orthopaedic Surgery
Hospital Universitario Vall d'Hebron
Barcelona, Spain

James Fountain, MB ChB, FRCS (Tr & Orth)
Cavendish Hip Fellow
Sheffield Teaching Hospitals Trust
Sheffield, England

Kevin Fricka, MD
Clinical Instructor
Adult Reconstruction Fellowship
Anderson Orthopaedic Clinic
Alexandria, Virginia

Daniel Fritschy, MD
Head of the Ambulatory Orthopaedic Unit
University Hospital of Geneva
Geneva, Switzerland

Bruno Fuchs, MD, PhD
Professor of Skeletal Tumor Surgery and Head of the Laboratory of Orthopaedic Research
Department of Orthopaedic Surgery
Balgrist University Hospital
University of Zurich
Zurich, Switzerland

Kishor Gandhi, MD, MPH
Director, Regional Anesthesia
Assistant Professor
Department of Anesthesiology
Jefferson Medical College
Philadelphia, Pennsylvania

Sean Garvin, MD
Clinical Assistant Professor of Anesthesiology
Weill Cornell Medical College
New York, New York
Assistant Attending Anesthesiologist
Hospital for Special Surgery
New York, New York

Dustin Gay, MD
Meadows Regional Medical Center
Department of Orthopedics
Vidalia, Georgia

Thorsten Gehrke, MD
ENDO Klinik Hamburg
Hamburg, Germany

Daniel T. Goldstein, MD
Department of Orthopaedic Surgery
Albert Einstein Medical Center
Philadelphia, Pennsylvania

Andreas H. Gomoll, MD
Assistant Professor of Orthopaedic Surgery
Harvard Medical School
Cambridge, Massachusetts
Cartilage Repair Center
Department of Orthopaedic Surgery
Brigham and Women's Hospital
Boston, Massachusetts

Allan E. Gross, MD, FRCSC
Associate Professor
University of Toronto
Division of Arthroplasty
Orthopaedic Department
Mount Sinai Hospital
Toronto, Ontario, Canada

Steven C. Gross, MD
Resident
Department of Orthopaedic Surgery
NYU Hospital for Joint Diseases
New York, New York

Shane Guerin, MB, BCh, BAO, MCh, MEng, FRCS (Tr & Orth)
Division of Orthopaedics
Dalhousie University
Halifax, Nova Scotia, Canada

Ernesto Guerra, MD
Septic and Reconstructive Surgery Unit
Department of Orthopaedic Surgery
Hospital Universitario Vall d´Hebron
Barcelona, Spain

Christina Gutowski, MD, MPH
Orthopaedic Surgery Resident
Thomas Jefferson University Hospital
Philadelphia, Pennsylvania

Steven B. Haas, MD
Hospital for Special Surgery
Department of Adult Reconstruction and Joint Replacement
New York, New York

William G. Hamilton, MD
Anderson Orthopaedic Clinic
Alexandria, Virginia

Erik N. Hansen, MD
Clinical Fellow
Adult Reconstruction
Rothman Institute
Thomas Jefferson University Hospital
Philadelphia, Pennsylvania

Arlen D. Hanssen, MD
Professor
Department of Orthopedic Surgery
Mayo Clinic College of Medicine
Rochester, Minnesota

Curtis W. Hartman, MD
Assistant Professor
Department of Orthopaedic Surgery and Rehabilitation
University of Nebraska Medical Center
Omaha, Nebraska

James B. Hept, MBA
Primary Knee Group Product Manager
Stryker Orthopaedics
Mahwah, New Jersey

Florian Hess, MD
Department of Orthopaedic Surgery
Balgrist University Hospital
University of Zurich
Zurich, Switzerland

Carlos A. Higuera, MD
Orthopaedic Surgery Clinical Fellow
Adult Reconstruction
Rothman Institute
Thomas Jefferson University Hospital
Philadelphia, Pennsylvania

Pierre Hoffmeyer, MD
Professor of Orthopaedic Surgery
Chief, Division of Orthopaedic Surgery and Musculoskeletal Traumatology
University Hospital of Geneva
Geneva, Switzerland
Chair, Department of Surgery
Faculty of Medicine
University of Geneva
Geneva, Switzerland

Stephen M. Howell, MD
Professor of Mechanical Engineering
Member of Biomedical Graduate Group
University California at Davis
Davis, California
Orthopedic Surgeon
Private Practice
Methodist Hospital
Sacramento, California

William J. Hozack, MD
Professor
Orthopaedic Surgery
Rothman Institute
Thomas Jefferson University Hospital
Philadelphia, Pennsylvania

Thomas Huff, MD
Assistant Professor
Adult Reconstruction
Hip and Knee Surgery
Department of Orthopaedics and Rehabilitation
Oregon Health and Sciences University
Portland, Oregon

Ali Hussam, PhD
CEO
Universal Research Solutions, LLC
Columbia, Missouri

Amir A. Jamali, MD
Clinical Associate Professor of Orthopaedics
UC Davis Medical Center
Department of Orthopaedics
Medical Director
Joint Preservation Institute
Sacramento, California

Aaron J. Johnson, MD, MS
Rubin Institute for Advanced Orthopedics
Center for Joint Preservation and Reconstruction
Sinai Hospital of Baltimore
Baltimore, Maryland

Christopher Jones, MB, BS, FRACS
Division of Orthopaedics
Dalhousie University
Halifax, Nova Scotia, Canada

Gareth G. Jones, BSc (Hons), MB BS (Lon), MRCS (Eng)
Specialist Registrar in Trauma and Orthopaedics
Imperial College Healthcare
Academic Health Science Centre
Imperial College
London, United Kingdom

Bhaveen H. Kapadia, MD
Rubin Institute for Advanced Orthopedics
Center for Joint Preservation and Reconstruction
Sinai Hospital of Baltimore
Baltimore, Maryland

Joseph A. Karam, MD
Joint Research Fellow
Department of Orthopaedic Research
Rothman Institute
Thomas Jefferson University Hospital
Philadelphia, Pennsylvania

Eoin C. Kavanagh, MD
Department of Radiology
Mater Misericordiae Hospital
Dublin, Ireland
Faculty of Radiology
Royal College of Surgeons in Ireland
Dublin, Ireland

Daniel Kendoff, MD
ENDO Klinik Hamburg
Hamburg, Germany

Barry E. Kenneally, MD
Sports Medicine Specialist
Rothman Orthopaedic Institute
Philadelphia, Pennsylvania

James F. Kennedy, MB, BCh, BAO, BEng, MCh
Specialist Registrar Trauma and Orthopaedic Surgery
Irish Higher Surgical Training Program
Dublin, Ireland

Robert M. Kenyon, MB, BCh, BAO
Department of Orthopaedics
Mater Misericordiae University Hospital
Dublin, Ireland
Cappagh National Orthopaedic Hospital
Dublin, Ireland

Constantinos Ketonis, MD, PhD
Orthopaedic Surgery Resident
Rothman Institute
Department of Orthopaedic Surgery
Thomas Jefferson University Hospital
Philadelphia, Pennsylvania

David Hyung Kim, MD
Attending Anesthesiologist
Hospital for Special Surgery
Clinical Instructor in Anesthesiology
Weill Cornell Medical College
New York, New York

Kang-Il Kim, MD, PhD
Professor and Chairmen
Department of Orthopaedic Surgery
Center for Joint Diseases and Rheumatism
Kyung Hee University Hospital
Gangdong, Seoul, South Korea

Raymond H. Kim, MD
Colorado Joint Replacement
Adjunct Associate Professor of Bioengineering
Department of Mechanical and Materials Engineering
University of Denver
Clinical Co-Director
Rocky Mountain Musculoskeletal Research Laboratory
Denver, Colorado

Yair Kissin, MD, FAAOS
Clinical Attending
Department of Orthopedic Surgery and Sports Medicine
Insall Scott Kelly Institute of Orthopaedic Surgery and Sports Medicine
Hackensack University Medical Center
Hackensack, New Jersey

Brian A. Klatt, MD
Assistant Professor
Joint Reconstruction
University of Pittsburgh
Physicians Department of Orthopaedic Surgery
Pittsburgh, Pennsylvania

Gregg R. Klein, MD
Vice-Chairman
Department of Orthopaedic Surgery
Hackensack University Medical Center
Hackensack, New Jersey

Yona Kosashvili, MD, MHA
Assistant Professor
University of Tel Aviv
Division of Arthroplasty
Orthopedic Department Beilinson Campus
Rabin Medical Centre
Petach Tikva, Israel

Andrzej Kotela, MD
Clinic of Orthopedic Surgery and Traumatology
Central Clinical Hospital of the Ministry of the Interior and Administration
Warsaw, Poland

Ireneusz Kotela, MD, PhD
Professor of Orthopedic Surgery
Clinic of Orthopedic Surgery and Traumatology
Central Clinical Hospital of the Ministry of the Interior and Administration
Warsaw, Poland
Department of Physiotherapy
Jan Kochanowski University of Humanities and Sciences
Kielce, Poland

Kenneth A. Krackow, MD
Professor and Vice Chairman
Department of Orthopaedic Surgery
State University of New York at Buffalo
Buffalo, New York
Clinical Director
Department of Orthopaedic Surgery
Kaleida Health
Buffalo, New York

Jacek Kruczyński, MD
Professor of Orthopaedics
Department of Orthopaedics
Poznan University of Medical Sciences
Poznan, Poland

James C. Kudrna, MD, PhD
Associate Clinical Professor
University of Chicago
Pritzker School of Medicine
Division of Orthopaedic Surgery
Chicago, Illinois

Gwo-Chin Lee, MD
Assistant Professor
Department of Orthopaedic Surgery
University of Pennsylvania
Philadelphia, Pennsylvania

Sang Hak Lee, MD, PhD
Assistant Professor in Orthopaedic Surgery
Center for Joint Diseases and Rheumatism
Kyung Hee University Hospital at Gangdong
Seoul, South Korea

Jess H. Lonner, MD
Attending Orthopaedic Surgeon
Rothman Institute
Bryn Mawr Hospital
Philadelphia, Pennsylvania
Associate Professor
Department of Orthopaedic Surgery
Thomas Jefferson University
Philadelphia, Pennsylvania

Anne Lubbeke, MD, DsC
Division of Orthopaedics and Trauma Surgery
Geneva University Hospitals
Geneva, Switzerland

Tad M. Mabry, MD
Assistant Professor of Orthopedics
Department of Orthopedic Surgery
Mayo Clinic
Rochester, Minnesota

Steven J. MacDonald, MD, FRCSC
Chief of Surgery
London Health Sciences Centre
University Hospital
London, Ontario, Canada

Junaid Makda, MD
Dupage Orthopedics
Bloomingdale, Illinois

Henrik Malchau, MD, PhD
Professor
Harvard Medical School
Co-Director
The Harris Orthopaedic Laboratory
Vice Chief of Orthopedics (Research)
Attending Physician
Adult Rcconstructive Unit
Orthopedic Department
Massachusetts General Hospital
Boston, Massachusetts

Paweł Małdyk, MD
Professor of Surgery and Head
Rheumoortopaedic Department
Institute of Rheumatology
Warsaw, Poland

Gregary D. Marhefka, MD, FACC
Assistant Professor of Medicine
Associate Director of Coronary Care Unit
Jefferson Medical College
Thomas Jefferson University Hospital
Philadelphia, Pennsylvania

Marta Massada, MD
Department of Orthopaedics
Centro Hospitalar do Porto–Hospital Santo António
Oporto, Portugal

Laura Matsen Ko, MD
Resident
Department of Orthopaedics and Rehabilitation
Oregon Health and Sciences University
Portland, Oregon

Andreas F. Mavrogenis, MD, PhD
First Department of Orthopaedics
Athens University Medical School
Attikon University Hospital
Athens, Greece

David J. Mayman, MD
Hospital for Special Surgery
Department of Adult Reconstruction and Joint Replacement
New York, New York

Alex C. McLaren, MD
Assistant Professor of Clinical Orthopaedic Surgery
University of Arizona College of Medicine
Phoenix, Arizona
Program Director
Banner Good Samaritan Orthopaedic Residency
Phoenix, Arizona

Ryan McLemore, PhD
Orthopaedic Research Specialist
Banner Good Samaritan Orthopaedic Residency
Phoenix, Arizona
Adjunct Professor
Bioengineering Department
Arizona State University
Phoenix, Arizona

Morteza Meftah, MD
Hospital for Special Surgery
New York, New York

Geno J. Merli, MD
Chief Medical Officer and Senior Vice President
Hospital Administration
Thomas Jefferson University Hospital
Philadelphia, Pennsylvania

William M. Mihalko, MD, PhD
Campbell Clinic Orthopaedics
Professor and JR Hyde Chair
Department of Orthopaedic Surgery and Biomedical Engineering
University of Tennessee
Memphis, Tennessee

Amer Mirza, MD
Assistant Professor
Orthopaedic Trauma
Department of Orthopaedics and Rehabilitation
Oregon Health and Sciences University
Portland, Oregon

Reza Jamei Moayedi, MD
Resident of Orthopaedic Surgery
Department of Knee Surgery
Shafa Rehabilitation and Orthopaedic Hospital
Tehran University of Medical Science
Tehran, Iran

Michael A. Mont, MD
Co-Director
Rubin Institute for Advanced Orthopedics
Center for Joint Preservation and Reconstruction
Sinai Hospital of Baltimore
Baltimore, Maryland
Associate Professor
Department of Orthopaedic Surgery
The Johns Hopkins Medical Institutions
Baltimore, Maryland

Bernard F. Morrey, MD
Professor of Orthopedic Surgery
Mayo Graduate School of Medicine and University of Texas Health Science Center
San Antonio, Texas

Mark E. Morrey, MD, MS
Assistant Professor of Orthopedic Surgery
Department of Orthopedic Surgery
Mayo Clinic
Rochester, Minnesota

Brian D. Murphy, MD
Department of Radiology
Mater Misericordiae Hospital
Dublin, Ireland
Faculty of Radiology
Royal College of Surgeons in Ireland
Dublin, Ireland

Trevor G. Murray, MD
Department of Orthopaedic Surgery
Adult Reconstruction Section
Cleveland Clinic
Cleveland, Ohio

Syed Soulat Naim, MS, MCh, FRCS (Trauma & Orth)
Knee Fellow
Exeter Knee Reconstruction Unit
Princess Elizabeth Orthopaedic Centre
Royal Devon & Exeter NHS Trust
Exeter, United Kingdom

Denis Nam, MD
Hospital for Special Surgery
Department of Adult Reconstruction and Joint Replacement
New York, New York

Sam Nasser, MD, PhD
Professor
Department of Biomedical Engineering
Wayne State University College of Engineering
Detroit, Michigan
Clinical Professor
Department of Orthopaedic Surgery
Wayne State University School of Medicine
Detroit, Michigan
Professor of Orthopaedic Surgery
Oakland University
William Beaumont School of Medicine
Rochester, Michigan

Dinesh K. Nathwani, MBChB, MSc, FRCSI (Tr & Orth)
Consultant and Honorary Senior Lecturer
Department of Trauma & Orthopaedic Surgery
Imperial College Healthcare Trust
Academic Health Science Centre
Imperial College
London, United Kingdom

Douglas D. R. Naudie, MD, FRCSC
Associate Professor
Department of Surgery
Division of Orthopaedic Surgery Schulich School of Medicine and Dentistry
The University of Western Ontario Consultant Surgeon
Joint Replacement Institute
London Health Sciences Center
University Campus
London, Ontario, Canada

David G. Nazarian, MD
Clinical Assistant Professor of Orthopaedics
University of Pennsylvania Health System
Pennsylvania Hospital
Philadelphia, Pennsylvania

Qais Naziri, MD
Rubin Institute for Advanced Orthopedics
Center for Joint Preservation and Reconstruction
Sinai Hospital of Baltimore
Baltimore, Maryland

Vassilios S. Nikolaou, MD, PhD
Clinical Fellow in Lower Extremity Adult Reconstruction
Division of Orthopaedic Surgery
Mt. Sinai Hospital
Toronto, Ontario, Canada

John M. O'Byrne, MCh, FRCSI, FRCS (Orth), FFSEM, FFSEM (UK)
Consultant Orthopaedic Surgeon at Cappagh National Orthopaedic Hospital
Dublin, Ireland
The Mater Private Hospital
Dublin, Ireland
The Sport Surgery Clinic
Dublin, Ireland
Abraham Colles Professor of Trauma & Orthopaedic Surgery
Royal College of Surgeons in Ireland
Dublin, Ireland
Honorary Consultant Orthopaedic Surgeon to The Football Association of Ireland – Senior Soccer Team
Dublin, Ireland

Mary I. O'Connor, MD
Chair
Department of Orthopedic Surgery
Mayo Clinic
Jacksonville, Florida
Associate Professor
Mayo Clinic College of Medicine
Jacksonville, Florida

Ali Oliashirazi, MD, FAAOS
Chairman and Professor
Department of Orthopaedic Surgery
Marshall University School of Medicine
Huntington, West Virginia

Alvin Ong, MD
Atlanticare Regional Medical Center
Mainland/City Division, Pomona
Atlantic City, New Jersey
Thomas Jefferson University Hospital
Philadelphia, Pennsylvania
Betty Bacharach Rehabilitation Hospital
Pomona, New Jersey
Rothman Specialty Hospital
Bucks County, Pennsylvania
Kennedy Health Systems
Washington Township, New Jersey

Fabio Orozco, MD
Atlanticare Regional Medical Center
Mainland/City Division, Pomona
Atlantic City, New Jersey
Thomas Jefferson University Hospital
Philadelphia, Pennsylvania
Betty Bacharach Rehabilitation Hospital
Pomona, New Jersey
Rothman Specialty Hospital
Bucks County, Pennsylvania
Kennedy Health Systems
Washington Township, New Jersey

Michael R. Pagnotto, MD
Tri-State Orthopaedics & Sports Medicine, Inc.
Pittsburgh, Pennsylvania

Henrik Palm, MD
Orthopaedic Specialist
Copenhagen University
Hvidovre Hospital
Copenhagen, Denmark

Panayiotis J. Papagelopoulos, MD
Professor and Chairman
Department of Orthopaedics
Athens University Medical School and Attikon University General Hospital
Athens, Greece

Sebastien Parratte, MD, PhD
Aix-Marseille University
Department of Orthopedic Surgery
Institute for Locomotion
Hospital Sainte-Marguerite
Marseille, France

Sadegh Parvizi, PhD, CEng, MIM3
Principal Materials Technology Specialist
CB&I Lummus
London, United Kingdom

Vincent D. Pellegrini, Jr., MD
James L. Kernan Professor and Chair
Department of Orthopaedics
University of Maryland Medical Center
Baltimore, Maryland

Krushen Pillay, MS
Research Associate
Joint Preservation Institute
Sacramento, California

Danielle M. Pineda, MD
General Surgery Resident
Department of Surgery
Thomas Jefferson University Hospital
Philadelphia, Pennsylvania

Michael S. Pinzur, MD
Professor of Orthopaedic Surgery and Rehabilitation
Loyola University Medical Center
Maywood, Illinois

Manny Porat, MD
Adult Reconstruction Specialist
Reconstructive Orthopedics
Lumberton, New Jersey

Amar S. Ranawat, MD
Hospital for Special Surgery
New York, New York

Chitranjan S. Ranawat, MD
Hospital for Special Surgery
New York, New York

Atul Rao, MD
Assistant Professor of Surgery
Division of Vascular and Endovascular Surgery
Thomas Jefferson University Hospital
Philadelphia, Pennsylvania

Nalini Rao, MD, FACP, FSHEA, FIDSA
Chief
Division of Infectious Diseases
UPMC Shadyside Clinical Professor of Medicine and Orthopedics
University of Pittsburgh School of Medicine
Pittsburgh, Pennsylvania

Glen Richardson, MD, FRCSC
Division of Orthopaedics
Dalhousie University
Halifax, Nova Scotia, Canada

Michael D. Ries, MD
Professor and Chief of Arthroplasty
Department of Orthopaedic Surgery
University of California
San Francisco, California

Merrill A. Ritter, MD
Center for Hip & Knee Surgery
Mooresville, Indiana

Steve Rocha, MD
Consultant Hand Surgeon
Head, Research and Academics
Sancheti Institute of Orthopaedics and Rehabilitation
Maharashtra, India

Michael G. Rock, MD
Professor of Orthopedic Surgery
Mayo Clinic College of Medicine
Consultant
Department of Orthopedic Surgery
Mayo Clinic
Rochester, Minnesota

Carlo Luca Romano, MD
Director
Centro di Chirurgia Ricostruttiva e delle Infezioni Osteo-articolari
Istituto Ortopedico I.R.C.C.S. Galeazzi
Milano, Italy

Francine Touzard Romo, MD
Section of Infectious Diseases
Rush University Medical Center
Chicago, Illinois

Vasileios I. Sakellariou, MD, PhD
Postdoctoral Research Fellow, Orthopaedic Surgery
Biomechanics Lab
First Department of Orthopaedics
Attikon University Hospital
Athens, Greece

Jonathon Salava, MD
Resident
Department of Orthopaedic Surgery
Marshall University School of Medicine
Huntington, West Virginia

Meghan Sampson, BS
Research Associate
Joint Preservation Institute
Sacramento, California

Parag Sancheti, MD
Professor and Chairman
Department of Orthopaedics
Sancheti Institute of Orthopaedics and Rehabilitation
Maharashtra, India

Joaquin Sanchez-Sotelo, MD, PhD
Consultant and Associate Professor
Director
Shoulder and Elbow Fellowship Program
Mayo Clinic
Department of Orthopedic Surgery
Rochester, Minnesota

Arjun Saxena, MD
Anderson Orthopaedic Research Institute
Alexandria, Virginia

Adam J. Schwartz, MD
Assistant Professor of Orthopaedic Surgery
Mayo Clinic College of Medicin
Phoenix, Arizona

Giles R. Scuderi, MD
Director
Insall Scott Kelly Institute for Orthopedics and Sports Medicine
New York, New York
Vice President
Orthopedic Service Line
Northshore LIJ Health System
Long Island, New York

John Segreti, MD
Professor of Internal Medicine
Section of Infectious Diseases
Rush University Medical Center,
Chicago, Illinois

Ari Seidenstein, MD
Orthopaedic Surgeon
Hartzband Center for Hip & Knee Replacement
Paramus, New Jersey

Peter F. Sharkey, MD
Professor of Orthopaedic Surgery
Thomas Jefferson University Hospital
Riddle Memorial Hospital and the Rothman Institute
Media, Pennsylvania

Rajrishi Sharma, MD, FRCSC
Arthroplasty Fellow
London Health Sciences Centre
University Hospital
London, Ontario, Canada

Eoin Sheehan, FRCS(Orth) MD
Consultant Trauma & Orthopaedic Surgeon
Senior Clinical Lecturer University of Limerick
Honorary Research Fellow
Materials Research
Athlone Institute of Technology
Co. Offaly, Ireland

Neil P. Sheth, MD
Attending Orthopaedic Surgeon
Orthocarolina
Charlotte, North Carolina

M. Wade Shrader, MD, FAAP
Clinical Assistant Professor of Orthopaedic Surgery
University of Arizona College of Medicine
Phoenix, Arizona
Pediatric Orthopaedic Surgeon
Director of Research
Center for Pediatric Orthopaedic Surgery
Phoenix Children's Hospital
Phoenix, Arizona

Ashok Shyam, MD
Consultant
Orthopaedic Surgeon, and Chief Researcher
Sancheti Institute for Orthopaedic and Rehabilitation
Maharashtra, India

John Siemon
Medical Student
Drexel University College of Medicine, East Falls
Philadelphia, Pennsylvania

Rafael J. Sierra, MD
Associate Professor and Consultant
Fellowship Director Adult Reconstruction
Department of Orthopedic Surgery
Mayo Clinic
Mayo College of Medicine
Rochester, Minnesota

Franklin H. Sim, MD
Professor of Orthopedic Surgery
Mayo Clinic
Rochester, Minnesota

Gautam Siram, MD
Summit Orthopedics
Chevy Chase, Maryland

Iwona Słowińska, MD
Orthopaedic Surgeon
Rheumoortopaedic Department
Institute of Rheumatology
Warsaw, Poland

Eric B. Smith, MD
Assistant Professor of Orthopaedic Surgery
Rothman Institute
Thomas Jefferson University Hospital
Philadelphia, Pennsylvania

Sang Jun Song, MD, PhD
Associate Professor
Department of Orthopaedic Surgery
Kyung Hee University Hospital
Seoul, South Korea

Alex Soriano, MD, PhD
Senior Specialist
Department of Infectious Diseases
Hospital Clinic of Barcelona
Barcelona, Spain

Ricardo Sousa, MD
Department of Orthopaedics
Centro Hospitalar do Porto–Hospital Santo António
Oporto, Portugal

Mark J. Spangehl, MD, FRCS(C)
Assistant Professor of Orthopaedics
Department of Orthopaedics
Mayo Clinic Arizona
Phoenix, Arizona

Scott Sporer, MD, MS
Associate Professor
Orthopaedic Surgery
Rush University Medical Center
Chicago, Illinois

Bryan D. Springer, MD
Fellowship Director
OrthoCarolina Hip and Knee Center
Charlotte, North Carolina

Ian Stockley, MB, ChB, MD, FRCS
Professor and Consultant Orthopaedic Surgeon
Honorary Professor
Sheffield Teaching Hospitals NHS Trust
Sheffield, United Kingdom

Hasan M. Syed, MD
Assistant Professor
Sports Medicine
Loma Linda University
Department of Orthopaedic Surgery
Loma Linda, California

Keith A. Synnott, MB, BCh, BAO, FRCSI (Tr&Orth)
Consultant Orthopaedic Surgeon
Department of Orthopaedics
Mater Misericordiae University Hospital
Dublin, Ireland
Cappagh National Orthopaedic Hospital
Dublin, Ireland

Michael J. Taunton, MD
Clinical Instructor
Department of Orthopedic Surgery
Mayo Clinic College of Medicine
Rochester, Minnesota

Emmanuel Thienpont, MD, MBA
University Hospital Saint Luc
Brussels, Belgium

Nicholas T. Ting, MD
Resident Physician
Orthopaedic Surgery
Cleveland Clinic
Cleveland, Ohio

Andrew D. Toms, FRCS, MSc, FRCS (Trauma & Orth)
Consultant Orthopaedic Surgeon
Exeter Knee Reconstruction Unit
Princess Elizabeth Orthopaedic Centre
Royal Devon & Exeter NHS Trust
Exeter, United Kingdom

Alfred Tria, Jr., MD
Clinical Professor of Orthopaedics
Department of Orthopaedic Surgery
Robert Wood Johnson Medical School
New Brunswick, New Jersey
Chief of Orthopaedics
St. Peter's University Hospital
New Brunswick, New Jersey

Mohan S. Tripathi, MD
Jefferson Medical College
Thomas Jefferson University
Philadelphia, Pennsylvania

Joel A. Tucker, MD
Bienville Orthopaedic Specialists
Biloxi, Mississippi

Gary A. Tuma, MD, FACS
Director of Plastic Surgery Capital Health
Plastic Surgery Associates of New Jersey
Pennington, New Jersey

Miraude E.A.P.M. Adriaensen van Roij, MD, PhD
Radiologist
Atrium Medical Center
Parkstad Heerlen, The Netherlands

Edward M. Vasarhelyi, MD, MSc, FRCSC
Fellow
Department of Surgery
Division of Orthopaedic Surgery
Schulich School of Medicine and Dentistry
The University of Western Ontario Joint Replacement Institute
London Health Sciences Center
University Campus
London, Ontario, Canada

David N. Vegari, MD
Chief Resident
Orthopaedic Surgery
Rothman Institute
Thomas Jefferson University Hospital
Philadelphia, Pennsylvania

Joseph V. Vernace, MD
Instructor
Thomas Jefferson University
Philadelphia, Pennsylvania
Co-Director Joint Replacement Program
Bryn Mawr Hospital
Main Line Orthopaedics, PC
Bryn Mawr, Pennsylvania

Jan Victor, MD, PhD
Professor of Orthopedics
Ghent University
Chair of Department of Orthopedics and Traumatology
University Hospital Ghent
Ghent, Belgium

Eugene R. Viscusi, MD
Director
Acute Pain Management
Department of Anesthesiology
Jefferson Medical College
Philadelphia, Pennsylvania

Peter C. Vitanzo, Jr., MD
Sports Medicine Specialist
Director
Division Non-Surgical Sports Medicine
Rothman Orthopaedic Institute
Philadelphia, Pennsylvania

Torrance Walker, MD
Adult Reconstructive Surgery Fellow
Campbell Clinic Orthopaedics
University of Tennessee
Memphis, Tennessee

Yan Wang, MD
Professor in Orthopedics
Chairman 301 Orthopedic Hospital
PLA Hospital
President of Chinese Orthopedic Association (COA)
Beijing, China

Heinz Winkler, MD
Consultant Orthopaedic Surgeon
Osteitis Centre
Privatklinik Doebling
Vienna, Austria

Laura E. White, MD
Baptist Hospital of South Florida
Miami, Florida

Leo A. Whiteside, MD
Director
Missouri Bone and Joint Center
Director
Missouri Bone and Joint Research Foundation
St. Louis, Missouri

Anthony C. Wong, BsC
Hospital for Special Surgery
New York, New York

Justin C. Wong, MD
Resident
Thomas Jefferson University Hospital
Department of Orthopedic Surgery
Philadelphia, Pennsylvania

Andrea Wood, BS
Universal Research Solutions, LLC
Columbia, Missouri

Charlie C. Yang, MD
Colorado Joint Replacement
Denver, Colorado

Hamidreza Yazdi, MD
Assistant Professor of Orthopaedic Surgery
Department of Knee Surgery
Shafa Rehabilitation and Orthopaedic Hospital
Tehran University of Medical Science
Tehran, Iran

Piotr Żbikowski, MD
Clinic of Orthopedic Surgery and Traumatology
Central Clinical Hospital of the Ministry of the Interior and Administration
Warsaw, Poland

Dedications

To my many mentors and friends whose guidance and support has paved my professional journey. To my wife, Fariba, whose endless dedication, devotion, and love is the essential sustenance for my life. To my fun and loving children, Niosha and Cyrus. And, mostly, to my patients, who are my teachers and companions in the gratifying practice of orthopaedics.

Javad Parvizi

I wish to acknowledge the contribution of all who have supported me by training and development as an orthopaedic surgeon. I hope that this book will advance the knowledge of others, the way that working on this book has added to mine. I want to thank my wife, Fiona, for her help and patience through the years.

James Cashman

To my parents, Vinod and Radha Goyal, who instilled in me the values of education and continuous learning, as well as a love for reading. To my beautiful wife, Rachna, who makes me a better person each and every day and always reminds me of what is most important in life. Finally, to my mentor, Javad Parvizi, for teaching me to critically question each study and inspiring me to constantly search for questions left unanswered.

Nitin Goyal

To my parents, who have been supportive of all of my endeavors; To Dr. Parvizi for allowing me the opportunity to contribute to the field; To Audrey – without her love and support none of this could have ever been accomplished.

Matthew Morrey

To my wife, Lisa, and my son, Santiago, for their endless love and understanding. To Richard Rothman, MD, William Hozack, MD, and especially to Javad Parvizi, MD, who have helped pave this path in my career.

Camilo Restrepo

Preface

Performing total knee arthroplasty (TKA) is a relatively easy operation in the majority of patients. There are, however, patients for whom this procedure requires special attention to preoperative optimization (such as patients with bleeding disorders or vascular disease) or a special set of instruments or alterations in surgical techniques (such as patients with gross deformities or Paget's disease). There are also patients for whom the type of prosthesis may need to be altered to accommodate the anatomical aberration (such as patients with posttraumatic arthritis).

Despite its lauded success, TKA does occasionally fail, leading to a need for revision arthroplasty. Knowledge of how to prevent failures such as infection, periprosthetic fractures, and instability is critical for enhancing the success and longevity of TKA. The ability to deal with these complications, when they occur, and to perform reconstructive procedures in patients with failed TKA is also an essential part of training of any reconstructive joint surgeon.

The Knee: Reconstruction, Replacement, and Revision has been written with one and only one objective in mind. This book intends to contain relevant, practical, and important information related to disorders of the knee that a reconstruction surgeon needs to know. It is the practical manual for the practicing or training orthopaedic surgeon who treats patients with disorders of the knee. The book, written by hip and knee reconstruction experts from around the world, provides step-by-step practical guidance and relevant information for treatment of each knee disorder. There are numerous chapters on the basic fundamentals of knee surgery that aim to help surgeons prevent complications of TKA and optimize the outcome of this procedure. The nonreplacement joint preservation options for treatment are also provided whenever appropriate. Each chapter is richly illustrated by figures, diagrams, and tables to impart the important information visually whenever possible.

The section editors and I decided to write this book when we became aware of the vacuum in orthopaedics and the need for such a text. Numerous meetings were held to ensure that the text being written is comprehensive, reader friendly, and useful to the practicing orthopaedic surgeon. I owe a huge debt of gratitude to my section editors, Drs. Cashman, Goyal, Morrey, and Restrepo, for their invaluable assistance in putting this project together. They have been involved with every step of the project and weighed in on an almost daily basis to ensure success of this project. I am most grateful to all the authors, who despite their immense commitment, took on the task of writing a comprehensive, evidence-based, and illustrated text in such a short notice. Their wisdom, expertise, and commitment were simply spectacular.

Last, but not least, I want to thank Kimberly Collignon from Data Trace for her organizational skill and leadership of the project. We could have certainly not pulled this project through without her. I am also grateful to Herb Fried and other members of Data Trace for their commitment to this massive project and for executing it in such an expeditious manner.

Javad Parvizi, MD, FRCS

Foreword

The Knee: Reconstruction, Replacement, and Revision is a wonderful book that has been compiled expeditiously so as to be current and relevant. All chapters are written by international experts in the field, and these experts all have published experience with their topic. As such, the book focuses on evidence-based information. Chapters that cover classifications are all written by the authors who originally have described these classifications. A distinctive feature of this book is its comprehensive coverage of joint preservation procedures for knee arthritis. It also has comprehensive coverage of the pertinent basic science topics, such as metal hypersensitivity and the molecular basis for arthrofibrosis. The book is very richly illustrated and, when appropriate, the details of the surgical procedure are effectively described. Even the minutiae of topics are covered. There are a number of chapters on total knee arthroplasty in patients with peculiar yet not uncommon situations, such as cancer, bleeding disorders, Paget's disease, and extreme limb deformity. Congratulations to Javad Parvizi and the Section Editors who have accomplished this difficult task!

William Hozack, MD

The Knee: Reconstruction, Replacement, and Revision

SECTION ONE: ARTHROPLASTY FUNDAMENTALS

SECTION TWO: PREVENTION AND MANAGEMENT OF COMPLICATIONS

SECTION FIVE: REVISION KNEE ARTHROPLASTY

SECTION SIX: SALVAGE PROCEDURES

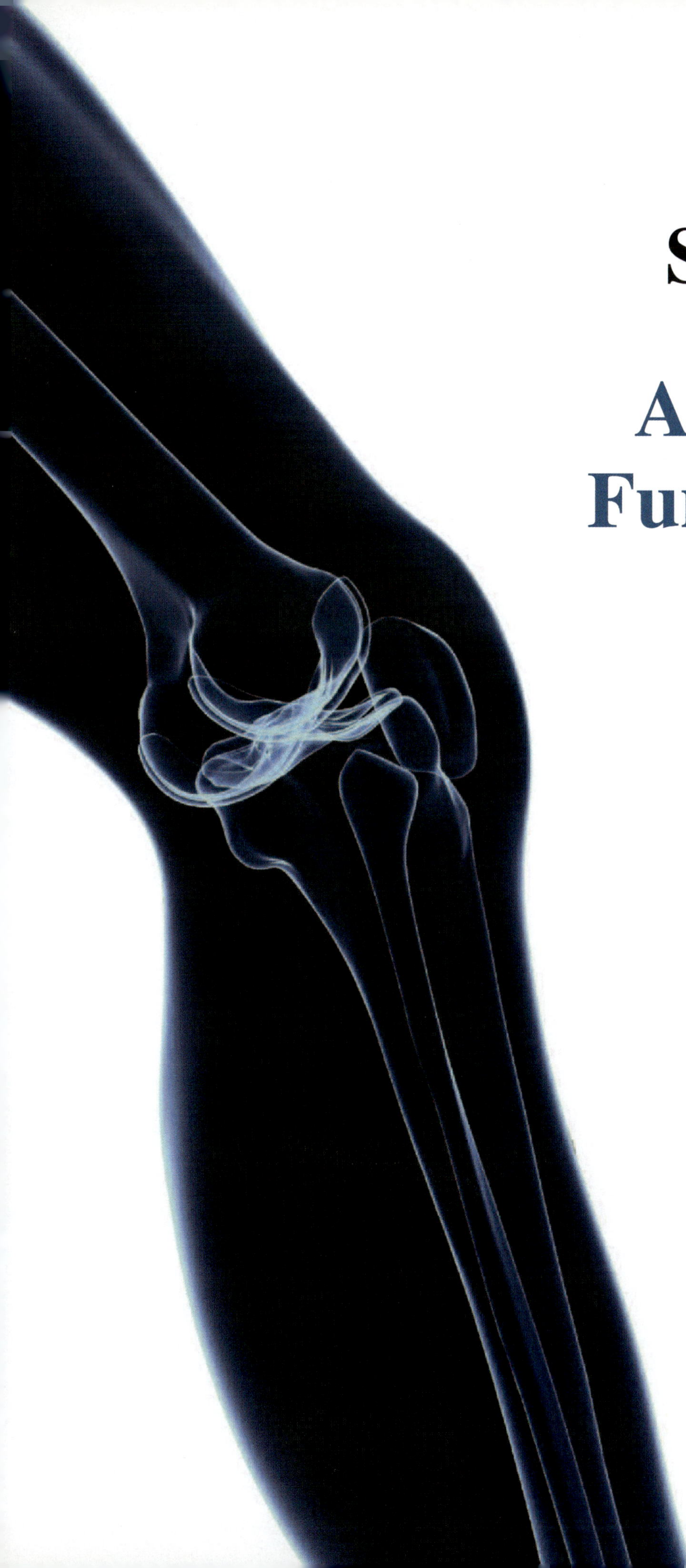

Section One

Arthroplasty Fundamentals

1

History of Knee Replacement

Bernard F. Morrey

Growing interest in the history of knee replacement has been evident from several recent reviews. Documentation of the history of knee joint replacement by Heaton and Dorr[1] and an interesting "modern history" focusing on individual surgeon contributions by Robinson[2] and others[1,3,4-6] have been helpful in developing this review.

A true history of knee joint replacement requires consideration of early efforts to reconstruction this joint. As with other procedures to alter joint pathology, most were functionally disabling salvage procedures: resection or fusion. Functionally restoring salvage operations appeared as some form of interposition arthroplasty, which eventually gave way to prosthetic replacements. Early efforts were custom hemi devices or linked implants, primarily employed for devastating bone loss, such as after trauma. The earliest replacements of both sides of the joint were linked hinged devices, and Shiers was one of the first to document the concept and results.[7] Once again, as with other joints, the early failures of these prosthetic implants were related to deficiencies in the understanding of the biomechanics of the joint and limitations in materials, instrumentation, and technique. In the knee, the major advance was understanding the mechanical axis and the gliding motion of the joint. Application of principles derived from biomechanical analysis led to the breakthrough concept of the unlinked total condylar implant.

Although there are a number of perspectives one might develop, this chapter first depicts the history of knee joint replacement based on the major philosophic approaches to the problem expressed over time (Table 1-1). The chapter then focuses on specific contributions to the development of prosthetic knee replacement as we know it today (Table 1-2).

THE PRECURSOR: RESECTION AND INTERPOSITION ARTHROPLASTY

Ferguson is given credit for the first knee resection arthroplasty performed in 1861.[22] This of course represents a nonfunctional salvage effort for an uncontrollable disease process. The other early "reconstructive" procedure was that of fusion. This also limited rather than restored function. The real forerunner of prosthetic replacement arthroplasty is that of interposition arthroplasty. In 1890, Gluck described a relatively large series of patients with ivory interposed between the distal femur and the proximal tibia.[23] Other tissues used in years past include fascia lata,[24] bursal tissue,[25] and fat along with fascia,[1] and these provide a colorful history for the first functional restoring salvage procedure at the knee. As expected, the biologic materials, such as fascia lata, bursa,[26] and skin,[27] have outperformed nonbiologic tissues, such as cellophane and nylon (Fig. 1-1).

As early as 1918, Henderson reported on a series of 43 interposition arthroplasties performed at the Mayo Clinic combined with 395 cases gathered from other centers.[28] Of the 438 cases, 126 (29%) involved the elbow and 117 (27%) involved the knee. The best results were of the temporomandibular joint, followed by the elbow and then the knee. Specifically, only 40% of the knees were considered good or fair at review.

TABLE 1-1. Phases of Knee Reconstruction

Period	Technique	Period	Status
Phase 1	Resection	1860	Remain as current salvage reconstruction options
	Fusion		
	Interposition	1880	
Phase 2	Hemireplacement Metallic	1940–1965	
Phase 3	Hinged replacement	1950–1970	
Phase 4	Unlinked, cemented	1970	Current
Phase 5	Multiple options of condylar replacement	1970 (see Table 1-2)	Current

TABLE 1-2. Evolution Subsequent to Total Condylar Device

Year[a]	Innovation/Issue	Author
1972	Total condylar replacement with patellar resurfacing	Insall,[8] Townley[9]
1972	Cruciate-sacrificing implant	Insall[10]
1973	Unireplacement	Marmor[11]
1976	Mobile bearing hemi	Goodfellow[12]
	Mobile bearing total	Buechel[13]
1978	Cruciate-substituting design	Walker,[14] Insall[8,15]
1979	Metal-backed tibial tray	Sledge,[16] Walker[14]
1980	Precise instrumentation/alignment	Whiteside,[17] Hungerford[18]
1980	Uncemented fixation	Hungerford[19]
1982	Modular implant	Bartell[20]
2000	Trabecular metal	Meneghini et al[21]
2000	Navigation/limited incision	

[a]Approximations.

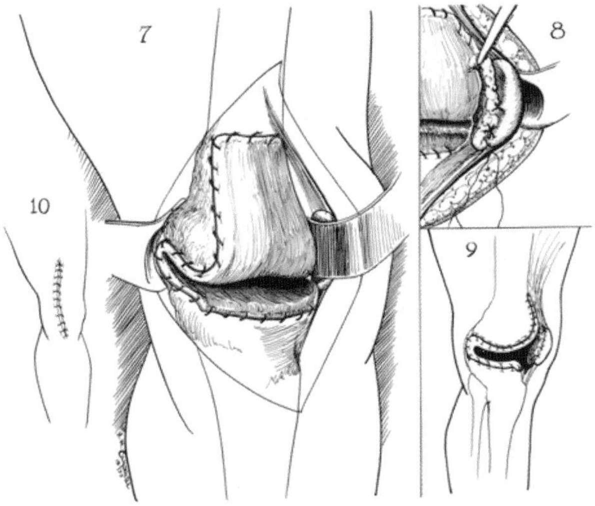

FIGURE 1-1. *Early reconstruction of the knee was the same form of interposition arthroplasty such as illustrated here and developed by Meyerding in 1939. (Reprinted with permission, Mayo Foundation)*

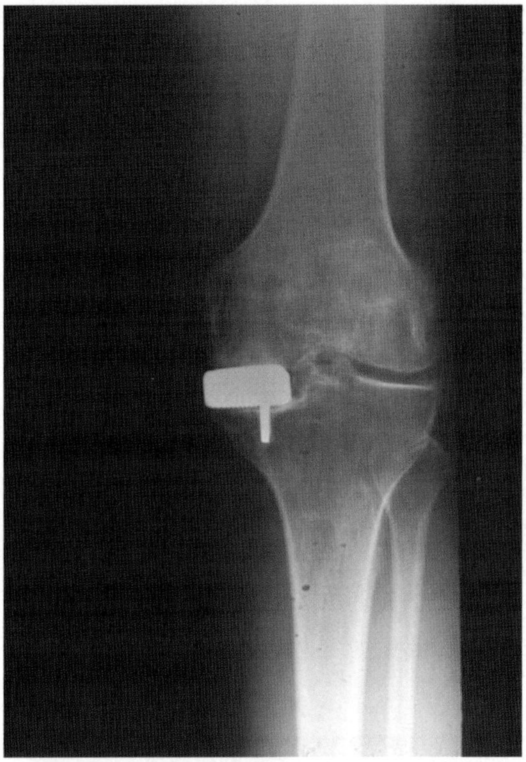

FIGURE 1-2. *A version of an early prosthetic intervention consisted of partial uncemented replacement such as that designed by McKeever to replace the diseased tibial plateau. Radiograph of implant serving as a spacer, not fixed to the bone.*

The era of interposition arthroplasty occurring during the first half of the 20th century was characterized with predictably unpredictable results. In some instances excellent outcomes were realized and in others the outcome was a total failure.[26,29,30] To make matters worse, one could not predict which would occur. Hence other solutions were appropriately sought.

Partial Arthroplasty

More formal anatomic metallic interposition efforts were undertaken as early as 1938 to address traumatic deficiencies.[25] In 1950, Aufranc adopted the concept of mold arthroplasty from the hip and applied it to the distal femur.[31] Also in the 1950s, a tibial articular surface replacement was developed. These efforts included an acrylic implant replacement in 1958 by Jensen, as reported by Heaton and Dorr,[1] and metallic replacements developed independently by MacIntosh from Canada[32] and McKeever from Kansas.[33] These metallic interposition "discs" replaced the diseased tibial articulation (Fig. 1-2) but were not secured to the underlying bone. As such, they tended to subside. Although some patients had outstanding outcomes, overall these efforts, once again, were quite unpredictable.

The first reference that I could find to an anatomic type of metallic resurfacing of both medial and lateral tibial plateaus is that of Townley in 1964.[34] In my opinion, Townley has been underrecognized as an innovator in joint replacement and is arguably the father of knee joint replacement. As with other implants, the problem that Townley faced was tibial fixation. His device was stabilized with screws, while the McKeever and the MacIntosh replacements were simply inserted to serve as loose spacers.

Linked Prosthetic Replacement

The above efforts were principally directed at arthritic conditions and required a certain amount of ligamentous stability and osseous integrity. In the same time frame, efforts to manage more significant bone deficiency resulting from posttrauma, infection, or tumor were undertaken with the first linked implants. Judet in 1947 described a linked hinged type of knee joint replacement stabilized in the shafts of the femur and tibia with screws.[35] Over the next 5 to 10 years, there was a flurry of activity to address a knee joint pathology for which there were few options. The first hinged implant design by Judet in France was followed by one designed by Magnoni d'Intignano in Italy.[36] The most popular hinged implant design of this era was probably that of Walldius from Scandinavia in 1951.[37] These were followed by several design modifications, including one designed by Shiers and one designed by Herm Young from the Mayo Clinic (Fig. 1-3).[38] All of these concepts were characterized by a rigid metal-on-metal hinge mechanism with mechanical fixation of the stem to the shaft of both the femur and the tibia. Overall, these linked devices demonstrated a marked improvement over the interposition procedures, but the good early outcome was often followed by failure due to implant loosening, which was ultimately the consequence of the poor restoration of function of the rigid hinged device and poor stem fixation. Even if fixed with cement, loosening was predictable with these hinged devices.

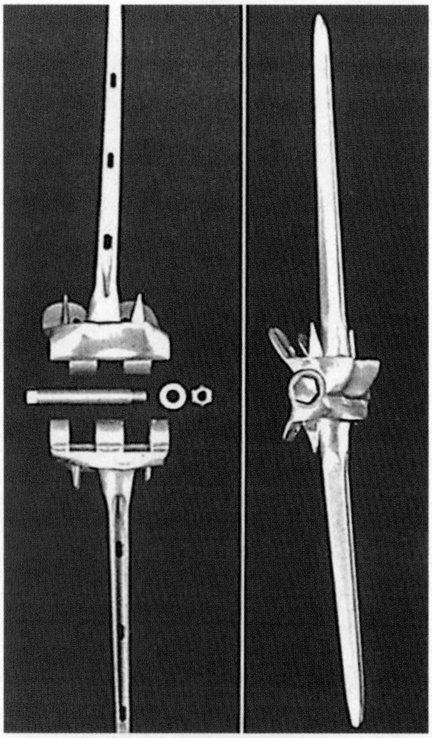

FIGURE 1-3. *Linked implants were a precursor to the current joint replacement designs. This implant was designed by Doctor Herm Young of the Mayo Clinic in 1960.*

THE MODERN ERA

Fixation

In my opinion, the modern era of knee joint replacement began in 1970 with the use of polymethacrylate as a means of component fixation. Historically, the most successful hinged implant was probably the GUEPAR.[39] This device became particularly successful when it was stabilized to the bone with methylmethacrylate as documented by Casagrande and Turner.[40] Charnley's demonstration of the effectiveness of methylmethacrylate spawned an explosion of subsequent knee joint designs. In the early 1970s, the incorporation of a patella component added further sophistication to the hinged joint replacement concept.[41] While polymethylmethacrylate was a true historical breakthrough, subsequent consideration has prompted some to revisit the issue of uncemented fixation.[42,43]

Unlinked Devices

The second breakthrough of the modern era was that of the unlinked implant. Gunston, a student of Charnley from Winnipeg, Manitoba, conceived and designed the four-part Polycentric joint replacement in 1971.[44] This unlinked device employed up to four components to replace the diseased femoral and tibial articular surfaces (Fig. 1-4). Since this was a four-part unlinked implant, of all the joint replacements it was one of the most difficult to accurately implant and instrumentation was rudimentary. Furthermore, this implant suffered the fate of poor mechanical support offered by the soft bone distal to the subchondral plate and consequently virtually all the tibia elements would eventually subside. This design also, by its very nature, prompted the first "hemireplacement," which became a common procedure at the Mayo Clinic and elsewhere in the 1970s (Fig. 1-4).[45] In the early 1970s, Coventry from the Mayo Clinic led a design team that included Lee Riley, Rod Turner, Jerry Finerman, and Jackson Upshaw to develop the so-called Geometric total knee arthroplasty (Fig. 1-5).[46,47] The design concept replaced the weight-bearing but not the patellar articular surfaces with a single femoral and a single tibial component that did not rely on long stems for fixation.

The real breakthrough in knee joint designs came in the early 1970s with the contributions of Townley[9] and Insall[15] to introduce and popularize the concept of a "condylar replacement." I personally recognize Townley as the first surgeon to introduce and popularize what might be termed a "generic condylar implant." Continuing his 1964 work of

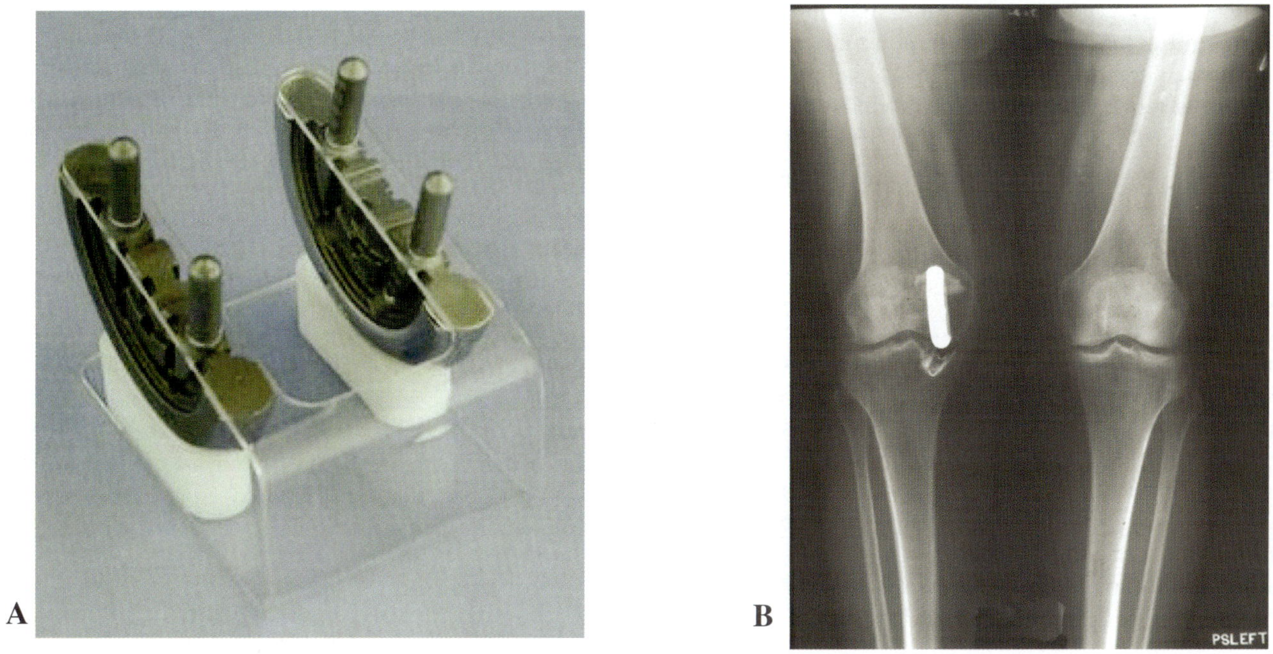

FIGURE 1-4. *The introduction of the four-part polycentric total knee arthroplasty (**A**) was a challenging technical procedure (**B**), but allowed the surgeon to apply judgment in those with limited disease and was the precursor of the current hemi-replacements.*

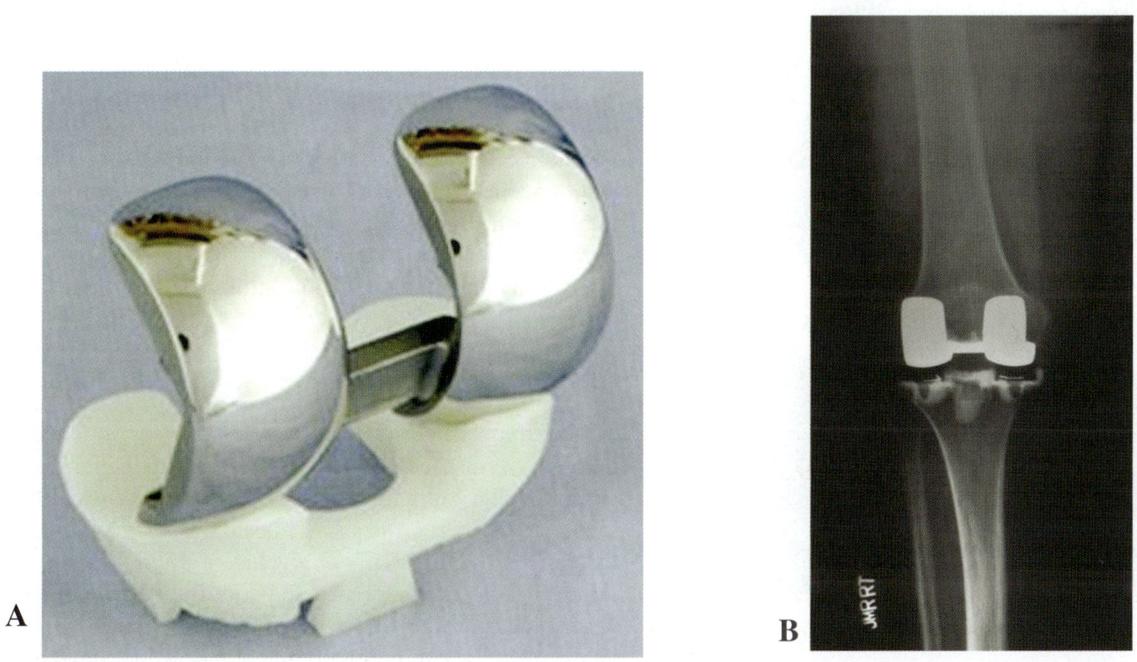

FIGURE 1-5. *The Geometric total knee arthroplasty was designed by Coventry and a team of investigators in the early 1970s (**A**). This device linked the medial and lateral components but did not address the patellar/femoral articulation (**B**).*

resurfacing the proximal tibia with a contoured metallic device,[34] Townley substituted a thin, flat, polyethylene implant to articulate with an anatomic replicating device applied to the femur.[9] The point of departure was that this condylar device allowed articulation with a patella implant. Thus, the 1972 total condylar design of Townley was, in my opinion, the precursor of modern knee replacement. Insall and colleagues are generally given credit for at least popularizing the total condylar concept, the Total Condylar, which was distinguished by enhanced fixation (Fig. 1-6). The tibia had a central peg, which proved to be of greater value than the simple resurfacing concept of Townley. These two contributions mark the sentinel breakthrough, at least in my judgment, in the history of knee joint replacement. Many variations of the condylar design quickly developed.[16,48] The essential design concept that gave the foundation to current successful knee replacement had appeared. Details of the history of knee replacement since this breakout condylar design has been nicely reviewed and illustrated by Robinson (Fig. 1-7).[2]

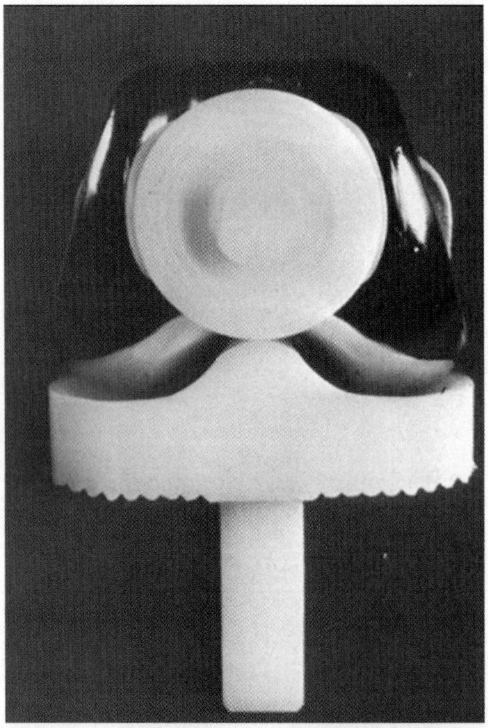

FIGURE 1-6. *The "Total Condylar" implant was a breakthrough from the perspective of concept, outcome, and marketing. (Compliments, C. Ranawat)*

Subsequent Contributions

As might be expected and as is the case with other joint replacements, a flurry of modifications sought to improve on the basic concept. With the advent of cement fixation and the acceptance of the condylar design concept, modifications and variations ensued on several fronts.

Patella resurfacing

Patellar resurfacing was initially described by McKeever as an isolated procedure in 1955.[49] In 1973, Hanslik adapted a patella implant to the hinged device,[41] but Insall and Townley are given credit for patella resurfacing as a standard element with the condylar type knee joint replacement. If this component were added, one would truly consider this to be a total knee arthroplasty. Various aspects of patellofemoral replacement have been a major focus in subsequent designs.

Modularity

Tibial component modularity was introduced in a number of early designs.[6,16,48,50] The superiority of a metal-backed tibial tray was demonstrated on a theoretical basis giving rise to numerous modular designs. By the early 1980s, virtually all the knee systems boasted modularity, principally related to the tibial baseplate. James Rand, working in conjunction with Raymond Gustillo and M. Reiss, designed the popular Genesis I and II knee replacement systems[51] (Fig. 1-8). The characteristics of this system were that it was modular with specific anatomic shape of the tibia respecting the differences between the medial and lateral tibial plateau contours. This implant did provide for a patellar replacement and, most important, reflecting Rand's interest and practice of complex revision surgery, this system offered several stem options and special inserts for bone deficiency in the revision setting.

Alignment

The importance of alignment also became increasingly recognized in the late 1970s. Before this time, accurate extramedullary alignment in the frontal plane was difficult to attain on a regular basis. Whiteside was arguably the first to recognize and discuss the value of alignment using the femoral canal as a reference and contributed several articles describing intramedullary alignment strategies. Over the years, medullary femoral alignment has been a standard, but intramedullary tibial alignment has proved to be of much less value. However, real risks from fat embolization were

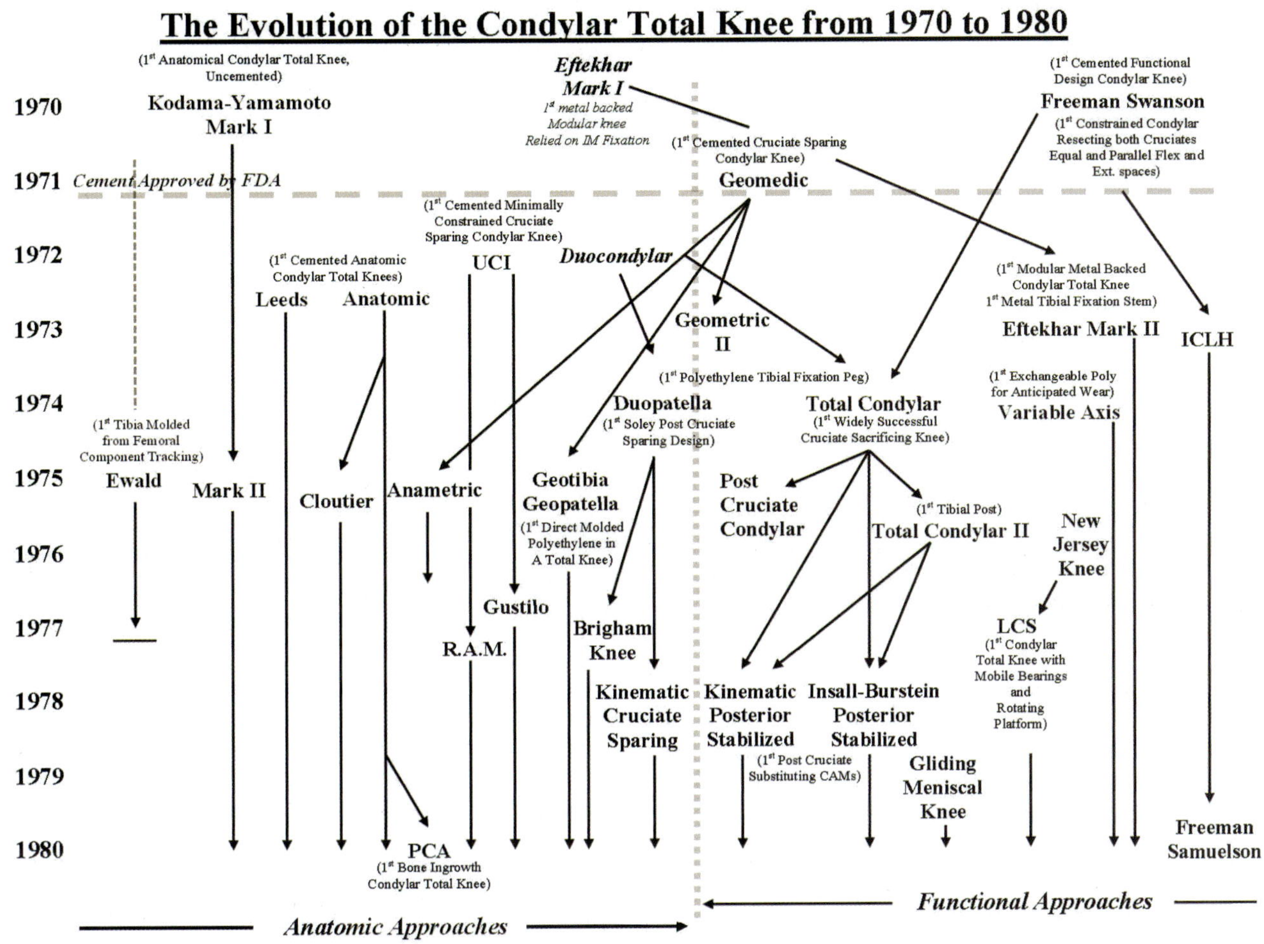

FIGURE 1-7. *Historic development of the "generic" condylar knee. (Reprinted with permission, Robinson[50].)*

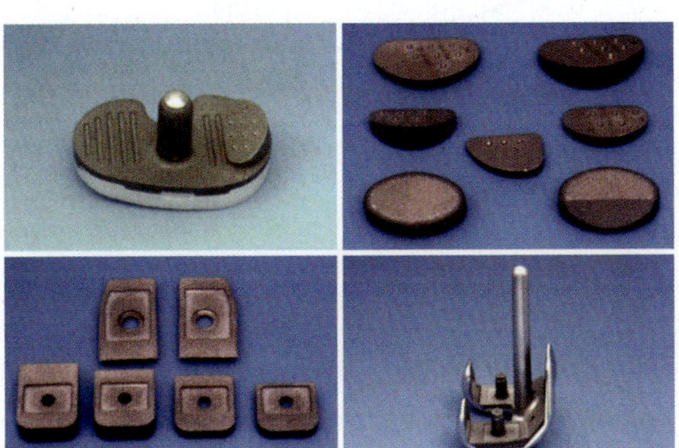

FIGURE 1-8. *The Genesis total knee arthroplasty was designed by Rand and Gustillo and represented an effort at a more anatomic replication of the tibial contour as well as introduced more extensive modularity to allow transition from a primary to a revision implant.*

documented with medullary manipulation. Yet, with continued innovations such as overdrilling and aspiration of the medullary canal, the risks documented with the early experience of intramedullary alignment have been dramatically lessened, except possibly if employed during simultaneous procedures.

Cruciate ligaments

The significance of the presence or absence of the cruciate ligament was an early point of contention and remains so. The controversy started 30 years ago in 1978 when the concept of removing both cruciate ligaments was introduced with the Total Condylar knee. Cloutier, however, advocated replicating normal kinematics and designed an implant that preserved both ligaments.[52] The idea of using a posterior cruciate-substituting device is attributed to Peter Walker. The clever addition of a prominent tibial spine allows stability of the femoral tibial articulation while the contour of the tibial surface allows for the physiologic roll-back phenomenon. Regardless, this is probably the most hotly contested and least resolved issue in knee replacement design philosophy today. I continue to use a posterior cruciate-sparing implant and Mayo Clinic data clearly show superior survival with the cruciate-retaining device (Fig. 1-9).[53] So, from my personal perspective, "QED" (Latin–*quod erat demonstrandum* = which was to be demonstrated. Used after a mathematical principle, theory, or hypothesis has been proven or demonstrated).

Partial replacements

As early as 1972, the use of Gunston's polycentric device to replace only the compartment most involved was regularly performed at the Mayo Clinic (see Fig. 1-4C). Marmor is credited with popularizing and documenting the first comprehensive experience with uni-joint replacement in 1973. He continued to favor this approach throughout his career.[11]

Mobile bearing implant

The concept of a mobile bearing implant was felt by the author and others[12] to offer the first true innovation in knee replacement since the introduction of the "generic" condylar design. This idea remained largely ignored until Buechel and Pappas introduced a mobile bearing total knee replacement designed in the 1980s.[13] The prospect of decreasing wear debris and improving motion, promised by this design philosophy, was very attractive to the orthopaedic community. By the early 2000s, the orthopaedic world was exploring the merits of the mobile bearing knee in its various forms in an aggressive fashion. However, neither the anticipated improvement in motion nor the improved wear characteristics have been realized in clinical practice and the enthusiasm for mobile bearing knees has dramatically waned. The jury is out, but it appears the current generation of mobile bearing knees are as good but no better than fixed articulations.

Fixation

Because the failure mode of most early cemented implants was one of cement failure, the weak link of cement fixation was addressed with uncemented designs with special surface characteristics to provide osseous fixation. The success of osseous incorporation by the dental profession[54] prompted efforts to adapt this technology to orthopaedic implants.[1] Toward this end in 1980, Hungerford, Krachow, and colleagues introduced the concept of porous-coated arthroplasty (PCA) both at the hip and at the knee.[19,55]

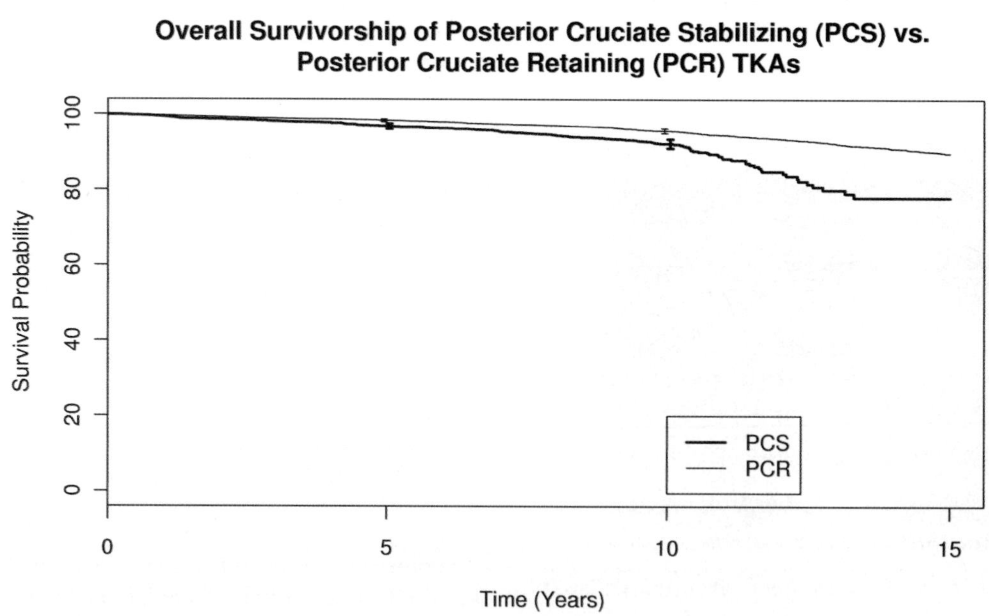

FIGURE 1-9. *Kaplan-Meier survival curves free of revision for patients undergoing cruciate-retaining or cruciate-substituting joint replacements at the Mayo Clinic.*

While the concept was a real innovation, this particular design for the hip or knee implant has not stood the test of time. However, at the knee there were two lasting contributions of this effort: (1) it introduced the concept of uncemented fixation at the knee, and (2) it emphasized the importance of precise alignment and instrumentation.[19] At the hip, the uncemented concept has become the standard of fixation. At the knee, some favor uncemented application, but the majority does not.

Precise instrumentation

Probably the most lasting benefit of Hungerford et al's contributions with the PCA philosophy was that of precise instrumentation based on fixation to the bone and alignment (Fig. 1-10).[18] The instrumentation employed by the PCA used the concept of rigid fixation to bone with pins or drill bits. This was a major departure to the hand-held alignment jigs that had been favored and used before the introduction of the PCA system. This is now the standard approach used by all knee systems. Intramedullary alignment was also introduced at this time,[17] and has proved to be the standard for femoral but not tibial alignment.[17]

Today, refinement of alignment using navigation systems is one of the most active avenues of investigation. Again, the jury is out. The verdict will pivot on documented cost-effectiveness.

Trabecular metal

The history of knee joint replacement would not be complete without recognizing the current and emerging value of trabecular metal in the reconstruction of the knee (Fig. 1-11).[21,56] Its utility has been extensively evaluated and explored by Hanssen, Lewallen, and other Mayo surgeons.[21,56,57] This innovation allows augmentation for osseous deficiency seen in revision settings. Early efforts to render the knee stable employed stems and linkage, but long-term results were not reliable.[58]

Currently, this remains an active and promising avenue of further design improvement, particularly for the devastating osseous deficiency observed in revision procedures. The trabecular metal also lends itself to adaptation with the polyethylene surface that would provide an attractive uncemented primary implant. The creative application of trabecular metal in design and practice is an unfinished chapter in the history of knee replacement.

Technique

Unquestionably, the surgical technique for knee implantation has dramatically evolved and improved. The aforementioned instrumentation introduced by Hungerford and associates is considered to be a major innovation. Limited exposures and subvastus deep exposures have been explored and recommended by some, but have proved to be of little or no added value.[59] Aggressive soft tissue release has allowed a reliable replacement, even in grossly deformed knee

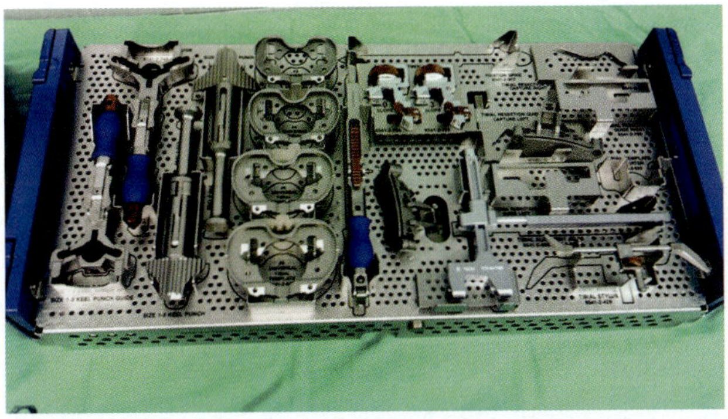

FIGURE 1-10. *The author credits Hungerford and Krackow for introducing the value and need for precise instrumentation and technique leading to proper alignment and soft tissue balance. The original instrumentation was the precursor for the modern instrumentation designs as pictured above.*

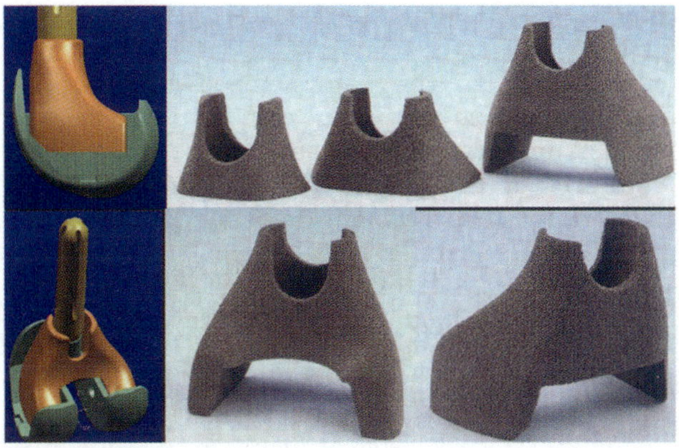

FIGURE 1-11. *Trabecular metal represents a real advance in the ability to reliably augment patients with difficult revision circumstances due to extensive osseous deficiency.*

joints. Although the posterior cruciate-substituting design is widely accepted today, there is concern that this may not be truly needed as often or be of value as is currently accepted.

THE FUTURE

The future of knee joint replacement is indeed quite bright, not from anticipated innovation but from much needed documentation. The success rate of modern generic condylar implants that are properly implanted exceeds 90% at 10 years. The ability to revise a failed implant also is quite reliable and approaches 90% for a successful first revision outcome. The history of knee joint replacement, therefore, is a true success story. The major responsibility of the profession at this time is to define those incremental opportunities that will truly improve the outcome from 95% to one that approaches 100%. Lacking that, the most important contribution in my mind in the future will be to accurately document those subtle differences in the currently available implants that distinguish long-term performance (see Fig. 1-9). It is also possible that some designs may be more effective in certain circumstances, such as in the morbidly obese patient or with gross deformity. Overall, I believe that the improvements will be more in surgical technique, such as with cost-effective navigation strategies, than with further implant design changes. Finally, the winner in the future will hopefully be one that optimizes reliability, reproducibility, and simplicity and is truly cost-effective.

REFERENCES

1. Heaton KT, Dorr LD. History of total knee arthroplasty. In: Callaghan JJ, Rosenberg AG, Rubash HE, Simonian PT, Wickiewicz TL, eds. *The Adult Knee.* Vol. I. Philadelphia, PA: Lippincott Williams & Wilkins, Wolters Kluwer Co.; 2003:15-24.
2. Robinson RP. The early innovators of today's resurfacing condylar knees. *J Arthroplasty.* 2005;20(1 suppl 1):2-26.
3. Cowell R. Early history of knee surgery. In: Callaghan JJ, Rosenberg AG, Rubash HE, Simonian PT, Wickiewicz TL, eds. *The Adult Knee.* Vol. I. Philadelphia, PA: Lippincott Williams & Wilkins, Wolters Kluwer Co.; 2003:1-13.
4. Cracchiolo A. Newer knowledge of total knee replacement. *Clin Orthop Relat Res.* 1979;145:2-3.
5. Kettlekamp DB, Leech RB. Total knee replacement. *Clin Orthop Relat Res.* 1973;94.
6. Ranawat CS, Shine JJ. Duo-condylar total knee arthroplasty. *Clin Orthop Relat Res.* 1973;94:185.
7. Shiers LGP. Arthroplasty of the knee: preliminary report of a new method. *J Bone Joint Surg Br.* 1954; 36:553.
8. Insall JN, Ranawat CS, Aglietti P, et al. A comparison of four models of total knee replacement prostheses. *J Bone Joint Surg Am.* 1975;58:754.
9. Townley CO. The anatomic total knee resurfacing arthroplasty. *Clin Orthop Relat Res.*1985;192:82.
10. Insall J, Ranawat CS, Scott WN, et al. Total condylar knee replacement: preliminary report. Symposium: Long-term followup of total knee arthroplasty. *Clin Orthop.* 2001;388:3-6.
11. Marmor L. The modular knee. *Clin Orthop Relat Res.* 1973;94:242-248.
12. Goodfellow J, O'Connor J. The mechanics of the knee and prosthesis design. *J Bone Joint Surg Br.* 1978;60:358-369.
13. Buechel FF, Keblish PA, Lee JM, et al. Low contact stress meniscal bearing unicompartmental knee replacement: long-term evaluation of cemented and cementless results. *J Orthop Rheum.* 1994;7:31-41.
14. Walker PS, Shoji H. Development of a stabilizing knee prosthesis employing physiological principles. *Clin Orthop Relat Res.* 1973;94:222-233.
15. Insall J, Ranawat CS, Scott WNS, et al. Total condylar knee replacement: preliminary report. *Clin Orthop Relat Res.* 1976;120:149-154.
16. Sledge CB, Ewald FC. Total knee arthroplasty exposure at the Robert Breck Brigham Hospital. *Clin Orthop Relat Res.* 1979;145:78-84.
17. Whiteside LA, Summers RG. Anatomical landmarks for an intramedullary alignment system for total knee replacement. *Orthop Trans.* 1983;793:546-547.
18. Hungerford DS, Krackow KA, Kenna RV. *Total Knee Arthroplasty: A Comprehensive Approach.* New York: Williams & Wilkins; 1983.
19. Hungerford DS, Kenna RV. Preliminary experience with a total knee prosthesis with a porous coating used without cement. *Clin Orthop Relat Res.* 1983; 176:95-107.
20. Bartel DL, Burstein AH, Santavicca EA, et al. Performance of the tibial component in total knee replacement. *J Bone Joint Surg Am.* 1982;64:1026.

21. Meneghini RM, Lewallen DG, Hanssen AD. Use of porous tantalum metaphyseal cones for severe tibial bone loss during revision total knee replacement. *J Bone Joint Surg Am*. 2008;90(1):78-84.
22. Fergusson W. Excision of the knee joint—recovery with a false joint and useful limb. *Med Times Gazette*. 1861;1:601.
23. Gluck T. Die invaginationsmethode der osteo- und arthroplastik. *Berliner Klinische Wochenschrift*. 1890; 27:732-736.
24. Murphy JB. Ankylosis, arthroplasty: clinical and experimental. *JAMA*. 1905;44:1573, 1671-1794.
25. Campbell WC. Arthroplasty of the knee—report of cases. *J Orthop Surg*. 1921;3:430-436.
26. Kuhns JG, Potter TA. Nylon arthroplasty of the knee. A follow-up study. *J Bone Joint Surg Br*. 1949;31:53-60.
27. Brown JE. Use of cutis as an interposing membrane in arthroplasty of the knee. *J Bone Joint Surg Am*. 1958; 40:1003-1018.
28. Henderson MS. What are the real results of arthroplasty? *Am J Orthop Surg*. 1918;16:30-33.
29. Albee FH. Original features in arthroplasty of the knee with improved prognosis. *Surg Gynecol Obstet*. 1928;47:312.
30. Baer WS. Arthroplasty with the aid of animal membrane. *Am J Orthop Surg*. 1918;16:171.
31. Aufranc OE, Jones WN. Mold arthroplasty of the knee. *J Bone Joint Surg Am*. 1958;40:1431.
32. MacIntosh DL. Hemiarthroplasty of the knee using a space occupying prosthesis for painful varus and valgus deformities. *J Bone Joint Surg Am*. 1958;40: 1431.
33. McKeever DC. Tibial plateau prosthesis. *Clin Orthop Relat Res*. 1960;18:86-95.
34. Townley CO. Articular-place replacement arthroplasty for the knee joint. *Clin Orthop Relat Res*. 1964;36:77.
35. Judet J, Judet R, Crepin GT. Essais de prosthese osteso-articulaire. *Presse Med*. 1947;52:302.
36. Magnoni d'Intignano JM. Genou en resine acrylique. *Rev Orthop*. 1949;35:556.
37. Walldius B. Arthroplasty of the knee joint employing an acrylic prosthesis. *Acta Orthop Scand*. 1954;23: 121-131.
38. Young H. Use of a hinged Vitallium prosthesis for arthroplasty of the knee. A preliminary report. *J Bone Joint Surg Am*. 1963;45:1627-1642.
39. Deburge A, Aubriot JH, Genet JP. Current status of a hinge prosthesis (GUEPAR). *Clin Orthop Relat Res*. 1979;145:91.
40. Casagrande PA, Turner RR. Total knee replacement. A preliminary report using methylmethacrylate cement in 38 consecutive knees. *Clin Orthop Relat Res*. 1972;89:150-159.
41. Hanslik L. First experience on knee joint replacement using the young hinged prosthesis combined with a modification on the McKeever patella prosthesis. *Clin Orthop Relat Res*. 1973;94:115-121.
42. London GC, Galante JO, Maley MM. Non-cemented total knee arthroplasty. *Clin Orthop Relat Res*. 1986; 205:49-57.
43. Whiteside LA. Clinical results of the Whiteside Ortholoc total knee replacement. *Orthop Clin North Am*. 1987;20:113-124.
44. Gunston FH. Polycentric knee arthroplasty. Prosthetic simulation of normal knee movement. *J Bone Joint Surg Br*. 1971;53:272-277.
45. Bryan RS, Peterson LFA, Combs JJ Jr. Polycentric knee arthroplasty: a preliminary report of postoperative complications in 450 knees. *Clin Orthop*. 1973; 94:148-152.
46. Coventry MD, Finerman GA, Riley LH, et al. A new geometric knee for total knee arthroplasty. *Clin Orthop Relat Res*. 1972;83:157-162.
47. Coventry MB, Upshaw JE, Riley LH, et al. The Geometric total knee arthroplasty. I. Conception, design, indications and surgical technic. *Clin Orthop Relat Res*. 1973;94:171-176.
48. Evanski PM, Waugh TR, Orofino CF, et al. UCI knee replacement. *Clin Orthop Relat Res*. 1976;120:33-38.
49. McKeever DC. Patellar prosthesis. *J Bone Joint Surg Am*. 1955;37:1074-1084.
50. Murray DG, Webster DA. The variable-axis knee prosthesis. A two-year follow-up study. *J Bone Joint Surg Am*. 1981;63:687-694.
51. Rand JA, ed. *Total Knee Arthroplasty*. New York: Raven Press Ltd; 1993:1-7.
52. Cloutier JM. Results of total knee arthroplasty with a non-constrained prosthesis. *J Bone Joint Surg*. 1983;65:906.
53. Abdel M, Morrey M, Jenson M, et al. Long-term survival of cruciate retaining and cruciate substituting knee replacements. *J Bone Joint Surg Am*. 2011; 93(22):2072-2078.
54. Branemark PI, Breine U, Adell R, et al. Intra-osseous anchorage of dental prostheses. I. *Scand J Plast Reconstr Surg*. 1969;3:81.

55. Hungerford DS, Krackow KA, Kenna RV. Two to five year experience with a cementless porous-coated total knee prosthesis. In: Rand JA, Dorr LD, eds. *Total Knee Arthroplasty: Proceedings of the Knee Society, 1985-1986*. Rockville, MD: Aspen Publishers; 1987.

56. Mabry TM, Hanssen AD. The role of stems and augments for bone loss in revision knee arthroplasty. *J Arthroplasty.* 2007;22(4 suppl 1):56-60.

57. Mittal Y, Fehring TK, Hanssen A, et al. Two-stage reimplatnation for periprosthetic knee infection involving resistant organisms. *J Bone Joint Surg Am.* 2007;89(6):1227-1231.

58. Noiles DG. Prosthetic knee joint. US patent 4,219,893, Sept. 2, 1980.

59. Pagnano MW, Argenson JN, Parratte S, et al. Minimally invasive total knee arthroplasty meets computer navigation. *J Bone Joint Surg Am.* 2009;91(suppl 5):56-58.

2 Joint Registries

Henrik Palm and Henrik Malchau

"Registries can identify otherwise hidden clinical problems – but not define future solutions."

The purpose of a joint registry is to track patients' results over time, helping to detect ineffective surgical practices and faulty devices and ultimately improving on the outcome of total knee arthroplasty. Registries provide large-scale epidemiological data concerning patients, implants, and procedures that are not otherwise accessible. By supplying this information, registries are expected to further improve an overall 10-year implant survival rate of greater than 95%.

HISTORY

National joint registries first started in Sweden in the 1970s with the purpose of quality measurement of recently introduced arthroplasty implants.[1] Quickly Norway and later Denmark followed suit. Nordic health care systems provide an optimal environment for epidemiological studies because they are dominated by public hospitals treating government-registered individuals. In the past decades, several larger countries have initiated national registries or have plans for doing so (Table 2-1). Within a few years of the establishment of these registries, researchers now have a substantial number of patients in their databases and a creditable compliance record.

National registries have begun to collaborate, providing even higher patient numbers, allowing for the analysis of smaller subgroups. The Nordic Arthroplasty Register Association (NARA) was established in 2007 for the purpose of improving and facilitating the Nordic research concerning implant surgery.[2]

LOGISTICS

The early registries were initiated by a local group of individual surgeons.[1] Today registries are most often run in close collaboration with the national orthopaedic societies and national health services providing the crucial economical support, although some registries still rely on grants. Registries are headed by a team of highly respected surgeons supported by statisticians and data technicians. Supplemental studies on subgroups are often conducted by research assistants.[1,3]

When registries are established, trials are normally performed in a smaller controlled environment. National coverage is then attempted based on this experience.[1] The registry must have support from the surgeons as well as other health care members, and data registration approval and individual patient consent might be needed.[3]

Until the past decade, data were reported on paper forms that were later merged into a computer database. Today data are most often reported directly into the electronic database.[1] Individual passwords are given, so that users can be identified as surgeon, staff, or even patient. Subjective patient data are assessed by asking specific questions with multiple answer choices in a scroll down window. Extra comments are limited but possible.

TABLE 2-1. Major National Registries for Knee Implants or with Knee Implants Included

Country	Name	Acronym	Homepage	Established	Total Patients	Annual Patients	Latest Completeness
Australia	National Joint Replacement Registry	AOA NJRR	dmac.adelaide. edu.au/aoanjrr/	1999	289,000	41,000	≈100
Canada	Joint Replacement Registry	CJRR	cihi.ca/cjrr	2000	200,000[a]	47,000[a]	41
England and Wales	National Joint Registry	NJR	njrcentre.org. uk	2003	239,000	78,000	98
New Zealand	National Joint Register	NJR	cdhb.govt.nz/ njr	1999	46,000	6,000	98
Denmark	Danish Knee Arthroplasty Register	DKR	dkar.dk	1997	60,000	10,000	91
Norway	Norwegian Arthroplasty Register	NAR	nrlweb.ihelse.n et	1994	42,000	5,000	≈100
Sweden	Swedish Knee Arthroplasty Register	SKAR	knee.se	1975	150,000	13,000	≈100

NOTE: Year of establishment is for total knee replacement. Patient numbers are for total knee replacement including revision procedures.

[a]Estimated number.

Results are published in an annual report and could be tailored to the participating hospitals or surgeons. Individual surgeons and hospitals are often able to identify their own procedures and outcomes in comparison with the overall results, and this may ultimately lead to improved patient care.

DATA

Demands for Data

Data should be differentiable and reproducible as well as prospectively entered into the database before outcome knowledge. A high compliance rate gives the registry credibility and the possibility for high-quality research. Ideally, the registry cohort should include procedures and follow-ups. In smaller geographic areas with minimal population emigration this is easily done; larger areas with a more transient population provide a greater challenge. Although debatable, a 90% fulfillment rate is normally considered acceptable.

An ideal registry should have 100% participation, most often based on hospital willingness, but participation could be made mandatory by health care authorities. Compliance could be increased by patient record audits and reimbursement for outcome measures for the individual hospitals. For optimal compliance, data should be easily recorded by the different people who are capable of capturing the data.

Type of Data

All types of data could, in principle, be recorded in a registry. For practical reasons, data are divided into four main levels (Table 2-2).

TABLE 2-2. The Four Levels of Register Data

Level I	Level II	Level III	Level IV
Patient identifier Age Side Gender Diagnosis (ICD) Procedure (ICD) Implant (type) Cement (type) Hospital (type and volume) Surgeon (volume)	Patient Height, weight, and BMI Comorbidities: ASA/Charlson Cardiac Diabetes Osteoporosis Process of care Operation environment Surgical technique Pain treatment Prophylaxis: Antibiotic Thromboembolic	Patient satisfaction and clinical outcome tools: EQ-5D WOMAC SF-36 Oxford Knee Score UCLA Others	Radiographs/CT scans: Anatomic configuration Implant positioning Implant movement Bone structure

Level I data represent the basic parameters such as identification of the patient, procedure, and implant type. These parameters are present and essential in all registries for analysis of the cohort, stratification possibilities, and subgroup studies.

Level II data represent the perioperative data. Medical comorbidities could be assessed based on overall scales (eg, ASA) or presence of specific illnesses (eg, diabetes). Level II data can allow the convalescence period for infection rates, pain management, and so forth to be intensively studied.

Level III data represent patient satisfaction and clinical outcome. Before the surgery, a baseline level is recorded so that future years' assessments can be compared. Different tools for clinical outcome and patient satisfaction can be used. Depending on the chosen tools, either the surgeon or the patient (Patient Reported Outcome Measure) can be responsible for assessment.

Level IV data represent radiographic data. The anatomic configuration of the joint and surrounding bone can be registered as angles and distances. Implant position and movement results from different tools and software programs (eg, Radio Stereofotometric Analysis) could be assessed. Also alterations in the surrounding bone structure could be registered for preoperative cysts and for postoperative development of radiolucency and radiolysis. Assessment of such information is time consuming but could provide possibilities for a more in-depth analysis of how and why a failure occurred.

RESULTS

Outcome Parameters

The most frequently utilized outcome parameters are the number of procedures, implant survival, and patient scores. The number of procedures is analyzed for the individual level I data groups. Monitoring the number of procedures is an important health care tool for quantifying diagnosis, treatment, and costs; analysis of the number of procedures could also identify local, regional, and national trends. Implant survival can be based on any cause for revision or based solely on revision with or without infection or death of the patient. Specific implants can be compared, as can overall implant design or different techniques (eg, cemented vs. uncemented). Patient-derived scores of mobility, pain, and satisfaction are studied by comparing the preoperative baseline to postoperative scores. Outcome can be compared in subgroups based on patient demographic, comorbidities, or implant design. Serious medical complications, such as thromboembolic events, cardiac events, or death, are often collected even if considered due to unrelated causes.

Special focus could be drawn to so-called "outliers," which are performances outside the expected. Positive outliers can serve as models and negative outliers can be further investigated and addressed. However, it should be remembered that identification of negative outliers can cause concern to the surgeon or patient and reduce overall compliance to a registry.

Outcome Presentation

Diagnosis, demographics, and procedure numbers are normally presented in tables or as a bar graph. Implant survival or revision rates are most often presented as survival curves with 2 or more years of follow-up. Differences within groups are studied with the use of a Cox regression analysis, in which demographic parameters, loss to follow-up, and death are taken into account. Figure 2-1 shows typical forms of presenting data.

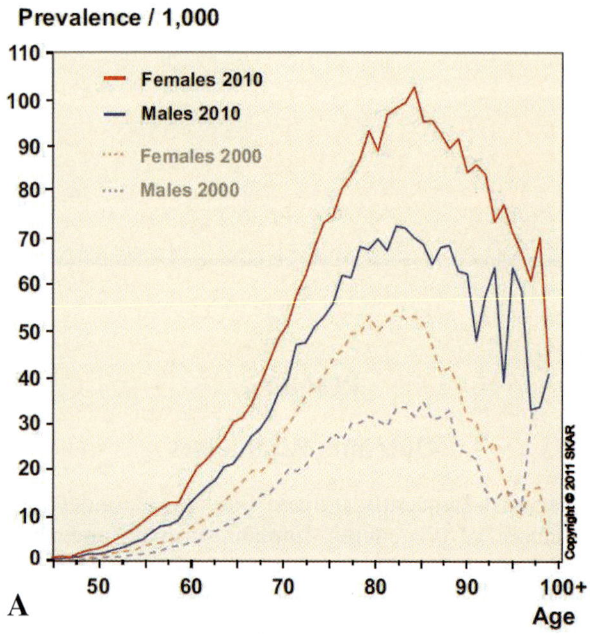

A

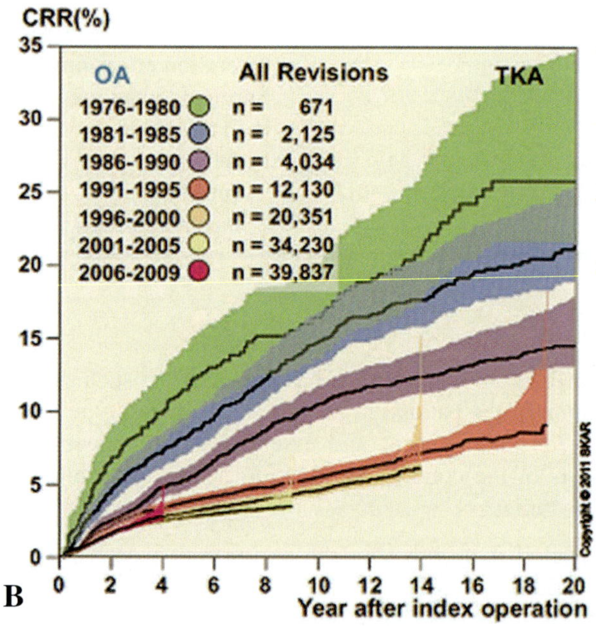

B

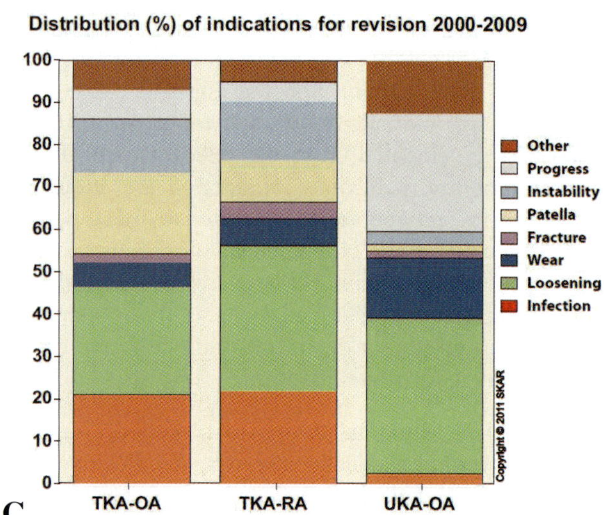

C

FIGURE 2-1. *Typical data presenting diagrams in joint registries: (**A**) Prevalence curves, here of knee arthroplasties in 2000 and 2010 distributed by gender and age. (**B**) Implant revision rate, here showing the cumulative revision rates (CRR%) with 95% confidence intervals for total knee arthroplasty (TKA) for osteoarthritis (OA) distributed by period of insertion — showing a constant reduction in risk of revision since 1976. (**C**) Bar graphs, here with indications for revision in three types of primary operations: total knee arthroplasty for osteoarthritis (TKA-OA), total knee arthroplasty for rheumatoid arthritis (TKA-RA) or unicompartmental knee arthroplasty for osteoarthritis (UKA-OA). (Reprinted with permission from The Swedish Knee Arthroplasty Register, www.knee.se.)*

Interaction with Other Research Methods

Registries can provide critical information on demographics and identify clinical problems, which enable improved planning of future studies. Registries cannot, however, directly develop new solutions, because only the present treatment is registered. Registries should therefore not be seen as an alternative, but rather as a supplement, to randomized studies.

The interaction between registries and other study types is especially indicated when introducing new implants. Here a critical stepwise evaluation is necessary for preventing large-scale clinical failures. Only when favorable results are obtained in one level should the next level be initiated (Fig. 2-2).

After initial preclinical testing and permission for human use, the first clinical step should be a prospective randomized study utilizing the minimum number of patients sufficient to obtain a valid evaluation in primary outcome measurements versus the gold standard procedure. This first step would often be performed by industry or the implant developer. The next step should be a multicenter study, preferably randomized with a substantial number of patients in order to expose the implant to a broader variety of surgeons and techniques.

With modern long-term implant survival rates, even a very ambitious randomized multicenter study would not necessarily identify certain failures. Continued quality control is therefore needed and is augmented by the large regis-try studies. Based on the actual patient population within an area in the national registries, even unusual complications can be visualized and potential catastrophic situations identified quickly.

Level of Evidence

Registry studies use scientific methods to collect and analyze data. Results are the actual outcome on the whole cohort of patients, and the high statistical power makes it possible to perform adequate analyses of even uncommon complications. A registry study is, however, not a scientifically performed trial, and confounders and bias are not controlled by randomization. Overall, registry studies are cohort studies and thus are given a 1b level of evidence if a follow-up above 80% is achieved.[4]

FUTURE OF REGISTRIES

There is an increased acknowledgment of the necessity of registries.[1] Due to cost considerations and quality concerns over new implants, groups such as health care politicians, insurance companies, journalists, and patient groups have been advocating for the creation of a registry that specifically looks at the annual number of inserted implants and surgical indications. Also, registries are seen as an instrument for developing health care payment systems focusing on quality of treatment. During the past decade, published registry results on individual implant survival and patient satisfaction have also gained popularity in industry marketing. Registries can provide an opportunity for industry product testing, but could also highlight industry products that are outdated or new and promising, but expensive, implants with suboptimal designs.

Currently many new national registries for knee implants are in the planning stage. Depending on the health care system, registries could be initiated by doctors, health care officials, politicians, or industry. The setup is demanding and, for objectivity, registries are probably best conducted by a research-educated doctoral staff. With the expected increasing number of large national registries, individual or multinational large registry studies are becoming an increasingly effective tool for providing evidence for treatment of knee implant patients.

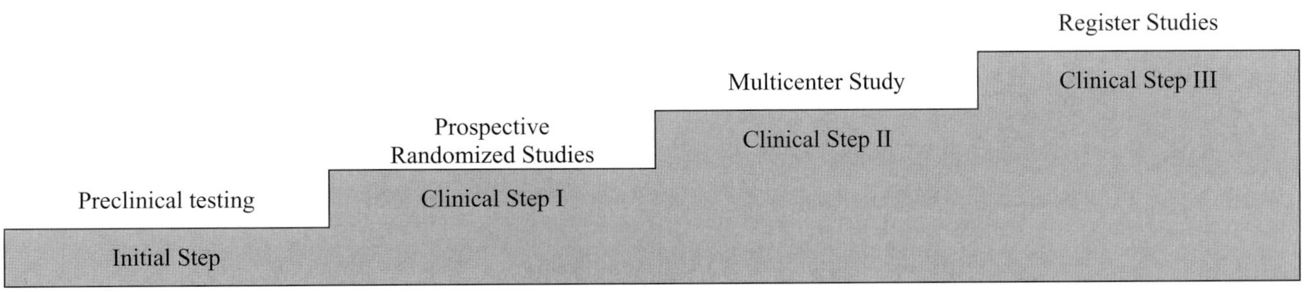

FIGURE 2-2. *Algorithm for the stepwise introduction of new implants into clinical praxis.*

REFERENCES

1. Knutson K, Robertsson O. The Swedish Knee Arthroplasty Register (www.knee.se). The inside story. *Acta Orthop*. 2010;81(1):5-7.
2. Nordic Arthroplasty Register Association. http://www.nordicarthroplasty.org/. Accessed July 11, 2011.
3. Bohm ER, Dunbar MJ, Bourne R. The Canadian Joint Replacement Registry—what have we learned? *Acta Orthop*. 2010;81(1):119-121.
4. Oxford Centre for Evidence-Based Medicine Levels of Evidence, March 2009. http://www.cebm.net/index.aspx?o=1025. Accessed July 11, 2011.

3 Study Design and Basic Statistics

Parag Sancheti and Steve Rocha

With rapid advancements made in techniques of knee surgery and the evolvement of new implants, the need for constant evaluation of results of surgery becomes crucial to the surgeon and investigator. The medical personnel are forced to deal with large quantities of relevant research findings in order to maximize health care. Evidence-based medicine is a systematic approach to finding and analyzing published data as the basis of clinical decision making. The hierarchy of evidence is important because it allows for clearer communication when discussing studies, and it also helps show the relative strengths of the types of research. In general, different systems rank 1 as high-quality evidence, while a rank of 4 or 5 indicates low-quality evidence. Figure 3-1 shows the hierarchy of evidence where randomized controlled trials (RCTs) rank as the highest level of evidence.

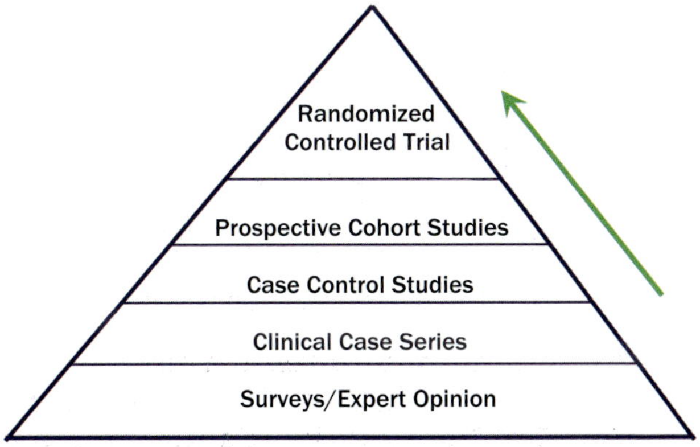

FIGURE 3-1. *Hierarchy of evidence.*

Before the levels of evidence are discussed, it is important to understand the different types of study design. In general, there are two broad classifications of study designs: analytic studies and descriptive studies.[1]

Analytic studies focus on the causes of a disease through testing the outcome of a particular exposure. Specifically, there are two types of analytic studies: observational studies include case-control and cohort studies, whereas experimental studies include randomized control trials.[1]

Descriptive studies focus on the distribution of a disease in relation to factors such as age, location, and sex. Studies that fall into this category include cross-sectional studies and case reports.[1]

It is important to distinguish between retrospective and prospective studies as well. Retrospective studies involve patient follow-up after the desired outcome, whereas prospective studies involve following up on patients before the desired outcome.[1]

CLINICAL STUDY DESIGNS

Clinical Case Series

Case reports and case series are descriptive studies, and, therefore, they are uncontrolled and retrospective in nature. Case reports are clinical observations of events that have been observed in a single patient.[1] Expansion of the individual case report to include multiple patients with an outcome of interest is a case series. Various factors that may have caused the specified outcome are studied backwards in time. Case series do not have a comparison group and therefore the data derived from such studies are prone to bias if data or follow-up of the patient are incomplete. Such studies are considered the lowest forms of evidence and are often underestimated in their ability to serve as valuable sources of information.[1] However, case series offer several advantages; they allow for the evaluation of new techniques or procedures on rare or unusual conditions.[1] For example, a researcher wishes to conduct a case series on patients who underwent total knee replacement just a month after it was initially introduced. The researcher can obtain valuable information by recording knee score and function score, range of motion, and postoperative anterior knee pain by enrolling these patients in a case series and collecting descriptions of postsurgery follow-up details and adverse effects. Therefore, case series serve as an easy alternative to investigate outcomes of new techniques. Apart from this, the simplicity of the design makes it less costly and less time consuming than other study designs.[1]

Case Control Studies

Case-control studies involve the comparison of a group of people with a certain disease state or condition (ie, cases) with a group of people without the disease or condition (ie, controls). They are considered retrospective in nature because the cases already have the disease or condition of interest and the researcher looks back in time to ascertain the factors that are associated with this outcome.[1] The relationship between a particular intervention or prognostic factor and the outcome of interest is examined by comparing the number of individuals with each intervention or prognostic factor in the cases and controls. For example, case-control studies can be used to compare the prognostic factors in patients with nonhealing fractures with a similar group of patients with well-healed fractures to see whether the patients with nonhealing fractures are more likely to be smokers.

The case-control study can be useful in studying rare outcomes, outcomes with multiple potential etiologic factors, and conditions with long latency periods, and for generating hypotheses or preliminary data.[1] Moreover, case-control studies can be conducted in a short time with small sample sizes and for less money than other types of studies. However, data may be inaccurate because the information usually is collected from patients or their hospital records.

Prospective Cohort Studies

Cohort is defined as a population or group of patients or healthy individuals who are followed over time to see if a specific, desired outcome arises.[2] Ideally this group meets a level of certain predetermined criteria that represent the population of interest and is followed with well-defined outcome variables. In a cohort study, patients are not randomly assigned to a specific treatment or group before the study.[2] One example of a large cohort study is the Framingham, Massachusetts, community involving residents with identifiable cardiovascular risk factors being followed up for cardiovascular events.[2] This group of cases is compared with a control population selected on the presence or absence of exposure to a factor of interest. The purpose of cohort studies is to describe the occurrence of certain outcomes with time and to analyze associations between prognostic factors and those outcomes.

Cohort studies can be prospective or retrospective or a combination of both. Prospective studies begin at a specific point and are followed forward in time to evaluate the influence of certain factors or interventions on the desired outcomes.[1] The control group (ie, control cohort) is similar to the study group except for the exposure being studied, or data from the general population may be used as control.[1] An example of cohort studies is the evaluation of refractures in patients initially treated for a fracture. The advantages of cohort studies include the ability to study several outcomes over time and to ensure that the data collected are relevant. The disadvantages are that it is difficult to address rare events, ample time is required, the studies are expensive, and only a single question or hypothesis may be addressed in most studies.[1]

A retrospective cohort study uses historical data; therefore, the outcomes are already available. Patients are followed backward in time from the present to the past records. These studies are less time consuming as compared with prospective studies.[1] The problem with these studies is that they lack the ability to control the selection of subjects and they lack control over outcome measurements.

Randomized Control Trials

The RCT is often considered as the gold standard for the assessment of treatment efficacy. RCTs provide the strongest evidence due to their strong methodology, randomization and blinding intervention, and outcome. Therefore, RCTs are considered as level 1 evidence.[1] Randomization is an important characteristic of RCTs in which patients are randomly assigned to a treatment or control group. Randomization ensures that the factors affecting the outcome of the study result are equally distributed among the treatment groups.[1] The control group receives the standard treatment or no treatment and the treatment group receives specific intervention of interest. Blinding is another unique feature of high-quality RCTs wherein the treatment group to which the patient is assigned is not revealed to the patient (single-blinded) or both the investigator and patient (double-blinded).[1]

An RCT offers several advantages; it can clearly show a cause–effect relationship since it controls all other factors that may affect the outcomes and can eliminate biases by the process of randomization and blinding of subjects. The drawbacks of RCTs are the ethical concerns raised due to the use of a placebo group. Additionally, there are practical issues such as time constraints and limited finances.[1]

There are four basic RCT designs: parallel study design, crossover design, factorial designs, and *n*-of-1 designs. These designs are discussed below.

Parallel group designs

A parallel group design is the most common design for confirmatory trials as stated in the ICH E9 guideline "*Statistical Principles for Clinical Trials*." In this design, each patient is randomized to receive one of the two treatments. The patient may be assigned to one of the two or more treatment arms. The strengths of a parallel design are that it is robust and tolerant to many kinds of problems, it is easy to implement, analysis is less complicated, it is cost-effective, and interpretation of results is straightforward. Hence it is applicable to most experimental situations and is considered the gold standard.[3,4]

The major drawback of using a parallel design is that intrasubject variability cannot be measured because the subjects are allocated to one treatment group only throughout the study. The two types of parallel designs are group comparison (or parallel group) designs and matched pair's parallel design. The simplest example of group comparison parallel group design is a two-group parallel design that compares two treatments, namely, treatment group and control group. In this design, first a homogenous group of subjects is selected, and then from this group, subjects are randomly assigned to one of the two treatment groups. Figure 3-2 shows the different group comparison parallel group designs that can be used. The parallel group design requires more patients as compared to other designs, and it is by far the most commonly used design in phase II and phase III studies.[4]

The matched pair design is comprised of pairs of patients identical with respect to all relevant factors who are then assigned randomly to two groups. One patient is randomized to receive treatment A and the other is randomized to receive treatment B. It requires a smaller patient population and can reduce variability from treatment comparison. However, the disadvantages are that patient recruitment is slow and all relevant factors may not be known.[3]

Crossover designs

In this design, each patient or a group of patients receives more than one treatment at different dosing periods. Therefore, each patient serves as his or her own control and this gives a within-patient comparison between treatments. Before the patient is switched over to the next treatment, each subject is brought back to the original or baseline status of the disease that was present at the time of initiation of treatment. This period between the two treatments to achieve the baseline status is called a "washout" period. This washout period between two treatments is necessary to rule out any carryover effect between the two treatments. The advantages with the use of this design are that it requires a smaller sample size because of its increased sensitivity and smaller variability and removes the interpatient variability. However, it is affected by patient dropouts and missing data.[3,5]

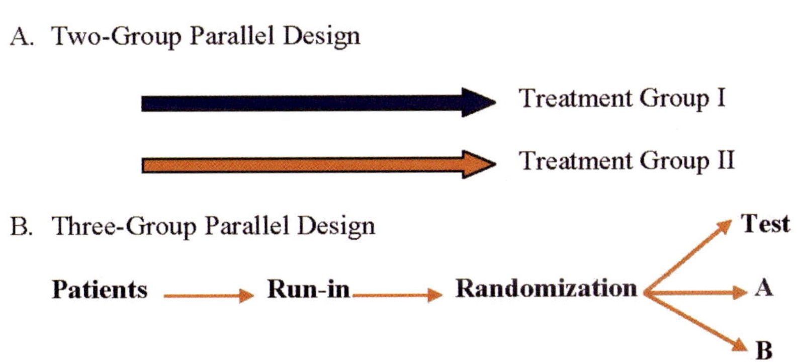

FIGURE 3-2. *Parallel group designs.*

Crossover studies are most appropriate where the effects of the treatment(s) are short-lived and reversible and are best suited to trials related to symptomatic but chronic conditions or diseases. A crossover design should not be used when the condition of interest is unstable and may change regardless of interventions.

Factorial designs

A factorial design is often used to understand the effect of two or more independent variables on a single dependent variable. In factorial designs, two or more interventions are evaluated simultaneously by using varying combinations of treatments.[6] The simplest example of factorial design is the 2 × 2 design. In this, there are two treatments (treatment A and treatment B) and there are four different combinations of these treatments: only A, only B, A + B, and no A no B. Patients are randomly assigned to one of the four groups so that they have an equal chance of being in any of the four groups. These designs are primarily used where it is possible to give the treatments together without modification (ie, they do not interfere with each other or potentiate each other's toxicity).[3]

Factorial designs are extremely useful to judge whether there is a link between variables, while reducing the possibility of experimental error and confounding variables. They allow for many levels of analysis. The major drawback of this design is the difficulty of experimenting with more than two factors or many levels. Other than these slight detractions, a factorial design is a mainstay of many scientific disciplines, delivering great results in the field.

Group sequential designs

Group sequential designs are used to facilitate the conduct of interim analysis.[6] With this design, a number of patients are enrolled, and studied. Then an interim analysis of data is conducted, and if the data are significant, the trial is stopped. If the results are not significant, another group of patients is enrolled and randomized as the original group.[3] An independent data and monitoring committee is usually set up to review or perform the interim analysis with group sequential designs. They are the most commonly used designs as it is feasible to assess the outcome of grouped subjects at periodic intervals during the trial rather than on a continuous basis as data from each subject become available.[6] The statistical methods to be used for interim analysis should be clearly specified in advance before the availability of information on treatment outcomes.

STATISTICS

Statistics play an important role in research, and to understand the statistical considerations for study designs, one must first understand the parameters that govern the use of these tests, such as the type of data generated (ie, nominal, ordinal, interval, and ratio data) and variables involved (dependent or independent). Nominal data are observations that fit into categories that have no intrinsic gradient in between them, such as yes/no or male/female. These data are often referred to as qualitative data. Ordinal data consist of categories with some meaningful scale between them. For example, open fractures are graded from type 1 to 3 in order of severity.[1] Nominal and ordinal data are nonparametric and do not assume any particular distribution.

Interval data (also sometimes called integer) are measured along a scale in which each position is equidistant from one another. Interval data cannot be multiplied or divided. Ratio data can be multiplied and divided. Interval and ratio data measure quantities and hence, are quantitative. Interval and ratio data are parametric and are used with parametric tools in which distributions are predictable (and often normal).

There are different statistical tests for analysis with different types of data, such as parametric tests and nonparametric tests. Parametric means that it meets certain requirements with respect to parameters of the population (eg, the data will be normal; the distribution parallels the normal or bell curve). Parametric statistics are considered more powerful than nonparametric statistics. Nonparametric data are lacking those same parameters and cannot be added, subtracted, multiplied, and divided. A nonparametric test is distribution free, which means that the data are not assumed to come from any specific distributions.

The following tests are discussed: *t* test, Mann-Whitney *U* test, χ^2 test, Fisher exact test, analysis of variance (ANOVA), and Kruskal-Wallis test. The chosen univariable statistical tests are applied to verify the trial primary hypothesis. The choice of the appropriate test is influenced by a number of statistical issues.

t Tests

The *t* test is a parametric test used in case of small sample size and it is applied to find the significance of difference between two means: as unpaired *t* test and as paired *t* test. The criteria for applying the *t* test are random samples, quantitative data, variable normally distributed, and sample size less than 30.[7]

For a comparison of the means of two independent samples of normally distributed continuous data, the appropriate test statistic is called t, hence, the t test. For large sample size (ie, >30 patients per group), the assumption of normality can be reasonably relaxed (the t test is then equivalent to a z test). For example, a randomized trial comparing fixation of fractures of the shaft of the humerus by dynamic compression plate (DCP) and intramedullary nail (IMN) was conducted by McCormack et al. One of the primary outcomes measured was function recorded via the American Shoulder and Elbow Surgeons (ASES) shoulder score ranging from 0 (worst score) to 52 points (best possible score).[8]

There was no significant difference in ASES function scores ($p = .71$) between the implants after the two-tailed t test was applied. Mean scores for the DCP and IMN groups were 48 and 47 points, respectively. However, samples sizes were small with 22 and 11 patients in the DCP and IMN groups, and no indication was provided in the paper regarding the distribution of the scores with each group.[2]

With small sample sizes and where the distribution of values are far from the normal distribution (eg, it is skewed), then it is better either to transform the values so that they look reasonably normally distributed (eg, by log transformation) or to use a nonparametric test such as the Wilcoxon rank sum test.[8]

Mann-Whitney *U* test

The Mann-Whitney U test is used to test whether two independent samples of observations are drawn from the same or identical distributions. This test offers the advantage that the two samples under consideration may not necessarily have the same number of observations.

It is a nonparametric test that can be applied to ordinal and continuous data without assuming normality. This test is an alternative to the independent two-sample t test when the assumption of normality is not met. Let us consider a hypothesis where H_0 (the mean change in knee flexion in group A) equals the mean change in knee flexion in group B versus H_1 (the means are different). We will assume the number of samples in group A and B as n_A and n_B, where the samples are equally distributed in both the groups. In order to calculate the test statistic U, the combined set of data is first arranged in ascending order with the smallest value receiving a rank of 1 and tied scores receiving a rank equal to the average position of those scores in the ordered sequence. The test statistic U is a function of these ranks[9]:

$$U = n_A n_B + \frac{n_A(n_A + 1)}{2} - R_A$$

where R_A is the sum of ranks for group A. The two important assumptions of the test are (1) the two samples are random and independent of each other, as are the observations within each sample, and (2) the observations are numeric or ordinal (arranged in ranks).

Chi-Square Test

The chi-square test is a simple method for testing the association between the row and column variables in a two-way table (contingency table). Contingency tables are used when analysis of categorical data is concerned with more than one variable.

The null hypothesis H_0 assumes that there is no association between the variables (in other words, one variable does not vary according to the other variable), while the alternative hypothesis H_a claims that some association does exist.[10] The chi-square test is based on a test statistic X^2 that measures the divergence of the observed data from the values that would be expected under the null hypothesis of no association. This requires calculation of the expected values based on the data. The expected value for each cell in a two-way table is equal to (row total * column total)/N, where N is the total number of observations included in the table:

$$e_{A,B} = \frac{\text{row } A \text{ total} \times \text{column } B \text{ total}}{\text{total } (N)}$$

Let us discuss an example where the frequency of three types of acromion shapes (flat, curved, or hooked) are reviewed in 33 cadaveric specimens with rotator cuff tears. H_0 represents the acromion shape that has no relation to rotator cuff tears and the expected or theoretical frequency of specimens with rotator cuff tears should be the same with each type of acromion (ie, 11 specimens should be found in each of the 3 groups). The data collected show a higher incidence of rotator cuff tears in specimens with curved acromiae, and an even higher incidence in specimens with hooked acromion types, with 3 specimens with flat acromiae, 8 with curved acromiae, and 22 with hooked acromiae (Table 3-1).

The chi-square test is used to evaluate these data and to derive a p value. The p value for this χ^2 statistic (17.636) is less than .005. A test statistic, χ^2 is computed from the data, and then the probability is calculated that the same or higher χ^2 value would be observed if the null hypothesis of equal proportions were true.[11]

TABLE 3-1. Frequency of Acromion Shapes in Specimens with Rotator Cuff Tears

Frequency	Acromion Morphology		
	Flat	Curved	Hooked
Observed	3	8	22
Expected	11	11	11

Fisher Exact Test

The chi-square test loses its power with small sample size, and it becomes more appropriate to apply the Fisher exact test that produces an accurate p value whatever the counts in any of the cells of a contingency table. It corrects for smaller numbers of observations and is used when the number of observations in a given grouping is less than 10 and the data may be arranged into a 2×2 table.[11]

As an example, in a study that compares the mortality rates between groups of patients undergoing unilateral and bilateral knee replacement, the incidence of death is very low, and this results in unbalanced distribution of data in the cells of the table. In such a case, the Fisher exact test is a suitable alternative to the X^2 test.

Kruskal-Wallis Test

The Kruskal-Wallis test is most commonly used when there is one nominal variable and one measurement variable, and the measurement variable does not meet the normality assumption of an ANOVA. The Kruskal-Wallis test does not make assumptions about normality. Like most nonparametric tests, it is performed on ranked data, so the measurement observations are converted to their ranks in the overall data set: the smallest value gets a rank of 1, the next smallest gets a rank of 2, and so on. The loss of information involved in substituting ranks for the original values can make this a less powerful test than an ANOVA, and ANOVA should be used if the data meet the assumptions.[12]

For example, H_0 assumes that the samples are from identical populations and H_A assumes that the sample comes from different populations. To calculate the value, apply the following formula:

$$H = \frac{12}{n(n+1)} \sum_{i=1}^{k} \frac{R_i^2}{n_i} - 3(n+1)$$

where H is the Kruskal-Wallis test, n is the total number of observations in all samples, and R_i is the rank of the sample.

The Kruskal-Wallis test statistic follows a chi-square distribution under the null hypothesis with k–1 degree of freedom where n_i should be greater than 5. The p value can be obtained from the X^2 distribution table.

ANOVA Test

ANOVA is one of the most common statistical tools used to identify differences between experimental group means. It allows performing hypotheses tests of significance to determine which factors influence the outcome of the experiment. ANOVA is commonly performed on the data coming from multicenter placebo-controlled clinical trials in order to evaluate the size of the difference in efficacy between the study medication and placebo.

One-way ANOVA

This test measures significant effects of one factor only and is an alternative to the independent two-sample t test for testing the equality of three or more means by use of variances. For example, an experiment might be defined by two parameters, such as treatment and time point. A one-way ANOVA would be able to assess only one parameter (ie, treatment effect or time effect), whereas a two-way ANOVA would assess both the treatment and time effect simultaneously and also assess whether there is an interaction between the parameters. A two-way ANOVA test generates three p values, one for each parameter and one for the interaction between the two parameters.

The null hypothesis will be that all population means are equal; the alternative hypothesis is that at least one mean is different. The whole idea behind the analysis of variance is to partition the total variation into "between-group variance" and "within-group variance" and compare the ratio (F statistic) of the two.

$$F \text{ Ratio} = \frac{\text{Between-group variance}}{\text{Within-group variance}}$$

$$= \frac{\text{Between-group mean square}}{\text{Within-group mean square}}$$

When the F ratio is close to 1, the estimates of variance are similar. This shows that the null hypothesis is not rejected, and the means came from the same population.[13] These terms are defined as follows. The grand mean is the average of all sample values.

TABLE 3-2. Two-Way ANOVA

Source	Sum of Squares	Degrees of Freedom	Mean Squares = SS/*df*	F Statistic
Main effect A	SS*A*	*A*, *a* – 1	MS*A*	MS(*A*) / MS(E)
Main effect B	SS*B*	*B*, *b* – 1	MS*B*	MS(*B*) / MS(E)
Interaction	SS*AB*	*A***B*, (*a* – 1)(*b* – 1)	MS*AB*	MS(*A***B*) / MS(E)
Error	SSE	*N* *ab*, *ab*(*n* – 1)	MSE	
Total	SST	*N* 1, *abn* – 1		

The within-group variation is the sum of squares within each treatment group. The within-group variance is the within-group variation divided by its degrees of freedom. If there are *k* samples, the total degrees of freedom are *k* less than the total sample size: $df = N–k$, where *N* is the total sample size.

Between-group variation is the sum of squared differences between each group mean and the grand mean. The between-group variance is the between-group variation divided by its degrees of freedom. If there are *k* groups, the degrees of freedom are then equal to $k–1$. The total variation (not variance) comprises the sum of the squares of the differences of each mean with the grand mean.

Two-way ANOVA prerequisites

Unlike the one-way ANOVA, which tests the effects of only one variable on equality of population means, the two-way ANOVA is designed to assess the effects of two or more variables or factors on population means. The assumptions in both the versions remain the same (ie, normality, independence, and equality of variance). The null hypothesis (H_0) in a two-way ANOVA includes the following:

- Main Effect: The main effect involves the independent variables one at a time. The population means of each factor are equal.
- Interaction Effect: The interaction effect is the effect that one factor has on the other factor. There is no interaction between the two factors.

In Table 3-2, it is assumed that main effect *A* has "*a*" levels (and $A = a - 1$ *df*), main effect *B* has "*b*" levels (and $B = b - 1$ *df*), *n* is the sample size of each treatment, and $N = abn$ is the total sample size. Notice the overall degree of freedom is once again one less than the total sample size.

The two-way ANOVA also divides the total variation into two main effects: between-group variation and within-group variation and interaction effects between the two factors. The *F* statistic is for two main effects and interaction effects.[14]

REFERENCES

1. Bhandari M, Sancheti P. *Clinical Research Made Easy.* New Delhi, India: Jaypee Brothers Medical Publishers; 2009.
2. Spilker B. Classification and description of phase IV postmarketing study designs. In: *A Guide to Clinical Trials.* New York: Raven Press; 1991:44-58.
3. Spilker B. Classification and description of phases I, II and III clinical trial designs. In: *A Guide to Clinical Trials.* New York: Raven Press; 1991:27-43.
4. Chow SC, Lui JP. Designs for clinical trials. In: *Design and Analysis of Clinical Trials: Concepts and Methodologies.* 2nd ed. Hoboken, NJ: John Wiley & Sons; 2004:167-214.
5. Sibbald B, Roberts C. Understanding controlled trials: crossover trials. *BMJ.* 1998;316:1719-1720.
6. ICH E9 Guideline: Statistical Principles for Clinical Trials. *Fed Register.* 1998;63(179):49583.
7. Mahajan BK. Significance of difference of means. In: *Methods in Biostatistics.* 6th ed. New Delhi, India: Jaypee Brothers Medical Publishers; 1997:130-155.
8. McCormack RG, Brien D, Buckley RE. Fixation of fractures of the shaft of the humerus by dynamic compression plate or intramedullary nail: a prospective randomised trial. *J Bone Joint Surg Br.* 2000;82:336-339.

9. Cooper DR, Schindler PS. Appendix B: Non-parametric significance test. In: *Business Research Methods*. 8th ed. New York: McGraw-Hill; 2009:662-668.
10. Walker G. The Chi Square Test. In: *Common Statistical Methods for Clinical Research: With SAS Examples*. 2nd ed. Cary, NC: SAS Publishing; 2002:265-279.
11. Kuhn JE, Greenfield VH. Statistical tests for discrete data. *Am Sports Med*. 1997;25:4.
12. McDonald JH. Tests for one measurement variable. In: *Handbook of Biological Statistics*. 2nd ed. Baltimore, MD: Sparky House Publishing; 2009:118-201.
13. Jekel JF. Multivariate analysis. In: *Epidemiology, Biostatistics & Preventive Medicine*. 3rd ed. New York: Elsevier Health Sciences; 2007:213-224.
14. Stephens LJ. Analysis of variance (ANOVA). In: *Beginning Statistics*. 2nd ed. New York: McGraw-Hill; 2009:299-338.

4

Knee Society Score

Jess H. Lonner and Giles R. Scuderi

In 1989, The Knee Society Clinical Rating System was developed as a simple, but objective scoring system to rate both the knee itself and functional abilities in terms of patients' abilities to walk and climb stairs after total knee arthroplasty.[1] This scoring system has been the most popular method of tracking and reporting outcomes after total and partial knee arthroplasty in the United States. However, it became clear over time that there were ambiguities and deficiencies with the original Knee Society scoring system that challenged its utility and validity in our contemporary patients, who often have different expectations, demands, and functional requirements than prior generations of knee replacement patients. The original Knee Society score was not validated and recently its reliability and responsiveness have been called into question.[2,3] It allowed a rather rudimentary assessment of stair climbing ability and walking ability (in terms of blocks) as well as use of assistive devices (Fig. 4-1). There is often inconsistency, however, with that score between its objective measures and the clinical and functional experiences of patients. Liow et al performed a study of 29 subjects assessed by six observers. The authors found high inter- and intraobserver variations of the Knee Society score, calling into question its reliability.[2] Another study by Lingard et al performed a prospective observational study of the outcomes of primary total knee arthroplasty for the treatment of osteoarthritis from a total of 12 centers in the United States, United Kingdom, and Australia. Nearly 700 patients completed preoperative and 12-month follow-up data using Knee Society clinical data, compared to Western Ontario and McMaster Universities Osteoarthritis Index (WOMAC), SF-36, patient satisfaction, and demographic data. The authors identified low correlations of the knee and function scores at both assessment times, and the Knee Society pain and function scores had moderate to strong correlations with the corresponding pain and function domains of the WOMAC and SF-36 ($R = 0.31–0.72$). The Knee Society knee score was highly responsive, in fact more responsive than the WOMAC or SF-36; however, the Knee Society function score component was the least responsive measure. Additionally, the authors found that correlation of changes in scores at 12 months with patient reports of satisfaction and improvement in health status were less responsive using the Knee Society scores than the WOMAC and SF-36 scores.[3]

While total and partial knee arthroplasty are highly successful interventions for knee arthritis, the defining parameters of success may vary depending on who is asked (ie, patient or physician), what defines success, and what variables are used to measure success. Certainly, more than 90% of patients at follow-up periods of 10 to 15 years have successful outcomes after total and partial knee arthroplasties based on implant survivorship. However, perception of outcomes will differ depending on whether objective or subjective measures are utilized, whether they are patient or clinician derived, and according to the parameters that are being measured. For instance, if implant survivorship is the ultimate outcome measure, then success may be unparalleled. Additionally, functional outcomes, patient satisfaction, and meeting patient expectations may be most important in determining whether an outcome is deemed successful or not.[4] Functional outcomes have been shown to vary with demographic and patient characteristics, such as body mass index, emotional health, sex, age, and severity of preoperative pain.[5] Furthermore, there is poor correlation between objective physician-assessed knee scores and patient-derived satisfaction scores, highlighting a discrepancy between physicians and patients in the interpretation and prioritization of outcomes.[6]

Given these concerns, it was important for the Knee Society to reevaluate its method of evaluating patients after both partial and total knee arthroplasty and to develop a new Knee Society Scoring System that integrates patient- and surgeon-derived outcomes assessments by means of a validated measure that is relevant to today's patients. Heeding the advice of statisticians, it was critical that this new score has adequate validity (ie, it measures what it is designed to measure), reliability (ie, it consistently produces the same score given the equivalence of status of the element), and responsiveness (ie, it assesses changes in a particular parameter at all stages of measurement).[7]

The new Knee Society Scoring System (Figs. 4-2 and 4-3), copyrighted in 2011, is a validated system that combines an objective component as well as a subjective patient-derived component that evaluates pain relief, functional abilities, satisfaction, and fulfillment of expectations.[7] This score, with its component elements, was validated in a thoughtful and methodical fashion. A multicentered study was undertaken over a several-year period capturing regionally diverse patients and physicians, with over 500 patients examined and surveyed both preoperatively and postoperatively. Objective and subjective data were captured and compared to the KOOS and SF-12 scores for validation. Using statisticians and epidemiologists, each question was analyzed to detect differential item functioning. A subgroup of cases was selected to evaluate and retest responses for internal reliability. The new updated Knee Society Scoring System has been proven to be broadly applicable across gender, age, activity level, and implant type. Given the diverse activity profiles of many contemporary patients, the functional component of the score was improved to include a patient-specific survey, which evaluates features such as standard activities of daily living as well as patient-specific sports and recreational activities, patient satisfaction, and patient expectations. Change in scores from preoperative to postoperative will indicate functional outcomes achieved by the procedure. Portions of the original Knee Society Scoring System have been integrated into the new version to try to maintain integrity of the prior version of the Knee Society score.[8]

The new Knee Society score is shown in Figures 4-2 and 4-3. It includes an initial assessment of demographic details, including the Charnley functional classification. The objective knee score, completed by the surgeon, includes a visual analog score of pain walking on level ground and on stairs or inclines, as well as an assessment of alignment, collateral, and cruciate stability, range of motion, and deductions for flexion contractures or extensor lags. Patient satisfaction, functional activities, and patient expectations are then recorded by patients and are considered a crucial component of the Knee Society Clinical Scoring System.

In conclusion, the new Knee Society Clinical Scoring System is a validated and responsive method for assessing objective and subjective outcomes after partial and total knee arthroplasty, without the ambiguities of the previous system. As physicians, clinical practices, and health systems become increasingly more responsible for tracking outcomes, the clear value of the updated Knee Society Clinical Rating System will become more apparent in years to come. *Figures continue on page 4-3.*

FIGURE 4-1. *Knee Society score (original method).*

Patient category

A. Unilateral or bilateral (opposite knee successfully replaced)
B. Unilateral, other knee symptomatic
C. Multiple arthritis or medical infirmity

Objective Scoring

Pain	Points
None	50
Mild or occasional	45
Stairs only	40
Walking & stairs	30
Moderate	
Occasional	20
Continual	10
Severe	0

Range of motion

(5º = 1 point)	25

Stability
(maximum movement in any position)

Anteroposterior

<5 mm	10
5-10 mm	5
10 mm	0

Mediolateral

<5º	15
6º -9º	10
10º -14º	5
15º	0

Flexion contracture

5º -10º	-2
10º -15º	-5
16º -20º	-10
>20º	-15

Extension lag

<10º	-5
10º -20º	-10
>20º	-15

Alignment

5º -10º	0
0º -4º	3 points each degree
11º -15º	3 points each degree

Functional Scoring

Walking	50
Unlimited	40
>10 blocks	30
5-10 blocks	20
<5 blocks	10
Housebound	0

Stairs

Normal up & down	50
Normal up,down with rail	40
Up & down with rail	30
Up with rail; unable down	15
Unable	0

Functional Deductions

Cane	-5
Two canes	-10
Crutches or walker	-20
Other	20

Knee Score
(If total is a minus number, score is 0)

FIGURE 4-2. *Knee Society score: preoperative. (Reprinted with permission, © 2011 The Knee Society.)*

KNEE SOCIETY SCORE: PRE-OP

DEMOGRAPHIC INFORMATION (To be completed by patient)

1- Today's date

☐☐ / ☐☐ / ☐☐☐☐

Enter dates as: mm/dd/yyyy

2- Date of birth

☐☐ / ☐☐ / ☐☐☐☐

3- Height (ft' in")

☐ ☐☐

4- Weight (lbs.)

☐☐☐

5- Sex

O Male O Female

6- Side of this (symptomatic) knee

O Left O Right

If both knees will be operated on, please use a different form for each knee

7- Ethnicity

O Native Hawaiian or other Pacific Islander O American Indian or Alaska Native O Hispanic or Latino

O Arab or Middle Eastern O African American or Black O Asian O White

8- Please indicate the expected date and surgeon for your knee replacement operation

Date

☐☐ / ☐☐ / ☐☐☐☐

Enter dates as: mm/dd/yyyy

Name of Surgeon

☐

9- Will this be a primary or revision knee replacement?

O Primary O Revision

To be completed by surgeon

10- Charnley Functional Classification (Use Code Below) ☐

A	Unilateral Knee Arthritis	C1	TKR, but remote arthritis affecting ambulation
B1	Unilateral TKA, opposite knee arthritic	C2	TKR, but medical condition affecting ambulation
B2	Bilateral TKA	C3	Unilateral or Bilateral TKA with Unilateral or Bilateral THR

FIGURE 4-2 Continued.

OBJECTIVE KNEE INDICATORS (To be completed by surgeon)

ALIGNMENT

1- Alignment: measured on AP standing Xray (Anatomic Alignment) **25 point max**

Neutral: 2-10 degrees valgus (25 pts)
Varus: < 2 degrees valgus (-10 pts)
Valgus: > 10 degrees valgus (-10 pts)

INSTABILITY

2- Medial / Lateral Instability: measured in full extension **15 point max**

None (15 pts)
Little or < 5 mm (10 pts)
Moderate or 5 mm (5 pts)
Severe or > 5 mm (0 pts)

3- Anterior / Posterior Instability: measured at 90 degrees **10 point max**

None (10 pts)
Moderate < 5 mm (5 pts)
Severe > 5 mm (0 pts)

JOINT MOTION

4- Range of motion (1 point for each 5 degrees)

Deductions

Flexion Contracture **Minus Points**
1-5 degrees (-2 pts)
6-10 degrees (-5 pts)
11-15 degrees (-10 pts)
> 15 degrees (-15 pts)

Extensor Lag **Minus Points**
<10 degrees (-5 pts)
10-20 degrees (-10 pts)
> 20 degrees (-15 pts)

FIGURE 4-2 Continued.

SYMPTOMS

(To be completed by patient)

1- Pain with level walking **(10 - Score)**

0	1	2	3	4	5	6	7	8	9	10

none **severe**

2- Pain with stairs or inclines **(10 - Score)**

0	1	2	3	4	5	6	7	8	9	10

none **severe**

3- Does this knee feel "normal" to you? **(5 points)**

O Always (5 pts) O Sometimes (3 pts) O Never (0 pts)

Maximum total points (25 points)

PATIENT SATISFACTION

1- Currently, how satisfied are you with the pain level of your knee while sitting? **(8 points)**

O Very Satisfied (8 pts) O Satisfied (6 pts) O Neutral (4 pts) O Dissatisfied (2 pts) O Very Dissatisfied (0 pts)

2- Currently, how satisfied are you with the pain level of your knee while lying in bed? **(8 points)**

O Very Satisfied (8 pts) O Satisfied (6 pts) O Neutral (4 pts) O Dissatisfied (2 pts) O Very Dissatisfied (0 pts)

3- Currently, how satisfied are you with your knee function while getting out of bed? **(8 points)**

O Very Satisfied (8 pts) O Satisfied (6 pts) O Neutral (4 pts) O Dissatisfied (2 pts) O Very Dissatisfied (0 pts)

4- Currently, how satisfied are you with your knee function while performing light household duties? **(8 points)**

O Very Satisfied (8 pts) O Satisfied (6 pts) O Neutral (4 pts) O Dissatisfied (2 pts) O Very Dissatisfied (0 pts)

5- Currently, how satisfied are you with your knee function while performing leisure recreational activities? **(8 points)**

O Very Satisfied (8 pts) O Satisfied (6 pts) O Neutral (4 pts) O Dissatisfied (2 pts) O Very Dissatisfied (0 pts)

Maximum total points (40 points)

FIGURE 4-2 Continued.

PATIENT EXPECTATIONS (To be completed by patient)

What do you expect to accomplish with your knee replacement:

1- Do you expect your knee joint replacement surgery will relieve your knee pain? **(5 points)**

O no, not at all (1 pt)
O yes, a little bit (2 pts)
O yes, somewhat (3 pts)
O yes, a moderate amount (4 pts)
O yes, a lot (5 pts)

2- Do you expect your surgery will help you carry out your normal activities of daily living? **(5 points)**

O no, not at all (1 pt)
O yes, a little bit (2 pts)
O yes, somewhat (3 pts)
O yes, a moderate amount (4 pts)
O yes, a lot (5 pts)

3- Do you expect you surgery will help you perform leisure, recreational or sports activities? **(5 points)**

O no, not at all (1 pt)
O yes, a little bit (2 pts)
O yes, somewhat (3 pts)
O yes, a moderate amount (4 pts)
O yes, a lot (5 pts)

Maximum total points (15 points) [ ]

FIGURE 4-2 Continued.

FUNCTIONAL ACTIVITIES (To be completed by patient)

WALKING AND STANDING (30 points)

1 - Can you walk without any aids (such as a cane, crutches or wheelchair)? **(0 points)**

O Yes O No

2 - If no, which of the following aid(s) do you use? **(-10 points)**

O wheelchair (-10 pts) O walker (-8 pts) O crutches (-8 pts) O two canes (-6 pts) ☐

O one crutch (-4 pts) O one cane (-4 pts) O knee sleeve / brace (-2 pts)

O other ☐☐☐☐☐☐☐☐☐☐☐☐☐☐☐☐☐☐☐☐

3 - Do you use these aid(s) because of your knees? **(0 points)**

O Yes O No

4 - For how long can you stand (with or without aid) before sitting due to knee discomfort? **(15 points)**

O cannot stand (0 pts) O 0-5 minutes (3 pts) O 6-15 minutes (6 pts) ☐

O 16-30 minutes (9 pts) O 31-60 minutes (12 pts) O more than an hour (15 pts)

5 - For how long can you walk (with or without aid) before stopping due to knee discomfort? **(15 points)**

O cannot walk (0 pts) O 0-5 minutes (3 pts) O 6-15 minutes (6 pts) ☐

O 16-30 minutes (9 pts) O 31-60 minutes (12 pts) O more than an hour (15 pts)

Maximum points (30 points) ☐

FIGURE 4-2 Continued.

STANDARD ACTIVITIES (30 points)

How much does your knee bother you during each of the following activities?	no bother 5	slight 4	moderate 3	severe 2	very severe 1	cannot do (because of knee) 0	I never do this	
1 - Walking on an uneven surface	○	○	○	○	○	○	○	☐
2 - Turning or pivoting on your leg	○	○	○	○	○	○	○	☐
3 - Climbing up or down a flight of stairs	○	○	○	○	○	○	○	☐
4 - Getting up from a low couch or a chair without arms	○	○	○	○	○	○	○	☐
5 - Getting into or out of a car	○	○	○	○	○	○	○	☐
6 - Moving laterally (stepping to the side)	○	○	○	○	○	○	○	☐

Maximum points (30 points) ☐

ADVANCED ACTIVITIES (25 points)

1 - Climbing a ladder or step stool	○	○	○	○	○	○	○	☐
2 - Carrying a shopping bag for a block	○	○	○	○	○	○	○	☐
3 - Squatting	○	○	○	○	○	○	○	☐
4 - Kneeling	○	○	○	○	○	○	○	☐
5 - Running	○	○	○	○	○	○	○	☐

Maximum points (25 points) ☐

FIGURE 4-2 Continued.

DISCRETIONARY KNEE ACTIVITIES (15 points)

Please check 3 of the activities below that you consider *most important* to you.
(Please do not write in additional activities)

Recreational Activities

- ☐ Swimming
- ☐ Golfing (18 holes)
- ☐ Road Cycling (>30mins)
- ☐ Gardening
- ☐ Bowling
- ☐ Racquet Sports (Tennis, Racquetball, etc.)
- ☐ Distance Walking
- ☐ Dancing / Ballet
- ☐ Stretching Exercises (stretching out your muscles)

Workout and Gym Activities

- ☐ Weight-lifting
- ☐ Leg Extensions
- ☐ Stair-Climber
- ☐ Stationary Biking / Spinning
- ☐ Leg Press
- ☐ Jogging
- ☐ Elliptical Trainer
- ☐ Aerobic Exercises

Please copy all 3 checked activities into the empty boxes below.

How much does your knee bother you during each of these activities?

Activity (Please write the 3 activites from list above)	no bother 5	slight 4	moderate 3	severe 2	very severe 1	cannot do (because of knee) 0	
1.	○	○	○	○	○	○	☐
2.	○	○	○	○	○	○	☐
3.	○	○	○	○	○	○	☐

Maximum points (15 points) ☐

Maximum total points (100 points) ☐

FIGURE 4-3. *Knee Society score: postoperative. (Reprinted with permission, © 2011 The Knee Society.)*

KNEE SOCIETY SCORE: POST-OP

DEMOGRAPHIC INFORMATION **(To be completed by patient)**

1- Today's date

☐☐ / ☐☐ / ☐☐☐☐

Enter dates as: mm/dd/yyyy

2- Date of birth

☐☐ / ☐☐ / ☐☐☐☐

3- Height (ft' in")

☐ ☐☐

4- Weight (lbs.)

☐☐☐

5- Sex

O Male O Female

6- Side of this (surgically treated) knee

O Left O Right

If both knees have been operated on, please use a different form for each knee

7- Ethnicity

O Native Hawaiian or other Pacific Islander O American Indian or Alaska Native O Hispanic or Latino

O Arab or Middle Eastern O African American or Black O Asian O White

8- Please indicate date and surgeon for your knee replacement operation

Date

☐☐ / ☐☐ / ☐☐☐☐

Enter dates as: mm/dd/yyyy

Name of Surgeon

☐

9- Was this a primary or revision knee replacement?

O Primary O Revision

To be completed by surgeon

10- Charnley Functional Classification **(Use Code Below)** ☐

A	Unilateral Knee Arthritis	C1	TKR, but remote arthritis affecting ambulation
B1	Unilateral TKA, opposite knee arthritic	C2	TKR, but medical condition affecting ambulation
B2	Bilateral TKA	C3	Unilateral or Bilateral TKA with Unilateral or Bilateral THR

FIGURE 4-3 Continued.

OBJECTIVE KNEE INDICATORS (To be completed by surgeon)

ALIGNMENT

1- Alignment: measured on AP standing Xray (Anatomic Alignment) — **25 point max** ☐

Neutral: 2-10 degrees valgus	(25 pts)
Varus: < 2 degrees valgus	(-10 pts)
Valgus: > 10 degrees valgus	(-10 pts)

INSTABILITY

2- Medial / Lateral Instability: measured in full extension — **15 point max** ☐

None	(15 pts)
Little or < 5 mm	(10 pts)
Moderate or 5 mm	(5 pts)
Severe or > 5 mm	(0 pts)

3- Anterior / Posterior Instability: measured at 90 degrees — **10 point max** ☐

None	(10 pts)
Moderate < 5 mm	(5 pts)
Severe > 5 mm	(0 pts)

JOINT MOTION

4- Range of motion (1 point for each 5 degrees) ☐

Deductions

Flexion Contracture — **Minus Points** ☐

1-5 degrees	(-2 pts)
6-10 degrees	(-5 pts)
11-15 degrees	(-10 pts)
> 15 degrees	(-15 pts)

Extensor Lag — **Minus Points** ☐

<10 degrees	(-5 pts)
10-20 degrees	(-10 pts)
> 20 degrees	(-15 pts)

FIGURE 4-3 Continued.

SYMPTOMS

(To be completed by patient)

1- Pain with level walking **(10 - Score)**

0	1	2	3	4	5	6	7	8	9	10

none **severe**

2- Pain with stairs or inclines **(10 - Score)**

0	1	2	3	4	5	6	7	8	9	10

none **severe**

3- Does this knee feel "normal" to you? **(5 points)**

O Always (5 pts) O Sometimes (3 pts) O Never (0 pts)

Maximum total points (25 points)

PATIENT SATISFACTION

1- Currently, how satisfied are you with the pain level of your knee while sitting? **(8 points)**

O Very Satisfied (8 pts) O Satisfied (6 pts) O Neutral (4 pts) O Dissatisfied (2 pts) O Very Dissatisfied (0 pts)

2- Currently, how satisfied are you with the pain level of your knee while lying in bed? **(8 points)**

O Very Satisfied (8 pts) O Satisfied (6 pts) O Neutral (4 pts) O Dissatisfied (2 pts) O Very Dissatisfied (0 pts)

3- Currently, how satisfied are you with your knee function while getting out of bed? **(8 points)**

O Very Satisfied (8 pts) O Satisfied (6 pts) O Neutral (4 pts) O Dissatisfied (2 pts) O Very Dissatisfied (0 pts)

4- Currently, how satisfied are you with your knee function while performing light household duties? **(8 points)**

O Very Satisfied (8 pts) O Satisfied (6 pts) O Neutral (4 pts) O Dissatisfied (2 pts) O Very Dissatisfied (0 pts)

5- Currently, how satisfied are you with your knee function while performing leisure recreational activities? **(8 points)**

O Very Satisfied (8 pts) O Satisfied (6 pts) O Neutral (4 pts) O Dissatisfied (2 pts) O Very Dissatisfied (0 pts)

Maximum total points (40 points)

FIGURE 4-3 Continued.

PATIENT EXPECTATION (To be completed by patient)

Compared to what you expected before your knee replacement:

1- My expectations for pain relief were... **(5 points)**

- O Too High- "I'm a lot worse than I thought" (1 pt)
- O Too High- "I'm somewhat worse than I thought" (2 pts)
- O Just Right- "My expectations were met" (3 pts)
- O Too Low- "I'm somewhat better than I thought" (4 pts)
- O Too Low- "I'm a lot better than I thought" (5 pts)

2- My expectations for being able to do my normal activities of daily living were... **(5 points)**

- O Too High- "I'm a lot worse than I thought" (1 pt)
- O Too High- "I'm somewhat worse than I thought" (2 pts)
- O Just Right- "My expectations were met" (3 pts)
- O Too Low- "I'm somewhat better than I thought" (4 pts)
- O Too Low- "I'm a lot better than I thought" (5 pts)

3- My expectations for being able to do my leisure, recreational or sports activities were... **(5 points)**

- O Too High- "I'm a lot worse than I thought" (1 pt)
- O Too High- "I'm somewhat worse than I thought" (2 pts)
- O Just Right- "My expectations were met" (3 pts)
- O Too Low- "I'm somewhat better than I thought" (4 pts)
- O Too Low- "I'm a lot better than I thought" (5 pts)

Maximum total points (15 points) ☐

FIGURE 4-3 Continued.

FUNCTIONAL ACTIVITIES (To be completed by patient)

WALKING AND STANDING (30 points)

1 - Can you walk without any aids (such as a cane, crutches or wheelchair)? **(0 points)**

O Yes O No

2 - If no, which of the following aid(s) do you use? **(-10 points)**

O wheelchair (-10 pts) O walker (-8 pts) O crutches (-8 pts) O two canes (-6 pts) ☐

O one crutch (-4 pts) O one cane (-4 pts) O knee sleeve / brace (-2 pts)

O other ☐☐☐☐☐☐☐☐☐☐☐☐☐☐☐☐☐☐☐☐

3 - Do you use these aid(s) because of your knees? **(0 points)**

O Yes O No

4 - For how long can you stand (with or without aid) before sitting due to knee discomfort? **(15 points)**

O cannot stand (0 pts) O 0-5 minutes (3 pts) O 6-15 minutes (6 pts) ☐

O 16-30 minutes (9 pts) O 31-60 minutes (12 pts) O more than an hour (15 pts)

5 - For how long can you walk (with or without aid) before stopping due to knee discomfort? **(15 points)**

O cannot walk (0 pts) O 0-5 minutes (3 pts) O 6-15 minutes (6 pts) ☐

O 16-30 minutes (9 pts) O 31-60 minutes (12 pts) O more than an hour (15 pts)

Maximum points (30 points) ☐

FIGURE 4-3 Continued.

STANDARD ACTIVITIES (30 points)

How much does your knee bother you during each of the following activities?	no bother 5	slight 4	moderate 3	severe 2	very severe 1	cannot do (because of knee) 0	I never do this	
1 - Walking on an uneven surface	○	○	○	○	○	○	○	☐
2 - Turning or pivoting on your leg	○	○	○	○	○	○	○	☐
3 - Climbing up or down a flight of stairs	○	○	○	○	○	○	○	☐
4 - Getting up from a low couch or a chair without arms	○	○	○	○	○	○	○	☐
5 - Getting into or out of a car	○	○	○	○	○	○	○	☐
6 - Moving laterally (stepping to the side)	○	○	○	○	○	○	○	☐

Maximum points (30 points) ☐

ADVANCED ACTIVITIES (25 points)

Activity	5	4	3	2	1	0	I never do this	
1 - Climbing a ladder or step stool	○	○	○	○	○	○	○	☐
2 - Carrying a shopping bag for a block	○	○	○	○	○	○	○	☐
3 - Squatting	○	○	○	○	○	○	○	☐
4 - Kneeling	○	○	○	○	○	○	○	☐
5 - Running	○	○	○	○	○	○	○	☐

Maximum points (25 points) ☐

FIGURE 4-3 Continued.

DISCRETIONARY KNEE ACTIVITIES (15 points)

Please check 3 of the activities below that you consider *most important* to you.
(Please do not write in additional activities)

Recreational Activities

☐ Swimming
☐ Golfing (18 holes)
☐ Road Cycling (>30mins)
☐ Gardening
☐ Bowling
☐ Racquet Sports (Tennis, Racquetball, etc.)
☐ Distance Walking
☐ Dancing / Ballet
☐ Stretching Exercises (stretching out your muscles)

Workout and Gym Activities

☐ Weight-lifting
☐ Leg Extensions
☐ Stair-Climber
☐ Stationary Biking / Spinning
☐ Leg Press
☐ Jogging
☐ Elliptical Trainer
☐ Aerobic Exercises

Please copy all 3 checked activities into the empty boxes below.

How much does your knee bother you during each of these activities?

Activity (Please write the 3 activites from list above)	no bother 5	slight 4	moderate 3	severe 2	very severe 1	cannot do (because of knee) 0	
1.	○	○	○	○	○	○	☐
2.	○	○	○	○	○	○	☐
3.	○	○	○	○	○	○	☐

Maximum points (15 points) ☐

Maximum total points (100 points) ☐

REFERENCES

1. Insall JN, Dorr LD, Scott RD, et al. Rationale of the Knee Society Clinical Rating System. *Clin Orthop Relat Res.* 1989;248:13-14.
2. Liow RY, Walker K, Wajid MA, et al. The reliability of the American Knee Society score. *Acta Orthop Scand.* 2000;71:603-608.
3. Lingard EA, Katz JN, Wright RJ, et al. Validity and responsiveness of the Knee Society Clinical Rating System in comparison with the SF-36 and WOMAC. *J Bone Joint Surg Am.* 2001;83:1856-1864.
4. Scott WN, Booth RE, Dalury DF, et al. Efficiency and economics in joint arthroplasty. *J Bone Joint Surg.* 2009;suppl 5:33-36.
5. Franklin PD, Li W, Ayers DC. Functional outcome after total knee replacement varies with patient attributes. *Clin Orthop Relat Res.* 2008;466:2597-2604.
6. Kreibich DN, Vaz M, Bourne RB, et al. What is the best way of assessing outcome after total knee replacement? *Clin Orthop Relat Res.* 1996;331:221-225.
7. Noble PC, Scuderi GR, Brekke AC, et al. Development of a new Knee Society Scoring System. *Clin Orthop Relat Res.* 2012;470(1):20-32.
8. Scuderi GR, Bourne RB, Noble PC, et al. The new Knee Society Knee Scoring System. *Clin Orthop Relat Res.* 2012;470(1):3-19.

5 A Tool for Measuring Lower Extremity Activity: A Well-Validated, Simple, One-Page, One-Mark Questionnaire

Kenneth A. Krackow, Laura E. White, and Cathy Buyea

The task of stratifying an individual patient's actual activity level has been recognized as an appropriate effort for many years. My own (KAK) interest in this occurred at the 1979 American Academy of Orthopaedic Surgeons meeting in San Francisco, California. Hugh Chandler, a well-known orthopaedic surgeon from the Massachusetts General Hospital, presented his paper on the high rate of failure within 5 to 10 years after total hip replacement in a group of patients with developmental dysplasia of the hip. The patients were 20 to 30 years of age, and in discussion the assumption was that the young age group was more active and therefore experiencing shortened survivorships.[1] I immediately questioned that explanation. It seemed to me that this population could easily have been troubled by technical issues of deficient bone stock, highly more complicated previous operations, and so forth.

CREATING A TOOL TO MEASURE ACTIVITY LEVEL

The question was, how does one put together a useful, inexpensive, reliable activity score? It appeared excessively daunting to consider a patient who sits all day in an office and does very little walking—to car and home—yet on the weekends is involved in very strenuous activity. The task at first seemed only possible by instrumenting a person's foot or leg not only to count steps, but also to judge mechanical force (ie, velocity, impact) about any kind of biomechanical variable that might be relevant.

It was necessary to think back on simpler methods of assigning categories. Clearly, scoring systems that exist within orthopaedic surgery are highly problematic if they involve too much detail. The task involved first categorizing a patient in rather broad choices or categories of overall activity. The first category would include patients who are the least active, essentially those who are non-ambulatory. The second category would include patients who are household ambulatory and the third category would include those who are community ambulatory. The final category would include all levels of training and athletic activity as well as occupational activity beyond normal.

It then became possible within these categories to create statements that reflected additional partitioning of activity levels. The formulated scale, as presented in Figure 5-1, has different levels of activity within each of the broader categories just mentioned.

LOWER EXTREMITY ACTIVITY SCALE

Kenneth A. Krackow, MD
Kaleida Health – The Buffalo General Hospital
State University of New York at Buffalo

Patient Name: ______________________________ Date:______________

Please read through each description given below, pick the ONE description that best describes your regular daily activity and put a check in that box. (Check only one box.)

1. ☐ I am confined to bed all day.

2. ☐ I am confined to bed most of the day except for minimal transfer activities (going to the bathroom, etc).

3. ☐ I am either in bed or sitting in a chair most of the day.

4. ☐ I sit most of the day, except for minimal transfer activities, no walking or standing.

5. ☐ I sit most of the day, but I stand occasionally and walk a minimal amount in my house. (I may rarely leave the house for an appointment and may require the use of a wheelchair or scooter for transportation.)

6. ☐ I walk around my house to a moderate degree but I don't leave the house on a regular basis. I may leave the house occasionally for an appointment.

7. ☐ I walk around my house and go outside at will, walking one or two blocks at a time.

8. ☐ I walk around my house, go outside at will, and walk several blocks at a time without any assistance (weather permitting).

9. ☐ I am up and about at will in my house and can go out and walk as much as I would like with no restrictions (weather permitting).

10. ☐ I am up and about at will in my house and outside. I also work outside the house in a ____**minimally** ____**moderately** _____**extremely** active job.

(Please circle the best description of your work level.)

11. ☐ I am up and about at will in my house and outside. I also participate in relaxed physical activity such as jogging, dancing, cycling, swimming ____**occasionally (2-3 times per month)** ____**2-3 times per week** ____**daily**.

(Please circle the best description of how often you participate in this activity.)

12. ☐ I am up and about at will in my house and outside. I also participate in vigorous physical activity such as competitive level sports ____**occasionally (2-3 times per month)** ____**2 –3 times per week** ___**daily**.

Please circle the best description of how often you participate in this activity.

FIGURE 5-1. *The Krackow Lower Extremity Activity Scale.*

VALIDATION

The validation process includes the following steps. First, agreement on the ordering of the questions was ascertained by printing each single activity level statement onto a single card and then shuffling that pile of cards into a random order. That random order was duplicated for a test involving 18 orthopaedic surgeons. These lower extremity reconstruction surgeons were directed to take this pile of cards with the described activity levels and to lay the cards out across a surface. Then they could decide the rank order of the cards (ie, placing each card in order with respect to the other cards above and below). After rearranging in ascending order, the surgeon would then reassemble the pile and present it back for evaluation. Out of all of the participating lower extremity reconstruction surgeons, there was only one person who had an exchange of two originally adjacent activity levels. The two cards were just rearranged one to the other. It is of note that this surgeon's primary language was Spanish. One can conclude from this particular validation process that an agreed upon ascending scale of activity had been constructed.

Second, patients filled in the activity survey at differing points in time, approximately 3 to 4 weeks apart, when there were no major changes in the patient's health situation. There was extremely close agreement for the repeated measurements. Furthermore, the activity form was provided to a close person—a spouse, parent, or others who lived directly with the patient. That person would grade the patient independently, and the results from that exercise also had very strict agreement.

Third, we developed a pedometer study including both patients and other volunteers of ages ranging from the late teenage years to the late 70s. The correlation coefficient between activity level and steps per week was 0.792 for all (a very high correlation).

The final step involved two more elements. First of all, we compared the patient's preoperative activity score to the 6- and 12-month postoperative activity score. The patients clearly improved by at least one or more category levels, sometimes substantially more. Next, the activity levels were correlated with other validated outcome measures as published in an article by Saleh et al.[2] This article has an extremely thorough explanation of all aspects of the validation process.

Following all of this work, which was presented at several meetings and is represented in some publications, this score has enjoyed some popularity under the designation LEAS (Lower Extremity Activity Scale). The scale is also referenced with my name as well.

Over the period of time during which we were working on this and up to the present day, a more widely utilized scale, the UCLA Activity Score, has received attention. One can agree that this is a simple, well-composed activity scale. That rating system differs from ours in that it is investigator determined and based on highest-rated activity, regardless of frequency or intensity.[3]

Furthermore, we noted by applying the UCLA score to all of our test patients during this period that the distinctions here were not very discriminating or widespread. That is to say, the overwhelming majority of patients fit only within two different and adjacent levels of the UCLA score.

We have used our Lower Extremity Activity Scale for more than 10 years. Its administration is quick, inexpensive, and thoroughly validated. Feel free to use it with no fees regarding copyright or other issues. The activity scale was designed by Kenneth A. Krackow, the studies and reviews were performed by Laura E. White, and the statistical methods were selected and executed by Cathy Buyea.

REFERENCES

1. Chandler HP, Reineck FT, Wixson RL, et al. Total hip replacement in patients younger than thirty years old. A five-year follow-up study. *J Bone Joint Surg Am.* 1981;63(9):1426-1434.
2. Saleh SJ, Mulhall KJ, Bershadsky B, et al. Development and validation of a lower extremity activity scale. *J Bone Joint Surg Am.* 2005;87(9):1985-1994.
3. Zahiri CA, Schmalzried TP, Szuszczewicz ES, et al. Assessing activity in joint replacement patients. *J Arthroplasty.* 1998;13(8):890-895.

6

Knee Outcome Questionnaires

Ali Hussam, Andrea Wood, and Christina Dorey

The purpose of this chapter is to provide an easy interpretation of common knee outcome questionnaires used in the health professions: Cincinnati, International Knee Documentation Committee (IKDC), Knee Injury and Osteoarthritis Outcome Score (KOOS), Knee Society score (KSS), Lysholm, Western Ontario and McMaster Universities Index of Osteoarthritis (WOMAC), Oxford, Activities of Daily Living (ADL), SF-12v1, and SF-36v1. The chapter provides doctors with a unique overview of each questionnaire by providing the following key information: questionnaire description, subscales, scoring description, required questions, minimum score, and maximum score (Table 6-1). In addition to their individual characteristics, the instruments are cross-referenced with each other and with important activities involving the knee. This reveals commonalities and differences among the questionnaires to further aid in understanding the alternatives available.

Information was gathered on each questionnaire from the available literature. Since many of the questionnaires have multiple versions, the most recent version was used for each questionnaire.

The information provided here is not readily available elsewhere. It promises to provide doctors with an efficient means to choose the most appropriate instrument for obtaining feedback from their patients.

CINCINNATI

- **Questionnaire Description**: A short patient knee questionnaire that consists of six multiple-choice questions and is not difficult to fill out. The questionnaire was created to assess athletic participation pre- and postsurgery and treatment.[1]
- **Subscales**:
  - **Walking**—One multiple-choice question with four possible answer responses with a scoring range from 0 to 40 (0 = most disabled, 40 = least disabled). This is the only form with this subscale.
  - **Using Stairs**—One multiple-choice question with four possible answer responses with a scoring range from 0 to 40 (0 = most disabled, 40 = least disabled). This subscale is also present in Lysholm.
  - **Squatting and Kneeling**—One multiple-choice question with four possible answer responses with a scoring range from 0 to 40 (0 = most disabled, 40 = least disabled). This subscale is also present in Lysholm.
  - **Straight Running**—One multiple-choice question with four possible answer responses with a scoring range from 40 to 100 (40 = most disabled, 100 = least disabled). This is the only form with this subscale.
  - **Jumping and Landing**—One multiple-choice question with four possible answer responses with a scoring range from 40 to 100 (40 = most disabled, 100 = least disabled). This is the only form with this subscale.

TABLE 6-1. Questionnaire Characteristics

Knee Questionnaire	Description of Use	Subscales	Scoring Description	Required Questions	Min Score	Max Score
Cincinnati	Pre/postop	Walking, Using Stairs, Squatting/Kneeling, Straight Running, Jumping/Landing, & Hard Twist Cuts and Pivots	Sum	6/6	120 (Most disabled)	420 (Least disabled)
IKDC	Variety of knee problems	Symptoms, Sports Activities, & Function	[Sum/Max possible score] × 100	16/19	0 (Most disabled)	87 (Least disabled)
KOOS	Knee ligament injuries	Pain, Symptoms, ADL, Sports/Recreation, & QOL	Scoring for each subscale: 100 [(Total score of section × 100)/ Max possible score for section]	40/42	0 (Most disabled)	100 (Least disabled)
KSS	Patients perception on knee function	Pain, ROM, & Stability	Sum	7/7	0 (Most disabled)	100 (Least disabled)
Lysholm	Knee ligament surgery	Instability, Pain, Catching/Locking, Swelling, Stair Climb, Squat, Limp, & Support	Sum	8/8	0 (Most disabled)	100 (Least disabled)
WOMAC	Hip/knee osteoarthritis	Pain, Stiffness, & Physical Function	Sum	N/A	0 (Least disabled)	96 (Most disabled)
Oxford	Post knee surgery	Pain & Function	Sum	12/12	12 (Least disabled)	30 (Most disabled)
ADL	Variety of knee problems	Symptoms & Functional Disability	(Sum/80) × 100	17/17	0 (Most disabled)	80 (Least disabled)
SF-12v1	Generic health form	Physical Health & Mental Health	Sum	12/12	12 (Least disabled)	47 (Most disabled)
SF-36v1	Generic health form	Physical Functioning, Physical Role limitations, Bodily Pain, General Health, Vitality, Social Functioning, Emotional Role Limitations, & Mental Health	Sum	36/36	0 (Most disabled)	100 (Least disabled)

QOL, quality of life; ROM, range of motion.

- **Hard Twist Cuts and Pivots**—One multiple-choice question with four possible answer responses with a scoring range from 40 to 100 (40 = most disabled, 100 = least disabled). This is the only form with this subscale.

- **Scoring Description**: Sum (points for all six activities)[2]
- **Required Questions**: 6/6
- **Minimum Score**: 120 (most disabled)[2]
- **Maximim Score**: 420 (least disabled)[2]

IKDC

- **Questionnaire Description**: A knee questionnaire that consists of 14 multiple-choice questions, four visual analog scale (VAS) questions, and one true/false question that concentrates on knee deformities. This questionnaire concentrates on symptoms, function, and sports activity that affect patients' everyday activities with a variety of knee problems.[3]
- **Subscales**:
  - **Symptoms**—Seven multiple-choice questions that consist of four multiple-choice questions (16 points max), two VAS questions (20 points max), and one true/false question (1 point max).This section has a maximum score of 37 and a minimum of 0 (0 = most disabled, 37 = least disabled). This subscale is also present in the KOOS.
  - **Sports Activities**—Ten multiple-choice questions with a maximum score of 40 points and a minimum of 0 points. (0 = most disabled, 40 = least disabled). This subscale is also present in the KOOS.
  - **Function**—Two VAS questions. The first VAS question (10a) is a nonscored item. This section has a maximum of 10 points and a minimum of 0 points (0 = most disabled, 10 = least disabled). This subscale is also present in the WOMAC, Oxford, ADL, SF-12v1, and SF-36v1.
- **Scoring Description**: [Sum of items/maximum possible score] × 100 (Do not score question 10A.)[4]
- **Required Questions**: 16/19[4]
- **Minimum Score**: 0 (most disabled)[4]
- **Maximum Score**: 87 (least disabled)[4]

KOOS

- **Questionnaire Description**: A knee questionnaire that consists of 42 multiple-choice questions that have a response scale from 0 to 4 (0 = no disability; 4 = severe disability). This questionnaire was created to focus on knee ligament injuries and to evaluate the course of a knee injury and the quality of treatment outcome.[5]
- **Subscales**:
  - **Pain**—Nine multiple-choice questions that have a maximum score of 36 and a minimum score of 0 (0 = least disabled, 36 = most disabled). This subscale is also present in the KSS, Lysholm, WOMAC, SF-12v1, Oxford, and SF-36v1.
  - **Symptoms**—Seven multiple-choice questions that have a maximum score of 28 and a minimum score of 0 (0 = least disabled, 28 = most disabled). This subscale is also present in the IKDC.
  - **Activities of Daily Living**—Seventeen multiple-choice questions that have a maximum score of 68 and a minimum score of 0 (0 = least disabled, 68 = most disabled). This is the only form with this subscale.
  - **Sports and Recreation**—Five multiple-choice questions that have a maximum score of 20 and a minimum score of 0 (0 = least disabled, 20 = most disabled). This subscale is also present in the IKDC.
  - **Quality of Life**—Four multiple-choice questions that have a maximum score of 16 and a minimum score of 0 (0 = least disabled, 16 = most disabled). This is the only form with this subscale.
- **Scoring Description**:
  - **Pain**: 100 [(Total score P1–P9 × 100)/36][6]
  - **Symptoms**: 100 [Total score S1–S7 × 100)/28][6]
  - **ADL**: 100 [Total score A1–S17 × 100)/68][6]
  - **Sports and Recreation**: 100 [Total score SP1–SP5 × 100)/20][6]

- **Quality of Life**: 100 [Total score Q1–Q4 × 100)/16][6]
- **Required Questions**: 40/42 (If more than two questions are omitted, then the response is considered invalid and no subscale score is calculated.[6])
- **Minimum Score**: 0 (extreme disability) (Each section is turned into a normalized score.[6])
- **Maximum Score**: 100 (no problems) (Each section is turned into a normalized score.[6])

KSS

- **Questionnaire Description**: A knee questionnaire consisting of six multiple-choice questions and one fill-in-the-blank question concentrating on the thoughts of how the patient perceives his or her knee function with specific activities.[7]
- **Subscales**:
  - **Pain**—Two multiple-choice questions with a maximum score of 50 and a minimum of 0 (0 = most disabled, 50 = least disabled). This subscale is also present in the KOOS, Lysholm, WOMAC, Oxford, SF-12v1, and SF-36v1.
  - **Range of Motion**—Fill-in-the-blank question with a maximum score of 25 and a minimum of 0 (0 = most disabled, 25 = least disabled). This is the only form with this subscale.
  - **Stability**—Two multiple-choice questions with a maximum score of 25 and a minimum of 10 (10 = most disabled, 25 = least disabled). This is the only form with this subscale.
- **Scoring Description**: Sum of three subscores[7]
- **Required Questions**: 7/7[7]
- **Minimum Score**: 0 (most disabled)[7]
- **Maximum Score**: 100 (least disabled)[7]

LYSHOLM

- **Description**: This form consists of eight multiple-choice questions which concentrate on disabilities of the knee. This questionnaire was created to evaluate the effectiveness of knee ligament surgery by concentrating on symptoms and instability of the knee pre- and postsurgery.[8]
- **Subscales**:
  - **Instability**—A multiple-choice question that has a maximum score of 25 and a minimum score of 0 (0 = most disabled, 25 = least disabled). This is the only form with this subscale.
  - **Pain**—A multiple-choice question that has a maximum score of 25 and a minimum score of 0 (0 = most disabled, 25 = least disabled). This subscale is also present in the KOOS, KSS, WOMAC, Oxford, SF-12v1, and SF-36v1.
  - **Catching/Locking**—A multiple-choice question that has a maximum score of 15 and a minimum score of 0 (0 = most disabled, 15 = least disabled). This is the only form with this subscale.
  - **Swelling**—A multiple-choice question that has a maximum score 10 and a minimum score of 0 (0 = most disabled, 10 = least disabled). This is the only form with this subscale.
  - **Stair Climb**—A multiple-choice question that has a maximum score of score 10 and a minimum score of 0 (0 = most disabled, 10 = least disabled). This subscale is also present in the Cincinnati form.
  - **Squat**—A multiple-choice question that has a maximum score of 5 and a minimum score of 0 (0 = most disabled, 5 = least disabled). This subscale is also present in the Cincinnati form.
  - **Limp**—A multiple-choice question that has a maximum score of 5 and a minimum score of 0 (0 = most disabled, 5 = least disabled). This is the only form with this subscale.
  - **Support**—A multiple-choice question that has a maximum score of 5 and a minimum score of 0 (0 = most disabled, 5 = least disabled). This is the only form with this subscale.
- **Scoring Description**: Sum of assigned scores of all responses[9]
- **Required Questions**: 8/8[9]
- **Minimum Score**: 0 (most disabled)[9]
- **Maximum Score**: 100 (least disabled)[9]

WOMAC

- **Description**: This form consists of 24 multiple-choice questions that concentrate on hip and knee osteoarthritis. This questionnaire has been modified to reduce the number of items to provide an increase in efficiency and compliance.[10]
- **Subscales**:
  - **Pain**—Consists of five multiple-choice questions with a maximum score of 20 and a minimum of 0 (0 = least disabled, 20 = most disabled). This subscale is also present in the KOOS, KSS, Lysholm, Oxford, SF-12v1, and SF-36v1.
  - **Stiffness**—Consists of two multiple-choice questions with a maximum score of 8 and a minimum of 0 (0 = least disabled, 8 = most disabled). This is the only form with this subscale.
  - **Physical Function**—Consists of 17 multiple-choice questions with a maximum score of 68 and a minimum score of 0 (0 = least disabled, 68 = most disabled). This subscale is also present in the IKDC, Oxford, ADL, SF-12v1, and SF-36v1.
- **Scoring Description**: Sum of assigned scores of all responses for each subscale[11]
- **Required Questions**: Not applicable[11]
- **Minimum Score**: 0 (least disabled)[11]
- **Maximum Score**: 96 (most disabled)[11]

OXFORD KNEE FORM

- **Description**: A knee questionnaire that consists of 12 multiple-choice questions. This questionnaire was created for administration to patients after they had a total knee replacement. The form is short and is not difficult to complete.[12]
- **Subscales**:
  - **Pain**—Consists of six multiple-choice questions with a maximum score of 30 and a minimum score of 6 (6 = least disabled, 30 = most disabled). This subscale is also present in the KOOS, KSS, Lysholm, WOMAC, SF-12v1, and SF-36v1.
  - **Function**—Consists of six multiple-choice questions with a maximum score of 30 and a minimum score of 6 (6 = least disabled, 30 = most disabled). This subscale is also present in the IKDC, WOMAC, ADL, SF-12v1, and SF-36v1.
- **Scoring Description**: Sum of all responses[12]
- **Required Questions**: 12/12[12]
- **Minimum Score**: 12 (least disabled)[12]
- **Maximum Score**: 30 (most disabled)[12]

ACTIVITIES OF DAILY LIVING SCALE

- **Description**: This questionnaire is a combination of activities of daily living and a sports activity scale that concentrates on the knee. It contains 17 multiple-choice questions that ask patients to concentrate on how well they can perform everyday activities and perform specific functional tasks.[13]
- **Subscales**:
  - **Symptoms**—Consists of seven multiple-choice questions with a maximum score of 35 points and a minimum of 0 (0 = most disabled, 35 = least disabled). This is the only form with this subscale.
  - **Functional Disability**—Consists of 10 multiple-choice questions with a maximum score of 45 and a minimum score of 0 (0 = most disabled, 45 = least disabled). This subscale is also present in the IKDC, WOMAC, Oxford, SF-12v1, and SF-36v1.
- **Scoring Description**: (Sum/80) × 100[13]
- **Required Questions**: 17/17[13]
- **Minimum Score**: 0 (most disabled)[13]
- **Maximum Score**: 80 (least disabled)[13]

SF-12V1

- **Questionnaire Description**: A generic health questionnaire that contains 12 short multiple-choice questions and was created by condensing the SF-36v1. This questionnaire combines the patients' input on physical and mental health concerning their disability.[14]

- **Subscales**:
  - **Physical Health**—Six multiple-choice questions with a maximum score of 20 and a minimum score of 6.
    - **General Health**—One multiple-choice question that has a maximum value of 5 and a minimum of 1. This subscale is also present in the SF-36v1.
    - **Physical Functioning—**Two multiple-choice questions that have a maximum score of 6 and a minimum of 2. This subscale is also present in the IKDC, WOMAC, Oxford, ADL, and SF-36v1.
    - **Physical Role Limitations**—Two multiple-choice questions that have a maximum score of 4 and a minimum of 2. This subscale is also present in the SF-36v1.
    - **Bodily Pain**—One multiple-choice question that has a maximum score of 5 and a minimum score of 1. This subscale is also present in the KOOS, KSS, Lysholm, WOMAC, Oxford, and SF-36v1.
  - **Mental Health**—Six multiple-choice questions with a maximum score of 27 and a minimum score of 6.
    - **Emotional Role Limitations**—Two multiple-choice questions with a maximum score of 4 and a minimum score of 2. This subscale is also present in the SF-36v1.
    - **Social Functioning**—One multiple-choice question with a maximum score of 5 and a minimum score of 1. This subscale is also present in the SF-36v1.
    - **Vitality/Mental Health**—Three multiple-choice questions with a maximum score of 18 and a minimum score of 3. This subscale is also present in the SF-36v1.
- **Scoring Description**: Sum of all responses (unless uses interpretation chart to convert each item response into both physical and mental standardized values[15])
- **Required Questions**: 12/12[15]
- **Minimum Score**: 12 (least disabled)[15]
- **Maximum Score**: 47 (most disabled)[15]

SF-36V1

- **Questionnaire Description**: A general medical questionnaire that contains seven yes/no questions and 29 multiple-choice questions and was created to go across age, disease, and treatment groups to make it a nonspecific disease questionnaire. It can be self-administered or can be administered in an interview manner.[16]
- **Subscales**:
  - **Physical Functioning**—Ten multiple-choice questions with a maximum score of 30 and a minimum score of 10 (10 = most disabled, 30 = least disabled). This subscale is also present in the IKDC, WOMAC, Oxford, ADL, and SF-12v1.
  - **Physical Role Limitations**—Four yes/no questions with a maximum score of 8 and a minimum score of 4 (scoring is varied). This subscale is also present in the SF-12v1.
  - **Bodily Pain**—Two multiple-choice questions that have a maximum score of 11 and a minimum score of 2 (2 = least disability, 11 = most disability). This subscale is also present in the KOOS, KSS, Lysholm, WOMAC, Oxford, and SF-12v1.
  - **General Health**—Five multiple-choice questions that have a maximum score of 32 and a minimum of 5 (scoring is varied). This subscale is also present in the SF-12v1.
  - **Vitality**—Four multiple-choice questions with a maximum score of 20 and a minimum score of 4 (scoring is varied). This subscale is also present in the SF-12v1.
  - **Social Functioning**—Two multiple-choice questions with a maximum score of 10 and a minimum score of 2 (2 = least disability, 10 = most disability). This subscale is also present in the SF-12v1.
  - **Emotional Role Limitations**—Three multiple-choice questions with a maximum score of 6 and a minimum score of 3 (3 = most disability, 6 = least disability). This subscale is also present in the SF-12v1.
  - **Mental Health**—Five multiple-choice questions with a maximum score of 30 and a minimum score of 6 (scoring is varied). This subscale is also present in the SF-12v1.

- **Scoring Description**: Sum of all responses (scores are normalized using a chart provided[16])
- **Required Questions**: 36/36[16]
- **Minimum Score**: 0 (most disability)[16]
- **Maximum Score**: 100 (least disability)[16]

ANALYSIS OF SIMILARITIES

- **Walking**
  - **Cincinnati**: Question 1 (Ability to walk)
  - **KSS**: Question 1 (Ability to walk)
  - **IKDC**: Questions 1, 5, 7, and 8 answers (Pain with walking, swelling while walking, giving way while walking, and highest level of activity is walking)
  - **Lysholm**: Question 1 answer (Limp when walking)
  - **WOMAC**: Question 1 Section 1 (Pain with walking) and Question 6 Section 3 (Ability to walk)
  - **KOOS**: Question 6 Section 1 (Pain while walking) and Question 6 Section 3 (Ability to walk)
  - **SF-36v1**: Questions 9, 10, and 11 (Ability to walk)
  - **ADL**: Question 8 (Ability to walk)
  - **Oxford**: Question 4 (Pain while walking)
- **Stairs**
  - **Cincinnati**: Question 2 (Ability to climb stairs)
  - **KSS**: Question 2 (Ability to climb stairs)
  - **IKDC**: Questions 9a and 9b (Ability to climb stairs)
  - **Lysholm**: Question 7 (Ability to climb stairs)
  - **WOMAC**: Questions 1 and 2 Section 1 (Pain while climbing stairs) and Questions 1 and 2 Section 3 (Ability to climb stairs)
  - **KOOS**: Questions 5 and 6 Section 1 (Pain while climbing stairs) and Questions 1 and 2 Section 3 (Ability to climb stairs)
  - **SF-12v1**: Question 3 (Ability to climb stairs)
  - **SF-36v1**: Questions 6 and 7 (Ability to climb stairs)
  - **ADL**: Questions 11 and 12 (Ability to climb stairs)
  - **Oxford**: Question 12 (Ability to climb stairs)
- **Squatting & Kneeling**
  - **Cincinnati**: Question 3 (Ability to squat and kneel)
  - **IKDC**: Questions 9c and 9b (Ability to squat and kneel)
  - **Lysholm**: Question 8 (Ability to squat)
  - **KOOS**: Questions 1 and 5 Section 5 (Ability to squat and kneel)
  - **SF-36v1**: Question 8 (Ability to kneel)
  - **ADL**: Question 14 (Ability to kneel) and Question 15 (Ability to Squat)
  - **Oxford**: Question 7 (Ability to kneel)
- **Running**
  - **Cincinnati**: Question 4 (Ability to run)
  - **IKDC**: Questions 1, 5, 7, and 8 answers (Pain with running, swelling while running, giving way while running, and highest level of activity is running) and Question 9g (Ability to run)
  - **KOOS**: Question 2 Section 5 (Ability to run)

  SF-36v1: Question 3 (Ability to run)
- **Jumping and Landing**
  - **Cincinnati**: Question 5 (Ability to jump and land)
  - **IKDC**: Questions 1, 5, 7, and 8 answers (Pain with jumping, swelling while jumping, giving way while jumping, and highest level of activity is jumping) and Question 9h (Ability to jump)
  - **KOOS**: Question 3 Section 5 (Ability to jump)
- **Twist/Pivot**
  - **Cincinnati**: Question 6 (Ability to twist/pivot)
  - **KOOS**: Question 2 Section 1 (Pain while twisting/pivoting)

- **Pain**
  - **IKDC**: Question 1 (Pain with what level of activity), Question 4 (Amount of pain), Question 3 (Severity of pain)
  - **Lysholm**: Question 5 (Amount of pain)
  - **WOMAC**: Questions 1–5 Section 1 (Amount of pain during certain activities)
  - **KOOS**: Question 1 (Frequency of pain), Questions 1–9 Section 1 (Amount of pain during certain activities
  - **SF-12v1**: Question 8 (Amount of pain)
  - **SF-36v1**: Question 21 (Amount of pain) and Question 7 (Pain interfered with pain)
  - **ADL**: Question 1 (Pain with what level of activity)
  - **Oxford**: Question 1 (Amount of pain), Question 4 (Pain with walking), Question 8 (Pain while lying in bed), Question 9 (Pain interfering with work)
- **Stiff/Swollen**
  - **IKDC**: Question 4 (Stiffness/Swollenness of knee) and Question 5 (Level of activity that causes stiffness)
  - **Lysholm**: Question 6 (Amount of swelling in knee)
  - **WOMAC**: Questions 1 and 2 section 2 (Occurrence of Stiffness)
  - **KOOS**: Questions 1 and 2 Section 2 (Occurrence of Swelling) and Question 3 Section 2 (Amount of swelling)
  - **ADL**: Question 3 (Stiffness affecting ADL) and Question 4 (Swollenness affecting ADL)
- **Locking/Catching**
  - **IKDC**: Question 6 (Does knee lock/catch)
  - **Lysholm**: Question 3 (Does knee lock/catch)
  - **KOOS**: Question 5 Section 3 (Does knee lock/catch)
- **Giving Way**
  - **IKDC**: Question 7 (Level of activity without giving way)
  - **Lysholm**: Question 4 (Level of activity without giving way)
  - **Oxford**: Question 10 (Giving way)
- **Highest Level of Activity**
  - **IKDC**: Question 8 (Highest level of activity)
  - **SF-12v1**: Questions 2 and 3 Section 2 (Highest level of activity)
  - **SF-36v1**: Questions 3–12 (Highest level of activity)
- **Ability to Perform Activities**
  - **IKDC**: Questions 10a and 10b
  - **SF-12v1**: Question 5
  - **SF-36v1**: Questions 15 and 16
- **Rising from Sitting**
  - **IKDC**: Question 9f (Ability to rise from sitting)
  - **WOMAC**: Question 3 Section 3 (Ability to rise from sitting)
  - **KOOS**: Question 3 Section 3 (Ability to rise from sitting)
  - **ADL**: Question 17 (Ability to rise from chair)
  - **Oxford**: Question 5 (Ability to rise from chair)
- **Standing**
  - **WOMAC**: Question 4 Section 3
  - **KOOS**: Question 4 Section 3
  - **ADL**: Question 13
- **Bending to Floor**
  - **WOMAC**: Question 5 Section 3
  - **KOOS**: Question 5 Section 3
- **Getting in and out of Car**
  - **WOMAC**: Question 7 Section 3
  - **KOOS**: Question 7 Section 3
  - **Oxford**: Question 3
- **Going Shopping**
  - **WOMAC**: Question 8 Section 3
  - **KOOS**: Question 8 Section 3
  - **Oxford**: Question 11
- **Putting on Socks**
  - **WOMAC**: Question 9 Section 3
  - **KOOS**: Question 9 Section 3

- **Rising from Bed**
  - **WOMAC**: Question 10 Section 3
  - **KOOS**: Question 10 Section 3
- **Taking off Socks**
  - **WOMAC**: Question 11 Section 3
  - **KOOS**: Question 11 Section 3
- **Lying in Bed**
  - **WOMAC**: Question 12 Section 3
  - **KOOS**: Question 12 Section 3
- **Sitting**
  - **WOMAC**: Question 13 Section 3
  - **KOOS**: Question 14 Section 3
- **Getting on/off Toilet**
  - **WOMAC**: Question 15 Section 3
  - **KOOS**: Question 15 Section 3
- **Heavy Domestic Duties**
  - **WOMAC**: Question 16 Section 3
  - **KOOS**: Question 16 Section 3
- **Light Domestic Duties**
  - **WOMAC**: Question 17 Section 3
  - **KOOS**: Question 17 Section 3
- **Grinding**
  - **KOOS**: Question 4 Section 2
  - **ADL**: Question 2
- **Using Crutch or Cane**
  - **Lysholm**: Question 2
  - **ADL**: Question 9
- **Sit with Knee Bent**
  - **IKDC**: Question 9e
  - **ADL**: Question 16
- **Limp**
  - **ADL**: Question 10
  - **Oxford**: Question 6
- **Bathing/Dressing**
  - **SF-36v1**: Question 12 (Bathing and dressing yourself)
  - **Oxford**: Question 2 (Bathing yourself)

(All questions in the SF-12v1 are included in the SF-36v1)

ANALYSIS OF DIFFERENCES

- **Stop and Start Quickly**
  - **IKDC**: Question 9i
- **Range of Motion**
  - **KSS**: Question 3
- **Straighten Knee Fully**
  - **KOOS**: Question 6 Section 2
- **Bend Knee Fully**
  - **KOOS**: Question 7 Section 2
- **Getting in/out of Bath**
  - **KOOS**: Question 13 Section 3
- **Awareness of Knee Problem**
  - **KOOS**: Question 1 Section 5
- **Modified Lifestyle to Avoid Damage**
  - **KOOS:** Question 2 Section 5
- **Troubled/Lack of Confidence**
  - **KOOS**: Question 3 Section 5
- **Amount of Difficulty With Knee**
  - **KOOS**: Question 4 Section 5
- **Health Compared to a Year Ago**
  - **SF-36v1**: Question 2
- **Emotions Affect ADLs**
  - **SF-36v1**: Questions 17–19
- **Vitality**
  - **SF-36v1**: Questions 33–36
- **Full of Pep**
  - **SF-36v1**: Question 23
- **Nervous Person**
  - **SF-36v1**: Question 24

- **Down in the Dumps**
  - **SF-36v1:** Question 25
- **Worn Out**
  - **SF-36v1**: Question 29
- **Happy Person**
  - **SF-36v1**: Question 30
- **Feeling Tired**
  - **SF-36v1**: Question 31
- **Slipping**
  - **ADL**: Question 5
- **Buckling**
  - **ADL**: Question 6
- **Lack of Strength**
  - **ADL**: Question 7

REFERENCES

1. Noyes FR, Barber SD, Mooar LA. A rationale for assessing sports activity levels and imitations in knee disorders. *Clin Orthop Relat Res.* 1989;246:238-249.
2. Marx RG. ISAKOS scientific committee report: knee rating scales. *Arthroscopy.* 2003;19(10):1103-1108.
3. Irrgang JJ, Anderson AF, Boland AL, et al. Development and validation of the International Knee Documentation Committee Subjective Knee Form. *Am J Sports Med.* 2001;29:600-613.
4. http://www.sportsmed.org/Medical-Professionals/Research/Grants/IKDC-Forms.
5. Roos EM, Roos HP, Lohmander LS, et al. Knee Injury and Osteoarthritis Outcome Score (KOOS)—development of a self-administered outcome measure. *J Orthop Sports Phys Ther.* 1998;28:88-96.
6. *A User's Guide to Knee Injury and Osteoarthritis Outcome Score (KOOS).* 2003:1-9.
7. Insall JN, Dorr LD, Scott RD, et al. Rationale of the Knee Society Clinical Rating System. *Clin Orthop Relat Res.* 1989;248:13-14.
8. Lysholm J, Gillquist J. Evaluation of knee ligament surgery results with special emphasis on use of a scoring scale. *Am J Sports Med.* 1982;10:150-154.
9. Ciconelli R, Cohen M, Peccin MS. Specific questionnaire for knee symptoms—the Lysholm Knee Scoring Scale. Translation and validation into Portuguese. *Acta Orthop Bras.* 2006;14(5):268-272.
10. Bellamy N, Buchanan WW, Goldsmith CH, et al. Validation study of WOMAC: a health status instrument for measuring clinically important patient relevant outcomes to antirheumatic drug therapy in patients with osteoarthritis of the hip or knee. *J Rheumatol.* 1988;15:1833-1840.
11. The WOMAC (Western Ontario and McMaster Universities) Index of Osteoarthritis. https://www.cebp.nl/vault_public/filesystem/?ID=1482.
12. Dawson J, Fitzpatrick R, Murray D, et al. Questionnaire on the perceptions of patients about total knee replacement. *J Bone Joint Surg Br.* 1998;80:63-69.
13. Irrgang JJ, Snyder-Mackler L, Wainner RS, et al. Development of a patient-reported measure of function of the knee. *J Bone Joint Surg Am.* 1998;80:1132-1145.
14. Ware J Jr, Kosinski M, Keller SD. A 12-item short-form health survey: construction of scales and preliminary tests of reliability and validity. *Med Care.* 1996;34(3):220-233.
15. Ware JE Jr, Snow KK, Kosinski M, et al. *SF36 Health Survey Manual and Interpretation Guide.* Positive Aging Resource Center; 1997.
16. Ware JE Jr, Sherbourne CD. The MOS 36-item short-form health survey (SF-36). I. Conceptual framework and item selection. *Med Care.* 1992;30(6):473-483.

7 Economic Aspects of Total Knee Arthroplasty

Christina Gutowski and Kevin J. Bozic

For decades, the rising cost of health care has been a topic of much debate in government as well as in the private sector. It is estimated that half of all growth in health care expenditures has been associated with advances in technology.[1] In light of this, diagnostic and therapeutic procedures such as total knee arthroplasty (TKA) have begun to undergo rigorous examination into not only their clinical implications, but the economic considerations of their utilization, and health care policymakers, payers, and providers have begun to factor these matters into decisions concerning patients' treatment. The economic implications of medical interventions will play an increasing role in health care debates in the future, at both the individual and societal level.

There has been a significant increase in the number of TKAs in the United States over recent decades,[2] and by 2030 it is projected that this number will increase by over 673% to 3.48 million.[3] Corresponding national annual hospital charges for primary total knee arthroplasty are expected to rise by 450% by year 2015.[4] Given these unprecedented expenditures for TKA (both already realized as well as projected), the economics surrounding this procedure has recently come under increased scrutiny. Total joint arthroplasty has been shown to be one of the most successful and cost-effective interventions in medicine, being one of the most successful surgical procedures for arthritis of the hip and knee and costing significantly less for a given improvement in quality of life as compared to many other surgical or medical interventions.[5,6] However, many factors influence the results of these cost-effectiveness analyses, including the methodology used in the analysis, the input values into these calculations, and the competing treatments with which a procedure is being compared in the analysis. It is therefore important that the consumer of this information think critically about results found in the literature and also understand the complex interplay of economic aspects surrounding TKA.

AN APPROACH TO COST-EFFECTIVENESS ANALYSIS

Evaluation of the cost-effectiveness analysis of a medical intervention often involves the calculation of the incremental cost-effectiveness ratio (ICER). This ratio represents the increase in cost associated with an incremental improvement in quality of life provided by an intervention. The improvement is often quantified in quality-adjusted life years (QALYs), which combine quality and duration of life into a single metric. The formula for ICER is $(\text{costs}_{\text{intervention}} - \text{costs}_{\text{comparator}}) / (\text{QALY}_{\text{intervention}} - \text{QALY}_{\text{comparator}})$,[7] and frequently a new technology, procedure, or technique (the "intervention") will be assessed compared to the traditional standard of care (the "comparator") with this calculation. All four of these inputs are derived from estimations of many parameters, leading to a degree of uncertainty in the final calculated value.

Utilizing its ICER, one can gauge an intervention's value and make comparisons across various interventions for various conditions. A lower ICER corresponds to greater cost-effectiveness, because the intervention is associated with less cost for gaining an additional QALY. From a health policy standpoint, four value-defining categories have been generally accepted for this measurement in the literature. Interventions that cost less than $20,000 per QALY are deemed very cost-effective; interventions costing $20,000–100,000 per QALY are considered moderately cost-effective, and interventions costing more than $100,000 per QALY are considered expensive and, while possibly effective, inefficient.[5,8] More commonly, a $50,000–$100,000 ICER threshold is used as a general touchstone for gauging an intervention's cost-effectiveness,[9] and an ICER of less than or equal to $0 is considered cost saving. While this ratio is not used as a criterion for governmental or institutional decision making in any direct sense (ie, in Medicare coverage decisions), it is a useful tool to provide an additional framework for the assessment of new technologies. Additionally, physicians can benefit from increased transparency regarding the cost and effectiveness of the interventions they are performing. If current trends continue, economic analyses will gain importance in discussions at all levels of the health care system, and a foundational understanding of this critical cost–utility ratio will be essential for the physician to possess.

Another important element of cost-effectiveness research is the sensitivity analysis, which examines the impact of uncertain parameters on the incremental cost-effectiveness ratio. Considering the uncertainty that exists in estimation of each parameter's value (e.g., complication and revision rates), the sensitivity analysis is helpful in identifying thresholds for each variable at which the intervention would be considered to be cost saving (providing an ICER of $0) or cost-effective (providing an ICER of $50,000, $100,000, etc.) Policymakers and providers can apply these results to inform their decisions depending on their individual input values for the parameters; for example, the cost-effectiveness of a procedure may vary with patient age,[10,11] or the purchase of new technology may only be cost-effective for a medical center of a certain size.[12]

Sensitivity analysis implicitly underscores the presence of uncertainty in the ICER calculation. In appreciation of this uncertainty, analysts encourage the results of cost-effectiveness analysis being used to inform and provide a framework for policymaking and clinical practice. However, they warn against these data entirely dictating decision making, without consideration of other clinical and situation-specific factors. While increasing emphasis is being placed on economic data in health care, the appropriate role of cost-effectiveness analysis in decisions of clinical practice, as well as in institutional and societal policymaking, has yet to be clearly defined in America. The cost-effectiveness of total knee arthroplasty has been well documented in the literature.[5,13] Several parameters, including patient age, individual risk of complications, the medical center's arthroplasty volume, price of the implant and surgical supplies, postoperative life expectancy and quality of life, and so forth, influence the procedure's calculated cost–benefit ratio, and the interplay of these many factors will continue to affect the economics of this procedure as new technology continues to develop.

REIMBURSEMENT POLICY FOR TOTAL KNEE REPLACEMENT

Currently, approximately 60% of total joint arthroplasty (TJA) procedures in the United States are reimbursed through Medicare's case-rate reimbursement structure.[14] These procedures have been grouped into one of several Medicare severity diagnosis-related groups (MS-DRGs) based on severity of the patient's illness and comorbidities, as well as whether primary or revision TJA is being performed.[15] Several factors influence the amount a hospital is reimbursed for a given MS-DRG, including geographic location, public/private/teaching status of the hospital, length of stay (LOS), and patient discharge disposition.[16] The patient's LOS is compared to the national geometric mean LOS, and reimbursement is adjusted accordingly. If the patient's LOS is equal to the mean, the hospital is reimbursed the full case-rate amount contingent on geography, teaching status, and so forth. If the patient is discharged earlier than the average LOS would suggest, and without any postdischarge services [eg, a home health aid, physical therapy, or transfer to a skilled nursing facility (SNF) or inpatient rehab facility (IRF)], the hospital receives the same full case-rate reimbursement. This paradigm represents an opportunity for the hospital to financially take advantage of an efficient inpatient stay and early discharge, because the institution would still be paid the full DRG payment for a shorter (therefore presumed less costly) inpatient stay. However, if the patient is discharged early with any postdischarge services ordered or is transferred to a post–acute care facility (eg, SNF or IRF, as is often the case in the Medicare population), the hospital reimbursement structure is shifted to a per-diem rate and the opportunity to take advantage of the early discharge is lost.[16] Given the propensity for the latter situation to occur, the disincentive for improving efficiency and thereby shortening LOS is apparent under this reimbursement structure.

The majority of non-Medicare TJA patients are insured by commercial payers. Hospital reimbursement for these patients either follows a case-rate model similar to Medicare or a per-diem payment structure in which differential amounts are paid to the hospital per day of inpatient stay.

The first day of hospital admission tends to be the most expensive,[17] since it is when elective TJA occurs and the most intensive (including operative) care is provided. To account for this, the per-diem reimbursement for hospital day 1 is the greatest, with a sequential decline in reimbursement for subsequent days. This per-diem structure is designed such that the total reimbursement for a patient with a mean LOS will approximately equal the amount reimbursed through a market-appropriate case-rate structure; inpatient days prolonging LOS past the average length are reimbursed with a per-diem maintenance rate that once again provides financial disincentive against swift discharge.[16]

Medicare reimbursement policy for TJA has evolved significantly over the past decade and will continue to be revised as economic pressures on the health care system escalate. Understanding and alignment of financial incentives on the part of the physician, hospital, patient, and payer will be critical in promoting safe, efficient, and clinically efficacious care, and arthroplasty surgeons are encouraged to think critically about the implications that reimbursement structure has on their patients' hospital experience.

ECONOMICS OF COMPUTER-ASSISTED TOTAL KNEE ARTHROPLASTY

Implant malalignment is a common cause of early failure of total knee arthroplasty, especially when it occurs in the coronal plane.[18,19] Computer-assisted navigation systems can improve accuracy and precision of component alignment, as compared with traditional mechanically guided methods.[20-22] While long-term improvements in implant survivorship resulting from computer-assisted surgery have yet to be proven, restoration of neutral alignment in the coronal plane has been shown to positively affect both functional success and component longevity, decreasing failure and subsequent revision rates.[18,23] Proponents of this new technology argue that forthcoming long-term outcome studies will show decreased revision rates associated with computer-assisted total knee replacement, as result of its consistent facilitation of improved alignment.

While per-patient costs of this technology vary somewhat with an institution's volume, region, type of navigation system used, and type of contract with the system manufacturer, computer-assisted arthroplasty comes at an increased cost as compared to the currently utilized mechanical alignment systems: an estimated per-case increase of \$600–\$2000 currently.[24,25] Lacking results of long-term outcome studies on this technology, economic models have been employed to evaluate the cost-effectiveness of computer-assisted knee arthroplasty and to estimate the impact that this new technology will have in the economics of total joint replacement.

A Markov decision model and Monte Carlo sensitivity analysis can be used to find the incremental cost-effectiveness ratio for computer navigation, as well as to identify thresholds for cost savings and cost-effectiveness dependent on a defined set of input variables.[24] After making evidence-based assumptions on probability of alignment, revision rates, quality of life, and the costs of computer-assisted surgery and mechanical guides, research supports the economic benefits of navigation systems in TKA.[24] However, specific clinical and financial factors must be considered, which may modify the calculated ICER for an individual medical center.[7-9] The sensitivity analysis discussed below highlights this concept.

Each of the variables affecting the cost-effectiveness calculation can be represented as a probability distribution of expected values. These variables include probability of malalignment and revision, procedure cost, and quality of life measures for mechanical and computer-assisted systems. The time to follow-up is another parameter to be varied. A Monte Carlo sensitivity analysis identifies cost savings and cost-effectiveness thresholds for these variables as they rise and fall in their respective values, using the accepted ICER threshold of \$50,000 per quality-adjusted life-year for "cost-effectiveness," and an incremental cost of zero as definition of "cost savings." Understanding the relationship that the variables have with each other within the model is critical to comprehending the sensitivity analysis. For example, as the cost of computer-assisted surgery increases, a higher probability of achieving neutral alignment with the technology would be required to achieve cost-effectiveness or cost savings.[24] Likewise, as the probability of achieving neutral alignment with computer-assisted navigation increases as compared to mechanical guides, cost savings would be achieved at a lower threshold of the probability of revision surgery secondary to malalignment. Table 7-1 illustrates thresholds that each variable needs to meet to achieve cost-effectiveness and cost savings, determined by one-way sensitivity analysis (assuming other parameters being held equal to the mean value of their respective distributions.)

There is considerable uncertainty in these calculations, in appreciation of the probability distributions characterizing the input variables. When investigating the magnitude of this uncertainty, it was found that only 54% of the Monte Carlo simulations had an ICER of less than \$50,000 per quality-adjusted life-year, and 74% had an ICER of less than \$100,000 per quality-adjusted life-year.[24] The high

TABLE 7-1. One-Way Sensitivity Analysis Thresholds for Achieving Cost-Effectiveness and Cost Savings with Computer-Assisted Navigation in TKA

	Cost-Effective: ICER < $50,000 per QALY	Cost Savings: Incremental Cost < $0
Additional cost of navigation	$1585	$629
Cost of revision TKA	$12,043	$33,190
Probability of neutral alignment with computer-assisted navigation	0.9	No threshold
Probability of neutral alignment with mechanical guide	0.77	0.57
Probability of revision @15 years after neutral alignment	0.069	No threshold
Probability of revision @15 years after malalignment	0.509	No threshold

Adapted from Novak EJ, Silverstein MD, Bozic KJ. The cost-effectiveness of computer-assisted navigation in total knee arthroplasty. *J Bone Joint Surg.* 2007;89:2389-2397.

probability simulations utilizing each variable's mean value suggest achievement of cost-effectiveness within 12.3 years, but many possible paradigms exist in which the outcome would not be as favorable. If incremental cost of the technology is underestimated or if its ability to achieve improved rates of alignment are overestimated, its cost-effectiveness will be valued too highly by these models.[26]

There are several implications for these data, the majority of which support computer-assisted arthroplasty being most cost-effective in high-volume centers.[12] By nature of their large volume of joint replacements, the per-case incremental costs of computer navigation are lowest, and the technology's reduction in annual revision rate necessary to deem computer-assisted navigation cost-effective is a modest one. At a smaller-volume hospital, fewer primary total joint procedures are being performed to offset the navigation system's annual cost; therefore, the long-term savings enjoyed by way of reduction in revision rate must be more substantial.

However, an interesting paradigm exists involving hospital volumes. Ignoring recent introduction of computer-assisted surgery, high-volume joint replacement centers have been shown to achieve lower complication rates in primary total knee arthroplasty,[27] with smaller hospitals experiencing relatively high rates of malalignment and subsequent need for revision. Significant room for improvement exists at these smaller centers, while arthroplasty service lines in large centers are already functioning at near-maximal clinical efficiency. Therefore, computer-assisted surgery may clinically benefit these small centers significantly more at the margin. This paradox presents an interesting decision for low-volume institutions. While cost-effectiveness analysis suggests that investment in navigation is not prudent within the low-volume setting due to the associated high cost per case, the possibility of computer-assisted surgery having a remarkable impact on an individual patient treated in that small hospital is great. Furthermore, the possibility of achieving a considerable reduction in aggregate revision rate—needed to achieve cost-effectiveness—could exist.

Implementing computer-assisted arthroplasty at an institution has operational implications to both the surgeon and hospital. Costs associated with training the surgical staff, increased procedure time, and potential for complications are not insignificant, although the "learning curve" may be temporary.[25] As the duration of each case increases, the surgeon's daily operative volume becomes limited. This productivity loss may not be compensated for by additional reimbursement for using computer assistance (which only recently received a separate CPT code, reimbursed in 2011 by Medicare for $164.16[28]). Concurrently, computer-assisted surgery may increase the total market size by inducing demand for arthroplasty, and it also tends to attract better-educated patients with private insurance, allowing a hospital to potentially capture a greater share of the market.

The financial considerations surrounding computer-assisted total joint replacement will continue to evolve as results on implant survival and revision rates become available. Especially given the sensitivity of this technology to incremental cost of the navigation equipment, the comparative probabilities of malalignment with the two methods, and the subsequent revision rates, modeling can provide a framework for considering the adoption of this new technology and how to optimize its cost-effectiveness. As the financial impact of revision arthroplasty on hospital resource utilization continues to grow,[12] the potential for cost savings by way of computer-assisted surgery will become increasingly significant.

ECONOMICS OF MINIMALLY INVASIVE TOTAL KNEE ARTHROPLASTY

Unresolved controversy remains among arthroplasty surgeons over minimally invasive surgical approaches to total knee replacement. Many studies have shown decreases in postoperative pain, shorter LOS, and earlier return to function to be associated with minimally invasive TKA (MITKA).[29-31] In light of these promising clinical results, the potential for cost reduction in TKA exists. However, the favorable economic implications of these clinical advantages may be offset by longer operative times, increased utilization of radiographic studies, different rehabilitation protocols, and concern for earlier revision with the MITKA technique.[32] Similarly to economic analyses of computer-assisted navigation in TKA, long-term data on rates of malalignment and ensuing revision associated with MITKA are unavailable; therefore, assumptions are necessary in conducting cost-effectiveness analysis of this new technique. There are several factors to bear in mind when considering its economic implications.

An early steep learning curve associated with the surgical technique has been shown, estimated to last the duration of a surgeon's first 50 cases.[31,32] This learning curve can result in longer operative times, increased complication rate, and potentially higher risk of component malalignment, which can have significant consequences vis-à-vis future revision arthroplasty.[31] While this (approximate) 50-case learning period may pass relatively quickly for a high-volume arthroplasty surgeon, it may be unacceptably long for a physician performing MITKA less frequently, especially considering that reimbursement for TKA has fallen in recent years.[14] Since conflicting data exist[31,33] regarding the risk of malalignment with this technique, the economic implications of this learning curve are not fully understood; it represents a potential disadvantage to MITKA in financial analysis.

Examination of direct cost centers contributing to total inpatient hospital costs demonstrates that the only cost center in which the minimally invasive technique was more expensive was operating room cost, secondary to prolonged operative time.[32] All other cost centers studied (eg, acute postoperative care, pharmacy, and physical therapy) showed a decrease in direct cost associated with MITKA as compared to traditional TKA. Additionally, a significantly lower proportion of MITKA patients are discharged to a skilled nursing facility as compared to traditional TKA patients, which would contribute further to societal cost savings.[32] Earlier return to function has also been shown to be associated with this technique[34]; thus less outpatient physical therapy may be required by MITKA patients, further decreasing costs associated with postdischarge care and rehabilitation.

Market forces and societal costs associated with MITKA should be considered as well.[16] Today's TJA patients are more involved in their care than ever, with greater financial resources, more widely accessible information, and pervasive direct-to-consumer marketing. They also have higher expectations of their medical care. These facts, compounded with insurance shielding the patient from bearing the true cost of their surgical procedure, have led to patients specifically requesting MITKA at an escalating rate.[16] Especially since MITKA tends to attract a younger and healthier patient population, who tend to be commercially insured and therefore attractive to hospitals, pressures on the surgeon and his or her institution to adopt this new technique are considerable. The dilemma posed by this novel procedure to a hospital operating in a competitive market is similar to that posed by surgical navigation systems: the new technique induces increased demand and offers an opportunity for the institution to capture market share, but at a considerable cost that must be carefully weighed against these benefits.

The opportunity cost of training the operating room staff in the MITKA procedure is considerable. Aforementioned costs associated with the learning curve, such as increased operative time and complication rate, may also be experienced. Additionally, current Medicare reimbursement policy discussed in a previous section largely disincentivizes procedures such as minimally invasive surgery, which either increase procedure costs or decrease length of stay.[16] In order for hospitals to support the implementation of this technique from a fiscal standpoint, reimbursement policy must be reformed such that a hospital's financial incentives are more closely aligned with clinical efforts to improve efficiency and shorten inpatient length of stay.

To date, no comprehensive cost-effectiveness analysis has been conducted on the minimally invasive approach to total knee replacement. As aforementioned, long-term data on differential revision rates experienced with this technique will be important in driving these studies. While available results tend to favor minimally invasive surgery from an economic standpoint, the improvements to date have been modest and insufficient to pose a compelling financial argument for widespread adoption of this approach. Instead, the decision should be made by the surgeon on clinical grounds, using the economic data to supplement the decision-making process.

ECONOMIC CONSIDERATIONS IN REVISION TOTAL KNEE ARTHROPLASTY

Mirroring the dramatic rise in primary total knee arthroplasty procedures anticipated in the future, the number of revision surgeries are also expected to increase significantly.[35] Hospital charges for revision procedures are projected to rise 450% to $4.1 billion by 2015,[4] and this growth in resource utilization will become an increasing burden on hospitals, payers, surgeons, and society.

Revision total knee arthroplasty is a more costly, complicated, and time-consuming surgery than primary TKA.[36] Revision TKA operative times are significantly longer, employing more expensive implants[35] and more frequently utilizing allograft bone.[36] Patients undergoing all types of revision surgery except isolated patellar component revision have been found to have higher severity of illness scores, indicating more significant comorbidities at the time of surgery, and this index has been shown to be an independent predictor of resource use.[15] Compared to primary TKA patients, revision patients experience significantly longer length of stay in hospital and a higher proportion of them are discharged to an extended care facility, which contributes significantly to this procedure's overall economic impact on the health care system.[36]

Considerable differences in resource consumption exist between groups of revision TKA patients, as depicted in Table 7-2.[35] In general, higher costs tend to be driven by longer length of stay, increased complication rate, and costlier implants. Risk factors for greater resource consumption include three-component exchange, two-stage procedures, and utilization of hinged implants,[35] and these expensive subtypes can be up to five times more expensive than standard subtypes of revision surgeries. Additionally, as the primary indication for revision TKA, periprosthetic joint infection (PJI) is associated with significantly higher cost, leading septic revision arthroplasty to be one of the highest resource consumption procedures in orthopaedic surgery.[37]

TABLE 7-2. Characteristics of Procedure Associated with High and Low Cost Levels

	Higher Cost	Lower Cost
Revision subtype	3-component	< 3 component
	2-stage	Isolated liner exchange
		Removal without reimplantation
Implant subtype	Hinged	Standard
		Constrained condylar
		Tibial insert only
Reason for revision	Deep joint infection	Aseptic loosening

Based on Lavernia C, Lee DJ, Hernandez VH. The increasing burden of knee revision surgery in the US. *Clin Orthop Relat Res.* 2006;446:221-226.

Despite the characteristics of revision surgery that make it much more resource intensive than primary total knee arthroplasty, until 2005 these procedures were coded identically and reimbursed equally by Medicare.[15] Changes to reimbursement policy in 2005 separated the two procedures into different DRGs for coding purposes, resulting in more equitable reimbursement for institutions that perform these complex revision surgeries. Two years later, further changes were made to Medicare reimbursement policy to reflect the association of severity of illness scores with greater hospital resource utilization, with the creation of different codes indicating a patient's medical complexity.

While no definite ICER threshold exists, interventions costing less than $50,000 per quality-adjusted life-year are widely considered to be of excellent value by most health economists.[8] Available studies estimate revision knee arthroplasty to be approximately 65% as cost-effective as primary total knee replacement,[38-40] still qualifying it as "excellent" in terms of cost-effectiveness and quality of life. As of 2011, the body of cost-effectiveness literature on revision TKA is not as robust as that for primary TKA, and published decision analysis models do not exist. In appreciation of the many changing parameters that contribute to a thorough analysis, conclusions on cost-effectiveness research on this procedure will continue to evolve as reimbursement policy, procedure efficacy, and cost continue to change. High-volume centers may have an advantage in this regard, with lower complication rates,[41] better negotiating power for implant price, and so forth, allowing for the most clinically efficacious and financially efficient revision procedure possible. As demand for this expensive procedure grows and the resulting economic burden on hospitals continues to spiral upward, the field may see a shift in the market toward these high-volume institutions attracting a larger market share. In order to accommodate the increase in patient demand for revision TKA, reimbursement policy for this expensive procedure will need to evolve in such a way as to financially support these large-volume centers that will likely bear a greater proportion of the caseload.

ECONOMIC CONSIDERATIONS OF VENOUS THROMBOEMBOLISM PHARMACOPROPHYLAXIS

Total joint arthroplasty is a high-risk procedure for venous thromboembolism (VTE),[42,43] and as the number of these procedures grows in the future, the economic burden of deep vein thrombosis (DVT) and pulmonary embolism (PE) will correspondingly increase. Prophylaxis guidelines published in 2008 by the American College of Chest Physicians recommend using potent anticoagulation regimens with agents such as fondaparinux, low-molecular-weight heparins (LMWH), and warfarin (target INR 2–3), discouraging aspirin alone.[43] Guidelines published by the American Academy of Orthopaedic Surgeons support the use of aspirin or a lower-potency warfarin regimen (INR < 2) as additional options to fondaparinux or LMWH.[44] In appreciation of the several options available and the conflicting opinions that exist, cost-effectiveness research will play an increasingly important role in identifying the safest, most efficient prophylaxis options. In addition to the direct costs of diagnosing and treating an acute postoperative DVT or PE, the economic burden of prolonged hospital stay and long-term morbidity associated with the event must be considered. It is therefore important in cost-effectiveness research to include long time horizons and the costs associated with the chronic sequelae of VTE, including recurrent DVT, postthrombotic syndrome, recurrent skin ulceration, impaired mobility, and excess mortality.[45]

Low-Molecular-Weight Heparin and Warfarin

The literature strongly shows that compared to no prophylaxis or aspirin alone, both LMWH and warfarin lead to a reduction in VTE events and total costs in TJA patients.[43,46-48] However, widespread consensus does not exist concerning the comparison of warfarin and LMWH, from both a clinical efficacy as well as cost-efficiency perspective. Sensitivity analysis has found the ICER calculation to be most sensitive to the two alternatives' DVT rates, as well as the incidence of long-term sequelae of these events. Since great variability exists in documented clinical efficacy rates of the two drugs, calculated ICERs for LMWH as compared to warfarin vary in the literature from approximately $2000 per VTE avoided[47,49] to over $100,000 per VTE avoided.

The acquisition cost of injectable LMWH is greater than that of oral warfarin.[45] Resource utilization is considerably higher if the patient requires daily nursing supervision for home injections, especially if compounded with a longer-term prophylaxis regimen; patients on warfarin only require weekly phlebotomy for INR monitoring.[50] Many studies have found LMWH to be slightly more effective at preventing VTE in the immediate postoperative and postacute phases, which compensates for its increased cost enough such that it falls within the acceptable range to be considered a cost-effective alternative to oral warfarin.[45,47,49,51,52] When the costs of long-term consequences of DVT are included in these models, some studies demonstrate that cost savings can be achieved with LMWH, because the avoidance of these sequelae allows for net decrease in lifetime cost combined with increased QALY.[45] However, studies also exist that demonstrate warfarin's superiority over LMWH in VTE prevention, suggesting it to be the dominant strategy based on its superiority of both efficacy and cost.[53,54] In light of these conflicting results, no definitive recommendation can be made and despite its increase in short-term expenditure, LMWH is generally considered to be a cost-effective alternative option to warfarin in VTE prophylaxis in total joint arthroplasty.

Fondaparinux

Fondaparinux is a factor Xa inhibitor that has shown very positive results in cost-effectiveness analysis compared to LMWH.[42] Over both short and long time horizons, the available literature strongly supports fondaparinux's dominance (higher clinical efficacy at lower cost) or at least cost-effectiveness (less than or equal to $1300 per VTE avoided) as compared to LMWH.[55-58] Some reports have found a slightly higher bleeding risk associated with this drug, but despite this these studies have still maintained its cost-effectiveness.[59] Having a higher acquisition cost, fondaparinux has been found by some studies to be associated with slightly increased cost during the inpatient period (which is shown to be partly offset by the drug's reduction in direct cost of treating VTE during hospital stay). As the time horizon extends further, fondaparinux becomes cost neutral and then cost saving, as the economic benefit of fondaparinux's improved VTE prevention is fully realized.[57] This temporal paradigm is an excellent example of a modest rise in short-term costs for effective prevention, being justified by significant long-term cost savings.

It should be noted, however, that some of the literature supporting fondaparinux's efficacy utilizes comparative rates of asymptomatic venographic DVT and extrapolates this to an expected rate of symptomatic DVT, suggesting a significant improvement with this drug. However, studies utilizing comparisons of solely the rates of symptomatic DVT associated with LMWH and fondaparinux yield slightly less impressive results.[42,55] Additionally, it is important to note that the cost-effectiveness of fondaparinux is sensitive to the price difference between the drug and LMWH, as well as variation in the rate of late DVT.[57,60] Many international studies support the economic value of fondaparinux,[57,61] but they may utilize different price estimates for the two drugs, leading to an analysis that may not be internationally generalizable given U.S. pharmaceutical pricing structure and the ICER's sensitivity to price variation. The subset of American studies that exist also support the superior cost-effectiveness of fondaparinux,[62,63] but U.S. reimbursement policy for brand-name and generic drugs will affect the price of the two options in the future; this may subsequently affect the cost-effectiveness analysis.

New Oral Anticoagulants: Dabigatran Etexilate and Rivaroxaban

New oral anticoagulants dabigatran etexilate (a direct thrombin inhibitor) and rivaroxaban (a factor Xa inhibitor) have been approved for VTE prophylaxis in patients undergoing TJA.[64] Practically and economically, these drugs are advantageous because they require no INR monitoring and are administered orally; home nursing visits for injections are unnecessary, plus the absence of daily injections may improve quality of life after surgery as well.[65] Recent studies have convinced overseas governing bodies to recommend these agents as cost-effective options for prevention of VTE.[66,67] Many have demonstrated the same time-dependent trend of cost-effectiveness that has been shown with fondaparinux; dabigatran has been found to be cost-effective compared to LMWH in the immediate postoperative hospital admission, with slightly higher cost and slightly higher bleeding rates, but associated with a significantly lower rate of lifetime VTE events which results in long-term cost savings.[65] Canadian,[68] Irish,[69] and British[65] data have supported rivaroxaban's superior clinical efficacy as compared to enoxaparin, and several of these studies have also shown achievement of cost savings associated with rivaroxaban after assuming equal acquisition prices of the two drugs.[65,68] However, these results are not entirely able to be translated to the United States, where this assumption cannot be made because the tiered pricing scheme of the American pharmaceutical market produces large price differences between competitors. The cost–utility calculation is very sensitive to variation in the price parameter; therefore, studies using American price points are needed to offer results applicable to the U.S. market. The literature admits to the high price of rivaroxaban and dabigatran and indicates this as a potential barrier to their widespread use despite clinical efficacy advantages.[70]

Long-Term Pharmacoprophylaxis

The risk of postoperative VTE is not eliminated when a patient is discharged from the hospital.[71] As the duration of hospital stay shortens, extending the duration of antithrombotic prophylaxis with an at-home pharmacologic regimen has been seriously considered. While many reports have shown decreased rates of subacute VTE events with extended-duration prophylaxis to 5 weeks postsurgery,[72,73] a few clinical trials have found negative results,[74,75] and the efficacy of such a regimen is still scrutinized by many arthroplasty surgeons. American College of Chest Physicians guidelines "recommend" extension of prophylaxis for total hip replacement and "suggests" it for TKA, despite arguably higher risk of bleeding associated with long-term anticoagulation.[69] A few studies to date examine the cost-effectiveness of this practice, with some conflict concerning cost of the improved prophylaxis it achieves.[50,69]

One systematic review of both LMWH and warfarin in total hip arthroplasty (THA) finds that extended prophylaxis with warfarin is much more cost-effective than it is with LMWH despite increased bleeding rates with warfarin.[50] This is largely due to the price difference between the two, which is especially significant with prolonged administration. The high costs of the LMWH regimen are also driven by the proportion of patients requiring daily home visits by a nurse; in light of this, limiting prescription of extended LMWH to patients who can self-manage their daily injections would ensure more efficient utilization of resources.[76] It has been suggested that the cost-effectiveness of LMWH crosses the "threshold of acceptability" between postoperative day 14 and 31 (dependent somewhat on price, etc)[77]; therefore, another more economical strategy would be to slightly shorten the extended regimen. As warfarin is a much cheaper drug to acquire, the key cost driver in these patients is the risk of a bleeding event.[50] From both a clinical and economic perspective, the physician should be aware of a patient's risk for falls before prescribing extended warfarin prophylaxis.

Slightly conflicting and nuanced results are found by other studies. Strong evidence is offered by one report for extended LMWH prophylaxis in THA, but a much less favorable ICER is found in the study's TKA cohort (the TKA ICER was 10 times greater than that for THA).[77] The lower benefit of extended prophylaxis in TKA (versus THA) may be due to the natural history and clinical severity of calf DVT as it differs from that of proximal thrombosis. Proximal DVT, more frequently seen in THA, is associated with increased rates of PE and postthrombotic syndrome, while calf DVT is more often associated with TKA and is more likely to be clinically silent. For this reason, the authors suggest that greater gains in QALY are seen with antithrombotic prophylaxis in THA patients, while these gains are not achieved as readily in TKA patients.[78]

While the clinical effectiveness of extended prophylaxis with LMWH and warfarin has been demonstrated by the literature, the cost-effectiveness of these strategies remains less certain. An individual patient's comorbidities, hospital course, risk of falls, and ability to self-inject will determine the safest and most economically justifiable regimen for their VTE prevention. The physician should utilize the concepts explained above as a framework in considering the pharmacologic management of each of his or her patients.

CONCLUSION

As pressures to control expenditures in health care continue to rise, the economic implications of clinical decision making will become increasingly important to consider on an individual and aggregate level. Being one of the most successful, yet financially burdensome, operations in the health care system, TKA will continue to be scrutinized in attempts to maximize its efficiency. It is critical that arthroplasty surgeons understand and advocate for cost-effective strategies to employ TKA and continue to investigate the long-term impacts of recent technological developments. It will also be valuable for physicians to grasp the economic considerations of future advances in TKA technology, as the procedure continues to evolve and improve.

REFERENCES

1. Technological Change and the Growth of Health Care Spending. US Congressional Budget Office. January 2008.
2. Kurtz S, Mowat F, Ong K, et al. Prevalence of primary and revision total hip and knee arthroplasty in the United States from 1990 to 2002. *J Bone Joint Surg Am.* 2005;87:1487-1497.
3. Kurz S, Ong K, Lau E, et al. Projections of primary and revision hip and knee arthroplasty in the United States from 2005 to 2030. *J Bone Joint Surg Am.* 2007;89:780-785.
4. Kurtz S, Ong K, Schmier J, et al. Future clinical and economic impact of revision total hip and knee arthroplasty. *J Bone Joint Surg Am.* 2007;89:144-151.
5. Lavernia CJ, Guzman JF, Gachupin-Garcia A. Cost effectiveness and quality of life in knee arthroplasty. *Clin Orthop Relat Res.* 1997;345:134-139.
6. Chang R, Pellissier J, Hazen G. A cost-effectiveness analysis of total hip arthroplasty for osteoarthritis of the hip. *JAMA.* 1996;275:858-865.
7. Center for the Evaluation of Value and Risk in Health. *The Cost-Effectiveness Analysis Registry.* Boston, MA: Tufts-New England Medical Center. Available at: http://www.tufts-nemc.org/cearegistry. Accessed June 2, 2011.
8. Laupacis A, Feeney DH, Detsky AS, et al. How attractive does new technology have to be to warrant adoption and utilization? Tentative guidelines for using clinical and economic evaluation. *J Can Med Assoc.* 1992;146:473-481.
9. Brauer CA, Rosen AB, Olchanski NV, et al. Cost-utility analysis in orthopaedic surgery. *J Bone Joint Surg Am.* 2005;87:1253-1259.

10. Bozic KJ, Morshed S, Silverstein MD, et al. Use of cost-effectiveness analysis to evaluate new technologies in orthopaedics. The case of alternative bearing surfaces in total hip arthroplasty. *J Bone Joint Surg Am.* 2006;88:706-714.
11. Rissanen P, Aro S, Sintonen H, et al. Costs and cost-effectiveness in hip and knee replacement: a prospective study. *Int J Technol Assess Health Care.* 1997;13: 574-588.
12. Slover JD, Tosteson ANA, Bozic KJ, et al. Impact of hospital volume on economic value of computer navigation for total knee replacement. *J Bone Joint Surg Am.* 2008;90:1492-1500.
13. Losina E, Walensky RP, Kessler CL, et al. Cost-effectiveness of total knee arthroplasty in the United States: patient risk and hospital volume. *Arch Intern Med.* 2009;169(12):1113-1121.
14. Mendenhall S. 2006 Hip and knee implant review. *Orthop Network News.* 2006;17:1-16.
15. Bozic KJ, Rubash HE, Sculco TP, et al. An analysis of Medicare payment policy for total joint arthroplasty. *J Arthroplasty.* 2008;23(6 suppl 1):133-138.
16. Bozic KJ, Beringer D. Economic considerations in minimally-invasive total joint arthroplasty. *Clin Orthop Relat Res.* 2007;263:20-25.
17. Bozic KJ, Katz P, Cisternas M, et al. Hospital resource utilization for primary and revision total hip arthroplasty. *J Bone Joint Surg Am.* 2005;87:570-576.
18. Ritter MA, Faris PM, Keating EM, et al. Postoperative alignment of total knee replacement: its effect on survival. *Clin Orthop Relat Res.* 1994;299:153-156.
19. Moreland JR. Mechanisms of failure in total knee arthroplasty. *Clin Orthop Relat Res.* 1988;226:49-64.
20. Bathis H, Perlick L, Tingart M, et al. Alignment in total knee arthroplasty. A comparison of computer-assisted surgery with the conventional technique. *J Bone Joint Surg Br.* 2004;86(5):682-687.
21. Mason JB, Fehring TK, Estok R, et al. Meta-analysis of alignment outcomes in computer-assisted total knee arthroplasty surgery. *J Arthroplasty.* 2007;22(8): 1097-1106.
22. Haaker RG, Stockheim M, Kamp M, et al. Computer-assisted navigation increases precision of component placement in total knee arthroplasty. *Clin Orthop Relat Res.* 2005;433:152-159.
23. Berend ME, Ritter MA, Meding JB, et al. Tibial component failure mechanisms in total knee arthroplasty. *Clin Orthop Relat Res.* 2004;428:26-34.
24. Novak EJ, Silverstein MD, Bozic KJ. The cost-effectiveness of computer-assisted navigation in total knee arthroplasty. *J Bone Joint Surg Am.* 2007;89:2389-2397.
25. Beringer DC, Patel JJ, Bozic KJ. An overview of economic issues in computer-assisted total joint arthroplasty. *Clin Orthop Relat Res.* 2007;463:26-30.
26. Dong H, Buxton M. Early assessment of the likely cost-effectiveness of a new technology: a Markov model with probabilistic sensitivity analysis of computer-assisted total knee replacement. *Int J Technol Assess Health Care.* 2006;22:191-202.
27. Katz JN, Barrett J, Mahomed NN, et al. Association between hospital and surgeon procedure volume and the outcomes of total knee replacement. *J Bone Joint Surg Am.* 2004;86:1909-1916.
28. American Medical Association. CPT Code Search. Available online: http://catalog.ama-assn.org/catalog/cpt /cpt_search_results.jsp?_requestid=21264.) Accessed May 26, 2011.
29. Bonutti PM, Mont MA, McMahon M, et al. Minimally invasive total knee arthroplasty. *J Bone Joint Surg Am.* 2004;86(2 suppl):26-32.
30. Berger RA, Sanders S, Gerlinger T, et al. Outpatient total knee arthroplasty with a minimally invasive technique. *J Arthroplasty.* 2005;20(73):33-38.
31. King J, Stamper DL, Schaad DC, et al. Minimally invasive total knee arthroplasty compared with traditional total knee arthroplasty. Assessment of the learning curve and the postoperative recuperative period. *J Bone Joint Surg.* 2007;89(7):1497-1503.
32. King JC, Manner PA, Stamper DL, et al. Is minimally invasive total knee arthroplasty associated with lower costs than traditional total knee arthroplasty? *Clin Orthop Relat Res.* 2011;469:1716-1720.
33. Lee MS, Yim MC, Wages JJ, et al. Component alignment with minimally invasive total knee arthroplasty: results of the first 100 cases performed. *J Arthroplasty.* 2010; E pub. Available online: http://www.sciencedirect.com.libproxy3.umdnj.edu/science/article/pii/S0883540310004985. Accessed June 21, 2011.
34. Han I, Seong SC, Lee S, et al. Simultaneous bilateral MIS-TKA results in faster functional recovery. *Clin Orthop Relat Res.* 2008;466(6):1449-1453.
35. Lavernia C, Lee DJ, Hernandez VH. The increasing burden of knee revision surgery in the US. *Clin Orthop Relat Res.* 2006;446:221-226.
36. Bozic KJ, Durbhakula S, Berry DJ, et al. Differences in patient and procedure characteristics and hospital resource use in primary and revision total joint arthroplasty. a multicenter study. *J Arthroplasty.* 2005;20(7 suppl 3):17-25.

37. Barrack RL. Economics of the infected knee replacement. *Orthopaedics.* 1998;19:780-782.
38. Burns AWR, Bourne RB, Chesworth BM, et al. Cost effectiveness of revision total knee arthroplasty. *Clin Orthop Relat Res.* 2006;446:29-33.
39. Vince, KG. Results of revision TKA. *Tech Orthop.* 2011;26:111-118.
40. Rorabeck CH, Murray P. The cost benefit of total knee arthroplasty. *Orthopedics.* 1996;19:777-779.
41. Katz JN, Losina E, Barrett J, et al. Association between hospital and surgeon procedure volume and outcomes of total hip replacement in the United States Medicare population. *J Bone Joint Surg Am.* 2001;83(11):1622-1629.
42. Kapoor A, Chuang W, Radhakrishnan N, et al. Cost-effectiveness of venous thromboembolism pharmacological prophylaxis in total hip and knee replacement. A systematic review. *Pharmacoeconomics.* 2010;28(7):521-538.
43. Geerts WH, Pineo GF, Height JA, et al. Prevention of venous thromboembolism: the Eighth ACCP Conference on Antithrombotic and Thrombolytic Therapy. *Chest.* 2008;133(suppl 3):S381-453.
44. American Academy of Orthopaedic Surgeons. *American Academy of Orthopaedic Surgeons Clinical Guideline on Prevention of Pulmonary Embolism in Patients Undergoing Total Hip and Knee Arthroplasty.* Rosemont, IL: AAOS; 2007. Available at: http://www.aaos.org/Research/guidelines/PE_guideline.pdf. Accessed June 11, 2011.
45. Botteman MF, Caprini J, Stephens JM, et al. Results of an economic model to assess the cost-effectiveness of enoxaparin, a low molecular-weight heparin, versus warfarin for the prophylaxis of DVT and associated long-term complications in total hip replacement surgery in the United States. *Clin Ther.* 2002;24(11):1960-1986.
46. Abdool-Carrim T, Adler H, Becker P, et al. The cost and benefit of prophylaxis against deep vein thrombosis in elective hip replacement. DVT/PE Prophylaxis Consensus Forum. *S Afr Med J.* 1997;87(5):594-600.
47. Sarasin FP, Bounameaux H. Out of hospital antithrombotic prophylaxis after total hip replacement: low-molecular-weight heparin, warfarin, aspirin, or nothing? A cost-effectiveness analysis. *Thromb Haemost.* 2002;87(4):586-592.
48. Anderson DR, O'Brien BJ. Cost effectiveness of the prevention and treatment of deep vein thrombosis and pulmonary embolism. *Pharmacoeconomics.* 1997;12:17-29.
49. Hull RD, Raskob GE, Pineo GF, et al. Subcutaneous low-molecular-weight heparin vs. warfarin for prophylaxis of deep vein thrombosis after hip or knee implantation: an economic perspective. *Arch Intern Med.* 1997;157(3):298-303.
50. Skedgel C, Goeree R, Pleasance S, et al. The cost-effectiveness of extended-duration antithrombotic prophylaxis after total hip arthroplasty. *J Bone Joint Surg.* 2007;89(4):819-828.
51. Sullivan SD, Kahn SR, Davidson BL, et al. Measuring the outcomes and pharmacologic consequences of venous thromboembolism prophylaxis in major orthopaedic surgery. *Pharmacoeconomics.* 2003;21(7):477-496.
52. Friedman RJ, Dunsworth GA. Cost analyses of extended prophylaxis with enoxaparin after hip arthroplasty. *Clin Orthop Relat Res.* 2000;370:171-182.
53. Anderson DR, O'Brien B, Nagpal S. *Economic Evaluation Comparing Low Molecular Weight Heparin With Other Modalities for the Prevention of Deep Vein Thrombosis and Pulmonary Embolism Following Total Hip or Knee Arthroplasty.* Ottowa, Ontario, Canada: Canadian Coordinating Office for Health Technology Assessment (CCOHTA); 1998.
54. Wade WE, Hawkins DW. Cost effectiveness of outpatient anticoagulant prophylaxis after total hip arthroplasty. *Orthopedics.* 2000;23(4):335-338.
55. Turpie AG, Bauer KA, Eriksson BI, et al. Fondaparinux vs. enoxaparin for prevention of VTE in major orthopaedic surgery: a meta-analysis of four randomized double-blind studies. *Arch Intern Med.* 2002;162(16):1833-1840.
56. Bauer KA, Eriksson BI, Lassen MR, et al. Steering Committee of the Pentassacharide in Major Knee Surgery Study. Fondaparinux compared with enoxaparin for the prevention of VTE after elective major knee surgery. *N Engl J Med.* 2001;345(18):1305-1310.
57. Gordois A, Posnett J, Borris L, et al. The cost-effectiveness of fondaparinux compared with enoxaparin as prophylaxis against thromboembolism following major orthopaedic surgery. *J Thromb Haemost.* 2003;1:2167-2174.
58. Spruill WJ, Wade WE, Leslie RB. A cost analysis of fondaparinux versus enoxaparin in total knee arthroplasty. *Am J Ther.* 2004;11(1):3-8.
59. Dranitsaris G, Kahn SR, Stumpo C, et al. Pharmacoeconomic analysis of fondaparinux compared with enoxaparin as prophylaxis against thromboembolism following major orthopaedic surgery. *J Thromb Haemost.* 2003;1(10):2167-2174.

60. Bjorvatn A, Kristiansen F. Fondaparinux sodium compared with enoxaparin sodium: a cost-effectiveness analysis. *Am J Cardiovasc Drugs.* 2005;5(2): 121-130.
61. Annemans L, Minjoulat-Rey MC, De Knock M, et al. Cost consequence analysis of fondaparinux versus enoxaparin in the prevention of venous thromboembolism after major orthopaedic surgery in Belgium. *Acta Clin Belg.* 2004;59(6):346-357.
62. Sullivan SD, Kwong L, Nutescu E. Cost-effectiveness of fondaparinux compared with enoxaparin as prophylaxis against venous thromboembolism in patients undergoing hip fracture surgery. *Value Health.* 2006;9(2):68-76.
63. Sullivan SD, Davidson BL, Kahn SR, et al. A cost-effectiveness analysis of fondaparinux sodium compared with enoxaparin sodium as prophylaxis against venous thromboembolism. Use in patients undergoing major orthopaedic surgery. *Pharmacoeconomics.* 2004;22(9):605-620.
64. Stassen JM, Hauel NH, Nar H, et al. Identification and in vitro characterization of BIBR 953 ZW, a novel synthetic low molecular weight direct thrombin inhibitor. Presented at 28th Congress of the International Society on Thrombosis and Haemostasis, Paris, France; July 6-12, 2001.
65. Wolowacz SE, Roskell NS, Maciver F, et al. Economic evaluation of dabigatran etexilate for the prevention of venous thromboembolism after total knee and hip replacement surgery. *Clin Ther.* 2009;31 (1):194-212.
66. Stevenson M, Scope A, Holmes M, et al. Rivaroxaban for the prevention of VTE: a single technology appraisal. *Health Tech Assess.* 2009;13(S-3):43-48.
67. Holmes M, Carroll C, Papioannou D. Dabigatran etexilate for the prevention of VTE in patients undergoing elective hip and knee surgery: a single technology appraisal. *Health Tech Assess.* 2009;13(suppl 2):55-62.
68. Diamantopoulos A, Lees M, Wells PS, et al. Cost-effectiveness of rivaroxaban versus enoxaparin for the prevention of postsurgical venous thromboembolism in Canada. *J Thromb Haemost.* 2010;104:760-770.
69. McCullagh L, Tilson L, Walsh C, et al. A cost-effectiveness model comparing rivaroxaban and dabigatran etexilate with enoxaparin sodium as thromboprophylaxis after total hip and total knee replacement in the Irish healthcare setting. *Pharmacoeconomics.* 2009; 27(10):829-846.
70. Mannucci PM, Franchini M. Old and new anticoagulations: a minireview. *Ann Med.* 2011;43:116-123.
71. White RH, Romano PS, Zhou H, et al. Incidence and time course of thromboembolic outcomes following total hip or knee arthroplasty. *Arch Intern Med.* 1998;158:1525-1531.
72. Elkelboom JW, Quinlan DJ, Douketis JD. Extended-duration prophylaxis against venous thromboembolism after total hip or knee replacement: a meta-analysis of the randomised trials. *Lancet.* 2001; 358:9-15.
73. Comp PC, Spiro TE, Friedman RJ, et al. Enoxaparin Clinical Trial Group. Prolonged enoxaparin therapy to prevent venous thromboembolism after primary hip or knee replacement. *J Bone Joint Surg Am.* 2001;83:336-345.
74. Heit JA, Elliott CG, Trowbridge AA, et al. Ardeparin sodium for extended out-of-hospital prophylaxis against venous thromboembolism after total hip or knee replacement. A randomized, double-blind, placebo-controlled trial. *Ann Intern Med.* 2000;132:853-861.
75. O'Donnell M, Linkins LA, Kearon C, et al. Reduction of out-of-hospital symptomatic venous thromboembolism by extended thromboprophylaxis with low-molecular-weight heparin following elective hip arthroplasty: a systematic review. *Arch Intern Med.* 2003;163:1362-1366.
76. Dranitsaris G, Stumpo C, Smith R, et al. Extended dalteparin prophylaxis for venous thromboembolic events: cost-utility analysis in patients undergoing major orthopedic surgery. *Am J Cardiovasc Drugs.* 2009;9(14):45-48.
77. Haentjens P, DeGroote K, Annemans L. Prolonged enoxaparin therapy to prevent VTE after primary hip or knee replacement. A cost-utility analysis. *Arch Orthop Trauma Surg.* 2004;124:507-517.
78. Prandoni P, Lensing AW, Cogo A, et al. The long-term clinical course of acute deep venous thrombosis. *Ann Intern Med.* 1996;125(1):1-7.

8 Anatomy: Description of Structures

Mohan S. Tripathi, Arjun Saxena, and Javad Parvizi

The knee is the largest and most superficial joint in the human body. It is comprised of the distal femoral condyles, proximal tibia, patella, and head of the fibula. The knee is primarily a hinge-type synovial joint that permits extension and flexion, but also allows for small degrees of medial and lateral rotation. This chapter focuses on the gross anatomic structures and the relationships that comprise the knee.

SURFACE ANATOMY

The bony landmarks and soft tissue structures that contribute to the surface anatomy of the knee are helpful during physical examination and surgery (Fig. 8-1). Careful examination combined with appropriate knowledge of anatomic structures aid the physician to assess for normal development, detect and evaluate fractures and/or dislocations, and help locate vital structures such as nerves or blood vessels.

The femoral epicondyles are subcutaneous and are easily palpated medially and laterally in either flexion or extension (Fig. 8-2). Anteriorly, the patella is subcutaneous. The superior margin of the patella is attached to the palpable quadriceps tendon while the inferior margin is connected to the tibial tuberosity via the patellar ligament approximately 4 to 5 cm from the inferior pole of the patella (Fig. 8-3). The fibular head is palpable at the inferolateral aspect of the knee, directly inferior to the lateral condyle of the tibia.

BONY ANATOMY

Femur

The femur is the longest and heaviest bone in the human body. It functions to transmit weight from the hip joint to the tibia during standing and also serves as the attachment site for numerous ligaments and tendons. This discussion will be limited to the distal aspect of the femur.

Distally, the femur is characterized by the medial and lateral femoral condyles. These condyles are the attachment sites for numerous ligaments and tendons and form the superior or proximal articular surface of the knee. The femoral articular surface is convex, and this convexity increases as one descends the anterior surface to the inferior surface of the condyles. When in an anatomic position, the two femoral condyles are on the same horizontal level, but the lateral femoral condyle has a more sharply increasing radius of curvature posteriorly and is slightly shorter and wider than the medial condyle at the intercondylar notch.

The medial and lateral femoral epicondyles, prominent features of the medial and lateral femoral condyles, serve as attachments for the collateral ligaments of the knee. The lateral epicondyle, slightly less prominent than the medial epicondyle, is the proximal attachment site of the lateral head of the gastrocnemius and popliteus muscle and the lateral collateral ligament (LCL). The medial epicondyle is the proximal attachment site of the medial collateral ligament (MCL).

The femoral condyles are separated by the intercondylar fossa. The fossa is narrowest at the distal end and widens

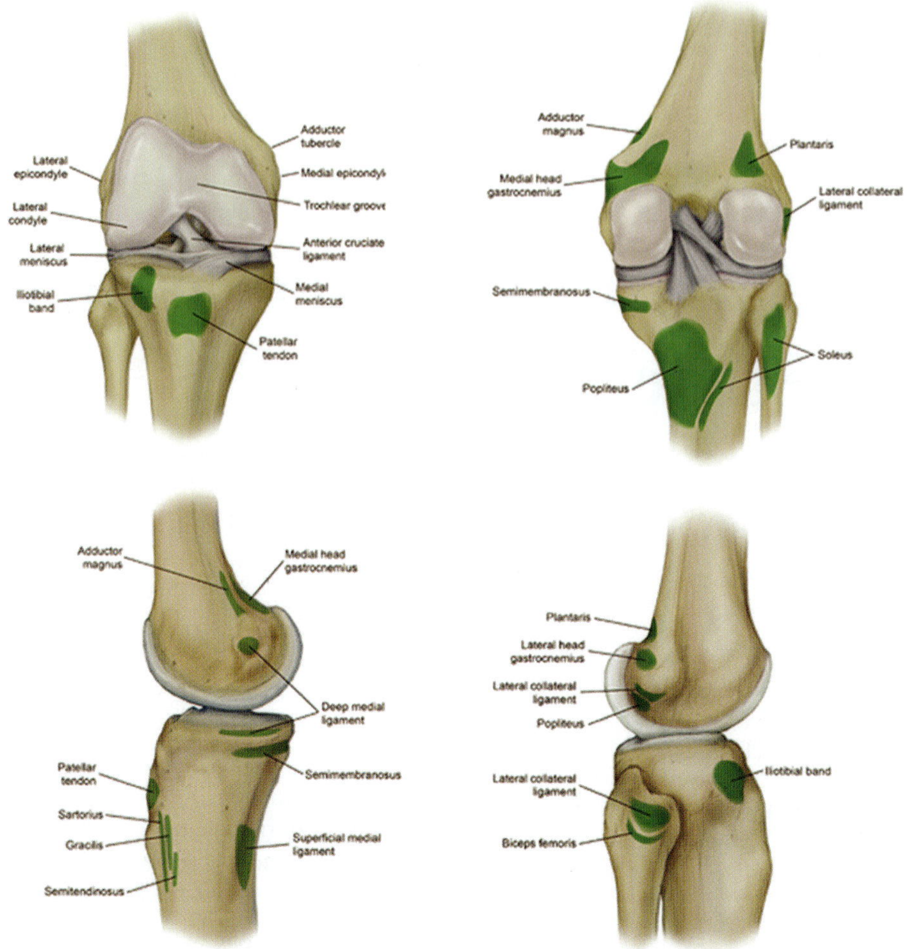

FIGURE 8-1. *Bony landmarks with ligament and tendon attachment sites. (Courtesy of Matthew Morrey, MD.)*

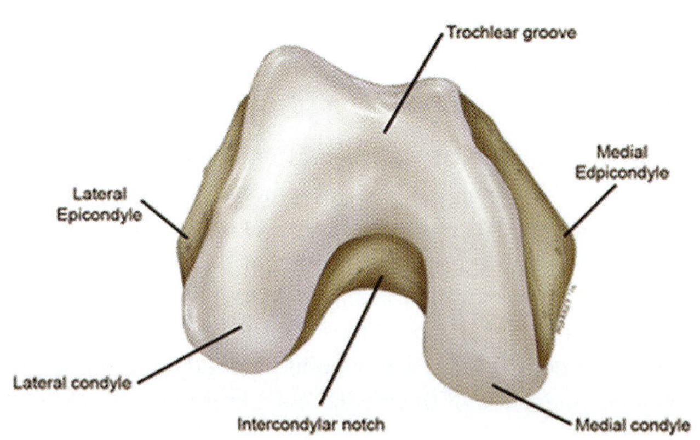

FIGURE 8-2. *Bony architecture of the distal femur. (Courtesy of Matthew Morrey, MD.)*

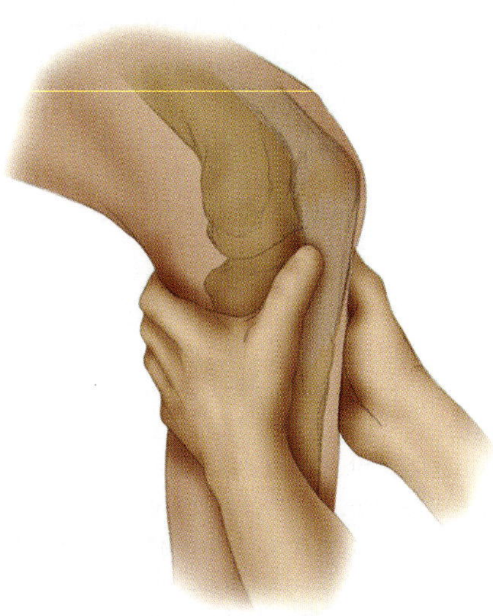

FIGURE 8-3. *Palpation of the patella tendon. (Courtesy of Matthew Morrey, MD.)*

proximally. The mean width of the intercondylar fossa is greatest at its midportion (2.4 cm) and decreases both proximally (1.3 cm) and distally (1.8 cm). The walls of the intercondylar fossa bear facets for the attachments for the cruciate ligaments. Anteriorly, the condyles merge to form a shallow, V-shaped depression referred to as the femoral trochlea, which articulates with the patella. In the native knee, the patella fits imperfectly within the trochlea, and the area of contact between patella and distal femur varies with position. The sulcus represents the deepest portion of the trochlea and lies slightly laterally relative to the midplane between the two femoral condyles.

Tibia

The tibia is the second longest bone in the body. Proximally, the tibia widens in a transverse plane to form medial and lateral condyles, forming a relatively flat surface that articulates with the femur. The tibial plateau is defined by the lateral and medial articular surfaces. The medial plateau is somewhat larger and slightly concave and is placed more directly over the shaft of the tibia. The lateral plateau is slightly circular and has a smaller articular surface than the medial plateau. Both articular surfaces are characterized by a slight posterior inclination of 10° relative to the tibial shaft.

On the medial aspect of the plateau, the articular surfaces of the tibia are separated by an intercondylar eminence (tibial spine) formed by the medial and lateral intercondylar tubercles. These tubercles fit into the intercondylar fossa found between the femoral condyles. A depression known as the anterior intercondylar fossa lies directly anterior to the medial and lateral intercondylar tubercles; it provides attachments sites for the menisci and the anterior cruciate ligament (ACL). Anterior to posterior, the anterior horn of the medial meniscus, the ACL, and the anterior horn of the lateral meniscus attach to this depression. Posterior to the medial and lateral intercondylar tubercles, a depression called the posterior intercondylar fossa provides additional attachment sites for the posterior cruciate ligament (PCL) and menisci of the knee. Anterior to posterior, this posterior depression affixes the posterior horn of the lateral meniscus, the posterior horn of the medial meniscus, and PCL. Gerdy's tubercle, the distal attachment site for the iliotibial (IT) band, is located on the anterolateral aspect of the proximal tibia. The lateral tibial condyle also bears the fibular articular facet, which is on the posterolateral aspect of the tibial metaphysis.

Fibula

The fibula is the long, slender bone posterolateral to the tibia. A synovial membrane lines the proximal tibiofibular joint and also possesses a capsule fortified by ligaments anteriorly and posteriorly. The fibula does not contribute any weight-bearing function and serves mainly as an attachment site for several muscles. The fibular head contains a circular facet on its superomedial surface that articulates with the fibular facet of the tibia, as described above. The styloid process of the fibular head, found on the posterolateral surface, is the insertion site of the LCL, patellofibular ligament, and arcuate ligament and also serves as an attachment site for the biceps femoris muscle.

Patella

The patella is the largest sesamoid bone in the body. It is formed within the tendon of the quadriceps femoris as it crosses anterior to the knee joint. Triangular in shape, the patella consists of an inferior apex, at which the patellar ligament connects the patella to the tibia, and a superior base, which serves as the attachment site for the quadriceps femoris tendon. The posterior surface of the patella articulates with the femoral trochlea; this articulation forms the patellofemoral compartment. There are seven facets on the posterior surface of the patella: three medial facets, three lateral facets, and one odd facet. The odd facet lies along the extreme medial border of the patella and only articulates with the femoral trochlea in extreme flexion. The articular surface of the patella is covered by the thickest hyaline cartilage in the body.

COLLATERAL LIGAMENTS

The collateral ligaments function to stabilize the knee by resisting medial and lateral displacement of the tibia on the femur (Fig. 8-4). Generally, these ligaments are taut during knee extension and contribute to knee stability in a standing person. During knee flexion, the ligaments become increasingly lax, allowing for a limited amount of joint rotation.

Lateral Collateral Ligament (Fibular Collateral Ligament)

The LCL (fibular collateral ligament) has its origin at the lateral femoral epicondyle and extends distally to the lateral surface of the fibular head. It is separated from the fibrous joint capsule via a bursa. The popliteus tendon passes deep to the LCL, separating the LCL from the lateral meniscus.

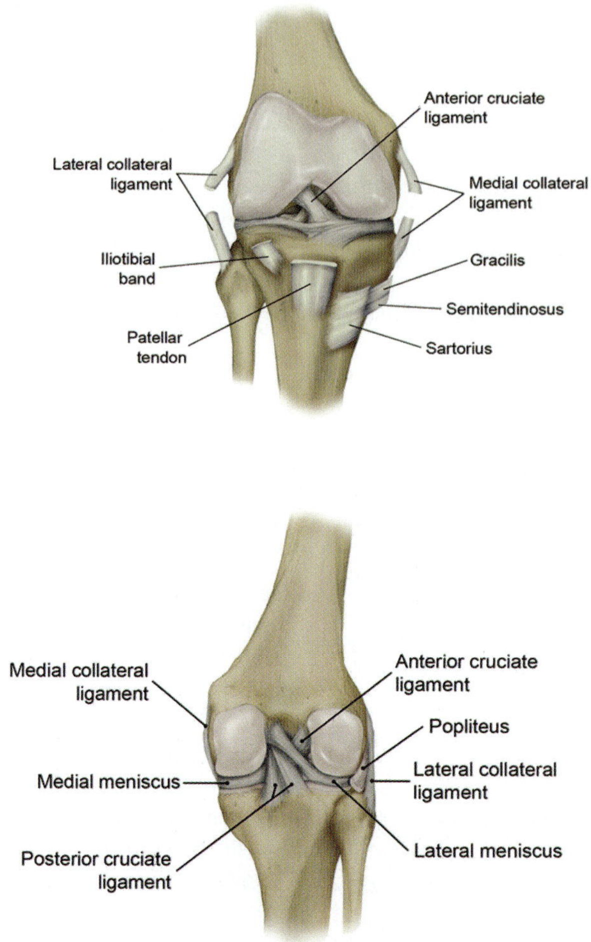

FIGURE 8-4. *Ligaments and tendons of the knee. (Courtesy of Matthew Morrey, MD.)*

Medial Collateral Ligament (Tibial Collateral Ligament)

The superficial fibers of the MCL (tibial collateral ligament) consist of parallel and oblique portions; the parallel fibers, consisting of vertically oriented fibers, arise from the medial femoral epicondyle and run distally to the medial tibial condyle and the medial tibal surface above and behind the pes anserinus (the distal attachment site of the gracilis, sartorius, and semitendiosus tendons). The oblique fibers originate at the medial femoral epicondyle and merge distally into the posteromedial joint capsule. The MCL, which is weaker than the LCL, is a broad and flat ligament, with much of its deep surface attaching to the underlying fibrous medial joint capsule. Midway through its course distally, the deepest fibers of the MCL directly attach to the medial meniscus.

CRUCIATE LIGAMENTS

The cruciate ligaments stabilize the knee by preventing anterior-posterior displacement of the tibia relative to the femur. These ligaments contain nerve endings that relay proprioceptive information back to the central nervous system. Blood supply is primarily via the middle geniculate artery.

Anterior Cruciate Ligament

The ACL arises from the posteromedial surface of the lateral femoral condyle, within the intercondylar fossa. It courses anteriorly and distally toward the tibia, with its fibers undergoing slight external rotation during their course. At the tibia, the ACL attaches to the anterior intercondylar fossa. Girgis et al measured the average length of the ACL at 38 mm and its average width at 11 mm.[1] The ACL functions as the primary stabilizer against anterior translocation of the tibia on the femur; several studies have shown that the ACL accounts for up to 86% of the total resistive force in an anterior drawer test.[2-5]

Posterior Cruciate Ligament

The origin of the PCL is at the posterior aspect of the lateral surface of the medial femoral condyle, within the intercondylar fossa. Distally, it attaches to a depression posterior to the intra-articular surface of the tibia. The average length of the PCL is 38 mm and its width is 13 mm.[1] During its course posteriorly, the fibers of the PCL experience slight internal rotation. The PCL is twice as strong as the ACL and is located close to the central axis of rotation of the knee joint.[6-10] Butler et al demonstrated that the PCL contributes nearly 95% of the total restraint to posterior dislocation of the tibia relative to the femur.[2]

MENISCI

Menisci are fibrocartilaginous structures that deepen the articular surface of the tibia (Fig. 8-5). The proximal surface of each meniscus is concave and receives the femoral condyles. In contrast, the distal surfaces of the menisci are relatively flat and rest firmly on the tibial plateau. The peripheral border of each meniscus is thick and convex and attaches to the joint capsule, whereas the central portion tapers into a thin, free edge in the interior of the knee joint. Each meniscus covers approximately the peripheral two-thirds of the articular surface of the tibia. Menisci function to transmit body weight across the knee joint. Furthermore, they serve to enhance articular conformity and increase the surface area of load transmission, while preventing soft tissue impingement during joint motion.

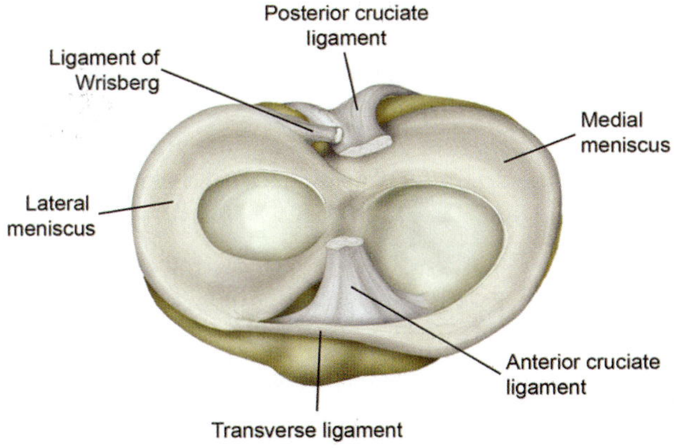

FIGURE 8-5. *Drawing of the superior aspect of the tibial plateau. (Courtesy of Matthew Morrey, MD.)*

Medial Meniscus

The semicircular medial meniscus is wedge-shaped in cross section. The anterior and posterior horn attachments of the medial meniscus have been described previously. The peripheral edge of the medial meniscus is continuous with the joint capsule and is also attached to the MCL. Posteromedially, the meniscus receives fibers from the insertion of the semimembranosus tendon via the joint capsule. A fibrous band called the transverse intermeniscal ligament connects the anterior horn of the medial meniscus with the anterior horn of the lateral meniscus. The coronary ligament creates an attachment between anterior horn and the tibial margin a few millimeters distal to the articular surface. At its midpoint, the medial meniscus attaches to the femur via a condensation of fibers in the joint capsule known as the deep medial ligament. Due to its numerous attachments to surrounding structures, the medial meniscus is less mobile than the lateral meniscus.

Lateral Meniscus

Circular in shape, the lateral meniscus is larger than the medial meniscus and therefore covers a larger portion of the articular surface. The anterior and posterior horn attachments have been described previously. Peripherally, the lateral meniscus' attachment to the capsule is interrupted by the popliteus hiatus, which allows the passage of the popliteal tendon. The meniscofemoral ligaments connect the posterior horn of the lateral meniscus to the intercondylar surface of the medial femoral condyle; the ligament of Humphrey passes anterior to the PCL, and the ligament of Wrisberg passes posterior to the PCL. Several studies have demonstrated that most patients will have one ligament or the other, while a smaller percentage will have both.[9,11,12]

NERVES ABOUT THE KNEE

Significant variation exists in the descriptions of the innervation of the various structures surrounding the knee joint. Gardner[13] and Kennedy et al[14] have separately described the predominant innervation of the knee. There are two groups of afferent nerve fibers. The anterior group consists of articular branches from the femoral, common peroneal, and saphenous nerves. The posterior group includes nerve fibers from the posterior articular branch of the tibial nerve and the obturator nerve.

Nerves of the Popliteal Fossa

Of the structures within the popliteal fossa, nerves are the most superficial of neurovascular structure, while arteries are the deepest. At the superior edge of the popliteal fossa, the sciatic nerve divides into the tibial nerve and common peroneal nerve.

Tibial nerve

The tibial nerve consists of afferent nerve fibers from the anterior rami of L4–S3. As it courses through the popliteal fossa, the tibial nerve extends motor branches to the soleus, gastrocnemius, plantaris, and popliteus muscles. In addition it gives rise to the medial sural cutaneous nerve, which descends the leg on the surface of the gastrocnemius muscle and receives the sural communicating branch of the common peroneal nerve to form the sural nerve.

Gardner described the largest and most consistent branch of the tibial nerve that supplies the joint: the posterior articular nerve.[13] This nerve, variable in origin, courses laterally around the popliteal vessels before passing deep to join the popliteal plexus. The popliteal plexus then sends penetrating fibers through the oblique popliteal ligament to innervate the posterior and perimeniscal capsule, as well as the synovial covering of the cruciate ligaments. A terminal branch of the posterior division of the obturator nerve also contributes to the popliteal plexus. This branch generally follows the course of the femoral artery into the popliteal fossa.

Common peroneal nerve

The common peroneal nerve, a terminal branch of the sciatic nerve derived from the anterior rami of L4–S2, forms at the superolateral edge of the popliteal fossa and runs close to the medial border of the biceps femoris muscle and its tendon. As it passes superficial to the lateral head of the gastrocnemius muscle, the common peroneal nerve leaves the popliteal fossa and courses around the posterior aspect of the fibular head and then winds around the neck of the fibular. It then penetrates the fibers of the peroneus longus muscle and subsequently divides into its terminal branches: the superficial peroneal and deep peroneal nerves. The common peroneal nerve also contributes to two articular branches: the lateral articular nerve and recurrent peroneal nerve. The lateral articular nerve arises at the level of the joint line and innervates the inferior lateral joint capsule and LCL. The recurrent peroneal nerve ascends the anterior surface of the tibia within the peroneus longus muscle and then enters the joint.[14]

Femoral Nerve

The femoral nerve contributes articular branches to nerves that innervate the joint capsule and the ligaments of the anteromedial and anterolateral knee. The articular branch that supplies the anteromedial capsule arises from the branch of the femoral nerve that innervates the vastus medialis muscle. The branch of the femoral nerve that supplies the vastus lateralis muscle also innervates the superolateral capsule.

The saphenous nerve arises from the posterior division of the femoral nerve and pierces the deep fascia on the medial side of the knee. The infrapatellar branch of the saphenous nerve traverses the sartorius muscle and joins the patellar plexus to provide innervation of the anteromedial capsule, patellar tendon, and anteromedial skin.[15] This patellar plexus lies anterior to the patella and patellar tendon. It is formed by numerous communications between the infrapatellar branch of the saphenous nerve and numerous divisions of cutaneous branches to the thigh. The medial cutaneous branch of the saphenous nerve runs along with the great saphenous vein, which runs along the medial aspect of the leg; the nerve innervates the skin of the medial leg and foot.

BLOOD SUPPLY

Femoral Artery

The superficial femoral artery is the main vessel that supplies oxygenated blood to the lower extremity. Before traversing the adductor hiatus, the superficial femoral artery gives off the descending geniculate artery, which divides into the saphenous branch, an articular branch, and a deep oblique branch. The saphenous branch courses distally with its like-named nerve and anatomoses with the medial inferior geniculate artery, while the deep oblique branch travels along the medial border of the femur and supplies the supracondylar aspect of the femur. The articular branch travels distally within the fibers of the vastus medialis muscle. After anastomosing with the lateral superior geniculate artery, it contributes to the geniculate anastomosis (Fig. 8-6).

Popliteal Artery

The popliteal artery begins immediately after the femoral artery courses through the adductor hiatus. It courses closely to the joint capsule and is the deepest (therefore, most anterior) structure in the popliteal fossa (Fig. 8-7). It is

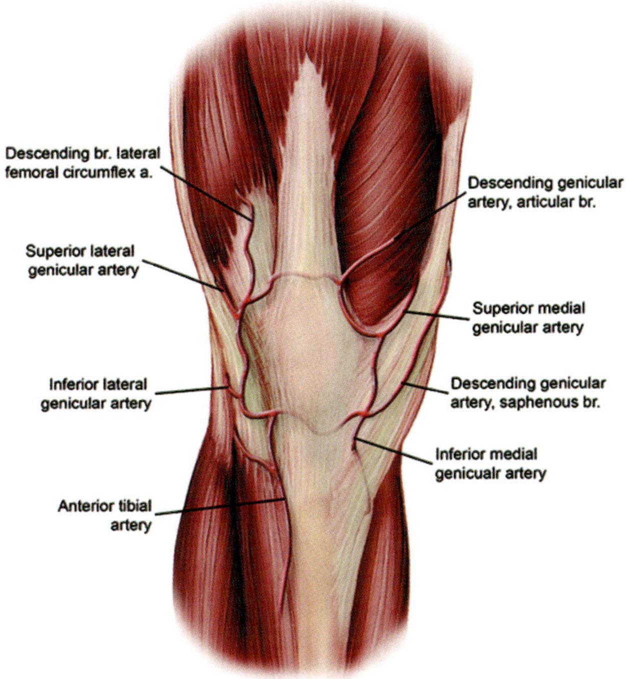

FIGURE 8-6. *Superficial vascular structures. (Courtesy of Matthew Morrey, MD.)*

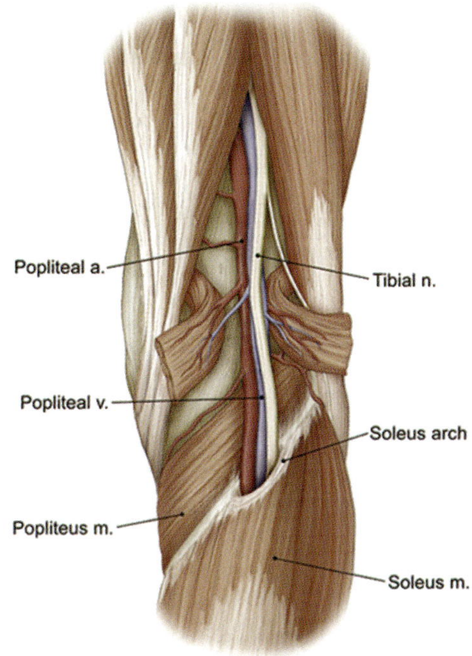

FIGURE 8-7. *Popliteal artery, vein, and nerve in popliteal fossa. (Courtesy of Matthew Morrey, MD.)*

separated from the femur by a fat pad proximally. Distally it descends in the popliteal fossa running superficial to the popliteus fascia. The artery ends as it divides into the anterior and posterial tibial arteries at the inferior border of the popliteus muscle.

During its relatively short course, the popliteal artery gives off numerous muscular and articular branches. Its muscular branches include vessels that supply the hamstrings, gastrocnemius, soleus, and plantaris muscles. There are five total articular branches of the popliteal artery (see Table 8-1 for a description of the arteries, their course, and the structures they supply).

The four superior and inferior geniculate arteries anastomose with the middle geniculate artery to form the genicular anastomosis. This anastomosis is a network of vessels that surrounds the knee and provides collateral blood circulation capable of maintaining blood supply to the leg during full knee flexion, during which the popliteal artery may kink. Furthermore, this anastomosis forms an anterior vascular circle around the patella to supply blood to the patella. The medial patellar retinaculum also derives its blood supply from this anterior anastomosis. The lateral patellar retinaculum derives its blood supply from the anastomosis of the superior and inferior lateral geniculate arteries.

JOINT CAPSULE

The joint capsule is a fibrous membrane comprised of an external fibrous layer and an internal synovial membrane; this synovial membrane lines the entirety of the interior surfaces of the articular cavity not covered by articular cartilage. The fibrous portion of the capsule contains areas of thickening that may progress into distinct ligaments, but generally the capsule remains thin and may be incomplete in some areas. The anterior capsule is relatively thin and is continuous anteriorly with the medial and lateral margins of the patellar ligament, patella, and quadiceps tendon. The fibrous layer attaches proximally to the femur, just proximal to the condylar articular margins. Distally, the capsule attaches circumferentially to the tibial plateau except in one area, the popliteal hiatus. The popliteal hiatus is a gap in the fibrous capsule through which the popliteus tendon enters the joint. This hiatus is posterior to the lateral tibial condyle and allows the popliteus muscle to pass out of the joint capsule. At the hiatus, the capsule is directed slightly inferiorly, toward the head of the fibula. A continuation of the capsule on the fibular head forms the arcuate ligament, found between the lateral meniscus and fibular styloid.

TABLE 8-1. Articular Branches of the Popliteal Artery

Artery	Origin	Course	Distribution
Middle geniculate artery	Anterior aspect of popliteal artery	Arises from anterior aspect of popliteal artery and pierces the posterior oblique ligament	1. Supplies the posterior joint capsule and posterior horns of both menisci 2. Gives rise to a ligamentous branch that traverses the synovium for form a vascular plexus covering the ACL and PCL
Lateral superior geniculate artery	Posterior aspect of popliteal artery superior to the joint line	Winds around the femur directly proximal to the lateral femoral condyle and then passes deep to the biceps femoris tendon	1. Anastomoses with descending branch of lateral femoral circumflex artery and medial superior geniculate artery 2. Supplies vastus lateralis
Medial superior geniculate artery	Posterior aspect of popliteal artery superior to the joint line	Winds around the femur directly proximal to the medial femoral condyle and then courses anteriorly deep to the semimembranosus and semitendinosus muscles and proximal to the origin of the medial head of the gastrocnemius	1. Supplies vastus medialis 2. Anastomoses with lateral superior geniculate artery
Lateral inferior geniculate artery	Posterior aspect of popliteal artery inferior to the joint line	Lies adjacent to the joint line and passes deep to the LCL and then traverses anteriorly to join the anterior anastomosis	Branches from both arteries converge to form a capillary complex in the anterior fat pad, supplying blood to the fat pad, patellar tendon, and synovial cavity
Medial inferior geniculate artery	Posterior aspect of popliteal artery inferior to the joint line	Passes 2–3 cm distal to the medial joint line, deep to the MCL	

The posterior portion of the fibrous joint capsule encloses the condyles and femoral intercondylar fossa. The capsule accepts fibers of the oblique popliteal ligament, which is derived from the semimembranosus tendon. This oblique ligament attaches to the proximal margin of the intercondylar fossa and forms part of the floor of the popliteal fossa.

SYNOVIUM

The synovial membrane lines the surfaces of the articular cavity that is not covered by articular cartilage. Its attachments include the periphery of the articular cartilage covering the femoral and tibial condyles and the posterior surface of the patella and the edges of the menisci. Furthermore, the synovium reflects onto the lateral and medial aspects of the inner surface of the joint capsule. Proximally, the synovium extends to the suprapatellar pouch (bursa), a synovial reflection located above the patella. This bursa is separated from the anterior femoral surface by a fat pad.

Intra-articularly, the synovium reflects anteriorly from the posterior joint line. The synovium extends beyond the intracondylar region and covers the cruciate ligaments, popliteal tendon, and the infrapatellar fat pad. An anterior intra-articular reflection creates a medial infrapatellar synovial fold that approaches the anterior aspect of the tibia. This synovial reflection essentially subdivides the articular cavity into right and left femorotibial articular cavities.

Anteriorly, the infrapatellar fat pad separates the synovial membrane and the patellar ligament. On either side of the pad, the synovial membrane reflects and creates an alar fold beneath the menisci.

MUSCULATURE

Anterior Aspect

The musculature of the anterior aspect of the thigh and knee consists of the quadriceps muscle group. The muscles that comprise the quadriceps include the rectus femoris, vastus lateralis, vastus medialis, and vastus intermedius (Table 8-2).

The rectus femoris muscle has two distinct heads that arise from the ilium, which join to form a muscle belly in the anterior aspect of the thigh. The rectus muscle is the only muscle in the quadriceps group that crosses both the hip and the knee joint; thus it functions to flex the thigh at the hip and can also extend the knee at the knee joint. The vastus lateralis muscle has its origin at the proximal end of the trochanteric line; some fibers also originate from the linea aspera on the femoral shaft. Near the distal end of the muscle, the muscle blends into the lateral patellar retinaculum, through which the vastus lateralis directly attaches to the patella. The vastus medialis originates from the trochanteric line, but distal to the origin of the vastus lateralis. This muscle is characterized by a unique group of fibers, collectively known as the vastus medialis obliquus. These most distal fibers of the vastus medialis arise from the tendon of the adductor magnus and pass horizontally anterior to the insertion into the common tendon. The medial most fibers of the vastus medialis blend with the medial patellar retinaculum. The vastus intermedialis has its origin on the lateral and anterior aspects of the femoral shaft. Medially, its fibers blend with those of the vastus medialis.

Distally, the four muscles of the quadriceps group merge to form the quadriceps tendon. This tendon extends anteriorly and inferiorly around the patella and becomes the patellar tendon. Hubbard et al[16] and Reider et al[17] separately described that fibers from the rectus femoris and vastus intermedialis insert almost perpendicularly into the superior patellar pole, whereas the fibers from the vastus medialis and lateralis insert obliquely. In the majority of patients, only fibers from the rectus femoris extend distally over the patella.

The patellar tendon has its origin at the apex of the patella superiorly and inserts onto the tibial tuberosity distally. The medial and lateral fibers from the quadriceps tendon extend beyond the patella to insert at the edges of the tibial tuberosity and merge into the capsule to become the medial and lateral patellar retinacula; these retinacula function to reinforce the joint capsule on either side of the knee joint.

TABLE 8-2. Quadriceps Muscles: Quadriceps Femoris

Muscle	Innervation	Proximal Attachment	Distal Insertion	Action
Rectus femoris	Femoral nerve (L2–L4)	Anterior inferior iliac spine and ilium superior to acetabulum		
Vastus lateralis	Femoral nerve (L2–L4)	Proximal end of greater trochanter and lateral lip of linea aspera	Attaches via common quadriceps tendon	Extend leg at the knee joint. Rectus femoris crosses both hip and knee joint, thus serving to stabilize the hip joint and assists in flexion at the hip.
Vastus medialis	Femoral nerve (L2–L4)	Distal part of intertrochanteric line and medial lip of linea aspera		
Vastus intermedius	Femoral nerve (L2–L4)	Anterior and lateral surfaces of femoral shaft		

Posterior Aspect

As previously described, the popliteal fossa is bordered proximally by the hamstring muscles (Table 8-3); the biceps femoris is lateral and the semimembranosus and the tendons of the pes anserine are medial. The distal border consists of the two heads of the gastrocnemius. The deep fascia of the leg forms the roof, while the posterior femoral surface, the posterior knee joint capsule, and the popliteus fascia that covers the popliteus muscle form the floor of the popliteal fossa.

The biceps femoris lies posterior to the IT tract. The fusiform muscle is comprised of two heads: a long head and short head. Inferiorly, the long head becomes tendinous and joins the short head to form a common tendon that inserts onto the head of the fibula.

The semitendinosus is a broad, membranous muscle that originates from the ischial tuberosity; it courses distally and medially on the surface of the semimembranosus to insert onto the posterior aspect of the medial tibial condyle. The semimembranosus muscle has its origin at the ischial tuberosity and passes deep to the semitendinosus. This muscle forms the superomedial border of the popliteal fossa and inserts into the posteromedial aspect of the tibia. Fibers from the semimembranosus insertion, known as the oblique popliteal ligament, are reflected laterally to superolaterally to the femoral condyle and function to reinforce the intercondylar portion of the joint capsule.

The gastrocnemius muscle is the most superficial muscle in the posterior aspect of the leg (Table 8-4). Its lateral head arises from the lateral femoral condyle, while its medial head arises from the popliteal surface of the femur and medial aspect of the medial femoral condyle. The two heads merge at the inferior border of the popliteal fossa. The soleus muscle's origins are multiple. They include the posterior aspect of the fibular head, the soleal line on the posterior surface of the tibia, and the tendinous arch that crosses the posterior tibial vessels and nerve, connecting the tibia and fibula. The soleus merges with the gastrocnemius fibers distally to insert into the calcaneous via the calcaneal tendon. The plantaris muscle is a small muscle that arises from the lateral supracodylar line of the femur, deep to the lateral head of the gastrocnemius muscle. It is a vestigial muscle and may be absent in 5% to 10% of humans. The popliteus muscle has its proximal attachment at the lateral surface of the lateral femoral condyle and lateral meniscus. It inserts into the posterior tibial surface, just superior to the soleal line. It passes deep to the arcuate ligament and the semimembranosus muscle expansion.

TABLE 8-3. Hamstring Muscles

Muscle	Innervation	Proximal Attachment	Distal Insertion	Action
Semitendinosus	Tibial division of sciatic nerve (L5, S1, S2)	Ischial tuberosity	Medial surface of proximal tibia	Extend thigh and flex leg. Also aids in medial rotation when leg is flexed.
Semimembranosus	Tibial division of sciatic nerve (L5, S1, S2)		Medial tibial condyle	
Biceps femoris	Long Head: tibial division of sciatic nerve (L5, S1, S2) Short Head: common fibular division of sciatic nerve (L5, S1, S2)	Long Head: ischial tuberosity Short Head: linea aspera, lateral supracondylar femoral line	Lateral aspect of fibular head	Flexion of leg and lateral rotation of knee when leg is flexed.

TABLE 8-4. Posterior Muscles of the Leg

Muscle	Innervation	Proximal Attachment	Distal Insertion	Action
Gastrocnemius	Tibial nerve (S1, S2)	Lateral Head: lateral femoral condyle Medial Head: popliteal surface of medial femoral condyle	Posterior aspect of calcaneus via calcaneal tendon	Plantarflexion of ankle when knee is extended; flexion of knee joint
Soleus	Tibial nerve (S1, S2)	Posterior aspect of fibular head; soleal line of fibula		Plantarflexion of ankle independent of knee position
Plantaris	Tibial nerve (S1, S2)	Inferior edge of lateral supracondylar femoral line		Weak plantarflexion
Popliteus	Tibial nerve (L4, L5, S1)	Lateral aspect of lateral femoral condyle and lateral meniscus	Posterior aspect of tibia	Weak flexion of knee and medial rotation of knee of non-weight-bearing limb

REFERENCES

1. Girgis FG, Marshall JL, Monajem A. The cruciate ligaments of the knee joint: anatomical, functional and experimental analysis. *Clin Orthop Relat Res.* 1975; 106:216-231.
2. Butler DL, Noyes FR, Grood ES. Ligamentous restraints to anterior-posterior drawer in the human knee: a biomechanical study. *J Bone Joint Surg Am.* 1980;62(2):259-270.
3. Furman W, Marshall JL, Girgis FG. The anterior cruciate ligament: a functional analysis based on postmortem studies. *J Bone Joint Surg Am.* 1976; 58(2):179-185.
4. Hsieh HH, Walker PS. Stabilizing mechanisms of the loaded and unloaded knee joint. *J Bone Joint Surg Am.* 1976;58(1):87-93.
5. Kennedy JC, Fowler PJ. Medial and anterior instability of the knee: an anatomical and clinical study using stress machines, 1971. *Clin Orthop Relat Res.* 1995; 321:3-9.
6. Clancy WG Jr, Shelbourne KD, Zoellner GB, et al. Treatment of knee joint instability secondary to rupture of the posterior cruciate ligament: report of a new procedure. *J Bone Joint Surg Am.* 1983;65(3):310-322.
7. Hughston JC, Andrews JR, Cross MJ, et al. Classification of knee ligament instabilities. Part I. The medial compartment and cruciate ligaments. *J Bone Joint Surg Am.* 1976;58(2):159-172.
8. Kennedy JC, Hawkins RJ, Willis RB, et al. Tension studies of human knee ligaments: yield point, ultimate failure, and disruption of the cruciate and tibial collateral ligaments. *J Bone Joint Surg Am.* 1976;58(3):350-355.
9. Van Dommelen BA, Fowler PJ. Anatomy of the posterior cruciate ligament: a review. *Am J Sports Med.* 1989;17(1):24-29.
10. Welsh RP. Knee joint structure and function. *Clin Orthop Relat Res.* 1980;147:7-14.
11. Renstrom P, Johnson RJ. Anatomy and biomechanics of the menisci. *Clin Sports Med.* 1990;9(3):523-538.
12. Wan AC, Felle P. The menisco-femoral ligaments. *Clin Anat.* 1995;8(5):323-326.
13. Gardner E. The innervation of the knee joint. *Anat Rec.* 1948;101(1):109-130.
14. Kennedy JC, Alexander IJ, Hayes KC. Nerve supply of the human knee and its functional importance. *Am J Sports Med.* 1982;10(6):329-335.
15. Hunter LY, Louis DS, Ricciardi JR, et al. The saphenous nerve: its course and importance in medial arthrotomy. *Am J Sports Med.* 1979;7(4):227-230.
16. Hubbard JK, Sampson HW, Elledge JR. Prevalence and morphology of the vastus medialis oblique muscle in human cadavers. *Anat Rec.* 1997;249(1):135-142.
17. Reider B, Marshall JL, Koslin B, et al. The anterior aspect of the knee joint. *J Bone Joint Surg Am.* 1981; 63(3):351-356.

9

Biomechanics of the Knee

Jan Victor and Emmanuel Thienpont

The knee is the largest joint in the human body, with an intricate asymmetric three-dimensional anatomy, and has been the subject of many studies for a long time. These studies of the knee joint were exemplary in the scientific development of biomechanics. Many biomechanical concepts were first applied to the knee. Understanding biomechanics has direct consequences to the daily practice of orthopaedic surgeons, in diagnosing, explaining, or treating knee pathology.

The basic patterns of human posture and locomotion have remained unchanged for many centuries, although exposure to physical activity at work has probably decreased in favor of sports and leisure-time activities. Biomechanics is traditionally described as the study of kinetics (forces and moments) and kinematics (relative motion of rigid bodies). In vivo experiments are difficult to conduct because invasive techniques are required for accurate measurements. In vitro work is mostly limited to the single knee joint, reducing the natural mechanical environment of hip–knee–ankle. Ideally the knee joint should be studied in relation to body posture, hip, and ankle joint. For instance, all muscles attached and acting around the knee joint, except the popliteus muscle, bridge two joints: hip and knee or knee and ankle. Obtaining relevant knowledge from animal models is limited too, since most are not bipedal or plantigrade and do not extend the knee during gait. Despite all these limitations of our research possibilities, new medical imaging techniques open doors for better research.

This chapter presents an introduction to the kinematics and kinetics of the knee joint with a special emphasis on disclosing the relation between alignment and kinematics. The human knee joint consists of three articulations: the tibiofemoral, the patellofemoral, and the tibiofibular joint. Because the mobility of the latter is very limited, it is not further mentioned and only the tibiofemoral and patellofemoral articulations are discussed.

KINEMATICS OF TIBIOFEMORAL JOINT

Kinematics is the description of the relative motion between rigid bodies. This relative motion is governed by surface geometry, ligaments, muscle action, and body inertia. Close to the knee joint, the bone architecture changes. The thick cortical bone, found in the diaphysis of the tibia and femur, changes to a thin-layered plate, filled with cancellous bone. At these periarticular areas, the bone becomes more elastic, providing a dampening effect to peak forces that act upon the joint. This progressive widening of the bones also increases the articular contact area. The articular surfaces of the femur and tibia are incongruent, thus using only a limited contact area at the time. This contact area will change with increasing flexion (Fig. 9-1). The menisci increase this articulating area but tend to be squeezed out by the spherical femoral condyles. Tensile stress (hoop) within the meniscus resists such forces. The ligaments serve multiple tasks: they act as proprioceptive stress transducers, allow motion, and limit motion. The range of motion of the knee joint has important individual variability and changes often with age.

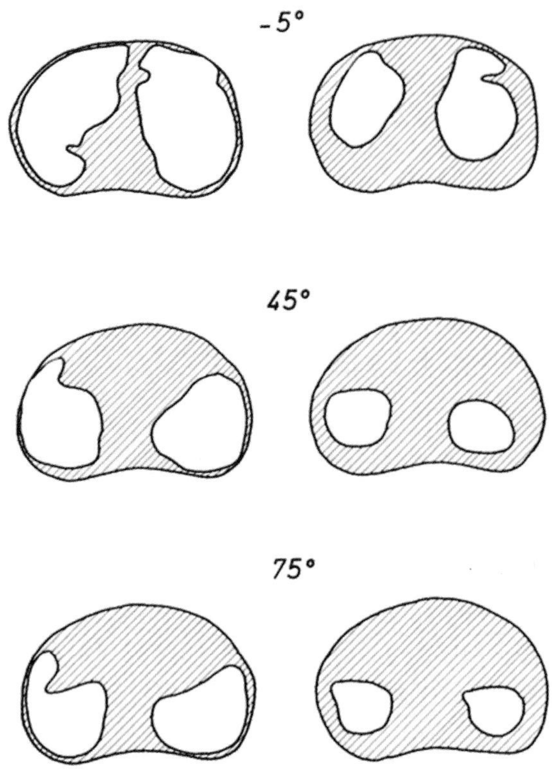

FIGURE 9-1. *Tibiofemoral contact areas according to flexion angle. Left, with menisci; right, without. (After Maquet, Biomechanics of the Knee, Springer-Verlag, Berlin, 1984.)*

The most widely accepted model of knee kinematics describes a posterior translation of the femoral condyles relative to the tibia with increasing flexion. This posterior translation is greater on the lateral than on the medial side, leading to relative internal rotation of the tibia with increasing flexion. However, different methodologies reveal different kinematic patterns and the existing literature is not unanimous in the description of "normal" knee kinematics.

History of Knee Kinematics

The study of how the femur moves on the tibia has a long history.[1] The first known description dates back to 1836 when Weber and Weber described the movement on the medial side to be "like a cradle." Since that first description, based on direct visual observation of a cadaveric specimen, several methods have been used to examine the kinematics of the human knee. The first radiological study was performed by Zuppinger,[2] who stated that the femur rolled back across the tibia during flexion as a result of the so-called rigid four-bar link mechanism provided by the two cruciate ligaments. In 1971, Frankel[3] introduced the concept of the instant center of rotation. He emphasized that as one link (rigid body) rotates around the other, there is at any given moment in time a point with zero velocity. That point is called the instant center of rotation (Fig. 9-2). He concluded that "due to the shapes of the bones and the restraints on motion imposed by the ligaments, capsule, and muscles, the instantaneous centers for successive positions of the links of the knee move." The initial work by Frankel was carried out by taking "true lateral" X-rays of the knee in patients lying on the side, at discrete intervals of 10° to 20° in the range of full extension to 90° of flexion. The knee was treated as if it were a "planar mechanism." In other words, the movement of the knee was reduced to a two-dimensional projection of a three-dimensional reality (Fig. 9-3). Menschik introduced in 1974 the concept of the four-bar linkage, representing the cruciate ligaments in two dimensions as two rigid bars and the lines connecting their insertion points on femur and tibia as the two other rigid bars.[4] The instant center of rotation is located at the point of intersection of the cruciate ligaments. This principle of "rigid four-bar linkage" was later widely popularized by Müller.

In the following years, the limitations of this two-dimensional methodology became clear, with the major flaws being the inability to ascertain the location of the axes of rotation before performing kinematic analyses.[5] In 1983, Grood and Suntay presented a joint coordinate system providing a geometric description of the three-dimensional rotational and translational motion between two rigid bodies, applied to the knee joint. The main step forward was the definition of a "floating axis." With this model, the described joint displacements became independent of the order in which the component rotations and translations occur.[6]

The new mathematical insights led to the concept of the helical axis and opened the door for a correct scientific description of the kinematics of the knee.[7] However, as the mathematical accuracy improved, the complexity increased and the model appeared to be impractical and difficult to apply to the clinical setting; the clinicians failed to understand the engineers.

Hollister, and later Churchill, tried to bridge the gap.[8,9] Hollister's model essentially described knee motion as pure rotations occurring around two axes: the so-called "flexion-extension axis" and the so-called "longitudinal rotation axis," with the understanding of the flexion-extension axis not being exactly located in the coronal plane and the longitudinal axis not being exactly located in the sagittal plane.[8]

A 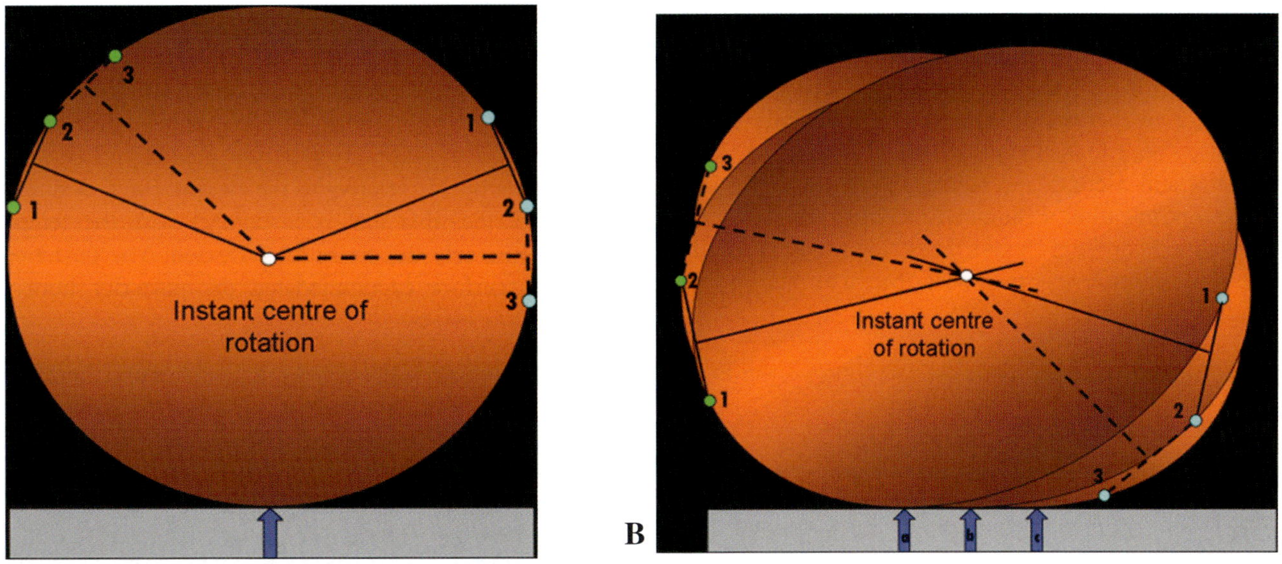

B

C 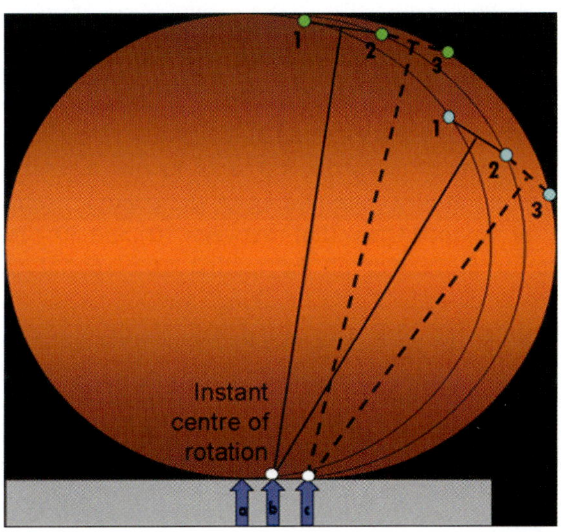

FIGURE 9-2. *The instant center of rotation determined with the method of Reuleaux.[3] The points on the body move from position 1 to position 2 and from 2 to 3.The perpendicular bisector for a pair of displacement points is drawn. The intersection of the bisectors is the point with zero velocity, called the instant center of rotation. The contact point is represented by the blue arrow. (**A**) For a circular body undergoing rotation with gliding, the instant center of rotation and the contact point remain fixed. (**B**) For a noncircular body undergoing rotation with gliding, the instant center of rotation remains fixed but the contact point shifts. (**C**) For a circular body undergoing rotation with rolling, the instant center of rotation coincides with the contact point and moves accordingly.*

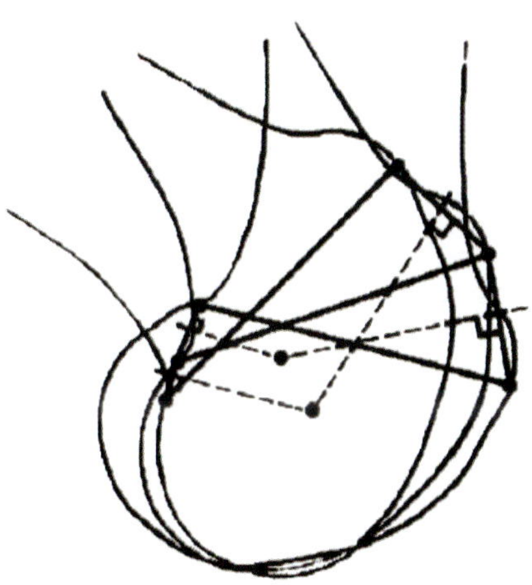

FIGURE 9-3. *The moving instant center of rotation of the knee, as described by Frankel[3] in a two-dimensional model.*

As a consequence, these mathematical "simple rotations" meant in reality flexion-extension, varus-valgus, and internal-external rotation of the knee joint, once again confusing the clinician trying to apply this knowledge to the practical setting. Churchill addressed this problem by allowing a mathematical error in the kinematic description, based on a loaded rig experiment with an ankle load of 100 N and a combined hamstrings load of 30 N.[9] He used an optimization technique to identify the locations of the so-called "optimal flexion" and "longitudinal rotation" axes. Knee motion was then described with the following formula:

$$K = \theta_{OF} + \theta_{LR} + R_\theta + R_X + R_Y + R_Z,$$

where

K = complete three-dimensional motion,

θ_{OF} = rotation about the optimal flexion axis, and

θ_{LR} = rotation about the longitudinal rotation axis.

He concluded that the optimal flexion axis coincided with the transepicondylar axis if one accepts the following errors and limitations: residual rotation (R_θ) = 2.9°, residual translations ($R_X + R_Y + R_Z$) = 3.4 mm, and applicable motion range of 5° to 90° of flexion. Despite those limitations, the advantage of this approach was the link between the kinematic description and certain anatomical landmarks, allowing clinicians to apply this knowledge in practice.

In recent times, technological progress allowed more advanced tools to be used, including in vitro studies with magnetic resonance imaging (MRI) on cadaveric specimens,[10,11] in vivo analyses using two-dimensional fluoroscopy with shape-matching techniques, based on computed tomography (CT) models,[12-15] roentgen stereophotogrammetric analysis (RSA),[16] and open dual-coil MRIs.[17-19] These newer methods revealed a more complete, three-dimensional insight into the morphology and kinematic patterns of the normal knee in loaded and unloaded conditions.

MRI Studies of Knee Kinematics

Iwaki and coworkers applied MRI scans to six unloaded cadaver specimens for the description of the surface geometry and relative passive movements of the femur and the tibia.[10] They visualized an approximate midsagittal section of the medial and lateral femoral condyle and analyzed the contours of the bones.

On the medial side of the femur, in the midsagittal section, the arc of two circles was described: the anterior or extension facet and the posterior or flexion facet. In their description, the midsagittal section of the medial side of the tibia consisted of an extension facet, a flexion facet, and a posterior horizontal surface. The extension facet, accommodating the anterior horn of the medial meniscus, sloped upwards by 11° relative to the flexion facet, defined as the area of the tibia that is in contact with the femur from approximately 20° to 120° of flexion. The posterior horizontal surface accommodated the posterior horn of the medial meniscus.

The midsagittal section of the lateral femoral condyle was found to be circular in its posterior part as on the medial side with a radius being 1 mm smaller. No clear extension facet was described on the lateral femoral condyle. The midsagittal section of the lateral tibia plateau essentially revealed a central area of 24-mm depth, called the tibial articular facet. Anterior and posterior to this area, the tibia accommodated the anterior and posterior horn of the lateral meniscus.

The main kinematic observation was the center of the femoral flexion facet (medial condyle) remaining relatively constant along the *X-Y* axis in the sagittal plane, suggesting almost pure sliding of the condyle from 0° to 110° of flexion. The initial (between 10° and 30°) relative posterior movement of the medial tibiofemoral contact area was described as a "rocking" motion as the contact shifts from the tibial extension facet onto the flexion facet. From 110° to 120° of flexion, a posterior motion of the center of the femoral flexion facet of 2 mm was described. On the lateral side, rolling and sliding took place simultaneously, translating the lateral femoral flexion facet center 4 mm between full extension and 45° and 15 mm between 45° and 120°.

In a later paper in 2004, Pinskerova et al[20] reworked these findings with the focus on the different patterns of translation of the tibiofemoral surface contact points and the condylar centers. Limitations of these studies include the following: MRI does not yield a homogenous Cartesian coordinate set, the definitions of the flexion facet centers in two dimensions only, and the discrete measurements with the absence of data between 45° and 90° of flexion.

The same group studied MRI data of 13 knees in living volunteers performing unloaded flexion. On the medial side, the anteroposterior (AP) position of the femoral condyle remained relatively stable, from full extension to 110° of flexion, provided that adjustment was made for the

2-mm translation during the rocking motion on the extension facet between –5° and 30° of flexion. On the lateral side, 3-mm posterior motion was observed as the knee was released from the screw-home mechanism, 1-mm posterior motion between 0° and 60°, and 13 mm between 60° and 110° of flexion. It was concluded that the kinematics of unloaded flexion of the knees of the living subjects was comparable to the kinematics observed in the cadaver specimens. In four subjects only, a loaded flexion movement under form of a squat from 0° to 90° of flexion was examined. The main difference with the unloaded movement was the anterior translation of the medial femoral condyle by 4 mm. Two additional tests were performed: isometric hamstrings contraction at 90° of flexion caused no change medially and an anterior translation of the lateral femoral condyle of 2 mm. Forced internal rotation of the tibia did not change kinematics between 0° and 90° of flexion, whereas forced external rotation of the tibia suppressed the normal rotational kinematics and forced the knee to flex as would a hinge, without axial rotation. Limitations of this study are equal to the previous study with the additional drawback of the small sample size and limited flexion (up to 90° only) of the loaded flexion measurement.

Nakagawa and coworkers[18] completed the previously described work in the high flexion arc, studying unloaded flexion in 20 Japanese volunteers with an open MRI. Active flexion was measured from 90° to 133° and passive flexion from 90° to 162°. They found a mean posterior translation of the medial condyle and lateral condyle of 2 mm and 13 mm, respectively, from 90° to 130° of flexion. Pushing the knee further, from 133° to 162° of flexion, caused further posterior translation, medially by 4.5 mm and laterally by 15 mm, subluxing the femur behind the tibia.

Johal and coworkers[19] studied the full range of motion of a "loaded squat" (wall-supported squat sit) with 10 volunteers, using an interventional MRI. They observed posterior translation of the lateral femoral condyle of 22 mm from hyperextension to 120° of flexion. The medial condyle moved forward 1.7 mm from hyperextension to 30° of flexion and started translating posterior from 90° flexion onwards: 3.6 mm between 90° and 120° and an additional 8.4 mm from 120° to full flexion. This differential translation on the medial and lateral side led to an external rotation of 20° of the femur relative to the tibia during flexion. Beyond 120° of flexion, posterior translation was equal on the medial and lateral side and no further tibiofemoral rotation was occurring. The subluxing nature of the tibiofemoral articulation beyond 120° of flexion inspired the authors to "question the ability of total knee replacement prostheses of the condylar type to achieve ranges of flexion above 120° in a physiologic manner."

RSA Studies of Knee Kinematics

Karrholm et al[16] confirmed the data published by Hill in an in vivo RSA experiment where volunteers performed a step-up activity from 50° to 65° of flexion to full extension. They also found anterior translation of the femoral condyle in early flexion (3 mm from 0° to 50° of flexion). Forced external rotation of the foot suppressed physiologic internal rotation of the tibia with flexion. The main weakness of this study is the variability of the motion that was performed and the fact that they only studied a single motion from moderate flexion to full extension and not a full motion cycle.

Fluoroscopy Studies Based on CT Models

Fluoroscopy allows following knee motion in real time in vivo, with an obvious drawback of delivering two-dimensional images. A preliminary CT scan allows making a three-dimensional bone model that can convert the two-dimensional fluoroscopic image with a shape-matching technique.[12] Lu and coworkers studied active knee extension in open chain at fixed angular speed in eight subjects and found no difference between the "unloaded" (ankle free) and "loaded" (5 kg attached at ankle) setting. Half of the tibiofemoral rotation occurred between full extension and 30° of flexion.[14] Komistek and coworkers used this technology to study gait and deep flexion activities in five volunteers. They found significantly less translation and rotation of the femur during gait than during deep flexion[13] They confirmed previous findings of less translation on the medial side than on the lateral side, but the most important result of their work seems to be the impressive interindividual variability. For deep flexion, the medial condyle translation ranged from +3 mm to –9 mm versus +1.4 to –30 mm for the lateral condyle. The average tibiofemoral rotation during flexion was 13°.

Bank's group used CT-derived bone models for model registration and added MRI-derived articular surfaces for obtaining higher accuracy of the contact areas. They observed the greatest femoral external rotation during the squat activity, but reported no posterior subluxation of either femoral condyle in maximum knee flexion.[15] In comparing kneel, squat, and stair climb motions, they found knee kinematics to vary significantly by activity.

In Vitro Kinematic Knee Rig Studies

Several authors examined knee kinematics based on an experimental cadaver setup. The advantage of this technology is the potential for accurate measurement as invasive methods can be used for following the motion of the bones in real time.[9,21-30] Optical trackers can be fixed, forming a rigid body with femur, tibia, and patella. The fixation of the femur and tibia to the kinematic knee rig is such that no constraints are imposed on the specimen and all 6 *df* are maintained. The specimen can be loaded on the different muscle attachments to reproduce active motion. Feedback systems guide the actuators, based on the measured ankle load and hip position (Fig. 9-4). The main weakness of this methodology is our ignorance about the magnitude and exact timing of hamstrings cocontraction. This is reflected in the high variability of loads applied to the hamstrings in the different experiments, ranging from 10 to 120 N.

State-of-the-Art Description of Knee Kinematics

In the past decade, most clinically oriented publications described passive knee kinematics as tibial rotation around the mechanical axis as a function of flexion angle or anteroposterior position of the medial and lateral condyle as a function of the flexion angle. Alternatively, progression of the line connecting medial and lateral tibiofemoral contact points (centroids of pressure) or projected centers of the femoral condyles on the surface of the tibia, represented as a plane, is plotted in function of the flexion angle. This representation is not devoid of flaws and assumptions, but it allows a clinical and intuitive understanding of the motion occurring (Fig 9-5). An overview of recent papers describing passive knee kinematics, with the respective methodologies, is given in Table 9-1.

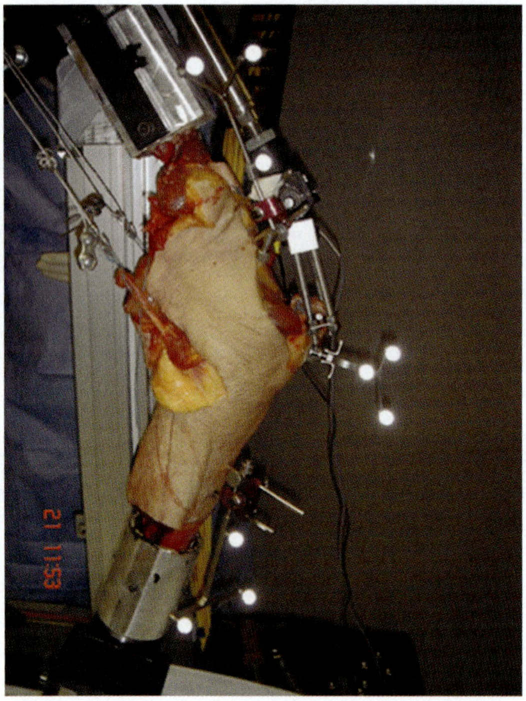

FIGURE 9-4. *Example of a cadaver specimen in a kinematic knee rig. Tibia and femur are fixed in containers. Two actuators control motion: vertical sliding of the "hip" will change the flexion angle and pulling the quadriceps will affect the ankle load, measured with a load cell under the tibia fixture.*

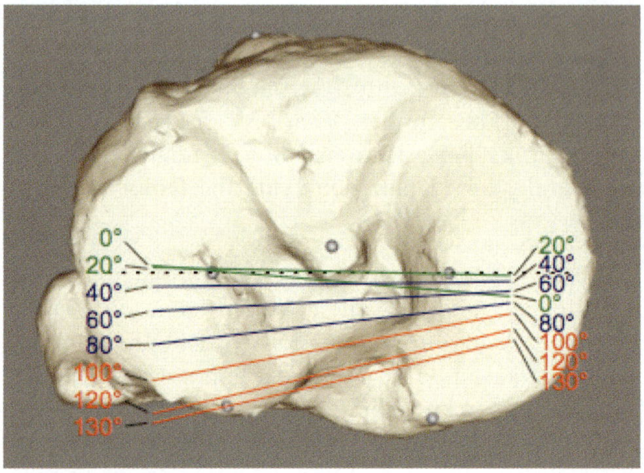

FIGURE 9-5. *Lines connecting the medial and lateral position of the femoral condyles, plotted on the axial plane of the tibia as a function of the flexion angle (mean positions taken from Fig. 9-6, B and C).*

TABLE 9-1. Recent Papers Describing Passive Knee Kinematics with Their Respective Methodologies

Author	Material	Motion	Load	Coord Frame	Technique
Hill[17]	6 Cadavers/ 13 living subjects	Series of static	No load, leg supported	AP position from ipsilateral posterior cortex	MRI, no 3D models
Iwaki[10]	6 Cadavers	Series of static	No load, leg on side	AP position from ipsilateral posterior cortex	MRI, no 3D models
Johal[19]	10 Living subjects	Series of static	No load	AP position from ipsilateral posterior cortex	MRI, no 3D models
Most[22]	6 Cadavers	Least resistance path, robot	No load or moment	Translation & rotation from value at 0° flexion	3D models based on digitization
Li[23]	13 Cadavers	Least resistance path, robot	No load or moment	Translation & rotation from value at 0° flexion	MRI, no 3D models
Lu[14]	8 Living subjects	Dynamic tests fluoroscopy	Active extension, no load	AP position from ipsilateral posterior cortex	3D models from CT
Wilson[21]	15 Cadavers	Dynamic tests with rig	No load	AP position from ipsilateral posterior cortex	MRI, no 3D models
Victor[46]	12 Cadavers	Continuous passive	No load, manual	AP position from projected femoral condyle center	CT, 3D models

The plots of medial and lateral condyle position and tibial rotation as a function of the flexion angle are shown in Figure 9-6. All studies report internal rotation of the tibia, relative to the femur with increasing flexion. The reported values range from –12° to –23°. Where all studies saw a gradual posterior translation of the lateral femoral condyle, from complete extension to maximum flexion, the motion of the medial condyle differs. Hill reports a very stable position of the medial femoral condyle, versus most describing initial anterior translation of the medial femoral condyle, reaching its most anterior position at 40° of flexion, followed by gradual posterior translation, but at a slower pace than the lateral femoral condyle.

One has to be aware that this well-accepted descriptive model only applies to passive knee kinematics. Muscle action will change kinematic behavior. Action of the quadriceps and the medial and lateral hamstrings has been examined in several experimental settings. In general, muscle loading reduces femoral translation, to a greater extent on the lateral than on the medial side, thus limiting or even reversing internal rotation with increasing flexion (Fig. 9-7).[21,22,24] The action of the muscles can in part be deducted from their attachment sites. Since the attachment from the biceps is farther away from the center of rotation around the vertical axis, its moment arm is greater than for the medial hamstrings. Probably, the greater natural laxity of the lateral compartment of the knee plays an equally important role in the greater effect of the hamstrings load on the lateral than on the medial side of the knee. The effect of the quadriceps load depends on the flexion angle (Fig. 9-8). Between full extension and 65° flexion, the patellar tendon angle is positive, and the resulting quadriceps load pulls the tibia forwards. Because the isolated quadriceps contraction can produce forces beyond those required for anterior cruciate ligament (ACL) tensile failure, it is clear that hamstrings cocontraction, especially on the lateral side, is an important protective mechanism for ACL integrity. Beyond 65° of knee flexion, the patellar tendon angle is negative, producing a posterior direction in the resulting horizontal component of the force vector acting on the tibia. This will, in synergy with the hamstrings, further reduce posterior translation of the femur with increasing flexion, as the tibia is pulled backwards.

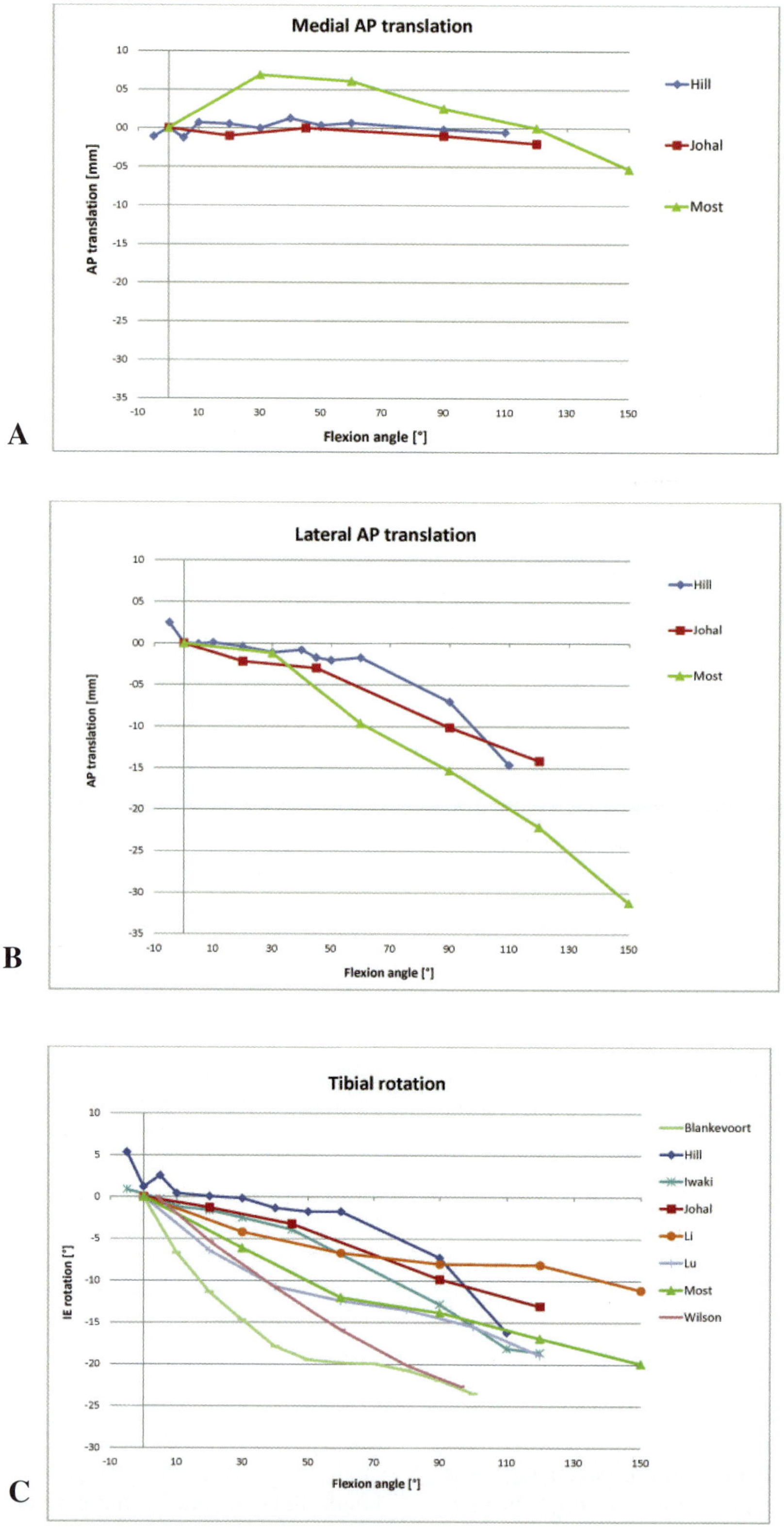

FIGURE 9-6. *Medial (**A**) and lateral (**B**) condyle position and tibial rotation (**C**) as a function of the flexion angle in the passive setting.*

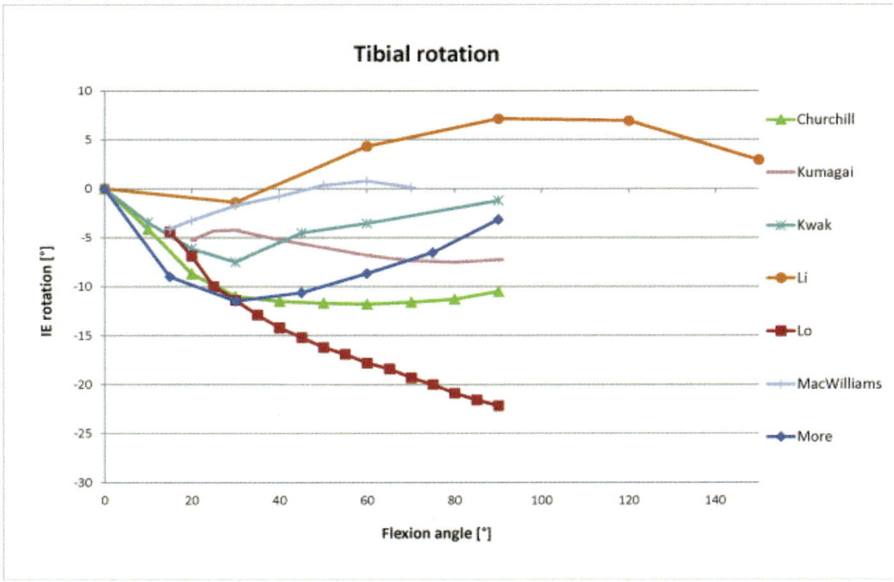

FIGURE 9-7. *Tibial rotation as a function of the flexion angle in the loaded (quadriceps and hamstrings) setting. Loading reverses the typical tibiofemoral rotation pattern in most published studies.*

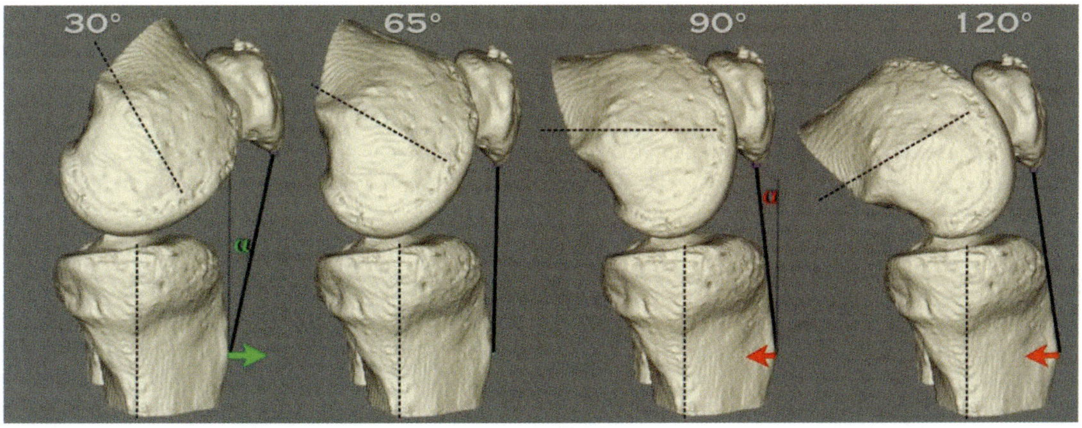

FIGURE 9-8. *Effect of the patellar tendon angle on the resulting AP force vector on the tibia. Below 65° flexion, the patellar tendon angle with the mechanical axis of the tibia is positive and the tibia is pulled anterior. Beyond 65° flexion, the angle is negative and the tibia is pulled posterior.*

KINEMATICS OF PATELLOFEMORAL JOINT

Motion of the patella relative to the femur is governed by different anatomical aspects of the knee joint: the shape of the patella, the geometry of the trochlear groove, the medial patellofemoral ligament, the lateral retinacular structures, the quadriceps muscle and its action on the different bones, and finally the patellar tendon angle in the coronal plane. The quadriceps acts along the axis of the femur and is resisted by the patellar tendon tension. Because these two forces are not collinear but diverge by 10° to 15° (Q-angle), a lateral directed force vector will act on the patella. The lateral facet of the femoral trochlea resists this force. The role of the surface geometry is less important from full extension to 30° of flexion because the compressive joint reaction force is low at these flexion angles and the trochlea is still very shallow. In this position, the medial patellofemoral ligament (MPFL) in conjunction with the vastus medialis muscle and vastus medialis obliquus function is paramount. Several studies have shown the MPFL to be most taut in the range between full extension and 30° flexion. With increasing flexion, the MPFL slackens and its role as a stabilizing structure against lateral patellar dislocation probably decreases.[31] The orientation of the trochlear groove in the coronal plane lies between the femoral mechanical and femoral anatomical axis.[32] With increasing knee flexion, the stabilizing role of the groove is emphasized, due to an increasing conformity and greater joint reaction forces. The angle formed between the line of action of the quadriceps and the patellar tendon is called the Q-angle. The magnitude of the lateral vector component of the force acting on the patellar tendon will increase with an increasing Q-angle, thus producing a higher shear force on the lateral patellofemoral articulation.

From full extension to deep flexion, the patella glides caudally, approximately 7 cm on both femoral condyles. The patella moves downwards with increasing tibiofemoral flexion, but at a lower rate. Nha et al measured patellar flexion at 0°, 30°, 90°, and 135° of knee flexion and reported, respectively, 8.1°, 21.7°, 66.1°, and 94.8° of patellar flexion around the epicondylar axis.[33] The patellar contact area is on its caudal part near full extension. With increasing flexion, the contact area moves cranial to the midportion of the patella to reach a broad area in the cranial half of the articular surface of the patella at 90° flexion.[34] The mean surface area in contact with the femur has been reported to be around 3.5 cm^2. With increasing flexion, this area remains fairly constant as the odd facet of the patella will contact the lateral border of the medial condyle and the lateral facet will largely contact the lateral femoral condyle. Near full passive flexion, the contact area decreases, but at angles beyond 130° flexion, the quadriceps tendon is wrapped around the distal femur and becomes a load-sharing structure. In addition, a large part of the fat pad is in contact with the tibia, playing a role in supporting the patella through its hydrostatic pressure.

Shift and tilt of the patella occur in the normal knee. Nha et al reported a mean shift of 3 mm and a mean tilt of 6° over the entire range of flexion. Between 0° and 75° flexion, the patella tilted laterally; between 75° and full flexion, the patella tilted medially.[33] During in vivo weight-bearing knee flexion, Li et al reported patellar tilt to be 16° over the flexion range. They demonstrated a strong correlation between patellar and tibiofemoral kinematics. When the knee moves from extension to flexion, the Q-angle will be reduced by the internal rotation of the tibia, relative to the femur. At the same time, the posterior movement of the lateral femoral condyle prevents excessive contact stress.[35]

KINETICS OF PATELLOFEMORAL JOINT

Imaging loads across the patellofemoral joint is a complex exercise. Three simplifications have been applied: (1) representation of the patellofemoral joint as a two-dimensional model in the sagittal plane only; (2) either a static model was used or (3) the patellofemoral joint was considered a frictionless pulley. More recent techniques using gait analysis, knee joint moments, and electromyography of various muscle groups have allowed building more representative three-dimensional models. Dynamic models show two peaks of force across this joint: the first occurs in the early stance phase and the second in the early swing phase.[36]

For the orthopaedic surgeon, basic understanding of the two-dimensional model and insight in the magnitude of forces and stresses is important. Forces across the patellofemoral joint are very high because of the short moment arm of the extensor mechanism. In cadaver experiments, the required quadriceps force for extending the knee is about 10 times the ankle load at 120° knee flexion.[37] The reported joint reaction forces range from 385 N for walking to 2500 N for stair climbing and descending, up to almost 6000 N when landing from a jump. Theoretically, pressures can be calculated by dividing the forces by the contact area between femur and patella. The resulting pressures for walking are in the range between 1.5 and 2.5 MPa. However, under load, the viscoelastic cartilage is deformed and the pressure-transmitting area increases. The pressure will be different for short-term and long-term loading; it can go up to 55 MPa for landing from a jump.[36] Muscle tightness will also increase joint reaction forces, specifically during sitting and resting activities. Given the magnitudes of the forces and pressures reported, it is clear that pathology of the patellofemoral joint will be strongly influenced by body weight, impact sports, and muscle tightness.

The two-dimensional model in the sagittal plane is useful for intuitive understanding and surgical consequences. A graphical representation of the force vectors is given in Figure 9-9. F_H represents the flexion force, resulting from body weight, hamstrings, and gastrocnemius force. This force is resisted by the quadriceps F_Q and patellar tendon F_p. The result of forces F_Q and F_p is R_p, the femoropatellar joint reaction force. The distance from F_p to the instant center of rotation C is d_p. The distance from F_h to the instant center of rotation C is d_h. When the system is in equilibrium, the moments are equal: $F_h \cdot d_h = F_p \cdot d_p$.

Following this equation, posterior sagging of the tibia or anterior sliding of the femur will decrease d_p and lead to higher quadriceps, patellar tendon, and patellofemoral joint reaction forces. This equation has consequences for total knee replacement and explains the advantages of a posterior-stabilized design for the extensor mechanism moment arm. Changes in patellar thickness equally affect the extensor mechanism moment arm: thinning will lead to higher quadriceps and patellar tendon forces; thickening will decrease those forces. However, the effect on the resulting patellofemoral joint reaction force R_p is counter-balanced by the opening or closing of the angle α between F_Q and F_p, leading to no significant change in R_p.[38]

ALIGNMENT OF THE KNEE

Alignment of the femur and tibia is defined in three planes: the frontal or coronal plane, the sagittal plane, and the horizontal or axial plane (Fig. 9-10). Each plane is defined by anatomically relevant points and axes. Definitions of axes and planes will affect description of knee motion and loading.

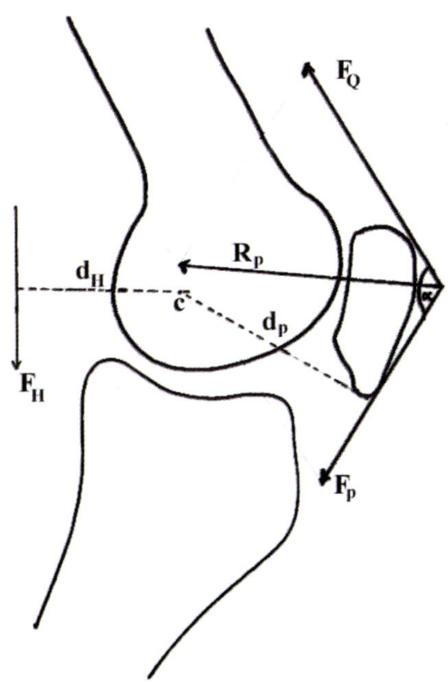

FIGURE 9-9. *Two-dimensional model in the sagittal plane representing force vectors acting on the patellofemoral joint. For abbreviations and symbols, see text.*

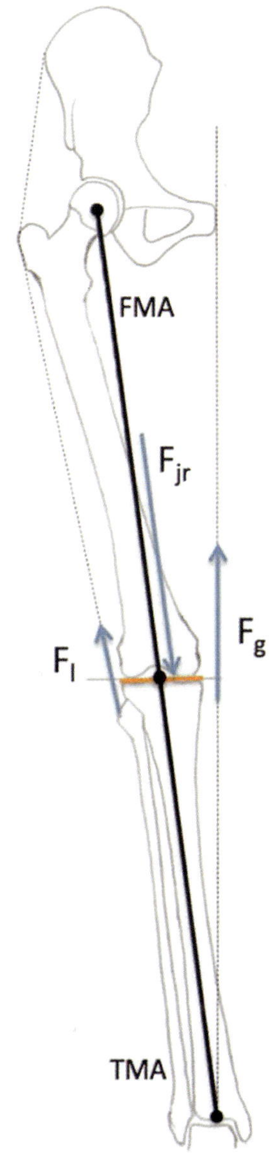

FIGURE 9-10. *Coronal alignment as it appears in a one-legged stance. The ground reaction force F_g has an equal magnitude and opposite direction to the gravitational force. It passes medial from the knee joint as the foot is positioned under the center of gravity of the body. F_l represents the combined force exerted by the iliotibial band and the gluteal muscles needed to stabilize the pelvis. F_{jr} represents the joint reaction force. Note that the joint line orientation (orange) is parallel to the floor and in relative varus position to TMA and that more load is taken by the medial than by the lateral compartment. When the knee deviates in varus, the moment arm of F_g will increase and a greater lateral reaction force F_l will be needed, causing a greater joint reaction force acting at a more medial position on the knee joint.*

Coronal Alignment

The femoral mechanical axis (FMA) runs from the center of the hip to the center of the knee (most anterior point of the femoral notch). The tibial mechanical axis (TMA) runs from the center of the knee (between the two tibial spines) to the center of the tibial plafond in the ankle.[39]

Coronal alignment of the lower extremity was described by Moreland et al.[40] They measured the limb alignment of 25 male volunteers and found a mean angle between FMA and TMA of 1.1° (left) to 1.5° (right) varus. Even as they excluded subjects with clinically obvious genu varum or valgum, there still was a range from 6.5° varus to 3° valgus with a standard deviation of 2.0°. This illustrates the large individual variability. The joint line orientation was not perpendicular to FMA or TMA but was at a mean angle of 3° varus.

Jenny et al[41] repeated the work of Moreland on a larger group of 100 normal volunteers of mixed gender. They reported a similar femorotibial angle of 1.4° but the range was even more impressive: from 12° varus to 5° valgus, yielding a standard deviation of 2.8°.

Only two cases met all the "normal" criteria on femorotibial alignment and joint line orientation. Sixty-six percent of the subjects had normal femorotibial alignment within a 2° varus or valgus range. Based on the two studies mentioned, one can conclude that the mean femorotibial alignment based on the mechanical axes is between 1° and 1.5° varus with an impressive individual variability leading to a significant number of outliers in the general population.

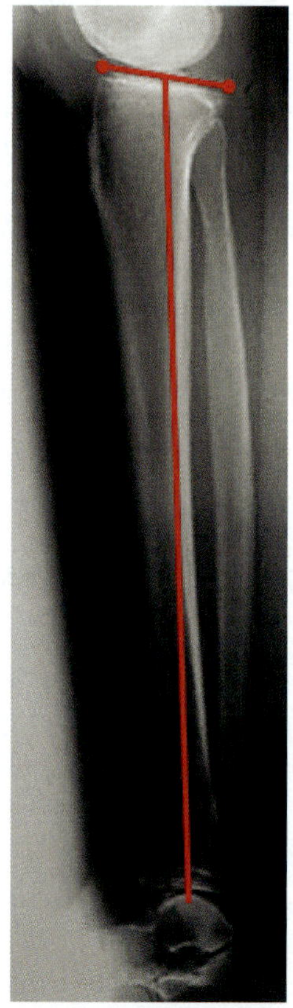

FIGURE 9-11. *The tibial mechanical axis and tibial slope of the medial compartment as measured on a lateral X-ray.*

Sagittal Alignment

In the sagittal plane too, the definition of the FMA is widely accepted. For the TMA, however, definitions are not unambiguous, and are often related to the type of imaging. Also, as the contact area between tibia and femur translates with the degree of flexion, as described in the section on kinematics, a general definition of the TMA applicable to the full range of motion is theoretically not possible.

On a long lateral radiograph of the tibia, the TMA is defined in the sagittal plane as the line connecting the midpoints of the medial tibial plateau and the tibial plafond (Fig. 9-11).[42] On three-dimensional imaging systems (CT or MRI), the tibial transverse axis accurately defines the proximal anteroposterior intersection of the TMA in the sagittal plane. The distal point is defined as the center of the tibial plafond.

The reference points for defining the tibial slope in the sagittal plane are usually the most anterior and posterior point of the medial plateau concavity for the medial compartment. In the lateral compartment, slope is hard to measure because the form of the tibial surface is convex and hard references anterior or posterior are lacking. In three-dimensional reconstructions, the relatively flat midportion of the lateral plateau is advocated.[43]

Yoo et al measured the slope of the medial tibial plateau on a lateral standard lateral radiograph, using the definitions given above. They reported a mean posterior slope of the medial tibial plateau of 10.6°, ranging from 1.9° to 19.6°, with a standard deviation of 3.5° in a Korean osteoarthritic population.[42] Han et al found similar values using three-dimensional reconstructions based on CT imaging. They reported similar values for the medial plateau: 8.7° ± 3.1°. The slope of the lateral plateau was reported to be 7.4°± 3.6°, using the definition of the tangent line to the relatively flat midportion of the lateral tibial plateau.[43] Tibial slope is important from a biomechanical standpoint because most of the motion in the knee occurs in the sagittal plane. With increasing slope, the resulting anterior component of the joint reaction force will increase, inducing anterior shear force on the tibia and higher forces on the anterior cruciate ligament. When tibial slope is decreased, femoral posterior translation with increasing flexion (the so-called rollback phenomenon) will be countered and anterior shear force on the tibia will be decreased.

Axial Plane

Axial plane alignment of the tibia and femur is most described in the literature. As for the coronal and sagittal plane, a mechanical or kinematic axis should serve as a reference. Studies focused initially on relative single-bone relationships of surface-derived axes of either the distal femur or the proximal tibia. These surface-derived axes for the femur include the surgical and anatomical transepicondylar axes (TEA), the posterior condylar axis, and the anteroposterior axis (Whiteside's line). Definitions and graphical illustration of these axes are given in Figure 9-12.

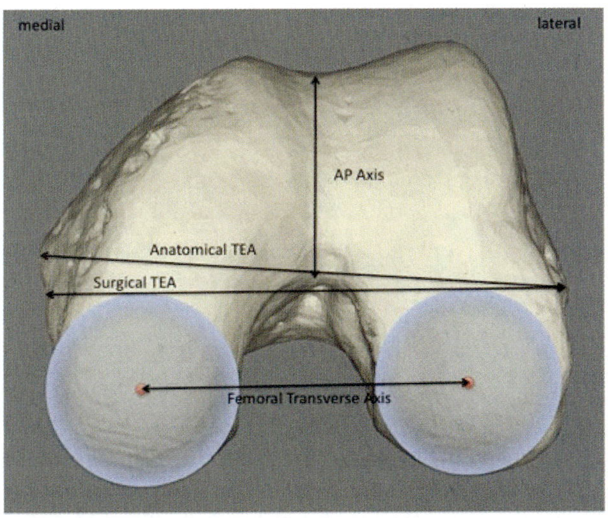

FIGURE 9-12. *Graphical illustration of rotational reference axes in the distal femur. The anteroposterior (AP) axis runs from the deepest point of the trochlea to the center of the femoral notch, with the femur viewed along its mechanical axis. The anatomical transepicondylar axis (TEA) runs from the medial to the lateral epicondyle. The surgical TEA runs from the medial sulcus to the lateral epicondyle. The posterior condylar line is the tangent line to the most posterior part of the femoral condyles with the femur viewed along its mechanical axis. The femoral transverse axis connects the centers of the two best-fit spheres to the femoral condyles. See also references 39, 46, and 47.*

The surface-derived axes of the tibia include the posterior condylar axis and Akagi's line. Recently, a functionally relevant axis was defined by Cobb et al.[44] The authors defined the tibial transverse axis (or "tibial anatomical axis") as the line connecting the two best-fit circles to the medial and lateral condyle of the tibia, at the level of 10 mm below the joint surface.[44] Eckhoff et al defined the "cylindrical axis" of the tibia as the coaxial line of the best-fit cylinders to the femoral condyles.[45] In analogy with Cobb, and based on the previous work by Eckhoff, Victor et al recently defined the "femoral transverse" axis as the line connecting the centers of the two best-fit spheres to the femoral condyles, using a three-dimensional reconstruction of the distal femur and proximal tibia. This axis was studied in its relation to the traditional surface-derived axes to describe a common reference frame.[46] The femoral transverse axis appeared to almost coincide with the tibial transverse axes when projected in the horizontal plane of the tibia with the knee in full extension. As such, both the tibial and femoral transverse axes can serve as a kinematic reference for describing rotation of the proximal tibia and the distal femur.

In a literature review, we compared previous papers describing the angular relationships between the different surface-derived axes of the distal femur.[47] Analysis of the different studies revealed the following relationships:

1. The posterior condylar axis (PCA) has a mean internal rotation relative to the surgical TEA of 3°, relative to the anatomical TEA of 5°, and relative to the trochlear AP axis of 4°.
2. The mean angle between the anatomical and surgical TEA is 2° with the anatomical TEA being more externally rotated.

Ranges and standard deviations were important across different studies. It is undeniable that a large morphotype variability exists among subjects, even in so-called homogeneous gender or racial populations. The mean values clearly fail to disclose the full story of natural variability and the traditional orthopaedic paradigm of aiming at "gold standards" could be discussed based on this knowledge.

Coronal and rotational malalignment have often been related to pathology as degenerative arthritis or patellofemoral instability. Other factors as genetically predisposed quality of articular cartilage and ligament laxity are probably the determinants for steering alignment variability toward functional coping or decompensation with subsequent clinical complaints and the need for surgical treatment. A good understanding of the three-dimensional alignment and the kinematic patterns of the knee is paramount.

REFERENCES

1. Pinskerova V, Maquet P, Freeman MAR. Annotation; writings on the knee between 1836 and 1917. *J Bone Joint Surg Br.* 2000;82:1100-1102.
2. Zuppinger H. *Die aktive flexion im unbelasten Kniegelenk: Züricher Habil Schr.* Wiesbaden, Germany: Bergmann; 1904:703-763.
3. Frankel VH, Burstein AH, Brooks DB. Biomechanics as determined by analysis of the instant centers of motion. *J Bone Joint Surg Am.* 1971;53:945-977.
4. Menschik A. Mechanik des Kniegelenks. *Teil 1 Z Orthop.* 1974;112:481-495.
5. Soudan K, Van Audekercke R, Martens M. Methods, difficulties and inaccuracies in the study of human joint kinematics and pathokinematics by the instant axis concept. Example: the knee joint. *J Biomech.* 1979;12:27–33.
6. Grood ES, Suntay WJ. A joint coordinate system for the clinical description of three-dimensional motions: application to the knee. *J Biomech Eng.* 1983;105:136-144.
7. Blankevoort L, Huiskes R, de Lange A. Helical axes of passive knee joint motions. *J Biomechan.* 1990;23:1219-1229.
8. Hollister AM, Jatana S, Singh AK, et al. The axes of rotation of the knee. *Clin Orthop Relat Res.* 1993;290:259-268.
9. Churchill DL, Incavo SJ, Johnson CC, et al. The transepicondylar axis approximates the optimal flexion axis of the knee. *Clin Orthop Relat Res.* 1998;356:111-118.
10. Iwaki H, Pinskerova V, Freeman MAR. Tibiofemoral movement 1: the shapes and relative movements of the femur and the tibia in the unloaded cadaver knee. *J Bone Joint Surg.* 2000;82:1189-1195.
11. Eckhoff DE, Hogan C, DiMatteo L, et al. Difference between the epicondylar and cylindrical axis of the knee. *Clin Orthop Relat Res.* 2007;461:238-244.
12. Banks SA, Hodge WA. Accurate measurement of three-dimensional knee replacement kinematics using single-plane fluoroscopy. *IEEE Trans Biomed Eng.* 1996;43:638-649.
13. Komistek RD, Dennis DA, Mahfouz M. In vivo fluoroscopic analysis of the normal human knee. *Clin Orthop Relat Res.* 2003;410:69-81.
14. Lu TW, Tsai TY, Kuo MY, et al. In-vivo three-dimensional kinematics of the normal knee during active extension under unloaded and loaded conditions using single-plane fluoroscopy. *Med Eng Phys.* 2008;30:1004-1012.
15. Moro-oka T, Hamai S, Miura H, et al. Dynamic activity dependence of in vivo normal knee kinematics. *J Orthop Res.* 2008;26:428-434.
16. Karrholm J, Brandsson S, Freeman MAR. Tibiofemoral movement 4: changes of axial rotation caused by forced rotation at the weight bearing knee studied by RSA. *J Bone Joint Surg Br.* 2000;82:1201-1203.
17. Hill PF, Vedi V, Williams A, et al. Tibiofemoral movement 2: the loaded and unloaded living knee studied by MRI. *J Bone Joint Surg Br.* 2000;82:1196-1198.
18. Nakagawa S, Kadoya Y, Todo S, et al. Tibiofemoral movement 3: full flexion in the living knee studied by MRI. *J Bone Joint Surg Br.* 2000;82:1199-1200.
19. Johal P, Williams A, Wragg P, et al. Tibio-femoral movement in the living knee. A study of weight bearing and non-weight bearing knee kinematics using "interventional" MRI. *J Biomech.* 2005;38: 269-276.
20. Pinskerova V, Johal P, Nakagawa S, et al. Does the femur roll-back with flexion? *J Bone Joint Surg Br.* 2004;86:925-931.
21. MacWilliams BA, Wilson DR, DesJardins JD, et al. Hamstrings cocontraction reduces internal rotation, anterior translation, and anterior cruciate ligament load in weight-bearing flexion. *J Orthop Res.* 1999; 17(6):817-822.
22. More RC, Karras BT, Neiman R, et al. Hamstrings—an anterior cruciate ligament protagonist. An in vitro study. *Am J Sports Med.* 1993;21(2):231-237.
23. Li G, Zayontz S, DeFrate LE, et al. Kinematics of the knee at high flexion angles: an in vitro investigation. *J Orthop Res.* 2004;22(1):90-95.
24. Kwak SD, Ahmad CS, Gardner TR, et al. Hamstrings and iliotibial band forces affect knee kinematics and contact pattern. *J Orthop Res.* 2000;18(1):101-108.
25. Kumagai M, Mizuno Y, Mattessich SM, et al. Posterior cruciate ligament rupture alters in vitro knee kinematics. *Clin Orthop Relat Res.* 2002;395:241-248.
26. Lo J, Müller O, Wünschel M, et al. Forces in anterior cruciate ligament during simulated weight-bearing flexion with anterior and internal rotational tibial load. *J Biomech.* 2008;41(9):1855-1861.
27. Coughlin KM, Incavo SJ, Churchill DL, et al. Tibial axis and patellar position relative to the femoral epicondylar axis during squatting. *J Arthroplasty.* 2003;18(8):1048-1055.
28. Browne C, Hermida JC, Bergula A, et al. Patellofemoral forces after total knee arthroplasty: effect of extensor moment arm. *Knee.* 2005;12(2):81-88.

29. D'Lima DD, Trice M, Urquhart AG, et al. Comparison between the kinematics of fixed and rotating bearing knee prostheses. *Clin Orthop Relat Res.* 2000;380:151-157.
30. Patil S, Colwell CW Jr, Ezzet KA, et al. Can normal knee kinematics be restored with unicompartmental knee replacement? *J Bone Joint Surg Am.* 2005;87(2):332-338.
31. Victor J, Wong P, Witvrouw E, et al. How isometric are the medial patellofemoral, superficial medial collateral, and lateral collateral ligaments of the knee? *Am J Sports Med.* 2009;37:2028-2036.
32. Eckhoff DG, Burke BJ, Dwyer TF, et al. Sulcus morphology of the distal femur. *Clin Orthop Relat Res.* 1996;331:23-28.
33. Nha KW, Papannagari R, Gill TJ, et al. In vivo patellar tracking: clinical motions and patellofemoral indices. *J Orthop Res.* 2008;26:1067-1074.
34. Nakagawa S, Kadoya Y, Kobayashi A, et al. Kinematics of the patella in deep flexion. *J Bone Joint Surg.* 2003;85:1238-1242.
35. Li G, Papannagari R, Nha KW, et al. The coupled motion of the femur and patella during in vivo weight-bearing knee flexion. *J Biomech Eng.* 2007;129:937-943.
36. Feller JA, Amis AA, Andrish JT, et al. Surgical biomechanics of the patellofemoral joint. *Arthroscopy.* 2007;23:542-553.
37. Victor J, Van Glabbeek F, Vander Sloten J, et al. An experimental model for kinematic analysis of the knee. *J Bone Joint Surg Am.* 2009;91(suppl 6):150-163.
38. Maquet PG. *Biomechanics of the Knee.* Berlin: Springer; 1976.
39. Victor J, Van Doninck D, Labey L, et al. How precise can bony landmarks be determined on a CT scan of the knee? *Knee.* 2009;16:358-365.
40. Moreland JR, Bassett LW, Hanker GJ. Radiographic analysis of the axial alignment of the lower extremity. *J Bone Joint Surg.* 1987;69:745-749.
41. Jenny JY, Boeri C, Ballonzoli L. Coronal alignment of the lower limb. *Acta Orthop.* 2005;76:403-407.
42. Yoo JH, Chang CB, Shin KS, et al. Anatomical references to assess the posterior tibial slope in total knee arthroplasty: a comparison of 5 anatomical axes. *J Arthroplasty.* 2008;23:586-592.
43. Han HS, Chang CB, Seong SC, et al. Evaluation of anatomic references for tibial sagittal alignment in total knee arthroplasty. *Knee Surg Sports Traumatol Arthrosc.* 2008;16:373-377.
44. Cobb JP, Dixon H, Dandachli W, et al. The anatomical tibial axis. *J Bone Joint Surg Br.* 2008;90:1032-1038.
45. Eckhoff DE, Hogan C, DiMatteo L, et al. Difference between the epicondylar and cylindrical axis of the knee. *Clin Orthop Relat Res.* 2007;461:238-244.
46. Victor J, Van Doninck D, Labey L, et al. A common reference frame for describing rotation of the distal femur: a CT-based kinematic study using cadavers. *J Bone Joint Surg Br.* 2009;91:683-690.
47. Victor J. Rotational alignment of the distal femur. A literature review. *Orthop Traumatol Surg Res.* 2009;95:365-372.

10

Biomaterials

James F. Kennedy, Keith A. Synnott, and John M. O'Byrne

The challenges facing knee arthroplasty surgeons are not to be underestimated. The demands in the United States for primary knee replacement surgery and revision knee replacement surgery are projected to rise by 673% and 601%, respectively, by 2030.[1] In order to successfully meet the projected requirement for primary knee replacement surgery and reduce the anticipated demand for revision knee replacement surgery, the operating surgeon should have a good working knowledge of biomaterials pertinent to the field. The aim of this chapter is to provide a brief but broad and up-to-date review of biomaterials in total knee replacement. This review is not intended to be all encompassing. For conciseness, some niche materials and theoretical advances have been purposefully omitted. Brief summaries of the key points are included at the end of each section.

METAL ALLOYS

The first unhinged total knee replacement was developed by Dr. Frank Gunston in 1970. Dr. Gunston was working in the same institution as Sir John Charley and thus chose to use arthroplasty materials familiar to him at the time. His knee consisted of stainless steel runners cemented into slots cut into the distal femur articulating on two polyethylene tibial bearing surfaces.[2] The modern condylar knee was first developed by Dr. Insall and colleagues in the early 1970s. They employed a cobalt chrome alloy femoral component articulating against a machined polyethylene tibial component.[3] Since Insall's innovation, the use of metallic alloys articulating against polyethylene has become standard in total knee replacement surgery. Metal alloys are formed from the amalgamation of metal and nonmetallic elements. Relative to other biomaterials, metals are stiff, ductile, and hard. No metal is completely biologically inert and all are subject to corrosion to one degree or another in the human body. Failure of metal alloy knee arthroplasty components is related to poor design or unanticipated biological interactions.

Structure and Fabrication

Metallic materials have a crystalline lattice microstructure, where the metal atoms are arranged in a repeating three-dimensional arrangement. The shapes of the crystals follow the theoretical arrangements for close-packed spheres, which were devised by the French mathematician Auguste Bravais in the 19th century. These three-dimensional crystalline arrangements are body center cubic (BCC), face center cubic (FCC), and hexagonal close packed (HCP). Each of the three crystalline arrangements has separate mechanical characteristics depending on the density of the packaging and the ability of the crystals to move relative to each other. Many alloys in common orthopaedic use can transform from one crystalline structure to another depending on temperature, manufacturing process, and varying alloy ingredients. The lattice have a tendency to perfectly arrange themselves into repeating groups of units known as grains. The grains are arranged together to make up the solid component.

Weakness within the material can arise from a number of sources. Macroscopic weaknesses such as voids and scratches are generally minimized by careful production and handling. Microscopic imperfections include granular boundaries, vacancies in the microstructure, and dislocations in the lattice microstructure.

Intergranular boundaries exist because the individual grains cannot achieve perfect three-dimensional alignment; reducing grain size reduces the size of the intergranular boundaries. Hence, material strength and fatigue resistance tend to increase with decreasing grain size. Mechanical properties of metal alloys can be altered in a number of ways. Strain hardening is a process by which dislocations in the crystalline lattice can be forced to accumulate by subjecting the material to an external stress (cold working). The defects in the lattice accumulate and interact with each other to form pinning points. These pinning points block the movement of further dislocations, increasing the amount of energy required to deform a material. With increasing stiffness, there is an accompanying loss of ductility. Strain hardening may be reversed at any stage by a process known as annealing. The process of annealing requires heating of the alloy above its recrystalization temperature followed by controlled cooling to restore the original crystalline lattice microstructure. Slow cooling allows larger crystals to form, while rapid cooling known as quenching leads to smaller grains sizes.

The mechanical properties of any base metal can also be tailored by altering the concentrations of nonmetallic solutes such as carbon to the crystalline microstructure. The solute atoms accumulate in the spaces between the metal atoms deforming the three-dimensional crystalline arrangements. In the case of carbon, the deformation results in the increased stiffness of high carbon steels.

The two most common metal alloys in total knee replacement are cobalt chrome alloys and titanium alloys. Cobalt chrome alloys are the most common material used to manufacture femoral components in total knee replacement. It is composed principally of cobalt and chromium with lesser amounts of nickel carbon, molybdenum, and tungsten. The principal advantage of cobalt chrome alloys is that they have little biological activity and are highly resistant to corrosion. Cobalt chrome alloys are relatively strong and have good surface properties, making them an ideal choice for bearing surfaces. Cobalt chrome alloys are manufactured by a number of different methods. Historically cobalt chrome alloys were cast in bars in prefabricated molds. The bars where then forged to restructure the crystalline microstructure so as to achieve a smaller grain size and the desired mechanical properties. The bars were subsequently machined to the required geometry for the femoral component. More recent production methods involve compression and sintering of a fine alloy powder. This allows smaller grain sizes to be achieved and reduces the requirement for further machining.

Common orthopaedic titanium alloys contain a mixture of titanium, vanadium, and aluminum. Due to the concerns in relation to the possible toxicity of vanadium, niobium-containing alloys are now being studied. Titanium is resistant to corrosion due a process known as passivation, where it forms a titanium oxide surface layer in oxygen-bearing environments. This titanium oxide layer is highly biocompatible and amenable to becoming incorporated into bone. Titanium alloys are used frequently to manufacture both patellar and tibial base plates in modular knee designs. They are not suitable for use as bearing surfaces because of low wear resistance. Titanium alloys are also highly notch sensitive. This means that titanium components are susceptible to crack propagation from surface flaws and subsequent brittle failure.

Failure in Metallic Implants

While comprehensive understanding of the material properties is useful in predicting outcomes from specific biomaterials in knee arthroplasty, unfortunately clinical trial and error is still a major source of information for the arthroplasty surgeon. Despite careful design, manufacture, and implantation of metallic components, the literature on knee replacement is still littered with reports of failures. Sometimes these failures are consequential to the patients' demands and requirements and fundamental biomechanics exceeding the constraints of current arthroplasty design, a good example of this being the hinged knee.[4] Other examples are attributable to immature designs and poor production techniques. This is illustrated by the fatigue failure of some porous-coated knee arthroplasty components because the sintering process used to attached the beads alters the granular microstructure of the component.[5-7]

Yet more failures are due to the biological response of the human knee to arthroplasty components. Review of failed metallic tibial base plates has shown component instability to be the dominant causative factor.[8] The instability was in most cases due to underlying osteolysis. Fatigue failure caused by the instability was the principal failure mode. It is thought that repetitive cantilever bending due to the instability as the joint is loaded leads to fatigue failure. Fatigue failure in metals involves three phases: crack initiation, crack propagation, and fracture of remaining undamaged material.[9] Instability-induced fatigue failure has also been reported in cobalt chrome femoral components due to both failure of osteointegration and aseptic loosening (Fig. 10-1).[10-12] That said, given the number of knee replacements performed worldwide, the reported incidence of metallic implant failure in nonhinged knee replacements is very low. Further advances in the composition and manufacturing of metallic knee arthroplasty components should suppress this further.

Metal Debris

While thankfully not as common as total hip replacement, granulonatous pseudotumor of the knee has been described.[13] Pseudotumors are likely less common in total knee replacement because of the lower volumes of metal debris. That said, dispersion of metal ions certainly occurs. Metal ions have been found in synovial fluid, blood, spleen, liver, and lymph nodes of patients with knee replacements.[14,15] Luetzner et al have attributed the dissemination of metal ions to corrosion from the surface of knee arthroplasty patients.[14]

The clinical effect of these metal ions within the human body is contentious. While not immune sensitizers on their own, metal ions can stimulate the immune system by forming a complex with native proteins.[16] These protein-bound metal ions are known to stimulate hypersensitivity reactions. The most common reactions are to cobalt and nickel, both of which are normally present in total knee replacement components. The incidence of metal hypersensitivity in the general population is approximately 15%, but this is doubled in patients who have received a metallic implant, and further increased where the implant is known to be failing.[17] It is not clear whether the failing metallic implant increases the likelihood of metal hypersensitivity or if a preexisting biological propensity to metal hypersensitivity has potentiated the failure. Clinically significant isolated negative effects attributed to metal released from a total knee replacement have been described.[18] High doses of metals used in knee replacement surgery are known to have toxic effects on the kidney, liver, heart, and nervous system.[19] There is an increase of chromosomal aberrations in lymphocytes of arthroplasty patients.[20,21] High concentration exposure to both vanadium and chromium is thought to be possibly carcinogenic.[22,23] While the significance of low-dose metal ion exposure in arthroplasty patients is not currently well understood, the individual risks to the recipient are probably low, but ultimately unquantifiable. Given the increasing numbers of ever-younger patients receiving total knee replacements, careful consideration should be given to this problem.

Key Points: Metals	
1.	*Mechanical properties of metal alloys are dependent on microstructure and manufacturing techniques.*
2.	*Cobalt chrome alloys are strong and corrosion resistant, making them ideal for bearing surfaces.*
3.	*There is a low reported incidence of knee arthroplasty implant failure. What failure exists is mostly attributed to instability-induced fatigue fractures.*
4.	*Both local and systemic metal ion levels are elevated in knee arthroplasty recipients.*
5.	*The long-term risks associated with elevated metal ions are thought to be low but are currently not fully understood.*

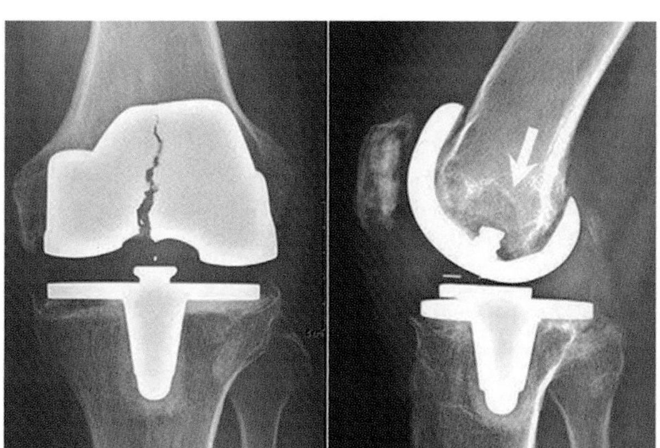

FIGURE 10-1. *Femoral component fracture due to osteolysis in the distal femur. (Reprinted with permission.[12])*

CERAMICS

Ceramics are compounds of metallic and nonmetallic elements. The first use of ceramic in knee arthroplasty was by Prof. G. Langer at the Klinikum Jena in 1972.[24] He successfully used ceramic implants in unicompartmental tibial resurfacing; however, the technique has fallen out of use with the development of modular size-specific implants.

Bioactivity

In the majority of ceramics, the metallic and nonmetallic elements are bound via an ionic bond where an electron is transferred to between the elements. A minority of ceramics are formed with a covalent bond where the electron is shared between elements. Due to the strength of the ionic or covalent bonds, ceramics are chemically stable and biologically inert. Systemic metal ion levels have been shown to be elevated in patients with a total knee replacement.[14] The clinical long-term implications of the presence of these metal ions is still unknown.[25] Nickel allergy has a reported prevalence of 14% in the general population.[26] Cross-sensitivity between nickel and cobalt is common.[17] The lack of bioactivity of ceramic materials and the absence of nickel from the prosthesis make ceramic implants a valid option for patients with a proven nickel allergy or for surgeons with concerns in relation to the long-term safety of metallic implants.

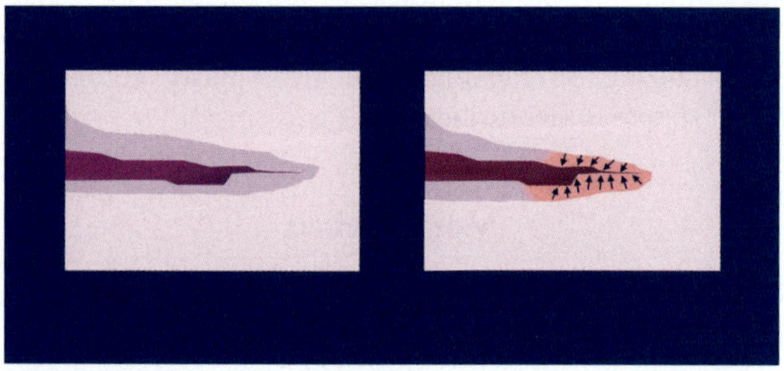

FIGURE 10-2. *Crack propagation along the intergranular plane is surpassed by strain-induced phase transformation in zirconium oxide ceramics. (Courtesy of Matthew Morrey, MD.)*

Mechanical Properties

The dominant motivation driving the development of ceramic arthroplasty components is a desire to develop longer lasting total knee replacements suitable for use in younger, more demanding patients. Relative to cobalt chrome, ceramic joint replacement surfaces are harder, smoother, scratch resistant, and more wettable (hydrophilic). The hydrophilic nature of ceramics has been shown in laboratory testing to confer advantages in lubrication when compared to conventional bearing surfaces.[27]

However, the extreme hardness of ceramic has raised concerns about the possibility of mechanical mismatch precipitating failure of the softer counter-surface in ceramic-on-polyethylene bearings in total hip replacement.[28] Similar to metal alloys, ceramics have a crystalline granular microstructure. The material properties of ceramics are dependent on the grain size and phase, which in turn are dependent on the particle size of the ingredient materials and manufacturing process used to construct the ceramic. Because of their crystalline microstructure, ceramics have a high resistance to plastic deformation. This stiffness comes at a price in that ceramic implants are prone to fail catastrophically and unexpectedly by brittle failure.[29-33] Brittle failure occurs with little or no preceding plastic deformation and occurs as a result of tensile stress acting normally to intergranular cleavage planes of low bonding (Fig. 10-2). Porosity, impurities, large grain size, and inadequate bonding all potentiate brittle failure. Debris from failed ceramic joint replacements is difficult to completely remove and potentially compromises revision surgery by acting as a third body, accelerating wear between the new bearing surfaces.

Composite Ceramics

A composite ceramic is a material in which a number of ingredients are combined to achieve optimal mechanical behavior. Composite ceramics of alumina and zirconium have been developed to increase the toughness of the material and reduce the thickness of the implants. Zirconium oxide ceramics exhibit the best initial material properties among medial grade ceramics. They are highly resistant to crack propagation due to a process know as phase transformation toughening. This process involves the transformation of the meta-stable tetragonal grain phase to the monoclinic phase due to stress at the crack tip.[34] This transformation is accompanied by an increase in volume, leading to local compression and a tendency to close the crack (Fig. 10-2).

Tetragonal zirconium oxide ceramic is the high-temperature phase. It is meta-stable solid and prone to transformation in the presence of water to the monoclinic phase, which has different material properties. This tendency for transformation has led to unacceptable failure rates in zirconium oxide femoral heads.[35] Yttria doping, which stabilizes the tetrahedral phase, and the use of composite alumina-yttria-doped zirconia ceramics open avenues for the advantageous mechanical properties of zirconium to be exploited.

Production

There are two ways of manufacturing surgical ceramics. The first involves mixing the powdered ingredients and pressing them together in prefabricated casts. The ceramic molds are then removed from the cast and sintered in high-temperature ovens so as to achieve a well-bonded high-density granular structure. The resulting solid is then machined to the final shape and surface quality. Alumina-based ceramic knee prostheses constructed in this fashion were first developed in Japan and implanted by Oonishi et al in 1982.[36] To avoid stress concentrations, early ceramic knee replacement prostheses were thicker than their metallic equivalents, necessitating larger bone resections. The composite ceramic Biolox Delta (Ceramatec AG, Germany), which is composed of 75% alumina oxide for hardness and wear resistance and 25% yttria-doped zirconium oxide for toughness, is now in clinical use in knee arthroplasty (Fig. 10-3). It is dimensionally similar to metallic arthroplasty components. This allows similar operative instrumentation and bone-sparing cuts. No clinical reviews of the outcomes with this novel material exist.

The second method of production of surgical ceramics is more common in total knee replacement and produces a metallic alloy with an oxidized ceramic surface. Zirconium oxide-surfaced ceramics are an example of this technology; they are manufactured from a wrought zirconium alloy (97.5% zirconium and 2.5% niobium) component that is subjected to thermal oxidation at temperatures greater than 500°C. At these temperatures, oxidative diffusion occurs, which transforms the outer surface of the alloy into a ceramic oxide. Cross-sectional studies have shown that the zirconium oxide ceramic has a stable monoclinic crystalline structure to a depth of approximately 5 μm.[37] The resulting oxidized ceramic layer is well bonded and has been shown to be resistant to delamination.[38,39] This method with the allows the manufacture of knee replacement components superior surface qualities of ceramic and equivalent thickness of metallic implants without the increased risk of brittle failure.

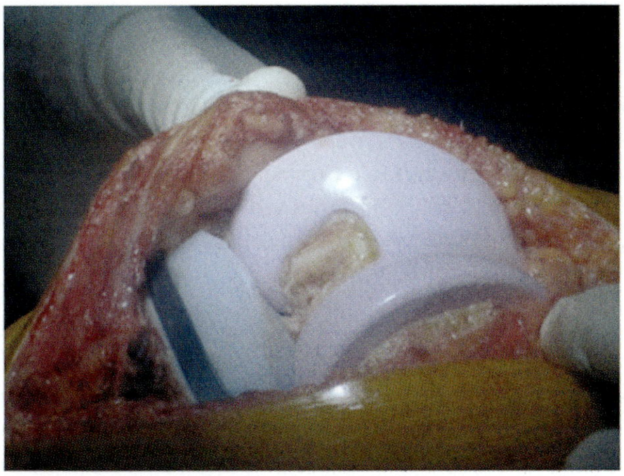

FIGURE 10-3. *Biolox Delta alumina–zirconia composite ceramic femoral implant. (Reprinted from European Musculoskeletal Review, Benazzo F et al., Ceramic Total Knee Arthroplasty – An Update, 2007;2:59-62, with permission from Touch Briefings Ltd.)*

Ceramic Results

Laboratory testing does support the hypothesis that ceramic biomaterials will result in a more long-lasting knee replacement; unfortunately, so far the outcome from clinical studies is more clouded. Ceramic femoral components in total knee replacement have been shown to substantially reduce the volume of polyethylene wear particles produced in knee simulator tests.[40,41]

Short- and medium-term clinical studies have demonstrated the safety of ceramic knee arthroplasty components. Despite the theoretical risk of brittle failure, unlike total hip replacement, there are no reports in the literature of catastrophic failure of a ceramic knee arthroplasty component; this, however, may reflect the relatively low numbers of patients receiving the implants.

Laskin describes improved functional outcomes at 2 years in patients who received an oxidized zirconium implant compared to a control group with a cobalt chrome alloy femoral component.[37] Hui et al performed a prospective randomized study to investigate the safety and effectiveness of zirconium oxide ceramic femoral components compared to conventional cobalt chrome implants. They recruited 40 patients who underwent simultaneous bilateral total knee replacement. Each patient received both a conventional femoral component and a ceramic oxide zirconium femoral component (Oxonium, Smith & Nephew, Memphis, TN). At 5 years, there was no significant difference in patient satisfaction or radiographic wear. Hui et al's study confirms the medium-term safety of the oxidized zirconium ceramic femoral component.[42] Contrary to Laskin's finding, Hui et al found no difference in patient satisfaction. The medium-term safety and survival of alumina oxide femoral components produced by isostatic compression and sintering is supported by Akagi et al, who found a 94% survival at a mean follow-up of 5.8 years.[43]

Minoda et al have demonstrated that lower numbers of rounder polyethylene wear particles are found in synovial fluid retrieved from knee implanted with an alumina ceramic prosthesis; however, this study is limited by the low numbers of patients who received ceramic components.[44] Kim et al published a larger cohort of 105 patients under the age of 60 years who received simultaneous bilateral total knee replacements where one knee of each patient was implanted with a zirconium oxide femoral component.[45] At

5 years, they could not detect any significant difference in patient satisfaction, knee function, or radiographic osteolyis. Interestingly, contrary to biomechanical studies and Minoda et al's clinical research, Kim et al found no difference in the quantity, size, or shape of polymer debris present in synovial fluid aspirated from ceramic implanted knees at 5 years. This indicates that the proposed improved clinical improvement in terms of reduced osteolysis and aseptic loosening from the superior surface qualities of the zirconium oxide components may not transpire.

Oonishi et al have published a long-term follow-up on alumina oxide ceramic knee arthroplasty components.[36] The Japanese experience with their first-generation alumina ceramic total knee replacements has led the designers to conclude that achieving stable cementless fixation can be difficult. They found unacceptably high rates of subsidence of tibial components.[46] This has driven the evolution of their designs with the substitution of titanium tibial base plates for the original alumina ceramic component and the development of hydroxyapatite coating and beaded surfaces for cementless alumina ceramic femoral components. Further longer-term studies are required to determine if the use of ceramic total knee arthroplasty components in patients without metal allergies is warranted.

Key Points: Ceramics

1. *Ceramics are compounds of metallic and nonmetallic elements.*
2. *Ceramics make ideal bearing surfaces because of their hardness, scratch resistance, and hydrophilic nature.*
3. *Laboratory wear testing suggests that ceramic-on-polyethylene bearing knee replacements have the potential for increased long-term joint survival, but this has yet to be borne out in clinical studies.*
4. *Composite aluminum-zirconium oxide ceramics offer improved fracture resistance.*
5. *The long-term value of the use of ceramic knee arthroplasty components, other than for patients with metal sensitivity, is unknown.*

POLYETHYLENE

Ultra-high-molecular-weight polyethylene (UHMWPE) has many desirable material properties, which have encouraged its common use in total knee replacement. It is chemically inert, amenable to being precisely formed into complex shapes, mechanically tough, and self-lubricating, demonstrating a low coefficient of friction allowing efficient articulation.

Structure

Polyethylene consists of repeating units of ethylene monomer. Polyethylene is formed by sequential addition of ethylene monomer units by a process known as condensation polymerization. Condensation polymerization is so named because it occurs when monomers with symmetrical ends liberate water or carbon dioxide during the polymerization reaction. Longer polymer chains and higher molecular weights are associated with improved mechanical properties. UHMWPE is by definition a polyethylene with at least 3 million monomer units.[47]

At room temperature, polyethylene exists as a mosaic of two distinct structural phases: the crystalline phase and the amorphous phase. The crystalline phase occurs when the individual polymer chains are folded into organized three-dimensional structures known as lamellae. These shapes allow the polymer chains to closely interact with each other, forming a high-density construct held together by van der Waals forces.

The second mode of structural organization is the amorphous phase, where the long polymer chains are randomly arranged and entangled. Polyethylene can therefore be considered to be a composite material composed of rigid crystalline lamella surrounded by a ductile amorphous matrix (Fig. 10-4). The mechanical properties of polyethylene are proportional to the degree of crystallinity present within the composite. Higher proportions of crystalline organization confer superior stiffness, strength, and fracture resistance to the material. This concept of the composite nature of polyethylene has clinical importance to total knee replacement because the processes involved in the manufacturing of implants have significant impacts on the proportion of cystallinity and thus clinical outcome.

UHMWPE is manufactured from a granular resin, which is heated and compressed to form a solid from which the arthroplasty components are produced. Most polyethylene used in knee arthroplasty today is manufactured from one of three commercially available polyethylene resins: GUR 1050 (Ticona, KY), GUR 1020 (Ticona, KY), and Montell 1900 (Hurcules Powder Company, Wilmington, DE).[48] Compression of resin produces a workable solid by two distinct mechanisms. The first method is physical compaction, where the heat and pressure melt the granules, causing them

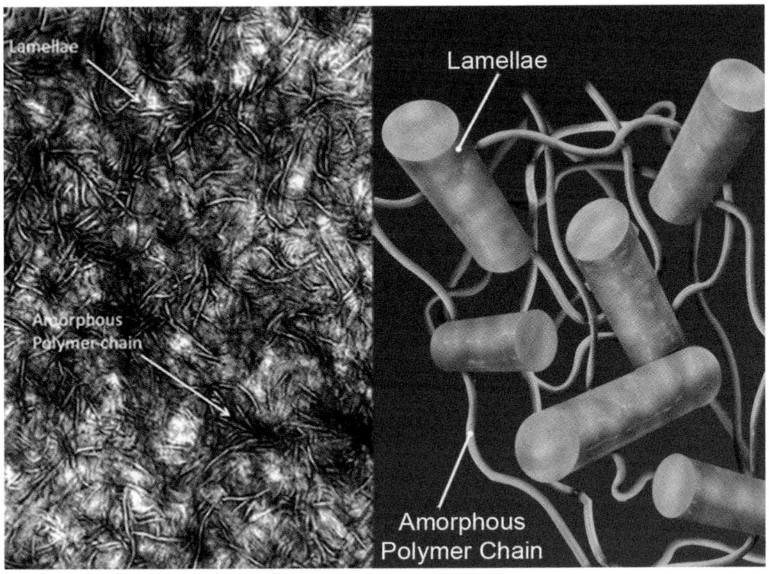

FIGURE 10-4. *Composite biphasic structure of polyethylene. (Reprinted with permission.[48] (Right figure portion redrawn courtesy of Matthew Morrey, MD.))*

to physically amalgamate. The second method is chemical compaction, which causes the polymeric chains to interpenetrate.

There are three methods of producing the solid polymer from the granular resin in common commercial use: ram extrusion, slab compression molding, and direct compression molding. Ram extrusion and slab compression molding are less costly but require more machining to create the finished geometry. Direct compression molding, while more expensive, requires less machining and has been shown to produce a more mechanically durable implant for total knee replacement.[49]

Historically, calcium stearate was added to the resin during production to act as a lubricant and reduce corrosion on tools. The addition of calcium stearate has been shown to be associated with the presence of fusion defects and to be more prone to oxidative degradation; therefore, calcium stearate is no longer added to polymers intended for arthroplasty implants.[50]

The temperatures and pressures occurring during the manufacturing process are critical to the mechanical properties and the durability of the UHMWPE produced. Production errors can lead to fusion voids within the polyethylene, which act as stress risers and which precipitate early failure. Tanner et al, in a study of 29 retrieved tibial liners, have demonstrated the clinical importance of manufacturing quality control in the outcome of total knee replacement.[51]

Wear

Wear is the single biggest challenge driving the optimization of UHMWPE as a biomaterial in knee arthroplasty. Wear is defined as the progressive loss of material due to mechanical or chemical action. Broadly speaking, polyethylene wear in total knee replacement can be divided into two categories: subsurface wear and surface wear. The distinction between the two types of wear is important in understanding the different mechanisms by which they contribute to poor clinical outcomes. Surface wear produces debris in the size range of 0.1 to 10 μm. Particles in this size have been shown to be biologically active and cause early joint replacement failure due to macrophage-mediated periprosthetic osteolysis.[52-54] Subsurface wear causes poor clinical outcomes due to fatigue failure of the tibial liner.[55]

Surface wear

Surface wear is due to a combination of adhesive and abrasive processes on the bearing surface. Abrasive wear is when an asperity in the counter-surface cuts a groove into the polyethylene, while adhesive wear is caused by physical bonding between bearing surfaces, causing material to be pulled away from the polyethylene as the surfaces move relative to each other.

Polyethylene is susceptible to both adhesive and abrasive wear because of its relative lack of surface hardness.

The rate at which damage occurs is related to surface smoothness, lubrication, and joint kinematics.[56] The generation of surface wear particles has been positively correlated with patient activity. Younger, more active patients are therefore at potentially higher risk of developing aseptic loosening.[57,58] Biomechanical studies have shown increased volumetric and gravimetric surface wear when the smoothness of the bearing surfaces within the knee replacement is reduced.[59,60]

Subsurface wear

Subsurface wear produces larger macroscopic debris. Subsurface polyethylene wear in total knee replacement is due to a process known as fatigue delaminating. Fatigue failure is a mechanical failure occurring under dynamic loads lower than the ultimate failure strength of the component. In total knee replacement, crack initiation begins in the polyethylene component in the zone of maximum stress, which has been shown to be located 1 to 2 mm below the contact point.[61,62] With cyclic loading during ambulation, the cracks propagate and eventually reduce the effective thickness of the material to a point where localized failure occurs. This causes the polyethylene to delaminate and the surface layer of the polyethylene to break away, releasing large macroscopic wear particles (Fig. 10-5). Fatigue wear of polyethylene is more common in total knee replacement than in total hip replacement because the joint is less conforming and, therefore, the polyethylene is more highly stressed. As fatigue delamination causes relatively large particles to be removed from the polyethylene component, the conformity and smoothness of the bearing surface is further degraded, accelerating both surface wear particle production and component failure. While surface wear is associated with physical conditions on the bearing surfaces, fatigue delamination is dependent on thickness, internal stress distribution, and manufacturing methods. Bartel et al have shown in their salient biomechanical investigations that tibial inserts with thicknesses of less than 8 to 10 mm are more prone to delaminating.[61,62] This is because as the thickness of the UHMWPE component is reduced, shear stress concentrations are increased.

It has also long been proposed that highly conforming knee designs would distribute the stresses over a larger area, leading to reduced fatigue failure.[62-64] Mobile bearing designs such as LCS have been shown in laboratory testing to be less susceptible to fatigue failure.[63,65] This is due to a decoupling of rotational forces, which decreases local stress concentrations.

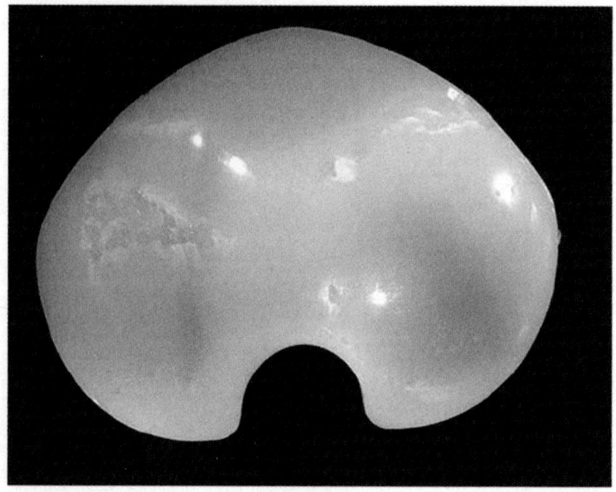

FIGURE 10-5. *Delaminating retrieved polyethylene component. (Reprinted with permission from The Journal of Bone and Joint Surgery, Muratoglu OK, Mark A, Vittetoe DA, et al., Polyethylene Damage in Total Knees and Use of Highly Crosslinked Polyethylene, 2003; 85-A (suppl 1):S7-S13.)*

Cross-Linking

Murotoglu et al have shown that the degree of cross-linking within UHMWPE is the dominant material factor influencing adhesive and abrasive wear.[66] The use of cross-linked polyethylene in arthroplasty is not novel, and the current clinical experience exceeds 40 years.[67] Increasing the amount of cross-linkage within a polymer is generally achieved by the use of an ionizing radiation source or by adding free radical-generating chemical additives, such as organic peroxides, to the polymer resin.[68] The use of ionizing radiation from either a gamma source or electron beam is the most common method in use today. There is some in vitro evidence that shows that cross-linked polyethylene produced using gamma ray irradiation has superior wear characteristics to cross-linked polyethylene produced with electron beam irradiation.[69]

Ionizing radiation has two chemical effects of the polyethylene molecules. The first is that it breaks the C–C bond in the polymer chains. This process is known as chain scission. The second effect of ionizing radiation is disruption of the C–H bonds. It is the disruption of these C–H bonds that allows the formation of cross-linkages between the chains.

Generally the energy level of the ionizing radiation used in sterilization is too low (2–4 MRads) to break the

C–H bonds and thus does not generate frequent cross-linkages, although free radicals are still produced.[68] The intensity of ionizing radiation required to break the C–H bonds is higher (>5 MRads), and while this does generate cross-linking, it also generates a higher number of free radicals. These free radicals and their subsequent oxidation effectively shorten the polymer chains, reducing the molecular weight and leading to substantial degradations in the mechanical properties of the UHMWPE. Free radicals created by ionizing radiation within the amorphous matrix are loosely arranged, they are therefore free to recombine or form cross-links.[70] Free radicals formed within the crystalline lamella are more constrained and therefore become trapped. The result is an accumulation of long-lived free radicals within the crystalline structure. These trapped free radicals are prone to oxidation, which in turn drives further chain scission and ongoing degradation of mechanical properties.[71]

So as to suppress the negative effects of radiation-induced oxidation, first-generation cross-linked polyethylene components have been subjected to post irradiation remelting or annealing, allowing the free radicals trapped in the crystalline phase to recombine. Unfortunately, as radiation-induced cross-link density within the UHMWPE increases, there is a corresponding reduction in crystallinity.[66] This reduced crystallinity leads to a theoretical reduction in other desirable mechanical properties, such a stiffness fatigue resistance and ultimate yield strength.[48] In vitro testing of standardized specimens of highly cross-linked polyethylene has shown there to be a reduction in toughness and resistance to fatigue failure.[72,73] Despite the theoretic concerns, the cross-link densities of commercially available components do not seem to cause a significant increase in susceptibility to fatigue delamination.[74]

There are concerns that the elongated shape and small size of the particulate wear debris produced by highly cross-linked polyethylene components have potentially higher bioactivity than debris from conventional UHMWPE. Fisher et al, in an in vitro study, investigated both cross-linked and conventional polyethylene tibial liners in mobile- and fixed-bearing knees.[75] They concluded that although cross-linked polyethylene components produced relatively fewer wear particles, a higher proportion of the particles produced were less than 0.1 μm. Fisher et al also investigated the biological activity of the particles as measured by the production of TNF-α from human macrophages cultured in the wear debris harvested from biomechanical testing. They noted a significant increase in TNF-α production from macrophages exposed to debris from cross-linked components.[75] Scott et al have also demonstrated a substantial increase in the proportion of smaller biologically active particles form cross-linked surfaces.[76]

Minoda et al studied joint fluid aspirated from 52 knees 9 to 12 months after implantation.[44] Four of these patients had received a highly cross-linked polyethylene tibial liner (Prolong, Zimmer, Warsaw, IN). They found fewer polyethylene wear particles in joint fluid aspirated from patients who had received cross-linked polyethylene arthroplasty components. They also noted, however, that the particles generated were relatively smaller and rounder in shape than wear debris generated from conventional UHMWPE. The reduced number and size and aspect ratio of wear particles found in joint fluid aspirated from knees implanted with highly cross-linked polyethylene inserts have also been noted by Iwakiri et al, working in the same group in Japan.[77]

While a randomized control trial on the use of highly cross-linked polyethylene in total hip replacement demonstrates a reduction in clinically apparent wear,[78] there is a paucity of published clinical experience with highly cross-linked tibial liners. Hodrick et al performed a retrospective review of 100 patients who had received highly cross-linked polyethylene liners (Durasal) and compared the outcomes to a similar cohort who received a non-cross-linked UHMWPE tibial insert.[79] The mean follow-up was 91 months. While they found reduced radiological evidence for osteolysis in those patients who had received a highly cross-linked component, there was no significant difference in the revision rate for aseptic loosening. Muratoglu et al studied 19 retrieved highly cross-linked tibial inserts and compared them to 16 retrieved conventional UHMWPE tibial components with similar duration of implantation.[80] They found evidence of reduced surface wear in the highly cross-linked components. Minoda et al have published on their experience with the highly cross-linked tibial liners (Prolong, Zimmer).[81] They report no significant difference in radiolucency in the 89 knees implanted with the highly cross-linked component when compared to 113 knees in which a conventional polyethylene component was used. This study is limited, however, by its relatively short 2-year follow-up.

There have been numerous laboratory analyses of the surface wearing properties of highly cross-linked tibial liners in comparison to conventional non-cross-linked components. On the whole, these evaluations of highly cross-linked components have significantly superior abrasive and cohesive wear characteristics.[74,82-87]

It is probable that cross-linked polyethylene components do generate less wear debris; however, the particles that are generated are smaller and potentially more destructive.[44,75,77] In the absence of long-term clinical follow-up, no strong recommendation on the use of cross-linked polyethylene can be given at this time.

Sterilization

Historically, polyethylene components in total knee replacement have been sterilized by gamma irradiations in air. This method has the advantage of being relatively cheap, microbiologically effective, and efficient from a manufacturing and package handling perspective. Fatigue wear has been shown to be accelerated in "gamma-in-air" sterilized polyethylene joint replacement components.[88] This is because the gamma ray sterilization process induces chain scission, generating free radicals and shortening the lengths of the polymer chains. In the presence of oxygen, the scission products do not recombine. Further oxidation of the chain scission products generates more free radicals which in turn induce further polymer chain scission. This process is known as oxidative chain scission. Oxygen has been shown to be able to defuse into the UHMWPE component both from air and at a slower rate from synovial fluid.[89,90] Thus, the process of oxidative chain scission can cause a progressive and long-term degradation in mechanical properties of polymer arthroplasty components and is known to be one of the factors leading to component failure. Currently gamma-in-air sterilization and storage in oxygen-bearing mediums have been substituted for gamma sterilization and storage in inert mediums or by chemical sterilization in ethylene oxide.

Vitamin E

Postradiation heating of first-generation highly cross-linked UHMWPE in a process known as annealing melts the polyethylene crystals and liberates the trapped free radicals. This increased cross-link density inhibits the folding of the polymer chains, impeding recrystallization. This resultant amorphous UHMWPE is known to have inferior resistance to fatigue delamination.[91-93]

Vitamin E (α-tocopherol) is a naturally occurring antioxidant. When added to UHMWPE, vitamin E neutralizes radiation-induced free radicals, avoiding the requirement for post-irradiation remelting. By maintaining crystallinity, the addition of vitamin E has been shown in laboratory studies to improve mechanical and fatigue properties.[94,95] The vitamin E-doped UHMWPE has been shown in laboratory testing to have superior mechanical properties to either virgin polymer or cross-linked and annealed polyethylene.[96]

Small animal models have demonstrated no adverse histological response from the addition of vitamin E to UHMWPE.[97] To date, no clinical studies of second-generation vitamin E-doped highly cross-linked UHMWPE have been made. Despite the encouraging biomechanical and animal studies, further investigation is required before the routine use of vitamin E-doped UHMWPE in total knee replacement can be recommended.

Key Points: Polyethylene
1. *Implant polyethylene exists as composite mosaic of both crystalline and amorphous phases.*
2. *The mechanical properties of polyethylene are dependent on molecular weight of polymer chains, proportion of crystallinity, cross-link density, and manufacturing technique.*
3. *Because polyethylene wear particles can trigger early implant failure, wear reduction is the driving force behind the refinement of surgical polymers.*
4. *Polyethylene is prone to both surface wear (which can trigger osteolysis) and subsurface wear known as fatigue delamination (which causes macroscopic failure).*
5. *Gamma-in-air sterilization triggers oxidative chain scission, accelerating both surface and subsurface wear.*
6. *Highly cross-linked polyethylene has been shown to produce less polymer wear debris in both laboratory and clinical studies. However, there are concerns that wear particles produced from highly cross-linked polyethylene may be more biologically destructive.*

REFERENCES

1. Kurtz S, Ong K, Lau E, et al. Projections of primary and revision hip and knee arthroplasty in the United States from 2005 to 2030. *J Bone Joint Surg Am.* 2007;89(4):780-785.

2. Gunston FH. Polycentric knee arthroplasty. Prosthetic simulation of normal knee movement. *J Bone Joint Surg Br.* 1971;53(2):272-277.

3. Ranawat CS, Flynn WF Jr, Saddler S, et al. Long-term results of the total condylar knee arthroplasty. A 15-year survivorship study. *Clin Orthop Relat Res.* 1993; (286):94-102.

4. Pour AE, Parvizi J, Slenker N, et al. Rotating hinged total knee replacement: use with caution. *J Bone Joint Surg Am*. 2007;89(8):1735-1741.
5. Pilliar RM. Powder metal-made orthopedic implants with porous surface for fixation by tissue ingrowth. *Clin Orthop Relat Res*. 1983;176:42-51.
6. Cook SD, Thomas KA. Fatigue failure of noncemented porous-coated implants. A retrieval study. *J Bone Joint Surg Br*. 1991;73(1):20-24.
7. Morrey BF, Chao EY. Fracture of the porous-coated metal tray of a biologically fixed knee prosthesis. Report of a case. *Clin Orthop Relat Res*. 1988;228:182-189.
8. Chatterji U, Ashworth MJ, Smith AL, et al. Retrieval study of tibial baseplate fracture after total knee arthroplasty. *J Arthroplasty*. 2005;20(1):101-107.
9. Callaghan JJ, Pellicci PM, Salvati EA, et al. Fracture of the femoral component. Analysis of failure and long-term follow-up of revision. *Orthop Clin North Am*. 1988;19(3):637-647.
10. Huang CH, Yang CY, Cheng CK. Fracture of the femoral component associated with polyethylene wear and osteolysis after total knee arthroplasty. *J Arthroplasty*. 1999;14(3):375-379.
11. Luring C, Perlick L, Schubert T, et al. A rare cause for knee pain: fracture of the femoral component after TKR. A case report. *Knee Surg Sports Traumatol Arthrosc*. 2007;15(6):756-757.
12. Han CD, Han CW, Yang IH. Femoral component fracture due to osteolysis after cemented mobile-bearing total knee arthroplasty. *J Arthroplasty*. 2009;24(2):323.e7-e12.
13. Griffiths HJ, Burke J, Bonfiglio TA. Granulomatous pseudotumors in total joint replacement. *Skeletal Radiol*. 1987;16(2):146-152.
14. Luetzner J, Krummenauer F, Lengel AM, et al. Serum metal ion exposure after total knee arthroplasty. *Clin Orthop Relat Res*. 2007;461:136-142.
15. Urban RM, Jacobs JJ, Tomlinson MJ, et al. Dissemination of wear particles to the liver, spleen, and abdominal lymph nodes of patients with hip or knee replacement. *J Bone Joint Surg Am*. 2000;82(4):457-476.
16. Yang J, Black J. Competitive binding of chromium, cobalt and nickel to serum proteins. *Biomaterials*. 1994;15(4):262-268.
17. Hallab N, Merritt K, Jacobs JJ. Metal sensitivity in patients with orthopaedic implants. *J Bone Joint Surg Am*. 2001;83(3):428-436.
18. Jacobs JJ, Urban RM, Wall J, et al. Unusual foreign-body reaction to a failed total knee replacement: simulation of a sarcoma clinically and a sarcoid histologically. A case report. *J Bone Joint Surg Am*. 1995;77(3):444-451.
19. Keegan GM, Learmonth ID, Case CP. Orthopaedic metals and their potential toxicity in the arthroplasty patient: a review of current knowledge and future strategies. *J Bone Joint Surg Br*. 2007;89(5):567-573.
20. Dunstan E, Ladon D, Whittingham-Jones P, et al. Chromosomal aberrations in the peripheral blood of patients with metal-on-metal hip bearings. *J Bone Joint Surg Am*. 2008;90(3):517-522.
21. Ladon D, Doherty A, Newson R, et al. Changes in metal levels and chromosome aberrations in the peripheral blood of patients after metal-on-metal hip arthroplasty. *J Arthroplasty*. 2004;19(8 suppl 3):78-83.
22. Cole P, Rodu B. Epidemiologic studies of chrome and cancer mortality: a series of meta-analyses. *Regul Toxicol Pharmacol*. 2005;43(3):225-231.
23. Leonard A, Gerber GB. Mutagenicity, carcinogenicity and teratogenicity of vanadium compounds. *Mutat Res*. 1994;317(1):81-88.
24. Langer G. Ceramic tibial plateau of the 70s. *Bioceramics in Joint Arthroplasty Proceedings 7th International BIOLOX Symposium*. March 15/16, 2002. Stuttgard: Thieme Verlag; 2002.
25. Jacobs JJ, Gilbert JL, Urban RM. Corrosion of metal orthopaedic implants. *J Bone Joint Surg Am*. 1998;80(2):268-282.
26. Basketter DA, Briatico-Vangosa G, Kaestner W, et al. Nickel, cobalt and chromium in consumer products: a role in allergic contact dermatitis? *Contact Dermatitis*. 1993;28(1):15-25.
27. Shrivastava S. Medical device materials. *Proceedings from the Materials & Processes for Medical Devices Conference 2003*. 8-10 September 2003. Anaheim, CA. Materials Park, OH: ASM International; 2004.
28. Needham J, Burns T, Gerlinger T. Catastrophic failure of ceramic-polyethylene bearing total hip arthroplasty. *J Arthroplasty*. 2008;23(4):627-630.
29. Simon JA, Dayan AJ, Ergas E, et al. Catastrophic failure of the acetabular component in a ceramic-polyethylene bearing total hip arthroplasty. *J Arthroplasty*. 1998;13(1):108-113.
30. Benazzo FM. Failure mechanisms of ceramic total hip arthroplasty. *J Bone Joint Surg Am*. 2007;89(5):1131-1132; author reply 2-3.

31. Park YS, Hwang SK, Choy WS, et al. Ceramic failure after total hip arthroplasty with an alumina-on-alumina bearing. *J Bone Joint Surg Am*. 2006;88(4):780-787.

32. Seidelmann U, Richter H, Soltesz U. Failure of ceramic hip endoprostheses by slow crack growth–lifetime prediction. *J Biomed Mater Res*. 1982;16(5): 705-713.

33. Hummer CD III, Rothman RH, Hozack WJ. Catastrophic failure of modular zirconia-ceramic femoral head components after total hip arthroplasty. *J Arthroplasty*. 1995;10(6):848-850.

34. Garvie RC, Hannink RH, Pascoe RT. Ceramic steel. *Nature*. 1975;258:703-704.

35. Masonis JL, Bourne RB, Ries MD, et al. Zirconia femoral head fractures: a clinical and retrieval analysis. *J Arthroplasty*. 2004;19(7):898-905.

36. Oonishi H, Aono M, Murata N, et al. Alumina versus polyethylene in total knee arthroplasty. *Clin Orthop Relat Res*. 1992;282:95-104.

37. Laskin RS. An oxidized Zr ceramic surfaced femoral component for total knee arthroplasty. *Clin Orthop Relat Res*. 2003;416:191-196.

38. Hunter G. Adhesion testing of oxidized zirconium. *Trans Soc Biomater*. 2001;24:540.

39. Hunter ML. Abrasive wear of oxidized Zr-2.5b, CoCrMo, and Ti-6Al-4V against bone cement. *Transactions of the Sixth World Biomaterials Congress*. Minneapolis: Society for Biomaterials; 2000.

40. Spector BM, Ries MD, Bourne RB, et al. Wear performance of ultra-high molecular weight polyethylene on oxidized zirconium total knee femoral components. *J Bone Joint Surg Am*. 2001;83(suppl 2 pt 2):80-86.

41. Ezzet KA, Hermida JC, Colwell CW Jr, et al. Oxidized zirconium femoral components reduce polyethylene wear in a knee wear simulator. *Clin Orthop Relat Res*. 2004;428:120-124.

42. Hui C, Salmon L, Maeno S, et al. Five-year comparison of oxidized zirconium and cobalt-chromium femoral components in total knee arthroplasty: a randomized controlled trial. *J Bone Joint Surg Am*. 2011;93(7):624-630.

43. Akagi M, Nakamura T, Matsusue Y, et al. The Bisurface total knee replacement: a unique design for flexion. Four-to-nine-year follow-up study. *J Bone Joint Surg Am*. 2000;82(11):1626-1633.

44. Minoda Y, Kobayashi A, Iwaki H, et al. In vivo analysis of polyethylene wear particles after total knee arthroplasty: the influence of improved materials and designs. *J Bone Joint Surg Am*. 2009;91(suppl 6):67-73.

45. Kim YH, Kim JS, Huh W, et al. Weight of polyethylene wear particles is similar in TKAs with oxidized zirconium and cobalt-chrome prostheses. *Clin Orthop Relat Res*. 2010;468(5):1296-1304.

46. Oonishi H, Kim SC, Kyomoto M, et al. PE wear in ceramic/PE bearing surface in total knee arthroplasty: clinical experiences of more than 24 years. In: Bennazo F, Falez F, Dietrich M, eds. *Ceramics in Orthopaedics. 11th BIOLOX® Symposium Proceedings*. Germany: Steinkopff Verlag Darmstad; 2006: 101-110.

47. Ramachandran M. *Basic Orthopaedic Sciences: The Stanmore Guide*. London: Hodder Arnold; 2007.

48. Kurtz SM, Muratoglu OK, Evans M, et al. Advances in the processing, sterilization, and crosslinking of ultra-high molecular weight polyethylene for total joint arthroplasty. *Biomaterials*. 1999;20(18):1659-1688.

49. Lombardi AV Jr, Ellison BS, Berend KR. Polyethylene wear is influenced by manufacturing technique in modular TKA. *Clin Orthop Relat Res*. 2008;466(11): 2798-2805.

50. Blunn G, Brach del Preva EM, Costa L, et al. Ultra high molecular-weight polyethylene (UHMWPE) in total knee replacement: fabrication, sterilisation and wear. *J Bone Joint Surg Br*. 2002;84(7):946-949.

51. Tanner MG, Whiteside LA, White SE. Effect of polyethylene quality on wear in total knee arthroplasty. *Clin Orthop Relat Res*. 1995;317:83-88.

52. Ingham E, Fisher J. Biological reactions to wear debris in total joint replacement. *Proc Inst Mech Eng H*. 2000;214(1):21-37.

53. Ingham E, Fisher J. The role of macrophages in osteolysis of total joint replacement. *Biomaterials*. 2005;26(11):1271-1286.

54. Tipper JL, Galvin AL, Williams S, et al. Isolation and characterization of UHMWPE wear particles down to ten nanometers in size from in vitro hip and knee joint simulators. *J Biomed Mater Res A*. 2006;78(3):473-480.

55. Jones SM, Pinder IM, Moran CG, et al. Polyethylene wear in uncemented knee replacements. *J Bone Joint Surg Br*. 1992;74(1):18-22.

56. Barnett PI, McEwen HM, Auger DD, et al. Investigation of wear of knee prostheses in a new displacement/force-controlled simulator. *Proc Inst Mech Eng H*. 2002;216(1):51-61.

57. Zahiri CA, Schmalzried TP, Szuszczewicz ES, et al. Assessing activity in joint replacement patients. *J Arthroplasty.* 1998;13(8):890-895.

58. Insall JN, Scott WN. *Surgery of the Knee.* 3rd ed. New York and London: Churchill Livingstone; 2001.

59. Fisher J, Firkins P, Reeves EA, et al. The influence of scratches to metallic counterfaces on the wear of ultra-high molecular weight polyethylene. *Proc Inst Mech Eng H.* 1995;209(4):263-264.

60. McNie C, Barton DC, Stone MH, et al. Prediction of plastic strains in ultra-high molecular weight polyethylene due to microscopic asperity interactions during sliding wear. *Proc Inst Mech Eng H.* 1998;212(1):49-56.

61. Bartel DL, Bicknell VL, Wright TM. The effect of conformity, thickness, and material on stresses in ultra-high molecular weight components for total joint replacement. *J Bone Joint Surg Am.* 1986;68(7):1041-1051.

62. Bartel DL, Rawlinson JJ, Burstein AH, et al. Stresses in polyethylene components of contemporary total knee replacements. *Clin Orthop Relat Res.* 1995;317:76-82.

63. McEwen HM, Barnett PI, Bell CJ, et al. The influence of design, materials and kinematics on the in vitro wear of total knee replacements. *J Biomech.* 2005;38(2):357-365.

64. Wright TM, Bartel DL. The problem of surface damage in polyethylene total knee components. *Clin Orthop Relat Res.* 1986;205:67-74.

65. McEwen HM, Fisher J, Goldsmith AA, et al. Wear of fixed bearing and rotating platform mobile bearing knees subjected to high levels of internal and external tibial rotation. *J Mater Sci Mater Med.* 2001;12(10-12):1049-1052.

66. Muratoglu OK, Bragdon CR, O'Connor DO, et al. Unified wear model for highly crosslinked ultra-high molecular weight polyethylenes (UHMWPE). *Biomaterials.* 1999;20(16):1463-1470.

67. Oonishi H, Kadoya Y. Wear of high-dose gamma-irradiated polyethylene in total hip replacements. *J Orthop Sci.* 2000;5(3):223-228.

68. Lewis G. Properties of crosslinked ultra-high-molecular-weight polyethylene. *Biomaterials.* 2001;22(4):371-401.

69. Hermida JC, Fischler A, Colwell CW Jr, et al. The effect of oxidative aging on the wear performance of highly crosslinked polyethylene knee inserts under conditions of severe malalignment. *J Orthop Res.* 2008;26(12):1585-1590.

70. Oral E, Malhi AS, Muratoglu OK. Mechanisms of decrease in fatigue crack propagation resistance in irradiated and melted UHMWPE. *Biomaterials.* 2006;27(6):917-925.

71. Costa L, Luda MP, Trossarelli L, et al. Oxidation in orthopaedic UHMWPE sterilized by gamma-radiation and ethylene oxide. *Biomaterials.* 1998;19(7-9):659-968.

72. Bradford L, Baker D, Ries MD, et al. Fatigue crack propagation resistance of highly crosslinked polyethylene. *Clin Orthop Relat Res.* 2004;429:68-72.

73. Cole JC, Lemons JE, Eberhardt AW. Gamma irradiation alters fatigue-crack behavior and fracture toughness in 1900H and GUR 1050 UHMWPE. *J Biomed Mater Res.* 2002;63(5):559-566.

74. Muratoglu OK, Bragdon CR, O'Connor DO, et al. Aggressive wear testing of a cross-linked polyethylene in total knee arthroplasty. *Clin Orthop Relat Res.* 2002;404:89-95.

75. Fisher J, McEwen HM, Tipper JL, et al. Wear, debris, and biologic activity of cross-linked polyethylene in the knee: benefits and potential concerns. *Clin Orthop Relat Res.* 2004;428:114-119.

76. Scott M, Morrison M, Mishra SR, et al. Particle analysis for the determination of UHMWPE wear. *J Biomed Mater Res B Appl Biomater.* 2005;73(2):325-337.

77. Iwakiri K, Minoda Y, Kobayashi A, et al. In vivo comparison of wear particles between highly crosslinked polyethylene and conventional polyethylene in the same design of total knee arthroplasties. *J Biomed Mater Res B Appl Biomater.* 2009;91(2):799-804.

78. Martell JM, Verner JJ, Incavo SJ. Clinical performance of a highly cross-linked polyethylene at two years in total hip arthroplasty: a randomized prospective trial. *J Arthroplasty.* 2003;18(7 suppl 1):55-59.

79. Hodrick JT, Severson EP, McAlister DS, et al. Highly crosslinked polyethylene is safe for use in total knee arthroplasty. *Clin Orthop Relat Res.* 2008;466(11):2806-2812.

80. Muratoglu OK, Greenbaum ES, Bragdon CR, et al. Surface analysis of early retrieved acetabular polyethylene liners: a comparison of conventional and highly crosslinked polyethylenes. *J Arthroplasty.* 2004;19(1):68-77.

81. Minoda Y, Aihara M, Sakawa A, et al. Comparison between highly cross-linked and conventional polyethylene in total knee arthroplasty. *Knee.* 2009;16(5):348-351.

82. Muratoglu OK, Burroughs BR, Bragdon CR, et al. Knee simulator wear of polyethylene tibias articulating against explanted rough femoral components. *Clin Orthop Relat Res*. 2004;428:108-113.

83. Muratoglu OK, Merrill EW, Bragdon CR, et al. Effect of radiation, heat, and aging on in vitro wear resistance of polyethylene. *Clin Orthop Relat Res*. 2003;417:253-262.

84. Muratoglu OK, Bragdon CR, O'Connor DO, et al. A novel method of cross-linking ultra-high-molecular-weight polyethylene to improve wear, reduce oxidation, and retain mechanical properties. Recipient of the 1999 HAP Paul Award. *J Arthroplasty*. 2001;16(2):149-160.

85. McKellop H, Shen FW, Lu B, Campbell P, et al. Development of an extremely wear-resistant ultra high molecular weight polyethylene for total hip replacements. *J Orthop Res*. 1999;17(2):157-167.

86. Wang A, Yau SS, Essner A, et al. A highly crosslinked UHMWPE for CR and PS total knee arthroplasties. *J Arthroplasty*. 2008;23(4):559-566.

87. Muratoglu OK, Bragdon CR, Jasty M, et al. Knee-simulator testing of conventional and cross-linked polyethylene tibial inserts. *J Arthroplasty*. 2004;19 (7):887-897.

88. Besong AA, Tipper JL, Ingham E, et al. Quantitative comparison of wear debris from UHMWPE that has and has not been sterilised by gamma irradiation. *J Bone Joint Surg Br*. 1998;80(2):340-344.

89. Costa L, Brach Del Prever E. *UHMWPE for Arthroplasty: Characterisation, Sterilisation and Degradation*. Torino, Italy: Minerva Medica; 2000.

90. Costa L, Luda MP, Trossarelli L, et al. In vivo UHMWPE biodegradation of retrieved prosthesis. *Biomaterials*. 1998;19(15):1371-1385.

91. Simis KS, Bistolfi A, Bellare A, et al. The combined effects of crosslinking and high crystallinity on the microstructural and mechanical properties of ultra high molecular weight polyethylene. *Biomaterials*. 2006;27(9):1688-1694.

92. Pruitt LA. Deformation, yielding, fracture and fatigue behavior of conventional and highly cross-linked ultra high molecular weight polyethylene. *Biomaterials*. 2005;26(8):905-915.

93. Ries MD, Pruitt L. Effect of cross-linking on the microstructure and mechanical properties of ultra-high molecular weight polyethylene. *Clin Orthop Relat Res*. 2005;440:149-156.

94. Oral E, Godleski Beckos CA, Lozynsky AJ, et al. Improved resistance to wear and fatigue fracture in high pressure crystallized vitamin E-containing ultra-high molecular weight polyethylene. *Biomaterials*. 2009;30(10):1870-1880.

95. Oral E, Christensen SD, Malhi AS, et al. Wear resistance and mechanical properties of highly cross-linked, ultrahigh-molecular weight polyethylene doped with vitamin E. *J Arthroplasty*. 2006;21(4): 580-591.

96. Bracco P, Oral E. Vitamin E-stabilized UHMWPE for total joint implants: a review. *Clin Orthop Relat Res*. 2011;469(8):2286-2293.

97. Jarrett BT, Cofske J, Rosenberg AE, et al. In vivo biological response to vitamin E and vitamin-E-doped polyethylene. *J Bone Joint Surg Am*. 2010;92(16): 2672-2681.

11 Metal Alloys

Vinay Aggarwal, Claudio Diaz, and Sadegh Parvizi

With the advent and further sophistication of aseptic surgical techniques in the late 1800s and into the 1900s, the relative decrease in postoperative infection allowed the once unfeasible possibility of using foreign biomaterials as implants in surgical procedures.[1] The science of biomaterials, which is the use of synthetic or treated natural materials in replacing or enhancing the function of human tissue or organs, has progressed exponentially from the 20th century and now into the 21st century.[2] In the field of orthopaedics, there still remains much room for improvement in the use of biomaterials, including in reducing prosthesis wear, promoting implant longevity, and reducing host responses to foreign material such as hypersensitivity and periprosthetic infection.[2,3]

For orthopaedic surgeons, knowledge of the different metal alloys used as biomaterials in joint reconstruction surgery is essential in guiding operative plans and is directly related to clinical results. This chapter is divided into three sections: a brief discussion regarding basic history and fundamentals of metals in total joint replacement surgery, an outline of the physical and chemical properties of different metal alloys, and finally a highlighting of several hot clinical topics regarding the use of different metals in total joint arthroplasty of the knee.

OVERVIEW OF METALS

Use in Total Knee Arthroplasty: A Brief History

Total joint arthroplasty is one of the most successful surgical endeavors in all of orthopaedics and much of the success of the procedure is due to the advancement of implant material and design over the decades. At its inception, total knee replacement lagged significantly behind total hip replacement in success because of problems with material selection leading to early implant loosening and wear.[4,5] In the past, materials as diverse as ivory, wood, rubber, and acrylic had been used in prosthetic implants. Metal alloys such as stainless steel and cobalt-chromium alloys used for bearing surface components were developed during the 1960s and 1970s. Then, during the late 1980s and for much of the 1990s, cobalt-chromium alloys used in conjunction with ultrahigh-molecular-weight polyethylene in articulating surfaces came into favor.[2] The highly polished metal against polyethylene proved to provide a lower level of friction and thus wear on weight-bearing joints including the hip and knee.

The balance between wear, longevity, and stability is of utmost important when choosing appropriate biomaterials for joint prostheses. As the 21st century progresses and younger patients comprise a higher proportion of the patients undergoing joint arthroplasty, more attention is being directed at longevity of implants and specific metal-on-metal surfaces. Nonetheless, it is important for both patients and orthopaedic surgeons to remember that the best bearing surface of all is natural, healthy, human articular cartilage because it provides friction levels of nearly zero and remains the ultimate benchmark for which all biomaterials must be compared.

General Metal Properties

Metals, which are made up of positively charged particles closely packed in nondirectional arrays within free-floating electron clouds, have traditionally been selected for structural implant purposes because of their superior strength.[6] Further, the nondirectional nature of the metallic bonds allows the property of ductility (ie, deformation without undergoing fracture), another important consideration when selecting material for weight-bearing joint replacement prostheses. In addition, the modulus of elasticity for metals is another property that must be examined when selecting an alloy's compatibility with the bone into which it is being implanted.[6,7] Although all metal alloys will be stiffer than bone, those with elastic moduli closer to bone will cause less stress shielding and better long-term results. Finally, due to the implantation of the metal alloy in body cavities bathed with body fluid, the alloy must have high resistance to corrosion in vivo.[6,8-10] These properties all in conjunction limit the possible choices of metal when manufacturers and subsequently surgeons choose a material for implantation during a joint replacement procedure.

Metal alloys are formed via combination of several metallic elements together and provide improved properties beyond those of a single element.[4] Three main alloy systems in particular are used in orthopaedic practice: cobalt-chromium alloys, titanium alloys, and stainless steel alloys comprised mostly of iron. These alloy systems have been selected for their optimum combination of the properties outlined above, including ultimate strength of implant, ductile behavior during weight-bearing loads to fracture, elastic modulus, and corrosion resistance within the joint.[2,6] In addition to in vivo performance, however, it is worth mentioning that an alloy must satisfy more than just physical and chemical properties to be considered successful in joint arthroplasty. There are practical manufacturing and marketing requirements, including the ability to engineer the prosthesis using the material, producing implants at a reasonable cost, and implanting the device with ease during surgery. Orthopaedic surgeons have the ultimate responsibility to understand the metallic biomaterials and their structural limitations and to maximize the success of their application.

SPECIFIC PROPERTIES OF METAL ALLOYS

Stainless Steel

While there are more than 50 commercially available alloys of stainless steel, W.O. Sherman is credited with first introducing use of the metal alloy in surgery via screws and plates during the early 20th century.[11] Type 316L iron-based stainless steel is the alloy most commonly used in orthopaedics today owing to its minimal corrosive carbon content and carefully manufactured inclusion of protective metals such as chromium (Cr), nickel (Ni), and molybdenum (Mo).[6-8] Stainless steel is both the cheapest and most easily manufactured alloy used in orthopaedic devices, and this form of type 316L stainless steel has considerable yield strength and a high elastic modulus.

The presence of carbon as well as impure nonmetallic inclusions characteristic of all steels are undesirable traits of this alloy; however, several alloy refinement processes, such as vacuum arc melting, are undertaken during manufacturing to optimize implant life span and performance.[6] Further efforts to prevent biodegradation and corrosive dissolution in vivo include a process termed passivation, or oxidation of surface particles via nitric acid exposure, and subsequent polishing.[6,12] This process removes surface iron particles and generates a thin chromium oxide film, which provides corrosion resistance. Nonetheless, due to the eventual fatigue failure and corrosive forces on stainless steel, the alloy is much more appropriately and heavily utilized in temporary fracture fixation devices rather than in permanent weight-bearing joint replacement implants.[13]

Cobalt-Chromium Alloys

The more expensive and difficult to manufacture cobalt-chromium alloys have several advantages over the stainless steel alloys. Cobalt-chromium-molybdenum alloys (referred to as ASTM F-75) have a particular role in joint arthroplasty surgery. Because of the chromium and molybdenum content, the surface film produced provides serious resistance to corrosion, which has been demonstrated via decreased electrolytic effects in bodily tissues and bone.[9] Further, this cast variety of the cobalt-based alloys has significant yield strength and cannot even be contoured at time of surgery, making it ideal for implantable joint prosthetics that can bear weight almost permanently.[6,13] Last, this alloy can be used in popular porous forms to allow for biologic fixation via bony ingrowth for hip and knee replacement.

Certain manufacturing processes including forging or hot isostatic pressing, both of which produce smaller, more compact grain sizes, can be used to create a stronger overall biomaterial that must be machine polished into a smooth bearing surface.[6] However, the very high elastic modulus of cobalt-based alloys has in some cases led to high stress shielding, leading to lower extremity pain in some patients with these implants.[14] A second variety of cobalt-chromium alloy is made with addition of nickel and tungsten (referred to as ASTM F-90) and is not as suitable for use as joint implants because of its decreased resistance to corrosion than the F-75 variety.[7] Its main use is in wiring and internal fixation devices such as plates, rods, and screws; however, because of high costs, it is still not used as commonly as stainless steel in this regard.

Titanium-Based Alloys

Titanium-based alloys also come in two main varieties: those referred to as commercially pure titanium (Ti) and common titanium-aluminum-vanadium alloy (referred to as Ti-6Al-4V). In the commercially pure form, titanium is only mixed with minute impurities of controlled amounts of dissolved oxygen to control yield strength and extremely trace amounts of hydrogen, carbon, nitrogen, and iron (less than 0.35% each). In the Ti-6Al-4V form, the alloy is mixed with approximately 6% aluminum (Al) and 4% vanadium (Va) to form a lightweight, ductile yet strong material.[6,7]

The advantages of titanium alloys include their incredibly superior biocompatibility (ie, titanium's significant ability to resist corrosion in vivo), a trait that has been confirmed in several human retrieval studies.[6] Further, titanium alloys have lower elastic moduli and allow for construction of modular implants with precise implant fit, especially in porous nonarticulating total joint prostheses.[13,15] Finally, titanium metals are usually materials of choice when patients are known to have previously infected or hypersensitive implant sites. The significant disadvantage of titanium alloys are the well-known poor wear properties of the material. The poor abrasion resistance is especially apparent when used in articulating surfaces with ultrahigh-molecular-weight polyethylene, such as in femoral heads or condyles.[16]

Tantalum and Composites

Tantalum is a metal that very recently has been studied for use in orthopaedic implants because of its remarkable resistance to corrosion. It is often manufactured in a highly porous form for bony ingrowth fixation, and it has a low modulus of elasticity, like titanium alloys, closer to that of bone than stainless steel or the cobalt-based alloys. Because of the high resistance to corrosion and bony ingrowth, it is being examined for long-term results in use of femoral stems as well as revision arthroplasty extended stems.[17-19]

The combination of metallic alloys with other biomaterials can result in implants with improved mechanical and physical properties. Current attempts in designing composite implants have not yielded highly successful results; however, the future possibilities for improvement are promising.

Ceramics: Alumina and Zirconia

It is worth briefly mentioning the growing use of ceramics, which utilize ionic rather than metallic bonding, in total joint reconstruction implants. The main reason for their use is the excellent wear resistance they provide, especially in bearing surfaces; however, their brittle nature makes them very susceptible to prosthetic fracture, especially in younger active patients.

Traditionally, alumina has had better wear properties and clinical results than zirconia implants in total hip prostheses. With the advent of oxidized zirconium (OxZr) alloy (marketed by Smith & Nephew as Oxinium), biomaterials researchers are aiming to utilize the metal–ceramic hybrid to improve upon ceramic properties even further. The initial wear results are positive; however, long-term results and effects of corrosion have yet to be fully documented.[20]

CLINICAL TOPICS: METAL ALLOYS IN TOTAL KNEE ARTHROPLASTY

Despite basic science studies supporting the use of metal alloys as biomaterials in knee arthroplasty, there are some relevant points that the clinician needs to know regarding their daily application.

Serum Metal Ions After Total Knee Arthroplasty

After recent studies with metal-on-metal total hip arthroplasty, there has been a growing interest regarding serum ion levels produced by metal alloys used in total joint arthroplasty. Even though total knee arthroplasty (TKA) does not utilize metal-on-metal bearings, Luetzner et al found that serum levels of metal ions, specifically Co, Cr, and Mo, have been found in both unilateral and bilateral TKA.[21] When comparing patients with and without TKA, there was no difference in Mo serum levels; however, the serum levels of Co and Cr were significantly higher among the TKA patient population. Of note, when comparing patients with unilateral to bilateral TKA, no differences were observed between the serum ion levels. Another study with 67-month follow-up showed that the serum levels of Co, Cr, and Mo in total knee megaprosthesis were all greater than the levels found in conventional TKA. Interestingly, these authors have proposed that the ions could be released not only from the weight-bearing surface, but also from the entire surface of the prosthesis.[22]

The issue of serum metal ion levels is a complex one, however, as demonstrated by a group who compared TKA patients with CoCr femoral components to those with OxZr femoral components. They found that after 3 years of follow-up, no statistical differences could be established when serum levels of Al, Co, Cr, and Mo were compared between the two groups, even though the OxZr implants did not contain a significant presence of those metals.[23] Thus, although no conclusion has been established on this topic, there appears to be sufficient evidence to demonstrate that TKA in general leads to increased metal ion serum levels, especially when CoCr is used.

Metal Allergies in Knee Arthroplasty

Materials used in knee arthroplasty are, in general, well tolerated by the human body. Regarding metal alloys, allergies associated with implants are a rare condition. Patient findings can include skin changes such as eczema, delayed wound and bone healing, recurrent effusion, pain, or implant loosening. Usually a thorough workup in the diagnosis of the allergic reaction relies primarily on skin patch testing after exclusion of other possibilities. Niki et al proposed a method for detection of metal sensitivity (MS) based on a modified lymphocyte stimulation test in TKA patients.[24] This test is performed in peripheral blood lymphocytes and is used to calculate the stimulation index (SI). In a subsequent publication, Niki et al established diagnostic criteria for MS in TKA patients: SI >200% in the modified lymphocyte stimulation test as well as the presence of eczematous dermatitis around the operative scar as determined by two dermatologists who have been blinded from the results of the lymphocyte stimulation test.[25] The results of these studies suggested that Cr is a potential cause of eczema following TKA, and Cr sensitivity may be a possible predictor for symptomatic MS.[24] Further, regarding the diagnosis of MS by studying joint fluid in TKA, a fluid sample with CD3(+)CD45RO(+) T cells is distinctive.[25] To date, the prevalence of MS has not been studied in a series of patients undergoing revision TKA, which would be interesting because MS has been known to mimic infection.[26]

In cases in which metal allergy is documented preoperatively, electing to use alternative biomaterials for implantation in total joint replacement has often been recommended but thus far is not routinely supported by evidence.[27] Granchi et al studied the frequency of sensitization to CoCrMo and TiAlV in patients who had undergone TKA, by using patch testing with haptens of CoCrMo and TiAlV and bone cements. The frequency of positive skin reactions to metals increased significantly after TKA, both with stable and unstable TKA fixation. Prior history of metal allergy seems to be a risk factor, because TKA failure was 4-fold more likely in patients who had symptoms of metal hypersensitivity before TKA in their series.[28]

Biomechanical Studies Comparing Metal Alloys in TKA

In biomechanical tests, the OxZr femoral component has been demonstrated to be more scratch resistant and 10 times less rough, and it produces a 78% reduction in wear of ultra-high-molecular-weight polyethylene over the CoCr femoral component in TKA patients.[29] In a recent study, Galetz et al compared the mechanical surface properties of an OxZr femoral component with those of cast and wrought CoCrMo and TiAlV6-4. The authors concluded that OxZr layer is very promising because of its high hardness, good bonding, and a modulus among the metal range. Unfortunately, the properties of the alloy underneath the surface are the poorest of all materials investigated.[30]

Bone–Metal Interface Versus Bone–Cement Interface for Tibial Fixation in TKA

Comparing the interface of bone–trabecular metal versus bone–cement in the tibial component in TKA, Minoda et al reported that the decrease in bone mineral density of the lateral tibial plateau was less in knees with a trabecular metal tibial implant than in knees with a cemented tibial CoCr component.[31] To date, however, there is no clinical evidence citing the benefits of using porous tantalum tibial components for TKA.

Use of Cemented Metal-Back Versus All Polyethylene Cemented Tibial Fixation in TKA

The use of metal-backed cemented tibial components has recently been compared with all polyethylene cemented tibial components in a randomized controlled trial (RCT). In terms of revision rate for any reason or revision for aseptic loosening, there is no difference at 10-year follow-up.[32] Despite this level I evidence, the historical preference among American surgeons for tibial fixation is for the cemented metal-back component.

Clinical Studies Regarding Different Metal Alloys as a Factor for Outcome in TKA

OxZr femoral component demonstrated a survivor rate of 98.7% at 7 years of follow-up, with one case of revision for aseptic loosening. Although this is a level IV study, the authors concluded that results justify pursuing the use of OxZr as an alternative bearing surface for a femoral component in TKA.[33]

In a RCT (level I evidence), OxZr femoral component did not demonstrate better clinical, subjective, and radiographic results than CoCr femoral component at 5-year follow-up.[34] In a retrieval analysis of 16 TKAs, the OxZr femoral component did not increase the polyethylene wear, measured using a wear and damage score. No failures associated with the OxZr femoral component were observed.[35]

Improving Image Analysis of TKA by Reducing the Metal Alloys Artifact

The Knee Society has proposed a standardized method for assessing radiological findings after TKA.[36] However, in some cases, the preoperative planning for a revision surgery (especially for aseptic loosening) includes other imaging modalities. Metal alloys produce image artifacts, altering visualization in computed tomography (CT) scans and magnetic resonance images (MRI). Lewis et al described reducing the metal artifacts to obtain the most accurate TKA assessment, using CT scans with 10° to 15° anteroinferior to posterosuperior angulation.[37] For MRI, the use of metal suppression software improves visualization of bone defects compared with X-rays in TKA, not only with a more accurate description of the defect size, but also by the diagnosis of defects previously undetected.[38]

Can Metal Alloys Make a Contribution in Preventing or Treating Infection in Knee Arthroplasty?

Implants made of copper (Cu) have been used for a long time in medicine.[39] Recently, Cu has demonstrated great antibacterial properties.[40] One study described its use in an orthopaedic animal model, as pins made from copper demonstrated high antimicrobial efficacy.[41] A more recent study showed that 317L stainless steel containing 4.5% copper alloy (317L-Cu) had strong antimicrobial activity and biocompatibility in vitro and in vivo; authors concluded that it could be used as a biomaterial to reduce implant-related infections.[42] More information is needed before proposing it as an alternative for treating or preventing infection in arthroplasty patients.

Another metal alloy that can be used for controlling infection is the nanoparticulate silver (Ar). The addition of this alloy to bone cement could be a good alternative, keeping in mind that NanoSilver-loaded cement showed better antimicrobial activity than gentamicin-loaded cement against multiresistant bacteria in vitro.[43] Additional research is needed.

Miscellaneous: Airport Metal Detectors and TKA Patients

Pearson and Matthews published a report stating that modern orthopaedic implants escape detection by airport metal detectors[44]; however, recent studies have described that patients with total knee implants could have up to 90% detection by airport security systems, especially those made of CoCr.[45] According to Abbassian et al, there is innate bias in these studies, however, because only a minority of the patients were actually asked for documentation of the implant.[46] Therefore, in the future, with security detection systems advancing, it may still be worthwhile to advise provision of implant documentation for TKA patients.

CONCLUSION

There is no question that the use of metal alloys by orthopaedic surgeons has rapidly advanced, especially in the past couple of decades. As the fields of materials science research and manufacturing progress at exponential rates, joint replacement surgery must aim to utilize the best metals available to promote implant longevity, reduce metal wear and complications, improve patient outcomes, and, most important, to best mimic natural articular cartilage and bone.

REFERENCES

1. Alexander JW. The contributions of infection control to a century of surgical progress. *Ann Surg*. 1985; 201(4):423-428.
2. Black J. *Orthopaedics Biomaterials in Research and Practice*. New York: Churchill Livingstone; 1988.
3. Von-Recum A. *Scientific, Technical and Clinical Testing of Implant Materials. Handbook of Biomaterials*. New York: Macmillan; 1986.
4. Bechtol CO, Laing PG. *Metals and Engineering in Bone and Joint Surgery*. Baltimore, MD: Williams & Wilkins; 1959.
5. Bertin K. *History of Joint Replacement*. [Cited 2011 September 16.] Available from: http://www.utahhipandknee.com/history.
6. Litsky AS. Biomaterials. In: Simon SR, ed. *Orthopedics Basic Science*. Columbus, OH: American Academy of Orthopaedic Surgeons; 1994:447-486.
7. American Society for Testing and Materials. *Standardization News: SN*. Philadelphia, PA: American Society for Testing and Materials; 1985:v.
8. Fontana MG, Greene ND. *Corrosion Engineering*. 2nd ed. New York: McGraw-Hill; 1978:xiii, 465.
9. Venable CS, Stuck WG, Beach A. The effects on bone of the presence of metals; based upon electrolysis: an experimental study. *Ann Surg*. 1937;105(6):917-938.

10. Jacobs JJ, Gilbert JL, Urban RM. Corrosion of metal orthopaedic implants. *J Bone Joint Surg Am.* 1998; 80(2):268-282.
11. Sherman WO. Vanadium steel plates and screws. *Surg Gyn Obstet.* 1912;14:629-634.
12. Yoo YR, Jang SC, Oh KT, et al. Influences of passivating elements on the corrosion and biocompatibility of super stainless steels. *J Biomed Mater Res B Appl Biomater.* 2008;86B(2):310-320.
13. Rubin LR. *Biomaterials in Reconstructive Surgery.* St. Louis, MO: Mosby; 1983:xviii, 1017.
14. Galante JO. Causes of fractures of the femoral component in total hip replacement. *J Bone Joint Surg Am.* 1980;62(4):670-673.
15. Jafari SM, Bender B, Coyle C, et al. Do tantalum and titanium cups show similar results in revision hip arthroplasty? *Clin Orthop Relat Res.* 2010;468(2): 459-465.
16. Engh CA Jr, Moore KD, Vinh TN, et al. Titanium prosthetic wear debris in remote bone marrow. A report of two cases. *J Bone Joint Surg Am.* 1997;79 (11):1721-1725.
17. Levine B, Sporer S, Della Valle CJ, et al. Porous tantalum in reconstructive surgery of the knee: a review. *J Knee Surg.* 2007;20(3):185-194.
18. Harrison AK, Gioe TK, Simonelli C, et al. Do porous tantalum implants help preserve bone?: evaluation of tibial bone density surrounding tantalum tibial implants in TKA. *Clin Orthop Relat Res.* 2010;468(10): 2739-2745.
19. Grelsamer RP. Applications of porous tantalum in total hip arthroplasty. *J Am Acad Orthop Surg.* 2007; 15(3):137, author reply 137-138.
20. Wright T, Elvin M. *Joint Replacement: Implant Bearing Surface Materials.* 2007 11/10/2009 [cited 2011 September 15]. Available from: http://www.hss.edu/conditions_Joint-Replacement-Implant-Bearing-Surface-Materials-History-Effectiveness-Future.asp.
21. Luetzner J, Krummenauer F, Lengel AM, et al. Serum metal ion exposure after total knee arthroplasty. *Clin Orthop Relat Res.* 2007;461:136-142.
22. Friesenbichler J, Maurer-Ertl W, Sadoghi P, et al. Serum metal ion levels after rotating-hinge knee arthroplasty: comparison between a standard device and a megaprosthesis. *Int Orthop.* July 14, 2011 [Epub ahead of print].
23. Garrett S, Jacobs N, Yates P, et al. Differences in metal ion release following cobalt-chromium and oxidized zirconium total knee arthroplasty. *Acta Orthop Belg.* 2010;76(4):513-520.
24. Niki Y, Matsumoto H, Otani T, et al. Screening for symptomatic metal sensitivity: a prospective study of 92 patients undergoing total knee arthroplasty. *Biomaterials.* 2005;26(9):1019-1026.
25. Niki Y, Matsumoto H, Otani T, et al. Five types of inflammatory arthritis following total knee arthroplasty. *J Biomed Mater Res A.* 2007;81(4):1005-1010.
26. Anand A, McGlynn F, Jiranek W. Metal hypersensitivity: can it mimic infection? *J Arthroplasty.* 2009; 24(5):826, e25-e28.
27. Thomas P, Schuh A, Ring J, et al. Orthopedic surgical implants and allergies. Joint statement by the Implant Allergy Working Group (AK 20) of the DGOOC (German Association of Orthopedics and Orthopedic Surgery), DKG (German Contact Dermatitis Research Group) and DGAKI (German Society for Allergology and Clinical Immunology). *Hautarzt.* 2008;59(3): 220-229.
28. Granchi D, Cenni E, Tigani D, et al., Sensitivity to implant materials in patients with total knee arthroplasties. *Biomaterials.* 2008;29(10):1494-1500.
29. Lee JK, Maruthainar K, Wardle N, et al. Increased force simulator wear testing of a zirconium oxide total knee arthroplasty. *Knee.* 2009;16(4):269-274.
30. Galetz MC, Fleischmann EW, Konrad CH, et al. Abrasion resistance of oxidized zirconium in comparison with CoCrMo and titanium nitride coatings for artificial knee joints. *J Biomed Mater Res B Appl Biomater.* 2010;93(1):244-251.
31. Minoda Y, Kobayashi A, Iwaki H, et al. Comparison of bone mineral density between porous tantalum and cemented tibial total knee arthroplasty components. *J Bone Joint Surg Am.* 2010;92(3):700-706.
32. Bettinson KA, Pinder IM, Moran CG, et al. All-polyethylene compared with metal-backed tibial components in total knee arthroplasty at ten years. A prospective, randomized controlled trial. *J Bone Joint Surg Am.* 2009;91(7):1587-1594.
33. Innocenti M, Civinini R, Carulli C, et al. The 5-year results of an oxidized zirconium femoral component for TKA. *Clin Orthop Relat Res.* 2010;468(5):1258-1263.
34. Hui C, Salmon L, Maeno S, et al. Five-year comparison of oxidized zirconium and cobalt-chromium femoral components in total knee arthroplasty: a randomized controlled trial. *J Bone Joint Surg Am.* 2011;93(7):624-630.
35. Heyse TJ, Davis J, Haas SB, et al. Retrieval analysis of femoral zirconium components in total knee arthroplasty: preliminary results. *J Arthroplasty.* 2011;26 (3):445-450.

36. Ewald FC. The Knee Society total knee arthroplasty roentgenographic evaluation and scoring system. *Clin Orthop Relat Res.* 1989;(248):9-12.

37. Lewis M, Toms AP, Reid K, et al. CT metal artefact reduction of total knee prostheses using angled gantry multiplanar reformation. *Knee.* 2010;17(4):279-282.

38. Vessely MB, Frick MA, Oakes D, et al. Magnetic resonance imaging with metal suppression for evaluation of periprosthetic osteolysis after total knee arthroplasty. *J Arthroplasty.* 2006;21(6):826-831.

39. Hofmeyr GJ, Singata M, Lawrie TA. Copper containing intra-uterine devices versus depot progestogens for contraception. *Cochrane Database Syst Rev.* 2010;(6):CD007043.

40. Grass G, Rensing C, Solioz M. Metallic copper as an antimicrobial surface. *Appl Environ Microbiol.* 2011;77(5):1541-1547.

41. Furkert FH, Sörensen JH, Arnoldi J, et al., Antimicrobial efficacy of surface-coated external fixation pins. *Curr Microbiol.* 2011;62(6):1743-1751.

42. Chai H, Guo L, Wang X, et al. Antibacterial effect of 317L stainless steel contained copper in prevention of implant-related infection in vitro and in vivo. *J Mater Sci Mater Med.* 2011;22(11):2525-2535.

43. Alt V, Bechert T, Steinrücke P, et al. Nanoparticulate silver. A new antimicrobial substance for bone cement. *Orthopade.* 2004;33(8):885-892.

44. Pearson WG, Matthews LS. Airport detection of modern orthopedic implant metals. *Clin Orthop Relat Res.* 1992(280):261-262.

45. Ramirez MA, Rodriguez EK, Zurakowski D, et al. Detection of orthopaedic implants in vivo by enhanced-sensitivity, walk-through metal detectors. *J Bone Joint Surg Am.* 2007;89(4):742-746.

46. Abbassian A, Datla B, Brooks RA. Detection of orthopaedic implants by airport metal detectors. *Ann R Coll Surg Engl.* 2007;89(3):285-287.

12 Surface Treatment to Foster Biological Incorporation

Matthew C. Morrey

Despite the excellent clinical results of current orthopaedic implant designs, further investigation into various surface and biological enhancement methods continue in an effort to further improve upon the success of total joint arthroplasty. Today, while several methods of surface treatment are currently being utilized, research continues to focus on design enhancements that allow the orthopaedic surgeon to achieve reliable osseous incorporation in a more rapid fashion with improved biocompatibility. This is typically accomplished by modifications that may be mechanical, chemical, physiological, or biological in nature. As with the initial application of advanced technology in this field, even today, many of the initiatives and research were made in the field of dentistry to which our specialty owes a debt of gratitude. In addition to what is discussed here, in recent years many of these surface treatments have been further altered by biologically active enhancements to facilitate the rate or quality of osseous incorporation. The realm of biological activation is extremely complex, is in the state of flux, and is only briefly mentioned here.

Various nonbiologically enhanced approaches to allow osseous incorporation may be classified as altering the substrate surface, modification of the substrate itself, or enhancement of the biological features of the substrate surface. Additional surface modifications have been introduced to enhance cement fixation, such as macrotexturing and molecular deposition of polymethylmethacrylate. Since cement fixation is much less employed today, this chapter reviews the basic approaches to enhance noncement fixation of the implant. Examples of these approaches are shown in Table 12-1.

TABLE 12-1. Strategies to Allow or Enhance Osseointegration

1. **Surface Modifications**
   - A. Grit blasting
   - B. Fiber mesh
   - C. Sintered bead coating
   - D. Plasma spray
   - E. Cast cobalt-chrome
2. **Substrate Modification**
   - A. Porous tantalum
   - B. Titanium foam
3. **Substrate Surface Treatment**
   - A. Hydroxyapatite
   - B. Growth factors
   - C. Type I collagen

SPECIFIC STRATEGIES

This section reviews these various fixation methods and their current relevance. It also briefly touches upon some of the ongoing research that may be clinically applied in the near future. It should be recognized that some designs may incorporate more than one of these surface modifications.

Hence the Mayo Conservative Hip (Zimmer, Warsaw, IN) has both fiber mesh pads and a corundumized surface treatment.

Surface Modifications

Surface enhancement to improve implant fixation was the first approach to improve the survivorship of early cemented implants. The effort to address the mechanical deficiencies of acrylic bone cement led to several lines of investigation. These included applying special surface treatments resulting in porous-coated implants with sintered metallic powders and the deposition of ceramic or metal coatings via plasma spray.[1-3] While these methods were deemed successful in terms of promoting integration and enhanced stability, in some instances substrate weakening occurred, making the implant vulnerable to fracture. Research is ongoing to improve the osseointegration of implants by making it faster and more predictable while avoiding unintended consequences such as substrate weakening. The goal of these processes is designed to allow osseous ingrowth or ongrowth. Characteristics are summarized in Table 12-2.

Grit blasting

Grit blasting is a process whereby small, hardened particles (grit) are propelled and bombard a metallic substrate, thereby creating a roughened surface. The grit is most often aluminum oxide or corundum, while the substrate is commonly titanium. The process is sometimes referred to as corundumization and the result is a textured surface that has demonstrated a reliable rate of osseous ongrowth.[4] This is of particular value with implants of smaller dimension, such as radial head implant stems. But it is readily applicable to larger hip or knee devices as well.

One concern regarding this technique is the introduction of contaminants within the grit, thereby potentially causing early third-body wear and the potential for subsequent loosening of the implant.[5] While still being utilized by some implant designs, the majority of newer options couple pure grit blasting with some form of adjuvant surface treatment to further enhance osseous incorporation.

Fiber mesh

Fiber mesh is a very early employed technology and is produced by a process in which fine metallic (titanium or cobalt-chrome) wires are woven and compressed into a thin layer that is then forged onto the surface of a metallic substrate either circumferentially or in pad form (Fig. 12-1). The process by which the metallic mesh is coupled to the substrate is called diffusion bonding. The typical porosity surface roughness ranges between 80 and 250 µm.

TABLE 12-2. Summary of Surface Modifications for Characteristics to Allow or Enhance Osseointegration

Characteristic	Finish/Coating			
	Grit Blast	Fiber Mesh	Sintered Beads	Plasma Spray
Process	Mechanical abrasion	Heat bonded	Metal sintering	Metal plasma spray
Typical roughness	6 µm	–250 µm	250 µm	–150 µm
Typical material	Any metal	Titanium	Co-Cr alloys	Titanium alloys

Adapted from Golish SR, Mihalko WM. *Orthopaedic Knowledge Online (AAOS): Orthopaedic Biomaterials: Part II. Metallurgy.* http://test2.aaos.org/oko/topicAuthors.cfm?topic=ADU0432008.

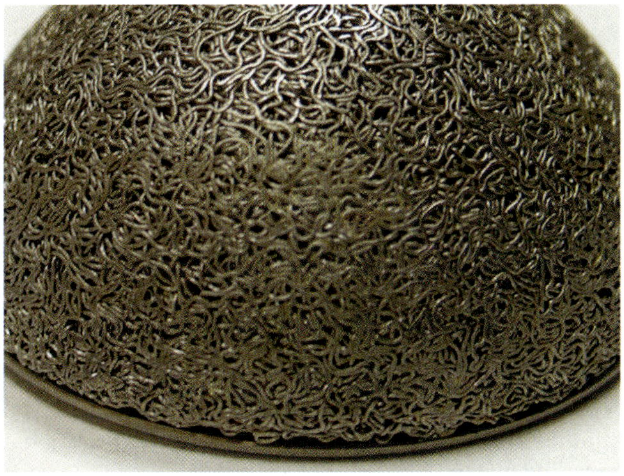

FIGURE 12-1. *Circumferential fiber mesh coating on acetabular component.*

Circumferential fiber mesh wrapping has demonstrated good results and is believed to function as a seal to prevent migration of wear particles. The use of bonded fiber mesh pads was the original application but this has been implicated in aseptic loosening thought to be the result of polyethylene wear particles migrating distally between the mesh pads.[6]

Sintered bead coating

Sintering describes a process whereby powdered objects are heated below their respective melting points until the particles adhere to one another.[7] The use of a sintering porous-coating process was developed for orthopaedic device use in the late 1970s and early 1980s. Metal alloy powders of cobalt-chromium-molybdenum (Co-Cr-Mo), 316L stainless steel, and titanium alloys (Ti6Al4V) were commonly utilized to form the porous surface layer on an implant substrate. While stainless steel demonstrated poor results, the Co-Cr-Mo and Ti6Al4V revealed reasonable bony ingrowth under ideal host conditions. It was determined that bone ingrowth was optimized with this surface treatment when pore sizes were greater than 100 μm, when relative motion of the implant–bone interface was minimal (maximum tolerable displacements of 50 μm), and in the presence of adequate vascularity, which promotes and supports the neogenesis of osseointegration.

Unfortunately the process of sintering requires a heat treatment that results in modifications of the microstructure of the metal substrate. Early application of this process involved temperatures of approximately 1300°. This resulted in implants that were susceptible to crack propagation and failure. It was subsequently discovered that utilization of specific heating and cooling schedules increased the ductility of the implant, thereby reducing the risk for crack propagation and ultimate failure.[8]

Currently, sintered porous coatings are formed on cast or wrought Co-Cr-Mo alloys as well as on Ti alloy implants (Fig. 12-2). The ideal porosity of this surface coating is roughly 100 to 400 μm with an average thickness of 300 μm to 1 mm.[9] This type of coating provides three-dimensional interlocking of the new bone, especially with multilayered coating. This does not occur with a single layered porous treatment. In general, the quality and depth of the osseointegration is dependent on the vascularity of the host bone as well as pore size and initial stability of the implant. Hence these physical properties are quite important.

A

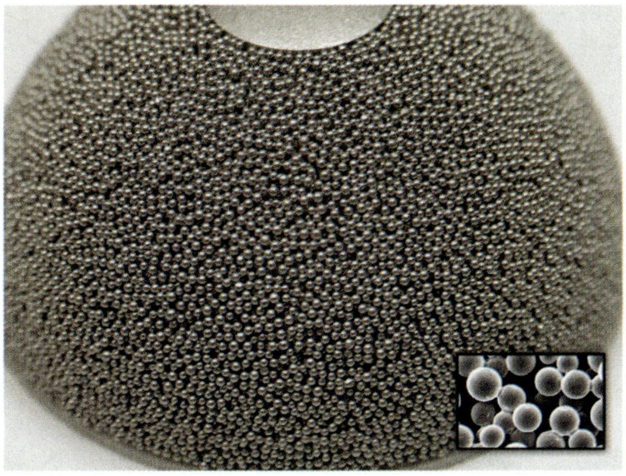

B

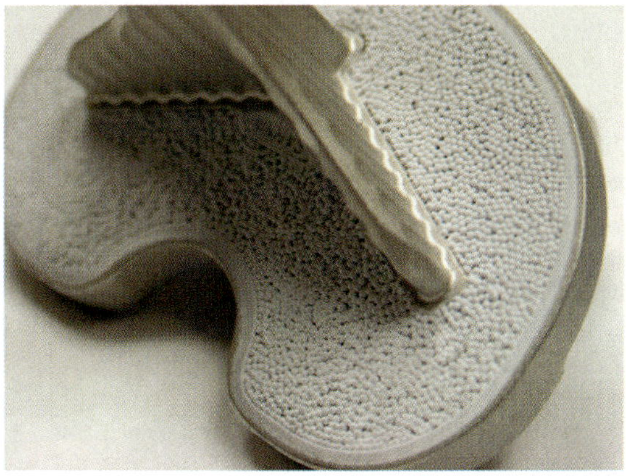

FIGURE 12-2. *(**A**) Sintered bead coating on acetabular component. (**B**) Hydroxyapatite-coated sintered beads on tibial baseplate.*

Plasma spray coating

Plasma spray coating was first introduced in the 1970s and has since become one of the main forms of surface treatment utilized in the manufacturing of orthopaedic implants. Excellent reviews of the current state of the science are available in the literature.[10] The process itself involves use of a high-temperature plasma jet with temperatures that exceed 10,000 K. These extreme temperatures facilitate the ability to spray refractory materials with high melting points, such as oxides and ceramics, onto a given substrate. However, unlike the sintering process, the extreme temperature is applied to the coating, not the substrate. It is for this reason that there is less substrate weakening by the plasma spray processes.

The macroscopic properties of plasma spray coating include porosity, hardness, and mechanical strength and are determined in large part by the microstructure of the deposited particles.[11] This in turn is determined by the actual shape of the material deposition and their interactions with one another, defining the overall properties of the substrate surface coating. Both metals and ceramics in the form of hydroxyapatite are applied as plasma spray. Details regarding the specifies of hydroxyapatite plasma spray coating are addressed later in the chapter.

Cast cobalt-chromium-molybdenum patterned surfaces

One notable concern with coated implants (sintered porous coating or plasma spray) is the potential for breakdown or delamination of the coated surface. This in turn can lead to particulate debris and foreign-body host reaction or even third-body wear if particles migrate into the joint articulation. In an effort to avoid this potential complication, direct casting methods of Co-Cr-Mo have been developed in an effort to enhance fixation and ingrowth. Originally introduced in the 1970s and 1980s, this technique produced implants with roughened, irregular textures of the substrate rather than true porous structures. Although clinical results are not as numerous as those for hydroxyapatite-coated implants (discussed below), the reported results do indicate successful osseointegration.[12]

Substrate Modification

This category defines a type of implant consisting of implant surface characteristics that are present throughout the implant.

Porous tantalum

In the mid-1990s, porous tantalum was introduced to the orthopaedic community as an alternative biomaterial with unique physical and mechanical properties.[13] This truly was a major advance. Tantalum demonstrates more porosity with more highly communicating pores and a higher coefficient of friction than other options. It is also able to be directly manufactured as the structure substrate of the implant without the need for an alternate supportive substrate while retaining the capacity as a unique surface coating.

Histologically, tantalum has been shown to promote both bone and fibrous tissue ingrowth.[14,15] In some recent reports, porous tantalum has been shown to promote or support an osteoblastic response, further validating it as a biocompatible material.[16]

Tantalum has been found to have a variety of uses in orthopaedic surgery. It has been demonstrated to be particularly beneficial in revision surgery where host bone is often less than ideal for implant fixation (Fig. 12-3). Recent reports suggest that tantalum may also function as a drug-delivery vehicle, allowing for various bone-stimulating agents to be eluded by the tantalum surface, thereby promoting a more profound bony response once implanted.[17]

Titanium foam

A foam is simply defined as a gas-filled substance. As such, the material is very porous: 75% to 95% by volume. The concept was developed in the early 1990s and in general there are two varieties: open and closed cells or pores. The dimension of the pore is between 1 and 8 mm. While much weaker than the solid material, it does possess the characteristics of the base metal (eg, it is noninflammatory). The manufacturing process is complex and expensive.

Titanium foam, as with other metal foams, is an example of a pure substrate modification that incorporates large volumes of gas-filled pores. The pores can be sealed (closed pore foam) or open, creating an interconnecting network. The unique characteristic of foam metals is their porosity, typically 75% to 90% of the substrate volume (Fig. 12-4). Recent animal studies have demonstrated that porous metal implants such as titanium foam allow for the formation of vascular systems, which integrate with the porous metal.[18] The porous nature of the titanium foam also allows for bony infiltration and osteoblast activity as well as soft tissue integration, similar to tantalum.

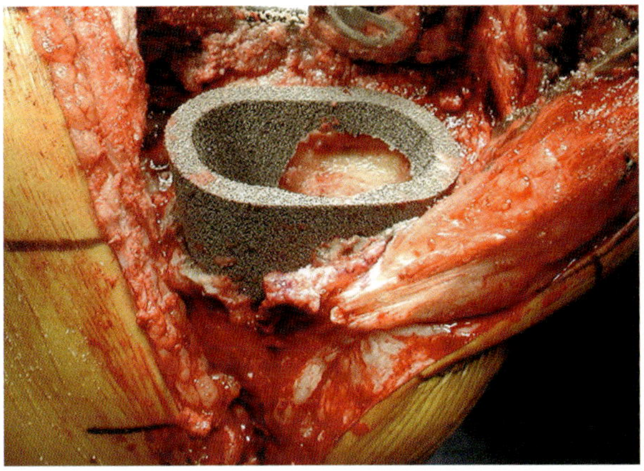

FIGURE 12-3. *Porous tantalum augment utilized in cavitary defect of the proximal tibia.*

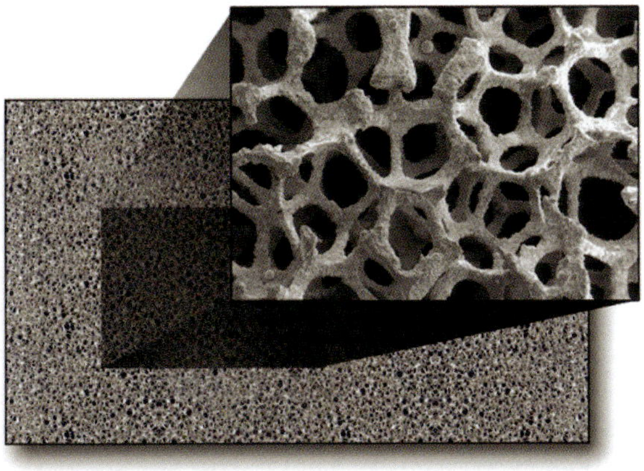

FIGURE 12-4. *Titanium foam; inset at 10× magnification.*

The surface treatment has found recent utilization in the orthopaedic arena as a scaffold in the setting of large bony defects requiring constructs of biologically active material designed to enhance reossification. Because of favorable mechanical properties and excellent biocompatibility, pure titanium foam has generated substantial interest as an alternative substrate to pure titanium and titanium alloys.[19]

Substrate Surface Treatment

Hydroxyapatite

Plasma-sprayed hydroxyapatite (HA) coatings have been utilized as surface treatment of metallic implants since the mid-1980s.[20] The process of plasma spraying results in a calcium phosphate treatment (HA over a Ti alloy substrate). This creates an irregular surface topography, allowing for mechanical interlocking of the bone to the implant during osseointegration. HA is an attractive surface coating because it is considered bioactive and has shown more rapid fixation and stronger bonding at the bone–implant interface.[21,22] HA coating has also been shown to promote bone growth across a gap of 1 mm between the bone and implant, as well as to offer a sealant against migration of polyethylene particles, which may decrease the potential for osteolysis and subsequent implant failure.[23,24]

The bioactivity of HA appears to be the result of its partial dissolution in vivo into the more soluble Ca-P phases. This amorphous phase has been attributed to faster bony incorporation because of more rapid dissolution.[25] Bone grows toward the implant, allowing for collagen to incorporate the HA crystals, forming a stronger bone–implant interface.

Plasma-spray coatings are typically 50 to 150 μm thick, have a highly irregular topography but do contain some voids and pores (Fig. 12-5). This surface irregularity provides an ideal condition for ingrowth, provided there is limited relative motion during early healing and adequate vascularity. The specific manufacturing process is important to avoid excess thickness and poor bonding to the substrate.

More recent advancements in the production of HA have demonstrated that silicate-modified HA particles may promote faster bone incorporation,[26] suggesting a possible advancement in the materials available for plasma spray coating and ultimately improved implant incorporation.

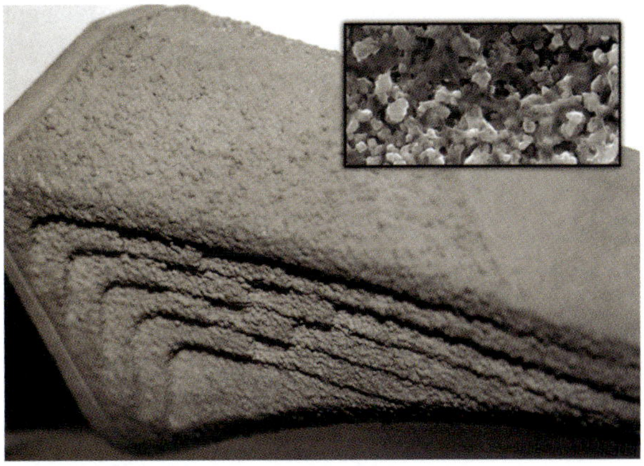

FIGURE 12-5. *Circumferential hydroxyapatite plasma spray coating on total hip femoral component.*

Growth factors

Growth factors such as bone morphogenic proteins (BMPs) and osteogenic protein-1 (OP-1) are cytokines that have been recognized as pivotal signaling molecules which orchestrate tissue modeling throughout the body, including cartilage and bone formation. BMPs and OP-1 have been investigated as a potential biocoating on orthopaedic implants in an effort to accelerate and enhance bone ingrowth as well as strengthen the osseous integration.[27,28]

One of the first studies looking at the potential role of BMPs as an adjuvant to promote osseointegration was in 1997 by Cole et al. They reported significantly more bone formation around titanium implants treated with BMP-2 versus the control in an animal model.[29] In 2000, Lind et al reported enhanced mechanical fixation and bony incorporation around uncoated, cementless implants when OP-1 was used as an adjuvant.[30] However, because of recently reported contradictory results,[31] further research regarding the use of BMP and OP-1 is needed to assess the overall efficacy, dosing, and cost.

Other growth factors that have been shown to improve osseointegration include platelet-derived growth factor (PDGF), insulin-like growth factor (IGF), and transforming growth factor beta-1 (TGFβ-1).[32,33] This is a complex area of investigation. As with BMPs and OP-1, further research is needed to ascertain appropriate dosing as well as justification of cost.

Type I collagen

A more recent, provocative, and interesting concept is the use of collagen as a surface enhancement. Type I collagen is the major collagen found in tendon and bone and is essential for the ultimate tensile strength of bone. It also demonstrates beneficial properties of bone remodeling, and it is this feature that has made it another potential adjuvant for osseointegration.

The use of collagen as a potential surface treatment was first reported in the late 1990s and early 2000s. In 2004, Rammelt et al reported a tendency for increased bone formation around titanium implants coated with type I collagen.[34] While novel in its concept, more research is required to ascertain whether or not collagen-coated implants would outperform the traditional noncemented implants as well as to justify the cost.

SUMMARY

The issue of surface enhancement is a complex and extremely interesting area of consideration that holds tremendous value to enhance the effectiveness of the currently used implants. As has been demonstrated, there are numerous strategies for improving and enhancing bony incorporation of orthopaedic implants. While the current generation of implants has an excellent clinical history, research is ongoing in an effort to improve upon these already well-reported results. Regardless, this is truly an important area of awareness and will be the source of substantive enhancement in the future.

REFERENCES

1. Pilliar RM. Porous-surfaced metallic implants for orthopaedic applications. *J Biomed Mater Res.* 1987; 21:1–33.
2. de Groot K, Geesink RGT, Klein CPAT, et al. Plasma-sprayed coatings of hydroxyapatite. *J Biomed Mater Res.*1987;21:1375–1381.
3. Judet R, Siguer M, Brumpt B, et al. A non-cemented total hip prosthesis. *Clin Orthop Relat Res.*1978;137: 76–84.
4. Aldinger PR, Jung AW, Pritsch M, et al. Uncemented grit-blasted straight tapered titanium stems in patients younger than fifty-five years of age: fifteen to twenty-year results. *J Bone Joint Surg Am.* 2009;91(6):1432-1439.
5. Schuh A, Holzwarth U, Kachler W, et al. Surface characterization of Al2O3-blasted titanium implants in total hip arthroplasty. *Orthopade.* 2004;33(8):905-910.
6. Maloney WJ , Woolson ST. Increasing incidence of femoral osteolysis in association with uncemented Harris-Galante total hip arthroplasty: a follow-up report. *J Arthroplasty.* 1996;11(2):130-134.
7. Grasso S, Sakka Y, Maizza G. (2009). Electric current activated/assisted sintering (ECAS): a review of patents 1906-2008. *Sci Technol Adv Mater.* 2009;10(5): 053001.
8. Kilner T, Pilliar RM, Weatherly GC, et al. Phase identification and incipient melting in a cast Co-Cr surgical implant alloy. *J Biomed Mater Res.* 1982;16:63-79.
9. Bobyn JD, Pilliar RM, Cameron HU, et al. The optimum pore size for the fixation of porous surfaced

metal implants by ingrowth of bone. *Clin Orthop Relat Res.* 1980;150:263-270.

10. Liang H, Shi B, Fairchild A. Application of plasma coatings in artificial joints, an overview. *Intl Symp Applied Plasma Sci.* 2004;73:317-326.
11. Furlong RJ, Osborn JF. Fixation of hip prostheses by hydroxyapatite ceramic coatings. *J Bone Joint Surg Br.* 1991;73:741-745.
12. Matsui M, Nakata K, Masuhara K, et al. The metal-cancellous cementless Lubeck total hip arthroplasty. Five to nine-year results. *J Bone Joint Surg Br.* 1998;80:404-410.
13. Black J. Biological performance of tantalum. *Clin Mater.* 1994;16:167-173.
14. Chan SP, Toh KK, Bobyn JD, et al. The osseous response to a new porous tantalum biomaterial. Presented at Triannual Meeting of the International Research Society of Orthopaedic Surgery and Traumatology; April 16-19, 1999; Sydney, Australia.
15. Bobyn JD, Stackpool GJ, Hacking SA, et al. Characteristics of bone ingrowth and interface mechanics of a new porous tantalum biomaterial. *J Bone Joint Surg Br.* 1999;81:907-914.
16. Findlay DM, Welldon K, Atkins GJ, et al. The proliferation and phenotypic expression of human osteoblasts on tantalum metal. *Biomaterials.* 2004; 25:2215-2227.
17. Tanzer M, Karabasz D, Krygier JJ, et al. Bone augmentation around and within porous tantalum implants by local bisphosphonate elution. *Clin Orthop Relat Res.* 2005;441:30-39.
18. Wen CE, Yamada, K, Shimojima, Y. Processing and mechanical properties of autogenous titanium implant materials. *J Mater Sci.* 2002;13(4):397-401.
19. Bettina M, Yang W, Kelly NH, et al. Osseointegration into a novel titanium foam implant in the distal femur of a rabbit. *J Biomed Mater Res Part A.* 2010;92:479-488.
20. Cook SD, Thomas KA, Dalton JF, et al. Hydroxyapatite coating of porous implants improves bone ingrowth and interface attachment strength. *J Biomed Mater Res.* 1992;26:989-1001.
21. Mostaghimi J, Chandra S. Splat formation in plasma-spray coating process. *Pure Appl Chem.* 2002;74(3):441-445.
22. Stephenson PK, Freeman MA, Revell PA, et al. The effect of hydroxyapatite coating on ingrowth of bone into cavities in an implant. *J Arthroplasty.* 1991;6:51-58.
23. Rahbek O, Overgaard S, Soballe K, et al. Hydroxyapatite coating might prevent peri-implant particle migration: a pilot study in dogs. *Acta Orthop Scand.* 1996;67(suppl 267):58-59.
24. Soballe K, Overgaard S. The current status of hydroxyapatite coating of prostheses. *J Bone Joint Surg Br.* 1996;78:689-690.
25. Ducheyne P, Hench LL, Kagan A, et al. The effect of hydroxyapatite impregnation on skeletal bonding of porous coated implants. *J Biomed Mater Res.* 1980;14:225-237.
26. Porter AE, Patel N, Skepper JN, et al. Effect of sintered silicate-substituted hydroxyapatite on remodeling processes at the bone-implant interface. *Biomaterials.* 2004;25:3303-3314.
27. Anitua E. Enhancement of osseous integration by generating a dynamic implant surface. *J Oral Implantol.* 2006;32:72-76.
28. Scheideler L, Geis-Gerstorfer J, Kern D, et al. Investigations of cell reactions to microstructured implant surfaces. *Mater Sci Eng.* 2003;23:455-459.
29. Cole BJ, Bostrom MP, Pritchard TL, et al. Use of bone morphogenetic protein 2 on ectopic porous coated implants in the rat. *Clin Orthop Relat Res.* 1997;345:219-228.
30. Lind M, Overgaard S, Song Y, et al. Osteogenic protein 1 device stimulates bone healing to hydroxyapaptite-coated and titanium implants. *J Arthroplasty.* 2000;15:339-346.
31. Salata LA, Burgos PM, Rasmusson L, et al. Osseointegration of oxidized and turned implants in circumferential bone defects with and without adjunctive therapies: an experimental study on BMP-2 and autogenous bone graft in the dog mandible. *Int J Oral Maxillofac Surg.* 2007;36:62-71.
32. Lynch SE, Buser D, Hernandez RA, et al. Effects of the platelet derived growth factor/insulin-like growth factor-I combination on bone regeneration around titanium dental implants. Results of a pilot study in beagle dogs. *J Periodontol.* 1991;62:710-716.
33. Sumner DR, Turner TM, Purchio AF, et al. Enhancement of bone ingrowth by transforming growth factor-beta. *J Bone Joint Surg Am.* 1995;77:1135-1147.
34. Rammelt S, Schulze E, Bernhardt R, et al. Coating of titanium implants with type-I collagen. *Orthop Res.* 2004;22(5):1025-1034.

13

Oxinium

Robert M. Kenyon and Keith A. Synnott

Total joint arthroplasty procedures are increasingly being performed in younger patients.[1] As a result, the expectations placed on arthroplasty prostheses are ever changing. Younger patients expect to return to a higher degree of functioning and at a faster rate than their older counterparts. Furthermore, there is greater expectation placed on the longevity of the prostheses. In the past, prosthetic joints may have only been intended to endure moderate levels of use and often a survival length of 10 to 15 years was entirely adequate for an older patient. Today, total knee arthroplasties (TKAs) are being placed under greater stresses for much greater durations. Traditionally, TKAs have generally been reserved for the older population (>65 years) and the rate of survival at 10 years has been reported as >97%; however, with patients less than 64 years of age a 3-fold higher rate of revision has been found.[1] The issue of prosthesis longevity and the complications that occur in association with revision surgery have come to the fore.

TKA prostheses generally consist of a femoral component (metal or ceramic) articulated with an ultra-high-molecular-weight polyethylene (polythene) component, which in turn is articulated with a metallic or ceramic tibial component. The dominant mode of failure of total joint replacements is aseptic loosening, which in many cases is caused by the osteolytic reaction of bone to the presence of implant debris generated from the polythene component.[2]

To simply eliminate the polythene from prostheses has not been widely considered as a viable design alternative because it limits the flexibility of the prosthesis. Furthermore, without the buffering effect of the polythene, a new problem is introduced, as fractures from ceramic-on-ceramic articulation could occur as well as metal ion release associated with metal-on-metal bearings.[3] Much work has been done instead to improve the quality of the polythene and thus increase the durability of the prosthesis. Increased cross-linking within the polythene structure does appear to increase the wear qualities of the material in total joint arthroplasty; however, the compromise is a reduced fracture toughness, which raises concerns about component failure under extreme stress or prolonged wear.[4] Second-generation highly cross-linked ultra-high-molecular-weight polythene has been developed in which a greater control of the degree of cross-linking during the manufacturing process has been achieved to optimize the qualities of the material.[1] Further advances continue to be made in this area.

Others have concentrated instead on producing bearing surfaces that minimize the volume of debris generated from the polythene component. Traditionally, cobalt-chromium (CoCr) has been used in the femoral component as the material with which the polythene articulates. Oxinium is the brand name of a material manufactured by the reconstructive orthopaedic surgery division of medical devices company Smith & Nephew for use in joint replacement.[3] It consists of a zirconium alloy metal substrate that transitions into a ceramic zirconium oxide outer surface. As a result, it displays the favorable wear qualities of the surface ceramic, but with the damage-resistant qualities of its metallic core. In addition, the biocompatible nature of its constituent metals gives it an advantage over traditional components in the context of metal allergy. Much research has been conducted to evaluate the safety and efficacy of this promising new material, yet its superiority is by no means proved.

CURRENT MANUFACTURING STATE OF THE ART

The manufacturing process of this material reveals much about its inherent advantage as an articulating surface. The Oxinium components are produced from a wrought zirconium alloy (Zr-2.5% Nb), by a process that heats the metal to a temperature of approximately 500°C under specific conditions, allowing oxygen to diffuse into the outer surface of the material. Oxygen is absorbed by the metal, transforming a thin outer layer of the substance (approximately 5 μm thick) to ceramic. The rest of the material remains in its original metallic form to retain its strength.[5] The result is a superior bearing surface that is part of the metal substrate rather than an external coating, making Oxinium very durable, but with an unusually high damage tolerance to its surface.

Oxinium components are currently used in total joint arthroplasy of both the hip and knee. They are indicated for patients undergoing primary or revision surgeries where other treatments or devices have failed, in rehabilitation of joints for trauma, and in inflammatory joint disease or non-inflammatory joint disease (eg, osteoarthritis, avascular necrosis, traumatic arthritis, etc). In particular, these components are recommended for use in younger patients because of the favorable wear properties of the material. The technology was first utilized in total hip arthroplasty prostheses in 1995 and in TKA prostheses in 1997.[5]

MECHANICAL PROPERTIES OF OXINIUM

Abrasion Resistance

Abrasion resistance is dependent on three principal factors: the smoothness of the surface, the hardness or scratch resistance of the material, and the strength of the adhesion between the surface coating and the substrate. The abrasion resistance qualities of Oxinium are well documented in the literature. One study has calculated that the surface of Oxinium is 160 times smoother than cobalt-chromium.[6] It has been demonstrated that Oxinium has levels of micro- and macrosurface hardness superior to both titanium alloys and cobalt-chromium alloys.[7] The results of an adhesion test in one study, which evaluated the strength of the bond between the surface material and the underlying substrate, demonstrated that Oxinium exhibits surface adhesion strength superior to cobalt-chromium and far superior to titanium alloy coated with a titanium nitrate plasma coating.[7] The surface hardness of the Oxinium component, coupled with the strong bonding that exists between the surface ceramic oxide and the metal substrate, help explain the superior abrasion resistance and thus the improved wear rates observed with this material, as compared to cobalt-chromium.

Friction

The coefficient of friction between Oxinium and polythene is significantly lower than that between cobalt-chromium and polythene. This may be partially attributable to the wettable nature of Oxinium. There is evidence to suggest that Oxinium surfaces in vivo tend to become more readily lubricated by synovial fluid, resulting in less friction.[8] The coefficient of friction between Oxinium and polythene was reported as 50% less than that between cobalt-chromium-molybdenum (CoCrMo) and polythene in one particular study which used deionized water as lubricant.[9] There is also evidence to suggest that in total joint arthroplasty the volume of synovial fluid can be significantly diminished and therefore it is conceivable that the wettable quality of Oxinium may confer an even greater improvement in wear characteristics in the context of relatively small volumes of lubricant.[10] One study by Patel and Spector placed a pin of bovine cartilage in contact with discs of both Oxinium and CoCr in constant motion within a bovine serum environment.[11] The paper cited a 30% reduced coefficient of friction for Oxinium compared with CoCr. Whether the Oxinium component is articulated with a polythene implant or with the native cartilage, a reduced rate of friction means less potential for wear and therefore a device that should last longer.

Damage Tolerance

Damage to the surface of femoral components is always a risk. When Oxinium components were subjected to two standard tests (crater and groove tests), they demonstrated an excellent damage tolerance. Absence of chipping or spalling of the surface material around the crater indentation implies strong adhesion of the surface ceramic layer to the underlying metal substrate. This ability to tolerate insults inflicted on the surface of the material ensures that even under extreme conditions, catastrophic failure will not result.[12]

Fatigue Strength

Ceramic materials have a favorable abrasion resistance profile, but ceramic components lack the fatigue strength of metal components. During the manufacture of Oxinium, only the surface of the material is converted to ceramic oxide. The core of the material remains in its metallic form and therefore retains its ability to withstand forces. Oxinium components have been found to support a minimum fatigue load of 1000 lb for 10 million cycles. This is equivalent to a cobalt-chromium femoral component of the same design.[13]

Metal Allergies and Biocompatibility

Between 3% and 8% of the population are estimated to have metal allergies.[14] A rise in the metal ion concentration in a patient's plasma occurs following the implantation of metal components in total joint arthroplasties. Sensitivity to nickel is the most commonly seen allergic complication following arthroplasty, and this is often associated with a cross-sensitivity to cobalt. Metal sensitivity may exclude a candidate for joint replacement with traditional prostheses because of risk of complications. The maximum nickel content of cobalt-chromium can be as high as 1%, whereas nickel levels in Oxinium are undetectable.[15] Oxinium contains 97.5% zirconium and 2.5% niobium, two of the most biocompatible metals available. The biocompatibility of an Oxinium component is considered to be comparable to those made from titanium alloy.[15]

CURRENT AREAS OF USE IN ORTHOPAEDICS

Oxidized zirconium has been adopted into many areas of medicine during the relatively short duration since the material was developed for use in medical instruments. Oxidized zirconium components are frequently utilized in dental implants and middle ear ossicular chain reconstruction. Zirconium compounds and zirconium-containing sorbents have also been widely used in nephrology, primarily for the purpose of filtration (eg, hemofiltration, hemodialysis, peritoneal dialysis, and in artificial kidneys). So far in orthopaedics the technology has only been adopted for hip and knee replacement.

Total Hip Arthroplasty

Although much evidence exists documenting the favorable wear rates of Oxinium in vitro, there are relatively few data on the performance of Oxinium in vivo. Because of the high mortality rate following fracture of the hip, it is difficult to elucidate the clinical benefits of Oxinium hemiarthroplasty. The first total hip arthroplasty (THA) that utilized an Oxinium component was in 1995. Preliminary clinical trials have demonstrated that Oxinium is safe for use in THA. There have been no incidents of accelerated wear or adverse events reported in short-term or mid-term follow-up studies of Oxinium prostheses.[16-18] The data that have been published to date, comparing Oxinium to cobalt-chromium in THA, have been somewhat conflicting. Some short-term and mid-term clinical trials have suggested that Oxinium confers no significant improvement of polythene wear performance.[17,18] There is consensus that Oxinium is a safe, effective alternative to traditional materials used in THA prostheses, but it is clear that further studies are necessary to evaluate the clinical performance of Oxinium in THA over longer periods of time.

Total Knee Arthroplasty

Oxinium components have been used clinically in TKA since 1997.[19] It has proved more difficult to adapt the technology for use in TKA than for THA. So far, the data collected regarding the in vivo effectiveness of Oxinium in TKA remain relatively limited. In particular, there have been no long-term trials published on the clinical efficacy of Oxinium in TKA. Preliminary clinical outcome studies have shown encouraging results. Oxinium has been shown to be safe for use in TKA, with no initial adverse effects observed following implantation.[20,21] The use of Oxinium components has not led to any increase in early failure rates due to early major wear. In one study that examined components retrieved from TKAs that had been revised due to infection, the wear damage in Oxinium knees was seen to be comparable to traditional metal-on-polythene implants.[19] There is evidence emerging from preliminary trials to suggest that, even in the short term, there is an improvement of the clinical performance observed with Oxinium compared to traditional prostheses. As with Oxinium in THA, the predicted advantage of Oxinium over traditional cobalt-chromium is the longevity of the replaced joint. Clinical trials that examine the performance of Oxinium over longer time periods must be performed before the use of this more expensive prosthesis in TKA can be comprehensively evaluated.

HISTORICAL RESULTS

In Vitro Studies

Reducing polythene wear is thought to decrease the risk of implant failure attributed to osteolysis. The abrasion-resistant qualities of Oxinium, coupled with the favorable friction levels when articulated with polythene components, likely contribute to the significantly lower polythene wear rates observed in simulator testing.

Much evidence exists to suggest that in vitro wear rates of Oxinium on polythene are superior to that of cobalt-chromium.[3,8,22,23] The difference is particularly pronounced when the surface of the femoral heads is deliberately abraded, reflecting a clinically relevant condition. In one particular in vitro study, which compared Oxinium femoral heads with cobalt-chromium femoral heads under similar conditions, the Oxinium head produced 27% less polythene wear when both heads were smooth and 61% less wear when both heads were in the roughened state.[3] The wear rates of roughened Oxinium femoral heads have been shown to be similar to the wear rates observed with undamaged cobalt-chromium heads.

Wear particles produced by articulating components within the joint may increase the potential for debris-induced osteolysis and aseptic loosening. It is believed that Oxinium components tend to produce less wear particles than cobalt-chromium. Other ceramic materials may have a similar effect in reducing wear, but unfortunately these materials are brittle and difficult to manufacture. Components made entirely of ceramic have been shown to be susceptible to catastrophic fracture.[17] The metal substrate of the Oxinium implant makes the component easier to manufacture and gives it greater toughness (a combination of strength and ductility). The advantages of this quality are certainly evident in THA, where it becomes possible to produce smaller femoral head components, which confer a direct improvement in wear performance.[16] In essence, this technology combines the abrasion resistance and low friction of a ceramic with the workability and toughness of a metal.

Given the increased looseness of the knee joint compared to the hip and the ploughing and rolling motion of knee kinematics, it is not unreasonable to doubt that the favorable results of Oxinium femoral heads in hip simulators might not be transferable to the knee. Spector et al compared the CoCr and Oxinium forms of the Genesis II prosthesis in a knee simulator for 6 million cycles, combining both gait and stair-climbing actions.[8] Polythene wear was evaluated via the weight loss experienced and through analysis of the particles produced. This study found an 85% reduced aggregate wear rate for Oxinium compared to CoCr. In addition, although it was not statistically significant, they found that Oxinium produced no more and perhaps fewer submicrometer-sized particles than CoCr, which has great implications for the rate of osteolysis in vivo. The authors also make the observation that whereas the CoCr femoral components demonstrated increasing number of scratches on inspection as the simulation proceeded, the Oxinium components remained visually pristine. This they felt reflected the superior counterface roughness of the material and was consistent with the posttest roughness of the components. Ezzet et al found similar results, with a 42% reduction in polythene wear with an Oxinium femoral component compared to a CoCr component.[24] The study also draws attention to the inherent difficulty in comparing the two materials in this manner. Although gravimetric estimates of polythene wear are straightforward, there is a danger of overestimating volumetric wear because of the phenomenon of volumetric creep (ie, the surface distortion of polythene inserts unique to each subject). Similarly, a study by White et al favored the wear-resistant qualities of Oxinium in comparison to traditional materials.[23] Again a significantly reduced level of polythene wear was reported following 2 million cycles in a knee simulator with varying axial loads. The surface of the cobalt-chromium became increasingly roughened as the simulation proceeded as expected, but the Oxinium components retained their hard ceramic surface. Another study by Ries et al compared femoral components that had been subjected to an abrasive tumbling procedure before testing in a knee simulator in order to resemble a clinically relevant condition. The findings showed a 44% reduction in the number of polythene particles produced by Oxinium relative to CoCr.[25]

In Vivo Studies

Despite favorable results of the Oxinium components in vitro, there is a relatively small body of data outlining the efficacy of Oxinium in TKA in vivo. Heyse et al published a study in 2009 on 16 femoral Oxinium components that had been retrieved from patients during revision for indications that included stiffness, infection, instability, and dislocation.[19] The authors report that there were no failures directly related to the implant in the cohort studied. The findings of the study are limited by the short duration that the components were in situ (mean duration 16.4 months); however, it was significant that even in components in which the zirconia on the femoral component had been damaged, the level of polythene abrasion and wear particle formation was much less than expected given the findings of similar studies which had looked exclusively at CoCr components. The data presented in the study demonstrated no increased levels of polythene wear compared to that of traditional prostheses. The authors highlight in their discussion the need for a comparative study with a matched group of traditional CoCr components.

In contrast to the findings of studies mentioned earlier regarding the production of polythene wear particles in vitro, a study by Kim et al disputes the transference of this quality in vivo. In Kim's study the polythene wear products produced in 100 patients who had received both a CoCr knee and an Oxinium knee were analysed using gravimetric analysis and scanning electron microscopy in vivo. The results revealed no significant difference between the weight, size, and shape of particles produced.[26] An important randomized control trial performed at an Australian institution compared Oxinium and CoCr components in 40 bilateral cruciate-retaining total knee arthroplasties. At 5 years there was no significant difference found between the Oxinium and CoCr either clinically or on radiological evaluation. However, of the four knees that were retrieved, the Oxinium components demonstrated significantly less wear than the CoCr components, as corelated with in vitro studies. The author concludes that routine use of the more expensive Oxinum component is not justified on the basis of these study findings, outside of the context of metal sensitivity.[27]

A prospective, randomized, controlled trial by Laskin in 2003 reported on the safety of the Oxinium at 2 years.[21] The author hypothesized that given the decreased coefficient of friction with Oxinium, a greater range of motion in the knee postarthroplasty may result. Although there was no significant difference found between the range of passive flexion reached by the Oxinium and CoCr components, a more rapid return of flexion as well as functional milestones were observed in the Oxinium knees. The study had also found that even when a strip of the oxidized surface was purposely removed before abrasion testing, the surrounding ceramic did not spall or chip away at an increased rate, reflecting the strong adherence between the surface and the substrate. An important paper from 2005 by Laskin and Davis demonstrated an encouraging 5-year survival rate that was comparable to traditional prostheses. Also, in the small cohort of patients who had reached the 6- and 7-year mark, the results were similarly positive.[28]

HISTORICAL COMPONENT FAILURE REVIEW

Catastrophic failure of ceramic components in total joint arthroplasty has been described in the literature.[17] The brittle nature of the ceramic belies an inherent weakness that, under extreme or persistent strain, has been shown to result in disruption of the integrity of the component. In Oxinium, this problem is believed to have been overcome by the favorable characteristics of the component imparted to it by its tough metallic core. And certainly in the short- to medium-term follow up, this does appear to be the case. A follow-up study by Bourne et al in 2007 demonstrated a Kaplan-Meier survivorship of 96% ± 2% at the 12-year mark in the first 100 consecutive TKRs that had utilized the Oxinium Genesis II prostheses.[29]

As of yet there are no published data outlining the failure of Oxinium components in TKA and there is a growing volume of data supporting the safety of the components in the short- to medium-term range. However, many papers have suggested a potentially worrying finding in Oxinium components used in THA.[30-32] Recurrent dislocation of the femoral head has been noted to result in visible damage to the zirconia surface, revealing the metallic core beneath. It appears that damage to Oxinium at the time of initial implantation could potentially result in a spoiled articulating surface prone to greatly increased wear. Similarly, in the study by Heyse et al that examined retrieved Oxinium components from TKA, a significant degree of damage was noted in the femoral components as a result of the retrieval process.[19] The authors note that this is a worrying finding and speculate on the danger of intraoperative metal-on-ceramic contact during the insertion of the prostheses.

Another in vitro study published by Burnell et al in 2011 presented the results of wear tests comparing retrieved CoCr and Oxinium TKA components.[33] The components in this case all had posterior condyle surface damage due to femoral and tibial bearing surfaces coming into direct contact. The findings of the paper again demonstrated the superior resistance of Oxinium to third-body abrasive wear in comparison to CoCr. Although on scanning electron microscopy the Oxinium components appeared to have incurred more damage than the CoCr components at the point of contact with the titanium tibial baseplates, the surface surrounding the initial scratch on the components showed far less secondary damage compared to CoCr. There was no evidence of the hypothesized delamination or chipping of the oxide along the edges of the scratches. As with other studies mentioned, the authors warn of the dangers of damage occurring from contact between the Oxinium surface and the other metal components or instruments at the time of insertion. Currently, Smith & Nephew recommend the use of a temporary plate cover to be placed over the tibial tray at the time of insertion of the Oxinium component to avoid such damage.[5]

CONCLUSION

Because of the superior wear properties of Oxinium, at least in vitro, this bearing surface has been considered ideal for young and active patients in whom wear is a very important issue. In addition, because of the absence of detectable nickel, Oxinium is thought to be an effective alternative to the traditional cobalt-chromium for patients with nickel (metal) allergy. It remains to be seen if the favorable mechanical properties of Oxinium will confer a significant improvement of longevity of the replaced joint in the clinical setting. The results of early trials confirm that Oxinium is a safe and effective material for use in total joint arthroplasty.

REFERENCES

1. Hidaka C, Maher S, Packer J, et al. What's new in orthopaedic research? *J Bone Joint Surg Am.* 2009;91: 2756-2770.
2. Cadambi A, Engh GA, Dwyer KA, et al. Osteolysis of the distal femur after total knee arthroplasty. *J Arthroplasty.* 1994;9:579-594.
3. Good V, Ries M, Barrack RL, et al. Reduced wear with oxidized zirconium femoral heads. *J Bone Joint Surg Am.* 2003;85:105-110.
4. Bradford L, Baker D, Ries MD, et al. Fatigue crack propagation resistance of highly crosslinked polyethylene. *Clin Orthop Relat Res.* 2004;429:68-72.
5. Oxinium. Surgeon information. Smith-Nephew.co.uk. 2003-2005.
6. Hunter G, Long M. Abrasive wear of oxidized Zr-2.5Nb, CoCrMo, and Ti-6Al-4V against bone cement. *6th World Biomaterials Congress Transactions.* Minneapolis, MN: Society for Biomaterials; 2000:835.
7. Galetz MC, Fleischmann EW, Konrad CH, et al. Abrasion resistance of oxidized zirconium in comparison with CoCrMo and titanium nitride coatings for artificial knee joints. *J Biomed Mater Res B Appl Biomater.* 2010;93(1):244-251.
8. Spector BM, Ries MD, Bourne RB, et al. Wear performance of ultra-high molecular weight polyethylene on oxidized zirconium total knee femoral components. *J Bone Joint Surg Am.* 2001;83(suppl 2):80-86.
9. Poggie RA, Wert JJ, Mishra AK, et al. Friction and wear characterization of UHMWPE in reciprocating sliding contact with Co-Cr, Ti-6Al-4V and zirconia implant bearing surfaces. In: Denton R, Keshavan MK, eds. *Wear and Friction of Elastomers*, ASTM STP 1145. Philadelphia, PA: American Society for Testing and Materials; 1992:65-81.
10. Mazzucco DC, McKinley GH, Scott RD, et al. Rheology of synovial fluid before and after total knee arthroplasty. *Trans Soc Biomater.* 2001;24:134.
11. Patel AM, Spector M. Tribiological evaluation of oxidized Zircinium using an articular cartilage counterface: a novel material for potential use in hemiarthroplasty. *Biomaterials.* 1997;18:441-447.
12. Hunter G. Adhesion testing of oxidized zirconium. *Trans. Soc. Biomater.* 2001;24:540.
13. Tsai S, Sprague J, Hunter G, et al. Mechanical testing and finite element analysis of oxidized zirconium femoral components. *Trans. Soc. Biomater.* 2001;24:163.
14. Hallab NJ, Merritt K, Jacobs JJ. Metal sensitivity in patients with orthopaedic implants. *J Bone Joint Surg Am.* 2001;83:428-436.
15. Hunter G, Jones WM, Spector M, et al., eds. Oxidized zirconium. In: *Total Knee Arthroplasty.* Heidelberg, Germany: Springer-Verlag; 2005:370-377.
16. Kim Y-H. Comparison of polyethylene wear associated with cobalt-chromium and zirconia heads after total hip replacement: a prospective, randomized study. *J Bone Joint Surg Am.* 2005;87:1769-1776.
17. Koshino T, Okamoto R, Takagi T, et al. Cemented ceramic YMCK total knee arthroplasty in patients with severe rheumatoid arthritis. *J Arthroplasty.* 2002; 17:1009.
18. Lewis PM, Moore CA, Olsen M, et al. Comparison of mid-term clinical outcomes after primary total hip arthroplasty with Oxinium vs cobalt chrome femoral heads. *Orthopedics.* 2008;31(12 suppl 2):ii. orthosupersite.com/view.asp?rID=37183.
19. Heyse TJ, Davis J, Haas SB, et al. Retrieval analysis of femoral zirconium components in total knee arthroplasty: preliminary results. *J Arthroplasty.* 2011;26 (3):445-450.
20. Innocenti M, Civinini R, Carulli C, et al. The 5-year results of an oxidized zirconium femoral component for TKA. *Clin Orthop Relat Res.* 2010;468(5):1258-1263.
21. Laskin RS, Davis J. Total knee replacement using the Genesis II prosthesis: a 5-year follow up study of the first 100 consecutive cases. *Knee.* 2005;12:163-167.
22. Bourne RB, Barrack R, Rorabec CH, et al. Arthroplasty options for the young patient: Oxinium on cross-linked polyethylene. *Clin Orthop Relat Res.* 2005;441:159-167.
23. White SE, Whiteside LA, McCarthy DS, et al. Simulated knee wear with cobalt chromium and oxidized zirconium knee femoral components. *Clin Orthop Relat Res.* 1994;309:176-184.
24. Ezzet KA, Hermida JC, Colwell CW Jr, et al. Oxidized zirconium femoral components reduce polyethylene wear in a knee wear simulator. *Clin Orthop Relat Res.* 2004;428:120-124.
25. Ries MD, Salehi A, Widding K, et al. Polyethylene wear performance of oxidized zirconium and cobalt-chromium knee components under abrasive conditions. *J Bone Joint Surg Am.* 2002;84:129-135.

26. Kim YH, Kim JS, Huh W, et al. Weight of polyethylene wear particles is similar in TKAs with oxidized zirconium and cobalt-chrome prostheses. *Clin Orthop Relat Res.* 2010;468(5):1296-304.
27. Hui C, Salmon L, Maeno S, et al. Five-year comparison of oxidized zirconium and cobalt-chromium femoral components in total knee arthroplasty: a randomized controlled trial. *J Bone Joint Surg Am.* 2011;93(7):624-630.
28. Laskin RS, Davis J. Total knee replacement using the Genesis II prosthesis: a 5-year follow up study of the first 100 consecutive cases. *Knee.* 2005;12:163-167.
29. Bourne RB, Laskin RS, Guerin JS. Ten-year results of the first 100 Genesis II total knee replacement procedures. *Orthopedics.* 2007;30(8 suppl):83-85.
30. Evangelista GT, Fulkerson E, Kummer F, et al. Surface damage to an Oxinium femoral head prosthesis after dislocation. *J Bone Joint Surg Br.* 2007;89(4):535-537.
31. Kop AM, Whitewood C, Johnston DJ. Damage of Oxinium femoral heads subsequent to hip arthroplasty diclocation. *J Arthroplasty.* 2007;22(5):775-779.
32. Jaffe WL, Strauss EJ, Cardinale M, et al. Surface oxidized zirconium total hip arthroplasty head damage due to closed reduction: effects on polyethylene wear. *J Arthroplasty.* 2009;24(6):898-902.
33. Burnell CD, Brandt JM, Petrak MJ, et al. Posterior condyle surface damage on retrieved femoral knee components. *J Arthroplasty.* 2011;26(8):1460-1467.

14 Ultra-High-Molecular-Weight Polyethylene

Luigi Costa and Elena M. Brach del Prever

Ultra-high-molecular-weight polyethylene (UHMWPE, also PE) was identified as possible bearing material and was subsequently introduced into total hip arthroplasty by Sir John Charnley in the 1960s, after catastrophic failures and early and excessive wear of the first polymer used, the polytetrafluoroethylene (PTFE), were reported. At the beginning of the third millennium, UHMWPE still represents the gold standard as an articulating counterface for total joint replacements (TJR). Because of its high molecular weight [in TJR usually 4 million amu (atomic mass unit)], it combines superior wear resistance along with high fracture toughness, good biocompatibility, and limited costs compared to other biomaterials. However, this is not a common feeling in the orthopaedic community, because in the recent past, in particular in the 1990s, numerous and unacceptable early failures of TJR due to severe wear and fracture of PE were observed. Now, it is clear that the main factor responsible for these catastrophic failures was not the insufficient mechanical properties of UHMWPE, but its oxidative degradation caused by final gamma sterilization in air. As has been well known from many years, high-energy radiation in air (gamma radiation and electron beam) causes excessive and unpredictable oxidation of the polymer, resulting in the scission of the chains, decreased molecular weight, insufficient mechanical properties, and consequent failure in vivo.[1,2] This is why ethylene oxide (EtO) and gas plasma-sterilized UHMWPE components maintain their chemical-physical properties, high biomechanical resistance, and good performance in vivo (Fig. 14-1).

During the 1990s, an effort to understand why UHMWPE was subject to failure was initiated via analysis of retrieved components. It was also during this time that many industries encouraged the orthopaedic surgeon to use alternative bearing materials such as ceramics and metals. These alternative bearing surfaces were associated with higher costs, different biomechanical characteristics, and new unknown problems in vivo. Furthermore, new UHMWPEs were subsequently introduced, such as highly cross-linked (X-PE) and vitamin E-stabilized UHMWPE (vitE-PE). However, once again it was demonstrated that the introduction of "new" biomaterials not supported by proper research can be negative for the patient and all the scientific community. In the recent past, a type of X-PE, unfortunately sterilized by gamma radiation in air, demonstrated failure similar to that observed with the previous version of standard UHMWPE.

The aim of this chapter is to define the standard UHMWPE and its new variants such as X-PE and vitE-PE, why and in which conditions they are good biomaterials for TJR, why some PE components failed in the past (or could still be at risk of failure at present, if not correctly processed), and where the research is heading. Our final goal is to help the orthopaedic surgeon choose the implants and PE components as well as properly educate the patient.

HISTORY

The first polyethylene was obtained in Great Britain in the early 1930s by radical polymerization of ethylene at high pressure (200–300 MPa) and high temperature

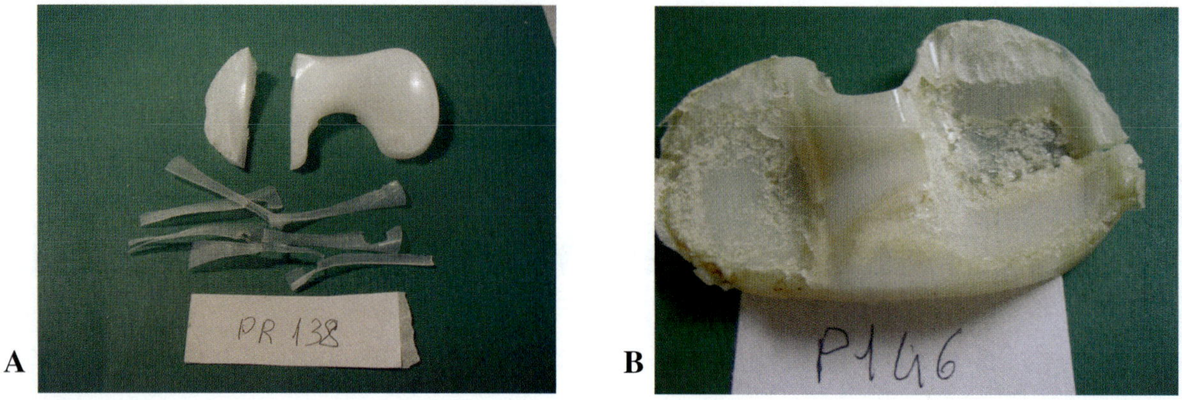

FIGURE 14-1. *(**A**) UHMWPE tibial plateau, EtO sterilized, retrieved after 16 years of service in vivo. Oxidation was absent. (**B**) UHMWPE tibial plateau sterilized by gamma ray in air retrieved after 6 years of service in vivo. Oxidative wear is clearly observed.*

(150°C–200°C). The resulting polymer had a high number of imperfections in the chain. Volumetric mass was low and density was 0.915 to 0.930 g/cc; to date, this type of polyethylene commercially is known as low-density polyethylene (LDPE). The first almost completely linear PE, with a density around 0.955 g/cc, was obtained by the Phillips Petroleum researchers. In the early 1950s, Ziegler and colleagues accidentally discovered that higher density PE (0.945–0.960 g/cc) could be obtained by using a catalytic system using titanium halides and alkyl aluminium, at low pressure and low temperatures (50°C–100°C). The name of this PE is high-density polyethylene (HDPE) or linear PE, with a molecular mass between 30,000 and 450,000 amu. If during polymerization with metallic catalysts a pure ethylene is used, the resulting polymer has a higher molecular mass as compared with that of HDPE, somewhere between 500,000 and 1,000,000 amu. This material is called high-molecular-weight polyethylene (HMWPE). If the molecular mass is more than 1,000,000 amu (generally it is more than 2,000,000 amu), then it takes the name of ultra-high-molecular-weight polyethylene.

UHMWPE is not only used in orthopaedics. It is found in industries that manufacture, among others items, screws, cogwheels, chain guides, pulleys, silo lining, ship-hold lining, and conveyor belts in mining. Thanks to the very high tensile yield strength of its fibers (obtained by gel spinning, which gives it a yield strength greater than steel wire), it is also used in military applications and as a liner for bulletproof jackets. All of these applications are based on the mechanical properties of UHMWPE as well as its resistance to abrasion.

Sir John Charnley, in the 1960s, used HDPE; in 1980 ASTM F648-80, the characteristic of UHMWPE for orthopaedic use, was defined. From then on, the UHMWPE has continued to be used all over the world. In the recent past, new modified and eventually improved UHMWPEs were introduced into the marketplace: X-PE and vitE-PE. Their clinical results are currently being compared to the original UHMWPE, still the golden standard for TJR.

MATERIAL USED IN UHMWPE

Polyethylene is a polymer obtained from ethylene polymerization, a gas produced by thermal decomposition of petroleum. The molecules of the ethylene monomer, joined to each other by a chemical process called polymerization, form the polymer chain of PE:

$$n\,CH_2{=}CH_2 \rightarrow \sim(CH_2{-}CH_2)_n\sim$$

The linear macromolecules of PE are generally described with the formula $\sim(CH_2{-}CH_2)_n\sim$ where n is the degree of polymerization (ie, the number of units of ethylene that make up the polymer chain). PE, like all polymeric materials, has a complex structure. Consider, for example, that in 1 g of UHMWPE there are slightly less than 10^{18} macromolecules, that is, a billion of billion big molecules. The degree of polymerization is not the same for each chain, but varies from chain to chain owing to the complexity of the polymerization process. Since there are numerous chains in the sample, the average degree of polymerization is defined.

This is characterized by a fairly broad distribution depending on the process that polymerized the monomer.

The word *polyethylene* is used in reference to quite a few polymeric materials, all characterized by the same structural unit, but having macromolecules of different lengths and different structures. The main characteristics that describe PE and, therefore, identify the type are molecular mass and crystallinity. The mechanical properties of the components under study depend on these chemical-physical aspects.

Molecular mass (MM), measured in amu, is the product of molecular mass of the structural unit [the ethylene residue in the polymeric chain, $(\sim CH_2–CH_2\sim)_n$, 28 amu] multiplied by the degree of polymerization n. Since n is an average value, the MM of the polymer is also an average value. The "plastic" bag used for shopping is composed of polyethylene of an average polymerization of about 2000, equivalent to an average molecular mass of about 56,000 amu. The polyethylene used in arthroprosthesis, UHMWPE, has an average molecular mass of 4 million amu.

Material crystallinity is defined as the percentage of weight of the crystalline phase as compared to the whole polymer (ie, compared to the sum of the amorphous and crystalline phases). At an equal percentage of crystallinity, the number of interactions for polymer molecules is a function of the molecular mass. The higher the molecular mass, the more numerous are the interactions between molecules for each individual polymer chain.

The crystallinity of UHMWPE, used in orthopaedics, varies between 45% and 60%. This value correlates to the difficulties encountered by the macromolecules in organizing themselves into crystallites during the cooling process owing to their length and, consequently, to their high viscosity.

In the crystalline phase, the macromolecules, packed into crystallites, take up less space than those in the amorphous state, when they are untidily laid out; therefore, the mass per unit of volume in the crystalline phase is greater than in the amorphous state. The chains are not well packed in the amorphous state so there is some uninterrupted free space (continuous free volume) within which the macromolecules can partially move.

During the amorphous phase, not only can small gaseous molecules diffuse, but also molecules of larger size having flexible linear chains. The diffusion penetration is a function of molecular mass and the temperature. It has been pointed out that the diffused products in the prosthetic components are mostly squalene (a cholesterol precursor), cholesterol, and cholesteryl esters with fatty acids and triglycerides, whose relative amount is highly variable depending on the patient.[3]

MECHANICAL PROPERTIES OF UHMWPE AND TESTING

The chemical-physical characteristics, in particular molecular mass and crystallinity, determine the mechanical properties of the polymeric material.[4] The mechanical properties of a material are evaluated experimentally, for instance, by traction tests: a sample is stretched at a predetermined stretching speed. UHMWPE samples react when they undergo stress by a variable load (eg, to supply a constant stretching speed). When a force or a load is applied to a material, an equally intense force is generated inside the material itself, but in the opposite direction, which opposes the former. Force applied to polyethylene causes the polymer to change its chemical-physical characteristics and, therefore, its mechanical properties. UHMWPE has a good tensile yield strength and ultimate tensile strength, optimum resilience, and high resistance to wear. It has optimum mechanical properties, which is why it has been chosen as the coupling material in TJR. The problem of friction between the two surfaces in contact (ie, the femoral head and the acetabular components or between the femoral component and the tibial component) is of utmost importance. Friction is correlated to material wear according to a complex process regulated by many factors.

Abrasion, or abrasion wear, is the complex process of removal of parts of polymeric prosthetic material from the surface during reciprocal movement against materials with greater hardness. Whereas the "oxidative wear" due to sterilization with high-energy radiation must be avoided (see section on sterilization), the abrasion wear can only be reduced but not eliminated because it is related to gravity and reciprocal movement.

UHMWPE abrasion occurs during joint movement: the PE liner is abraded by the metal or ceramic prosthetic femoral head or the PE tibial component is abraded by the metallic femoral condyle. Although the articular surfaces are processed and finished to the smoothest possible degree, there are still imperfections at micrometric level. Therefore, joint movement over time leads to the removal of parts of the material that have lower resistance to abrasion. The abrasion properties of polymeric materials depend on many factors, one of which is the molecular mass: the higher the molecular mass, the lower the abrasions. This is why X-PE has increased resistance to abrasion. The international standards governing the quality control and testing are directed at the chemical-physical and mechanical properties of the raw material and not aimed at the sterilized and finished product.

CURRENT MANUFACTURING STATE OF THE ART IN PROSTHETIC COMPONENTS

Process

Many companies produce UHMWPE, but today, Ticona is the exclusive producer of UHMWPE for orthopaedic use with the trade name GUR. UHMWPE leaves the factory in powder form. It cannot be press-molded in the normal manner used to work thermoplastic materials (LDPE, HDPE, polypropylene, polystyrene, etc) because, although it melts below 145°C, its melted form is highly viscose due to its very high molecular mass.

There are two techniques to work powdered UHMWPE, both of which use high pressure: compression molding and ram extrusion. The first can be carried out in two ways by synthesizing the powder into its final shape, first hot and then cold, and, if necessary, incorporating a machined finish. The second one is to compress the melted powder into large sheets by high-pressure compression following controlled heating and cooling cycles. Rectangular sectioned bars are cut out of the sheet, which are then machined to obtain the desired finished product. Ram extrusion of the melted powder produces circular sectioned bars that can be processed to obtain the finished prosthetic component.

The process to transform powder into sheets and bars for orthopaedic use is carried out at a worldwide level by a few specialized firms owing to the complexity of the process and the need to use UHMWPE having low pollutant values. Compression-molded prosthetic components in UHMWPE, usually tibial components, are produced directly by the firms that sell them.

The required characteristics of UHMWPE for use in orthopaedics are regulated by Standard ASTM F648-10a (Table 14-1). Except for the density, there are no prescribed maximum limits governing the other characteristics. As a result, the UHMWPE can have different initial characteristics, whether chemical-physical or mechanical. It must be noted, however, that determination is prescribed and carried out on the original material before it is either compressed or extruded and before sterilization.

Sterilization

Before in vivo implant, the material must be adequately sterilized on the surface. This limitation is irrelevant in the case of prosthetic PE, which does not require sterilization in depth since the components come from the sheets which have undergone treatment at temperatures higher than 200°C. Furthermore, because of their dimensions, bacteria cannot penetrate and spread into the polymeric mass. Sterilization by steam is not feasible since the treatment implies high temperatures (about 135°C), which would modify the piece dimension. The main processes used today employ ethylene oxide and gas plasma; until recently, sterilization was obtained by high-energy radiation (ie, gamma rays and electron beam).

TABLE 14-1. Requirements for UHMWPE Fabricated Forms

Properties	Type 1 (GUR 1020)	Type 2 (GUR 1050)
Density, kg/m^3	927–944	927–944
Ash, mg/kg (maximum)	125	125
Tensile strength 23°, MPa (minimum)		
Ultimate	40	40
Yield	21	19
Elongation, % (minimum)	380	340
Izod impact strength, kJ/m^2 (minimum)	126	73
Charpy impact strength, kJ/m^2 (minimum)	180	90

Sterilization using ethylene oxide

Prosthetic components in PE, stored in gas-permeable vacuum packages, are treated with EtO for as long as it takes the gas to diffuse inside the package. These now sterilized packages are left under vacuum to eliminate the ethylene oxide from the packages. At room temperature, ethylene oxide is a gas that quickly diffuses inside the container and into the interfaces of polyethylene, ceramics, and metal, with or without hydroxyapatite lining. It does not diffuse into the metallic and ceramic materials, but it slowly diffuses into the polymeric matrix; therefore, it only sterilizes the surface but does not interfere with the polyethylene molecules.

Sterilization with gas plasma

As in sterilization with EtO, the sterilization with gas plasma is done in permeable vacuum packages. Inside of the sterilization box, hydrogen peroxide or peracetic acid is introduced and, after diffusion in the prosthetic component box, is decomposed by plasma in free radicals OH°. These radicals react and inactivate the bacteria.

Sterilization using gamma rays

The lethal effect of high-energy radiation on microorganisms was immediately clear when Roentgen discovered X-rays in 1895. ^{60}Co is a radioisotope frequently used to make, even highly powerful, irradiators. The dose absorbed by the material during sterilization, according to ASTM and ISO norm, must be more than 25 kGy. Because the dose rate is of the order of some kGy/h, the total time of irradiation is generally more than 5 hours. The quantity absorbed depends on the geometry of the sample and on its position in relation with the source; therefore, it is common practice to submit the sample to more than one pass so as to reach as uniform absorption as possible.

Sterilization using electron beams (also incorrectly called "beta rays")

Electron beam (e-beam) sterilization is a fairly recent procedure. Electrons, produced by thermally exciting a tungsten filament, are accelerated by magnetic fields up to 10 MeV and then conveyed on the material to be sterilized. The advantages of this method are the fairly easy control of the apparatus and the very short period of treatment.

Sterilization by high-energy radiation (gamma ray and electron beam)

Gamma ray and e-beam produce energy at several orders of magnitude greater than that of the chemical bonds of polyethylene. Current literature has given ample demonstration that gamma ray and e-beam treatment triggers a degradation process which causes bond fragmentation and the formation of macroradicals. Degradation always brings variation to the mechanical properties of the polymeric material, easily observed when the degraded PE component is implanted in vivo under biomechanical stress. This is the reason why severe and unpredictable failures due to high-energy degradation (or oxidative wear) were observed in the recent past. To avoid this, the prosthetic components in UHMWPE are sterilized with EtO or gas plasma.

Unfortunately, in the recent past, the sterilization process was mainly based on the economic aspect (using gamma ray and electron beam), without any great consideration given to the likelihood that the chemical-physical characteristics of the material may undergo change. This lack of control was possible since the international standards governing this field are directed at the chemical-physical and mechanical properties of the raw material and not at the sterilized and finished product.

The macroradicals, produced by the high-energy radiation treatment, can react with the molecules (oxygen, chain defects, and additives) present into the amorphous phase of the UHMWPE. When alkyl macroradicals react with oxygen, they induce oxidation; with vinyl double bonds, they produce cross-linking; and with antioxidant additives (as vitamin E), they reduce the oxidation process (Scheme 14-1).

Oxidation Process and Critical Products

As already pointed out, polyethylenes are only partly crystalline polymeric materials. The crystalline portion is extremely compact, which is why it is highly unlikely that foreign molecules, other than very small ones such as hydrogen and helium whose molecular diameter is about 0.2 nm, may penetrate the space (about 0.45 nm) between the polymeric chains. The amorphous portion on the contrary is less compact and has continuous free volume between the different chain segments.

Oxygen, already present in the amorphous polymeric bulk, can only be eliminated by keeping the sample under high dynamic vacuum for the same amount of time as it took to saturate it. Therefore, oxygen is always present in the UHMWPE components.

The oxidation process is the reaction of alkyl macroradicals with oxygen. Many products are formed: ketones and hydroperoxides (ROOH) are the primary products of oxidation; hydroperoxides, being unstable, easily decompose giving rise to new macroradicals, which can continue the oxidation process.[2]

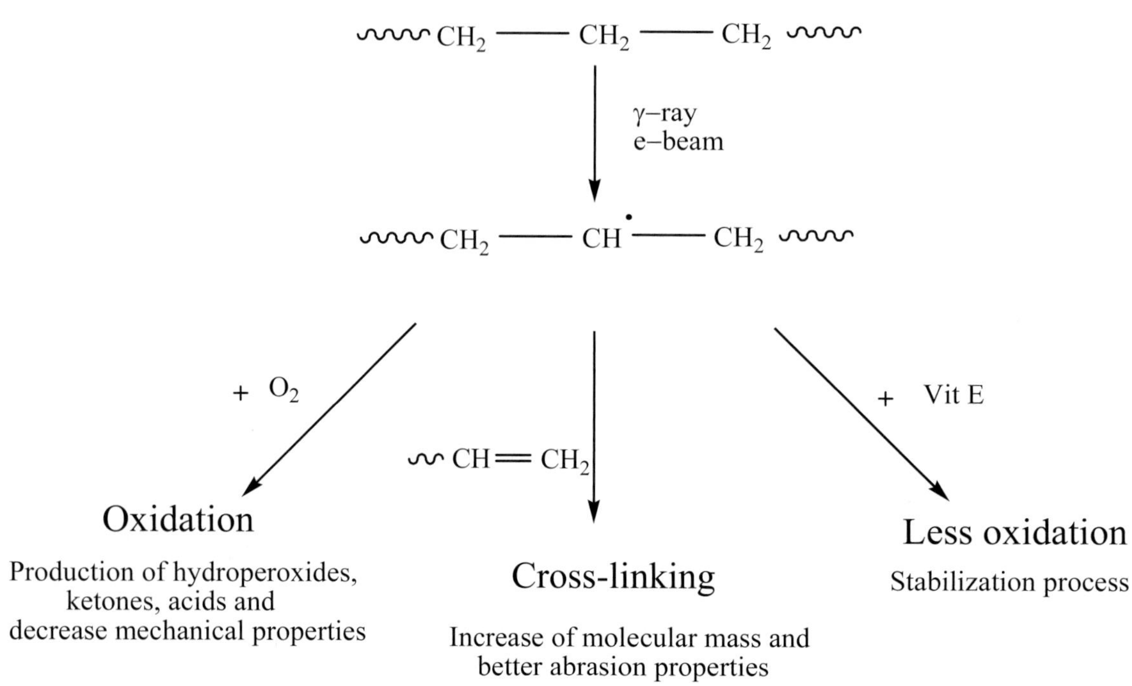

SCHEME 14-1. *Irradiation process of UHMWPE induced by gamma ray and e-beam treatment.*[2]

The orthopaedic literature in the 1990s reported the quantity of ketones present as an index of the degree of oxidation. It must be pointed out, however, that ketones, a product of the oxidative process, do not derive from polymeric chain splitting, and so consistent variations of the mechanical properties cannot be correlated with ketone content. From this perspective, ketones cannot be used as an index of variations in the mechanical properties of the material under investigation. Carboxylic acids (R-COOH) are the products arising from chain scission followed by oxidation. Their presence in the polymer confirms a decrease of its molecular mass and consequently a deterioration in the chemical, physical, and mechanical properties.

Cross-Linked UHMWPEs

The cross-linked UHMWPE is normal PE in which the polymeric chains are connected by a chemical bond, determining an infinite molecular mass. Cross-linking of UHMWPE is obtained by reaction between vinyl double bonds and alkyl macroradicals. Vinyl double bonds are present in virgin UHMWPE; macroradicals are produced by irradiation with high energy.

The chemical-physical characteristics of a cross-linked polymeric material, because of the chemical bonds linking the polymer chains together, are different from those of the analogous polymer composed of linear chains. The different mechanical properties are a function of the degree of cross-linking. With an increased degree of cross-linking, the tensile yield strength increases and the elongation at break point decreases; thus, the elastic modulus increases (ie, the material becomes more rigid).[4] This is why some authors have concerns regarding the use of some types of X-PE in the knee, where the biomechanics are more complex.

New UHMWPEs Stabilized to Oxidation: Vitamin E Added to PE

Most polymers are easily subjected to the oxidative processes, which strongly compromises their mechanical and aesthetic characteristics. In the first years of industrial production of polymers, one of the main goals of the manufacturers was the complete understanding of the mechanisms of oxidation, of polyolefins in particular, and the development of effective strategies of stabilization.[5]

To stabilize the polyethylene, the addition of a reactive species is required. The additive (ADH) reacts with the polymeric macroradical (alkyl or peroxy), giving a kinetically and thermodynamically stable radical (AD•) and a saturated macromolecule.

The more stable the AD• radical, the more the oxidation process is slowed down. Therefore, all commercial polyethylene is commonly stabilized to oxidation with specific additives for each application.

Despite this evidence, ASTM F648 and ISO 5834 standards forbid the use of any additive in orthopaedic UHMWPE. The ban dates back to the early 1980s, when some of the additives used in polymer stabilization were suspected carcinogenic products (eg, aromatic amines for ultraviolet stabilization). The choice to forbid dangerous substances into medical UHMWPE was obviously understandable because the additives can potentially diffuse into the human body during in vivo implantation. It is worth mentioning that the first dramatic failures of UHMWPE components in the mid-1980s were attributed to inadequate mechanical properties of the original polymer, despite the evidence that these properties, in pristine UHMWPE, were much better than those required by ASTM F648.

In the 1990s, some researchers showed that a biocompatible stabilizer could have been useful, or even necessary, to stabilize orthopaedic UHMWPE. α-Tocopherol (synthetic vitamin E) is the most widely used among natural stabilizers. Its mechanisms of stabilization have been widely studied in polymers processing, and it has been shown to be more effective when compared with other commercial additives. Vitamin E, an apolar molecule that is the most important lipid-soluble antioxidant in humans, is not synthesized in the human body, but it is acquired by nourishment. Vitamin E is emulsified together with the fat-soluble components of the food and transported in the body. Lipolysis and emulsification of the formed lipid droplets then lead to the spontaneous formation of mixed micelles.[6]

Vitamin E is soluble in UHMWPE (around 3% by weight at room temperature), while it is insoluble in water and in the synovial fluid, and therefore it cannot be drawn out from the UHMWPE prosthetic components. UHMWPE films with 0.5% of vitamin E irradiated in air at 100 kGy after 60 days in water at 70°C do not show loss of vitamin E or degradation products. This behavior is similar, but in an opposite way, to the diffusion of the apolar products present in the synovial fluid.

According to the results obtained using norms EN 30993-5, DIN UA 12, and in vivo animal tests reported in the literature,[7] vitamin E and its products of oxydegradation are biocompatible and not cytotoxic. In the 2007 ASTM designation (F2695-07), the use of vitamin E as an additive of UHMWPE is introduced. There are two methods of incorporating vitamin E into the UHMWPE. One is to blend vitamin E powder before consolidation at a concentration around 0.1%. Once consolidated, the blend can be cross-linked using high-energy radiation. The presence of vitamin E in UHMWPE during irradiation protects the polymers from oxidation but reduces the efficiency of the cross-linking while the vitamin E itself is reacted; therefore, the vitamin E concentration and the subsequent radiation dose can be optimized to obtain a simultaneously wear- and oxidation-resistant UHMWPE. The alternative method is the diffusion of vitamin E into UHMWPE after the irradiation cross-linking. The cross-linking efficiency is not adversely affected in this method, since vitamin E is not present during irradiation. The polymer remains unprotected against oxidation during irradiation and after storage, until vitamin E is incorporated. Furthermore, a homogenization step is required after incorporation to obtain adequate antioxidant concentration throughout the implants.

CURRENT USE

UHMWPE and its variants are used all over the world for articulating counterfaces in all TJR: in the hip, the PE acetabular liner remains the gold standard; in the knee, the tibial insert is universally manufactured from PE. UHMWPE is also used for shoulder, wrist, and small articular replacements of the hand and ankle.[8]

According to international rules, UHMWPE and its variants such as X-PE and vitamin E-blended PE can be implanted. Any new biomaterial, with different chemical-physical characteristics, should be proven to be at least comparable to standard UHMWPE starting from in vitro testing and then in vivo evaluation according to international rules.[8]

HISTORICAL RESULTS IN VITRO AND IN VIVO AND HISTORICAL COMPONENT FAILURES

Whereas UHMWPE showed and continues to show good mechanical resistance and biocompatibility in vitro, in the past, particularly in the 1990s as already mentioned above, catastrophic failures were observed in vivo due to severe PE oxidative wear induced by high-energy radiation sterilization. The PE oxidative degradation due to inadequate sterilization was the first and main cause of its failure in vivo, with production of aggressive PE debris and consequent periprosthetic osteolysis and implant aseptic loosening.

This oxidative wear must be separated from the classical abrasion wear, commonly called "wear," which is the process of removal of parts of a material from the surface during reciprocal movement along another surface with greater hardness (Fig. 14-1). In TJR, the UHMWPE is removed because the interactions of its chains are weak compared to those between metal or ceramic atoms of the femoral heads and femoral knee components.

The abrasion and the production of abraded particles are a time-dependent phenomenon and remain a problem in young active patients with high life expectancy. This is why current research continues to try to increase the abrasion resistance of articulating biomaterials: in polymers by increasing the molecular weight and in ceramics and metals by improving the surface quality and decreasing the roughness.

The PE wear particles, usually named "debris," in vivo cause a foreign-body granulomatous response, which is a nonspecific chronic inflammatory reaction, with the participation of activated mononucleated macrophages, fibroblasts, and a few T lymphocytes. Historically, the activation of macrophages has been related to the size, shape, volume, and number of UHMWPE debris. Particles with a size of 0.3 to 10 μm are phagocytable and are, therefore, the more biologically active compared to larger particles. Unfortunately, the biological reaction in vivo to PE debris has been related to the type of implanted PE only a few times in the literature. Often the authors do not report if the failed PE component was oxidized or not (ie, if the main cause of PE debris was oxidative wear or abrasive wear). Many factors could be responsible for different debris reactivity: the composition of the surface of the particles themselves (superficial reactivity) and therefore the level of oxidation (oxidized particles from gamma-irradiated UHMWPE inserts would be more effective in activating the macrophages, compared to the nonoxidized particles from EtO-sterilized UHMWPE). Furthermore, the surface reactivity of the particles could be also related to absorbed molecules, the hydrophilic and hydrophobic characteristics, and the release of radicals that could react with human tissues.

The biological reaction to wear particulate generated by X-PEs compared to those generated by conventional UHMWPE is not yet clearly understood. X-PE would generate a larger percentage of small particles, which would lead to a higher release of tumor necrosis factor-alpha (TNF-) and therefore to a higher reactivity, but similar levels of cytokines, IL-6, IL-1, IL-1, and TNF-. The final result is a reduced periprosthetic osteolysis compared to the conventional PE-related reaction.

FUTURE RESEARCH

UHMWPE is a good biomaterial for counterface in total knee replacement when not degraded by high-energy radiation sterilization (gamma ray and electron beam).

Whereas the oxidative wear due to sterilization can be easily avoided, the abrasion wear due to reciprocal movement between the tibial plateau and the femoral component subject to gravity can not be eliminated, but only reduced. This is why current research is going in two directions:

1. To improve the counterface in order to have "new" surfaces processed and finished to the smoothest possible degree with consequent decreased number of PE debris: new metallic and ceramic surfaces are being tested to improve the femoral component.
2. To improve the UHMWPE resistance to abrasion increasing the molecular mass, one of many factors that influence the abrasion: X-PE decreases the quantity of debris weight, the dimension, and biological reactivity of PE-abraded particles.

The abrasion resistance is not the only problem that needs to be addressed: PE oxidation is still a major concern. UHMWPE is partly crystalline and partly amorphous. Whereas the crystalline portion is extremely compact, the amorphous portion has continuous free volume between the chains, allowing oxygen penetration and reaction. Stabilization of UHMWPE with antioxidants, such as vitamin E, in both in vitro and in vivo animal tests has been shown to decrease the oxidation to clinically irrelevant levels; furthermore, vitamin E products of oxydegradation are biocompatible and not cytotoxic, and the abraded particles (debris) are few, small, not oxidized, and with low biological reaction.[9] Which of the two methods of incorporating vitamin E into the UHMWPE (blending vitamin E powder before consolidation or diffusion of vitamin E into UHMWPE after the irradiation cross-linking) is better remains unclear.

As a final consideration, according to Standard ASTM F648-10a, except for the density, there are no prescribed maximum limits governing the chemical-physical-mechanical characteristics. This means that the UHMWPE can have different initial characteristics. As already discussed, the quality tests are carried out on the original material, before any processing (compression, extrusion, sterilization, cross-linking, stabilization with vitamin E) has occurred. Furthermore, the polymeric chain configuration allows diffusion of oxygen as well as molecules from synovial fluid into the material. Whereas metallic prosthetic components are "stable" materials, UHMWPE is an interesting "living" biomaterial, changing its characteristics during the in vivo service.

Further studies are mandatory to improve our knowledge on this fascinating polymer.

CONCLUSION

The success of a prosthetic implant depends on many factors, varying from patient characteristics to implant design and surgical technique. The type and quality of the UHMWPE is one of the factors to be considered. If severe errors in processing are avoided, such as oxidative wear secondary to improper sterilization, UHMWPE and its variants are good materials to be considered for the present and the future.

Let us conclude with the words of Primo Levi in order to remember and emphasize the role of polymers in our human history:

> Now, at that time, there did not exist polyethylene, which would have suited me perfectly since it is flexible, light, and splendidly impermeable: but it is also a bit too incorruptible, and not by chance God Almighty himself, although he is a master of polymerization, abstained from patenting it: he does not like incorruptible things. (Primo Levi, from Cerium in *The Periodic Table*, New York: Schocken Books; 1984.)

SUGGESTED READING

Costa L, Brach del Prever EM. *UHMWPE for Arthroplasty.* Turin, Italy: Edizioni Minerva Medica; 2000.

Kurtz SM. *UHMWPE Biomaterials Handbook.* New York: Elsevier; 2009.

Willert HG, Buchhorn GH, Eyerer P. *Ultra-High Molecular Weight Polyethylene as Biomaterial in Orthopedic Surgery.* Toronto, Ontario, Canada: Hogrefe & Huber Publishers; 1991.

www.UHMWPE.org.

REFERENCES

1. Costa L, Luda MP, Trossarelli L, et al. Oxidation in orthopaedic UHMWPE sterilised by gamma-radiation and ethylene oxide. *Biomaterials.* 1998;19:659-668.
2. Costa L, Bracco P. Mechanism of crosslinking and oxidative degradation and stabilization of UHMWPE. In: Kurtz S, ed. *UHMWPE Biomaterial Handbook.* New York: Academic Press; 2009:309-322.
3. Costa L, Bracco P, Brach del Prever EM, et al. Analysis of products diffused in UHMWPE prosthesis components in vivo. *Biomaterials.* 2001;22:307-315.
4. Lewis G. Properties of crosslinked UHMWPE. *Biomaterials.* 2001;22:371-401.
5. Bracco P, Oral E. Vitamin E-stabilized UHMWPE for total joint implants: a review. *Clin Orthop Relat Res.* 2011;469:2286-2293.
6. Bracco P, Brach del Prever EM, Dalla Pria R, et al. Can incorporation of Vitamin E be an alternative to remelting of radiation crosslinked UHMWPE? *Journal of Biomedical Materials Research Part B; Applied Biomaterials.* Accepted 2012.
7. Wolf C, Lederer K, Müller U. Tests of biocompatibility of α-tocopherol with respect to the use as a stabilizer in ultrahigh molecular weight polyethylene for articulating surfaces in joint endoprostheses. *J Mater Sci Mater Med.* 2002;13(7):701-705.
8. Brach del Prever EM, Bistolfi A, Bracco P, et al. UHMWPE for arthroplasty: past or future? *J Orthop Traumatol.* 2009;10:1-8.
9. Brach del Prever EM, Costa L, Bistolfi A, et al. The biological reactivity of polyethylene wear debris is related with sterilization methods of UHMWPE. *Chir Organ Mov.* 2003;LXXXVIII:291-304.

15

Polymethylmethacrylate

Alex C. McLaren and Ryan McLemore

Acrylic bone cement, polymethylmethacrylate (PMMA), is a five-carbon synthetic polymer of methacrylate $(C_5O_2H_8)_n$. PMMA is a strong, lightweight thermoplastic with a 40- to 50-year history in orthopaedic surgery. It has two main uses: (1) fixing implants to bone and (2) local antimicrobial delivery.

The methylmethacrylate ester of methacrylic acid was first polymerized into polymethylmethacrylate in 1877 by the German chemists Fittig and Paul.[1] Commercial production of PMMA did not occur until 1928. PMMA is clear, hard, and brittle, transmitting up to 92% of visible light. Recognizing its potential as acrylic glass, German chemist Otto Röhm patented PMMA in 1933. PMMA was commercialized as Plexiglas. Acrylic glass was extensively used in aviation, leading to unintended biocompatibility testing in World War II when acrylic shrapnel was found to be nonreactive in pilots.

The medical and dental use of PMMA came in 1936 after it was discovered that a moldable dough could be formed by mixing ground PMMA powder, liquid methacrylate monomer, and benzoyl peroxide (BPO), an initiator. The free radical polymerization that follows requires heating to 100°C, resulting in hard PMMA. Because of the high temperature, applications were ex vivo. The first medical use in 1938 was to fabricate custom cranial segments in monkeys. Shortly thereafter, cranial defects in humans were closed with custom PMMA plates made from the heat-cured product known as Paladon 65.[2] In 1943 Paladon 65 was modified by adding tertiary aromatic amine co-initiators and accelerators (eg, *N,N*-dimethyl-*p*-toluidine), which caused the polymerization reaction to occur without being heated.[2] Room temperature cured PMMA is the basis for acrylic bone cement in clinical use today.

Orthopaedic applications began with articular resurfacing of the femoral head by Kaier in 1951, followed by femoral head replacement by Judet in 1956. These implants were abandoned because of mechanical failure. Based on its use in dentistry, PMMA was first used to fix orthopaedic implants to bone by E. J. Haboush at the Hospital for Joint Diseases in New York in 1953.[3,4] Sir John Charnley developed the first reproducible surgical technique to use PMMA for fixation of implants in 1958, solving one of the key impediments to durable total hip arthroplasty. In 1968, Frank Gunston, a Canadian working with Charnley, used PMMA fixation for his polycentric total knee arthroplasty (TKA).[5] The prototype design for modern cemented TKA followed in 1970 as a collaboration between Insall and Walker at the Hospital for Special Surgery in New York and Freeman and Swanson in London.[5] Since the early 1970s, many design advances in TKA have occurred, improving both the implant and fixation.

In the area of antimicrobial delivery, the concept of antimicrobial-loaded bone cement (ALBC) began in 1969 by Bucholtz in Germany. ALBC has received a considerable amount of resources and effort over the ensuing four decades to understand and optimize its use.

PMMA for orthopaedic use is currently manufactured by emulsion polymerization of methylmethacrylate producing microspheres of PMMA ranging in diameter from 10 to 60 μm. When entrapped by polymerized methylmethacrylate monomer, the composite becomes an amorphous radiolucent thermoplastic with physical properties that have led to its orthopaedic applications. The clinical formulations available today are two-part, self-curing formulations. The powder component is over 95% PMMA with various copolymers, initiators and accelerators, and radio-opacifiers. The liquid component consists of methylmethacrylate monomer, polymerization-inhibiting free radical scavengers, and coloring agents (Table 15-1). The powder-to-monomer ratio is 2:1 wt/vol. Small variations in constituents result in specific variations in mixing and handling characteristics (set time, maximum setting temperature, shrinkage, strength, microporosity, crack propagation, solubility). Higher powder-to-monomer ratio increases the viscosity, causing stiffer dough and decreased workability; a lower ratio increases the maximum setting temperature and leads to more unpolymerized monomer. At the time of this writing, there are a minimum of 34 different acrylic cement formulations marketed by at least 12 companies, manufactured by various manufacturing companies. Manufacturing and marketing details have changed over time for cements that maintain the same name. As with most orthopaedic products, all cements are not equal; minor differences are associated with different properties.

Most important, PMMA is a thermoplastic. Thermoplastics are elastic and flexible above their glass transition temperature T_g and, at their melting temperature T_m, they do not have a phase change (melt); they just decrease viscosity, allowing them to be molded. For PMMA, T_g is typically 100° to 120°C and T_m is 130° to 140°C. At room temperature and body temperature, PMMA is in its glass phase, hard and brittle compared to ultra-high-molecular-weight polyethylene (UHMWPE) ($T_g = -160°C$). PMMA is amorphous, not crystalline, in its glass phase. Amorphous thermoplastics are susceptible to environmental stress cracking (ESC) (ie, crazing). ESC is an important phenomenon. Fifteen percent to thirty percent of all domestic and industrial plastic component failures start from ESC.[6] ESC breaks the secondary linkages between polymer chains, not the polymer bonds. Minute cracks in the polymer propagate to form crazing. Furthermore, PMMA has hydrolyzable ester groups that are susceptible to chemical degradation. Exposure to organic fluids accelerates ESC at lower stresses. ESC initiation and propagation in PMMA are caused by the combined action of functional stress and a corrosive environment.[7,8] Lower-molecular-weight PMMA is more sensitive to organic fluids

TABLE 15-1. Components of PMMA

Powder	Liquid	Radio-opacifier	Antimicrobial
Polymethylmethacrylate	Methylmethacrylate	Barium sulfate	Gentamicin sulfate
Copolymers:	Butylmethacylate (comonomer)	Zirconium dioxide	Clindamycin hydrochloride
Polymethylacrylate	*N*-decylmethacrylate (comonomer)		Erythromycin-gluco heptonate
Poly(methylmethacrylate-ethylmethacrylate-styrene)	4*N*, *N*-(Dimethylamino) phenylethanol (accelerator)		Colistin-methane sulfonate-sodium
Poly(butyl methacrylate-methylmethacrylate			
Ethylexyl methacrylate, Co(methylmethacrylate-styrene), Ethyl methacrylate, Polymethylacrylate *n*-BUMA	*N,N*-dimethyl-4-toluidine (accelerator, initiates BPO dissociation into free radicals) Hydroquinone (inhibitor – free radical scavenger prevents self-polymeration)		
Benzoyl peroxide (initiator) Tri-*n*-butylborane (initiator) Di-cyclohexylphthalate (plasticizer) Chlorophyllin (natural green 3, color)	Ethylene glycol dimethacrylate (EGDMA) (cross-linker)		

All of the clinically available acrylic bone cements are made up of combinations of constituents including powder: PMMA, various copolymers, initiator, co-initiator; liquid monomer, comonomer, accelerator, inhibitor, and a radio-opacifier. Antimicrobial additives are limited to a few commercially prepared ALBCs.

than higher-mass grades of PMMA. Crazing in PMMA creates a diffusion path, perpetuating crazing and providing routes for antimicrobial release. Solubility of PMMA in water (how much water it will absorb) is extremely low with a diffusion coefficient of 10^{-11} m^2/s, leading to water absorption of only 2% to 3%.[9]

The physical properties that determine the performace of PMMA are affected by multiple factors: composition of copolymers, additives, radio-opacifiers, initiators and accelerators, molecular weight,[10] porosity,[11] sterilization,[12] and mixing method[13] (Table 15-2). When PMMA fails, microcracks in the newly polymerized PMMA (between the prepolymerized PMMA microspheres) propagate and coalesce to form structural fracture lines (Fig. 15-1). Residual stress from temperature shifts and shrinkage during polymerization, stress risers from inclusion particles (radio-opacifiers, poragens, antimicrobials) and stress risers around pores all contribute to crack initiation and propagation.[13,14]

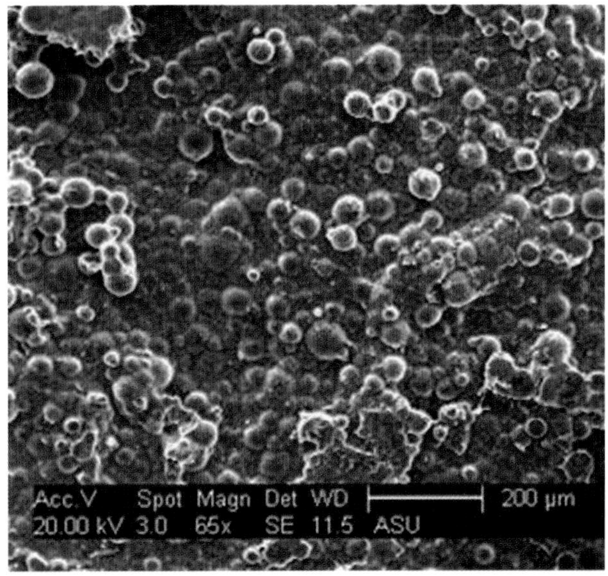

FIGURE 15-1. *Scanning electron microscopic image of polymethylmethacrylate bone cement. Fracture surface showing intact prepolymerized spheres at the fracture surface with polymerized methylmethacrylate between them.*

TABLE 15-2. Physical Properties of PMMA

Property	Value
Density	~1.18 g/cm^3
Compressive strength	80–100 MPa (ISO 5388 minimum–70 MPa)
Tensile strength	24–50
Shrinkage[55]	7%
Water absorption[15]	2.1–2.9
Diffusion coefficient in water[15]	0.1–0.2 $10^{<11}$ m^2/s
Fracture toughness	1.93 MPa–$m^{1/2}$ (low-dose cement)
Fatigue	1,000,000–5,000,000 cycles 4 Hz, 15 MPa
Young's modulus (tension)	1500–4000 MPa[18]
Young's modulus (compression)	2500–3000 MPa[18]
T_g	100°–120°C
T_m	130°–140°C

POLYMERIZATION

Curing is an exothermic reaction that proceeds by free radical vinyl polymerization initiated by benzoyl peroxide splitting into free radicals. As polymerization progresses, the monomer is consumed, generating PMMA chains, engulfing the prepolymerized PMMA microspheres and particulate additives (BaSO, antimicrobial powder, poragen). Viscosity increases, diffusion of the constituents decreases, chain propagation slows, and the reaction stops. Polymerization never completely consumes all the reagents. Toxic reagents leach out of the cement over the ensuing weeks and months. About 2% to 6% of the monomer is left unpolymerized.[15] Most of the unpolymerized monomer is released in a few weeks, but up to 0.5% remains for years. Vacuum mixing decreases free monomer released after polymerization.[16]

Methylmethacrylate is systemically and locally toxic[17,18] and is known to cause hypercoagulation with the potential for intravascular clotting.[19] *N,N*-dimethyl-4-toluidine[20] is locally toxic and detectable for years. The free radicals produced by BPO are present long term with concerns for genotoxicity.[21] In spite of these documented toxicities, in situ polymerization of PMMA has excellent long-term durability with close tissue apposition. Wound healing and local necrosis are not identified problems.

MIXING

When the liquid components are added to the powder components, gentle stirring is required to wet the powder with the liquid (mixing phase, typically about 1 to 2 minutes). This varies considerably from formulation to formulation. Once the powder and liquid are completely mixed, the PMMA is sticky and one must wait before it can be handled (waiting phase, typically 3 to 4 minutes). It is during this phase that low-viscosity cements can be injected through narrow cement syringes into narrow cavities. This is also the optimal time to apply the cement to any implant surface that will benefit from optimal adhesion, such as the tibial base plate.[22] When the cement is not sticky to the touch, it can be molded by hand and applied to cancellous bone surfaces by hand (working phase, typically 5 to 8 minutes). When the cement becomes too stiff to effectively flow or mold, its temperature rises, contained air and vaporized monomer expand, and polymerization finishes, leading to cooling and shrinkage (hardening phase, typically 2 to 3 minutes). PMMA is known to shrink about 7% during the hardening phase.[23] It is important to maintain compression on the implant–cement–bone complex to prevent separation of the cement from the implant.

Dough time is the time it takes to reach the working phase and working time starts when the cement is no longer sticky and lasts until its temperature is halfway to the maximum setting temperature, giving a measurable end to the working phase. Setting time is dough time plus working time.[13]

Increased ambient temperature, increased storage temperature (monomer and/or polymer temperature), and containment of the generated heat all decrease setting time and increase the maximum setting temperature. Prechilling the monomer to 4° to 5°C prolongs the setting time and improves handling, especially for centrifugation and for injection into narrow cavities.

Maximum setting temperature is expected to be 70° to 110°C in bulk cement,[24] although fixation of metal implants does not typically achieve such high temperatures or induce tissue injury in vivo.[18,25-27] This is likely due to the thin cement mantle, conduction by the implant, and heat dissipation into the tissue.

PMMA has macroporosity (pores > 1.0 mm) and microporosity (pores < 0.1 mm). Vigorous stirring is known to trap air in the cement, causing voids. Mixing under vacuum and centrifugation decrease macroporosity. Both improve its mechanical properties, with centrifugation being somewhat more effective.[13] Microporosity is likely due to entrapped air around powder particles that were not wetted by the monomer during mixing and also caused by vaporization of the monomer during polymerization. Vacuum reduces microporosity in high-viscosity cement but increases microporosity in low-viscosity cement, especially when the monomer is chilled. Although vacuum mixing improves the mechanical properties of the cement, the molecular weight of the polymer is a far more important determinant of strength than microporosity.[10]

CEMENT TECHNIQUE

Cement fixation for TKAs is reliable and durable,[28-34] continuing as the dominant fixation method for TKA[35–38] even when noncemented fixation dominates total hip arthroplasty and there are reports of successful noncemented technology for TKA.[29,31,34,39] Since initially described by Charnley, cement technique has been refined to ensure direct apposition against clean bone with penetration into empty irregularities and interstices, surrounding the first few trabeculae in cancellous bone. Modern cement technique includes plugging any cavities beyond where cement fixation is intended (eg, intramedullary canals); high-pressure, pulsatile lavage to remove all bone debris, fat, and marrow; and retrograde filling of cavities to prevent air entrapment. Pressurizing cement in the waiting phase with a cement gun or by finger in the early working phase improves cement penetration. Secondary pressurization at the time of implant insertion through containment of cement in the interval between the implant and bone is also very effective. Maintaining clean, dry implant surfaces improves adhesion to the implant. Maintaining a constant load on the cement mantle until the hardening phase is complete is also important to prevent the PMMA from pulling away from the implant surfaces due to shrinking.[40]

Considerable improvement in results for cemented total hip arthroplasty have been achieved over time. While these basic principles apply, TKA fixation is mostly on large, flat, uncontained surfaces. Recesses for short pegs and stems are filled without voids because of the ease with which air and fluid are pushed into the large volume of cancellous bone, and osseous blood flow is eliminated by the use of a tourniquet. Contours on the cementing surfaces of the implants ensure a minimum, even layer of cement. Consequently cementing tends to be by hand application of cement to the bone or implant surfaces in the working phase for primary TKA. Containment under broad implant surfaces has been shown to have excellent intrusion into well-prepared cancellous bone.[41-43] When intramedullary stems are used in complex or revision TKA cases, they can be cemented using the technique described for femoral hip stems. More commonly, a hybrid technique is used. The stems are press-fitted without cement and the broad surfaces in the meta-epiphyseal region of the implant are cemented, achieving durable fixation with 90% survival at 10 years.[44]

Penetration into cancellous bone increases interface strength and stiffness.[41,43] High-viscosity cement may produce a more durable interface for implant stems but it is not determined how viscosity effects the broad flat interfaces about TKA implants.[45]

While sufficient interface strength and stiffness are necessary for stable, pain-free fixation, rigid fixation may not be desirable. Metal implants essentially carry all of the load from the first point of fixation. As such, there is a potential for extreme bone resorption from stress shielding under the implant.[46] Bone ingrowth into porous implant surfaces can achieve this level of fixation but cement fixation does not. Postmortem analysis of well-fixed cemented TKA implants reveals a more compliant, lower strength interface due to interposed soft tissue at the bone–cement interface.[47] Serendipitously, the implant–cement interface is protected from loads that would separate the cement from the implant and the underlying bone experiences less stress shielding.[46]

CEMENT ADHESION

Commonly considered a gap filler or grout achieving fixation by macromechanical interlock, PMMA is actually a true adhesive. The adhesive mechanism is mechanical, without any chemical molecular bonds. Before PMMA hardens, it can work its way into microirregularities in the implant surface. If left undisturbed until it hardens, flow out of or away from these irregularities cannot occur without fracturing the material. A bond results by capturing surface disparities.[22] Metal implant surfaces are highly wettable by methylmethacrylate monomer, allowing very small irregularities to be completely apposed with PMMA after polymerization. Maintenance of the implant–cement interface allows the bone–cement interface to remodel based on physiologic loads. Increasing compliance at the bone–cement interface decreases the stress at the implant–cement interface, resulting in durable implant–cement interfaces. Implant stems are surrounded by cement and gain interface strength through hoop stresses as the cement shrinks. The cement–implant interface along flat surfaces under knee implants is subject to tension during shrinkage. It is therefore important to maximize the cement–metal contact by continuously loading the implant during hardening and by applying the PMMA early[48] when as much monomer as possible is available to wet the surface. The cement–implant interface must be held absolutely motionless during hardening to establish the mechanical adhesion. This is especially true for the tibial cementing surfaces because there is no cement containment from the geometry of the implant site or the implant. The contours and recesses on the implant cementing surface can sustain sheer stress, but tension is carried by adhesion at the interface. When hip implants were industrially precoated with PMMA, the bond was durable. Fixation failed clinically at the cement–bone interface due to the lack of compliance at the cement–implant interface. Loading conditions for TKA components are different than seen by hip stems. Precoating knee implants with PMMA has not been explored.

ADDITIVES

Acrylic bone cement functions extremely well for fixation of implants. Current cement techniques and implant designs appear to be outperforming the technology that has led to survival of 95% at 15 years and 90% at 20 years.[28,30,32] Many cases have greater than 30-year survival or outlast the patient. Improving on PMMA for fixation may prove to be a difficult task, with the obligation of proving that a change is an improvement before it is released for general use. Nevertheless, attempts continue to improve the mechanical performance of PMMA by adding 1 to 2 vol% of structural fibers (carbon, graphite, aramid, polyethelene, PMMA, Kevlar, titanium) or adding materials to improve incorporation at the bone–cement interface (bone, hydroxyapatite), decrease its brittleness, or increase its toughness (rubber).[13] None of these have gained regulatory approval or are expected to be available for clinical use in the foreseeable future.

Improvement in the radio-opacifing agent has justification. Both barium sulfate and zirconium dioxide increased osteolysis associated with particulate PMMA and zirconium dioxide has been associated with radioactive contaminants.[49] Using alternate radio-opacifiers will require that the mechanical performance is not unfavorably affected.[13,24]

OSTEOLYSIS

Osteolysis associated with TKA is currently attributed to small particles from UHMWPE wear[50,51]; however, PMMA can contribute to osteolysis.[52] When the cement–implant interface fails, interface motion can lead to the generation of PMMA particles.[22] When PMMA particles (<12 μm) undergo phagocytosis by macrophages, a cascade of cellular and molecular events ensues, leading to lysis, similar to the response seem with polyethylene wear particles. Aggravating the process are the radio-opacifying agents. Both barium sulfate and zirconium dioxide particles are toxic,[53,54] increasing the inflammatory response and osteolysis.

Before osteolysis was understood, it was attributed to fragmented cement and was called "cement disease." Attention was directed to developing noncemented fixation to avoid the use of cement.[52] Lysis in the absence of cement led to intense investigations delineating the cellular and molecular mechanisms now understood to be associated with lysis. Improved cementing techniques led to sealed bone–cement interfaces, durable fixation, and a reduction in aseptic loosening. Osteolysis from polyethylene wear was felt to be associated with noncemented implants. However, cases of osteolysis are encountered in cemented TKA that are not loose,[55,56] and it is now recognized that osteolysis does occur in cemented TKA.[57] The occurrence of osteolysis in stable cemented TKA has a later onset, probably due to the cement restricting migration of the wear particles into the adjacent bone.

PMMA AS A LOCAL ANTIMICROBIAL DELIVERY VEHICLE

Since its use was first published by Bucholtz in 1970, ALBC has been used for both the prevention of prosthetic joint infections and the treatment of established infections. Consensus has not been reached about the use of ALBC in TKA for routine prophylaxis or for high-risk cases.[58–62] There is, however, uniform agreement that local antimicrobial delivery is effective in the management of established infections and for fixation in revision cases.

The need for local antimicrobial delivery is based on the antimicrobial resistance that exists in bacteria once they have established a biofilm. All prosthetic joint infections are biofilm based. Bacteria in biofilm express a distinct phenotype with lower metabolic activity, decreased replication, and altered surface structure, rendering them unidentified by host defenses and unaffected by antimicrobials in usually effective concentrations. Extremely high levels, 100 to 1000 times the usual mean inhibitory concentration for most antimicrobials, are needed to kill bacteria in biofilm[63,64]—levels that are frequently associated with unacceptable toxicity. Local delivery can achieve these levels with little systemic exposure.

ANTIMICROBIAL LOAD

Gentamicin, tobramycin, vancomycin, cefuroxime, and cefazolin are the antimicrobial agents most commonly used in ALBC. Essentially all powder antimicrobials have been added to cement at some point, often with limited data guiding the amount. The in vitro pattern of release for most water-soluble antibacterial powders tends to be similar with the majority of the release occurring during the first 7 to 30 days.[65] This pattern of release behavior does not predict how much of the antimicrobial load will be released, what the local wound and tissue levels will be, how long the local levels will be present, the distribution of the local levels, or any potential local tissue toxicity.

To understand the release behavior for any antimicrobial–bone cement combination, the specific ALBC formulation needs to be studied. Currently there is no method to determine the in vivo distribution following local release in clinical use.[66] Prudence must be exercised when applying the available data to determine type and load of antimicrobial for clinical use. Even the commonly used antimicrobials can have different release behaviors if the ALBC formulation and method of use are changed. Antimicrobial release from ALBC is dependent on the amount (volume percent) of antimicrobial powder loaded into the cement, the interaction between the bone cement and the antimicrobial, the fluid dynamics (volume and flow) of the environment, the type of antimicrobial that is being released, the interaction between the antimicrobial agent and the fluid (eg, solubility), and the permeability (porosity) of the ALBC. The volume of distribution and the flow rate for local delivery are extremely small compared to systemic delivery, leading to extremely high levels based on wound fluid level measurements from case reposts and animal studies. It is therefore not recommended to experiment with new antimicrobial formulations in clinical practice. However, when clinical need dictates a specific therapeutic requirement, a prudent approach might be to load an amount of antimicrobial powder corresponding to a 24-hour systemic dose into acrylic bone cement that is made porous using a poragen. One hundred percent of the antimicrobial load is never released in the first 24 hours, ensuring the maximum release to be systemically acceptable. As a general guide, 10 g of cefazolin is a reasonable choice to use as a poragen (create pores). It is available, inexpensive, and has enough volume to render bone cement porous. Caution must be exercised. Even in experienced hands, unexpected results can occur, as illustrated by attempts to use amphotericin B or daptomycin before adequate data are available.

LOW-DOSE VERSUS HIGH-DOSE ALBC

Porosity is the key determinant for ALBC permeability, which in turn, determines the dissolution, diffusion, and release of antimicrobials. Native porosity of the PMMA varies (micro- and macroporosity) based on the PMMA formulation and mixing conditions. Antimicrobial release therefore varies among the available cements. When soluble particulate materials (including antimicrobials) are added to PMMA, they act as poragens, creating interconnecting pores as the material dissolves.[67] It is the amount of poragen that determines the classification of ALBC as low dose or high dose. The native porosity and microcracks become much less important when high-dose poragens are added. Frequently enough antimicrobial powder is used so that an inert poragen is not needed.

Porosity is the volume of the voids (pores) compared to the volume of the material. Unfortunately, antimicrobials and other inert powders are quantified by weight, not volume, leading to misleading quantification of the antimicrobial load. Formulations of different drugs can vary greatly in density, usually based on the carrier with which they are formulated. When the antimicrobial density is near 1 g/cc, the weight percent and volume percent are nearly equal; however, for lower-density drugs, such as generic tobramycin, voriconazole and liposomal amphotericin, the weight of the drug needed for high-dose ALBC is 3.5 times, 40 times, and 50 times less, respectively.

Up to 3 vol% is considered low dose, producing noninterconnecting pores and minimal mechanical effect. The commercial preparations with 0.5 to 1.0 g of antimicrobial powder per batch of PMMA (40 g of polymer powder and ~20 mL of monomer liquid) fall within this range, as does 1 to 2 g of most water-soluble antibacterial powders. A 10 vol% or greater is considered high dose, achieving a highly permeable ALBC with interconnecting pores. Ten or more grams of most antibacterial powders per batch of bone cement falls in this range. An example of a low-density antimicrobial powder that requires less drug mass is the antifungal voriconazole, requiring only 250 mg for high-dose formulation.

ANTIMICROBIAL RELEASE

Antimicrobial release at the macrolevel is related to surface area. The more surface exposed to the surrounding fluid (eluate), the greater is the release. Surface area is determined by the geometry (external surface area) and the interconnecting porosity (internal surface area). Traditionally ALBC has been made into spherical beads; however, alternate shapes with greater surface area to contained volume are favored to increase the release with the same amount of ALBC; thin layers of ALBC (ALBC chips: often 1–2 cm × 3–4+ cm × 1 mm thick) have a considerably larger surface-to-volume ratio for use in large wounds (Fig. 15-2). ALBC rods for intramedullary sites and ALBC chips are also considerably easier to retrieve at the time of removal, if that is required. When an ALBC spacer is used to meet a structural need, the surface-to-volume issue is addressed by using porous high-dose ALBC where the internal surface area is massively greater than the external surface.

Elution studies are performed to characterize the relative performance of local delivery vehicles, not to determine what the antimicrobial levels will be in clinical use. These studies are designed to measure the maximum release possible (amount over time) using accepted controlled release engineering principles.[68] The in vitro testing conditions are not related or even similar to the clinical release environment, which is generally unquantified and poorly understood.[66] The antimicrobial must be soluble in the eluate; the concentration of antimicrobial in the eluate must not be high enough to inhibit continuing diffusion (infinite sink), and enough time must be taken to allow release of all the available antimicrobial. Not all the load is available for release. For PMMA, when the rate approaches zero, often by 30 days, an insignificant amount of the available antimicrobial

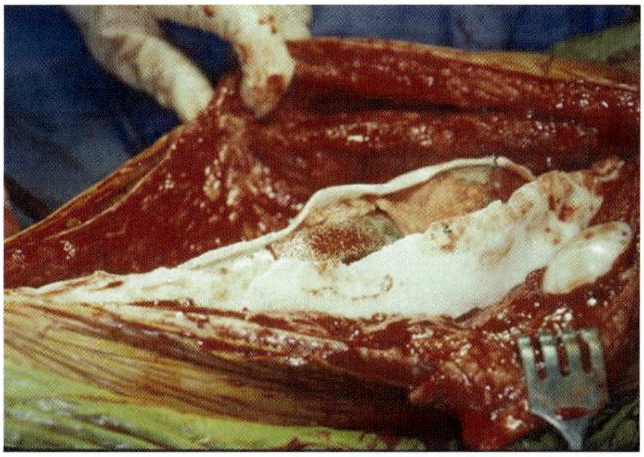

FIGURE 15-2. *ALBC "chips." Postdebridement wound with ALBC chips layered along the medial and lateral gutters of a case with a successfully retained implant; proximal is right, distal is left, anterior is top, and the patella can be seen near the right side of the image. (Reprinted with permission from McLaren AC, Gutierrez FN, Martin M, McLemore R: Local Antimicrobial Treatment, in Cierny G III, McLaren AC, Wongworawat MD, eds: Orthopaedic Knowledge Update Musculoskeletal Infection. Rosemont, IL, American Academy of Orthopaedic Surgeons, 2009:104-105.)*

load remains unreleased. The total amount of recovered antimicrobial is determined and expressed as an absolute amount at a specific time (M_t, where M is the mass of drug and t is the time) or, more appropriately, as a percentage of the available antimicrobial load.[65]

MECHANICAL PROPERTIES OF ALBC

Implant fixation must withstand functional loads. The minimum mechanical properties of PMMA necessary to meet the functional demands are given in ISO 5833. When 4.5 g of antimicrobial powder are loaded in PMMA, its compressive strength falls below the minimum 70 MPa.[69,70] Unfortunately very few data in the literature are presented in volume percent. In general, 1 to 2 g of most antibacterial powders are in the low-dose range and do not cause weakening of the ALBC below 70 MPa. For essentially all high-dose ALBC formulations, the compressive strength falls meaningfully below 70 MPa, with greater loss for higher doses.[71] Interestingly the extent to which the compressive strength is decreased is not seen until after at least a week of elution. Of note are recent data on liposomal amphotericin and voriconazole that show much larger losses in strength: 600 mg of voriconazole (24 vol%) led to compressive strength of 20 MPa[72]; 800 mg of liposomal amphotericin (47 vol%) led to compressive strength of 36 MPa[73]; and 800 mg of amphotericin B deoxycholate (10 vol%) led to compressive strength of 101 MPa.[73] The amphotericin B data further illustrate the complexity of ALBC formulations. Free amphotericin B increases the strength of ALBC,[74] mitigating loss due to porosity.

High-dose ALBC is intended for local delivery from beads, chips rods, and spacers. The minimum mechanical properties that are required for these functions are unknown. Beads, chips, and rods do not bear load. The requirement for these implants is that they remain intact for removal. Spacers can have mechanical function other than maintaining a working space. Spacers made with high-dose antibacterial ALBC are reinforced with a metal core. Mechanical failure is an unusual problem. The extreme strength loss from the antifungals may pose a risk for load- bearing spacers.

ALBC SPACERS

ALBC spacers are made with high-dose ALBC. They provide drug delivery, dead space management, limb stability, pain control, and sedentary function. High-dose ALBC is intended to deliver antimicrobials. Fabrication of an ALBC spacer should not compromise that function. Some postresection wounds have dead space that can be managed with nonstructural high-dose ALBC. For infected TKA, there is usually an associated mechanical instability causing tissue shear and functional limitation. An ALBC spacer can be fabricated to replace the mechanical function without compromising its local drug delivery. In addition to its drug delivery and structural functions, a spacer and additional nonstructural ALBC should occupy the entire dead space to maintain the collateral ligaments at length and fill the volume of resected tissue. This provides the working space needed for the implant and graft material that will be used during the second-stage reimplantation. It must be emphasized that local antimicrobial delivery and spacer fabrication should never substitute for complete resection of all the infected tissues, including the intramedullary canals.

Static ALBC spacers, the author's preferred method at the knee, are equivalent to a temporary ALBC fusion (Fig. 15-3). They minimize tissue shear and maximize wound healing. The temporary absence of motion is well tolerated by patients and knee motion reliably recovers after reimplantation without the need for a quadricepsplasty. If good stability cannot be achieved or patient compliance is in doubt, an alternative method, possibly an articulating spacer, should be considered to gain stability. Metal reinforcement, usually a ¼-inch rush rod, is required to prevent fracture in the tibiofemoral gap. Medullary extensions are required to prevent instability at the ALBC–bone interface, a potential cause of catastrophic bone loss. The intramedullary portions should extend a couple of bone diameters into sound diaphyseal bone with late working phase ALBC used to fill the metaphyseal and epiphyseal osseous dead space, thereby providing secure interface stability and knee stability.

Articulating spacers allow movement at the joint. Soft tissue protection needed for more severe soft tissue involvement is not provided; however, articulating spacers are often acceptable and associated with good results.[75-78] Freehand fabrication is difficult to get right. Silicone molds (StageOne Knee Cement Sparer Molds, Biomet, Warsaw, IN) produces much more accurate articulation surfaces, but some variation in the shape and size can occur. While the prosthesis of antimicrobial-loaded acrylic cement (PROSTALAC, DePuy, Warsaw, IN) molding system is readily available for the hip, the knee PROSTALAC is not.[79] Commercially prefabricated ALBC spacers (Spacer K, Tecres, Verona, Italy) (Fig. 15-4) can be used, although antimicrobial selection cannot be individualized with these. Custom molds[80] are also an option for the resourceful few.

The use of a mold requires the ALBC to be workable. High-dose ALBC may be too stiff for some molds and intermediate-dose ALBC (eg, 3.6 g of tobramycin and 1.5 g of

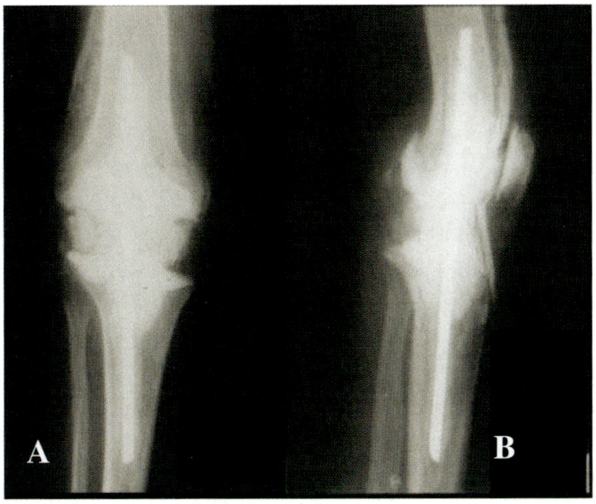

FIGURE 15-3. *Anteroposterior (**A**) and lateral (**B**) radiographs of a static ALBC spacer. Note the "chips" of ALBC in the gutters and suprapatellar pouch layered on the posterior condyles and rolled up in the voids around the bulk ALBC in the tibiofemoral interval. (Figure 15-3b is reprinted with permission from McLaren AC, Gutierrez FN, Martin M, McLemore R: Local Antimicrobial Treatment, in Cierny G III, McLaren AC, Wongworawat MD, eds: Orthopaedic Knowledge Update Musculoskeletal Infection. Rosemont, IL, American Academy of Orthopaedic Surgeons, 2009:105.)*

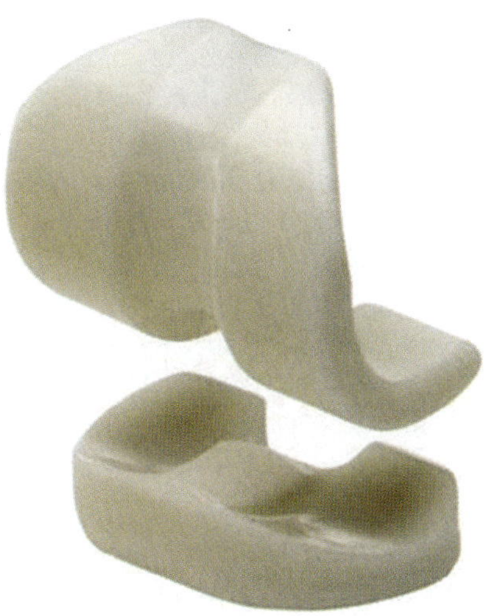

FIGURE 15-4. *Articulating spacer. Commercially made ALBC Spacer K by Tecres (Verona, Italy). Following removal of the infected implant and debridement of all infected bone and soft tissue, the Space K is "cemented" onto the residual bone using late working phase ALBC, so that the collateral ligaments are normally tensioned and normal joint kinematics can occur. (Reprinted with permission from Tecres SPA.)*

vancomycin per batch) is used. This intermediate ALBC formulation in PROSTALAC hip spacers maintains synovial fluid concentrations above the break point susceptibility limit for several weeks.[81]

ADVERSE RESPONSES

Local delivery of antimicrobials from ALBC rarely causes adverse reactions. There are isolated reports of renal toxicity to aminoglycosides,[82-85] but rate-dependent responses, such as redman syndrome (vancomycin) and reaction to formulation impurities, generally do not occur because of the nature of the controlled release. Interestingly, allergic responses are also unusual, possibly due to the slow uninterrupted rise from undetectable levels, similar to rapid desensitization.[86,87]

Local toxicity is an issue that has not been adequately addressed. Many of the antibacterials used have significant systemic toxicity. Drain fluid levels of aminoglycosides and vancomycin have been measured in excess of 2000 μg/mL, 100 times systemic targets, indicating local tissue exposure can be at least this high. There have been no in vivo studies looking at the tissue and cellular response to specific antimicrobials at these levels. However, clinical experience has not identified a problem with wound healing, fracture healing, implant ingrowth, or bone graft incorporation. Empirically no news seems to be good news. Cell culture studies on fibroblasts and osteoblasts cultured in gentamicin, tobramycin, cefazolin, and amphotericin B suggest that toxicity does exist, particularly for amphotericin B.[88-92] Further knowledge about the concentration, distribution, and tissue response to locally delivered antimicrobials is required.

Antimicrobial resistance is a significant concern. Gentamicin-resistant organisms have been cultured from the surface of gentamicin-ALBC,[93,94] even when there is no other indication that bacteria are present. It may be prudent to use a different antimicrobial for future ALBC in situations such as revision of a TKA that was fixed with prophylactic gentamicin-ALBC.

Methicillin-resistant *Staphylococcus aureus* (MRSA) and *Staphylococcus epidermidis* are encountered at an increasing rate. Vancomycin is appropriate for these infections if one accepts that its penetration into bone is not optimal. However, routine use of vancomycin for prophylaxis is unacceptable. Vancomycin-resistant organisms are emerging in part related to injudicious use of vancomycin, and vancomycin is not adequate coverage for the more common pathogens. Vancomycin-ALBC is appropriate for active or past MRSA infection, MRSA carriers, and high-risk institutions. Daptomycin-ALBC has been used for vancomycin-resistant infections. There are limited data showing good release when 1 to 2 g of daptomycin are loaded in PMMA with a poragen.[95-99] Clinical success for controlling these infections has been reported.[95-99] However, concerns about renal function secondary to rhabdomyolysis from the constant exposure of muscle to high local levels of daptomycin remain.

CLINICAL RESULTS

Prophylaxis

Low-dose ALBC in the index procedures is generally reported to decease the deep infection rate by about 0.5% to 1%[59,60,62]; however, some studies reported no improvement [58,61] and some of the trends in large registries lack significance.[61,100] Revision surgery for aseptic loosening has reported infection rates that are 2% to 3% lower when low-dose ALBC is used (eg, a decrease from 4% to 2%).[61,100,101] Revision for aseptic loosening may be a one-stage exchange for unrecognized infection in some cases, so fixation with low-dose ALBC in revisions for aseptic loosening is considered appropriate treatment by many surgeons.

Treatment

For the second-stage reimplantation, low-dose ALBC is used for fixation. Recurrence rates are decreased by 10% to 20% with the use of low-dose ALBC.[61,100,101] Results from direct exchange for prosthetic joint infections using low-dose ALBC are similar to two-stage treatment with careful patient selection and surgical technique.[61]

Lack of consistency in treatment protocols prohibits rigorous analysis of results from the use of high-dose ALBC. Consensus is that there is a therapeutic benefit from high antimicrobial levels delivered locally. The data are largely from level 3 or 4 observational studies reporting approximately 90% infection control.[13,59,61,75,79,80,100-102]

SUGGESTED READING

Review publications provide more detailed information on material properties,[18] local delivery,[65] ALBC,[61,102] spacers,[101] and comprehensive related topics.[13]

REFERENCES

1. Anon. Acrylic plastic: how products are made. Available at: http://www.enotes.com/how-products-encyclopedia/acrylic-plastic. Accessed October 4, 2011.
2. Kuhn K-D. What is bone cement? In: Breusch SJ, Malchau H, eds. *The Well-Cemented Total Hip Arthroplasty: Theory and Practice*. New York: Springer; 2005.
3. Gomez PF, Morcuende JA. Early attempts at hip arthroplasty—1700s to 1950s. *Iowa Orthop J*. 2005;25:25-29.
4. Haboush EJ. A new operation for arthroplasty of the hip based on biomechanics, photoelasticity, fast-setting dental acrylic, and other considerations. *Bull Hosp Joint Dis*. 1953;14(2):242-277.
5. Shetty A, Tindall A, Ting P, Heatley F, et al. The evolution of total knee arthroplasty. Part III: surface replacement. *Curr Orthop*. 2003;17(6):478-481.
6. Mark H. *Encyclopedia of Polymer Science and Technology, Part 3*. 3rd ed. Hoboken, NJ: Wiley-Interscience; 2003.
7. Arnold JC. The effects of diffusion on environmental stress crack initiation in PMMA. *J Mater Sci*. 1998;33(21):5193-5204.
8. Ezrin M, Lavigne G. Unexpected and unusual failures of polymeric materials. *Eng Failure Anal*. 2007;14(6):1153-1165.
9. Migliaresi C, Fambri L, Kolarik J. Polymerization kinetics, glass transition temperature and creep of acrylic bone cements. *Biomaterials*. 1994;15(11):875-881.
10. Lewis G. Relative roles of cement molecular weight and mixing method on the fatigue performance of acrylic bone cement: Simplex P versus Osteopal. *J Biomed Mater Res*. 2000;53(1):119-130.
11. Jasty M, Davies JP, O'Connor DO, et al. Porosity of various preparations of acrylic bone cements. *Clin Orthop Relat Res*. 1990;259:122-129.
12. Lewis G, Mladsi S. Effect of sterilization method on properties of Palacos R acrylic bone cement. *Biomaterials*. 1998;19(1-3):117-124.
13. Serbetci K. *Biomaterials in Orthopedics*. Yaszemski MJ, ed. Boca Raton, FL: CRC Press; 2004.
14. Lennon A, Prendergast P. Residual stress due to curing can initiate damage in porous bone cement: experimental and theoretical evidence. *J Biomech*. 2002;35(3):311-321.
15. Vallo C. Residual monomer content in bone cements based on poly(methyl methacrylate). *Polymer Int*. 2000;49:831-838.

16. Bettencourt A, Calado A, Amaral J, et al. The influence of vacuum mixing on methylmethacrylate liberation from acrylic cement powder. *Int J Pharm.* 2001; 219(1-2):89-93.
17. Kindt-Larsen T, Smith DB, Jensen JS. Innovations in acrylic bone cement and application equipment. *J Appl Biomater.* 1995;6(1):75-83.
18. Lewis G. Properties of acrylic bone cement: state of the art review. *J. Biomed. Mater. Res.* 1997;38(2): 155-182.
19. Gaszyński W, Lewicki R, Pruszyńska-Bednarek A. The effect of bone cement used for stabilization of endoprostheses on blood clotting system activity. *Anaesth Resusc Intensive Ther.* 1976;4(4):237-244.
20. Boesch P, Herms H, Lintner F. Detection of the catalytic constituents of dimethyl-p-toluidine even after long-term implantation. *Arch Toxicol.* 1982;51:157-166.
21. Ciapetti G, Granchi D, Stea S, et al. In vitro testing of ten bone cements after different time intervals from polymerization. *J Biomater Sci Polym Ed.* 2000;11 (5):481-493.
22. Crowninshield RD, Jennings JD, Laurent ML, et al. Cemented femoral component surface finish mechanics. *Clin Orthop Relat Res.* 1998;355:90-102.
23. Gilbert JL, Hasenwinkel JM, Wixson RL, et al. A theoretical and experimental analysis of polymerization shrinkage of bone cement: a potential major source of porosity. *J Biomed Mater Res.* 2000;52(1):210-218.
24. Lewis G. Alternative acrylic bone cement formulations for cemented arthroplasties: present status, key issues, and future prospects. *J. Biomed Mater Res Part B.* 2008;84(2):301-319.
25. Eriksson RA, Albrektsson T. The effect of heat on bone regeneration: an experimental study in the rabbit using the bone growth chamber. *J Oral Maxillofac Surg.* 1984;42(11):705-711.
26. Morberg P, Johansson CB, Malchau H. No biological advantage with a low temperature curing versus a conventional bone cement: an experimental, mechanical and histomorphometrical study in the rabbit tibia. *J Mater Sci Mater Med.* 1999;10(6):329-331.
27. Jaeblon T. Polymethylmethacrylate: properties and contemporary uses in orthopaedics. *J Am Acad Orthop Surg.* 2010;18(5):297-305.
28. Robertsson O, Knutson K, Lewold S, et al. The Swedish Knee Arthroplasty Register 1975-1997: an update with special emphasis on 41,223 knees operated on in 1988-1997. *Acta Orthop Scand.* 2001;72(5):503-513.
29. Baker PN, Khaw FM, Kirk LMG, et al. A randomised controlled trial of cemented versus cementless press-fit condylar total knee replacement: 15-year survival analysis. *J Bone Joint Surg Br.* 2007;89(12):1608-1614.
30. Font-Rodriguez DE, Scuderi GR, Insall JN. Survivorship of cemented total knee arthroplasty. *Clin. Orthop. Relat. Res.* 1997;345:79-86.
31. Gandhi R, Tsvetkov D, Davey JR, et al. Survival and clinical function of cemented and uncemented prostheses in total knee replacement: a meta-analysis. *J Bone Joint Surg Br.* 2009;91(7):889-895.
32. Rand JA, Ilstrup DM. Survivorship analysis of total knee arthroplasty. Cumulative rates of survival of 9200 total knee arthroplasties. *J Bone Joint Surg Am.* 1991;73(3):397-409.
33. Ranawat CS, Flynn WF Jr, Saddler S, et al. Long-term results of the total condylar knee arthroplasty. A 15-year survivorship study. *Clin Orthop Relat Res.* 1993;286:94-102.
34. Gao F, Henricson A, Nilsson KG. Cemented versus uncemented fixation of the femoral component of the NexGen CR total knee replacement in patients younger than 60 years: a prospective randomised controlled RSA study. *Knee.* 2009;16(3):200-206.
35. Phillips AM, Goddard NJ, Tomlinson JE. Current techniques in total knee replacement: results of a national survey. *Ann R Coll Surg Engl.* 1996;78(6): 515-520.
36. Lutz MJ, Halliday BR. Survey of current cementing techniques in total knee replacement. *ANZ J Surg.* 2002;72(6):437-439.
37. Debakanta J, Ng B, Courtman N, et al. Current attitudes to cementing techniques in total knee replacement: a national survey. Available at: http:// ista.confex.com/ista/2003/techprogram paper_1227. htm. Accessed September 11, 2011.
38. Phillips AM, Goddard NJ, Tomlinson JE. Current techniques in total knee replacement: results of a national survey. *Ann R Coll Surg Engl.* 1996; 78(6): 515-520.
39. Blaha JD, Insler HP, Freeman MA, et al. The fixation of a proximal tibial polyethylene prosthesis without cement. *J Bone Joint Surg Br.* 1982;64(3):326-335.
40. Scott S, McCaskie AW, Calder SJ, et al. Current cementing techniques in hip hemi-arthroplasty. *Injury.* 2001;32(6):461-464.
41. Waanders D, Janssen D, Mann KA, et al. The mechanical effects of different levels of cement pene-

tration at the cement-bone interface. *J Biomech*. 2010; 43(6):1167-1175.

42. Ritter MA, Herbst SA, Keating EM, et al. Radiolucency at the bone-cement interface in total knee replacement. The effects of bone-surface preparation and cement technique. *J Bone Joint Surg Am*. 1994; 76(1):60-65.
43. Bauze AJ, Costi JJ, Stavrou P, et al. Cement penetration and stiffness of the cement-bone composite in the proximal tibia in a porcine model. *J Orthop Surg (Hong Kong)*. 2004;12(2):194-198.
44. Sah AP, Shukla S, Della Valle CJ, et al. Modified hybrid stem fixation in revision TKA is durable at 2 to 10 years. *Clin Orthop Relat Res*. 2011;469(3):839-846.
45. Miller MA, Race A, Gupta S, et al. The role of cement viscosity on cement-bone apposition and strength: an in vitro model with medullary bleeding. *J Arthroplasty*. 2007;22(1):109-116.
46. Van Lenthe GH, de Waal Malefijt MC, Huiskes R. Stress shielding after total knee replacement may cause bone resorption in the distal femur. *J Bone Joint Surg Br*. 1997;79(1):117-122.
47. Miller MA, Eberhardt AW, Cleary RJ, et al. Micromechanics of postmortem-retrieved cement-bone interfaces. *J Orthop Res*. 2010;28(2):170-177.
48. Davies JP, Singer G, Harris WH. The effect of a thin coating of polymethylmethacrylate on the torsional fatigue strength of the cement-metal interface. *J Appl Biomater*. 1992;3(1):45-49.
49. Hopf W, Hopf CG, Glöbel B. About radioactivity in some PMMA bone cements. *Acta Orthop Belg*. 1990; 56(2):443-444.
50. Gupta SK, Chu A, Ranawat AS, et al. Osteolysis after total knee arthroplasty. *J Arthroplasty*. 2007;22(6): 787-799.
51. Naudie DDR, Ammeen DJ, Engh GA, et al. Wear and osteolysis around total knee arthroplasty. *J Am Acad Orthop Surg*. 2007;15(1):53-64.
52. Jacobs JJ, Roebuck KA, Archibeck M, et al. Osteolysis: basic science. *Clin Orthop Relat Res*. 2001;393: 71-77.
53. Ingham E, Green TR, Stone MH, et al. Production of TNF-alpha and bone resorbing activity by macrophages in response to different types of bone cement particles. *Biomaterials*. 2000;21(10):1005-1013.
54. Lazarus MD, Cuckler JM, Schumacher HR Jr, et al. Comparison of the inflammatory response to particulate polymethylmethacrylate debris with and without barium sulfate. *J Orthop Res*. 1994;12(4):532-541.
55. Griffin FM, Scuderi GR, Gillis AM, et al. Osteolysis associated with cemented total knee arthroplasty. *J Arthroplasty*. 1998;13(5):592-598.
56. Ries MD, Guiney W Jr, Lynch F. Osteolysis associated with cemented total knee arthroplasty. A case report. *J Arthroplasty*. 1994;9(5):555-558.
57. Lachiewicz PF, Soileau ES. Fifteen-year survival and osteolysis associated with a modular posterior stabilized knee replacement. A concise follow-up of a previous report. *J Bone Joint Surg Am*. 2009;91(6):1419-1423.
58. Namba RS, Chen Y, Paxton EW, et al. Outcomes of routine use of antibiotic-loaded cement in primary total knee arthroplasty. *J Arthroplasty*. 2009;24(suppl 6):44-47.
59. Diefenbeck M, Mückley T, Hofmann GO. Prophylaxis and treatment of implant-related infections by local application of antibiotics. *Injury*. 2006;37(suppl 2):S95-104.
60. Dunbar MJ. Antibiotic bone cements: their use in routine primary total joint arthroplasty is justified. *Orthopedics*. 2009;32(9). Available at: http://www.ncbi.nlm.nih.gov/pubmed/19751021. Accessed October 3, 2011.
61. Joseph TN, Chen AL, Di Cesare PE. Use of antibiotic-impregnated cement in total joint arthroplasty. *J Am Acad Orthop Surg*. 2003;11(1):38-47.
62. Parvizi J, Saleh KJ, Ragland PS, et al. Efficacy of antibiotic-impregnated cement in total hip replacement. *Acta Orthop*. 2008;79(3):335-341.
63. Chuard C, Vaudaux P, Waldvogel FA, et al. Susceptibility of *Staphylococcus aureus* growing on fibronectin-coated surfaces to bactericidal antibiotics. *Antimicrob Agents Chemother*. 1993;37(4):625-632.
64. Stewart PS, Costerton JW. Antibiotic resistance of bacteria in biofilms. *Lancet*. 2001;358(9276):135-138.
65. McLaren A, McLemore R, Gutierrez F, et al. *Orthopaedic Knowledge Update: Musculoskeletal Infection*. Rosemont, IL: AAOS; 2009:95-117.
66. Giers MB, Estes CS, McLaren A, et al. Jeannette Wilkins Award: MRI can image antimicrobial distribution after local delivery: a pilot study. *Clin Orthop Relat Res*. 2012;470-410.
67. Anagnostakos K, Kelm J. Enhancement of antibiotic elution from acrylic bone cement. *J Biomed Mater Res Part B*. 2009;90(1):467-475.
68. Kydonieus AF. *Treatise on Controlled Drug Delivery: Fundamentals, Optimization, Applications*. New York: Marcel Dekker; 1992.

69. Gambhlr A, Hanson B, Wroblewski B, et al. The mechanical properties of modern additional antibiotics in acrylic bone cement. *J Bone Joint Soc Br.* 2002; 84B:152-153.
70. Lautenschlager EP, Jacobs JJ, Marshall GW, et al. Mechanical properties of bone cements containing large doses of antibiotic powders. *J Biomed Mater Res* 1976;10(6):929-938.
71. Nugent M, McLaren A, Vernon B, et al. Strength of antimicrobial bone cement decreases with increased poragen fraction. *Clin Orthop Relat Res.* 2010;468 (8):2101-2106.
72. Miller R, McLaren A, Pauken C, et al. Voriconazole is delivered from ALBC. *Clin Orthop Relat Res.* 2013; accepted for publication.
73. Cunningham B, McLaren A, Pauken C, et al. Liposomal formulation increases local delivery of amphotericin from bone cement. *Clin Orthop Relat Res.* 2012; accepted for publication.
74. Kweon C, McLaren AC, Leon C, et al. Amphotericin B delivery from bone cement increases with porosity but strength decreases. *Clin Orthop Relat Res.* 2011; 469(11):3002-3007.
75. Shen H, Zhang X, Jiang Y, et al. Intraoperatively-made cement-on-cement antibiotic-loaded articulating spacer for infected total knee arthroplasty. *Knee.* 2010;17(6):407-411.
76. Evans RP. Successful treatment of total hip and knee infection with articulating antibiotic components: a modified treatment method. *Clin Orthop Relat Res.* 2004;427:37-46.
77. Fehring TK, Odum S, Calton TF, et al. Articulating versus static spacers in revision total knee arthroplasty for sepsis. The Ranawat Award. *Clin Orthop Relat Res.* 2000;380:9-16.
78. Hofmann AA, Kane KR, Tkach TK, et al. Treatment of infected total knee arthroplasty using an articulating spacer. *Clin Orthop Relat Res.* 1995;321:45-54.
79. Haddad FS, Masri BA, Campbell D, et al. The PROSTALAC functional spacer in two-stage revision for infected knee replacements. Prosthesis of antibiotic-loaded acrylic cement. *J Bone Joint Surg Br.* 2000; 82(6):807-812.
80. Kohl S, Krueger A, Roeder C, et al. An aluminium mold for intraoperative production of antibiotic-loaded PMMA knee prostheses. *Acta Orthop.* 2009; 80:389-391.
81. Masri BA, Duncan CP, Beauchamp CP. Long-term elution of antibiotics from bone-cement: an in vivo study using the prosthesis of antibiotic-loaded acrylic cement (PROSTALAC) system. *J Arthroplasty.* 1998; 13(3):331-338.
82. Dovas S, Liakopoulos V, Papatheodorou L, et al. Acute renal failure after antibiotic-impregnated bone cement treatment of an infected total knee arthroplasty. *Clin. Nephrol.* 2008;69(3):207-212.
83. Patrick BN, Rivey MP, Allington DR. Acute renal failure associated with vancomycin- and tobramycin-laden cement in total hip arthroplasty. *Ann Pharmacother.* 2006;40(11):2037-2042.
84. Wallenkamp G. *Gentamicin-PMMA Beads: A Clinical, Pharmacokinetic and Toxicological Study.* Darmstadt, FR Germany: E Merck; 1983.
85. Walenkamp GH, Vree TB, van Rens TJ. Gentamicin-PMMA beads. Pharmacokinetic and nephrotoxicological study. *Clin Orthop Relat Res.* 1986;205:171-183.
86. Castells M. Desensitization for drug allergy. *Curr Opin Allergy Clin Immunol.* 2006;6(6):476-481.
87. Tidwell B, Cleary J, Lorenz K. Antimicrobial desensitization: a review of published protocols. *Hospital Pharm.* 32:1362-1369.
88. Harmsen S, McLaren AC, Pauken C, et al. Amphotericin B is cytotoxic at locally delivered concentrations. *Clin Orthop Relat Res* 2011;469(11):3016-3021.
89. Wahlig H, Dingeldein E. Antibiotics and bone cements. Experimental and clinical long-term observations. *Acta Orthop Scand.* 1980;51(1):49-56.
90. Edin ML, Miclau T, Lester GE, et al. Effect of cefazolin and vancomycin on osteoblasts in vitro. *Clin Orthop Relat Res.* 1996;333:245-251.
91. Isefuku S, Joyner CJ, Simpson AHRW. Gentamicin may have an adverse effect on osteogenesis. *J Orthop Trauma.* 2003;17(3):212-216.
92. Miclau T, Edin ML, Lester GE, et al. Bone toxicity of locally applied aminoglycosides. *J Orthop Trauma.* 1995;9(5):401-406.
93. Neut D, van de Belt H, van Horn JR, et al. Residual gentamicin-release from antibiotic-loaded polymethylmethacrylate beads after 5 years of implantation. *Biomaterials.* 2003;24(10):1829-1831.
94. Thomes B, Murray P, Bouchier-Hayes D. Development of resistant strains of *Staphylococcus epidermidis* on gentamicin-loaded bone cement in vivo. *J Bone Joint Surg Br.* 2002;84(5):758-760.
95. McLaren AC, McLaren SG, Smeltzer M. Xylitol and glycine fillers increase permeability of PMMA to enhance elution of daptomycin. *Clin Orthop Relat Res.* 2006;451:25-28.

96. Weiss BD, Weiss EC, Haggard WO, et al. Optimized elution of daptomycin from polymethylmethacrylate beads. *Antimicrob Agents Chemother.* 2009;53(1): 264-266.
97. Baker K, Shorez J, Delandsheer T, et al. Elution kinetics and mechanical properties of bone cement loaded with daptomycin and tobramycin. 2010. Available at: http://www3.aaos.org/education/anmeet/anmt2010/poster/poster.cfm?Pevent=P055. Accessed October 3, 2011.
98. Smeltzer M, Weiss B, Haggard W, et al. Optimization of polymethylmethacrylate (PMMA) formulations for local delivery of antibiotics. Available at: http://www3.aaos.org/education/anmeet/anmt2008/poster/poster.cfm?Pevent=P203.
99. Montgomery C, Evans RP. Novel treatment of failed two-stage revision for periprosthetic MRSA sepsis. Available at: http://www3.aaos.org/education/anmeet/anmt2010/poster/poster.cfm?Pevent=P200.
100. Hanssen AD. Local antibiotic delivery vehicles in the treatment of musculoskeletal infection. *Clin Orthop Relat Res.* 2005;437:91-96.
101. Cui Q, Mihalko WM, Shields JS, et al. Antibiotic-impregnated cement spacers for the treatment of infection associated with total hip or knee arthroplasty. *J Bone Joint Surg Am.* 2007;89(4):871-882.
102. Lewis G. Properties of antibiotic-loaded acrylic bone cements for use in cemented arthroplasties: a state-of-the-art review. *J Biomed Mater Res Part B.* 2009; 89(2):558-574.

16 Individual Host Variation in Knee Arthroplasty

Matthew P. Abdel and Mark E. Morrey

With the advent of individualized medicine, the interaction between individual host variation and foreign bodies is becoming of increasing interest in orthopaedic surgery. Clinical observation of failed procedures about the knee strongly suggests some variation in the manner and extent to which individuals are influenced by, and react to, the presence of a foreign material, including orthopaedic implants and grafts.

The ultimate fate of a total knee arthroplasty (TKA) in some patients may be related to the individual host response to the implant, wear debris, allograft material, and/or biosynthetic material. With regard to total knee arthroplasties, it has been shown that biologic responses to particulate debris are dependent on the size, number, and surface morphology of debris particles, as well as the rate of accumulation in the periprosthetic tissues (Fig. 16-1).[1,2] Wear particles and implant materials have received considerable attention, while the host factors responsible for conditions such as osteolysis, pathogen-associated molecular patterns (PAMPs) in aseptic loosening, and aseptic lymphocytic-dominated vasculitis-associated lesions (ALVAL) in metal allergies have remained largely unknown. Knowledge of which genes and proteins are up- and down-regulated may provide keys to novel pathways of loosening and other mechanisms of failure. If bacterial antigens play a role in generating PAMPs, they may prove to be responsible for some of the aseptic loosening cases currently observed. As such, potential treatment options may focus on particular genes implicated in the pathogenesis of failures. Surprisingly, only a small number of genes and proteins have been investigated using animal models and human studies. For example, Gordon et al found that hosts with the *FRZB* 200T allele were negatively associated with osteolysis.[3]

Despite advances in orthopaedic surgery, postsurgical knee joint contractures remain a great challenge.[4,5] Intra-articular and periarticular injuries, including surgical intervention, can lead to restriction of joint motion, often significantly affecting daily activities. The knee joint is particularly prone to this complication.[6-12] Current therapeutic approaches, which include surgical correction and aggressive physical therapy, do not always prove to be effective, thus raising the question of developing new

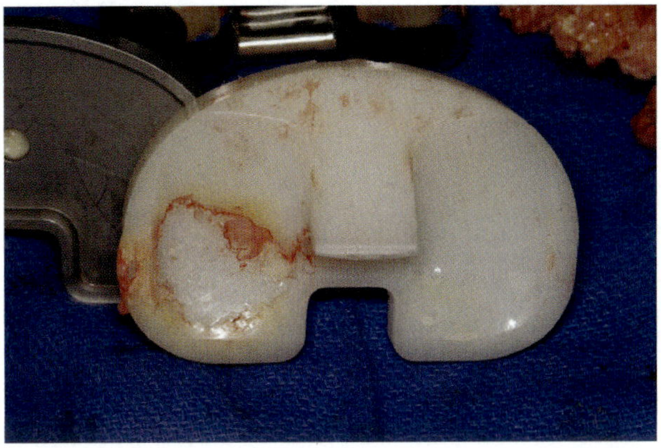

FIGURE 16-1. *Intraoperative photograph of an 84-year-old male with gross polyethylene wear at 4 years postoperatively.*

approaches tailored to the individual. Using pharmacologic agents appears to be a promising option, with recent advances in antifibrotic therapy providing new opportunities for treatment and prevention.[11,13-20]

Understanding the underlying pathology of arthrofibrosis is a crucial step to determining adequate therapies. Detailed descriptions of changes in gene transcription and protein levels in pathologically changed periarticular tissues can reveal potential molecular targets for pharmacological treatment. More important, they can identify genetic polymorphisms that will allow for screening of such conditions before surgical intervention.

In unpublished data from our laboratory at the Mayo Clinic, we have recently been able to identify the temporal mRNA relationship of over 300 genes in an animal knee model of arthrofibrosis.[21] At 2 weeks, caspase-10 and urokinase plasminogen activator were the most significantly increased genes, while the tenascin-X gene was most significantly decreased (Table 16-1). The genes for IL-1, LOX-1, and macrophage scavenger receptor type II were most significantly decreased at 8 weeks. At 24 weeks, neutrophil attractant/activation protein-1 (IL-8), α-3 type IV collagen, and aggrecanase-2 genes were most significantly decreased. The most significant change from 2 to 8 weeks was an increase in the calmodulin-dependent protein kinase II (CDPK-II) gene (Table 16-2). From 8 to 24 weeks, the most significant change was a decrease in the CDPK-II gene. When comparing 2 to 24 weeks, the most significant change was an increase in the tenascin-X gene. It is possible that these data will aid with the development of human screening and diagnostic tools. Furthermore, pharmacologic interventions may be created to complement current surgical treatment strategies.

IMMUNOLOGIC RESPONSE

Most clinicians have experienced uncommon host responses that lead to failures. Host response to a foreign stimulus can activate the acquired (or adaptive) and/or innate immune system (Fig. 16-2). The acquired immune system depends on T- and B-lymphocytes interacting with specific epitopes. Conversely, the innate immune system is nonepitope specific, but functions via other receptors and the complement system to activate phagocytic cells, primarily monocytes and macrophages.[22] This type of reaction is most often implicated in osteolytic lesions around total knee arthroplasties. Macrophages phagocytize particulate debris from implant wear, which causes subsequent granuloma formation and osteolysis.

Hypersensitivity Reactions

The host response to foreign bodies manifests as one of four hypersensitivity reactions. The types are (1) type I or anaphylactic hypersensitivity, (2) type II or cytotoxic hypersensitivity, (3) type III or immune complex (complement)

TABLE 16-1. Genes Most Up- or Down-Regulated Over Time

2 Weeks (Fold Change)	8 Weeks (Fold Change)	24 Weeks (Fold Change)
↑ Caspase-10 (1.7×)	↓ IL-1 (-1.2×)	↓ Neutrophil attractant/activation protein-1 (IL-8) (-2.5×)
↑ Urokinase plasminogen activator (2.1×)	↓ LOX-1 (-1.6×)	↓ α-3 type IV collagen (-2.1×)
↓ Tenascin-X (-1.6×)	↓ Macrophage scavenger receptor type II (-2.4×)	↓ Aggrecanase-2 (-1.6×)

TABLE 16-2. Genes with the Greatest Change Over Time

2 to 8 Weeks (Fold Change)	8 to 24 Weeks (Fold Change)	2 to 24 Weeks (Fold Change)
↑ Calmodulin-dependent protein kinase II (0.8×)	↓ Calmodulin-dependent protein kinase II (–1.2×)	↑ Tenascin-X (1.9×)
↑ Dystroglycan (1.4×)	↓ Caveolin (–0.8×)	↓ Neutrophil attractant/activation protein-1 (IL-8) (–1.9×)
↑ VEGF (1.2×)	↓ α-3 type IV collagen (–2.0×)	↓ Endothelial leukocyte adhesion molecule I (–3.0×)

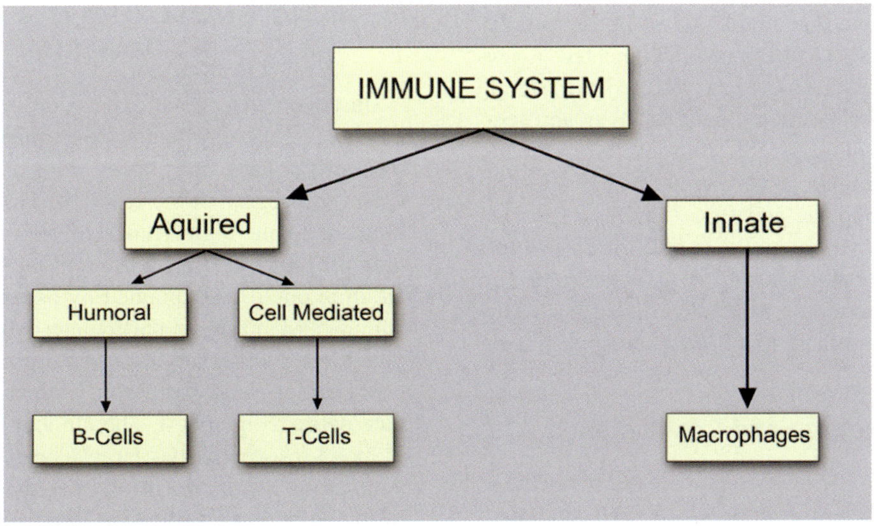

FIGURE 16-2. *The immune system is divided into the acquired (adaptive) and innate immune systems. The acquired immune system is further classified as either humoral or cell-mediated. Typically, B- and T-cells are the key mediators in the acquired immune system, whereas macrophages are essential to the innate immune system. (After Morrey, Joint Replacement Arthroplasty, 2010.)*

hypersensitivity, and (4) type IV or cell-mediated, delayed hypersensitivity. Types I, II, and III are usually immediate responses, whereas type IV reactions are delayed responses. Metal allergies and reactions to polyethylene debris are most comparable with a type IV hypersensitivity host response.[23-28] Types I, II, and III hypersensitivity reactions are rare with orthopaedic implants. The most clinically relevant hypersensitivity reaction is the cell-mediated, delayed type IV reaction.

Cell-Mediated, Delayed Hypersensitivity (Type IV)

Type IV hypersensitivity reactions are characterized by mononuclear cell infiltrates. Multiple assays of serum, blood, and urine have consistently revealed increased concentrations of metallic components in patients with metal-on-metal bearing surfaces.[23,29-31] Increased concentrations of virtually all of the metallic constituents of prosthetic devices have been reported, while nickel, cobalt, and chromium are most commonly involved.[32,33]

In type IV delayed hypersensitivity reactions that occur in those with metal allergies, sensitized T-lymphocytes recognize metal ions as antigens. Cytokines are then released and attract a variety of inflammatory cells. Macrophages can subsequently activate more T-cells through their unique ability to present class II major histocompatibility complexes (MHC). This response can lead to tissue damage and inflammation.[34] Furthermore, the activated cytokine cascade can overlap with inflammatory bone loss.[24-27] Goldring speculated that such a response may be the explanation of some cases of painful implants without an obvious source for the pain. He also hypothesized that such instances may eventually end in early loosening and revision.[35]

It is interesting to note that an allergic response to polymethylmethacrylate (PMMA) has been documented in several studies.[30,32,36-38] One study has detected an allergic response to *N,N*-dimethylparatoluidine (DMT), an accelerator utilized in bone cement.[37] This response was directly correlated to early loosening. In another study, patch testing and mononuclear lymphocyte cell subset analysis revealed PMMA lymphocyte hypersensitivity in 50% of 26 patients with a loose total joint arthroplasty.[36] Patch testing of 112 patients with a full-functioning implant revealed no hypersensitivity to PMMA, implicating a PMMA reaction.[39]

Clinical Expression and Implications

Some materials can elicit a reaction in the majority of patients. Conversely, many materials are well tolerated, except in those patients with a hypersensitivity to the agent. In this setting, the response can be so profound as to cause catastrophic failure.

There is no more pertinent example than metal sensitivities. The prevalence of metal sensitivity among the general population is noted to be approximately 10% to 15%.[33] In patients with well-functioning arthroplasties, the prevalence of metal sensitivity is roughly twice that of the general population (approximately 25%). Interestingly, the average prevalence of metal sensitivity among patients with a failed implant is about 60%.[33] Overall, the prevalence of metal sensitivity in patients with a failed implant is six times that of the general population and about two to three times that of all patients with a metal implant.[33] In a controlled assessment of 66 patients, 15% developed a positive patch test to one or more constituents of the prosthesis. Of the 10 who tested positive, one (10%) developed aseptic loosening. In the control group, 5% had evidence of allergy to the elements tested before the prosthesis was inserted.[32] In a larger sample of 220 implants, 6% of the patients developed sensitivity to nickel, cobalt, or chromium. Fourteen percent of those with failed devices had positive patch tests to one or more of the metallic constituents.

The issue is further clouded by the report of Rooker and Wilkinson, who observed that five of six patients with positive patch tests to either nickel, chromium, or cobalt before implantation had negative tests after the procedure.[40] None of the current diagnostic modalities, including the patch test, lymphocyte proliferation test (LTT), or leukocyte migration inhibition testing (MIF), used in isolation provide the definitive diagnosis, further complicating such investigation.[33]

INNATE HOST RESPONSE TO FOREIGN MATERIAL

Based on the above discussion, there is little question that host sensitivity to the constituent materials of a total knee arthroplasty does occur, with host variation playing a role in the degree of the reaction. There is, however, uncertainty as to the significance of this response. The clinical variability of implant failures raises the possibility that the variation could be explained by nonallergic host responses. Our understanding of particulate debris is developing, but radiographic observation of osteolysis is believed to be the most characteristic expression of the host response to particulate debris (Fig. 16-3). The clinical expression of osteolysis, bone resorption, has largely been suggested to occur as nonallergic granuloma formation that is dependent on the following: volume and rate of debris generation, size, shape, and composition of debris. Variable responses to similar radiographic expressions of wear are perplexing. Since the exact mechanism of osteolysis remains to be uncovered, orthopaedic surgeons should remain open to the possibility that individual response variation exists on a spectrum of particulate exposures.

Clinical Expression and Implications

Many of the osteolytic lesions seen in total knee arthroplasties today can be traced back to earlier sterilization tech-

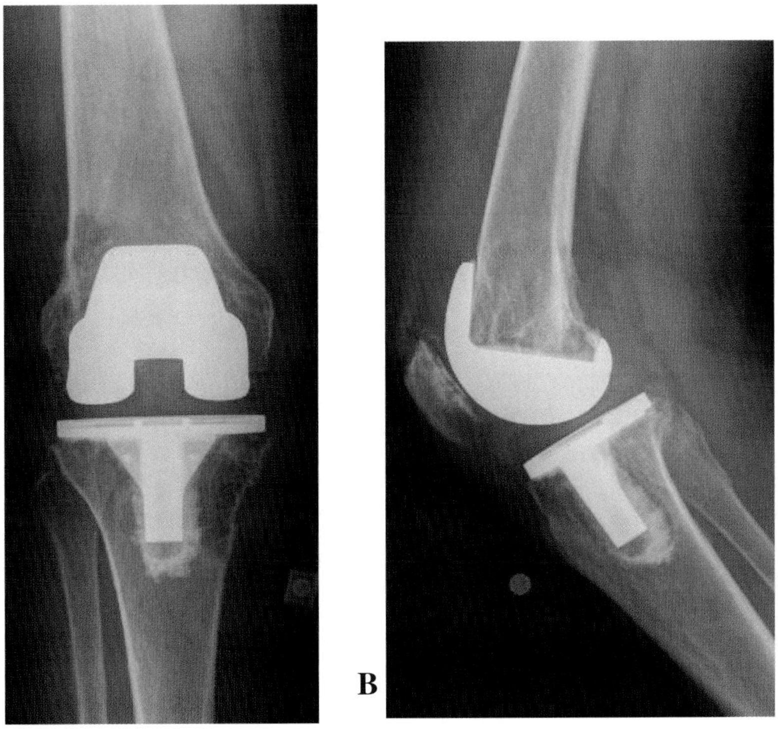

A B

FIGURE 16-3. *Anteroposterior (**A**) and lateral (**B**) radiographs of a 54-year-old male who developed massive osteolysis around both the femoral and tibial components at 5 years postoperatively.*

niques. However, despite newer procedures, these implants continue to fail.[41] Further, the number of implants in the 1990s, before the change in sterilization practices, did increase each consecutive year. Some investigators have observed debris production, tissue reaction, host foreign-body identification, and granuloma formation with osteolysis as a reproducible process.[27] Other investigators concur with this assessment and believe the variation is due to mechanical factors, such as the amount, type, and the size of the particles, rather than to individual host characteristics.[42] Because phagocytosis of the particulate matter is mediated by antibodies and complement, the conclusion was that all particles activate macrophages in a similar manner.[42] This line of reasoning supports the concept that the volume of wear particles is the major contributor to macrophage activation and eventually osteolysis (Fig. 16-1).

Others have suggested two different types of granuloma reaction to foreign material: nonimmune and immune. The immune granuloma is distinguished by B- and T-cell lymphocytes, whereas the nonimmune granuloma is a volumetric response to nondigestible particles. Concern that response to the wear debris may have individual host response features is supported by findings from our laboratory, which show regions of T-cell lymphocytes in the membranes of loose and reconstructed knee joints.[43] The central question remains as to whether granulomata form solely in response to the rate and size of debris particles, as most commonly suggested, or whether an individual host response contributes and modulates the reaction to debris at the molecular level.[35,42,44] The latter question is the topic of recent and ongoing investigations.

Given that most implants fail after 10 years, the number of revision surgeries for osteolysis is expected to increase.[45,46] Alternative bearing surfaces (ceramic-on-ceramic and metal-on-metal) were developed as a response to the dilemma of particulate wear. Nevertheless, while patients implanted with alternative bearing surfaces have a reduction in osteolysis, it is clear that they are not immune to the development of this disease (Fig. 16-4). As new data emerge, it is apparent that an even more profound issue may occur related to production of particulates.[26,27,47-52] Metal ions may be generated from metal-on-metal prostheses or metal-backed components. This supports the notion of an individualized host response.

Other more recent theories have suggested that bacterial by-products play a large role in the development of osteolysis. PAMPs have emerged as possible catalysts to increased osteolysis at the bone–implant interface.[53] Several sources exist for these PAMPs, including a bacterial biofilm that

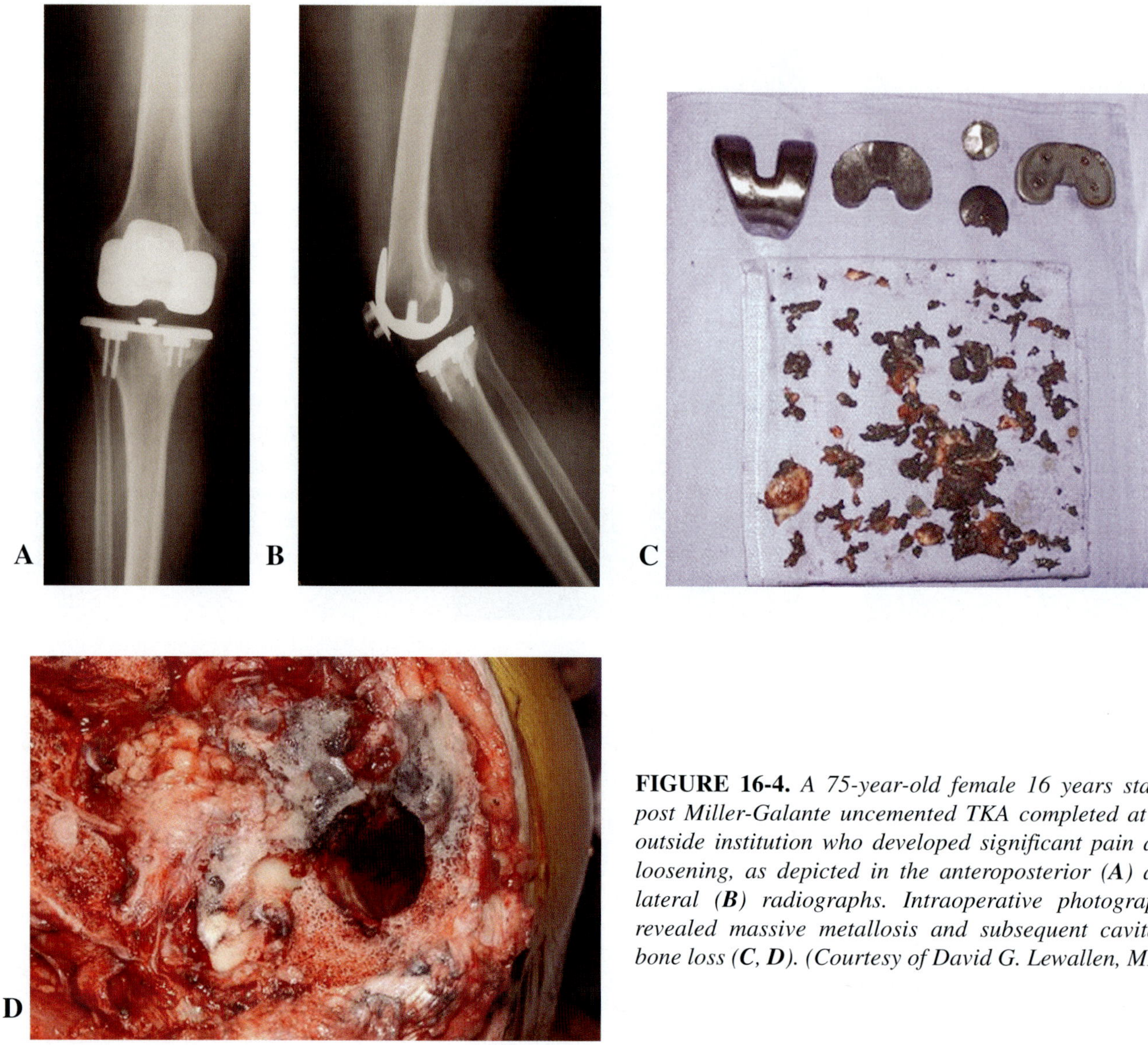

FIGURE 16-4. *A 75-year-old female 16 years status post Miller-Galante uncemented TKA completed at an outside institution who developed significant pain and loosening, as depicted in the anteroposterior (**A**) and lateral (**B**) radiographs. Intraoperative photographs revealed massive metallosis and subsequent cavitary bone loss (**C**, **D**). (Courtesy of David G. Lewallen, MD.)*

forms on the implants, accumulation of bacteria from the bloodstream into periprosthetic tissues, and bacterial debris on the implant before surgical implantation.[53] Regardless of the source, a challenge remains as to who is susceptible and how their host factors interact with an unknown pathogen, the wear debris itself, or a combination of the two to produce osteolysis.

SUMMARY

Most authorities believe there is a common final pathway whereby a similar sequence of events occurs to result in osteolysis, regardless of the precise particle or biologic agent mediating the reaction. As previously discussed, it is generally accepted that the chief variables accounting for the specific response are the rate of generation of the debris and the size and shape of the particle. Nevertheless, the host response to the implanted material may prove to play a greater role and allergic responses to implantable materials do account for a certain percentage of arthroplasty failures. This issue of individual host response will hopefully benefit from the exciting developments in genomic and proteomic research as it is applied to the musculoskeletal system.

REFERENCES

1. Jacobs JJ, Campbell PA, Konttinen Y. How has the biologic reaction to wear particles changed with newer bearing surfaces? *J Am Acad Orthop Surg*. 2008;6(suppl 1):S49-S55.
2. Shanbhag AS, Jacobs JJ, Black J, et al. Human monocyte response to particulate biomaterials generated in vivo and in vitro. *J Orthop Res*. 1995;13(5):792-801.
3. Gordon A, Southam L, Loughlin J, et al. Variation in the secreted frizzled-related protein-3 gene and risk of osteolysis and heterotopic ossification after total hip arthroplasty. *J Orthop Res*. 2007;25(12):1665-1670.
4. Trudel G, Laneuville O, Uhthoff HK. Joint contractures. *Clin Orthop Relat Res*. 2007;456:2.
5. Fergusson D, Hutton B, Drodge A. The epidemiology of major joint contractures: a systematic review of the literature. *Clin Orthop Relat Res*. 2007;456:22-29.
6. Morrey BF. The posttraumatic stiff elbow. *Clin Orthop Relat Res*. 2005;431:26-35.
7. Lindenhovius AL, Jupiter JB. The posttraumatic stiff elbow: a review of the literature. *J Hand Surg Am*. 2007;32(10):1605-1623.
8. Eckenrode BJ, Sennett BJ. Arthrofibrosis of the knee following anterior cruciate ligament reconstruction. *J Orthop Sports Phys Ther*. 2011;41(1):32.
9. Fitzsimmons SE, Vazquez EA, Bronson MJ. How to treat the stiff total knee arthroplasty?: a systematic review. *Clin Orthop Relat Res*. 2010;468(4):1096-1106.
10. Said S, Christainsen SE, Faunoe P, et al. Outcome of surgical treatment of arthrofibrosis following ligament reconstruction. *Knee Surg Sports Traumatol Arthrosc*. 2011;19(10):1704-1708.
11. Schiavone Panni A, Cerciello S, Vasso M, et al. Stiffness in total knee arthroplasty. *J Orthop Traumatol*. 2009;10(3):111-118.
12. Su EP, Su SL, Della Valle AG. Stiffness after TKR: how to avoid repeat surgery. *Orthopedics*. 2010;33 (9):658.
13. Naqvi T, Duong TT, Hashem G, et al. Relaxin's induction of metalloproteinases is associated with the loss of collagen and glycosaminoglycans in synovial joint fibrocartilaginous explants. *Arthritis Res Ther*. 2005;7(1):R1-R11.
14. Hashem G, Zhang Q, Hayami T, et al. Relaxin and beta-estradiol modulate targeted matrix degradation in specific synovial joint fibrocartilages: progesterone prevents matrix loss. *Arthritis Res Ther*. 2006; 8(4):R98.
15. Negishi S, Li Y, Usas A, et al. The effect of relaxin treatment on skeletal muscle injuries. *Am J Sports Med*. 2005;33(12):1816-1824.
16. Ferguson MW, O'Kane S. Scar-free healing: from embryonic mechanisms to adult therapeutic intervention. *Philos Trans R Soc Lond B Biol Sci*. 2004; 359(1445):839-850.
17. Franklin TJ. Current approaches to the therapy of fibrotic diseases. *Biochem Pharmacol*. 1995;49(3): 267-273.
18. Shah M, Foreman DM, Ferguson MW. Neutralising antibody to TGF-beta 1,2 reduces cutaneous scarring in adult rodents. *J Cell Sci*. 1994;107(pt 5):1137-1157.
19. Liu W, Wang DR, Cao YL. TGF-beta: a fibrotic factor in wound scarring and a potential target for anti-scarring gene therapy. *Curr Gene Ther*. 2004;4(1):123-136.
20. Badalamente MA, Hurst LC. Efficacy and safety of injectable mixed collagenase subtypes in the treatment of Dupuytren's contracture. *J Hand Surg Am*. 2007;32(6):767-774.
21. Abdel MP, Morrey ME, Steinmann SP, et al. Gene expression profiles over time of fibrosis in a rabbit knee model of joint contracture. Presented at Orthopedic Research Society Meeting 2011.
22. Tuan RS, Lee FY, Konttinen Y, et al. What are the local and systemic biologic reactions and mediators to wear debris, and what host factors determine or modulate the biologic response to wear particles? *J Am Acad Orthop Surg*. 2008;16(suppl 1):S42-S48.
23. Jacobs JJ, Urban RM, Hallab NJ, et al. Metal-on-metal bearing surfaces. *J Am Acad Orthop Surg*. 2009;17(2):69-76.

24. Korovessis P, Petsinis G, Repanti M, et al. Metallosis after contemporary metal-on-metal total hip arthroplasty. Five to nine-year follow-up. *J Bone Joint Surg Am*. 2006;88(6):1183-1191.
25. Milosev I, Trebse R, Kovac S, et al. Survivorship and retrieval analysis of Sikomet metal-on-metal total hip replacements at a mean of seven years. *J Bone Joint Surg Am*. 2006;88(6):1173-1182.
26. Park YS, Moon Y, Lim S, et al. Early osteolysis following second-generation metal-on-metal hip replacement. *J Bone Joint Surg Am*. 2005;87:1515-1521.
27. Willert HG, Buchhorn GH, Fayyazi A, et al. Metal-on-metal bearings and hypersensitivity in patients with artificial hip joints. A clinical and histomorphological study. *J Bone Joint Surg Am*. 2005;87(1):28-36.
28. Davies AP, Willert HG, Campbell PA, et al. An unusual lymphocytic perivascular infiltration in tissues around contemporary metal-on-metal joint replacements. *J Bone Joint Surg Am*. 2005;87(1):18-27.
29. Benson MK, Goodwin PG, Brostoff J. Metal sensitivity in patients with joint replacement arthroplasties. *Br Med J*. 1975;4(5993):374-375.
30. Deutman R, Mulder TJ, Brian R, et al. Metal sensitivity before and after total hip arthroplasty. *J Bone Joint Surg Am*. 1977;59(7):862-865.
31. Elves MW, Wilson JN, Scales JT, et al. Incidence of metal sensitivity in patients with total joint replacements. *Br Med J*. 1975;4(5993):376-378.
32. Cancilleri F, De Giorgis P, Verdoia C, et al. Allergy to components of total hip arthroplasty before and after surgery. *Ital J Orthop Traumatol*. 1992;18(3):407-410.
33. Hallab N, Merritt K, Jacobs JJ. Metal sensitivity in patients with orthopaedic implants. *J Bone Joint Surg Am*. 2001;83(3):428-436.
34. Hallab NJ, Anderson S, Stafford T, et al. Lymphocyte responses in patients with total hip arthroplasty. *J Orthop Res*. 2005;23(2):384-391.
35. Wang J, Goldring S. *The Role of Particulate Orthopaedic Implant Materials in Peri-Implant Osteolysis*. New York: Raven Press; 1993:119.
36. Gil-Albarova J, Lacleriga A, Barrios C, et al. Lymphocyte response to polymethylmethacrylate in loose total hip prostheses. *J Bone Joint Surg Br*. 1992;74(6):825-830.
37. Haddad FS, Cobb AG, Bentley G, et al. Hypersensitivity in aseptic loosening of total hip replacements. The role of constituents of bone cement. *J Bone Joint Surg Br*. 1996;78(4):546-549.
38. Wooley PH, Petersen S, Song Z, et al. Cellular immune responses to orthopaedic implant materials following cemented total joint replacement. *J Orthop Res*. 1997;15(6):874-880.
39. Carlsson AS, Magnusson B, Moller H. Metal sensitivity in patients with metal-to-plastic total hip arthroplasties. *Acta Orthop Scand*. 1980;51(1):57-62.
40. Rooker GD, Wilkinson JD. Metal sensitivity in patients undergoing hip replacement. A prospective study. *J Bone Joint Surg Br*. 1980;62(4):502-505.
41. Sutula LC, Collier JP, Saum KA, et al. The Otto Aufranc Award: impact of gamma sterilization on clinical performance of polyethylene in the hip. *Clin Orthop Relat Res*. 1995;319:28-40.
42. Murray DW, Rushton N. Macrophages stimulate bone resorption when they phagocytose particles. *J Bone Joint Surg Br*. 1990;72(6):988-992.
43. Witkiewicz H, Turner R, Rock M. *The Local Cellular Response of Components of Total Hip Arthroplasty Experiencing Osteologies*. New York: Raven Press; 1993:425.
44. Willert HG, Bertram H, Buchhorn GH. Osteolysis in alloarthroplasty of the hip. The role of bone cement fragmentation. *Clin Orthop Relat Res*. 1990;258:108-121.
45. Kurtz S, Mowat F, Ong K, et al. Prevalence of primary and revision total hip and knee arthroplasty in the United States from 1990 through 2002. *J Bone Joint Surg Am*. 2005;87:1487-1497.
46. Kurtz SM, Walker PS. How have new designs and new types of joint replacement influenced wear behavior? *J Am Acad Orthop Surg*. 2008;16(suppl 1):S107-S110.
47. Callaghan JJ, Cuckler JM, Huddleston JI, et al. How have alternative bearings (such as metal-on-metal, highly cross-linked polyethylene, and ceramic-on-ceramic) affected the prevention and treatment of osteolysis? *J Am Acad Orthop Surg*. 2008;16(suppl 1):S33-S38.
48. D'Antonio J, Capello W, Manley M, et al. Alumina ceramic bearings for total hip arthroplasty: five-year results of a prospective randomized study. *Clin Orthop Relat Res*. 2005;436:164-171.
49. Dietrich KA, Mazoochian F, Summer B, et al. Intolerance reactions to knee arthroplasty in patients with nickel/cobalt allergy and disappearance of symptoms after revision surgery with titanium-based endoprostheses. *J Dtsch Dermatol Ges*. 2009;7(5):410-413.

50. Frigerio E, Pigatto PD, Guzzi G, et al. Metal sensitivity in patients with orthopaedic implants: a prospective study. *Contact Dermatitis*. 2011;64(5):273-279.
51. Garrett S, Jacobs N, Yates P, et al. Differences in metal ion release following cobalt-chromium and oxidized zirconium total knee arthroplasty. *Acta Orthop Belg*. 2010;76(4):513-520.
52. Savarino L, Tigani D, Greco M, et al. The potential role of metal ion release as a marker of loosening in patients with total knee replacement: a cohort study. *J Bone Joint Surg Br*. 2010;92(5):634-638.
53. Greenfield EM, Bechtold J. What other biologic and mechanical factors might contribute to osteolysis? *J Am Acad Orthop Surg*. 2008;16(suppl 1):S56-S62.

17 Orthopaedic Implant Oncogenesis

Joseph F. Alderete, Jr., and Michael G. Rock

Prosthetic-derived metal wear debris is generated by mechanical wear, surface corrosion, or both, and consists of particulate and solid forms. The presence of particulate metal matter, polyethylene, and even fragments of polymethylmethacrylate in local tissues has been confirmed.[1-3] In spite of all the modifications made in implant composition, implant fixation, and articulation, corrosion of these products persists and such corrosion can lead to osteolysis and failure of the implant.[4-7] Corrosion occurs at all metal surfaces, yielding corrosion products consisting mainly of metal oxides (Cr_2O_3, CoO, TiO_2, Al_2O_3, etc) and hydroxides [$Cr(OH)_3$, $Co(OH)_2$, etc]. These corrosion products have the ability to produce different responses in the local environment than their parent particulate matter. The search for the ultimate frictionless bearing surface and strongest biocompatible fracture implant remains the focus of many biomechanical laboratories and orthopaedic literature to avoid osteolysis-related implant failure.[8] The ultimate question is: Can these corrosion products generate enough of an immune response to elicit oncogenesis?

The individual host response can be divided into three categories: (1) allergic hypersensitivity, (2) cell-mediated reaction, and (3) toxic response to the implant.[9] The local tissue response to wear particles is attributed to particle characteristics and the immunogenic response. Particle factors include composition, size, shape, volume, and bioreactivity. Metal-on-metal prostheses generate 6.7 × 10^12 to 2.5 × 10^14 particles per year which is significantly higher than the standard metal-on-polyethylene bearing.[10] Despite the larger number of particles, the absolute amount of debris, or volumetric wear, from a metal-on-metal articulation is much lower owing to the size of the particles (<50 nm) versus the 0.1-μm size observed in a metal-on-polyethylene articulation. Nevertheless, the surface area of released metal debris is much higher than that of polyethylene debris, leading to a greater potential for corrosion and bioreactivity.[11] This bioreactivity can take the form of osteolysis, pseudotumor, periprosthetic effusion, and the theoretic potential for malignancy.

Finally, the design of articular surfaces and their subsequent wear differ from hip to knee arthroplasty. Femoral head size, polyethylene thickness, and the effective joint space are factors that contribute to wear in hip arthroplasty. Surface conformation, polyethylene size and composition, and backside wear are factors significant to knee arthroplasty osteolysis. Wear, osteolysis, and tumorigenesis are therefore slightly different from hip to knee; however, the final common pathways are consistent and the potential for immune response is the same.

PHYSIOLOGIC RESPONSE TO DEBRIS

The body's response to the local presence of debris is dependent on the size and amount of debris, as well as the rate of accumulation. Endocytosis is the mechanism by which cells uptake metal nanoparticles (150 μm), whereas larger particles stimulate phagocytosis by macrophages.[10] The body attempts to neutralize these foreign particles by precipitating granulomatous foreign-body reactions and/or removing them through local lymphatic channels. If the local accumulation of debris exceeds the body's ability to neutralize or transport it, the debris migrates from the site to remote areas, including the bone–cement or bone–implant surfaces, possibly contributing to, if not initiating, the phenomenon of loosening and osteolysis.

Of equal or possibly even greater concern is the detection of metal ions, polyethylene, and even methylmethacrylate in areas remote from the implant, including serum, urine, and regional draining lymph nodes. Elevated serum levels of metal ions consistent with the composition of the implanted alloy have been confirmed in experimental models in animals and in humans after total hip arthroplasty identifying serum levels of chromium, nickel, and titanium that are 2- to 3-fold higher than preoperative determinations.[12,13] These figures are widely within the accepted normal range for these metallic ions in humans. Therefore, it is assumed that toxic levels of these foreign materials do not materialize. However, when the serum-to-urine concentration in patients subjected to conventional total hip arthroplasty is analyzed, it has become apparent that the urine concentration of chromate in particular does not rise with the same magnitude as the serum level. This would suggest that the rise in serum values of metal ions that occurs within the first several weeks postoperatively exceeds the urinary ability to excrete them; therefore, it is entirely plausible that metal ions can accumulate in organs and tissues remote from implantation and that these concentrations, unlike those in the systemic circulation, can increase as a result of the unidirectional, intracellular ingestion of these particles.

Evidence for metallic debris accumulating in distant organs has been confirmed by Langkamer et al, who identified widespread dissemination of particulate wear debris from hip prostheses to lymph nodes, liver, and spleen.[14,15] They reported increases above normal levels in these organs to 30-fold for aluminum, chromium, and iron in the lymphatics and 10-fold in the spleen and liver. This was previously suggested by Steineman, who calculated the potential release of metallic ions of 0.15 to 0.3 μg/cm^2/day, which would translate to between 11 and 22 mg/year in patients with total hip replacement.[16] This incidentally coincides with the total body burden of such metallic ions in a 70-kg man. These findings suggest that concentrations of metal ions at remote sites may reach such proportions as to precipitate altered cellular dynamics in organs principally of the lymphoreticular system. It would only be logical to assume that local concentrations of such debris at the site of implantation would be even higher, although attempts at quantifying local concentrations have been fraught with inaccuracies, mostly resulting from sampling error and the inability to measure bioavailable or nonbioavailable metal species.

What is potentially more disturbing is that these figures for serum concentrations and the identification of this debris in remote organs have come from patients who have been subjected to conventional cemented components. With the increasing use of uncemented porous-coated implants, particularly in younger patients, these figures would be expected to increase, creating the distinct possibility of toxic levels in the serum, tissues, and organs. These structures could respond with altered cellular dynamics and function.

At the cellular level, altered function of T cells, B cells, and macrophages in response to metal ions can result in altered cytokine release, immunogenic compounds, and direct cytotoxicity. Evidence of decreased lymphoproliferative cell lines has been observed in arthritis patients and lymphoid population decreases have been induced in experimental animals in response to metal implantation.[10] The systemic response can be divided into allergic hypersensitivity, cell-mediated reaction, and toxic response to the implant.[9] It has been observed that wear and osteolysis resulting in failure have a macrophage granuloma-mediated foreign-body reaction where one sees polyethylene-debris-laden histiocytes.[17] Metal-on-metal components have the potential to generate the same response or a vascular infiltrate of T-lymphocytes and plasma cells with increased vascularity, fibrin exudation, and necrosis. Willert et al observed this pattern to resemble a type IV hypersensitivity reaction and thus coined the term aseptic lymphocytic vasculitis and associated lesions (ALVAL).[18]

There has been great interest in the environment composed of the implant and the surrounding wear debris-generated pseudocapsule. When does the insult occur that transforms a benign granulomatous environment into neoplasia? Preneoplastic mesenchymal lesions have not been well defined or classified and their exact significance is unclear.[19] Nevertheless, there may be a spectrum from granulomatous masses seen around implants, such as in the 2007 report by Papagelopoulos et al, which at some point undergo subcellular tumorigenesis and become cancer.[20]

WEAR-ASSOCIATED SOFT TISSUE MASS OR PSEUDOTUMOR

There is considerable debate in the literature over whether early osteolysis and failure is a result of host hypersensitivity or a predictable response to excess wear particles and a primed immune system. Calcedo et al have proposed a mechanism by which there is a dose-related response and activation of cytokines IL-1b, TNF-alpha, and NFcB, which can lead to bone resorption and failure and a soft tissue response.[21] Bhandari et al, in a review of pseudotumor, described the spectrum of results from this process. The final common pathway can lead to ALVAL and soft tissue necrotic pseudotumors, wear particle granulomatous pseudotumor, effusion and bursal formation, infection, or allergy.[17] Where the end result is a mass around the implant, two entities are typically seen. The first is a solid or semi-solid structure consisting of necrosis, "ghost" spindle cells, aggregates of histiocytes, giant cells, and inflammatory cells (Figs. 17-1 to 17-3).[22,23] This large granuloma is thought to be a dose-related response to a poorly functioning arthroplasty, yielding many wear particles. This can happen with metal-on-metal articulations as well as conventional bearing surfaces. Another type of mass that can form around an implant is ALVAL. This pattern of mass is a description for a family of reactions for which metal-on-metal bearing failures have been associated with diffuse and perivascular T-lymphocyte and plasma cell invasion, increased endothelial vascularity, fibrin exudation, and necrosis.[22,23] With the presence of mesenchymal spindle cells, histiocytes, giant cells, and necrosis, this entity can be confused histologically with neoplasm or fungal infection. Morphologically ALVAL and associated necrotic granulomatous tumors are different from wear particle graulomatous pseudotumors by the absence of identifiable particulate matter in ALVAL-associated lesions and more frank necrosis.[22]

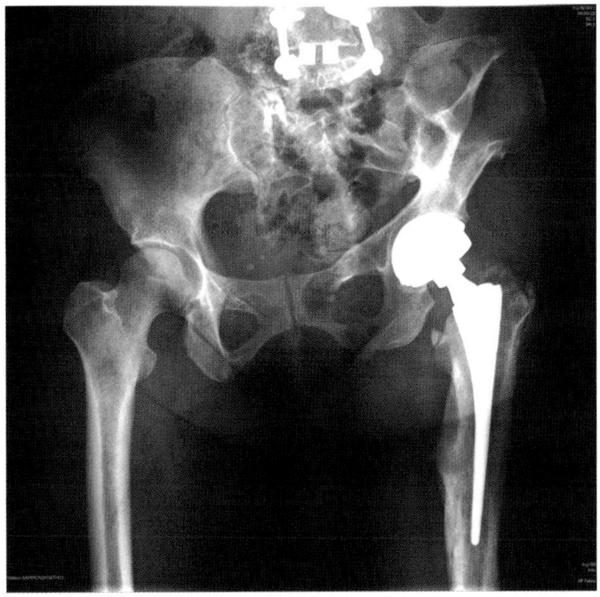

FIGURE 17-1. *Plain anteroposterior X-ray of the pelvis of a 47-year-old female with a painful metal-on-metal left total hip arthroplasty. Her workup was negative for infection and metal ion sensitivity.*

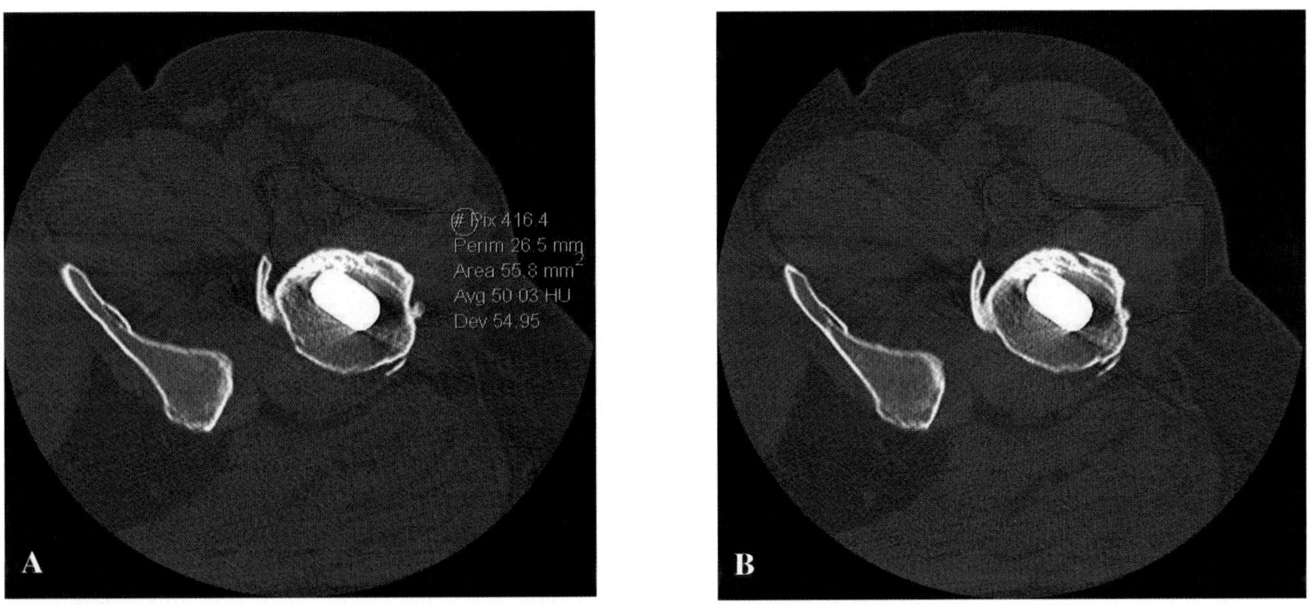

FIGURE 17-2. (*A* and *B*) *Computed tomography scan of left hip revealing a 2.6 × 2.1 × 2.0-mm mass with Hounsfield Unit (HU) measurement of 58 HU consistent with complex fluid collection with some semi-solid areas.*

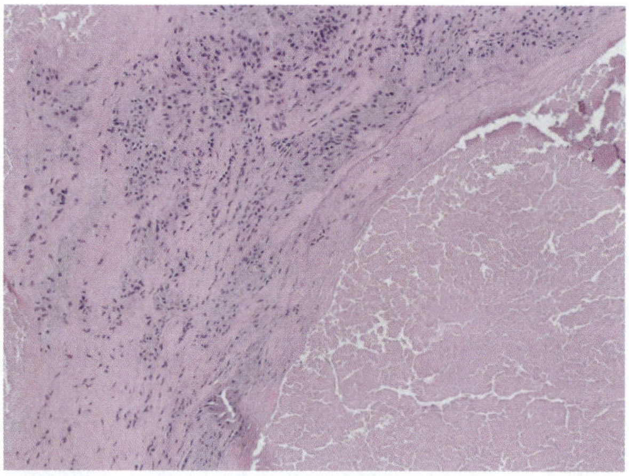

FIGURE 17-3. *Histology. Variable degree of peripheral dense fibroconnective tissue with scattered foci of predominantly chronic inflammation composed of lymphocytes and histiocytes. Of note, there are numerous histiocytes, confirmed by CD68 and fine, foreign particulate matter, which is nonpolarizable with polarized light. The histopathologic features are consistent with a foreign-body granulomatous mass (ie, a fibrinous exudative capsule surface, a variable chronic or granulomatous inflammatory infiltrate, and an accumulation of foamy macrophages).*

CARCINOGENIC POTENTIAL OF METALS AND POLYMERS

Perhaps one of the greatest concerns with debris dissemination locally and within the systemic circulation is the possibility of inducing carcinogenesis. This is thought to be possible by one of two mechanisms:

1. A "solid-state" mechanism has been proposed whereby a large foreign object implanted in vivo stimulates mutagenesis of local cells, creating a tumor by its mere presence. Most large foreign objects, on implantation, initiate a very marked fibrous reaction. The cells within this fibrous reaction ultimately mutate and become neoplastic.

2. The other inescapable possibility is that either particulate metal matter or other sources of debris have an innate capacity to promote oncogenesis.

Metal ions released from orthopaedic implants can induce apoptosis and necrosis with Co(II) and V(III) among the most cytotoxic. Corrosion products including CoO, Cr_2O_3, and $CrPO_4$ also show cytotoxicity.[10] Within a cell nucleus, these metal ions or corrosion products can cause mutation by forming adducts with DNA and DNA cross-links. Redox metals, such as Ni, Co, and Ti, can generate reactive oxygen species such as the superoxide radical and hydroxyl radical by reacting with hydrogen peroxide. Reactive oxygen species can induce oxidative damage to DNA. DNA repair impairment, altered signal transduction, and gene expression have all been observed in response to multiple implant ions, especially Ni(II), Cr(VI), and Co(II).[11]

Well-documented cases of carcinoma and sarcoma have developed in refinery workers who have inhaled nickel and chromium and in miners who were exposed to iron, or even at local injection sites of iron dextran.[24] Aluminum has been linked to a high rate of lung and bladder cancer in exposed individuals, and titanium has been associated with experimental induction of lymphoreticular tumors and leukemia. Although the results have not been universally accepted, many animal experiments have shown a direct correlation between the initiation of sarcomas and the injection of particulate metal debris. This appears to be related to concentration, as well as physical nature, of the metal implanted.[25,26]

Further refinement to the animal model has been presented in which a high incidence of malignant mesenchymal tumors arose around subcutaneously implanted biomaterials. Malignant tumors, such as malignant fibrous histiocytoma and pleomorphic sarcomas, were found in 25.8% of the implantation sites over a 6-month to 2-year period. What was unique about this study was the histologic confirmation of a spectrum of change within the capsule around the implanted biomaterials. This included changes from focal proliferation to preneoplastic proliferation and ultimate evolution into incipient sarcoma. This study afforded the opportunity to witness defined stages in the development of mesenchymal malignancies as a by-product of implanted biomaterials.

Furthermore, particulate metal matter may not be the only solid-form material that can be, and has been proven to be, carcinogenic in the environment. In 1954, long before the first total hip arthroplasty was performed, Laskin postulated the carcinogenic capability of polymethylmethacrylate after subcutaneous introduction of this material in mice.[27] His conclusions suggested similar occurrences of tumor in humans who were being treated at that time with methylmethacrylate for dental deficiencies and that this evolution of cancer may take up to 20 years of exposure, given the proportional time of exposure before tumors were seen in the mice. A similar conclusion was reached by Carter and Rowe, regarding the use of polyethylene plastics before it was conventional to use them in the management of arthritic joints.[28] Regardless of the form, whether powder or large segments, polyethylene plastic produced sarcomas in 25% and 30% of rats, respectively. Their conclusions also suggested that there is a latent period of 20 years in humans before such an event could be expected to occur.

It is therefore noteworthy that investigators were forewarning the medical community of the carcinogenic effect of metals and polymers years before the development and introduction of joint replacements using these very same materials. In 1969, Sir John Charnley introduced total hip arthroplasty as an alternative in the management of arthritic hips. No other orthopaedic procedure has been adopted with such enthusiasm. Forty years later, we are still witnessing an incremental increase in the yearly utilization of this operation, attesting to its obvious success. According to some investigators, we may be coming into an era of increased tumor activity in the vicinity of, or possibly remote from, implantation of these prostheses.

CASE REPORTS OF NEOPLASIA AT OR NEAR ORTHOPAEDIC IMPLANTS

The phenomenon of sarcoma at or near the site of an orthopaedic implant is most disconcerting. Neoplasia near an implant has been observed since 1956 when McDougall reported a histologically high-grade vascular lesion associated with a plate-and-screw construct for trauma.[29] Since the 1950s, masses around implants have taken two forms: granulomatous pseudotumor and frank malignancy (sarcoma, lymphoma, or carcinoma).

In 1976, Harris et al described an aggressive granulomatous lesion around a cemented femoral stem in a total hip replacement.[30] This was a condition of localized tumor-like bone resorption that appeared radiographically as large lytic defects within the femur, approximating the cement mantle of the implant. Initially thought to be neoplastic, these lesions were surgically biopsied and found to be consistent with well-organized connective tissue containing numerous histiocytes, monocytes, and fibroblastic reactive zones. Immunohistologic evaluation revealed multinucleated giant cells and nonspecific esterase-positive monocyte macrophages. These findings suggest a foreign-body type reaction, and, with the subsequent isolation of polyethylene, methylmethacrylate, and metal debris, it was theorized that these constituents of the construct likely migrated down around the implant cement mantle in cemented prostheses throughout the effective joint space. Such a reaction suggests an excessive accumulation of debris at the site of articulation that surpasses the body's ability to neutralize or transport the material, resulting in migration of debris to sites remote from the source. This rapid appearance of bone loss radiographically, which is often associated with a deteriorating clinical course, has been termed type II aseptic loosening. More recently Papagelopoulos et al described a pseudotumorous mass in the distal leg after wide resection for proximal tibial osteosarcoma and reconstruction with a knee megaprosthesis.[20] Seven years after reconstruction, an open biopsy for a palpable mass located in the leg distal to the operative site revealed dark amorphous metal debris with histology showing metal particle fibroblasts, osteoblasts, histiocytes, and macrophages. There was no evidence of recurrence.[20] This is characteristic of wear debris-associated masses that have no malignant features but represent the body's attempt to localize a tissue response to foreign-body accumulation.

Seventy-six cases of implant-associated malignancy have been reported over the past 50 years, 22 involving non-arthroplasty-associated hardware (plates and screws for trauma, staples for arthrodesis, etc) and 54 cases associated with hip or knee arthroplasty. Fifty-one sarcomas are associated with total hip arthroplasty[31-33] and three are associated with total knee arthroplasty (see Tables 17-1 to 17-3).[34-36] Forty-seven cases have appeared in published series around arthroplasty and seven in unpublished case forum. Reports in which there were obvious predisposing conditions complicating the association between the implant and tumorigenesis have not been included.

In a review of the most recent literature, several criteria emerge for implant-related sarcoma. These are by no means an agreed upon consensus but are more repetitive observations[26]:

1. The tumor must be in direct vicinity of the implant.
2. There must exist some latency period for tumorigenesis. Oppenheimer first observed that implants removed at 12 months did not induce sarcoma in experimental animals.[37] Since then we have not been able to agree upon a reasonable interval that represents an oncogenic event. Some have suggested that the latency should be 5 years corresponding to the agreed upon latency for postradiation sarcoma. Studies have been able to use spectroscopic trace metal analysis to identify statistically significant elevations in metal ion complexes, specifically vanadium, within an osteosarcoma at 3 years.
3. Finally, the patient should not have received a concomitant tumorigenic insult or have history of malignancy or predisposing condition (radiation therapy, Maffucci syndrome, or Ollier's disease, etc).

Observation of the potential for implant oncogenesis started with implants to treat fractures and, since McDougal's first report in 1956, 22 cases of tumors around nonarthroplasty hardware have been reported (Table 17-1).[29,38-40] The vast majority of malignancies both in the prosthetic and internal fixation groups have occurred in the vicinity of vitallium implants. This is not, however, to exonerate stainless steel, because tumors in the proximity of implants made of this alloy have been reported in the animal literature as well as the human experience utilizing stainless steel as fixation devices for traumatology. There have also been cases of sarcomas adjacent to titanium arthroplasty, fracture, and dental implants.[33,39,41] It is interesting to note that, in 1976, veterinarians were encouraged within their own literature to report similar experiences of tumors around implants, 8 years before such concern was voiced regarding the application of these metallic alloys in humans. Most recently, McDonald et al reported on two high-grade angiosarcomas of bone in association with a Sherman stainless steel plate for trauma.[39] Interestingly, both patients had an extraordinarily long latency period (40 years), and high-grade angiosarcoma of bone is extremely rare, comprising less than 1% of malignant bone tumors. There have been three other associations of high-grade vascular lesions around implants out of the total 74 cases.[29,39,42,43]

Since the introduction of the Charnley hip in the 1960s, joint replacement arthroplasty has changed a great many lives. However, with the increasing number of implant recipients and the increasing age of the general population,

TABLE 17-1. Malignancy Associated with Nonarthroplasty Implants

Author	Year	Age and Sex	Implant	Time Interval (yrs)	Tumor Type
McDougall-McNally	1956	42M	Stainless steel	30	Ewings
Delgado et al	1958	40M	Stainless steel	3	Undifferentiated
Dube-Fisher et al	1972	84M	Stainless steel	36	Angiosarcoma
Tayton et al	1980	11F	Vitallium	7.5	Ewings
McDonald et al	1981	48M	Vitallium	17	Lymphoma
Dodion et al	1982	49M	Vitallium	1.2	Lymphoma
Lee et al	1984	58M	Vitallium	14	Malignant fibrous histiocytoma
Hughes et al	1987	42M	Vitallium	29	Malignant fibrous histiocytoma
Ward et al	1990	65F	Stainless steel–Smith-Peterson	9	Osteosarcoma
Khurana et al	1991	39M	Stainless steel–Hansen-Street	13	Malignant fibrous histiocytoma
Radhi et al	1998	25M	Stainless steel	8	Non-Hodgkins lymphoma
Laffargue et al	2001	20M	NA	NA	MFH
McDonald et al	2002	70 M	Stainless steel	52	Angiosarcoma
McDonald et al	2002	71M	Stainless steel	41	Angiosarcoma
Keel et al	2001	18M	Stainless steel (staples for osteotomies)	10	OGS

Continued

TABLE 17-1. *Continued*

Author	Year	Age and Sex	Implant	Time Interval (yrs)	Tumor Type
Keel et al	2001	16F	Stainless steel (staples for osteotomies)	NA	OGS
Keel et al	2001	54M	IM nail for trauma (stainless steel)	14	MFH
Keel et al	2001	65F	IM nail for trauma (stainless steel)	9	OGS
Keel et al	2001	38M	IM nail for trauma (stainless steel)	20	OGS
Keel et al	2001	56M	IM nail for trauma (stainless steel)	15	OGS
Olmedo et al	2007	35F	Pin/screw fixation for arthrodesis	4	MFH
McGuff et al	2008	38F	Titanium maxillary implant	11 mos	Low-grade chondroblastic OGS

M, male; F, female; MFH, malignant fibrous histiocytoma (undifferentiated high-grade pleomorphic sarcoma); OGS, osteogenic sarcoma; IM, intramedullary; NHL, non-Hodgkins lymphoma; NA, not available.

there have been increasing reports of tumors around implants (Table 17-2). In 1978, only 2 years after the introduction of pseudotumors of bone induced by the components of total hip arthroplasty, Arden and Bywaters reported a case of a 56-year-old patient who developed a high-grade fibrosarcoma of soft tissue 2.5 years after receiving a metal-on-metal McKee-Farrar hip prosthesis.[44] The tumor apparently did not have any direct association with the underlying bone or any components of the total hip arthroplasty. No formal analysis of the tumor for debris products was performed. This case drew attention to the possibility of tumors being initiated in the presence of large orthopaedic appliances. It was not until 1984 that this concept became fashionable, in large part because of three articles that appeared simultaneously in the *Journal of Bone and Joint Surgery* recounting two malignant fibrous histiocytomas and one osteosarcoma at the site of a total hip arthroplasty.[12,45,46]

TABLE 17-2. Published Malignancies Associated with Arthroplasty

Author	Year	Implant	Age	Time Interval (yrs)	Tumor Type
Castleman	1965	Autin-Moore	56M	1	Malignant fibrous histiocytoma
Rushford	1974	McKee-Farrar	54M	0.5	Osteosarcoma
Arden & Bywaters	1978	McKee-Farrar	56M	2.5	Fibrosarcoma
Bago-Granell	1984	Charnley-Müller	77F	2	Malignant fibrous histiocytoma

Continued

TABLE 17-2. *Continued*

Author	Year	Implant	Age	Time Interval (yrs)	Tumor Type
Penman & Ring	1984	Ring	75F	5	Osteosarcoma
Swann	1984	McKee-Farrar	63M	4	Malignant fibrous histiocytoma
Weber	1986	Cemented TKA	81F	4.5	Epithelioid sarcoma
Ruy	1987	Ceramic + CrCo/AlO uncemented	40M	1.5	Malignant fibrous histiocytoma
Vives	1987	Charnley-Müller	69M	2	Malignant fibrous histiocytoma
Van der List	1988	Charnley-Müller	72F	12	Angiosarcoma
Lamovec	1988	Charnley-Müller	50M	12	Synovial sarcoma
Lamovec	1988	Charnley-Müller	65F	10	Osteosarcoma
Tait	1988	Charnley-Müller	56F	11	Malignant fibrous histiocytoma
Martin	1988	Charnley-Müller	66F	10.5	Osteosarcoma
Haag & Adler	1989	Weber-Huggier	69F	10	Malignant fibrous histiocytoma
Brien	1990	Charnley	60F	8	Osteosarcoma
Troop	1990	Charnley-Müller	39M	15	Malignant fibrous histiocytoma
Kolstad & Högstorp	1990	Freeman TKA	75M	0.25	Metastatic adenocarcinoma
Jacobs	1992	AML cementless	65M	0.5	Malignant fibrous histiocytoma
Solomon & Sekel	1992	Charnley-Müller	48F	7	MFH
Aboulafia et al	1994	CoCr	64F	1.5	MFH
Minami et al	1995	THA (bipolar)	NA	NA	NA
Theegarten et al	1995	Lord	63M	5	MFH
Mathiessen	1995	Charnley-Müller	74F	15	MFH
Bell et al	1997	Cemented, CrCo, THA	62F	4	MFH
Cole et al	1997	Previous Ti uncemented to CrCo	61F	2	MFH
Langkamer et al	1997	Charnley-Müller	77F	3	Leiomyosarcoma
Langkamer et al	1997	Charnley-Müller	75M	2	MFH
Langkamer et al	1997	Charnley-Müller	77F	20	Leiomyosarcoma
Langkamer et al	1997	Charnley-Müller	69M	4	MFH

Continued

TABLE 17-2. ***Continued***

Author	Year	Implant	Age	Time Interval (yrs)	Tumor Type
Radhi et al	1998	CrCo, THA, uncemented	63F	4	NHL
Stephensen et al	1999	Titanium cemented	57M	6	Liposarcoma
Ito & Shimizu	1999	Charnley, stainless steel	80F	8	NHL
Ganapathi et al	2001	Stainless steel	85F	12	NHL
Rana et al	2001	Howse I	66F	13	Spindle cell sarcoma
Keel et al	2001	NA	73F	2.5	OGS
Keel et al	2001	NA	85M	7	MPNST
Keel et al	2001	NA	75M	5	MFH
Keel et al	2001	Plate/screw fixation for fx then THR	50M	2.5 after THA; 33 after ORIF	MFH
Keel et al	2001	Ti Alloy Modular System	68M	3	OGS
Keel et al	2001	Cr Co	61M	6.5	MFH
Lucas et al	2001	Bipolar CrCo	77F	2	MFH
Lucas et al	2001	Bipolar then Osteonic Omnifit	67M	8	MFH
Prasad et al	2002	Howse II	70M	6.5	OGS
Syed et al	2002	Exeter	75F	8	NHL
Adams et al	2003	Harris-Galante	62M	3	OGS
Shuh et al	2004	Jorgensen Ti5A12, 5Fe	66F	8	MFH

M, male; F, female; MFH, malignant fibrous histiocytoma (undifferentiated high-grade pleomorphic sarcoma); OGS, osteogenic sarcoma; MPNST, malignant peripheral nerve sheath tumor; NHL, non-Hodgkins lymphoma; THA, total hip arthroplasty; TKA, total knee arthroplasty; THR, total hip replacement; NA, not available; ORIF, open reduction and internal fixation.

This sudden and rather unexpected evolution prompted an editorial in the same journal that addressed the issue of sarcoma and total hip arthroplasty and encouraged the orthopaedic community worldwide to report such cases to a central registry to obtain more accurate findings on the incidence of such a problem.[47] These tumors occurred 2, 4, and 5 years after hip replacement that was performed with various femoral and acetabular components, some with metal-on-metal articulations and others with metal-on-polyethylene. In two of these cases, the proximal femur was extensively involved with tumor that was in direct contact with the component. The remaining case was a soft tissue sarcoma not in direct approximation to the prosthesis. Two of these tumors were malignant fibrous histiocytomas, one of bone and one of soft tissue. The remaining tumor was an osteosarcoma. In this particular case, there was evidence of gray-brown pigmentation both intra- and extracellularly between the tumor and the femoral component. No formal metal analysis was performed. Three additional cases emerged before 1988 at 15 months, 4.5 years, and 2 years after implantation.[34,48,49]

In 1988, five cases were reported occurring at 10 years[50,51] and 11 years[12,43,52] after implantation. The sarcomas included two osteosarcomas, two malignant fibrous histiocytomas, and one synovial sarcoma. Two of these were of soft tissue in location with no direct association with the implant, yet in a case report by Tait there was evidence of nickel within the tumor cells.[52] In the remaining three patients, all sarcomas had direct contact with either the cement or implant, with the tumor originating in bone.

In 1990, there were three additional reports in the literature, which included an osteosarcoma that developed at the site of a Charnley total hip arthroplasty 8 years after implantation,[53] a malignant fibrous histiocytoma that developed 15 years after a Charnley-Müller total hip arthroplasty,[54] and metastatic adenocarcinoma that developed at the site of a Freeman total knee arthroplasty 3 months after implantation.[35] In 1992, Jacobs et al presented a malignant fibrous histiocytoma that developed 6 months after implantation of a cementless AML total hip arthroplasty.[55] In that same journal volume, unpublished but submitted reports of five tumors that occurred around implants were brought to orthopaedic attention.[56] These included two malignant fibrous histiocytomas around a Thompson-Müller total hip arthroplasty, an osteosarcoma around a Charnley total hip arthroplasty, a rhabdomyosarcoma of soft tissue in the vicinity of a Christiansen total hip arthroplasty, as well as a chondrosarcoma developing in a patient with Maffucci syndrome who had undergone a Charnley total hip arthroplasty. The intervals from implantation to tumor detection were 9, 3, 10, 9, and 1 years, respectively. More recently a liposarcoma has been identified in the vicinity of a total joint prosthesis.[57] To this, we add two additional patients, neither of whom had their joint replacement done at the Mayo Clinic (Table 17-3). The first is that of a 79-year-old man who, 9 months previously, had a total hip replacement with an uncemented Harris-Galante component; he was found to have a large malignant fibrous histiocytoma engulfing the proximal femur and extending to the implant. There was, however, no evidence of any particulate debris within the tumor cells removed. The second case was that of a 56-year-old man who developed a soft tissue osteosarcoma 14 months after a left total knee arthroplasty with conventional cemented components. The tumor extended down to both the femoral and patellar components.

Keel et al of Massachusetts General Hospital reported 12 cases of orthopaedic implant-associated neoplasia occurring in patients aged 18 to 85 (mean 55): 5 patients had a total hip arthroplasty, 4 patients had an intramedullary nail for trauma, 2 had staples for an osteotomy, and 1 patient had fracture fixation followed by a hip arthroplasty.[19] There were 2 soft tissue sarcomas and 10 bone tumors consisting of 7 osteosarcomas, 4 high-grade pleomorphic undifferentiated sarcomas (previously malignant fibrous histiocytomas, MFHs), and 1 malignant peripheral nerve sheath tumor. Other series include that by Rana et al, who presented a 79-year-old female with a high-grade spindle cell sarcoma 13 years after total hip arthroplasty with a stainless steel implant. Magnetic resonance imaging showed direct communication between the tumor and the intramedullary canal

TABLE 17-3. Unpublished Malignancies Associated with Arthroplasty

Author	Year	Implant	Time Interval (yrs)	Tumor Type
Harris	1992	Charnley	1	Chondrosarcoma
Surin	1992	Christiansen	9	Rhabdomyosarcoma
Lightowler	1992	Charnley	10	Osteosarcoma
Rees	1992	Thompson	3	Malignant fibrous histiocytoma
Nelson	1992	Müller	9	Malignant fibrous histiocytoma
Rock	1992	PCA ingrowth	8	Malignant fibrous histiocytoma
Rock	1992	PCA TKA	1.2	Osteosarcoma

PCA, porous-coated anatomic; TKA, total knee arthroplasty.

through a cortical breach.[58] Prasad et al reported an osteosarcoma occurring 6.5 years after a Howse II TiALV component total hip arthroplasty.[59] Adams et al observed an osteogenic sarcoma 3 years after implantation of a Harris-Galante Ti stem/CoCr head implant in a 62-year-old male. They used a detailed spectroscopic trace metal analysis to recover elevated vanadium and chromium, but not aluminum, nickel, or titanium, from the tumor.[60] Schuh et al reported a high-grade pleomorphic undifferentiated sarcoma in a 66-year-old female 8 years after total hip arthroplasty, discovered for increasing pain and loosening of the implant. This case is yet another illustration that new pain and severe osteolysis should prompt consideration of sarcoma in an evaluation. Of note, she had a history of rheumatoid arthritis and long-term steroid use, which has been suggested to be a risk factor for MFH.[32] Finally, our colleagues in dentistry and oral-maxillofacial surgery reported the first case of osteogenic sarcoma around a titanium dental implant 11 months after the index surgery. This tumor was located in the maxilla directly adjacent to the implant and there were no other identifiable predisposing factors (infection, etc). Osteogenic sarcoma of the mandible and maxilla make up only 10% of osteogenic sarcoma presentations.[41]

There is no direct correlation between the morphology of the sarcoma and biomaterial type in previous animal studies.[26,37] Likewise, there was no correlation between sarcoma type and implant makeup in the combined series above. There are some trends, however. Pure titanium, nickel chromium, cobalt chromium alloy, and aluminum oxide were less associated with proliferative and malignant changes, while polymethylmethacrylate, polyethylene, and silicone implants had a greater association with neoplasia.

A review of the published literature on the subject indicates that the diagnosis of a tumor superimposed on, or at least in proximity to, these replacements carries with it a dismal prognosis. Most are high grade at presentation and figures available suggest that a vast majority of patients succumb to disease within the first year after diagnosis and many within several weeks to months from the time of tumor detection and management.

CRITICAL ANALYSIS AND SIGNIFICANCE

As impressive as these cases may be, they must be put into a perspective given the global use of internal fixation and prosthetic devices. In a recent report, Iorio et al reported that approximately 285,000 hips were replaced and 523,000 knees were replaced in the United States to date.[61] We are approaching 1 million hip and knee replacements performed worldwide each year, not to mention the shoulder, elbow, wrist, and ankle arthroplasty performed. In another epidemiologic work, the American Academy of Orthopaedic Surgeons estimated that 9.65 million arthroplasties were performed in the United States between 1990 and 2002. Twenty patients were reported to have an implant-related sarcoma during that period. That provides an incidence of 1 implant sarcoma in 482,000 people. Now, there are approximately 3000 new primary bone tumors and 5000 soft tissue tumors in the United States per year. This would give an incidence of approximately 1 in 100,000 for the general population to develop a primary bone sarcoma and 1 in 40,000 to develop a soft tissue sarcoma per year. These figures obviously are not stratified for age, given that many primary bone tumors develop in the second and third generation of life; however, it does afford the opportunity to put this rather unusual event in perspective.

If one looks at tumor subtypes, MFH (now called high-grade pleomorphic undifferentiated sarcoma) was the most common diagnosis in both the arthroplasty and nonarthroplasty implant groups. Next in order of prevalence was osteosarcoma with the rest of the tumors occurring sporadically. MFH of soft tissue has been accepted as the most common soft tissue sarcoma ranging in incidence from 28% to 63%. The incidence among cases examined here is within accepted parameters for the general population.[33]

The prevalence of osteosarcoma among the osseous malignancies in this series is not entirely unexpected. Of the total number of cases of osteosarcoma, 15% to 20% occur in patients older than 50 years. Most of these cases are superimposed on Paget's disease or in previously irradiated tissue; however de novo cases of osteosarcoma do occur in this age group. There is also a strong association between osteosarcoma and bone infarct. Malignant fibrous histiocytoma of bone is somewhat less common than its soft tissue counterpart. A review of the Mayo Clinic files reveals 71 cases, with more than half occurring in individuals older than 55. Thus, the distribution of sarcomas in the combined series could have been predicted from general population data given the age of patients and the anatomic distribution.

One recent study suggests the possibility of metastasis as a cause of osteolysis and mechanical failure of implants precipitating revision surgery. In a series of 93 patients who underwent revision hip arthroplasty, 11.8% had a history of a previous malignancy. Two of these patients demonstrated obvious gross microscopic metastasis and were thought to have contributed to the mechanical failure of the original reconstruction. As such, when revision hip arthroplasty is considered, patients with a history of malignancy, particularly those who have had a predilection to bone metastasis including thyroid, lung, breast, kidney, and prostate, require additional preoperative assessment and appropriate biopsies at the time of revision arthroplasty to identify the possible occult disease.[62]

As surveillance for tumors related to orthopaedic implants increased, case reports increased as well, especially in the time period from 1985 to 1995. In an effort to understand the risk to the population, five separate reports critically analyzed the cancer risk among arthroplasty recipients.[51,63-66] The combined person-years of exposure after operation among these series were in excess of 500,000. The overall cancer incidence in the combined series did not appear to be any different from what was expected or anticipated in the general population. The cancer observed/expected ratio was especially low for the first 2 years after surgery, implying that patients undergoing these procedures are otherwise generally healthy.

Several papers in the late 1980s reported an increased association between orthopaedic implants and cancer, such as Gillespi et al in 1988. These authors reported a 75% excess incidence of lymphatic and hematopoietic tumors in patients undergoing hip replacement when compared to controls. Immunogenic upregulation in exposure to foreign bodies and the observed propensity for particulate matter to accumulate in the reticuloendothelial system[14,15] prompted the authors to conclude causal associations.[6] Multiple more recent reviews of the English literature have failed to show any association between hip or knee prostheses and malignancy of any kind.[10,67] In fact, more recent extensive analyses of the Finnish cancer database would suggest no increased risk of hematopoietic cancers after 31,651 total hip arthroplasties had been performed.[68] Visuri and colleagues followed their original paper from 2001 with a review of the literature and comparison with Nordic cohorts of the 46 tumors around hip prostheses in 2006. They observed only 1 sarcoma at the site of total hip arthroplasty in 3 Nordic cohorts of total hip arthroplasty and cancer with 268, 189 person-years of exposure yielding 0.37 cases per 100,00 person-years corresponding.[33,66,68,69] Their paper included the largest cohort to date, Signorello et al, who reported on the Swedish experience examining cancer incidence among 116,727 patients who underwent total hip replacements from 1965 to 1994.[69] Through record linkage to the Swedish Cancer Registry, they identified all cancer reports through 1995 yielding 693,954 person-years of observation. They observed no material increase risk for bone or connective tissue cancer for men or women in any follow-up period. A 2006 meta-analysis by Onega et al involving 175,166 patients and 1,435,356 person-years of follow-up found no overall increase in malignancy in arthroplasty patients as a whole. They noted a decrease in bone and soft tissue malignancies relative to the general population but noted an increase in melanoma and prostate cancer when one followed patients over 10 years. The authors were careful to note that this observation was likely linked to selection bias and age-related increases in some malignancies in the general population.[70,71]

SUMMARY

Our interpretation of the literature suggests that implants commonly used for fixation and reconstruction may not be entirely inert. Accumulation of particulate debris will to some extent occur in all patients who have large metallic implants, either for fracture or arthroplasty. This includes the distinct possibility of systemic exposure to these foreign objects and, as a by-product, a heightened immunologic sensitivity. At any point from exposure to immunologic response, a genetic event inciting oncogenesis can occur. We also observe a great range of immune responses among individuals, so defining a dangerously high immune response that would promote an oncogenic aberration would be difficult to say the least. In spite of these concerns and although theoretically possible, there is currently no convincing evidence to support the increased incidence of primary mesenchymal or lymphoproliferative malignancies as a by-product of biomaterials used for fixation and reconstruction in orthopaedic practice. Furthermore, the International Agency for Research on Cancer (IARC) recently evaluated carcinogenic risk to humans of surgical implants and other foreign bodies and concluded that orthopaedic implants including ceramics were not classifiable as to their carcinogenicity to humans.

REFERENCES

1. Coleman MP, Herrington J, Scales JT. Concentration of wear products in hair, blood, and urine after total hip arthroplasty. *Br Med J*. 1973;1:527.
2. Lux F, Zeisler R. Investigations of the corrosive deposition of components of metal implants and of the behavior of biologic trace elements in metallosis tissue by means of instrumental, multielement activation analysis. *J Radiol Anal Chem*. 1974;19:289.
3. Rock MG, Hardie R. Analysis of local tissue response in 50 revision total hip arthroplasty patients. Presented at the Symposium on Retrieval and Analysis of Surgical Implants and Biomaterials, Snowbird, UT; 1988.
4. Buchert BK, Vaughn BK, Mallory TH, et al. Excessive metal release due to loosening and spreading of sintered particles on porous coated hip prosthesis:

Report of two cases. *J Bone Joint Surg Am.* 1986; 68:606.

5. Agins HJ, Allock NW, Bansal M, et al. Metallic wear in failed titanium alloy total hip replacements: a histological and quantitative analysis. *J Bone Joint Surg Am.* 1988;70:347.
6. Jacobs JJ, Skipor AK, Black J, et al. Release in excretion of metal in patients who have a total hip replacement component made of titanium base alloy. *J Bone Joint Surg Am.* 1991;73:1475.
7. Witt JD, Swann M. Methyl wear in tissue response and failed titanium alloy total hip replacements. *J Bone Joint Surg Br.* 1991;73:559.
8. Callaghan JJ, Cuckler JM, Huddleston JI, et al. How have alternative bearings (such as metal on metal. highly cross linked polyethylene, and ceramic on ceramic) affected the prevalence and treatment of osteolysis. *J Am Acad Orthop Surg.* 2007;16(suppl 1):S33-38.
9. Abdel MP, Morrey ME, Morrey BF. Individual host response to foreign materials. In: Morrey BF, An K, Sperling JW, eds. *Joint Replacement Arthroplasty: Basic Science, Elbow, and Shoulder.* Philadelphia, PA: Lippincott Williams & Wilkins; 2010:47.
10. Keegan GM, Learmonth ID, Case CP. Orthopaedic metals and their potential toxicity in the arthroplasty patient. *J Bone Joint Surg Br.* 2007;89:567-573.
11. Keegan GM, Learmonth ID, Case CP. A systematic comparison of the actual, potential, and theoretical health effects of cobalt and chromium exposures from industry and surgical implants. *Crit Rev Toxicol.* 2008;38(8):645-674.
12. Penman HG, Ring PA. Osteosarcoma in association with total hip replacement. *J Bone Joint Surg Br.* 1984:66:632-634.
13. Bartolozzi A, Black J. Chromium concentrations in serum blood clot and urine from patients following total hip arthroplasty. *Biomaterials.* 1985;6:2.
14. Langkamer VG, Case CP, Heap P, et al. Systemic distribution of wear debris after hip replacement: a cause for concern? *J Bone Joint Surg Br.* 1992;74:831.
15. Case CP, Langkamer BG, James C, et al. Widespread dissemination of the metal debris from implants. *J Bone Joint Surg Br.* 1994;76:701.
16. Steineman SG. Corrosion of titanium and titanium alloys for surgical implant. In: Lutergering G, Swicker U, Bunk W, eds. *Titanium, Science, and Technology.* Berlin: Springer-Verlag; 1985:1373.
17. Quigley L, Sprauge S, Bhandari M. Pseudotumors following total hip and knee arthroplasty. *Joint Evidence.* 2010;1973-e:1-33.
18. Willert HG, Fayyazi A, Lohmann CH. Histopathological changes in tissue surrounding metal/metal joints—signs of delayed type hypersensitivity? In: Rieker C, Oberholzer C, Wyss U, eds. *World Tribology Forum in Arthroplasty.* Bern, Germany: Hans Huber; 2001:147-166.
19. Keel SB, Jaffe KA, Petur Nielsen G, et al. Orthopaedic implant-related sarcoma: a study of twelve cases. *Mod Pathol.* 2001;14(10):969-977.
20. Papagelopoulos PJ, Mavrogenis AF, Karamitros AE, et al. Distal leg wear debris mass from a rotating hinged knee prosthesis. *J Arthroplasty.* 2007;22(6): 909-915.
21. Calcedo MD, McAllister R, Reddy K, et al. Soluble and particulate Co-Cr-Mo alloy implants activate the inflammasome danger signaling pathway in human macrophages: a novel mechanism for implant debris reactivity. *J Orthop Res.* 2009;27(7):847-854.
22. Singh C, Kaplan A, Pambuccian SE. Necrotic granulomatous pseudotumor following metal-on-metal hip arthroplasty: a potential mimic of sarcoma on fine needle aspiration cytology. *Diagn Cytopathol.* December 30, 2010 [Epub ahead of print].
23. Walsh AJ, Nikolaou VS, Antoniou J. Inflammatory pseudotumor complicating metal-on-highly cross-linked polyethylene total hip arthroplasty. *J Arthroplasty.* April 15, 2011 [Epub ahead of print].
24. Doll R. Cancer of lung and the nose: nickel workers. *Br J Indian Med.* 1958;15:217.
25. Swanson SAV, Freeman MAR, Heath JC. Laboratory tests on total joint replacement prosthesis. *J Bone Joint Surg Br.* 1973;55:759.
26. Moizhess TG. Carcinogenesis induced by foreign bodies. *Biochemistry (Moscow).* 2008;73(7):763-775.
27. Laskin DM. Experimental production in sarcomas by methacrylate implant. *Proc Soc Exp Biol Med.* 1954; 87:329.
28. Carter RL, Rowe FJC. Induction of sarcomas in rats by solid and fragmented polyethylene: experimental observations and clinical implications. *Br J Cancer.* 1969;23:401.
29. McDougall A. A malignant tumor at site of bone plating. *J Bone Joint Surg Br.* 1956;38:709-713.
30. Harris WH, Schiller AL, Scholler JM, et al. Extensive localized bone resorption in the femur following total hip replacement. *J Bone Joint Surg Am.* 1976;58:612.
31. Lucas OR, Miller PR, Mott MP, et al. Arthroplasty associated malignant fibrous histiocytoma. Two case reports. *Histopathology.* 2001;39(6):620-628.

32. Shuh A, Zeiller G, Holzworth U, et al. Malignant fibrous histiocytoma at the site of a total hip arthroplasty. *Clin Orthop Relat Res.* 2004;425:218-222.

33. Visuri T, Pulkkinen P, Paavolainen P, et al. Malignant tumors at the site of total hip prosthesis. Analytic review of 46 cases. *J Arthroplasty.* 2006;21(3):311-323.

34. Weber PC. Epithelioid sarcoma in association with total knee replacement. *J Bone Joint Surg Br.* 1986; 68:824.

35. Kolstad K, Hogstrop H. Gastric carcinoma metastasis to a knee with a newly inserted prosthesis: a case report. *Acta Orthop Scand.* 1990;61:369.

36. Himmer O, Lootvoet L, Deprez C, et al. Angiosarcoma after total knee prosthesis: apropos of a case. *Rev Chir Orthop Reparatrice Appar Mot.* 1991;77: 125-129.

37. Oppenheimer BS, Oppenheimer ET, Stout AP, et al. The latent period in carcinogenesis by plastics in rats and its relation to the presarcomatous stage. *Cancer.* 1958;11:204-207.

38. Laffargue P, Hildebrand HF, Lecomte-Houcke M, et al. Malignant fibrous histiocytoma of bone 20 years after femur fracture treated by plate and screw fixation: analysis of corrosion products and their role in malignancy. *Rev Chir Orthop Reparatrice Appar Mot.* 2001;87(1):84-90.

39. McDonald DJ, Enneking WF, Sundaram M, et al. Metal-associated angiosarcoma of bone: report of two cases and review of the literature. *Clin Orthop Relat Res.* 2002;396:206-214.

40. Olmedo DG, Michanié E, Oivi L, et al. Malignant fibrous histiocytoma associated with coxofemoral arthrodesis. *Tumori.* 2007;93(5):504-507.

41. McGuff HS, Heim-Hall J, Holsinger FC, et al. Maxillary osteosarcoma associated with a dental implant: report of a case and review of the literature regarding implant-related sarcomas. *J Am Dental Assoc.* 2008; 139(8):1052-1059.

42. Dube VE, Fisher DE. Hemangioendothelioma of the leg following metallic fixation of the tibia. *Cancer.* 1972;30(5):1260-1266.

43. van der List JJ, van Horn JR, Slooff TJ, et al. Malignant epithelioid hemangioendothelioma at the site of a hip prosthesis. *Acta Orthop Scand.* 1988;59: 328-330.

44. Arden GP, Bywaters EGL. Tissue reaction. In: Arden GP, Ansel BM, eds. *Surgical Management of Juvenile Chronic Poly Arthritis.* London: Academic Press; 1978:269.

45. Bago-Granell J, Aguirre-Canyadell M, Nardi J, et al. Malignant fibrous histiocytoma of bone at the site of a total hip arthroplasty: a case report. *J Bone Joint Surg Br.* 1984;66:38.

46. Swann M. Malignant soft tissue tumor at the site of a total hip replacement. *J Bone Joint Surg Br.* 1984; 66:269.

47. Hamblen DL, Carter RL. Sarcoma and joint replacement (editorial). *J Bone Joint Surg Br.* 1984; 66:625.

48. Ryu RKN, Bovill EG Jr, Skinner HB, et al. Soft tissue sarcomas associated with aluminum oxide ceramic total hip arthroplasty: a case report. *Clin Orthop Relat Res.* 1987;216:207.

49. Vives P, Sevestre H, Grodet H, et al. Histiocytome fibreux malin du femur apres prostheses totale de hanche. *Rev Chir Orthop.* 1987;73:407.

50. Lamovec J, Zidar A, Cucek-Plenicar M. Synovial sarcoma associated with total hip replacement: a case report. Addendum: Osteosarcoma associated with a Charnley-Mueller hip arthroplasty. *J Bone Joint Surg Am.* 1988;70:1558.

51. Martin A, Bauer TW, Manley MT, et al. Osteosarcoma at the site of a total hip replacement. *J Bone Joint Surg Am.* 1988;70:1561.

52. Tait NP. Case reports, malignant fibrous histiocytoma occurring at the site of a previous total hip replacement. *J Bone Joint Surg Br.* 1988;55:759.

53. Brien WW, Salvati EA, Healey JH, et al. Osteogenic sarcoma arising in the area of a total hip replacement: a case report. *J Bone Joint Surg Am.* 1990;72:1097.

54. Troop JK, Mallory TH, Fisher DA, et al. Malignant fibrous histiocytoma after total hip arthroplasty: a case report. *Clin Orthop Relat Res.* 1990;253:297.

55. Jacobs JJ, Rosenbaum DH, Hay RM, et al. Early sarcomatous degeneration near a cementless hip replacement: a case report and review. *J Bone Joint Surg Br.* 1992;74:740.

56. Goodfellow J. Malignancy and joint replacement (editorial). *J Bone Joint Surg Am.* 1992;74:645.

57. Stephensen SL, Schwarz Lausten G, Thomasen HS, et al. Liposarcoma in association with a total hip replacement. *Int Orthop.* 1999;23:187-189.

58. Rana B, Shetty S, Grigoris P, et al. Sarcoma arising, adjacent to a total hip arthroplasty. *Scot Med J.* 2001;46(1):17-19.

59. Prasad PSV, Latham JB, Tucker JK, et al. Disseminated osteosarcoma arising in the pelvis after total hip arthroplasty. *J Arthroplasty.* 2002;17(3):373-378.

60. Adams JE, Jaffe KA, Lemons JE, et al. Prosthetic implant associated sarcomas: a case report emphasizing surface evaluation and spectroscopic trace metal analysis. *Ann Diagn Pathol*. 2003;7:35.
61. Iorio R, Robb WJ, Healy WL, et al. Orthopaedic surgeon workforce and volume assessment for total hip and knee replacement in the United States: preparing for an epidemic. *J Bone Joint Surg Am*. 2008;90: 1598-1605.
62. Salai M, Zippel D, Perelman M, et al. Revision hip arthroplasty in patients with a history of previous malignancy. *J Surg Oncol*. 1999;70:122.
63. Gillespie WJ, Frampton CMA, Henderson RJ, et al. The incidence of cancer following total hip replacement. *J Bone Joint Surg Br*. 1988;70:539.
64. Coleman MP. Cancer risk from orthopedic prostheses. *Ann Clin Lab Sci*. 1996;26:139.
65. Fryzek JP, Mellemkjaer L, McLaughlin JK, et al. Cancer risk among patients with finger and hand joint and temporomandibular joint prosthesis in Denmark. *Int Cancer*. 1999;81:723.
66. Paavolainen P, Pukkala E, Pulkkinen P, et al. Cancer incidence in Finnish hip replacement pateints from 1980 to 1995: a nation-wide cohort study involving 31,651 patients. *J Arthroplasty*. 1999;14:272.
67. Thurani R, Dorey FJ, Schmalzreid TP. Risk of cancer following total hip or knee arthroplasty. *J Bone Joint Surg Am*. 2001;83:774-780.
68. Visuri T, Pukkala E. Does metal-on-metal total hip prosthesis have influence on cancer? A long-term follow-up study. In: Rieker C, Oberholzer C, Wyss U, eds. *World Tribology Forum in Arthroplasty*. Bern, Germany: Hans Huber; 2001:181.
69. Signorello LB, Ye W, Fryzek JP, et al. Nationwide study of cancer risk among hip replacement patients in Sweden. *J Natl Cancer Inst*. 2001;93(18):1405-1410.
70. International Agency for Research on Cancer (IARC). Composite medical and dental implants. In: *IARC Monographs on the Evaluation of Carcinogenic Risks to Humans*. Lyon, France: IATC; 1999:102-108.
71. Onega T, Baron J, MacKenzie T. Cancer after total joint arthroplasty: a meta-analysis. *Cancer Epidemiol Biomarkers Prev*. 2006;15(8):1078.

18 Basic Science of Bacteria and Antibacterial Agents

Alex Soriano

Approximately 10% of patients receiving a joint prosthesis develop a complication during their lifetime. Although aseptic loosening is most common, infection is the most severe complication requiring sometimes multiple interventions, prolonged hospitalization, and large courses of antimicrobial therapy. Furthermore, the pathogenesis of aseptic loosening is not well established and some data suggest that a percentage of prosthetic failures considered aseptic are actually septic.[1] The postsurgical infection rate is about 1% to 3% in spite of correct surgical techniques, aseptic measures, and antibiotic prophylaxis.[2] Taking into account the increasing number of arthroplasties performed each year in the developed world, a parallel increase in the number of prosthetic joint infections is expected. The management of these infections is complex due to the progressive increase of antibiotic-resistant bacteria and the ability of bacteria to grow, forming biofilms on the implant surface. The aim of this chapter is to provide a general knowledge about the bacterial science (life cycle, structure, and virulence determinants) and the mechanism of action of the main antimicrobial agents.

BACTERIAL LIFE CYCLE AND IMPLICATIONS FOR ANTIBIOTIC PROPHYLAXIS

Bacteria face constant challenges in the environment and they have evolved in efficiency to rapidly use nutrients when they are available, in the ability to survive during periods lacking nutrients, and in resistance to life-threatening challenges including physical (heat, radiation) and chemical (antibiotics) agents. The small size (around 1 μm) and the machinery for rapidly converting nutrients to energy allow bacteria to grow extremely fast in the presence of nutrients. The different phases of bacterial growth in the laboratory are shown in Figure 18-1. When bacteria find themselves in a suitable environment, they first identify the available nutrients (lag phase) and, after several hours, start to exponentially grow (exponential phase). The time it takes for a bacterium to become two during the exponential phase is called the generation time or doubling time. For instance, *Escherichia coli* requires about 20 minutes to double in rich nutrient broth. Growth goes on until the population reaches a certain density, when the nutrients in the environmental become exhausted or toxic metabolites accumulate (stationary phase).

During the lag phase, bacteria sense the presence of nutrients in the environment; in the exponential phase, bacteria express in their surface a large number of adhesion molecules to bind matrix proteins such as fibrinogen or collagen that allow bacteria to colonize the tissue; and finally, in the stationary phase, bacteria synthesize exoproteins essential for invading the host. Since antibiotics block metabolic pathways that are active during the exponential phase but reduced during the lag and stationary phases, bacteria are more susceptible to antibiotics in the exponential phase than in the lag or stationary phase.

According to this life cycle, even a small bacterial inoculum (ie, contamination of surgical wound) could produce an infection; however, in the tissue of the body, bacteria is

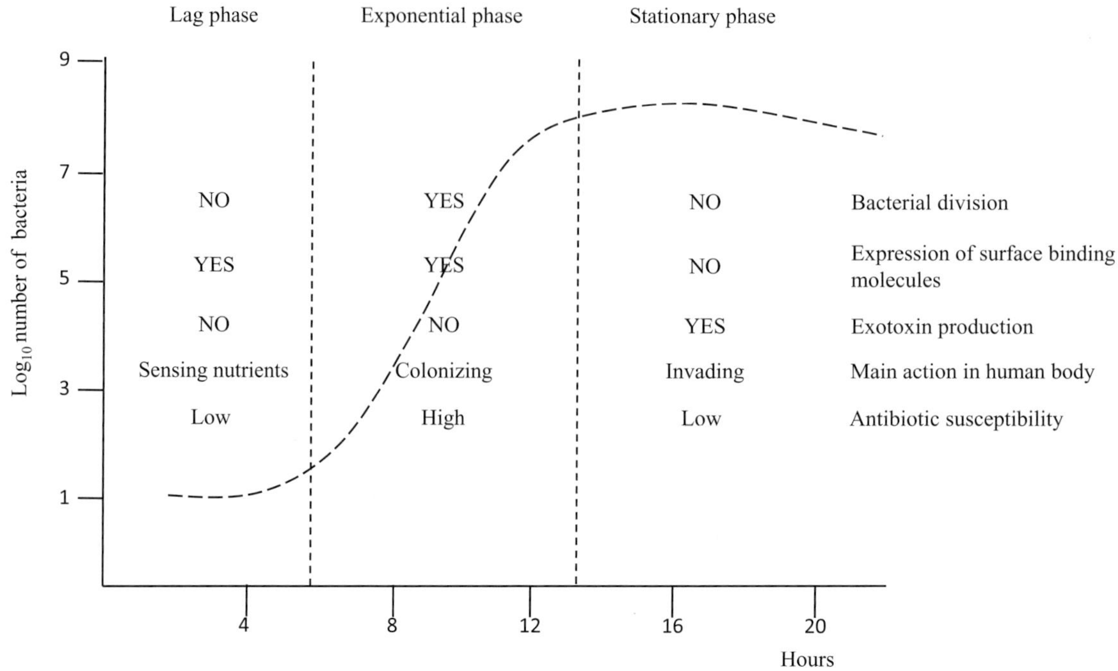

FIGURE 18-1. *The growth of bacteria in culture and features of bacteria in each growth phase.*

often stressed by the absence of nutrients and the action of defense mechanisms. During surgery, the balance between bacterial inoculum and bacterial virulence by one side and the host defenses and prophylactic antibiotics by the other will determine the development of a surgical site infection. Quantitatively, it has been shown that if a surgical site is contaminated with $>10^5$ microorganisms per gram of tissue, the risk of surgical site infection is markedly increased.[3] For clean surgery, like total knee arthroplasty, the bacterial load into the wound depends on (1) the correct application of barrier measures to avoid contamination from the skin of patients, surgeons, environment, or surgical material, and the duration of surgery; (2) the virulence of the microorganism; and (3) the host immune system (Fig. 18-2). However, it is well recognized from animal models that the bacterial load necessary to cause infections when a foreign body is present could be reduced 10,000-fold in comparison to those without implants (ie, 10^2 staphylococci per gram of tissue introduced on silk sutures are enough to cause infection). Local antisepsis reduces but does not eliminate the skin flora, since up to 20% of skin-resident bacteria is localized in appendages such as hair follicles and sebaceous glands (Fig. 18-3). This fact is associated with the impairment of phagocyte function on the inert surfaces and the ability of microorganisms to grow, forming a complex community embedded in a polysaccharide matrix called biofilm, which is characterized by a high resistance to phagocytosis and antibiotics.[4] Therefore, in clean surgery with foreign-body implantation, the use of antibiotic prophylaxis is always recommended.

According to the susceptibility to antibiotics described in Figure 18-1, the most reasonable moment to administer prophylactic antibiotics is 4 to 5 hours after bacterial contamination, when bacteria enter the exponential growth phase (Fig. 18-4). In contrast, research in antimicrobial prophylaxis has established that the efficacy of antibiotics in reducing the infection rate is higher when they are infused just before the intervention.[5,6] What is the explanation for this apparent contradiction? During surgery, there is a constant process of hematoma formation. These hematomas could be contaminated and microoganisms are entrapped in fibrin clots. Once the hematoma is organized, some hours after surgery, this cavity is excluded from the circulation and it is difficult to achieve high antibiotic concentrations even using high dosages. Therefore, during the process of hematoma formation, it is essential to reach the highest serum antibiotic concentration to obtain high concentrations within the hematoma in order to kill the potential contaminant microorganisms during the following 12 to 24 hours. To achieve this objective, it is necessary to infuse prophylactic antibiotics during the induction of

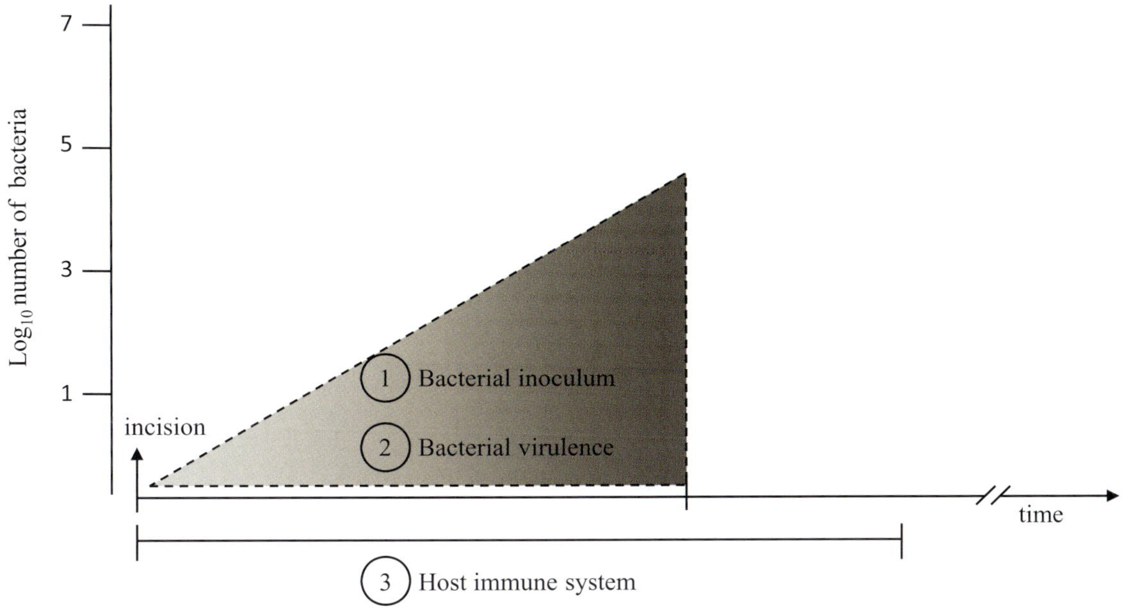

FIGURE 18-2. *Factors determining the development of surgical site infections.*

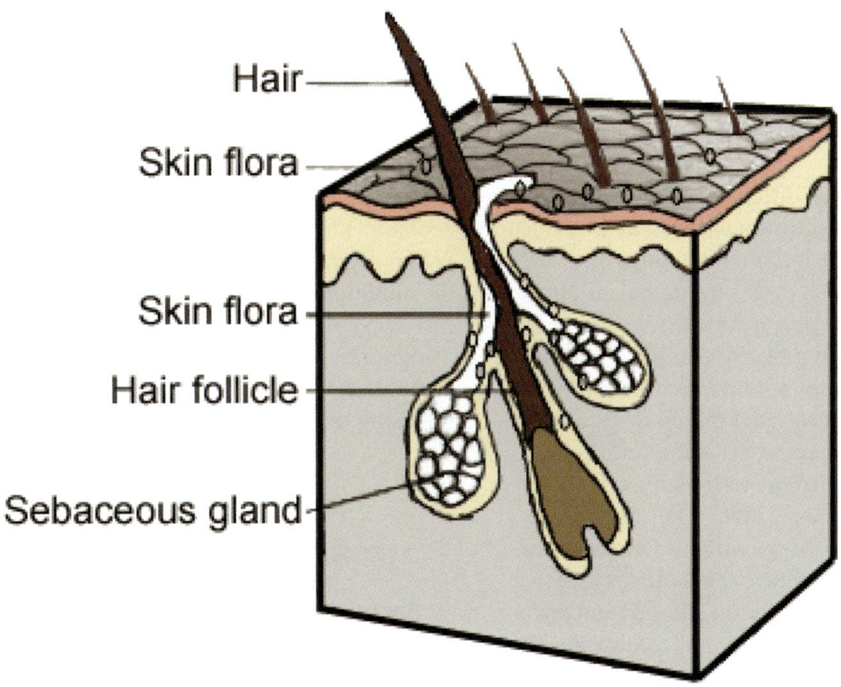

FIGURE 18-3. *Skin and soft tissue structure showing the distribution of bacteria. Up to 20% of the skin flora is in the hair follicle or sebaceous glands and they are not eliminated with skin disinfection.*

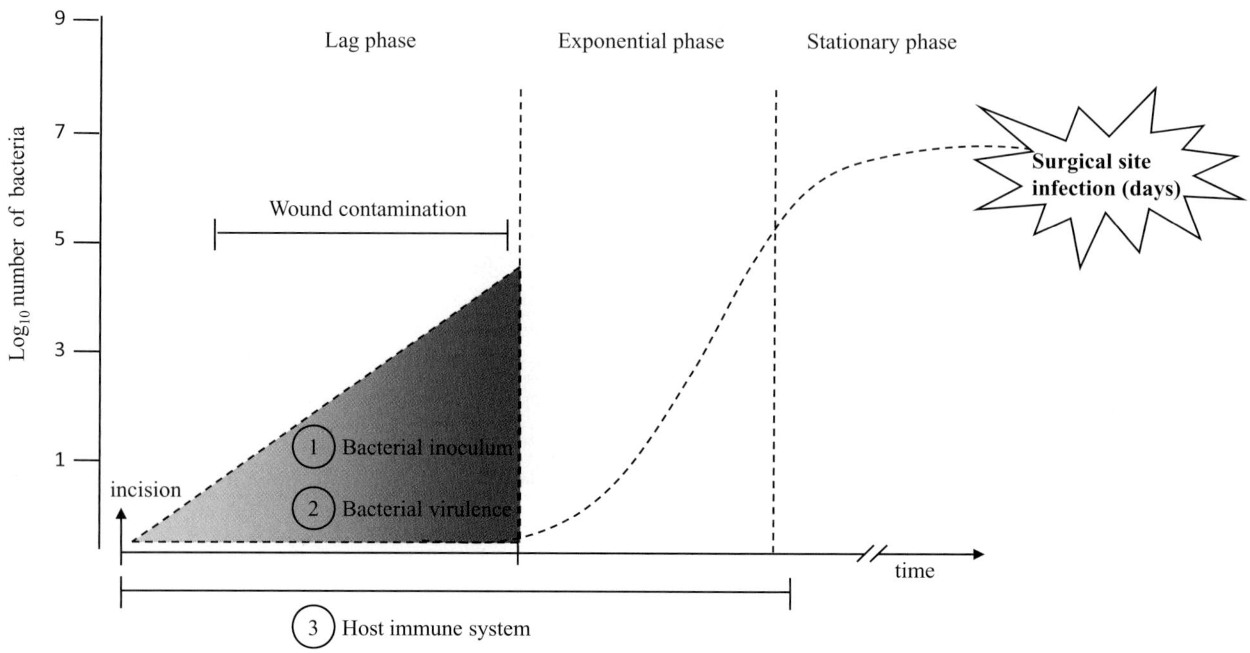

FIGURE 18-4. *Bacterial growth after contaminating the surgical wound.*

anesthesia. However, when the surgery is performed under ischemia (ie, total knee arthroplasty), the antibiotic is administered before inflating the tourniquet. The precise timing for infusing the antibiotic was established by several authors,[7,8] who measured the antibiotic concentration in bone and fat during total knee arthroplasty after administering the antibiotic at different intervals before inflating the tourniquet. The conclusion was that by infusing the antibiotic 10 minutes before inflating the tourniquet, the concentration in bone and fat was over the minimal inhibitory concentration of cephalosporins for the main pathogens. However, in spite of applying these precautions, some authors have observed a higher infection rate in knee arthroplasty than in hip arthroplasty. Furthermore, two pilot studies that compared the outcome of knee arthroplasty performed with or without tourniquet, or early release of tourniquet, observed a lower rate of infectious complications in the arm operated on without tourniquet or with early release of it.[9,10] A possible explanation is that the hematoma formed around the prosthesis should contain a high antibiotic concentration to kill the contaminant microorganisms. In the case of knee arthroplasty, the blood reaches the wound and forms a hematoma after the tourniquet release. This means a delay of about 60 to 80 minutes from the infusion of the antibiotic to the moment of tourniquet release. Therefore, if an antibiotic with a half-life of 1 hour is used, at the moment of tourniquet release the blood bathing the wound will have a low antibiotic concentration. Richardson et al[11] measured the concentration of cephamandole (a cephalosporin with an 0.8-hour half-life) in serum and drain fluid to determine the benefit of an intravenous dose of antibiotic at the time of tourniquet deflation in 32 knee replacement operations. The most important findings were (1) the concentration of cephamandole in drain fluid was directly proportional to the serum concentration at the time of tourniquet release and (2) the addition of a "tourniquet release" dose of antibiotic increased concentration in the drain fluid threefold. Therefore, some authors recommend the administration of an additional dose of prophylactic antibiotic just before releasing the tourniquet.[12]

MECHANISMS OF BACTERIAL VIRULENCE

Bacterial virulence factors include any component of a microbe that is required for or potentiates its ability to cause disease. The number and nature of virulence factors expressed by bacterial pathogens is wide, and they can be summarized in (1) mechanisms to adhere to and cross the human barriers, (2) mechanisms to invade the host tissue, (3) mechanisms to evade the action of host defenses, and (4) toxin production. The detailed description of each one of these mechanisms is beyond the scope of this chapter. We have focused on the revision in the virulence factors of the main bacteria producing infection in orthopaedic surgery, *Staphylococcus aureus*. About 30% of the general population carries *S. aureus* in the nares and this is a risk factor for developing an invasive infection due to the same strain when these people undergo an invasive procedure like joint arthroplasty.[13]

This pathogen causes a great diversity of infections through the expression of different virulence factors that are strictly coordinated by global regulators that help bacteria to adapt to the hostile environment by producing factors enabling them to survive and subsequently to cause infection at the appropriate time. The first step in the infectious process is binding to the cell or tissue surface, and *S. aureus* is particularly well prepared for this task by proteins anchored to the peptidoglycan called MSCRAMMS (microbial surface components recognizing adhesive matrix molecules). These proteins are responsible for attaching the bacterium to various extracellular matrices, such as collagen, fibronectin, or vitronectin. This avidity for matrix proteins could explain the findings of Murdoch et al,[14] who prospectively followed up 44 patients with a prosthetic joint who developed *S. aureus* bacteremia from a distal source, and 15 out of 44 prostheses (34%) became infected. For tissue invasion, *S. aureus* produces and secretes proteases, staphylokinase, lipases, and cytotoxins, such as hemolysins or leukocidins (Panton-Valentine leukocidine), implicated in the degradation of different host components and favoring the bacterial invasion.

One of the most important virulence factors of *S. aureus* is its ability to evade the immune system and to remain, in special circumstances, hidden but viable for a long period of time and causing recurrent relapses, as is the case in osteomyelitis. Protein A and capsule are the main factors expressed by this pathogen to avoid opsonophagocytosis and prevent the killing by neutrophils or macrophages. However, the mechanism for understanding the ability of *S. aureus* to persist within the host and to resist the action of antibiotics but ready to regain their fully virulent phenotype and to attack the host, is more complex. Chronic and therapy-refractory staphylococcal infections have been particularly associated with an altered bacterial phenotype, the small colony variants (SCVs).[15] SCVs form small colonies on agar plates (about 10 times smaller than the parent strain) due to their slow growth rate and reduced metabolism, which also explains their decreased susceptibility to a variety of antibiotics. SCVs are well adapted to the intracellular environment (Fig. 18-5) and recent data demonstrate that bacterial phenotype switching is an integral part of the infection process that enables the bacteria to hide inside host cells, which can be a reservoir for chronic and therapy-refractive infections.[16] This infection strategy relates to the intracellular location as a source for recurrent infections and most likely represents an important immune escape mechanism. Clinically, this can explain treatment failures in spite of sufficient activity of the antimicrobial substances in vitro, as SCVs usually have an increased antimicrobial resistance profile and many antimicrobial agents do not reach sufficient high doses intracellularly.

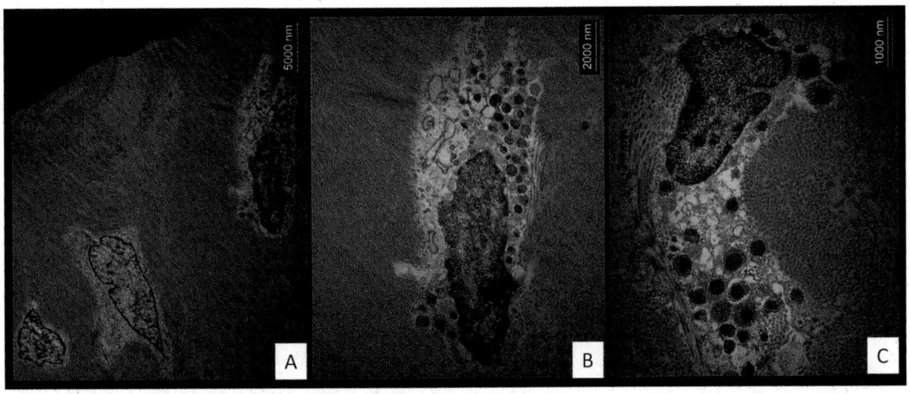

FIGURE 18-5. *Transmission electron micrography of a sample obtained from the hip joint capsule of a patient with prosthetic joint infection revealing three fibroblasts surrounded by collagen fibers (**A**). Intracellular cocci are shown in the right cell of panel **A** and in an enlarged image in panel **B**. Intracellular cocci in a fibroblast are shown in panel **C**. (Reprinted with permission from Sendi P, Rohrbach M, Graber P, et al. Clin Infect Dis. 2006;43:961-967. © 2006 by the Infectious Diseases Society of America.)*

Another important mechanism for explaining recalcitrant infections, especially when orthopaedic implants are involved, is the development of a biofilm on the inert surface. Infection after total joint arthroplasty is the result of a microorganism seeding on the prosthesis surface. Infections can be detected during the first 3 months after surgery or later than 3 months or even years after joint arthroplasty. Carlsson et al,[17] in a randomized, prospective, controlled study of antibiotic prophylaxis in hip arthroplasty, demonstrated that deep wound infections that developed 2.5 years after surgery were most likely to have occurred among placebo versus cloxacillin recipients (14% vs. 2%, respectively; $p < .05$). Other authors observed a decrease in the incidence rate of late infections when prosthetic joints were cemented with an antibiotic.[18] These data strongly suggest that bacteria inoculated into the wound at the time of surgery may lie dormant for years and be responsible for late chronic infections. Once the microorganisms achieve the prosthesis surface, they grow, forming biofilms. A biofilm is defined as a bacterial community embedded in a polysaccharide matrix where the cells are protected from the environment stresses. Biofilm formation is a three-step process. The initial stage is the adhesion of microorganisms to a surface. The second stage involves cell proliferation on the surface, the production of a polysaccharide matrix that facilitates intercellular aggregation, and the organization of encased bacteria into three-dimensional structures with channels through which nutrients and waste products can flow. The third stage involves the detachment of individual bacteria or fragments of biofilm that potentially could colonize distal surfaces or tissues (Fig. 18-6). The differentiation of mature biofilms is controlled by cell-to-cell communicating systems that detect the population density (quorum sensing) and stimulate or repress the transcription of target genes that promote biofilm formation.[19]

There are two important consequences of the biofilm mode of growth: (1) the clinical manifestations of these infections differ from typical suppurative infections since matrix-enclosed sessile bacteria elicit much less inflammatory response and, therefore, fever is infrequent and inflammatory markers are usually low; and (2) bacteria embedded in a biofilm show higher resistance to the host's defenses and higher tolerance to antibiotics than their planktonic counterpart.[20] Specific mechanisms can explain, in part, the phenomenon of tolerance showed by bacterial cells living in biofilms. Betalactamases accumulate in the biofilm matrix and hydrolyze the betalactams; negatively charged extracellular matrix binds to positively charged aminoglycosides, impeding its diffusion, and slime reduces the activity of glycopeptides through unknown mechanisms. However, the tolerance to antibiotics is not homogeneous in the biofilm; a top-to-bottom gradient of decreasing antimicrobial susceptibility has been described. In the deep strata, the bacteria find an adverse environment characterized by a poor nutritional supply and low oxygen concentration (Fig. 18-6).[21] This stressful situation turns on stress-response genes that decrease the metabolic activity and duplicative rate of bac-

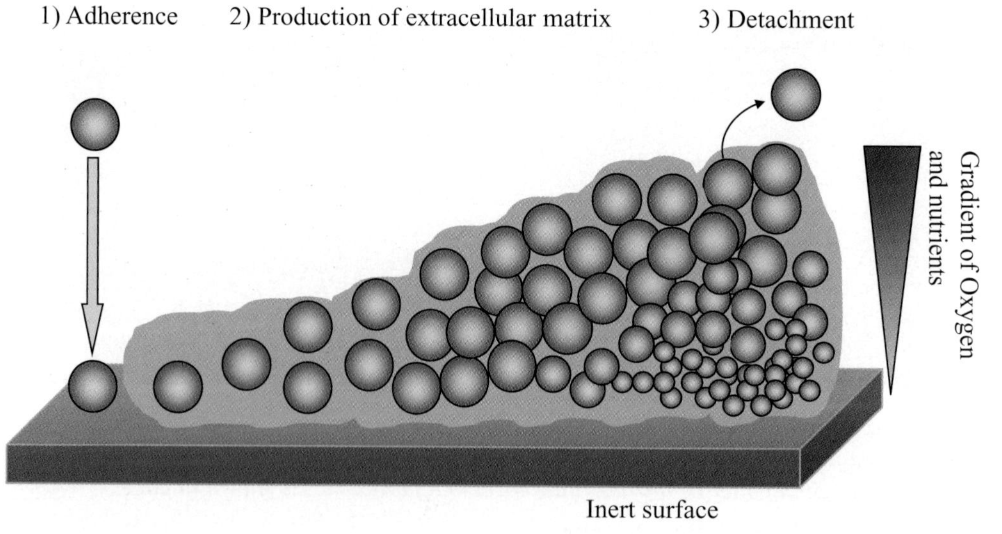

FIGURE 18-6. *Phases of biofilm formation and maturation.*

teria. The average specific growth rate of bacteria in biofilms was only 0.032 per hour compared to the specific growth rate of planktonic bacteria of 0.59 per hour, which means that sessile bacteria double their population every 31 hours and planktonic bacteria do so in 1.6 hours.[22] Since the antibiotics act best against rapidly dividing bacteria, these findings could explain the tolerance of biofilms and why antibiotics with a good performance against stationary phase bacteria in vitro (eg, rifampin) are more successful in clearing biofilms in vivo.[23] Recently, a novel mechanism to explain the tolerance of biofilms based on "persisters" has been proposed. In all bacterial populations there is a small fraction of essentially invulnerable cells, so-called persisters, that neither grow nor die in the presence of antibiotics, thus exhibiting a multidrug tolerance. In infections produced only by planktonic cells (eg, pneumonia), polymorphonuclear leukocytes kill persisters, but in a biofilm they are protected from phagocytosis and are able to repopulate the biofilm after withdrawal antibiotics.[24]

The complexity of the different strategies developed by staphylococci to persist in the human body and to defend against the activity of antibiotics makes the treatment of these infections a challenge. There is an intense investigation to find new targets to kill biofilm bacteria; however, up to now the only way is to use the combination of surgery and conventional antibiotics that are reviewed in the following section.

GENERAL CONCEPTS OF ANTIBACTERIAL AGENTS

The effectiveness of antibiotics depends on their in vitro activity well described by the minimum inhibitory concentration (MIC). The MIC is the minimal antibiotic concentration that inhibits the macroscopic growth of bacteria; therefore, the lower the MIC, the higher the activity. Based on this information, microbiologists inform about the susceptibility or resistance of bacteria to each antibiotic. Although MIC is a useful tool for predicting the efficacy of antibiotics, experience from animal models and clinical studies has shown that the information provided by the MIC is limited. This test is performed in the laboratory using low bacterial inoculum in the exponential growth phase and using static antibiotic concentrations, whereas in patients, bacterial inoculum could be significantly higher, part of the bacteria is in biofilms, intracellular, or in the stationary phase, and antibiotic concentration in serum and tissues is constantly changing. For this reason, during the past years, infectious disease physicians, microbiologists, and pharmacologists have investigated the relationship between measurements of drug exposure (pharmacokinetics: absorption, distribution, and elimination) and antimicrobial effect in animal models and human beings; this interaction is called "pharmacodynamics."[25] The development of pharmacodynamics has proven valuable for the design of appropriate regimens and to define more accurate susceptibility break points. It is possible to identify three patterns of antimicrobial activity:

1 Concentration-dependent antibiotics with prolonged postantibiotic effect. Higher concentrations of these antibiotics kill microorganisms more rapidly than lower levels and prolonged postantibiotic effect allows for infrequent administration of large doses. This pattern is observed with aminoglycosides, fluoroquinolones, or daptomycin. The goal of a dosing regimen of these drugs would be to maximize concentrations over the MIC (C_{max}/MIC index).

2 Time-dependent antibiotics with minimal or no postantibiotic effects. High antibiotic concentrations do not kill microorganisms better than lower levels and microorganisms regrow very soon after serum levels fall below the MIC. This pattern is typical of ß-lactams and the goal of a dosing regimen is to maintain serum levels two- to threefold over the MIC for the entire period between two doses. An excellent way to administer these antibiotics is continuous infusion ($T >$ MIC).

3 Global exposure-dependent antibiotics. These antibiotics are time dependent but they have prolonged postantibiotic effects, preventing regrowth during the interval when the serum concentration is below the MIC. This pattern is observed in macrolides, clindamycin, glycopeptides, oxazolidinones, and tetracyclines. The goal of a dosing regimen is to optimize the amount of drug to ensure that killing occurs, and the best parameter describing the global exposure is the area under the concentration curve for 24 hours at the MIC (AUC_{24}/MIC) (Fig. 18-7).

Classically antibiotics have been divided into bactericidal or bacteriostatic and, in general, cidal agents are preferable to static ones; however, this distinction should not be taken as absolute. The definition of cidality is again a laboratory concept. Bactericidal agents are those that kill bacteria rapidly (≥3 logarithms of colony forming units in 24 hours), while bacteriostatic also kill bacteria, but they do it slowly (Fig. 18-8). Bactericidal agents are preferred when the host's defenses are insufficient, such as in neutropenic patients or in meningitis. However, in other circumstances, a bacteriostatic agent is better; this is the case of necrotizing fasciitis due to *Clostridium perfringens* or *Streptococcus pyogenes*, where animal models and some clinical data

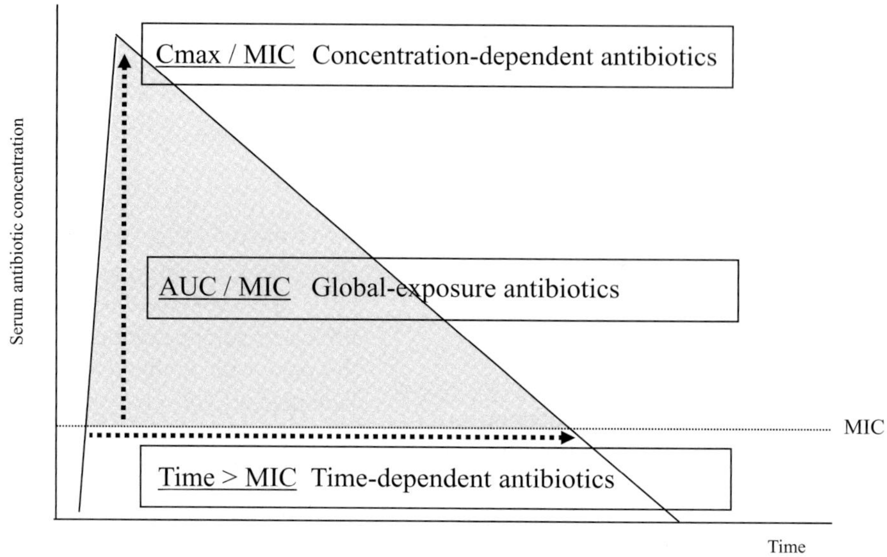

FIGURE 18-7. *Pharmacodynamic indexes that predict the effectiveness of antibiotics (see text for description).*

show that clindamycin or linezolid (static agents) prevent mortality better than ß-lactams (cidal agent). Protein synthesis inhibitors (clindamycin, linezolid) abruptly stop the production of toxins, critical in the pathogenesis of necrotizing fasciitis, while ß-lactams do not reduce or even increase the toxin production during the first 24 hours.[26] More recently, several clinical trials comparing linezolid with glycopeptides or ß-lactams showed similar results in skin and soft tissue infections, pneumonia, or bacteremia.[27] In special situations, such as patients with infected foot ulcers and skin abscess, linezolid was superior to cidal comparators,[28,29] probably because linezolid is a small and hydrophobic molecule with low protein binding, properties that give linezolid a good diffusion rate to poor vascularized tissues. These data suggest that in addition to MIC and the cidal activity, there are other aspects, including pharmacodynamics, mechanism of action, or tissue diffusion, that should be taken into account when selecting an antibiotic.

The main bacterial components whose synthesis or structure is inhibited or disrupted by specific antibiotics are (1) the cell wall (ß-lactams, glycopeptides), (2) the cytoplasmic membrane (daptomycin), (3) the single circular chromosome of double-stranded DNA and the specific enzymes involved in DNA synthesis and supercoiling (fluoroquinolones), (4) the synthesis of folic acid (cotrimoxazole), and (5) the protein and RNA synthesis machinery (linezolid, rifampin). However, bacteria have developed mechanisms to circumvent the action of antibiotics. These mechanisms can be divided into four groups:

1. Antibiotic modification by breaking down the molecule using enzymes. For instance, ß-lactamases hydrolyze the ß-lactam ring of penicilins and are responsible for high penicillin-resistance in *S. aureus* (>90%).

2. Modification of the target site preventing the binding of the antibiotic. An example is the acquisition of a protein-binding penicillin (PBP) with a mutation in the ß-lactam binding site that makes *S. aureus* resistant to all ß-lactams, including those resistant to the action of ß-lactamases like methicillin (MRSA).

3. Prevention of access to the target by inhibiting uptake. This mechanism is important for gram-negative bacteria since these bacteria have an outer membrane that has porins, which permit only the entry of small (≤700 Da) hydrophilic antibiotics (Fig. 18-9). By loosening these pores, bacteria become resistant to those antibiotics that use this channel.

4. Prevention of access to the target site by increasing export of the drug using efflux pumps. These pumps have been described in gram-positive and gram-negative bacteria and are responsible for resistance to fluoroquinolones or tetracyclines.

The principal antibiotics according to their mechanism of action, antibacterial spectrum, pharmacodynamic indexes, and the main resistant mechanisms are described in Table 18-1.

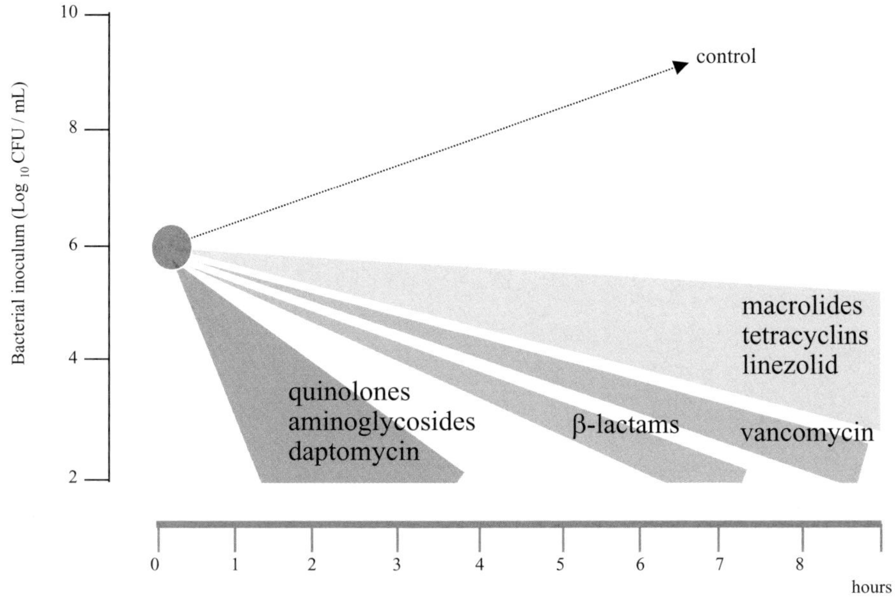

FIGURE 18-8. *Bactericidal activity of different antibiotics. All antibiotics kill bacteria, but some do it rapidly while others do it slowly.*

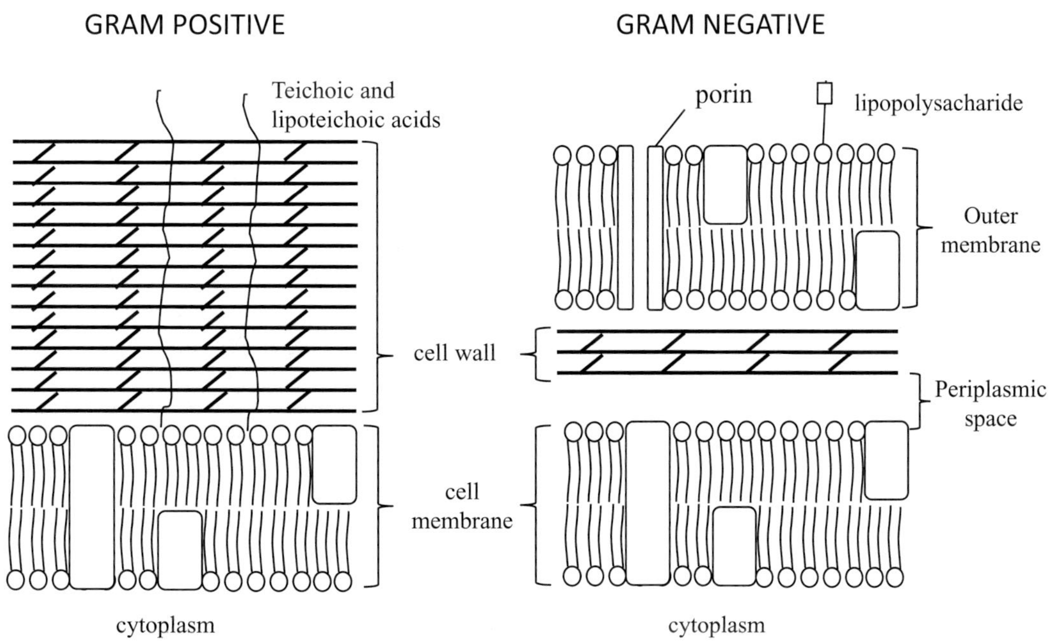

FIGURE 18-9. *The envelope structure of gram-positive and gram-negative bacteria.*

TABLE 18-1. Description of Antibiotics According to Their Mechanism of Action, Antibacterial Spectrum, Pharmacodynamic Predictor of Efficacy, and Main Resistance Mechanism

Mechanism of Action and Antibiotic	Activity for GP	Activity for GN	Pharmacodynamic Index	Main Resistance Mechanism
Cell wall inhibitors				
ß-lactams: penicilins, cephalosporins, carbapenems, monobactams	+	+	$T >$ MIC	Enzymatic modification of the drug, modification of the target site, and reduced access to the target
Glycopeptides: vancomycin, teicoplanin	+	–	AUC_{24} / MIC	Modification of the target site
Inhibitors of membrane function				
Lipopeptides: daptomycin	+	–	C_{max} / MIC	Modification of the target site
Polyene: colistin	–	+	AUC_{24} / MIC	Modification of the target site
DNA synthesis inhibitors				
Metronidazol	+[a]	+[a]	C_{max} / MIC	Reduced access to the target
Fluoroquinolones: ciprofloxacin, levofloxacin, moxiflaxacin, gatifloxacin, gemifloxacin	+	+	C_{max} / MIC	Modification of the target site and efflux pumps
Folate antagonists				
Sulfonamides: sulfamethoxazol, sulfadiazine	+	+	ND	Modification of the target site
Trimethoprim	+	+	ND	Modification of the target site
Protein and RNA synthesis inhibitors				
Aminoglycosides: gentamycin, tobramycin, amikacin	+	+	C_{max} / MIC	Enzymatic modification of the drug
Tetracyclines and glicilciclines: doxicyclin, minocycline, tigecycline	+	+	AUC_{24} / MIC	Efflux pumps
	+	–	AUC_{24} / MIC	Modification of the target site
Macrolides and lincosamides: erythromycin, clarythromycin, azithromycin, clindamycin	+	–	AUC_{24} / MIC	Modification of the target site
Oxazolidinones: linezolid	+		ND	Modification of the target site
Fusidic acid	+		C_{max} / MIC	Modification of the target site
Rifampin (RNA synthesis inhibitor)				

GP, gram-positive bacteria; GN, gram-negative bacteria; +, in vitro activity; -, no in vitro activity; MIC, minimal inhibitory concentration; *T*, time between two consecutive doses of the antibiotic; AUC_{24}, area under the serum concentration curve for 24 h; C_{max}, peak serum concentration; ND, no data.

[a]Only active against anaerobic GP or GN.

PARTICULAR ASPECTS OF ANTIBIOTIC SELECTION IN ORTHOPAEDIC IMPLANT INFECTIONS

The empirical antibiotic treatment in prosthetic joint infections should be active against the most common microorganisms according to the susceptibility of each area. Once the antibiogram of the pathogen is obtained, the antibiotic should be adapted. However, it has not been established which antibiotic or combination of antibiotics is the most appropriate and for how long it should be administered. The quality of the majority of the studies is limited for their small sample sizes. Clinical and experimental observations indicate a lack of correlation between the minimal bactericidal concentration (MIC) of a drug and its efficacy in device-related infections. Alternative in vitro tests indicate that the efficacy of a drug in an experimental implant-associated infection depends on its activity on nongrowing and adhering microorganisms.[30] This fact probably explains why the use of intravenous â-lactams or glycopeptides (only active against duplicating microorganisms) for 4 to 6 weeks have shown a low success rate in *S. aureus* prosthetic joint infections and osteomyelitis.[31,32] Conversely, the combination of rifampin with other antibiotics (ie, ofloxacin, levofloxacin, or fusidic acid) in orthopaedic implant infections has demonstrated a higher success rate.[33,34] Zimmerli et al[35] demonstrated in a randomized, double-blind study that in the acute staphylococcal orthopaedic implant infections an open debridement followed by the association of ciprofloxacin (750 mg/12 h) with rifampin (450 mg/12 h) administered for 3 months (hip prosthesis and orthopaedic implant infections) or 6 months (knee prosthesis infections) was more effective than ciprofloxacin alone (curing percentages of 100% and 53%, respectively, $p < .05$, after a follow-up of 35 months). Nowadays, levofloxacin is superior to ciprofloxacin due to levofloxacin's better therapeutic index as a consequence of a lower MIC against *S. aureus* and a high serum concentration (higher bioavailability). Furthermore, its once-a-day administration facilitates the adherence to long-term treatment. The experience from our group shows that prolonged oral regimen with levofloxacin plus rifampin is well tolerated and has good results in prosthetic joint infections due to gram-positive cocci.[36,37] Rifampin is a concentration-dependent antibiotic and the better pharmacodynamic parameter related to its activity is C_{max}/MIC. Administration in a 600-mg mono-dose is easier and also allows a higher C_{max}/MIC than the 450 mg/12 h dosage. In addition, taking into account the long duplicative rate of sessile bacteria (>1 day), the administration of rifampin once a day could be sufficient.

The incidence of methicillin-resistant (MR) staphylococci and enterococci is on the increase and the failure rate, using glycopeptides, is higher than in other microorganisms.[38] However, recent data using other antibiotics different from glycopeptides for treating MRSA infections do not show differences in the outcome of MRSA and susceptible *S. aureus*.[39] This finding suggests the need for alternatives to glycopeptides. High doses of cotrimoxazole[40] or linezolid[41] either alone or combined with rifampin[42,43] have shown good results. However, it is necessary to closely monitor its hematological (cotrimoxazole and linezolid) and neurological (linezolid) toxicity in prolonged treatments. Other alternative agents with shorter experience but with good results are tetracyclines and fusidic acid combined with rifampin.[44,45]

The experience in orthopaedic implant infections due to gram-negative bacteria is scarce but, in general, the outcome is considered to be poor. However, recent experience from our group suggests that when fluoroquinolones (ciprofloxacin or levofloxacin) are included in the antibiotic regimen and the gram-negative bacteria are susceptible, the success rate is higher.[46] Fluoroquinolones are probably efficacious for the treatment of implant infections and osteomyelitis due to gram-negative bacteria for two reasons: (1) their diffusion to synovial fluid and bone,[47] and (2) their activity against biofilms. In an in vitro model of a *Pseudomonas* biofilm, Tanaka et al[48] showed that the bactericidal action of â-lactams against biofilm cells was affected by the low rate of cell growth inside the biofilm, while that of fluoroquinolones was considerably greater and independent of the growth rate. Unfortunately, the resistance rate to fluoroquinolones in the *Enterobacteriaceae* family is increasing; therefore, it is necessary to further investigate new options for treating these infections.

REFERENCES

1. Tunney MM, Patrick S, Curran MD, et al. Detection of prosthetic hip infection at revision arthroplasty by immunofluorescence microscopy and PCR amplification of the bacterial 16S rRNA gene. *J Clin Microbiol*. 1999;37:3281-3290.
2. Schutzer SF, Harris WH. Deep-wound infection after total hip replacement under contemporary aseptic conditions. *J Bone Joint Surg Am*. 1988;70:724-727.
3. Krizek TJ, Robson MC. Evolution of quantitative bacteriology in wound management. *Am J Surg*. 1975; 130:579-584.
4. Falcieri E, Vaudaux P, Huggler E, et al. Role of bacterial exopolymers and host factors on adherence and phagocytosis of *Staphylococcus aureus* in foreign body infection. *J Infect Dis*. 1987;155:524-531.

5. Miles AA, Miles EM, Burke J. The value and duration of defence reactions of the skin to the primary lodgement of bacteria. *Br J Exp Pathol.* 1957;38:79-96.
6. Classen DC, Evans RS, Pestotnik SL, et al. The timing of prophylactic administration of antibiotics and the risk of surgical-wound infection. *N Engl J Med.* 1992;326:281-286.
7. Johnson DP. Antibiotic prophylaxis with cefuroxime in arthroplasty of the knee. *J Bone Joint Surg Br.* 1987;69:787-789.
8. Friedman RJ, Friedrich LV, White RL, et al. Antibiotic prophylaxis and tourniquet inflation in total knee arthroplasty. *Clin Orthop Relat Res.* 1990;260:17-23.
9. Abdel-Salam A, Eyres KS. Effects of tourniquet during total knee arthroplasty. A prospective randomised study. *J Bone Joint Surg Br.* 1995;77:250-253.
10. Barwell J, Anderson G, Hassan A, et al. The effects of early tourniquet release during total knee arthroplasty: a prospective randomized double-blind study. *J Bone Joint Surg Br.* 1997;79:265-268.
11. Richardson JB, Roberts A, Robertson JF, et al. Timing of antibiotic administration in knee replacement under tourniquet. *J Bone Joint Surg Br.* 1993;75:32-35.
12. Soriano A, Bori G, García-Ramiro S, et al. Timing of antibiotic prophylaxis for primary total knee arthroplasty performed during ischemia. *Clin Infect Dis.* 2008;46:1009-1014.
13. Kalmeijer MD, Nieuwland-Bollen E, Bogaers-Hofman D, et al. Nasal carriage of *Staphylococcus aureus* is a major risk factor for surgical-site infections in orthopedic surgery. *Infect Control Hosp Epidemiol.* 2000;21:319-323.
14. Murdoch DR, Roberts SA, Fowler JV, et al. Infection of orthopedic prostheses after *Staphylococcus aureus* bacteremia. *Clin Infect Dis.* 2001;32:647-649.
15. Sendi P, Rohrbach M, Graber P, et al. *Staphylococcus aureus* small colony variants in prosthetic joint infection. *Clin Infect Dis.* 2006;43:961-967.
16. Tuchscherr L, Medina E, Hussain M, et al. *Staphylococcus aureus* phenotype switching: an effective bacterial strategy to escape host immune response and establish a chronic infection. *EMBO Mol Med.* 2011; 3:129-141.
17. *Carlsson AK, Lidgren L, Lindberg L.* Prophylactic antibiotics against early and late deep infections after total hip replacements. *Acta Orthop Scand.* 1977;48:405-410.
18. Engesaeter LB, Lie SA, Espehaug B, et al. Antibiotic prophylaxis in total hip arthroplasty: effects of antibiotic prophylaxis systemically and in bone cement on the revision rate of 22,170 primary hip replacements followed 0-14 years in the Norwegian Arthroplasty Register. *Acta Orthop Scand.* 2003; 74(6):644-651.
19. Miller MB, Bassler BL. Quorum sensing in bacteria. *Ann Rev Microbiol.* 2001;55:165-199.
20. Ceri H, Olson ME, Stremick C, et al. The Calgary Biofilm Device: new technology for rapid determination of antibiotic susceptibilities of bacterial biofilms. *J Clin Microbiol.* 1999;37:1771-1776.
21. Huang CT, Yu FP, McFeters GA, et al. Nonuniform spatial patterns of respiratory activity within biofilms during disinfection. *Appl Environ Microbiol.* 1995;61:2252-2256.
22. Anderl JN, Zahller J, Roe F, et al. Role of nutrient limitation and stationary-phase existence in Klebsiellapneumoniae biofilm resistance to ampicillin and ciprofloxacin. *Antimicrob Agents Chemother.* 2003;47:1251-1256.
23. Zimmerli W, Frei R, Widmer AF, et al. Microbiological tests to predict treatment outcome in experimental device-related infections due to *Staphylococcus aureus*. *J Antimicrob Chemother.* 1994;33:959-967.
24. Lewis K. Persister cells. *Annu Rev Microbiol.* 2010; 64:357-372.
25. Craig WA. Pharmacodynamics of antimicrobials: general concepts and applications. In: Nightingale Ch, Ambrose PG, Drusano GL, et al, eds. *Antimicrobial Pharmacodynamics in Theory and Clinical Practice.* New York: Informa Healthcare; 2007:1-19.
26. Stevens DL, Ma Y, Salmi DB, et al. Impact of antibiotics on expression of virulence-associated exotoxin genes in methicillin-sensitive and methicillin-resistant *Staphylococcus aureus*. *J Infect Dis.* 2007;195:202-211.
27. Falagas ME, Siempos II, Vardakas KZ. Linezolid versus glycopeptide or beta-lactam for treatment of gram-positive bacterial infections: meta-analysis of randomised controlled trials. *Lancet Infect Dis.* 2008; 8:53-66.
28. Weigelt J, Itani K, Stevens DL, et al. Linezolid versus vancomycin in treatment of complicated skin and soft tissue infections. *Antimicrob Agents Chemother.* 2005;49:2260-2266.
29. Lipsky BA, Itani K, Norden C, et al. Treating foot infections in diabetic patients: a randomized, multicenter, open-label trial of linezolid versus ampicillin-sulbactam/amoxicillin-clavulanate. *Clin Infect Dis.* 2004;38:17-24.

30. Widmer AF, Frei R, Rajacic Z, et al. Correlation between in vivo and in vitro efficacy of antimicrobial agents against foreign body infections. *J Infect Dis.* 1990;162:96-102.
31. Brandt CM, Sistrunk WW, Duffy MC, et al. *Staphylococcus aureus* prosthetic joint infection treated with debridement and prosthesis retention. *Clin Infect Dis.* 1997;24:914-919.
32. Tice AD, Hoaglund PA, Shoultz DA. Risk factors and treatment outcomes in osteomyelitis. *J Antimicrob Chemother.* 2003;51:1261-1268.
33. Drancourt M, Stein A, Argenson JN, et al. Oral rifampin plus ofloxacin for treatment of Staphylococcus-infected orthopedic implants. *Antimicrob Agents Chemother.* 1993;37:1214-1218.
34. Widmer AF, Gaechter A, Ochsner PE, et al. Antimicrobial treatment of orthopedic implant-related infections with rifampin combinations. *Clin Infect Dis.* 1992;14:1251-1253.
35. Zimmerli W, Widmer AF, Blatter M, et al. Role of rifampin for treatment of orthopedic implant-related staphylococcal infections: a randomized controlled trial. *JAMA.* 1998;279:1537-1541.
36. Soriano A, Garcia S, Bori G, et al. Treatment of acute postsurgical infection of joint arthroplasty. *Clin Microbiol Infect.* 2006;12:930-933.
37. Vilchez F, Martínez-Pastor JC, Garcia-Ramiro S. Outcome and predictors of treatment failure in early post-surgical prosthetic joint infections due to *Staphylococcus aureus* treated with debridement. *Clin Microbiol Infect.* 2011;17:439-444.
38. Salgado CD, Dash S, Cantey JR, et al. Higher risk of failure of methicillin-resistant *Staphylococcus aureus* prosthetic joint infections. *Clin Orthop Relat Res.* 2007;461:48-53.
39. Senneville E, Joulie D, Legout L, et al. Outcome and predictors of treatment failure in total hip/knee prosthetic joint infections due to *Staphylococcus aureus*. *Clin Infect Dis.* 2011;53:334-340.
40. Stein A, Bataille JF, Drancourt M, et al. Ambulatory treatment of multidrug-resistant Staphylococcus-infected orthopedic implants with high-dose oral co-trimoxazole. *Antimicrob Agents Chemother.* 1998;42: 3086-3091.
41. Bassetti M, Vitale F, Melica G, et al. Linezolid in the treatment of gram-positive prosthetic joint infections. *J Antimicrob Chemother.* 2005;55:387-390.
42. Nguyen S, Pasquet A, Legout L, et al. Efficacy and tolerance of rifampicin-linezolid compared with rifampicin-cotrimoxazole combinations in prolonged oral therapy for bone and joint infections. *Clin Microbiol Infect.* 2009;15:1163-1169.
43. Soriano A, Gómez J, Gómez L, et al. Efficacy and tolerability of prolonged linezolid therapy in the treatment of orthopedic implant infections. *Eur J Clin Microbiol Infect Dis.* 2007;26:353-356.
44. Pavoni GL, Giannella M,Falcone M, et al. Conservative medical therapy of prosthetic joint infections: retrospective analysis of an 8-year experience. *Clin Microbiol Infect.* 2004;10:831-837.
45. Aboltins CA, Page MA, Buising KL, et al. Treatment of staphylococcal prosthetic joint infections with debridement, prosthesis retention and oral rifampicin and fusidic acid. *Clin Microbiol Infect.* 2007;13:586-591.
46. Martinez-Pastor JC, Muñoz-Mahamud E, Vilchez F, et al. Outcome of acute prosthetic joint infections due to gram-negative bacilli treated with open debridement and retention of the prosthesis. *Antimicrob Agents Chemother.* 2009;53:4772-4777.
47. Rimmele T, Boselli E, Breilh D, et al. Diffusion of levofloxacin into bone andsynovial tissues. *J Antimicrob Chemother.* 2004;53:533-535.
48. Tanaka G, Shigeta M, Komatsuzawa H, et al. Effect of the growth rate of Pseudomonas aeruginosa biofilms on the susceptibility to antimicrobial agents: beta-lactams and fluoroquinolones. *Chemotherapy.* 1999;45:28-36.

19

The Human Meniscus

Constantinos Ketonis

The menisci are two fibrocartilaginous tissues that lie in the knee joint and play a key role in joint stabilization,[1] shock absorption,[2,3] force dissipation, protection of articular cartilage from excessive stress, and joint lubrication.[4] This is partly achieved by increasing the load-bearing area in the joint, thereby "correcting" to a significant extent the incongruence of the femoral and tibial articular surfaces.[5,6] Removal of the meniscus drastically alters the mechanical function of the knee joint and leads to greater stress on the articular cartilage.

Meniscal lesions represent the most common intra-articular knee injury in the United States with a mean annual incidence of 66/100,000[7,8] and, according to the National Center for Health Statistics, over 600,000 surgeries each year are the result of complications with the meniscus.[9] Men tend to suffer meniscal injuries more than women, with the right knee being more often injured, and the overall incidence peaks at 20 to 29 years of age for both sexes.[10,11] The most common cause of meniscal lesion in young patients is sports related and specifically sports involving cutting or twisting, such as football, basketball, soccer, baseball, and skiing.[10,11] Consequently, these injuries are especially frequent in athletes who participate in high-demand sports and can cause a great deal of disability and morbidity.[12-14] With increasing age, injuries to the menisci tend to be more associated with degenerative changes.

Today a substantial amount of research is dedicated to new technologies to repair or regenerate the meniscus, but the importance and role of this tissue was not realized until the late 1940s when Fairbank described the radiographic changes that occur in the absence of the meniscus.[15] At the time, the meniscus was considered a vestigial tissue, but as the first disappointing long-term results following total meniscectomy began to surface, demonstrating a very high rate of osteoarthritis development, the mind-set in the medical community began to change. The need to shift away from total meniscectomies to more conservative clinical approaches to the management of meniscal tears became apparent, leading to the pursuit of new strategies for meniscal salvage.[15] With the advent of arthroscopy and newer surgical technologies available to surgeons, total meniscectomy is now considered only as a last resort and every effort is made to conserve as much meniscus as possible via partial meniscectomy and meniscal repair. Nonetheless, meniscal injuries still remain a challenge and can lead to long-term degenerative joint changes, articular cartilage degeneration, and osteoarthritis. A thorough understanding of meniscal anatomy and physiology is necessary in order to understand the function and mechanics of the knee as well as for the development of new tissue engineering solutions.

ANATOMY

The menisci are two semicircular fibrocartilaginous structures located in the medial and lateral compartments of the tibiofemoral articulation and are critical components of a healthy knee joint.[16,17] On gross inspection, the menisci are glossy, smooth white tissues that measure approximately 35 mm in diameter[18] and are attached to the joint capsule by their thick convex-shaped peripheral rim, which has a length of 110 mm including the length of the insertional ligaments.[16] The medial meniscus is smaller than its counterpart and it is semicircular or C-shaped, while the lateral one is nearly circular or O-shaped. The surface of the menisci in contact with the femoral condyles is concave, whereas the distal surface is flat or slightly convex as it lies on the tibial plateaus. On cross section, the menisci are wedge shaped and taper to a sharp tip oriented toward the center of the joint. This characteristic shape is attained early in the prenatal period and maintained throughout the adult life.[19]

The menisci are attached to the tibial plate mainly via insertional ligaments at their anterior and posterior horns.[20] It has been shown that there is variation in the exact location of these attachment sites between people, specifically the anterior horn, which may have clinical applications for patients with atypical anterior knee pain.[21] Other ligaments that attach to and stabilize the menisci include the deep medial collateral ligament (dMCL), the anterior intermensical (or transverse) ligament (AIL), which attaches the anterior lateral meniscus to the anterior medial meniscus,[18] and the two meniscofemoral (or coronary) ligaments (MFLs).[12,22,23] Although the anterior and posterior meniscofemoral ligaments, also known as the ligaments of Humphrey and Wrisberg, respectively,[24] are commonly referred to as ligaments, they in fact link bone to meniscus and not bone to bone.[23] Both ligaments transverse between the posterior horn of the lateral meniscus to a location near the posterior cruciate ligament (PCL) insertion site on the medial femoral condyle, though the ligament of Humphrey runs anteriorly to the PCL and the ligament of Wrisberg runs posteriorly[24] as shown in Figure 19-1. Everyone has at least one of the two ligaments, but only 46% of people have both of them.[23] When first described in 1899 by Poirier and Charpy, the MFL was thought to be a third cruciate ligament,[23] but more recently several investigators have suggested that the MFLs play a significant role in altering the position of the lateral meniscus to increase the congruity between the meniscotibial socket and the lateral femoral condyle.[22,24,25]

Blood supply to the meniscus is limited and varies with age. In an infant, the meniscus is fully vascularized, and as the infant starts bearing weight on his or her knees, the vessels in the inner portion of the menisci progressively close down under the body's weight and muscular forces. By age 9 months, the inner one-third is largely avascular, and at 10 years, the meniscus closely resembles the adult meniscus.[27] In the adult only the outer one- to two-thirds of the tissue is usually vascularized,[28] with the exception of the posterolat-

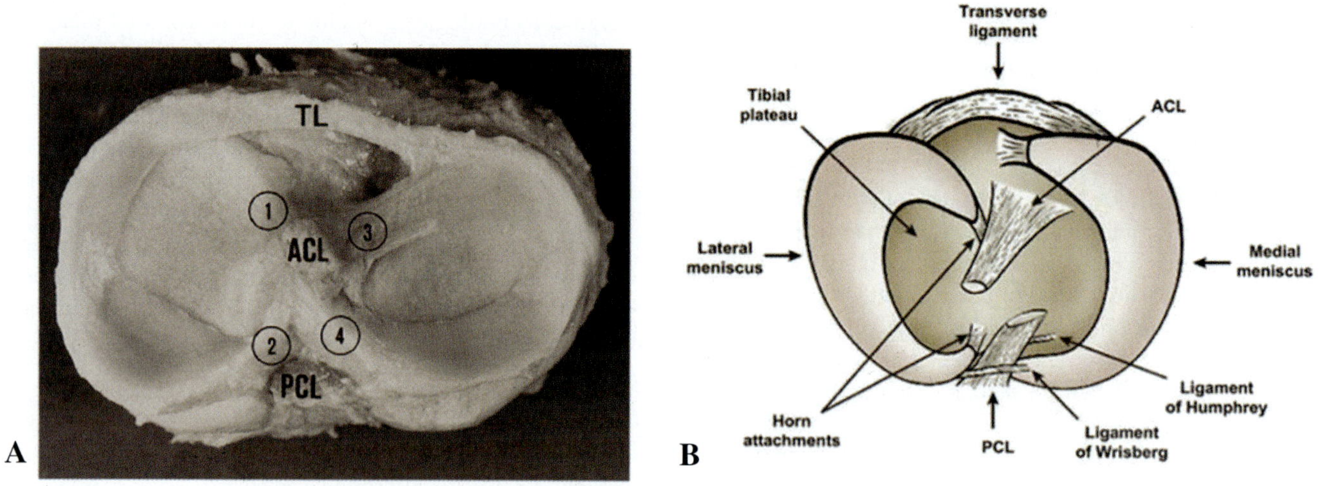

FIGURE 19-1. *Meniscus anatomy. (A) Right human knee joint from above (anterior is at the top of the photo). TL, transverse ligament; 1, anterior insertional ligament of the medial meniscus; 2, posterior insertional ligament of the medial meniscus; 3, anterior insertional ligament of the lateral meniscus; 4, posterior insertional ligament of the lateral meniscus; ACL, cross section of the anterior cruciate ligament; PCL, cross section of the posterior cruciate ligament. (Reprinted from Messner and Gao,[18] with permission from John Wiley & Sons, Inc.)* ***(B)*** *Diagrammatic anatomy of the human meniscus highlighting the relationship of the ligaments of Humphrey and Wrisberg. (Reprinted from Makris et al,[26] with permission from Elsevier.)*

eral aspect of the lateral meniscus, which also becomes relatively avascular. Perfusion to the menisci is predominantly supplied by the lateral and medial geniculate arteries (inferior and superior), which form a perimeniscal capillary plexus with radial branches that penetrate and supply the menisci.[28,29] The terminal branches of the penetrating blood vessels also supply the peripheral portion of the avascular areas, whereas central portions of the menisci are supplied by diffusion from the synovial fluid.[30,31]

Similarly, the innervation to the menisci is also limited to the outer one-third.[18] Large nerve fibers arising mainly from the posterior articular nerve (albeit innervation of the medial meniscus is also partly provided by branches of the medial articular nerve) enter through the attachment sites of the horns to the tibia and course circumferentially giving off smaller nerve fibers that are oriented radially toward the center.[32] The nerve supply as well as vascularity in the horns of the menisci appears to be more extensive than in the body,[30,31] a configuration that is conserved throughout life since these areas are never subjected to weight-bearing forces. The peripherally infiltrating capillaries and nerves only penetrate up to 10% to 30% of the meniscus width[29] and provide the basis for natural division of the menisci into sections and zones.

TISSUE SUBDIVISIONS

On an axial view, the meniscus can be generally divided into a central "body" and the terminal anterior and posterior "horns" that insert into the tibial spine centrally. On a coronal cut, the menisci are wedge-shaped and can be subdivided into an outer (red) zone, where blood vessels and nerve endings reside as they extend inwards from the synovium, an inner (white) zone that is devoid of vascularization and innervation, and a middle (red-white) zone that represents the transition from the outer to the inner zone.[33] The demarcation between these zones cannot be determined with gross inspection of the meniscus and thus cannot be distinguished, for example, at the time of surgery. However, the vascular and avascular zones of the meniscus can be differentiated histologically, not only by the presence or absence of vasculature but also by the remarkable variation in architecture, composition, and type of cells that can be found in these regions.[30]

COMPOSITION

Although the meniscus surface appearance grossly resembles that of articular cartilage, histologically, it is more typical of fibrocartilage.[34] It is principally composed of water, collagens, and proteoglycans in approximate bulk mass proportions of 72%:22%:1%.[35] These proportions vary with age and can be altered when subjected to previous injuries. A small quantity (0.6% dry weight) of elastin is also found within meniscus, although its exact function is still not known.

As in articular cartilage, collagen is a main constituent of the meniscus, but in contrast to articular cartilage, which contains principally type II collagen and an abundance of proteoglycan, the meniscal matrix collagen is approximately 98% type I, with smaller amounts of collagen types II, III, V, and VI.[36] Furthermore, the proteoglycan content of the meniscus is <1%, approximately one-tenth to one-eighth that of articular cartilage, but it plays an important role in its function. The main types of glycosaminoglycans (GAGs) that are found attached to the core protein of these proteoglycans in the normal human meniscal tissue are chondroitin-6-sulfate (60%), dermatan sulfate (20%–30%), chondroitin-4-sulfate (10%–20%), and keratin sulfate (15%).[35] The combination of these GAGs give rise to aggrecan, biglycan, and decorin, which enable the meniscus to absorb water—a property vital to the normal function of the meniscus because it provides support when the tissue is under compression.[37] Adhesion glycoproteins such as fibronectin, thrombospondin, and collagen VI[19] are also found in the meniscus matrix, and they serve as a link between extracellular matrix (ECM) components and cells. The organic matrix of the meniscus is permeable to fluid flow, although nearly sixfold less so than articular cartilage. Interestingly, despite its significant heterogeneity and differences with articular cartilage, the changes in composition of the meniscus with maturation and aging are similar to those seen with articular cartilage.[38,39]

HISTOLOGY

The arrangement, composition, and structure of the collagen fibrils have been found to vary in different regions of the meniscus. Most changes can be observed from the outer to the inner portions of the meniscus and from superficial to deep layers, defining the biomechanical properties of each portion and of the tissue as a whole.[40,41] For example, the outer two-thirds of the meniscus is both histologically and biochemically organized like fibrocartilage, whereas the inner one-third of the meniscus is arranged more like hyaline cartilage. This unique variable organization allows the meniscus to resist the large compressive forces it is subjected to in the inner portion while also withstanding the great tensile loads it experiences in the periphery.[5,19,42]

Collagen

Perhaps the most important feature of the human meniscus is the complex arrangement of the collagen that is believed to have a direct relationship to its load-bearing function. Scanning electron microscopy (SEM) studies reveal three distinct layers in the meniscus,[43] as demonstrated in Figure 19-2: (1) superficial layer—a thin fibril network (diameter ~ 30 nm) covering the femoral and tibial surfaces, showing no preferred orientation; (2) lamellar layer—lying beneath the superficial layer with radial fibrils in the external circumference so that they then intersect at random angles as they approach the central portion; and (3) central main layer—composed of circumferentially oriented fibril bundles along with a few radial collagen fibrils (radial tie fibers) interwoven with the circular fibril bundles in the region of the internal circumference that significantly increase the tissue tensile resistance.[44] In the middle of this layer, connective tissue from the joint capsule is also found to penetrate radially between the circular bundles.[45]

Cells

The characterization of the cellular component of the meniscus has been an area of debate. Many terms have been used to categorize these cells over the years, such as fibrocytes, fibroblasts, meniscus cells, and chondrocytes, but their exact identity still remains somewhat controversial in the literature today. Even though, during early development, all meniscus cells present the same cellular morphology in terms of both size and shape with no regional variations, it is now widely accepted that in the adult meniscus they differ depending on their location. In regards to the cellular population, the meniscus can be divided into two main zones: the superficial zone, which borders the articular surfaces, and the deep zone, which constitutes the majority of the meniscus substance. The cells in the superficial zone have been compared to the flattened chondrocytes akin to those found in the superficial zone of articular cartilage. They are usually, but not invariably, oval or fusiform with a few cell processes and a scant amount of cytoplasm, making the nucleus of the cell seem abnormally large.[17,46] In contrast, the cells in the deep zone are viewed as similar to the chondrocytes from the transitional and radial zones of articular cartilage that are more rounded or polygonal; they can be found alone or occasionally in pairs or in short longitudinal rows woven in bundles of dense collagen fibers. In reality these cells possess properties found both in fibroblasts and chondrocytes and the term "fibrochondrocytes" has been more commonly used to describe these unique cells.

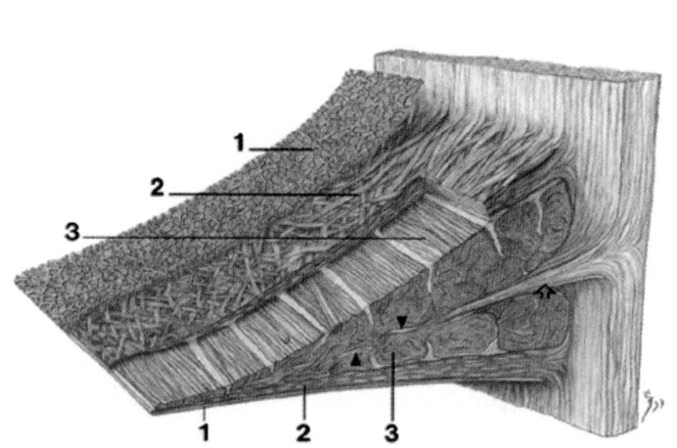

FIGURE 19-2. *Drawing demonstrating three distinct layers in the meniscus cross section: (1) the superficial network, (2) lamellar layer, and (3) central main layer. Arrowheads point to radial collagen fibrils and the arrow shows the loose connective tissue from the joint capsule penetrating the meniscus. (Reprinted from Petersen and Tillmann,[45] with permission from Springer.)*

More recently, Hellio Le Graverand et al[5] identified four major morphologically distinct classes of cells within the adult rabbit meniscus using antibodies to cytoskeletal proteins, two of which were found in the fibrocartilage region. The other two were found in the hyaline-like region and the superficial region, respectively, further subdividing the meniscus to even more zones. Other cell types that have been successfully isolated and characterized from canine and rabbit menisci by culturing in various growth media include occasional microvascular endothelial cells as well as myofibroblasts, which are more typically seen around injured tissue.[47] Nevertheless, these cells in general contain abundant endoplasmic reticulum and Golgi complex with only sparse mitochondria. This suggests that, much like articular chondrocytes, they mainly depend on anaerobic glycolysis as their major pathway for energy production.

MECHANICAL PROPERTIES

Perhaps the most important function that the menisci perform is to serve as shock absorbers and force dissipaters for the knee.[48,49] They enhance the ability of articular cartilage to provide a smooth, near-frictionless articulation and to distribute loads evenly to the underlying bone of the femur and tibia. This is mainly achieved by minimizing the impact of the incongruity between the semicircular-shaped femoral condyles and the comparably flat tibial plateau.[18,50] The stress or contact pressure experienced by the articulating surfaces is proportional to the load applied and inversely proportional to the contact area; in other words, the larger the contact area over which the load is distributed, the less the contact stresses on the contact area.[22] The intact menisci occupy 60% of the contact area between the tibial and femoral cartilage surfaces, absorbing some of the load and transmitting 50% of joint compressive forces in full extension and approximately 85% of the load in 90° of flexion.[51-53] The significance of the meniscus in the mechanics of the knee was recapitulated by Paletta et al,[54] who, after total removal of the lateral meniscus in 10 cadaveric knees, reported a 50% decrease in total contact area, which then resulted in a 235% to 335% increase in peak local contact loads.

The menisci are very efficient in their function both because of their intrinsic material properties and their architecture and shape. When a load is applied to the knee joint, the meniscus is compressed but is also displaced away from the center of the femoral condyles and extrudes radially out of the joint.[12] This is due to the unique wedge-shaped structure of the menisci and the insertional ligaments at their horns anteriorly and posteriorly, which allow displacement in all directions. This results in the transformation of part of the axial load into hoop stresses at the meniscal periphery. The degree of displacement varies depending on the load and the angle of the knee. Generally, compression of the tissue at angles of 15° and 30° flexion result in greater displacement when compared to direct perpendicular loads at 0°,[55] with the lateral meniscus experiencing a greater displacement than the medial meniscus (8.2 ± 3.2 mm and 3.3 ± 1.5 mm, respectively[56]). Conversely, the contact area is greatest when the knee is in full extension and decreases while also moving posteriorly on the tibial plate with flexion. For about every 30° of knee flexion, the contact surface between the femur and tibia decreases by 4%,[57] resulting in contact areas in deep flexion that are approximately 75% of those at full extension.[56] The areas that experience the highest pressures are located on the lateral meniscus as well as the areas that are not covered by the meniscus where direct articular cartilage contact takes place both in the medial and lateral compartments.[58]

The contact area as well as the distribution of load also varies with the total force being transmitted through the knee. Walker and Erkman[6] showed that under no load, only 10% of the cartilage makes direct contact, and thus the meniscus absorbs most of the load. As the load increases, direct articular contact on the medial side increases fairly proportionally, whereas the lateral meniscus preserves the articular coverage and continues to transmit the load. For example, under loads of 150 kg, the lateral meniscus still carries most of the load on that side, whereas at that same force, the medial meniscus shares the load equally 50/50 with the exposed articular cartilage. Interestingly, the area of cartilage that was found to be most frequently contacted was the medial tibial spine.

The mechanical properties of the meniscus have been extensively studied and it is known that they depend heavily on the collagen orientation and thus vary between portions of the meniscus. The coarse, circumferential type I collagen fiber bundles of the meniscus give the tissue great tensile stiffness, which is further increased by the radial tie fibers. The tensile modulus of the tissue is approximately 100 to 150 MPa in the circumferential direction and it is less than half of this radially.[59,60] Moreover, the tensile modulus does not only vary between the circumferential and radial direction, but also from anterior to the posterior of the meniscus, as seen in Table 19-1. The meniscus under load resists axial compression with an aggregate modulus of 100 to 150 kPa[61] and, as it is simultaneously deformed, shear forces develop between the collagen fibers. The shear modulus of the meniscus is approximately 120 kPa[59] and its relatively low circumferential shear strength is thought to be partly responsible for the occurrence of longitudinal tears.[12,62]

HEALING POTENTIAL

The overriding problem with meniscal injuries is that the meniscus has a limited ability to heal itself effectively.[12] It relies on penetrating arteries for its supply of nutrients and oxygen and thus for its healing. Only the peripheral one-third of the meniscus is vascularized and therefore able to repair itself.[12]

Etiologically, meniscal tears can result either from excessive application of force to a normal meniscus or from normal forces acting on a degenerative structure.[27] Most tears at a young age are traumatic, but with increasing age, degenerative complex tears are more frequently seen. Meniscal tears are most often classified according to their location, type, thickness, and resulting stability.[27,63-65] For injury localization, the meniscus can be generally divided into an anterior, middle, and posterior thirds as well as inner, middle, and outer thirds. Tears in the outer third or peripheral vascularized portion are denoted as red-red tears, in the middle third portion as red-white or white-white tears, and in the inner avascular portion as white-white tears. Tears in the red-white region, approximately 4 mm from the meniscal attachment, are considered to have partial vascular supply.[52] Tears are further characterized as partial or full thickness, and full-thickness injuries can be deemed stable

TABLE 19-1. Tensile Properties of Human Knee Meniscus

Direction	Location	Stiffness (± SD, MPa)	
		Lateral	Medial
Circumferential			
	Anterior	124.58 ± 39.51	106.21 ± 77.95
	Central	91.37 ± 23.4	77.95 ± 25.09
	Posterior	143.73 ± 38.91	82.36 ± 22.23
Radial			
	Anterior	48.47 ± 25.67	48.31 ± 24.35
	Central	45.86 ± 24.20	46.20 ± 27.56
	Posterior	29.85 ± 12.77	32.55 ± 11.27

Adapted from Tissakht and Ahmed.[60]

or unstable. Depending on the mechanism of injury, different patterns or types of meniscal tears can result, of which the most important are vertical/longitudinal (including bucket handle), flat/oblique, radial/transverse, and horizontal/complex (including degenerative).[26,66]

An accurate classification based on these descriptors and the assessment of any other concurrent intra-articular injuries (especially anterior cruciate ligament lesions, which can accompany meniscal tears in >80% of cases[67,68]) are paramount for the determination of a correct treatment plan and management.[51] Tears in the peripheral vascular zone, where healing potential is relatively high, have traditionally been repaired. Various approaches have been described using fixators, such as arrows,[69-71] staples,[72] and all-inside biodegradable screws[73,74]; however, arthroscopic-assisted suture repair remains the gold standard.[51] These approaches as well as the various arthroscopic-assisted techniques, such as inside-out, outside-in, and all-inside, and the indications and contraindications for each have been extensively studied and compared in the literature and are beyond the scope of this chapter.[9,26,33,63,75]

Tears that extend 4 to 5 mm beyond the peripheral meniscal rim and into the avascular zone tend to be more complex and broad and their repair has traditionally been discouraged because of the poor healing potential.[51] Repairs in this area have been associated with poor prognosis with a high possibility of retearing. Even though numerous investigators[68,75-78] have recently reported good results with repair of simple tears in the avascular region of select patients (see Gallacher et al[79] for criteria), the main strategy for treating such tears is still considered to be partial meniscectomy. This intervention can provide pain relief and improve function in the short run, but can result in long-term degeneration of the articular cartilage.[80,81] To that end, new methods of repair rather than excision and new techniques to increase healing in the avascular meniscus have been of particular interest and an area of active research in the past decade.

One popular strategy has been to promote healing by increasing the vascularity of the inner meniscus. The most notable techniques tried include trephination, which induces bleeding and creates access channels connecting the periphery to the central avascular portion and rasping of the vascularized parameniscal synovium to promote an injury response and thus assist healing. Another approach has been the application of a fibrin clot directly on the defect, which acts as a reparative scaffold supplying growth factors and promoting chemotaxis, cell proliferation, and matrix synthesis to the tear site.[9,82] Similarly, platelet-rich plasma has been tried, given recent evidence that it may stimulate chemotaxis, cell proliferation, and angiogenesis.[83] Even though numerous studies have been performed using these techniques, the results in the literature still seem conflicting.

More recently, tissue engineering of the meniscus has gained traction and many investigators have refocused their efforts on such technologies. Many cell sources and scaffold combinations have been tried, but the unique nature of the meniscal cells as well as the complex organization of its extracellular matrix make the meniscus a difficult tissue to engineer successfully.[12] Nevertheless, the use of autologous cells has been attempted, which involves a biopsy to isolate cells and their expansion in vitro. Extracting sufficient healthy cells and successful in vitro expansion are extremely challenging and investigators have resorted to more available allogeneic and xenogenic cell sources, with some success reported in pigs[84] and rabbit animal models.[85] Another emerging cell source has been human embryonic stem cells (hESCs), which due to their pluripotency and unlimited proliferative capacity have become very popular in the regeneration of not only the meniscus[86,87] but also articular cartilage, intervertebral disc,[88] and even heart muscle.[89,90] Since much controversy and politics surround the use of hESCs, many studies have now switched to adult mesenchymal stem cells (MSCs), which can be either expanded ex vivo and directly transplanted to the site of injury to replenish the local cell population or can be activated and differentiated in situ by using acellular scaffolds and administration of growth factors such as vascular endothelial growth factor (VEGF).

Finally, the successful engineering of an effective tissue construct requires the selection of an appropriate scaffold. There is a plethora of scaffolds in development today and many have been tried in the engineering of a meniscus, including synthetic polymer scaffolds, such as polyurethane and polylactic coglycolic acid; hydrogel scaffolds, which can be synthetic (poly *N*-isopropyl acrylamide) or natural (alginate); ECM component scaffolds, such as collagen meniscus implants; hyaluronan scaffolds; and, finally, tissue-derived scaffolds, such as small intestinal submucosa, decellularized tissue or ECM, and silk.

A different approach that has been considered, without much success, is meniscal prostheses. Prostheses have been developed using poly(tetrafluoroethylene) and Dacron, both plain and polyurethane-coated, but have typically exhibited inferior mechanical properties than native meniscal tissue[91-93] and have not gained much popularity. Currently, attempts for regeneration and tissue engineering of the meniscus remains a very active field of research and many new exciting developments are expected in the next few years.

REFERENCES

1. Shoemaker SC, Markolf KL. The role of the meniscus in the anterior-posterior stability of the loaded anterior cruciate-deficient knee. Effects of partial versus total excision. *J Bone Joint Surg Am*. 1986;68:71-79.
2. Hsu RW, Himeno S, Coventry MB, et al. Normal axial alignment of the lower extremity and load-bearing distribution at the knee. *Clin Orthop Relat Res*. 1990:215-227.
3. Voloshin AS, Wosk J. Shock absorption of meniscectomized and painful knees: a comparative in vivo study. *J Biomed Eng*. 1983;5:157-161.
4. Macconaill MA. The function of intra-articular fibrocartilages, with special reference to the knee and inferior radio-ulnar joints. *J Anat*. 1932;66:210-227.
5. Hellio Le Graverand MP, Ou Y, Schield-Yee T, et al. The cells of the rabbit meniscus: their arrangement, interrelationship, morphological variations and cytoarchitecture. *J Anat*. 2001;198:525-535.
6. Walker PS, Erkman MJ. The role of the menisci in force transmission across the knee. *Clin Orthop Relat Res*. 1975:184-192.
7. Morgan CD, Wojtys EM, Casscells CD, et al. Arthroscopic meniscal repair evaluated by second-look arthroscopy. *Am J Sports Med*. 1991;19:632-637; discussion 7-8.
8. Salata MJ, Gibbs AE, Sekiya JK. A systematic review of clinical outcomes in patients undergoing meniscectomy. *Am J Sports Med*. 2010;38:1907-1916.
9. Shybut T, Strauss EJ. Surgical management of meniscal tears. *Bull NYU Hospital Joint Dis*. 2011;69:56-62.
10. Steinbrück K. Epidemiology of sports injuries—25-year-analysis of sports orthopedic-traumatologic ambulatory care. *Sportverletz Sportsc*. 1999;13:38-52.
11. Steinbrück K. Epidemiology of sports injuries. A 15-year analysis of sports orthopedic ambulatory care. *Sportverletz Sportsc*. 1987;1:2-12.
12. Sweigart MA, Athanasiou KA. Toward tissue engineering of the knee meniscus. *Tissue Eng*. 2001; 7:111-129.
13. Baker P, Coggon D, Reading I, et al. Sports injury, occupational physical activity, joint laxity, and meniscal damage. *J Rheumatol*. 2002;29:557-563.
14. Neuman P, Englund M, Kostogiannis I, et al. Prevalence of tibiofemoral osteoarthritis 15 years after nonoperative treatment of anterior cruciate ligament injury: a prospective cohort study. *Am J Sports Med*. 2008;36:1717-1725.
15. Fairbank TJ. Knee joint changes after meniscectomy. *J Bone Joint Surg Br*. 1948;30:664-670.

16. Kohn D, Moreno B. Meniscus insertion anatomy as a basis for meniscus replacement: a morphological cadaveric study. *Arthroscopy.* 1995;11:96-103.
17. Ghadially FN, Thomas I, Yong N, et al. Ultrastructure of rabbit semilunar cartilages. *J Anat.* 1978;125:499-517.
18. Messner K, Gao J. The menisci of the knee joint. Anatomical and functional characteristics and a rationale for clinical treatment. *J Anat.* 1998;193(pt 2):161-178.
19. McDevitt CA, Webber RJ. The ultrastructure and biochemistry of meniscal cartilage. *Clin Orthop Relat Res.* 1990;252:8-18.
20. Ghosh P, Taylor TK. The knee joint meniscus. A fibrocartilage of some distinction. *Clin Orthop Relat Res.* 1987;224:52-63.
21. Berlet GC, Fowler PJ. The anterior horn of the medical meniscus. An anatomic study of its insertion. *Am J Sports Med.* 1998;26:540-543.
22. Masouros SD, McDermott ID, Amis AA, et al. Biomechanics of the meniscus-meniscal ligament construct of the knee. *Knee Surg Sports Traumatol Arthrosc.* 2008;16:1121-1132.
23. Kusayama T, Harner CD, Carlin GJ, et al. Anatomical and biomechanical characteristics of human meniscofemoral ligaments. *Knee Surg Sports Traumatol Arthrosc.* 1994;2:234-237.
24. Poynton AR, Javadpour SM, Finegan PJ, et al. The meniscofemoral ligaments of the knee. *J Bone Joint Surg Br.* 1997;79:327-330.
25. Gupte CM, Bull AM, Thomas RD, et al. A review of the function and biomechanics of the meniscofemoral ligaments. *Arthroscopy.* 2003;19:161-171.
26. Makris EA, Hadidi P, Athanasiou KA. The knee meniscus: structure-function, pathophysiology, current repair techniques, and prospects for regeneration. *Biomaterials.* 2011;32:7411-7431.
27. Greis PE, Bardana DD, Holmstrom MC, et al. Meniscal injury: I. Basic science and evaluation. *J Am Acad Orthop Surg.* 2002;10:168-176.
28. Arnoczky SP, Warren RF. Microvasculature of the human meniscus. A*m J Sports Med.* 1982;10:90-95.
29. Cipolla M, Cerullo G, Puddu G. Microvasculature of the human medial meniscus: operative findings. *Arthroscopy.* 1992;8:522-525.
30. Gray JC. Neural and vascular anatomy of the menisci of the human knee. *J Orthop Sports Phys Ther.* 1999;29:23-30.
31. Day B, Mackenzie WG, Shim SS, et al. The vascular and nerve supply of the human meniscus. *Arthroscopy.* 1985;1:58-62.
32. Freeman MA, Wyke B. The innervation of the knee joint. An anatomical and histological study in the cat. *J Anat.* 1967;101:505-532.
33. Rattner JB, Matyas JR, Barclay L, et al. New understanding of the complex structure of knee menisci: implications for injury risk and repair potential for athletes. *Scand J Med Sci Sports.* 2011;21:543-553.
34. Adams ME, Muir H. The glycosaminoglycans of canine menisci. *Biochem J.* 1981;197:385-389.
35. Herwig J, Egner E, Buddecke E. Chemical changes of human knee joint menisci in various stages of degeneration. *Ann Rheumat Dis.* 1984;43:635-640.
36. Eyre DR, Wu JJ. Collagen of fibrocartilage: a distinctive molecular phenotype in bovine meniscus. *FEBS Lett.* 1983;158:265-270.
37. Scott PG, Nakano T, Dodd CM. Isolation and characterization of small proteoglycans from different zones of the porcine knee meniscus. *Biochim Biophys Acta.* 1997;1336:254-262.
38. Inerot S, Heinegård D. Bovine tracheal cartilage proteoglycans. Variations in structure and composition with age. *Collagen Rel Res.* 1983;3:245-262.
39. Franzén A, Inerot S, Hejderup SO, et al. Variations in the composition of bovine hip articular cartilage with distance from the articular surface. *Biochem J.* 1981;195:535-543.
40. Shirazi R, Shirazi-Adl A, Hurtig M. Role of cartilage collagen fibrils networks in knee joint biomechanics under compression. *J Biomechan.* 2008;41:3340-3348.
41. Shirazi R, Shirazi-Adl A. Deep vertical collagen fibrils play a significant role in mechanics of articular cartilage. *J Orthop Res.* 2008;26:608-615.
42. Cheung HS. Distribution of type I, II, III and V in the pepsin solubilized collagens in bovine menisci. *Connective Tissue Res.* 1987;16:343-356.
43. Chevrier A, Nelea M, Hurtig MB, et al. Meniscus structure in human, sheep, and rabbit for animal models of meniscus repair. *J Orthop Res.* 2009;27:1197-1203.
44. Skaggs DL, Warden WH, Mow VC. Radial tie fibers influence the tensile properties of the bovine medial meniscus. *J Orthop Res.* 1994;12:176-185.
45. Petersen W, Tillmann B. Collagenous fibril texture of the human knee joint menisci. *Anat Embryol.* 1998;197:317-324.

46. Ghadially FN, Lalonde JM, Wedge JH. Ultrastructure of normal and torn menisci of the human knee joint. *J Anat.* 1983;136:773-791.
47. Webber RJ, Harris MG, Hough AJ. Cell culture of rabbit meniscal fibrochondrocytes: proliferative and synthetic response to growth factors and ascorbate. *J Orthop Res.* 1985;3:36-42.
48. Kurosawa H, Fukubayashi T, Nakajima H. Load-bearing mode of the knee joint: physical behavior of the knee joint with or without menisci. *Clin Orthop Relat Res.* 1980;149:283-290.
49. Wojtys EM, Chan DB. Meniscus structure and function. *Instruct Course Lect.* 2005;54:323-330.
50. Donahue TLH, Hull ML, Rashid MM, et al. A finite element model of the human knee joint for the study of tibio-femoral contact. *J Biomechan Eng.* 2002;124: 273-280.
51. Heckmann TP, Barber-Westin SD, Noyes FR. Meniscal repair and transplantation: indications, techniques, rehabilitation, and clinical outcome. *J Orthop Sports Phys Ther.* 2006;36:795-814.
52. Noyes FR, Barber-Westin SD. Repair of complex and avascular meniscal tears and meniscal transplantation. *J Bone Joint Surg.* 2010;92:1012-1029.
53. Ahmed AM, Burke DL. In-vitro measurement of static pressure distribution in synovial joints. Part I: Tibial surface of the knee. *J Biomechan Eng.* 1983;105:216-225.
54. Paletta GA, Manning T, Snell E, et al. The effect of allograft meniscal replacement on intraarticular contact area and pressures in the human knee. A biomechanical study. *Am J Sports Med.* 1997;25:692-698.
55. Bylski-Austrow DI, Ciarelli MJ, Kayner DC, et al. Displacements of the menisci under joint load: an in vitro study in human knees. *J Biomechan.* 1994;27:421-431.
56. Yao J, Lancianese SL, Hovinga KR, et al. Magnetic resonance image analysis of meniscal translation and tibio-menisco-femoral contact in deep knee flexion. *J Orthop Res.* 2008;26:673-684.
57. Walker PS, Hajek JV. The load-bearing area in the knee joint. *J Biomechan.* 1972;5:581-589.
58. Fukubayashi T, Kurosawa H. The contact area and pressure distribution pattern of the knee. A study of normal and osteoarthrotic knee joints. *Acta Orthop Scand.* 1980;51:871-879.
59. Fithian DC, Kelly MA, Mow VC. Material properties and structure-function relationships in the menisci. *Clin Orthop Relat Res.* 1990;252:19-31.
60. Tissakht M, Ahmed AM. Tensile stress-strain characteristics of the human meniscal material. *J Biomechan.* 1995;28:411-422.
61. Sweigart MA, Zhu CF, Burt DM, et al. Intraspecies and interspecies comparison of the compressive properties of the medial meniscus. *Ann Biomed Eng.* 2004;32:1569-1579.
62. Zhu W, Chern KY, Mow VC. Anisotropic viscoelastic shear properties of bovine meniscus. *Clin Orthop Relat Res.* 1994;306:34-45.
63. Noyes FR, Heckmann TP, Barber-Westin SD. Meniscus repair and transplantation: a comprehensive update. *J Orthop Sports Phys Ther.* 2011 Sep 4 [Epub ahead of print].
64. Noyes FR, Barber-Westin SD, Chen RC. Repair of complex and avascular meniscal tears and meniscal transplantation. *Instruct Course Lect.* 2011;60:415-437.
65. Noyes FR. *Noye's Knee Disorders: Surgery, Rehabilitation, Clinical Outcomes.* Philadephia, PA: Saunders; 2009.
66. Terzidis IP, Christodoulou A, Ploumis A, et al. Meniscal tear characteristics in young athletes with a stable knee: arthroscopic evaluation. *Am J Sports Med.* 2006;34:1170-1175.
67. Duncan JB, Hunter R, Purnell M, et al. Meniscal injuries associated with acute anterior cruciate ligament tears in alpine skiers. *Am J Sports Med.* 1995;23:170-172.
68. Rubman MH, Noyes FR, Barber-Westin SD. Arthroscopic repair of meniscal tears that extend into the avascular zone. A review of 198 single and complex tears. *Am J Sports Med.* 1998;26:87-95.
69. Ellermann A, Siebold R, Buelow JU, et al. Clinical evaluation of meniscus repair with a bioabsorbable arrow: a 2- to 3-year follow-up study. *Knee Surg Sports Traumatol Arthrosc.* 2002;10:289-293.
70. Lee GP, Diduch DR. Deteriorating outcomes after meniscal repair using the meniscus arrow in knees undergoing concurrent anterior cruciate ligament reconstruction: increased failure rate with long-term follow-up. *Am J Sports Med.* 2005;33:1138-1141.
71. Gill SS, Diduch DR. Outcomes after meniscal repair using the meniscus arrow in knees undergoing concurrent anterior cruciate ligament reconstruction. *Arthroscopy.* 2002;18:569-577.
72. Laprell H, Stein V, Petersen W. Arthroscopic all-inside meniscus repair using a new refixation device: a prospective study. *Arthroscopy.* 2002;18:387-393.

73. Hantes ME, Kotsovolos ES, Mastrokalos DS, et al. Arthroscopic meniscal repair with an absorbable screw: results and surgical technique. *Knee Surg Sports Traumatol Arthrosc*. 2005;13:273-279.

74. Petsche TS, Selesnick H, Rochman A. Arthroscopic meniscus repair with bioabsorbable arrows. *Arthroscopy*. 2002;18:246-253.

75. Kessler MW, Sgaglione NA. All-arthroscopic meniscus repair of avascular and biologically at-risk meniscal tears. *Instruct Course Lect*. 2011;60:439-452.

76. Scott GA, Jolly BL, Henning CE. Combined posterior incision and arthroscopic intra-articular repair of the meniscus. An examination of factors affecting healing. *J Bone Joint Surg Am*. 1986;68:847-861.

77. Fox DB, Warnock JJ, Stoker AM, et al. Effects of growth factors on equine synovial fibroblasts seeded on synthetic scaffolds for avascular meniscal tissue engineering. *Res Vet Sci*. 2010;88:326-332.

78. Hennerbichler A, Moutos FT, Hennerbichler D, et al. Repair response of the inner and outer regions of the porcine meniscus in vitro. *Am J Sports Med*. 2007;35: 754-762.

79. Gallacher PD, Gilbert RE, Kanes G, et al. White on white meniscal tears to fix or not to fix? *Knee*. 2010; 17:270-273.

80. Andersson-Molina H, Karlsson H, Rockborn P. Arthroscopic partial and total meniscectomy: a long-term follow-up study with matched controls. *Arthroscopy*. 2002;18:183-189.

81. Roos EM, Ostenberg A, Roos H, et al. Long-term outcome of meniscectomy: symptoms, function, and performance tests in patients with or without radiographic osteoarthritis compared to matched controls. *Osteoarth Cartilage*. 2001;9:316-324.

82. Port J, Jackson DW, Lee TQ, et al. Meniscal repair supplemented with exogenous fibrin clot and autogenous cultured marrow cells in the goat model. *Am J Sports Med*. 1996;24:547-555.

83. Ishida K, Kuroda R, Miwa M, et al. The regenerative effects of platelet-rich plasma on meniscal cells in vitro and its in vivo application with biodegradable gelatin hydrogel. *Tissue Eng*. 2007;13:1103-1112.

84. Weinand C, Peretti GM, Adams SB, et al. An allogenic cell-based implant for meniscal lesions. *Am J Sports Med*. 2006;34:1779-1789.

85. Ramallal M, Maneiro E, López E, et al. Xeno-implantation of pig chondrocytes into rabbit to treat localized articular cartilage defects: an animal model. *Wound Repair Regen*. 2004;12:337-345.

86. Baker BM, Gee AO, Sheth NP, et al. Meniscus tissue engineering on the nanoscale: from basic principles to clinical application. *J Knee Surg*. 2009;22:45-59.

87. Angele P, Johnstone B, Kujat R, et al. Stem cell based tissue engineering for meniscus repair. *J Biomed Mat Res A*. 2008;85:445-455.

88. Anderson DG, Risbud MV, Shapiro IM, et al. Cell-based therapy for disc repair. *Spine J*. 2005;5:297S-303S.

89. Flynn A, Brien T. Stem cell therapy for cardiac disease. *Expert Opin Biol Ther*. 2011;11:177-187.

90. Martinez EC, Kofidis T. Adult stem cells for cardiac tissue engineering. *J Mol Cell Cardiol*. 2011;50:312-319.

91. Johnson LL, Feagin JA. Autogenous tendon graft substitution for absent knee joint meniscus: a pilot study. *Arthroscopy*. 2000;16:191-196.

92. Messner K, Gillquist J. Prosthetic replacement of the rabbit medial meniscus. *J Biomed Mat Res*. 1993; 27:1165-1173.

93. Messner K. Meniscal substitution with a Teflon-periosteal composite graft: a rabbit experiment. *Biomaterials*. 1994;15:223-230.

20 Epidemiology and Pathogenesis of Knee Osteoarthritis

Alvin Ong and Fabio Orozco

Arthritis technically refers to the inflammation of the joint. However, not all arthritis is due to an inflammatory process. Knee arthritis is more accurately defined as a disease that leads to loss or damage to articular cartilage. It can be categorized as due to a noninflammatory or an inflammatory process and is a leading cause of disability in the United States. Noninflammatory arthritis is degenerative in nature and caused by mechanical injury to the joint. Inflammatory arthritis is caused by immunologically mediated damage to the joint. It is usually part of a systemic process and often an autoimmune disorder, in which the body views its own tissues as foreign and reacts with inflammation. This chapter reviews the etiology and pathogenesis of knee osteoarthritis and inflammatory arthritis with a brief overview of the pathogenesis, diagnosis, and treatment.

OSTEOARTHRITIS AND OSTEOARTHROSIS

Osteoarthritis (OA) of the knee affects over 10 million people in the United States. Its prevalence is increasing as the population ages. The Centers for Disease Control and Prevention has recently published the epidemiology of knee arthritis. Almost half (46%) of all people will develop painful knee arthritis over their lifetime. Moreover, nearly two-thirds (65%) of people who are obese will develop osteoarthritis. Osteoarthritis is a disease of cartilage. It is a process by which damage to and loss of hyaline cartilage occurs.

It is best to differentiate knee OA as primary or secondary OA. Primary OA is thought to be largely due to "wear and tear" of cartilage that occurs with aging. Its cause is idiopathic, not related to one known etiology. It is a degenerative disorder that results from the biochemical breakdown of articular (hyaline) cartilage in the synovial joints, involving not only the articular cartilage, but also the entire joint, including the subchondral bone and synovium. Secondary OA is damage to articular cartilage due a specific etiology, another disease or condition. Common causes of secondary OA include trauma, osteonecrosis, obesity, infection, abnormal development, or crystalline disease. Each of these processes can adversely affect the articular cartilage and subchondral bone of the affected joints. Secondary osteoarthritis often occurs in relatively young individuals.

Causes of Secondary Osteoarthritis

Trauma

Traumatic injury to the knee can be a single episode or repetitive in nature. Traumatic insults to the articular cartilage, ligaments, or menisci lead to abnormal biomechanics in the joints and to premature degeneration. The relationship of the meniscus and articular cartilage provides function in the complex biomechanics of the knee joint, including load distribution, shock absorption, viscoelasticity, a smooth low-friction gliding surface, and resilience to compression. Meniscectomy have been implicated in the destruction of cartilage and to subsequent osteoarthritis of the knee joint. Osteoarthritic changes after meniscectomy have been reported in up to 89% of patients.[1] This has been corroborated by other authors who have reported that surgical removal of a meniscus following knee injury represents a significant risk factor for radiographic tibiofemoral OA, with a relative risk of 14.0 after 21 years.[2]

The ligament-injured joint is also at high risk for osteoarthritis. Current conservative (eg, rehabilitation) and surgical (eg, reconstruction) treatment options appear not to reduce osteoarthritis following ligament injury. Mechanical instability is the likely initiator of osteoarthritis in the ligament-injured patient.[3] For instance, anterior cruciate ligament (ACL) deficiency is a well-recognized risk factor for the development of knee OA. Studies have shown that a torn ACL leads to OA in more than half of affected knees 5 to 15 years after injury.[4]

Osteonecrosis

Osteonecrosis (ON) is a condition in which the blood supply is interrupted to the subchondral bone leading to necrosis and collapse, which lead to secondary disruption of the overlying cartilage. The exact cause of ON of the knee is unknown. More than 3 times as many women than men are affected; most are over the age of 60 years. One theory is that a stress fracture, combined with a specific activity or trauma, results in an altered blood supply to the bone. Another theory supposes that edema within the bone increases the blood pressure within the bone, diminishing circulation. Osteonecrosis of the knee has been divided into two separate entities: spontaneous osteonecrosis of the knee (SPONK) and secondary osteonecrosis.[5]

SPONK, also known as Ahlbäck disease, occurs commonly in elderly females. Presentation is usually in the 6th or 7th decade of life. Clinical symptoms and signs vary in severity. The patient characteristically presents with acute onset of pain in the medial compartment of the knee without history of exacerbation or injury.[6] This condition often mimics other painful conditions of the knee, such as meniscal tears or OA.

A radiographically visible lesion typically develops within 6 months after onset of symptoms. Radionuclide scans can be used to differentiate between SPONK and other painful conditions of the knee.[7] The prognosis of SPONK is dependent on the size of the lesion. In knees with a lesion larger than 2.3 cm^2, osteoarthritis is likely to develop. Smaller lesions can be treated nonoperatively with analgesia, protected weight bearing, bracing, and exercise. Indications for surgical treatment include persistent severe pain despite conservative treatment. Surgery can also be considered for large osteonecrotic lesion with collapse of the condyle resulting in knee deformity. The best results were achieved with high tibial osteotomy and by knee arthroplasty.[8]

There are several causes of secondary ON. Excessive alcohol intake, corticosteroid use, trauma, and thalasemia or sickle cell disease, hypertension, vasculitis, radiation or chemotherapy, inflammatory and decompression sickness, and antiretroviral therapy have all been implicated. Secondary ON generally occurs in younger patients and frequently has an insidious onset with mild or vague pain. The lateral compartment of the knee is often involved, and the lesions are generally larger than lesions arising spontaneously. In the great majority of cases, they involve the femoral condyles and/or tibial plateaus. Bilateral distribution and multifocal involvement can also be seen in these forms.[9] Progression of joint collapse can occur because of the tendency for larger lesions. Surgical intervention may be necessary to prevent progression and treat symptoms of pain and disability.[10]

Obesity

Obesity has been implicated as a cause of the increased incidence of secondary OA in the United States. Obesity increases the mechanical stress in a weight-bearing joint. It has been strongly linked to osteoarthritis of the knees. In the Framingham study, obesity was associated with the risk of developing both symptomatic and asymptomatic osteoarthritis.[11] In a study of twins, obesity was shown to be an important risk factor for development of OA at the tibiofemoral and patellofemoral joints with significant increases of 9% to 13% in risk of OA per kg increase in body weight. This study emphasizes the potential importance of even minor weight loss in the prevention of the development of knee OA.[12] Moreover, one large study suggests that a large proportion of severe knee osteoarthritis is attributable to obesity and that risk is particularly high among obese people who also have other risk factors such as meniscal tear, injury, or previous surgery to the knee joint. There findings give strong support to public health initiatives aimed at reducing the burden of knee OA by controlling obesity.[13]

Infection

Septic arthritis is the inflammation of the joint caused by an infecting organism, of which the most common is the bacterial infection. Bacteria and the subsequent inflammatory response to the infection both contribute to articular cartilage damage and joint destruction. The bacterial source can be hematologic, contiguous, or direct inoculation via an injury or surgery. The age range of those affected is broad, extending from the neonatal period to advanced age. The most common bacteria include *Staphylococcus* and *Streptococcus* species. In certain high-risk individuals, other bacterial species may cause septic arthritis, such as *Escherichia coli*, *Salmonella*, and *Pseudomonas*. *E. coli* infections are more likely in the elderly, whereas *Salmonella* septic arthritis is more common in individuals with sickle cell disease. *Pseudomonas* septic arthritis may be seen in intravenous drug users. Chronic septic arthritis (which is less common) is caused by organisms such as *Mycobacterium tuberculosis* and *Candida albicans*. Other bacteria that can cause septic arthritis include *Mycobacterium tuberculosis* and the spirochete bacterium that causes Lyme disease.

The presentation of septic arthritis of the knee includes the inability to move the limb, intense joint pain, joint swelling, redness, and low-grade fever. With acute infection, symptoms present quickly. Often, patients will seek medical treatment because of the intensity of pain and swelling. Aspiration of the joint is diagnostic, although a negative aspiration does not rule out a septic joint. Normal synovial fluid contains <60 to 180 cells per mL. Cell count with leukocytosis of >50,000/mm^3 with a predominance of polymorphonuclear leukocytes (>75%) is diagnostic. Gram stain and culture can help identify the infecting organism.

Prompt treatment with antibiotics combined with irrigation and debridement of the joint is the treatment of choice for septic joint infection. Arthroscopic lavage[14] and formal open arthrotomy are both accepted treatment for septic arthritis, although one study reported better functional outcome with arthroscopic treatment.[15] The delay between the onset of symptoms and surgery was the major prognostic factor of success (p = .023) in one study. This delay was correlated with Gächter's staging of the intra-articular lesions.[16] Treatment delays can lead to osteoarthrosis and joint deformity. Thus, prompt treatment is integral in the treatment of the infection and to prevent joint destruction.[17]

Abnormal Development

Abnormal development of the knee has been implicated as a cause of secondary OA. Excessive varus or valgus deformity leads to abnormal distribution of weight across the joint, which leads to premature articular cartilage wear. Moreover, hypoplasia of the femur can lead to maltracking syndrome, which leads to subluxation and dislocation of the patella leading to patellofemoral OA. A study by Khan et al in patients with early symptomatic knee osteoarthritis showed a clear relationship between local knee alignment and severity of knee osteoarthritis. In this study, each degree of increase in the local varus angle was associated with a significantly increased risk of having predominantly medial compartment osteoarthritis, and a similar association was found between the valgus angulation and lateral compartment osteoarthritis.[18]

Usually, a genu valgum deformity is the result of a dysplastic lateral femoral condyle that contributes to pathologic loading of the lateral compartment and subsequent bone and cartilage destruction. Likewise, genu vara deformity leads to pathologic loading of the medial compartment. An experimental model has demonstrated that the mechanical overloading of a single compartment of the knee leads to degenerative change in that compartment.[19] Osteotomy of the femur in valgus deformity and osteotomy of the tibia in varus knees have been well described in the delay in progression and treatment of early OA by correcting deformity. In the normal knee, loads up to 2 to 4 times body weight are imparted on the tibiofemoral joint. In general, approximately 60% of the load is transmitted through the medial compartment with the remainder transmitted to the lateral side. In patients with abnormal development (excessive varus or valgus malalignment) the load distribution is abnormal, leading to deformity and premature articular cartilage wear. Osteotomy redistributes the load to the unaffected compartment, thereby improving symptoms and delaying progression of OA. Long-term follow-up studies have that concluded osteotomy allows for improved function and pain relief in properly selected young patients.[20]

Crystalline Disease

Crystalline arthropathy is caused by the abnormal deposition of crystals within the joint. These crystals can form as a result of defects in the absorption or metabolism of various natural substances such as uric acid (gout) and calcium pyrophosphate (pseudogout).

Gout

Gout is a disease arising from the deposition of monosodium urate crystals in the knee joint with accompanying inflammatory and degenerative consequences. Gout occurs when there is hyperuricemia or renal uric acid undersecretion. There are several causes of uric acid overproduction. Genetics play a significant role in some individuals. Other causes include excessive purine intake, alcohol use, certain drugs (nicotinic acid, warfarin, and chemotherapy), obesity, malignancy, hemolytic anemia, and tissue destruction (hypoxia, ischemia, and trauma). Undersecretion of uric acid can occur with decreased glomerular filtration rate, organic acidosis, lead nephropathy, and certain drugs.

Diagnosis is made by aspiration. The synovial fluid is evaluated microscopically for uric acid, which are negatively birefringent needle-shaped crystals. Treatment of gout can be accomplished with medication such as allopurinol, colchicines, and nonsteroidal anti-inflammatory drugs

(NSAIDs) such as indomethacin. Colchicine and NSAIDs are used for acute attacks, whereas allopurinol is used for prevention. Joint aspiration with glucocorticosteroid injection can be helpful.

Pseudogout

Pseudogout is a disease arising from the deposition of calcium pyrophosphate dihydrate (CPPD) crystals into the joint. Deposition of CPPD crystals lead to acute inflammatory attacks. Flare-ups affect large joints such as the knee. It occurs as commonly as gout and mimics it. Pseudogout attacks occurring before the age of 50 are uncommon. This disease is associated with aging. Diagnosis is made by aspiration of the joint. The synovial fluid is evaluated microscopically. CPPD crystals are rhomboid in shape and positively birefringent. Treatment includes use of NSAIDs such as indomethacin and intra-articular glucocorticosteroid injections.

INFLAMMATORY ARTHRITIS

Inflammatory arthritis refers to a class of arthritis that is immunologic response mediated. This form of arthritis is systemic in nature and thus, typically, polyarticular. In most instances, the immune system is triggered by normal tissue, such as cartilage, tendon, and ligaments, and responds with severe inflammatory reaction as if these normal tissues are foreign antigens. In other instances, an infection can trigger a similar autoimmune response. Examples of inflammatory arthritis include rheumatoid arthritis, psoriatic arthritis, systemic lupus erythematosus, and Reiter's syndrome.

Patients with inflammatory arthritis are a diagnostic and management challenge. When symptoms are of recent onset, they mimic other forms of illness or arthritis. The diagnosis of inflammatory arthritis should be considered for patients less than 50 years of age with joint pain and swelling lasting longer than 6 weeks.

The characteristic symptoms of inflammatory arthritis are pain and swelling of one or more joints. These symptoms may first appear after a minor illness such as a sore throat or a cold, or they may even be associated with a period of emotional stress. Patients with inflammatory arthritis usually have multiple joint involvements. Simultaneous bilateral knee joint symptoms are common.

Rheumatoid Arthritis

Rheumatoid arthritis (RA) is a relatively common disorder that affects men and women at any age. Most commonly patients are first affected in their 3rd to 6th decades. The prevalence of RA in the population is 0.5% to 1% and the annual incidence is variable (12–1200 per 100,000 population) depending on gender, race and ethnicity, and calendar year.[21] Both incidence and prevalence of rheumatoid arthritis are 2 to 3 times greater in women than in men. About 30% of the causes of rheumatoid arthritis can be attributed to genetic factors; the remaining are unknown.[22] Other factors have been suggested as important in the development or progression of RA. These include infectious agents, oral contraceptives, and smoking.

The main genetic risk factor of RA is the human leukocyte antigen (HLA) DRB1 alleles. Tumor necrosis factor alleles have also been linked with RA. However, it is estimated that these genes can explain only 50% of the genetic effect. A number of other genes have been investigated and linked with RA, including corticotrophin-releasing hormone, estrogen synthase, IFN-γ, and other cytokines.[23,24]

Environmental factors have also been implicated in the development of RA. Female sex hormones may play a protective role in RA; for instance, the use of the oral contraceptives and pregnancy are both associated with a decreased risk. On the contrary, exposure to infection may act as a trigger for RA. A number of virus and bacteria have been implicated. These include Epstein-Barr virus, parvovirus, Proteus, and Mycoplasma.[25]

There is no known cure for rheumatoid arthritis. The American College of Rheumatology in 2008 recommended earlier, more aggressive treatment of RA. This reflected heightened expectations of treatment effectiveness, including remission or substantial alleviation of symptoms for a rising percentage of patients.[26] The goal of treatment is twofold: alleviating symptoms and preventing the future destruction of the joint. Current treatment recommendation includes disease-modifying antirheumatic drugs (DMARDs) alone or in combination. There are several classes of drugs, including chemically synthesized DMARDs (azathioprine, cyclosporine, methotrexate, sulfasalazine), cytotoxic drugs (cyclophosphamide), biologic agents (TNF-alpha blockers, IL-1 blockers, monoclonal antibodies). Joint-related symptoms can be managed with anti-inflammatory agents (glucocorticoid, NSAIDs) and analgesics.

Late effects of RA can lead to disabling knee arthritis. Often the knee joint presents with severe deformity and instability. Total knee arthroplasty is often required to treat this disabling disease.

Psoriatic Arthritis

Psoriatic arthritis (PsA) is a unique chronic inflammatory arthritis that develops in about 30% of patients with psoriasis.[27] Its prevalence varies from 0.3% to 1% of the population. Initially, PsA typically presents as an oligoarticular and mild disease. However, with time, PsA becomes polyarticular, and it is a severe disease in at least 20% of patients. In the majority of the patients, PsA will appear several years after the onset of skin lesions. However, the arthritic disease can precede the skin lesion in approximately 13% to 17% of cases.[27]

The genetic epidemiology of PsA also supports its unique status. PsA has been associated with HLA class 1 alleles as opposed to the class 2 alleles associated with RA.[28] The linkage to the human leukocyte-associated antigen C gene (HLA C) has been reported consistently in psoriasis sibling pair families.[29]

Common symptoms of PsA include pain, swelling, and stiffness of one or more joints. Joints may become red and warm to touch. Psoriatic arthritis may remain mild or may progress to more destructive joint disease. Periods of active disease, or flares, will typically alternate with periods of remission. Because prolonged inflammation can lead to joint damage, early diagnosis and treatment to slow or prevent joint damage is recommended.[30]

Treatment strategy is similar to the management of RA. The goal of treatment is twofold: alleviating symptoms and preventing the future destruction of the joint. Current treatment recommendation includes DMARDs alone or in combination. Symptomatic treatment includes anti-inflammatory agents and analgesics. Surgery is reserved for chronic, severe disease. Total knee arthroplasty is recommended in end-stage disease with severe knee joint destruction.

Systemic Lupus Erythematosus

Systemic lupus erythematosus (SLE) is an autoimmune connective tissue disease that can lead to severe disabling knee arthritis. It is a type III hypersensitivity reaction caused by antibody-immune complex formation. The reported prevalence of SLE in the population is 20 to 150 cases per 100,000. The estimated incidence rates are 1 to 25 per 100,000 in the United States.[31]

Arthritis in SLE is one of the most common disease manifestations. Nearly all joints can be affected by SLE, but knee involvement is very common. Avascular necrosis of the knee can also occur. Unlike other forms of inflammatory arthritis, lupus arthritis is less disabling and usually does not cause severe destruction of the joints.

Diagnosis is obtained by serology. Antinuclear antibody testing and antiextractable nuclear antigen are the mainstay of diagnostic testing. Other tests routinely performed in suspected SLE are complement system levels (low levels suggest consumption by the immune system), electrolytes and renal function (disturbed if the kidney is involved), liver enzymes, and complete blood count.

Symptoms mimic other forms of inflammatory arthritis but to a lesser degree. There may be pain, with or without swelling. Stiffness and pain may be particularly evident in the morning. Arthritis may be a problem for only a few days or weeks or may be a permanent feature of the disease. Fortunately, the arthritis usually is not crippling.

Treatment strategy is similar to the management of other inflammatory arthritis. The goal of treatment revolves around alleviating symptoms and preventing systemic disease progression. Current treatment recommendation includes DMARDs alone or in combination. Symptomatic treatment includes anti-inflammatory agents and analgesics.

Reiter's Syndrome

Reiter's syndrome or reactive arthritis (ReA) is an inflammatory arthritis that is triggered by an infection. The type of infection is usually gastrointestinal (food poisoning) or genitourinary (sexual transmitted disease) in nature. Common infecting organisms include *Salmonella*, *Shigella*, *Yersinia*, *Campylobacter*, *Chlamydia*, and *Neisseria gonorrhea*. The classic triad of manifestation includes arthritis, conjunctivitis, and urethritis. ReA primarily affects young white men between the ages of 20 and 40, although it can occur in older people or children. About 75% of people with Reiter's syndrome are HLA-B27 positive. Urinary symptoms usually appear within days or weeks of an infection. Low-grade fever, inflammation of the conjunctiva of the eye (conjunctivitis), and arthritis develop over the next several weeks. The arthritis may be mild or severe and may affect only one side of the body or more than one joint.

The goal of treatment is to relieve symptoms and treat any underlying infection. Conjunctivitis and skin lesions associated with the syndrome do not require treatment and will go away on their own. The gastrointestinal or urinary infection should be treated with antibiotics. NSAIDS and pain relievers may be recommended for those with joint pain. Glucocorticoid injections can be utilized for painful, swollen knee joints. Immune suppressive medication may be considered for individuals with a severe case of the disease.[32]

Reactive arthritis may go away in a few weeks, but can last for a few months. Symptoms may return over a period of several years in up to half of these patients. The condition may also become chronic.

SUMMARY

The etiology of knee arthritis is varied. All types of arthritis lead to a process that creates loss or damage to articular cartilage. These processes can be categorized as noninflammatory or inflammatory arthritis. Accurate diagnosis is important to properly treat the patient and prevent progression. Ultimately, severe and chronic disease will require knee reconstruction procedures, including partial and total knee arthroplasty.

REFERENCES

1. Rangger C, Kathrein A, Klestil T, et al. Partial meniscetomy and osteoarthritis: implication of treatment for athletes. *Sports Med.* 1997;23(1):61-68.
2. Roos H, Lauren M, Jonsson K, et al. Knee osteoarthritis after meniscectomy: prevalence of radiographic changes after twenty-one years, compared to match controls. *Arthritis Rheum.* 1998;41(4):687-693.
3. Fleming B, Hulstyn M, Oksendahl, et al. Ligament injury, reconstruction and osteoarthritis. *Curr Opin Orthop.* 2005;16(5):354-362.
4. Neuman P, Englund M, Kostogiannis I, et al. Prevalence of tibiofemoral osteoarthritis 15 years after nonoperative treatment of anterior cruciate ligament injury. *Am J Sports Med.* 2008;3(9):1717-1725.
5. Zywiel MG, McGrath MS, Seyler TM, et al. Osteonecrosis of the knee: a review of three disorders. *Orthop Clin North Am.* 2009;40(2):193-211.
6. Aglietti P, Insall JN, Buzzi R, et al. Idiopathic osteonecrosis of the knee. Aetiology, prognosis and treatment. *J Bone Joint Surg Br.* 1983;65(5):588-597.
7. Lotke PA, Ecker ML, Alavi A. Painful knees in older patients. Radionuclide diagnosis of possible osteonecrosis with spontaneous resolution. *J Bone Joint Surg Am.* 1977;59(5):617-621.
8. Rozing P, Insall J, Bohne W. Spontaneous osteonecrosis of the knee. *J Bone Joint Surg Am.* 1980;62 (1):2-7.
9. Narvaez J, Narvaez A, Rodriguez-Moreno J, et al. Osteonecrosis of the knee: differences among idiopathic and secondary types. *Rheumatology.* 2000;39 (9):982-989.
10. Mont M, Tomek I, Hungerford D. Core decompression for avascular necrosis of the distal femur: long term followup. *Clin Orthop Relat Res.* 1997;334:124-130.
11. Felson D, Anderson J, Naimark A, et al. Obesity and knee osteoarthritis. The Framingham Study. *Ann Intern Med.* 1988;109(1):18-24.
12. Cicuttini F, Baker J, Spector T. The association of obesity with osteoarthritis of the hand and knee in women: a twin study. *J Rheumatol.* 1996;23:1221-1226.
13. Coggon D, Reading I, Croft P, et al. Knee osteoarthritis and obesity. *Intern J Obesity.* 2001;25(5):622-627.
14. Thiery J. Arthroscopic drainage in septic arthritis of the knee: a multicenter study. *Arthroscopy.* 1989;5(1): 65-69.
15. Wirtz D, Marth M, Miltner O, et al. Septic arthritis of the knee in adults: treatment by arthroscopy or by arthrotomy. *Int Orthop.* 2001;25(4):239-241.
16. Balabaud L, Gaudias J, Boeri C, et al. Results of treatment of septic knee arthritis: a retrospective series of 40 cases. *Knee Surg Sports Traumatol Arthrosc.* 2007; 15(4):387-392.
17. Stutz G, Kuster MS, Kleinstück F, et al. Arthroscopic management of septic arthritis: stages of infection and results. *Knee Surg Sports Traumatol Arthrosc.* 2000;8 (5):270-274.
18. Khan FA, Koff MF, Noiseux NO, et al. Effect of local alignment on compartmental patterns of knee osteoarthritis. *J Bone Joint Surg Am.* 2008;90(9):1961-1969.
19. Cooke TDV, Bryant JT, Scudamore RA. Biomechanical factors in alignment and arthritic disorders of the knee. In: Fu FH, Harner CD, Vince KG, eds. *Knee Surgery.* Baltimore, MD: Lippincott Williams & Wilkins; 1994:1061.
20. Preston CF, Fulkerson EW, Meislin R, et al. Osteotomy about the knee: applications, techniques, and results. *J Knee Surg.* 2005;18(4):258-272.
21. Alarcón GS. Epidemiology of rheumatoid arthritis. *Rheum Dis Clin North Am.* 1995;21(3):589-604.
22. Gabriel SE. The epidemiology of rheumatoid arthritis. *Rheum Dis Clin North Am.* 2001;27(2):269-281.
23. MacGregor AJ, Snieder H, Rigby AS, et al. Characterizing the quantitative genetic contribution to rheumatoid arthritis using data from twins. *Arthritis Rheum.* 2000;43(1):30-37.
24. Meyer JM, Evans TI, Small RE, et al. HLA-DRB1 genotype influences risk for and severity of rheumatoid arthritis. *J Rheumatol.* 1999;26(5):1024-1034.

25. Silman AJ, Hochberg MC. Rheumatoid arthritis. In: Silman AJ, Hochberg MC, eds. *Epidemiology of the Rheumatic Diseases*. Oxford, UK: Oxford University Press; 2001:31-71.

26. Saag KG, Gim GT, Nivedita M, et al. American College of Rheumatology 2008 recommendations for the use of nonbiologic and biologic disease-modifying antirheumatic drugs in rheumatoid arthritis. *Arthritis Rheum*. 2008;59(6):762-784.

27. Zachariae H. Prevalence of joint disease in patients with psoriasis: implications for therapy. *Am J Clin Dermatol*. 2003;4(7):441-447.

28. Rahman P, Elder JT. Genetic epidemiology of psoriasis and psoriatic arthritis. *Ann Rheum Dis*. 2005;64 (suppl II):ii37-ii39.

29. Nair RP, Henseler T, Jenisch S, et al. Evidence for two psoriasis susceptibility loci (HLA and 17q) and two novel regions (16q and 20p) by genome-wide scan. *Hum Mol Genet*. 1997;6:1349-1356.

30. Farragher TM, Lunt M, Plant D, et al. Benefit of early treatment in inflammatory polyarthritis patients with anti-cyclic citrullinated peptide antibodies versus those without antibodies. *Ann Rheum Dis*. 2010; 62(5):664-675.

31. Pons-Estel GJ, Alarcón GS, Scofield L, et al. Understanding the epidemiology and progression of systemic lupus erythematosus. *Semin Arthritis Rheum*. 2010;39(4):257-268.

32. Carter JD, Hudson AP. Reactive arthritis: clinical aspects and medical management. *Infect Dis Clin North Am*. 2009;35(1):21-44.

21

Surgical Exposures

Ari Seidenstein and Gregg R. Klein

Multiple treatments exist for osteoarthritis of the knee. However, the gold standard for treatment of end-stage knee arthritis continues to be total knee arthroplasty (TKA). Multiple studies report excellent long-term results in regard to both function and survivorship.[1,2] However, the procedure must be performed properly in order to see these results come to fruition and an adequate exposure is vital to doing so.

A multitude of surgical exposures are available to the orthopaedic surgeon when performing total knee arthroplasty. The most common approaches described in the literature are the medial parapatellar, lateral parapatellar, subvastus, and midvastus approaches. Minimally invasive modifications of all of these exposures have been described as well.[3] Regardless of which is chosen, the orthopaedic surgeon should use an approach that allows for an adequate exposure that can both be easily reproduced and extended if proven necessary.

SKIN INCISION

The anterior midline incision is the most commonly described skin incision among those that have been described. Depending on surgeon preference, it may be made directly midline, slightly medial to the midline, or mildline but with a slight medial curve. Some authors report the medial parapatellar incision leads to a more aesthetically pleasing scar because its path follows Langer's lines of the knee. Despite the cosmetic advantage, as well as its theoretical advantage of being subject to less tension with flexion of the knee,[4] few authors favor this incision. Both of these incisions commonly lead to numbness lateral to the skin incision due to either contusion or laceration of the infrapatellar branch of the saphenous nerve.[5,6]

Before making the incision, the surgeon should make note of the anatomic landmarks of the knee, including the four borders of the patella as well as the medial aspect of the tibial tubercle. The anterior midline incision should bisect the medial and lateral halves of the patella and lead distally just medial to the tibial tubercle. The incision is preferably made in flexion, thus preventing the possibility of the distal aspect of the incision translating laterally over the tibial tubercle as can be seen if made in extension.[7] This could become problematic as a scar over the tibial tubercle could become painful during kneeling. Adequate exposure dictates the length of any incision. Situations that could lead to the need for a larger incision are increased size of the patient, greater preoperative deformity, contracture, and less tensile soft tissues. An incision that is too small can lead to poor visualization and increases the chance of a poor outcome. Incision size usually decreases as the surgeon gains more experience. Generally speaking, the incision should extend from a given point proximal to the superior pole of the patella to the most distal aspect of the tibial tubercle (Fig. 21-1).

A challenge presents itself when previous competing incisions exist over the knee. Transverse incisions may be crossed perpendicularly without hesitation. However, crossing old transverse incisions at more acute angles may be

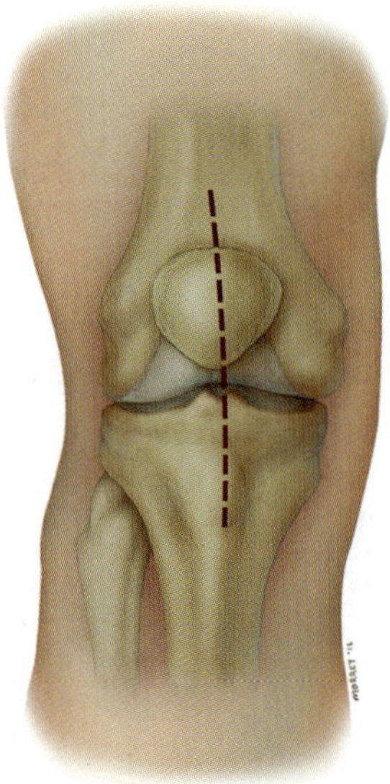

FIGURE 21-1. *Skin incisions for TKA. (Courtesy of Matthew Morrey, MD.)*

cause for concern because this might lead to avascular areas of skin. If presented with multiple longitudinal incisions, the lateralmost incision that will provide sufficient exposure should be used since the blood supply stemming from the saphenous and descending geniculate arteries is medial. However, the more medial incision may be used if it was made more recently and healed without complication. Finally, it is extremely important to avoid parallel incisions that create small skin bridges. A plastic surgeon should be consulted if there is any question regarding viability and healing potential of the skin and soft tissues.

Regardless of the incision that is chosen, undermining of the subcutaneous tissues must be minimized. Ideally, dissection should be carried out straight through the subcutaneous fat directly over the proposed arthrotomy. The blood supply to the skin arises from deep perforating vessels of the saphenous artery and the descending genicular artery, which anastomose just superficial to the fascia.[8] These vessels then penetrate the subcutaneous fat and proceed to the epidermal layer. Thus, any undermining superficial to the fascia puts the blood supply to the skin at risk and dissection should be limited to the tissues deep to the fascia.[9]

MEDIAL PARAPATELLAR APPROACH

The medial parapatellar approach is one of the most commonly used exposures because it is straightforward and both easily reproducible and extensile (Fig. 21-2). The starting point proximally is dictated by the required amount of exposure for the given procedure. The arthrotomy begins longitudinally at the medial quadriceps tendon, leaving 3 to 5 mm of tendon attached to the vastus medialis for repair during closure. The incision progresses distally through the extensor mechanism curving around the medial aspect of the patella through the medial retinaculum. Again, a few millimeters of retinaculum is left attached to the patella for repair. As the incision proceeds, it curves laterally around the inferior pole of the patella toward the patella tendon, running parallel to it as it proceeds to a point 5 mm medial to the distal aspect of the tibial tubercle. The dissection is carried down to the anterior cortex of the tibia, leaving a small cuff of tissue medially for later repair.

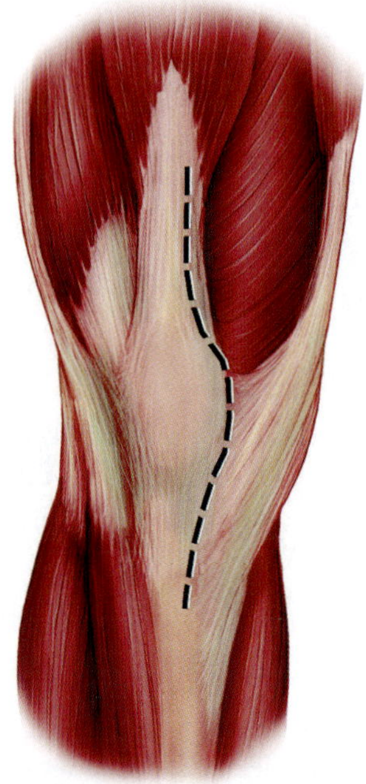

FIGURE 21-2. *Medial parapatellar approaches. (Courtesy of Matthew Morrey, MD.)*

Medially, a sleeve of soft tissue consisting of the deep medial collateral ligament (MCL) and medial capsule is released subperiosteally. This sleeve is extended posteromedially from the medial border of the patellar tendon to the midcoronal plane of the tibia. The release should not proceed more than 8 mm distal to the joint line because this is where the superficial MCL inserts. The lateral patellofemoral ligament is identified and released, if necessary.

Excision of the infrapatellar fat pad remains controversial. Lemon et al compared knees in which the fat pad was excised and those in which it was retained and found that the fat pad excision group showed significant patellar tendon shortening of 4.2%.[10] Conversely, Meneghini et al reviewed 1055 primary total knee replacements with and without fat pad excision and found that fat pad excision had no significant effect on patellar tendon contracture, range of motion, Knee Society score, or function scores.[11]

Although the patella has historically been everted during TKA, recent studies have reported patellar eversion to negatively affect functional recovery. Stoffel et al used laser Doppler flowmetry to quantify patella intraosseous blood flow and found that blood flow was preserved more significantly in patients with lateral patellar retraction as compared to patellar eversion.[12] Walter et al prospectively compared knees in which the patella was everted during exposure and found that avoiding patellar eversion enhanced return of quadriceps function.[13]

During closure, it is important to re-approximate the capsular closure to prevent patella baja. Studies are still inconclusive as to whether the position of the knee during closure affects outcome. Masri et al prospectively randomized knees closed in flexion or extension and concluded that the degree of flexion of capsular closure did not have an effect on early rehabilitation.[14] In contrast, Emerson et al have reported that knees closed in flexion demonstrated a statistically significant increase in postoperative motion at 1 year.[15]

MIDVASTUS APPROACH

In the 1990s, the midvastus approach was made popular by Engh (Fig. 21-3).[16] Similar to the medial parapatellar approach, an anterior midline incision is used. The arthrotomy is usually performed with the knee in 60° of flexion. The vastus medialis obliquus (VMO) insertion is identified medially at the superior pole of the patella. The VMO is bluntly split with a finger parallel to its fibers at its insertion and is carried out in a superior and medial direction for approximately 4 cm. The surgeon must make certain to maintain the full thickness of the muscle and to stay in line with its fibers. Neither the quadriceps tendon nor the VMO insertion is ever violated. The approach distal to the VMO insertion is identical to the medial parapatellar approach mentioned previously. The lateral patellofemoral ligament is released as well.

Closure is also performed in 60° of flexion. Although the muscle of the VMO is reattached to the capsule, the muscle itself is generally not repaired.

Dalury and his associates prospectively randomized 20 patients undergoing bilateral TKA for the treatment of one

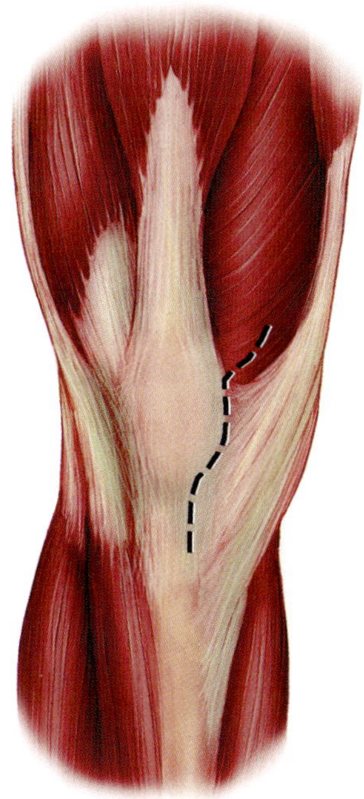

FIGURE 21-3. *Midvastus approach. (Courtesy of Matthew Morrey, MD.)*

knee with the midvastus approach and the other with the medial parapatellar approach.[17] After examining X-rays, electromographies, nerve conduction studies, range-of-motion tests, and Knee Society function and pain tests, the study showed the midvastus approach to be a safe alternative for knee arthrotomy for TKA without the concerns for damage to the vastus medialis obliquus.

Knees with less than 80° of flexion preoperatively, obesity, large muscular males, patients with previous high tibial osteotomies, and hypertrophic arthritis are all relative contraindications to performing this approach.[16]

SUBVASTUS APPROACH

Advocates of the subvastus approach describe it as being the more anatomic approach; however, it is still less commonly used (Fig. 21-4).[18] This approach also uses the anterior midline incision. The inferior border of the VMO is bluntly dissected free from the underlying periosteum as well as the intramuscular septum. It is then retracted anterolaterally, so that the joint capsule is exposed. Beginning medially, a transverse incision is made in the knee capsule proceeding toward the medial aspect of the patella. Again, the distal extent of the arthrotomy is performed in similar

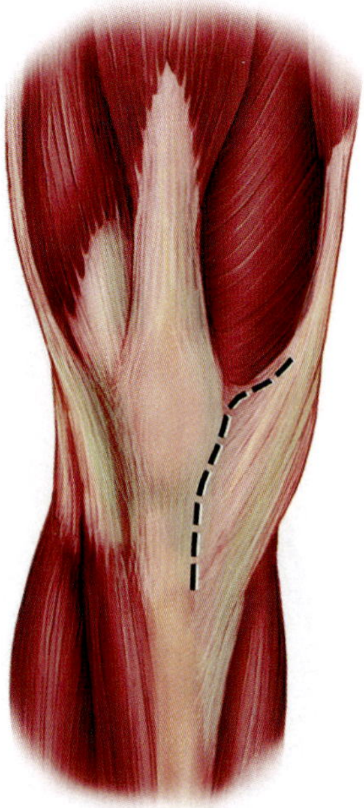

FIGURE 21-4. *Subvastus approach. (Courtesy of Matthew Morrey, MD.)*

fashion to the medial parapatellar approach. If necessary, the VMO can be further freed from the intermuscular septum. To do so, the patella must be subluxated while the knee in flexion. Although the entire arthrotomy must be closed, it is not necessary to repair the VMO to the intermuscular septum. Prior knee arthrotomy, morbid obesity, large thigh girth (>55 cm), previous high tibial osteotomy, and revision arthroplasty are all contraindications to this approach.[18,19]

Schroer et al retrospectively reviewed 150 TKAs done with the standard medial parapatellar approach and 150 TKAs done with the subvastus approach.[20] Comparisons showed no increase in the number or severity of complications and no difference in operating room time while achieving earlier straight leg raise and increased knee flexion.

In another study, Schroer and colleagues retrospectively reviewed 747 consecutive posterior-stabilized TKAs that were separated into three groups: those done with a medial parapatellar approach, those done with a mini-subvastus approach, and those done with a mini-subvastus approach but with a different femoral component that has a more posterior transition to the intercondylar notch.[21] They found that among the knees that used the same femoral component, those that were exposed with the subvastus approach and achieved increased knee flexion had a significantly higher incidence of patellar clunk syndrome. The knees that were exposed with the subvastus approach but with the femoral component with the more posteriorly placed notch did not have a clunk when achieving higher flexion.

LATERAL PARAPATELLAR APPROACH

First described by Kocher, this incision is rarely used today.[9] The arthrotomy is carried down the lateral edge of the quadriceps tendon, leaving a small cuff of tendon laterally. It proceeds distally around the lateral aspect of the patella, much like is done in a lateral retinacular release. It continues lateral to the patellar tendon, again leaving a few millimeters of soft tissue cuff for later repair.

One of the disadvantages of this approach is that the patella is not easily everted or subluxated medially. Additionally, although the approach has the potential to be extended, significant undermining of the subcutaneous tissues in the process and the patella may end up becoming devascularized as well. This approach may have a role in knees with severe fixed valgus deformity (>15°).

COMPARISON STUDIES

A true consensus does not exist as to which approach is best. Multiple comparison studies of different knee approaches have been performed using the medial parapatellar approach as the gold standard.

Juosponis et al prospectively randomized 70 knees into those undergoing a mini-midvastus approach and those undergoing a medial parapatellar approach.[22] The two groups were compared with respect to component position and functional results. The knees done with the mini-midvastus approach were associated with faster recovery but the same eventual function and the same accuracy in component positioning.

Nestor and colleagues performed a prospective, randomized, double-blinded study looking at 27 patients scheduled for bilateral TKA, each to undergo a mini-midvastus approach on one side and standard approach on the other.[23] The only significant difference in strength testing was increased isokinetic and isometric extension torque at 3 weeks postoperatively for the mini-midvastus approach. However, no differences were found for stride length, stance time, pain visual analog scale, or knee range of motion. Thus, they concluded that the mini-midvastus approach has limited benefit compared to the standard approach for TKA.

Floren and his group retrospectively reviewed 137 knees, one group having undergone a midvastus approach and the other a standard approach.[24] They found a significant decrease in the amount of patients with patella baja in the midvastus group. This finding was also related to reduced flexion as well as increased pain as early as 1 year after TKA.

White and associates compared 109 patients who underwent bilateral total knee arthroplasty with a medial parapatellar approach on one side and a midvastus approach on the other.[25] All other surgical aspects including implant choice and physical therapy protocols were identical. The authors found that the midvastus approach resulted in less postoperative pain, a quicker time to straight leg raise, and a lower incidence of lateral retinacular release. However, the clinical results at 6 months were identical.

Keating et al prospectively compared 100 bilateral total knee replacements with a midvastus approach on one side and a medial parapatellar approach on the other.[26] There were no differences in range of motion, ability to straight leg raise, or lateral release. There were two postoperative hematomas and one manipulation in the midvastus group and no complications in the medial parapatellar group. The authors did not recommend this approach over the medial parapatellar approach.

Kelly and associates prospectively randomized 51 knees undergoing total knee arthroplasty into either a medial parapatellar or midvastus approach.[27] The authors found no difference in functional parameters. However, there was a greater incidence of lateral release and blood loss in the medial parapatellar group. In addition, the authors found a 43% incidence of electromyographic (EMG) changes in the vastus splitting group. At 5 years follow-up, seven knees with abnormal EMG findings postoperatively had a normal EMG exam. Two knees had evidence of chronic changes without functional deficit. Interestingly in the two knees with chronic changes, the muscle was split with sharp dissection, while the seven knees that returned to normal were split with blunt dissection.

Varela-Egocheaga and his associates prospectively randomized 150 patients into undergoing a subvastus approach or a conventional medial parapatellar approach.[28] The subvastus approach resulted in improved long-term Knee Society scores and range of motion without the increased risk of component malalignment, surgical time, or complication rate.

Matsueda and Gustilo retrospectively reviewed 169 consecutive knee arthroplasties treated with a medial parapatellar approach and 167 arthroplasties treated with a subvastus approach and found no difference in functional parameters and range of motion.[29] There was a lower rate of lateral retinacular release in the subvastus group (37%) as compared to the medial parapatellar group (67%). However, the study was performed over a 9-year period and changing technique may have resulted in this decreased lateral release rate.

Jung and his colleagues prospectively randomized 40 knees into those undergoing a subvastus approach and those undergoing a medial parapatellar approach.[30] Although those undergoing the subvastus approach had better knee flexion at 10 days, that difference disappeared at 6 weeks postoperatively. Also, the improved patella tilt and shift seen with the subvastus approach in Matsueda and Gustilo's study was not seen in this study.

In a prospective, randomized, blinded study, Roysam and Oakley compared the results of a medial parapatellar approach to the subvastus approach and found that the subvastus group had a significantly earlier return of straight leg raise, lower consumption of opiates in the first week, less blood loss, and greater knee flexion at 1 week.[31] Weinhardt and colleagues randomized knees into either a medial parapatellar approach or a subvastus approach and found that the subvastus group attained full extension and 90° of flexion earlier.[32] However, there was not a significant difference in range of motion or function by the time patients were discharged from the hospital.

Pan and associates conducted a prospective randomized study comparing the clinical and radiological results of 88 primary TKAs using either a mini-subvastus approach or a standard medial parapatellar approach.[33] Patients undergoing the mini-subvastus approach experienced less pain 1 day postoperatively, achieved an active straight leg raise earlier, and underwent fewer lateral retinacular releases. Although the mini-subvastus knees showed better functional outcomes and range of motion 9 months postoperatively, there was no significant difference at 12 months. Five of the knees done with a medial parapatellar approach had malaligned tibial components compared to none in the mini-subvastus group.

Bridgman et al prospectively randomized 116 patients undergoing TKA to a subvastus approach and 115 to a medial parapatellar approach.[34] The subvastus approach was more effective with regard to range of motion, Knee Society scores as well as Western Ontario and McMaster Universities Osteoarthritis Index (WOMAC) and SF-36 scores. However, the surgeons reported a more difficult exposure with the subvastus approach.

Bonutti et al prospectively randomized 51 patients undergoing bilateral TKA, each patient having undergone the mini-subvastus approach in one knee and the mini-midvastus approach in the other.[35] There was no clinically relevant difference in operative times or total blood loss. Also, at 12 weeks postoperatively, there were no significant differences in isokinetic muscle strength, straight leg raise test, or range of motion. At 2 years postoperatively, there were no significant differences in outcome or, more important, patient preference between the two knees. It was recommended that the decision between these surgical approaches should be based on surgeon preference and experience.

Chang et al prospectively studied patients undergoing TKA by using either the midvastus or subvastus approach.[36] They found no significant differences in peak muscle torque or hamstring–quadriceps ratio between the two groups.

Berth and colleagues prospectively randomized the knees of 20 patients undergoing bilateral TKA, one knee undergoing a midvastus approach and the other a subvastus approach.[37] There were no differences between the two approaches with regard to both maximal voluntary contraction and voluntary activation. However, the knees that had undergone the subvastus approach did cause patients significantly more pain up until 6 months after surgery.

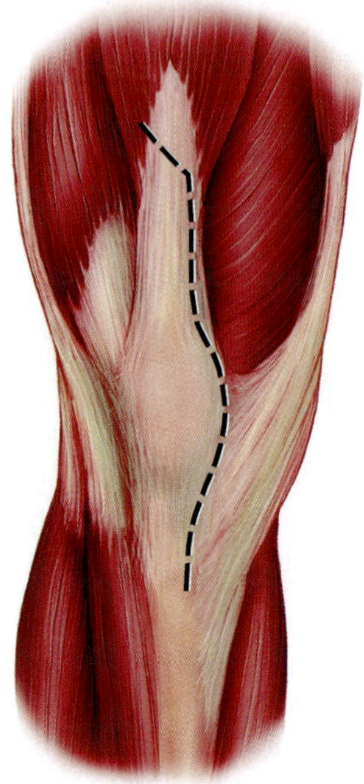

FIGURE 21-5. *Quadriceps snip. (Courtesy of Matthew Morrey, MD.)*

EXTENSILE APPROACHES

Occasionally a surgeon's approach may need to be extended in order to perform the TKA. This may occur in revision surgery, patients with prior tibial osteotomy, or in knees with severe flexion contractures, stiffness, and/or deformity. An extensile approach should also be considered if an inordinate amount of tension is being placed on the patellar tendon. The decision to extend one's approach may be made preoperatively or during the procedure.

The first option in extending the medial parapatellar approach is the quadriceps snip (Fig. 21-5).[38] At the apex of the medial arthrotomy, the quadriceps tendon is incised in a lateral oblique fashion from distal to proximal at a 45° angle splitting the vastus lateralis obliquus fibers. The quadriceps snip should exit the quadriceps tendon distal to the musculotendinous junction of the rectus femoris muscle. A lateral retinacular release placed 1 cm lateral to the lateral border of the patella may be performed to facilitate lateral dislocation of the patella. The lateral superior geniculate artery should be identified and preserved when possible.

Postoperative physical therapy can begin without delay and is not altered because of the surgical exposure. Patients are allowed unrestricted passive and active range of motion.[38]

If after performing a quadriceps snip and lateral release the exposure is still unsatisfactory, a tibial tubercle osteotomy (Fig. 21-6) may be indicated and should be performed.[39] If it has not been done already, the incision is extended distal to the tibial tubercle. The borders of the patella tendon insertion on the tibial tubercle are identified and an oscillating saw is used to osteotomize the tubercle medially, proximally, and distally. Although the thickness of the osteotomy varies based on the actual thickness of the tubercle and patella tendon, the length should be at least 8 cm. An osteotome is used to lift the tubercle laterally while attempting not to disrupt the soft tissue and periosteum sleeve laterally.

The osteotomy is most commonly repaired with three wires that are passed through drill holes. The most proximal wire is passed through the osteotomy fragment and the other two encompass the fragment. In order to tension the wires, they are angled distally from a lateral to medial direction. Again, postoperative rehabilitation is usually not altered. Potential complications include overlying skin necrosis, nonunion of the osteotomy, and tibial tubercle fracture.[40]

Nikolopoulos and colleagues prospectively randomized 44 knees with severe valgus deformity (15°–36°)

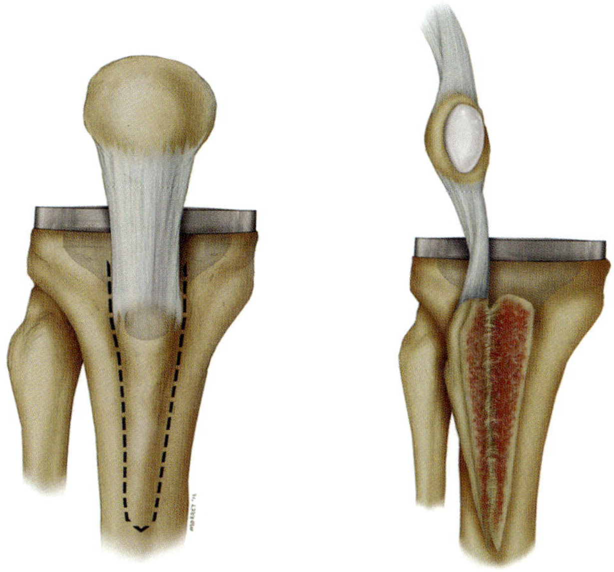

FIGURE 21-6. *Tibial tubercleosteotomy. (Courtesy of Matthew Morrey, MD.)*

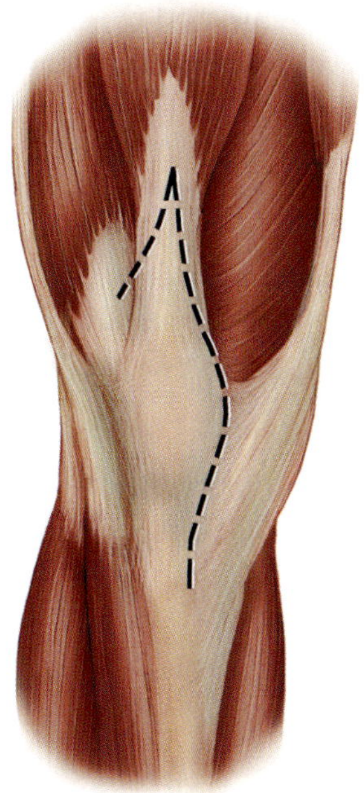

FIGURE 21-7. *Patella turndown. (Courtesy of Matthew Morrey, MD.)*

undergoing primary TKA to a group undergoing medial parapatellar arthrotomy and another undergoing a lateral parapatellar arthrotomy combined with a tibial tubercle osteotomy.[41] There was no significant difference in the clinical scores; however, residual valgus deviation occurred in 32% of the TKAs that underwent the standard approach compared to 9% in the group with the lateral parapatellar combined with the tibial tubercle osteotomy.

Rarely, a quadriceps turndown (Fig. 21-7) or V-Y quadricepsplasty[42] may be needed for the extremely stiff or ankylosed knee. This approach can only be extended from the medial parapatellar approach. If the surgeon anticipates that a quadriceps snip will not give enough exposure, the quadriceps incision can instead be continued distally and laterally, also at a 45° angle to the tendon. Depending on the amount of exposure needed, the incision can be continued distally through the vastus lateralis and the iliotibial band to varying extents.

Although this approach provides excellent exposure to the stiff knee, it does so at the possible cost of significant morbidity as well as an extensor lag. Postoperatively, motion should be restricted or at the very least limited for 6 weeks to allow adequate time for the arthrotomy to heal. Last, if the extensor mechanism is already chronically short, performing a V-Y quadricepsplasty can lengthen it.

An additional technique sometimes used in revision surgeries that further aids with exposure is the femoral peel.[42] Windsor and Insall first described the femoral peel in 1988.[9] After exposing the joint with the standard medial parapatellar approach, dissections around the lateral and medial aspects of the femur are continued subperiostally to include the origins of the MCL and lateral collateral ligament. The capsule posteriorly is then stripped off from the back of the femur as well. Although this results in complete exposure of the joint, the femoral peel may devascularize the distal femur as well.

The medial epicondylar osteotomy is another exposure technique that may be used during revision TKA.[9] It can be used in the setting of a medial parapatellar approach or a subvastus approach. The superficial MCL as well as the tissues superior to the medial epicondyle are raised as a flap. The medial epicondyle is osteotomized so that it lies as a bone fragment within the soft tissue flap. The dissection proceeds posterolaterally around the tibia and the femur while externally rotating the knee and applying a valgus stress to expose the knee. The osteotomy is repaired using a screw to reattach the epicondyle.

CONCLUSION

In order to achieve the goals of total knee arthroplasty, the surgeon must have adequate exposure. All of the aforementioned approaches have both their advantages and disadvantages (Table 21-1). The surgeon must take all of these factors into account when deciding which one to use. Controversy still exists over which is the best. Each surgeon must consider his or her level of comfort with whichever exposure is performed, also keeping in mind when a surgery may require a more extensile approach.

TABLE 21-1. Comparison of Different Exposures for Primary Total Knee Arthroplasty

Approach	Advantages	Disadvantages
Medial parapatellar	• Easy • Reproducible • Extensile	• Detachment of VMO • Disruption of patellar vascular supply
Midvastus	• VMO insertion on patella preserved • Avoid quadriceps tendon incision • Patella blood supply less interrupted	• Less extensile • Exposure more difficult in large patients with contractures
Subvastus	• Anatomic exposure • Extensor mechanism not violated	• Not extensile • Potential for neurovascular injury • Patella clunk with increased knee flexion
Lateral parapatellar	• May help in severe fixed valgus knees	• Patella is not easily everted • Extending the approach can devascularize the skin and patella
Quadriceps snip	• Provides additional exposure in stiff knees • Postoperative protocols not altered • Superior lateral geniculate artery spared	• Violation of quad tendon
Tibial tubercle osteotomy	• Wide exposure • May reposition tibial tubercle	• Nonunion • Osteotomy escape • Tendon rupture • Postoperative rehabilitation can be altered
Quadriceps turndown	• Widest exposure	• Extensor lag common • Avascular necrosis of patella • Blood supply violated • Rehabilitation delayed, range of motion restricted

REFERENCES

1. Ranawat CS, Flynn WF Jr, Saddler S, et al. Long-term results of the total condylar knee arthroplasty. A 15-year survivorship study. *Clin Orthop Relat Res.* 1993;286:94-102.
2. Scuderi GR, Insall JN, Windsor RE, et al. Survivorship of cemented knee replacements. *J Bone Joint Surg Br.* 1989;71:798-803.
3. Berger RA, Deirmengian CA, Della Valle CJ, et al. A technique for minimally invasive, quadriceps-sparing total knee arthroplasty. *J Knee Surg.* 2006;19:63-70.
4. Johnson DP, Houghton TA, Radford P. Anterior midline or medial parapatellar incision for arthroplasty of the knee. A comparative study. *J Bone Joint Surg Br.* 1986;68:812-814.
5. Chambers GH. The prepatellar nerve.A cause of suboptimal results in knee arthrotomy. *Clin Orthop Relat Res.* 1972;82:157-159.
6. Sundaram RO, Ramakrishnan M, Harvey RA, et al. Comparison of scars and resulting hypoaesthesia between the medial parapatellar and midline skin incisions in total knee arthroplasty. *Knee.* 2007;14:375-378.
7. Yacoubian SV, Scott RD. Skin incision translation in total knee arthroplasty: the difference between flexion and extension. *J Arthroplasty.* 2007;22:353-355.
8. Haertsch PA. The blood supply to the skin of the leg: a post-mortem investigation. *Br J Plast Surg.* 1981; 34:470-477.
9. Younger AS, Duncan CP, Masri BA. Surgical exposures in revision total knee arthroplasty. *J Am Acad Orthop Surg.* 1998;6:55-64.
10. Lemon M, Packham I, Narang K, et al. Patellar tendon length after knee arthroplasty with and without preservation of the infrapatellar fat pad. *J Arthroplasty.* 2007;22:574-580.
11. Meneghini RM, Pierson JL, Bagsby D, et al. The effect of retropatellar fat pad excision on patellar tendon contracture and functional outcomes after total knee arthroplasty. *J Arthroplasty.* 2007;22:47-50.
12. Stoffel KK, Flivik G, Yates PJ, et al. Intraosseous blood flow of the everted or laterally-retracted patella during total knee arthroplasty. *Knee.* 2007;14(6):434-438.
13. Walter F, Haynes MB, Markel DC. A randomized prospective study evaluating the effect of patellar eversion on the early functional outcomes in primary total knee arthroplasty. *J Arthroplasty.* 2007;22:509-514.
14. Masri BA, Laskin RS, Windsor RE, et al. Knee closure in total knee replacement: a randomized prospective trial. *Clin Orthop Relat Res.* 1996;331:81-86.
15. Emerson RH Jr, Ayers C, Higgins LL. Surgical closing in total knee arthroplasty. A series followup. *Clin Orthop Relat Res.* 1999;368:176-181.
16. Engh GA, Parks NL. Surgical technique of the midvastus arthrotomy. *Clin Orthop Relat Res.* 1998;351: 270-274.
17. Dalury DF, Snow RG, Adams MJ. Electromyographic evaluation of the midvastus approach. *J Arthroplasty.* 2008;23:136-140.
18. Hofmann AA, Plaster RL, Murdock LE. Subvastus (southern) approach for primary total knee arthroplasty. *Clin Orthop Relat Res.* 1991;269:70-77.
19. In Y, Kim JM, Choi NY, et al. Large thigh girth is a relative contraindication for the subvastus approach in primary total knee arthroplasty. *J Arthroplasty.* 2007; 22:569-573.
20. Schroer WC, Diesfeld PJ, Reedy ME, et al. Mini-subvastus approach for total knee arthroplasty. *J Arthroplasty.* 2008;23:19-25.
21. Schroer WC, Diesfeld PJ, Reedy ME, et al. Association of increased knee flexion and patella clunk syndrome after mini-subvastus total knee arthroplasty. *J Arthroplasty.* 2009;24:281-287.
22. Juosponis R, Tarasevicius S, Smailys A, et al. Functional and radiological outcome after total knee replacement performed with mini-midvastus or conventional arthrotomy: controlled randomised trial. *Int Orthop.* 2009;33:1233-1237.
23. Nestor BJ, Toulson CE, Backus SI, et al. Mini-midvastus vs standard medial parapatellar approach: a prospective, randomized, double-blinded study in patients undergoing bilateral total knee arthroplasty. *J Arthroplasty.* 2010;25(suppl):5-11.
24. Flören M, Davis J, Peterson MG, et al. A mini-midvastus capsular approach with patellar displacement decreased the prevalence of patella baja. *J Arthroplasty.* 2007;22(suppl):51-57.
25. White RE Jr, Allman JK, Trauger JA, et al. Clinical comparison of the midvastus and medial parapatellar surgical approaches. *Clin Orthop Relat Res.* 1999; 367:117-122.
26. Keating EM, Faris PM, Meding JB, et al. Comparison of the midvastus muscle-splitting approach with the median parapatellar approach in total knee arthroplasty. *J Arthroplasty.* 1999;14:29-32.
27. Kelly MJ, Rumi MN, Kothari M, et al. Comparison of the vastus-splitting and median parapatellar approaches for primary total knee arthroplasty: a pro-

spective, randomized study. *J Bone Joint Surg Am.* 2006;88:715-720.

28. Varela-Egocheaga JR, Suárez-Suárez MA, Fernández-Villán M, et al. Minimally invasive subvastus approach, improving the results of total knee arthroplasty: a prospective, randomized trial. *Clin Orthop Relat Res.* 2010;468:1200-1208.

29. Matsueda M, Gustilo RB. Subvastus and medial parapatellar approaches in total knee arthroplasty. *Clin Orthop Relat Res.* 2000;371:161-168.

30. Jung YB, Lee YS, Lee EY, et al. Comparison of the modified subvastus and medial parapatellar approaches in total knee arthroplasty. *Int Orthop.* 2009; 33:419-423.

31. Roysam GS, Oakley MJ. Subvastus approach for total knee arthroplasty: a prospective, randomized, and observer-blinded trial. *J Arthroplasty.* 2001;16:454-457.

32. Weinhardt C, Barisic M, Bergmann EG, et al. Early results of subvastus versus medial parapatellar approach in primary total knee arthroplasty. *Arch Orthop Trauma Surg.* 2004;124:401-403.

33. Pan WM, Tang TS, Qian ZL, et al. Mini-subvastus versus a standard approach in total knee arthroplasty: a prospective, randomized, controlled study. *J Int Med Res.* 2010;38:890-900.

34. Bridgman SA, Walley G, MacKenzie G, et al. Subvastus approach is more effective than a medial parapatellar approach in primary total knee arthroplasty: a randomized controlled trial. *Knee.* 2009;16:216-222.

35. Bonutti PM, Zywiel MG, Ulrich SD, et al. A comparison of subvastus and midvastus approaches in minimally invasice total knee arthroplasty. *J Bone Joint Surg Am.* 2010;92:575-582.

36. Chang CH, Yang RS, Chen KH, et al. Muscle torque in total knee arthroplasty: comparison of subvastus and midvastus approaches. *Knee Surg Sports Traumatol Arthrosc.* 2010;18:934-938.

37. Berth A, Urbacj D, Neumann W, et al. Strength and voluntary activation of quadriceps femoris muscle in total knee arthroplasty with midvastus and subvastus approaches. *J Arthroplasty.* 2007;22:83-88.

38. Garvin KL, Scuderi G, Insall JN. Evolution of the quadriceps snip. *Clin Orthop Relat Res.* 1995;321: 131-137.

39. Whiteside LA. Exposure in difficult total knee arthroplasty using tibial tubercle osteotomy. *Clin Orthop Relat Res.* 1995;321:32-35.

40. Piedade SR, Pinaroli A, Servien E, et al. Tibial tubercle osteotomy in primary total knee arthroplasty: a safe procedure or not? *Knee.* 2008;15:439-446.

41. Nikolopoulos DD, Polyzois I, Apostolopoulos AP, et al. Total knee arthroplasty in severe valgus knee deformity: comparison of a standard medial parapatellar approach combined with tibial tubercle osteotomy. *Knee Surg Sports Traumatol Arthrosc.* 2011; 19(11):1834-1842.

42. Scott RD, Siliski JM. The use of a modified V-Y quadricepsplasty during total knee replacement to gain exposure and improve flexion in the ankylosed knee. *Orthopedics.* 1985;8:45-48.

43. Lavernia C, Contreras JS, Alcerro JC. The peel in total knee revision: exposure in the difficult knee. *Clin Orthop Relat Res.* 2011;469:146-153.

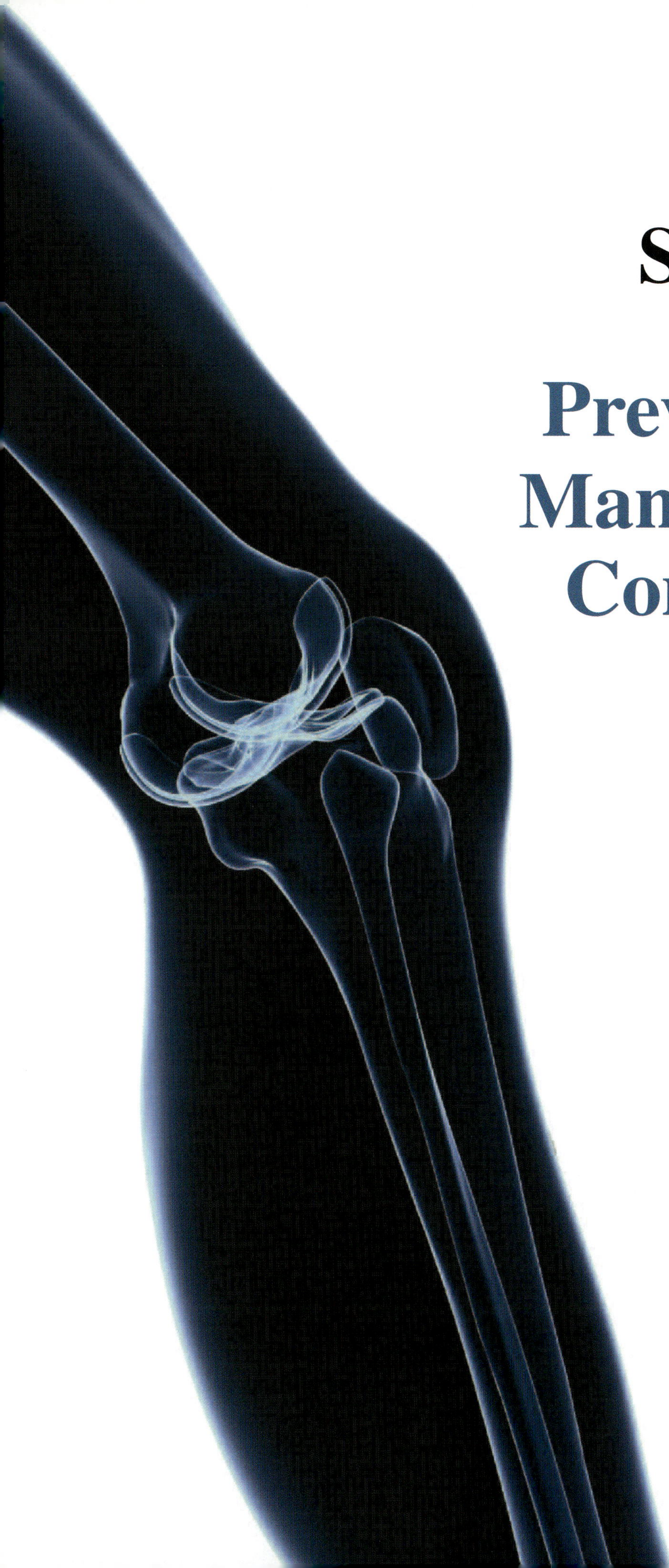

Section Two

Prevention and Management of Complications

22 Prevention of Complications: Venous Thromboembolism

Vincent D. Pellegrini, Jr.

Historically, total hip arthroplasty was known as an operation with a strong propensity for thromboembolic complications with potentially life-threatening consequences. Charnley and colleagues, in a series of 7959 total hip replacements performed from 1962 to 1973, identified the overall prevalence of pulmonary embolism as nearly 8%, with 1% being fatal.[1,2] Charnley stated, "The possibility of fatal pulmonary embolism after total hip replacement is a hip surgeon's constant worry … no matter how rare this might be."[3] During the same time period in North America, Coventry reported pulmonary embolism in 2.2% of 2012 consecutive total hip replacements; in a subset of patients who received no prophylactic anticoagulation, the prevalence of fatal pulmonary embolism was 3.4%.[4] With increasing attention attracted by thromboembolic disease, one decade later Insall likewise suggested that "prevention of thrombophlebitis and pulmonary embolism should be a major goal of every orthopaedic surgeon who performs total knee arthroplasty."[5] He and his colleagues documented an 84% prevalence of deep venous thrombosis in patients undergoing total knee replacement in the absence of any thromboembolism prophylaxis; there were no fatal pulmonary emboli and clinically evident pulmonary embolism occurred in 1.7% of patients. In what would become a controversial opinion, they concluded that, "the positive venogram, although not itself associated with local symptoms, is of clinical significance."[6] Such admonitions from our most respected teachers form the historical basis for the discussion of venous thromboembolism after total knee arthroplasty.

PATHOPHYSIOLOGY

While the components of Virchow's triad (stasis, intimal injury, and hypercoagulability) have not changed since their original description and remain relevant today, it is essential to recognize that the clinical presentation of thromboembolic disease following total hip and knee arthroplasty is different.[7-9] Moreover, the differential effects of stasis and intimal injury may logically explain the observed differences in clot prevalence and distribution after each of these two procedures. In the era before routine use of chemoprophylaxis, proximal deep venous thrombosis accounted for 50% to 60% of all observed thrombi after total hip arthroplasty, while 90% of deep vein thrombosis originated distally, primarily in the calf veins, after knee replacement (Fig. 22-1). Proximal vein thrombosis, defined as involving the popliteal vein or more proximally, occurs only infrequently after total knee replacement and accounts for less than 10% of all thrombi; when present, proximal thrombi are nearly always contiguous with more distal disease in the calf and rarely extend above the popliteal vein (Fig. 22-2). This regional distribution of deep venous thrombosis after knee replacement, with a predilection for distal clots, has remained unchanged despite the influence of modern antithrombotic agents. In contrast, with use of contemporary chemoprophylaxis after total hip arthroplasty, more than 90% of deep thrombi now occur in the calf with only rare appearance of primary proximal clots. These proximal thrombi are segmental in nature and appear in the femoral vein near the region of the lesser trochanter (Fig. 22-3). Similarly, the relative prevalence of pulmonary embolism

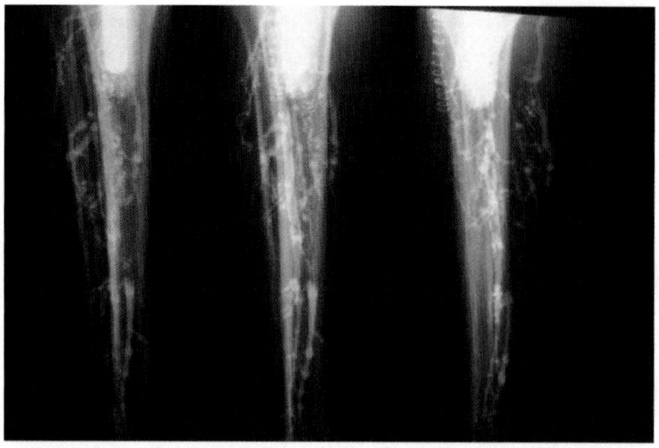

FIGURE 22-1. *Extensive venographic thrombosis in the deep veins of the calf following total knee arthroplasty. The patient was asymptomatic and had an uneventful course on 6 weeks of low-intensity (INR 2.0) warfarin therapy.*

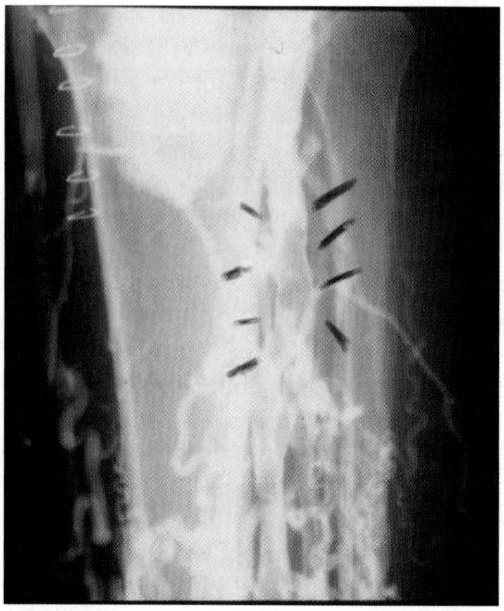

FIGURE 22-2. *Popliteal vein thrombus contiguous with distal thrombosis in the calf noted on screening venography after total knee arthroplasty. The patient was asymptomatic and had an uneventful course on 12 weeks of low-intensity (INR 2.0) warfarin therapy.*

has been historically greater after hip than knee replacement.[7-9] This follows the distribution of proximal clots as one might predict, since proximal thrombi are generally larger, more likely to embolize, and have greater hemodynamic consequences when they reach the lung. As suggested earlier, this natural propensity for proximal thrombi after hip replacement and more distal thrombi after knee arthroplasty may be explained by the predominance of different components of Virchow's triad after each procedure. Proximal clots are likely the result of intimal injury to the femoral vein, which is twisted during positioning of the lower limb for femoral preparation and component insertion regardless of the surgical approach.[10] Such intimal injury is best mitigated by potent anticoagulants, which have markedly decreased the prevalence of proximal thrombi after total hip replacement. Conversely, the prevalence of distal thrombi after knee replacement may be more likely the result of stasis secondary to folding and occlusion of the popliteal vein during shotgun exposure of the knee.[9] Interestingly, this clot distribution after knee arthroplasty has been historically unaffected by either use or avoidance of the tourniquet. Additionally, distal thrombi more likely resulting from stasis might be reasonably predicted to be more refractory to prophylaxis with potent anticoagulants alone. In some studies, deep vein thrombosis after total knee replacement has been shown to be uniquely preventable by use of intermittent pneumatic compression devices and/or regional anesthetic techniques that negate the effects of stasis on the lower limb. While substantially improved from the 80% to 90% rates observed before routine prophylaxis, the residual thrombosis prevalence after total knee arthroplasty has proven relatively refractory to solitary use of highly specific anticoagulants. Indeed, most surgeons use intermittent pneumatic compression devices alone or in combination with chemoprophylaxis after total knee replacement.

Likewise, in the setting of both hip and knee replacement, a systemic diathesis is evident.[8,9] Bilateral venogram end point trials have revealed a 10% to 15% prevalence of deep vein thrombosis in the nonoperative limb following each procedure (Fig. 22-4). It is unclear whether use of a tourniquet during knee replacement aggravates this clotting propensity by causing stasis in the leg or whether stimulation of endothelial cell-mediated fibrinolysis mitigates this effect and actually results in a lower prevalence of thrombosis than might be observed without a tourniquet.[11] An increased awareness of the intense activation of the clotting cascade that occurs during operation and persists for over 24 hours underscores the importance of intraoperative events. Specifically, it has been observed that activation of the clotting cascade occurs during instrumentation of the medullary canal in hip arthroplasty,[12] and one might logically expect a similar phenomenon with intramedullary instrumentation of the distal femur during knee replacement. Upon release of the tourniquet during total knee replacement, transesophageal echocardiography has demonstrated "noise" in the

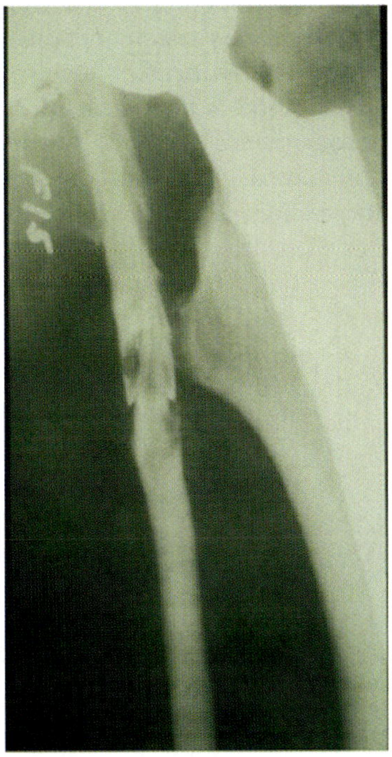

FIGURE 22-3. *Segmental femoral vein thrombosis in the region of the lesser trochanter seen on screening venography after total hip arthroplasty. The patient was asymptomatic and managed uneventfully with 12 weeks of low-intensity (INR 2.0) warfarin therapy.*

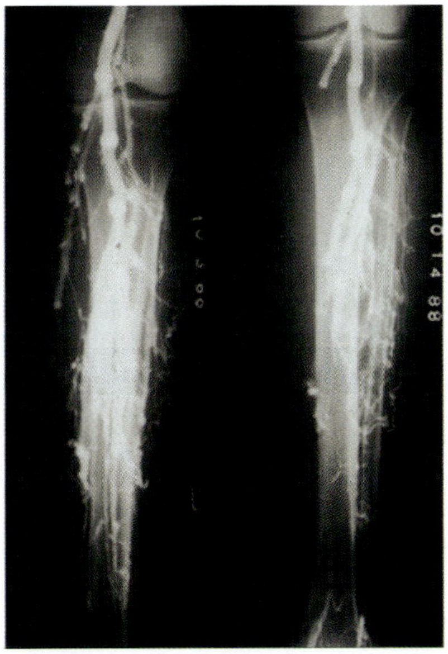

FIGURE 22-4. *Extensive deep calf vein thrombosis seen on screening venography in the nonoperative contralateral calf of an asymptomatic patient following elective total knee replacement.*

echo pattern from embolic material; marrow elements, fat, and thrombi have been recovered from aspirated femoral vein blood samples during the procedure (Fig. 22-5).[13] Most convincing of the ongoing intraoperative activation of the clotting cascade is the observation in one study that 70% of patients who ultimately developed deep vein thrombosis following total knee arthroplasty had positive contrast venography by 24 hours after operation.[14] The problem is compounded by stasis in the lower extremity caused by obstruction of femoral or popliteal venous outflow. Moreover, kinking of the femoral or popliteal veins can produce endothelial injury that provides a nidus for the formation and propagation of clots, particularly in an environment where stasis is substantial. Disturbance of the intramedullary canal with intravasation of marrow fat, resulting from both canal preparation and pressurization during stem cementation, is a potent stimulus of the clotting cascade.

A unique propensity for venous thromboembolic disease in the knee arthroplasty patient is the cumulative result. Specifically, the combined impact of greater efficacy of chemoprophylaxis in preventing thrombosis after hip replacement as compared with knee replacement along with the greater frequency of knee replacement procedures performed each year makes total knee arthroplasty responsible for a majority of the clinical venous thromboembolic events that the orthopaedic surgeon will see in practice.[15] This represents a notable change in the landscape of orthopaedic venous thromboembolism from four decades ago at the birth of hip arthroplasty.

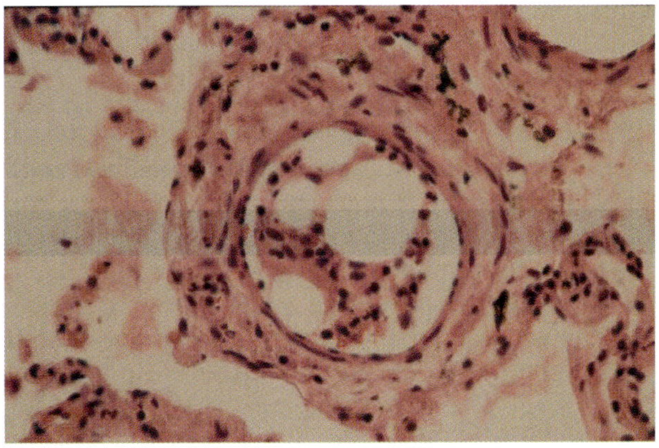

FIGURE 22-5. *Marrow fat and cellular elements embolic to the lung from peripheral blood after cementation of the intramedullary canal during total joint arthroplasty.*

EPIDEMIOLOGY AND CLINICAL CONTEXT

Likewise, the clinical management of arthroplasty patients has most certainly changed from the historical benchmark; some would contend that a concomitant reduction in the prevalence of venous thromboembolic disease has been the principal benefit of an expedited convalescence, improved anesthetic management with increasing use of regional techniques, multimodal pain control, and a dramatically shorter hospital stay.[7-9] Notwithstanding an apparent reduction in fatal thromboembolic disease coinciding with more widespread use of routine anticoagulant prophylaxis and faster rehabilitation, venous thromboembolism remains the most common reason for emergency readmission following total joint replacement.[8,9] Indeed, in one series of 1638 total joint arthroplasties managed with routine surveillance venography and warfarin treatment of all deep venous thromboses, the overall 6-month readmission rate was 1.3% (22/1638).[16,17] Of interest, readmission for symptomatic venous thromboembolic events after total hip arthroplasty (1.8%; 19/1079)[16] occurred more than three times as frequently as after total knee replacement (0.54%; 3/559; $p = .04$).[17] The overall 6-month mortality rate was 0.79% with two fatal pulmonary emboli (0.12%) accounting for 15% of deaths from all causes. More recent data from the Danish Knee Arthroplasty Registry, wherein 83% of 37,223 primary knee replacement patients received fractionated heparin or fondaparinux prophylaxis for a "short" perioperative period, demonstrate a 90-day readmission rate of 1.2% (441/37,223) at a median of 15 days following operation.[18] During this period, the rate of deep venous thrombosis was 0.9% compared with a rate of 0.3% for pulmonary embolism. All-cause mortality was 0.43% (161/37,223) with a presumed 90-day overall symptomatic venous thromboembolism rate of 1.6%.

Two caveats concerning differential clinical management of thromboembolic disease about the knee and hip deserve special mention at this time. With respect to bleeding complications related to anticoagulant prophylaxis, it should be noted that the skin envelope surrounding the knee is much less forgiving than that around the hip. Therefore, a wound hematoma is less well tolerated after knee replacement than following comparable surgery about the hip. It is also safe to say that calf thrombosis is generally a less feared complication than proximal deep venous thrombosis because of an implied lower risk of direct embolization. Nonetheless, in the postoperative patient, calf clots propagate to the thigh in 17% to 25% of cases and thereafter carry a substantial risk of embolization. Even though a large majority of thrombi after knee replacement are in the calf distal to the popliteal vein, compared with the more proximal clots historically seen after hip replacement, one should not be lulled into a state of nontreatment of distal thrombi in the postoperative setting. Specifically, there is a real risk of undertreating this condition if the literature from ambulatory medical patients, which is the basis for the well-intended advice of internal medicine colleagues, is referenced for guidance in clinical management.

Notwithstanding its clinical importance, the sociopolitical spotlight has sharpened its focus on venous thromboembolism in recent years. Under such scrutiny, the orthopaedic community has focused the emphasis of prophylaxis on prevention of clinical events, rather than a reduction in venographic disease, in an effort to balance the risks of bleeding with the positive benefits of anticoagulation. In the ensuing 25 years since the last National Institutes of Health (NIH) consensus conference on venous thromboembolic disease,[19] many new and more selective anticoagulant drugs have been introduced, but the evidence for prevention of fatal pulmonary embolism after total knee replacement has changed little. The Institute of Medicine has identified this issue as a priority for comparative effectiveness research and the Agency for Healthcare Research and Quality has an ongoing Evidence-Based Practice Center project in progress on the subject. The Joint Commission for Accreditation of Healthcare Organizations, the National Quality Forum, and the Centers for Medicare and Medicaid Services have joined forces to shepherd the establishment of "voluntary consensus standards" for venous thromboembolic disease prophylaxis and treatment. Moreover, it is likely that these consensus standards will serve as another benchmark for a federal "pay for performance" initiative. Hospital performance on these measures will become a matter of public record via the Health and Human Services website reporting. If the purpose of these standards is to raise awareness of hospital personnel to the risk of venous thromboembolism, certainly the orthopaedic community has long been preoccupied with the notion of venous thromboembolism risk and the possibility of fatal pulmonary embolism complicating total joint arthroplasty. Nevertheless, the Joint Commission and Surgical Care Improvement Project now mandate venous thromboembolism prophylaxis for hip and knee arthroplasty patients according to prevailing guidelines. The American College of Chest Physicians (ACCP) recommends prophylaxis based on the goal of reducing the frequency of deep vein thrombosis as a surrogate for fatal pulmonary embolism, with a relatively low concern for bleeding; they endorse use of fractionated heparins, full-intensity warfarin, and synthetic pentasaccharide as suitable chemoprophylaxis after total knee replacement for a duration of at least 10 days and consideration of 28 to 35 days (Fig. 22-6).[20] Moreover, the ACCP guidelines previously

ACCP GUIDELINES: 1992-2008 (8th Edition)

	Hip Replacement	Knee Replacement	Hip Fracture
Stockings	Against (1A)	Against (1A)	
Pneumatic Compression			
Aspirin	Against (1A)	Against (1A)	Against (1A)
LDUFH	Against (1A)	Against (1A)	yes, 1B
Warfarin	yes, 1A INR 2.5	yes, 1A INR 2.5	yes, 1B INR 2.5
LMWH	yes, 1A	yes, 1A	yes, 1B
Fondaparinux	yes, 1A	yes, 1A	yes, 1A

FIGURE 22-6. *ACCP guidelines for prophylaxis of orthopaedic venous thromboembolic disease after total hip and knee arthroplasty. Evidence database includes* ***only*** *level I randomized controlled studies with contrast venography as primary endpoint; recommended duration 10 to 35 days.*[20]

recommended against specific practices—namely, the use of aspirin as a prophylactic agent in any setting or the use of Doppler screening for deep vein thrombosis in asymptomatic patients at the time of hospital discharge. For the first time since their initial publication, the 2008 guidelines endorsed the solitary use of intermittent pneumatic compression devices in the acute perioperative setting if the bleeding risk is felt to be substantial, precluding the use of chemoprophylaxis agents.[20] The ACCP guidelines go on to suggest that chemoprophylaxis be instituted as soon as the elevated bleeding risk subsides; they do not endorse the solitary use of intermittent pneumatic compression devices as the sole and definitive means of thromboprophylaxis. Conversely, the American Academy of Orthopaedic Surgeons (AAOS) first promulgated guidelines in 2009 with the intent of reducing clinical pulmonary embolism[21] while maintaining vigilance to avoid bleeding that might result in wound hematoma, knee stiffness, wound breakdown, and secondary infection, all of which may require reoperation and ultimately removal of the joint prosthesis. The AAOS endorsed selective use of ACCP agents, as well as intermittent pneumatic compression devices, aspirin, or low-intensity warfarin (Fig. 22-7)[21]; the latter are associated with comparable rates of clinical pulmonary embolism and lesser rates of bleeding than some of the newer more potent agents. It is important that within the four quadrants of risk stratification implicit in the AAOS guidelines, it should be noted that an elevated risk of bleeding trumps an elevated risk of thrombosis. The recommended agents for patients with increased risk of both bleeding and thrombosis are identical as those for the group with an isolated increase in bleeding risk; both groups are suggested to receive either aspirin or warfarin, with the notable omission of the more potent contemporary anticoagulants because of their attendant bleeding risk. Randomized clinical trials have demonstrated a reduction in lower limb clots without similar reduction in fatal pulmonary embolism using these potent new agents. Yet, these trials have not been sufficiently powered to discern a difference in bleeding events and are conflicted by a bias related to industry funding.

VENOUS THROMBOEMBOLIC DISEASE
AAOS VTE Task Force – 2009

"Standard" Risk of VTE *"Standard" Risk of Bleed*	*Elevated Risk of VTE* *"Standard" Risk of Bleed*
Aspirin LMWH Fondaparinux Warfarin (INR 2.0)	(***NO Aspirin***) LMWH Fondaparinux Warfarin (INR 2.0)
"Standard" Risk of VTE *Elevated Risk of Bleed*	*Elevated Risk of VTE* *Elevated Risk of Bleed*
Aspirin Warfarin (INR 2.0) NONE	Aspirin Warfarin (INR 2.0) NONE

FIGURE 22-7. *Original AAOS guidelines for prophylaxis of pulmonary embolism after total hip and knee arthroplasty.*

Disagreement between prior guidelines had been highlighted by endorsement of aspirin by the AAOS for "standard risk" patients and specific "recommendation against" use of aspirin by the ACCP. This apparent schism was predicated upon the surgical community's concern over bleeding in the perioperative period coupled with observational data that suggested aspirin's efficacy in preventing clinical pulmonary embolism despite its failure to reduce radiographic thrombosis in venogram end point trials. Within the 6 months prior to the publication of this text, new guidelines appeared from both camps; the AAOS released a second edition in the Fall of 2011 and the ACCP released a belated 9th edition in early 2012. Interestingly, each organization has moved toward a middle ground; the AAOS stopped specifically *endorsing* aspirin, while the ACCP stopped specifically recommending *against* aspirin. Both sets of guidelines now provide a similar strength endorsement to *all* agents based on evidence with a clinical thromboembolic event end point, primarily pulmonary embolism, balanced by a new valuation by the ACCP of the patient's perceived importance of bleeding. The absence of a clear endorsement of a preferred chemoprophylaxis regimen by either set of guidelines, and specifically the acceptance of aspirin by both groups, calms the turbulent medicolegal environment surrounding pulmonary embolism after total joint replacement. This development of equipoise is a welcome reprieve for surgical practitioners. Nonetheless, in their generic recommendations, the new guidelines leave open for debate, and further focused study, the choice of a preferred prophylaxis strategy. Clearly, controversy persists and the ideal prophylaxis is yet to be determined. It must represent a balance between the risk of fatal pulmonary embolism and the morbidity of bleeding associated with anticoagulation.[22] Never before have medical and social forces been so focused on the issue of venous thromboembolism nor has it even been so critical for the orthopaedic practitioner to have an appreciation of what is and is not considered appropriate management, in the public's eye, of this often silent, but occasionally fatal, disease. *What is increasingly evident is that little short of an independently funded, large-scale, randomized clinical trial will end this debate with any degree of conviction and a sense of what is genuinely in the best interests of the patient.*

PROPHYLAXIS OF VENOUS THROMBOEMBOLISM

Regional Anesthesia

In several randomized clinical trials with total hip replacement, spinal or epidural anesthesia has consistently reduced venographic deep vein thrombosis by approximately 50% compared with general anesthesia. The data are slightly less compelling after total knee arthroplasty; extended epidural anesthesia has been shown to reduce proximal thrombosis rates by 50% and calf clots by 20%.[23] The mechanism of action is thought to be related to an augmentation of venous return as a result of venodilatation secondary to the sympathectomy effect of epidural anesthesia. There is no evidence for any influence of regional anesthesia on intraoperative thrombogenesis, but intimal stimulation of fibrinolysis may be enhanced by vasodilatation.[24] In general, regional anesthetic techniques are preferred for total knee replacement for many reasons, one of which is a clear beneficial effect on the reduction of deep vein thrombosis.

Notwithstanding these advantages of regional anesthesia, when combined with potent anticoagulants for thromboembolism prophylaxis following total knee arthroplasty, such as fractionated heparins, there have been reports of bleeding complications at the spinal puncture site. Accordingly, effective anticoagulation should not be present at the time of institution of neuraxial anesthesia and catheter removal should be performed with care in between dosing intervals of anticoagulants or with an international normalized ratio (INR) of less than 1.5 in the setting of warfarin use.[25]

Pneumatic Compression

Intermittent pneumatic compression devices, in the form of plantar foot pumps, calf sleeves, or sequential compression sleeves for the entire lower limb, have gained great popularity in the orthopaedic arena of venous thromboembolism prophylaxis on the basis of their lack of associated bleeding complications. The intent of these devices is to substitute for the normal physiologic muscle pump during ambulation and their mechanism of action is largely via enhancement of venous return from the capacitance vessels of the lower extremity, thereby mitigating the effects of stasis in Virchow's triad. As such, mechanical compression further augments the venous flow enhancement of regional anesthesia and some have suggested a synergistic effect with combined use of these two modalities. Moreover, there is a theoretical basis for mechanical stimulation of the fibrinolytic activity of the vessel intima, which may further potentiate the effects of pneumatic compression devices.[26-28]

Unlike after total hip arthroplasty, where pneumatic compression alone has been associated with a decrease in calf thrombi accompanied by a reciprocal increase in segmental proximal thrombi, intermittent pneumatic compression devices have been shown to reduce both proximal and distal thrombosis after total knee replacement. In one study in which all patients received regional anesthesia for total knee arthroplasty, the addition of plantar foot pumps to standard aspirin prophylaxis resulted in more than a 50% reduction in overall thrombi from 59% (49/83) to 27% (22/81; $p < .001$).[29] In this trial there were no proximal clots in any patient using pneumatic compression compared with 14% (12/83; $p < .0003$) proximal thrombosis in those receiving aspirin prophylaxis alone. Similarly, in a meta-analysis involving total knee replacement, Westrich and colleagues suggested that intermittent pneumatic compression and fractionated heparin were comparable in reducing deep venous thrombosis (17% and 29%, respectively) and significantly better than warfarin or aspirin.[30] However, in one total knee replacement trial comparing warfarin and pneumatic compression boots, the use of a general rather than a regional anesthetic was the strongest predictor of proximal thrombosis and had greater influence than either method of prophylaxis.[31] One might reasonably conclude that after total knee replacement the combination of mechanical compression and chemical anticoagulant appears to be superior to the isolated use of either method alone, but the optimal combination remains to be determined and the anesthetic technique plays an equally important role as does the method of prophylaxis.

Aspirin

In 1986 the NIH Consensus Conference concluded that aspirin "has not been shown to be beneficial"[19] with respect to venous thromboembolism prophylaxis after hip and knee arthroplasty. This statement, coupled with conventional wisdom among thrombosis experts that antiplatelet agents were ineffective on the venous side of the circulation, all but eliminated any enthusiasm for aspirin in orthopaedic thromboembolism prophylaxis. However, during the 1990s aspirin enjoyed renewed popularity among orthopaedic surgeons,[32,33] likely because of its greater safety profile compared with the increased bleeding observed with use of the fractionated heparins, which were introduced during the same decade. Indeed, one large meta-analysis compared all-cause mortality after total hip and knee replacement in patients who had been given low-molecular-weight heparin or another potent new anticoagulant (12,291 patients) compared with those who had received either warfarin (4370 patients) or multimodal thromboprophylaxis (7193 patients), which was defined as a combination of aspirin, pneumatic compression devices, and regional anesthesia.[34] Both the randomized trial and consecutive cohorts were included in the analysis as long as they provided 6-week or 3-month mortality rates. Eighteen publications were identified: 10 using low-molecular-weight heparin, ximelagatran, or fondaparinux (group A); 6 with a protocol utilizing regional anesthesia (epidural or spinal), with or without intraoperative heparin, pneumatic compression, and aspirin (group B); and 4 using warfarin (group C). There were 12,291, 7193, and 4370 patients included in these groups, respectively. The rate of clinical nonfatal pulmonary embolism (0.65% vs. 0.35%; $p = .008$) as well as all-cause mortality (0.47% vs. 0.19%; $p = .003$) was significantly higher with the newer anticoagulants than with multimodal aspirin prophylaxis. Rates for nonfatal pulmonary embolism and all-cause mortality were 0.5% and 0.41%, respectively, for the warfarin group. Indeed, in the absence of convincing data for preventing clinically meaningful pulmonary embolism, a steady 15% of orthopaedic surgeons continue to prefer aspirin for inpatient prophylaxis and more than one-third use aspirin for extended prophylaxis following hospital discharge.[35,36]

Nevertheless, observational data from three large single-center studies (two involving total knee arthroplasty) and a national joint replacement registry support the notion that aspirin may effectively prevent clinical pulmonary embolism (PE) after total knee replacement, especially when used in conjunction with regional anesthesia. In more than 3400 total knee replacements performed with extended (36 hours) regional anesthesia followed by 325 mg bid of aspirin for 6 weeks, fatal PE was observed in 0.1% of patients with an overall venous thromboembolism (VTE) readmission rate of 0.5%, half of which were for nonfatal pulmonary embolism.[37] It should be noted that 2% of patients in this study were classified as "high risk" and received warfarin VTE prophylaxis. A mixed hip and knee series from Ireland consisted of over 4200 consecutive primary arthroplasties (hip 2203; knee 2050) performed at a single center under spinal anesthesia with aspirin 150 mg given daily for 6 weeks; here again approximately 2% of patients were deemed to be at high risk and received warfarin or fractionated heparin prophylaxis.[38] The fatal PE rate in this aggregate group was 0.07% with an overall VTE-related readmission rate of 1.1%, which included 0.7% nonfatal PE. Most notable is an analysis of the 2009 National Joint Registry data from the United Kingdom, wherein 20% of surgeons were seen to utilize aspirin as their primary VTE prophylaxis after hip and knee replacement.[39] A matched cohort subanalysis compared 22,942 patients receiving aspirin with an identical number receiving fractionated heparin; there were no differences in 90-day outcomes for clinically evident pulmonary embolism (0.7%), deep vein thrombosis (0.95%), stroke or gastrointestinal bleed (0.75%), and reoperation (0.35%). However, fractionated heparin patients enjoyed a 25% risk reduction in all-cause mortality compared with those on aspirin (0.49% vs. 0.65%; RR 0.75; $p = .02$).

It is important to recognize that these data were not previously considered by the ACCP guideline committee because they are not from level I clinical studies. Moreover, a more generous reassessment of the Pulmonary Embolism Prevention Trial[33] by the ACCP resulted in an interpretation that allowed pooling of hip fracture and arthroplasty patients to arrive at an overall 43% reduction in clinical pulmonary embolism and a 29% reduction in symptomatic venous thrombosis. This was accompanied by prevention of 4 PE related deaths in 1000 patients. Accordingly, there is both evidence and momentum growing to justify a randomized clinical trial comparing aspirin, warfarin, and the newer agents in conjunction with regional anesthesia for venous thromboembolism prophylaxis after total joint arthroplasty.

Chemoprophylaxis

While symptomatic, and indeed fatal, pulmonary embolism was recognized early on as occurring far less commonly following total knee than after total hip arthroplasty. It is interesting to note that the residual venographic prevalence of deep venous thrombosis has been greater after total knee than after total hip arthroplasty. This observation is predicated on the fact that prevention of deep venous thrombosis after total knee replacement has been far more refractory to both traditional and contemporary pharmacologic prophylaxis. Over the past three decades the prevention of venous thromboembolic disease after total hip and knee arthroplasty has become the center of considerable discussion and debate in the orthopaedic community, as well as the focus of substantial drug development efforts in the pharmaceutical industry. Conventional warfarin prophylaxis following total hip replacement has resulted in venographically documented deep vein thrombosis in 9% to 26% of patients, with proximal thrombosis rates of approximately 2% to 5%.[8,9] Comparable figures after knee replacement with warfarin prophylaxis reveal a persistent overall prevalence of deep vein thrombosis of 35% to 55% with proximal thrombosis rates of 2% to 14%.[9] Nevertheless, extended low-intensity warfarin (INR 2.0) prophylaxis for 6 weeks after operation reduced 6-month VTE-related readmission rates to 0.6% (8/1321) following total knee replacement with 3 pulmonary emboli and 5 symptomatic proximal thromboses.[17] Moreover, 6 weeks of low-intensity warfarin eliminated readmission for pulmonary embolism in a combined series of 3293 total hip and knee arthroplasties. One intracranial bleed on warfarin was fatal in this series.[16,17]

The development of the low-molecular-weight or fractionated heparins, a family of compounds having greater specificity for binding with anti-thrombin III than conventional heparin, led to a much larger reduction in the venographic prevalence of thrombosis after total hip than after total knee arthroplasty.[40-42] With use of enoxaparin or dalteparin, overall residual clot rates after hip replacement fell to less than 10%, while venographic evidence of thrombosis remained identifiable in more than 30% of patients after total knee arthroplasty. Heparin-induced thrombocytopenia (HIT) is an uncommon but potentially devastating complication encountered with all naturally occurring heparins[43]; its incidence is estimated to be 2.6% in patients on conventional unfractionated heparin compared with 0.2% in patients on low-molecular-weight heparin prophylaxis.[44] ACCP recommends a baseline platelet count and repeat platelet count within 24 hours of starting prophylaxis.

Only after the subsequent introduction of fondaparinux, a synthetic pentasaccharide that binds specifically and only to the anti-thrombin III heparin site (and therefore has theoretically no risk of HIT), did residual venographic clot rates fall to 12.5% after total knee arthroplasty, representing an overall 63% relative risk reduction in venous thromboembolism.[45] By comparison, overall venous thromboembolism rates fell to 6% after total hip arthroplasty for a 28% relative risk reduction over North American enoxaparin prophylaxis.[46-48] Most recently, in July 2011, the Food and Drug Administration approved the use of rivaroxaban in the United States. This direct activated factor X inhibitor has achieved overall venous thromboembolism plus all-cause mortality rates under 7% in 3148 patients undergoing total knee arthroplasty in the RECORD4 trial, for a 31.4% relative risk reduction compared with the North American regimen of enoxaparin started postoperatively.[49] By way of comparison, rivaroxaban achieved overall venous thromboembolism plus all-cause mortality rates of 1.1% in 4541 patients undergoing total hip replacement compared to 3.7% with once daily enoxaparin prophylaxis administered for 35 days.[50,51] Rivaroxaban requires no monitoring, is administered orally and metabolized in the liver, and has been used at a fixed 10 mg once daily dosing in nearly 13,000 patients enrolled in the four RECORD total hip and knee replacement trials.[49-52] However, pooled analysis of the RECORD trials demonstrated a statistically greater risk of aggregated major and nonmajor clinically evident bleeding with rivaroxaban than with enoxaparin.

Careful study of the comparative efficacy of thromboprophylaxis after total hip and knee replacement over the past two decades illustrates the relatively recalcitrant nature of venous thromboembolism after total knee as compared with total hip replacement. Nevertheless, it is undeniable that the sequential development and use of newer highly selective antithrombotic agents has relentlessly and dramatically reduced the rates of residual venographic thrombosis after total knee replacement. The remaining task is to balance the relative reduction in clinically evident pulmonary embolism with the risk of bleeding that is attendant with use of any anticoagulant agent so that guidelines for chemotherapeutic regimens that optimize clinical and functional outcomes can be established. In view of the tenuous soft tissue envelope surrounding the knee and its intolerance of postoperative bleeding, finding the balance between efficacy and safety of thromboprophylaxis methods is arguably even more critical after total knee than it is after total hip replacement.

TREATMENT OF VENOUS THROMBOEMBOLISM

Therapeutic anticoagulation for documented venous thromboembolism remains the standard of care. While most frequently delegated to the medical service, the operating surgeon should be sufficiently knowledgeable to remain involved in the anticoagulation management of the postoperative patient so as to advocate for the mitigation of bleeding risk in this vulnerable population. Traditionally, perioperative calf vein thrombosis was managed with 6 weeks of warfarin, proximal deep vein thrombosis with 12 weeks of warfarin, and patients who suffered a pulmonary embolism received 3 to 6 months of therapeutic (INR 2.0–3.0) warfarin after initial anticoagulation with parenteral unfractionated heparin. Experience after total hip replacement has shown that bolus dosing of heparin to achieve rapid anticoagulation within the first week of operation is fraught with untoward bleeding complications in approximately one-third of patients. Accordingly, institution of heparin anticoagulation in the early perioperative period is more safely accomplished by starting a continuous drip without an accompanying bolus. More recently, in the era of fractionated heparins, immediate outpatient treatment of venous thromboembolism has become popular. However, in the postoperative patient with a substantial attendant risk of bleeding, initiation of anticoagulation as an inpatient followed by outpatient therapy after anticoagulant dosing and intensity have been stabilized is a more prudent approach.

REFERENCES

1. Johnson R, Carmichael JHE, Almond HGA, et al. Deep venous thrombosis following Charnley arthroplasty. *Clin Orthop Relat Res.* 1978;132:24-30.
2. Johnson R, Green JR, Charnley J. Pulmonary embolism and its prophylaxis following the Charnley total hip replacement. *Clin Orthop Relat Res.* 1977;127:123-132.
3. Charnley J. *Low Friction Arthroplasty of the Hip: Theory and Practice.* Berlin, Germany: Springer-Verlag; 1979.
4. Coventry MB, Beckenbaugh RD, Nolan DR, et al. 2,012 total hip arthroplasties. A study of postoperative course and early complications. *J Bone Joint Surg Am.* 1974;56:273-284.
5. Insall JN. *Surgery of the Knee.* New York: Churchill Livingstone; 1984:646-647.
6. Stulberg BN, Insall JN, Williams GW, et al. Deep-vein thrombosis following total knee replacement: an analysis of six hundred and thirty-eight arthroplasties. *J Bone Joint Surg Am.* 1984;66:194-201.
7. Pellegrini VD Jr, Clement D, Lush-Ehmann C, et al. The natural history of thromboembolic disease following hospital discharge after total hip arthroplasty. *Clin Orthop Relat Res.* 1996;333:27-40.
8. Salvati EA, Pellegrini VD Jr, Sharrock NE, et al. Recent advances in venous thromboembolic prophylaxis during and after total hip replacement. *J Bone Joint Surg Am.* 2000;82:252-270.
9. Sculco TP, Colwell CW, Pellegrini VD, et al. Prophylaxis against venous thromboembolic disease in patients having a total hip or knee arthroplasty. *J Bone Joint Surg Am.* 2002;84:466-477.
10. Binns M, Pho R. Femoral vein occlusion during hip arthroplasty. *Clin Orthop Relat Res.* 1990;255:168-172.
11. Aglietti P, Baldini A, Vena LM, et al. Effect of tourniquet use on activation of coagulation in total knee replacement. *Clin Orthop Relat Res.* 2000;371:169-177.
12. Sharrock NE, Go G, Harpel PC, et al. Thrombogenesis during total hip replacement. *Clin Orthop Relat Res.* 1995;319:16-27.
13. Berman AT, Parmet JL, Harding SP, et al. Emboli observed with use of transesophageal echocardiography immediately after tourniquet release during total knee arthroplasty with cement. *J Bone Joint Surg Am.* 1998;80:389-396.
14. Maynard MJ, Sculco TP, Ghelman B. Progression and regression of deep vein thrombosis after total knee arthroplasty. *Clin Orthop Relat Res.* 1991;273:125-130.
15. Kurtz S, Ong K, Lau E, et al. Projections of primary and revision hip and knee arthroplasty in the United States from 2005 to 2030. *J Bone Joint Surg Am.* 2007;89:780-785.
16. Pellegrini VD Jr, Donaldson CT, Farber DC, et al. The John Charnley Award. Prevention of readmission for venous thromboembolic disease after total hip arthroplasty. *Clin Orthop Rel Res.* 2005;441:56-62.
17. Pellegrini VD Jr, Donaldson CT, Farber DC, et al. The Mark Coventry Award. Prevention of readmission for venous thromboembolic disease after total knee arthroplasty. *Clin Orthop Rel Res.* 2006;452:21-27.
18. Pedersen AB, Mehnert F, Johnsen SP, et al. Venous thromboembolism in patients having knee replacement and receiving thromboprophylaxis: a Danish population-based follow-up study. *J Bone Joint Surg.* 2011;93:1281-1287.
19. NIH Consensus Development Conference Statement. *Prevention of Venous Thrombosis and Pulmonary Embolism.* Vol. 6, No. 2. Bethesda, MD: U.S. Department of Health and Human Services; March 24-26, 1986.
20. Geerts WH, Bergqvist D, Pineo GF, et al. Prevention of venous thromboembolism: American College of Chest Physicians evidence-based clinical practice guidelines (8th ed.). *Chest.* 2008;133(suppl 6):381S-453S.
21. Johanson NA, Lachiewicz PF, Lieberman JR, et al. Prevention of symptomatic pulmonary embolism in patients undergoing total hip or knee arthroplasty. AAOS Work Group. 2007. www.aaos.org/Research/guidelines/PE_guideline.pdf. *J Am Acad Orthop Surg.* 2009;17:183-196.
22. Eikelboom JW, Karthikeyan G, Fagel N, et al. American Association of Orthopaedic Surgeons and American College of Chest Physicians guidelines for venous thromboembolism prevention in hip and knee arthroplasty differ: what are the implications for clinicians and patients? *Chest.* 2009;135:513-520.
23. Sharrock NE, Haas SB, Hargett MJ, et al. Effects of epidural anesthesia on the incidence of deep-vein thrombosis after total knee arthroplasty. *J Bone Joint Surg Am.* 1991;73:502-506.
24. Sharrock NE, Go G, Williams-Russo P, et al. Comparison of extradural and general anaesthesia on the fibrinolytic response to total knee arthroplasty. *Br J Anaesth.* 1997;79:29-34.

25. Horlocker TT, Wedel DJ, Benzon H, et al. Regional anesthesia in the anticoagulated patient: defining the risks (the second ASRA Consensus Conference on Neuraxial Anesthesia and Anticoagulation). *Reg Anesth Pain Med.* 2003;28:172-197.
26. Knight MT, Dawson R. Effect of intermittent compression of the arms on deep venous thrombosis in the legs. *Lancet.* 1976;2:1265-1268.
27. Jacobs DG, Piotrowski JJ, Hoppensteadt DA, et al. Hemodynamic and fibrinolytic consequences of intermittent pneumatic compression: preliminary results. *J Trauma.* 1996;40:710-716.
28. Comerota AJ, Chouhan V, Harada RN, et al. The fibrinolytic effects of intermittent pneumatic compression: mechanism of enhanced fibrinolysis. *Ann Surg.* 1997;226:306-313.
29. Westrich GH, Sculco TP. Prophylaxis against deep venous thrombosis after total knee arthroplasty. Pneumatic plantar compression and aspirin compared with aspirin alone. *J Bone Joint Surg Am.* 1996;78:826-834.
30. Westrich GH, Haas SB, Mosca P, et al. Meta-analysis of thromboembolic prophylaxis after total knee arthroplasty. *J Bone Joint Surg Br.* 2000;82:795-800.
31. Pellegrini VD, Rubash HE, Parrish WM, et al. Plantar pneumatic compression versus warfarin for prevention of deep venous thrombosis after total knee arthroplasty. AAOS 68th Annual Meeting Proceedings, San Francisco, CA. February 28-March 2, 2001:556-557.
32. Antiplatelet Trialists' Collaboration. Collaborative overview of randomized trials of antiplatelet therapy. III. Reduction in venous thrombosis and pulmonary embolism by antiplatelet prophylaxis among surgical and medical patients. *BMJ.* 1994;308:235-246.
33. Pulmonary Embolism Prevention (PEP) Trial. Prevention of pulmonary embolism and deep venous thrombosis with low dose aspirin. *Lancet.* 2000;355: 1295-1302.
34. Sharrock NE, Della Valle AG, Go G, et al. Potent anticoagulants are associated with a higher all-cause mortality rate after hip and knee arthroplasty. *Clin Orthop Relat Res.* 2008;466:714-721.
35. Markel DC, York S, Liston MJ, et al, AAHKS Research Committee. Venous thromboembolism (VTE): management by American Association of Hip and Knee Surgeons. *J Arthroplasty.* 2010;25:3-9.
36. Anderson FA, Huang W, Friedman RJ, et al. Prevention of venous thromboembolism after hip or knee arthroplasty. Findings from a 2008 survey of US orthopaedic surgeons. *J Arthroplasty.* 2012;27 (5):659-666.
37. Lotke PA, Lonner JH. The benefit of aspirin chemoprophylaxis for thromboembolism after total knee arthroplasty. *Clin Orthop Relat Res.* 2006;452:175-180.
38. Cusick LA, Beverland DE. The incidence of fatal pulmonary embolism after primary hip and knee replacement in a consecutive series of 4253 patients. *J Bone Joint Surg Br.* 2009;91:645-648.
39. Jameson S, Gregg PJ, Charman S, et al. Thromboprophylaxis in primary hip arthroplasty: low molecular weight heparin versus aspirin. Presented at AAOS Annual Meeting, San Diego, CA. February 18, 2011.
40. Bergqvist D, Benoni G, Björgell O, et al. Low molecular weight heparin (enoxaparin) as prophylaxis against venous thromboembolism after total hip replacement. *N Engl J Med.* 1996;335:696-700.
41. Colwell CW Jr, Collis D, Paulson R, et al. Comparison of enoxaparin and warfarin for the prevention of venous thromboembolic disease after total hip arthroplasty: evaluation during hospitalization and three months after discharge. *J Bone Joint Surg Am.* 1999;81:932-940.
42. Francis CW, Pellegrini VD Jr, Totterman S, et al. Prevention of deep-vein thrombosis after total hip arthroplasty: comparison of warfarin and dalteparin. *J Bone Joint Surg Am.* 1997;79:1365-1372.
43. Warkentin TE, Greinacher A. Heparin-induced thrombocytopenia recognition, treatment, and prevention. *Chest.* 2004;126S:311-337.
44. Martel N, Lee J, Wells PS. Risk for heparin-induced thrombocytopenia with unfractionated and low molecular weight heparin thromboprophylaxis: a meta-analysis. *Blood.* 2005;106:2710-2715.
45. Bauer KA, Eriksson BI, Lassen MR, et al. Fondaparinux compared with enoxaparin for prevention of venous thromboembolism after elective major knee surgery. *N Engl J Med.* 2001;345:1305-1310.
46. Lassen MR, Bauer KA, Eriksson BI, et al. Postoperative fondaparinux versus preoperative enoxaparin for prevention of venous thromboembolism in elective hip replacement surgery: a randomized double blind trial. Lancet 2002;359:1715-1720.
47. Turpie AGG, Bauer KA, Eriksson BI, et al. Postoperative fondaparinux versus postoperative enoxaparin for prevention of venous thromboembolism in elective hip replacement surgery: a randomized double blind trial. *Lancet.* 2002;359:1721-1726.
48. Lassen MR, Bauer KA, Eriksson BI, et al. Postoperative fondaparinux versus preoperative enoxaparin for

prevention of venous thromboembolism in hip fracture surgery. *N Engl J Med.* 2001;345:1298-1304.

49. Turpie AG, Lassen MR, Davidson BL, et al. Rivaroxaban versus enoxaparin for thromboprophylaxis after total knee arthroplasty (RECORD4): a randomized trial. *Lancet.* 2009;373:1673-1680.
50. Eriksson BI, Borris LC, Friedman RJ, et al. Rivaroxaban versus enoxaparin for thromboprophylaxis after hip arthroplasty. *N Engl J Med.* 2008;358:2765-2775.
51. Kakkar AK, Brenner B, Dahl OE, et al. Extended duration rivaroxaban versus short term enoxaparin for the prevention of venous thromboembolism after total hip arthroplasty: a double-blind, randomized controlled trial. *Lancet.* 2008;372:31-39.
52. Lassen MR, Ageno W, Borris LC, et al. Rivaroxaban versus enoxaparin for thromboprophylaxis after total knee arthroplasty. *N Engl J Med.* 2008;358:2776-2786.

23 Perioperative Cardiovascular Management in Reconstructive Knee Surgery

Gregary D. Marhefka and Geno J. Merli

In the United States, patients with degenerative joint diseases, rheumatoid arthritis, or other rheumatic disorders frequently undergo total knee replacement surgery. In addition, better preventative health care and new innovations in medical management have increased the longevity of this population, which has resulted in joint replacement surgery well into the 70- to 90-year-old age range. It is important for orthopaedic surgeons and medical consultants to be familiar with the assessment and management of the patient with cardiovascular disease scheduled for total knee replacement surgery. Appropriate care of patients with cardiovascular disorders, which may include hypertension, coronary artery disease, atrial fibrillation, and heart failure, requires a systematic evaluation and management in the perioperative period. In this chapter the assessment and management in the perioperative period of the most common cardiovascular problems are reviewed.

EPIDEMIOLOGY

The 2009 American College of Cardiology (ACC) Foundation/American Heart Association (AHA) guidelines on perioperative cardiovascular care of noncardiac surgical patients classify orthopaedic surgery as intermediate risk, portending a 1% to 5% incidence of postoperative cardiovascular complications.[1] Myocardial infarction (MI) is by far the most concerning complication, followed by heart failure (HF) and arrhythmias.

The European Society of Cardiology (ESC), ACC, AHA, and the World Heart Federation (WHF) define MI as a rise and fall of troponin with at least one value above the 99th percentile of the upper reference limit (URL) plus at least one of the following: symptoms of ischemia, dynamic electrocardiographic (ECG) ST-T wave changes or new left bundle branch block, development of pathologic ECG Q waves, and imaging evidence of new loss of viable myocardium or a new segmental wall motion abnormality.[2] Typically postoperative MIs are non-ST elevation and are often not accompanied by angina.[3] In a 2004 prospective study from Brigham and Women's Hospital, Boston, Massachusetts, 4315 patients were followed after major noncardiac surgery (defined as procedures with an expected length of stay of 2 or more days). Ischemic postoperative ECG changes were associated with MI, pulmonary edema, cardiac arrest, ventricular fibrillation, and complete heart block in 6.7% versus 1.9% in patients without ECG changes.[4] This difference was maintained even when stratified by the established Revised Cardiac Risk Index described later in this chapter.[5] Thus, monitoring for intra- and postoperative ST segment changes is generally recommended in patients with known significant coronary artery disease (CAD) or multiple risk factors.[1] Recent data (Table 23-1) on the epidemiology of MIs following total joint arthroplasty suggest an incidence as low as 0.1% to 1%, with higher rates in patients who are older (particularly > 80 years of age) and undergo revision and bilateral procedures. MIs typically occur from 1 to 4 days postoperatively.[6-12] Preexisting anemia (hemoglobin <12 g/dL in females and <13 g/dL in males) does not appear to be a risk factor in a

Mayo Clinic retrospective cohort study that identified 391 patients with postoperative death or MI following total hip or knee arthroplasty from 1987 to 2006, though only 4% of the controls and 6% of the index cases had severe anemia defined as hemoglobin < 10 g/dL.[13]

The incidence of HF in noncardiac surgery has been reported to be from 1% to 6%,[14] though in reconstructive knee surgery the incidence has not been specifically defined. Postoperatively, HF may occur immediately due to a prolonged procedure, hypertension, myocardial ischemia, and/or rapid fluid shifts or in the days following surgery due to atrial fibrillation, renal failure, or third-spaced fluid reabsorption.[15]

Pre-existing CAD and HF are well known to be major risk factors for perioperative cardiovascular events, but pre-existing atrial fibrillation may also be an important risk factor. In a recent Canadian population-based cohort study conducted from 1999 to 2006 involving 38,047 patients undergoing noncardiac surgery (10% were orthopaedic surgery patients), the overall 30-day mortality was higher in the patients with a history of HF and atrial fibrillation than with CAD: 9.3% in nonischemic HF, 9.2% in ischemic HF, 2.9% in CAD, and 6.4% in atrial fibrillation (each versus CAD, p < .0001).[16] In looking specifically at the small number of patients who underwent elective orthopaedic surgery, the 30-day mortality was not trivial: 6.5% in nonischemic HF, 5.1% in ischemic HF, 1.4% in CAD, and 1.5% in atrial fibrillation.

TABLE 23-1. Death and Myocardial Infarction Rates in Joint Replacement Surgeries[6-12]

Author	Publication Year	Patients	Death	MI	Time to MI
Mantilla	2002	10,244 total joint arthroplasty (3601 unilateral TKA)	0.5%	0.4% (♀ age 60–69: 0.1%) (♂ age 60–69: 0.4%) (♀ age ≥ 80: 1.3%) (♂ age ≥ 80: 2.2%)	1d (83% <3d)
Bullock	2003	514 unilateral TKA 255 bilateral TKA		Unilateral 0.39% (age 80: 1.7%) Bilateral 2% (age 80: 11.5%)	
Mahomed	2005	124,986 primary TKA 11,726 revision TKA	Primary TKA: 0.7% Revision TKA: 1.1%	Primary TKA: 0.8% Revision TKA: 1%	
Gandhi	2006	3471 total joint arthroplasty (1992 TKA)		1.8%	3d
Parvizi	2007	1636 unilateral LE arthroplasty (670 TKA)	0.06%	0.37%	< 4d
Khatod	2008	15,943 primary TKA 1137 revision TKA	Primary TKA: 0.3% Revision TKA: 0.6%	Both: 0.1%	
Pulido	2008	15,383 total joint arthroplasty (7153 TKA)		0.2%	

MI, myocardial infarction; TKA, total knee arthroplasty; ♀, female; ♂, male.

PREOPERATIVE EVALUATION

Cardiovascular Status and Consultation

The major focus of preoperative evaluation of the orthopaedic patient is to determine the patient's current cardiovascular status. In the absence of a rare, orthopaedic surgical emergency, there are four active cardiac conditions that are surgical contraindications and mandate urgent consultative evaluation and treatment before proceeding.[1] The first condition is acute coronary syndrome, which includes unstable angina, non- ST elevation, and ST elevation MI. Acute MI is defined as occurring within the past 7 days and recent MI as having occurred after 7 days but within 30 days. Elective surgery should be done no sooner than 1 month after an MI in a stable, treated patient without any further active cardiac conditions. Unstable angina is new rest angina usually lasting >20 minutes within the past week or new onset angina or increasing angina that occurs with minimal activity within the past 2 months.[17] The second active condition is decompensated HF, a clinical syndrome characterized by acute onset of dyspnea, fatigue, edema, and rales.[18] The third condition involves unstable arrhythmias, such as symptomatic bradycardia, high-grade or third-degree heart block, newly recognized or symptomatic ventricular arrhythmias, and uncontrolled atrial arrhythmias such as rapid atrial fibrillation. The fourth condition is severe valvular disease, including symptomatic severe aortic or mitral stenosis.

Patients who should have elective consultation with a family medicine physician, internist, or cardiologist are those who already carry a diagnosis of stable CAD (including prior MI, coronary artery stents, or bypass surgery), HF, arrhythmias (including pacemakers and implantable cardioverter defibrillators), or valvular disease (including previous valve replacement).[1] Consultation is also suggested for those with suspected cardiovascular disease: previously unevaluated angina or anginal equivalents, dyspnea, presyncope or syncope, patients older than 50 with reduced exercise tolerance independent of the knee pathology, an uncharacterized murmur, or abnormal ECG. Following the 2009 ACC Foundation/AHA guidelines on perioperative cardiovascular care of noncardiac surgical patients, the consultant will first assess functional status (again independent of the knee pathology)[1] (Figure 23-1). If the patients are able to perform more than 4 metabolic equivalents of task (METs) of activity (such as climbing up a flight of stairs or walking up a hill) without limitation or symptoms, then typically they can proceed to surgery without further cardiovascular testing (Fig. 23-2). If they are unable to perform 4 METs, even if the knee is the limiting factor, then their Revised Cardiac Risk Index factors are identified: history of ischemic heart disease, compensated or prior HF, cerebrovascular disease, diabetes mellitus, and renal insufficiency[5] (Table 23-2). If there are no factors present, patients may generally proceed to surgery without further cardiovascular testing. If the patient has one or more risk factors, then the consultant may consider noninvasive stress testing if it will change management. Stress testing will assess the burden of ischemia and may lead to further evaluation with cardiac catheterization. Decisions about revascularization with coronary artery stenting or bypass surgery

1 MET ↓ 4 METs	Can you . . . Take care of yourself? Eat, dress, or use the toilet? Walk indoors around the house? Walk a block or 2 on level ground at 2 to 3 mph (3.2 to 4.8 kph)? Do light work around the house like dusting or washing dishes?	4 METs ↓	Can you . . . Climb a flight of stairs or walk up a hill? Walk on level ground at 4 mph (6.4 kph)? Run a short distance? Do heavy work around the house like scrubbing floors or lifting or moving heavy furniture? Participate in moderate recreational activities like golf, bowling, dancing, doubles tennis, or throwing a baseball or football?
		Greater than 10 METs	Can you . . . Participate in strenuous sports like swimming, singles tennis, football, basketball, or skiing?

FIGURE 23-1. *Metabolic equivalents of task (MET) of certain activities. (Reprinted with permission from Fleisher LA, Beckman JA, Brown KA, et al. Circulation 2009;120(21):e169-276.)*

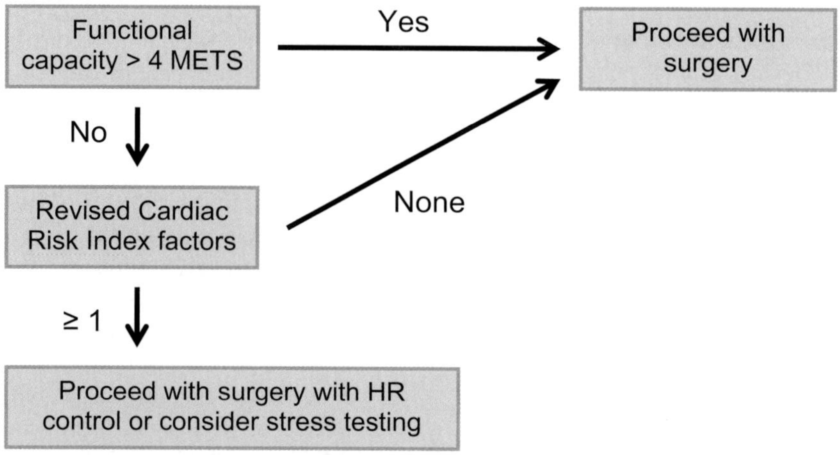

FIGURE 23-2. *Perioperative cardiac risk evaluation algorithm for intermediate-risk orthopaedic surgery, in the absence of need for rare emergent surgery or active cardiac conditions (acute coronary syndrome, decompensated heart failure, unstable arrhythmias, or severe valvular disease). HR, heart rate. See Figure 23-1 for metabolic equivalents of task (MET) definition. See Table 23-2 for revised cardiac risk index. (Reprinted with permission from Fleisher LA, Beckman JA, Brown KA, et al. Circulation 2009;120(21):e169-276.)*

TABLE 23-2. Revised Cardiac Risk Index Factors

Number of Factors	Major Cardiac Complication Rate
0	0.4%
1	0.9%
2	7%
≥3	11%

Revised cardiac risk index factors are history of (1) ischemic heart disease, (2) compensated or prior heart failure, (3) cerebrovascular disease, (4) diabetes mellitus, and (5) renal insufficiency (creatinine > 2 mg/dL). Major cardiac complications are myocardial infarction, pulmonary edema, ventricular fibrillation or primary cardiac arrest and complete heart block. (Reprinted with permission from Lee TH, Marcantonio ER, Mangione CM, et al. *Circulation* 1999;100(10):1043-1049.)

are then made depending on the history and coronary anatomy, independent of the planned noncardiac surgery. For example, findings of significant left main coronary artery disease (defined as a stenosis > 50%), even in the asymptomatic patient, would be an indication for coronary artery bypass surgery independent of the planned noncardiac surgery.[19] Furthermore, patients with stable angina and 3-vessel disease or 2-vessel disease that includes proximal left anterior descending artery disease [particularly with left ventricular dysfunction (ejection fraction < 50%)] may also benefit from revascularization with coronary artery bypass surgery or possibly coronary artery stenting, again independent of the planned noncardiac surgery.[19,20] However, newer data (unrelated to noncardiac surgery) suggest that even in the chronic stable angina patient with an ejection fraction of more than 30% (of which one-third had significant proximal left anterior descending artery disease), revascularization with coronary artery stenting did not reduce the risk of death, myocardial infarction, or other major cardiovascular events when added to optimal medical therapy.[21] In the absence of significant left main coronary artery disease, coronary artery revascularization to "get a stable cardiac patient through noncardiac surgery" has never been shown to be beneficial.

Hypertension

Uncontrolled hypertension is best managed preoperatively to avoid lability that often occurs during induction of anesthesia, which may lead to ischemia. According to the Seventh Report of the Joint National Committee on Prevention, Detection, Evaluation, and Treatment of High Blood Pressure,[22] deferring elective surgery for blood pressure > 180/110 mm Hg is recommended, though no data exist to suggest that control modifies perioperative risk. However, hypertension identified in the preoperative period can sometimes be the first indicator of this diagnosis for a patient, providing a unique opportunity to initiate general management of this cardiovascular risk factor.[1] Controlled hypertensive patients should be maintained on their outpatient regimen, including on the day of surgery, particularly if they are on a beta-blocker or clonidine to avoid withdrawal. Postoperative hypertension is common, secondary to pain, increased intravascular volume, sympathetic tone, and vascular resistance.[22] Resumption of outpatient medications as soon as possible postoperatively is essential.

Antiplatelet and Anticoagulation Management

As many patients undergoing reconstructive knee surgery have concomitant coronary artery disease, these patients are often prescribed aspirin. Though there are no data specifically addressing the bleeding risk of aspirin in reconstructive knee surgery, one trial in 1996 suggested an increased requirement for blood transfusions in total hip arthroplasty patients.[23] Cessation of aspirin in patients without a coronary artery stent or bypass surgery is individualized and at the discretion of the consultant and surgeon based on the risks of perioperative bleeding. Patients with coronary artery stents, however, need to be carefully assessed for the timing and type of stent placed (bare metal or drug eluting). Data show that about 5% of patients who have undergone coronary artery stenting will undergo elective noncardiac surgery within 1 year.[24]After coronary artery bypass surgery or coronary artery stenting, aspirin is recommended indefinitely. Following coronary artery bypass surgery, aspirin reduces the risk of saphenous vein graft closure. After coronary artery stenting, aspirin plus clopidogrel or prasugrel reduce the risk of acute stent thrombosis (a potentially life-threatening condition). In any revascularized patient, aspirin (at least 81 mg) should be continued if at all possible perioperatively, especially after a drug-eluting stent (due to delayed endothelialization, which can act as a trigger for acute stent thrombosis). In addition to aspirin, clopidogrel or prasugrel should be continued for a minimum of 1 month (but preferably for 1 year) following a bare metal stent, and for a minimum of 1 year (and possibly longer) after a drug-eluting stent.[25] If clopidogrel or prasugrel must be stopped, it is recommended that elective reconstructive knee surgery not be scheduled within 1 month of a bare metal stent or 1 year of a drug-eluting stent. To allow time for recovery of platelet activity, clopidogrel should be held 5 days before noncardiac surgery and prasugrel for 7 days, and both should be restarted as soon as it is deemed safe postoperatively.

Warfarin and dabigatran are prescribed for stroke prevention in high-risk atrial fibrillation and atrial flutter patients (dabigatran for nonvalvular atrial fibrillation only). Interruption of anticoagulation for nonvalvular atrial fibrillation for a period of up to 1 week for procedures is acceptable. However, in high-risk patients (prior stroke, transient ischemic attack, systemic embolization, or mechanical valves), therapeutic intravenous unfractionated heparin or subcutaneous low-molecular-weight heparin should be administered in the perioperative period when the international normalized ratio (INR) is subtherapeutic.[26] Dabigatran is a new direct thrombin inhibitor approved by the Food and Drug Administration in 2010, which was found to be superior to warfarin in nonvalvular atrial fibrillation stroke reduction with the advantage of not requiring dose changes based on blood draws and less drug–drug interactions.[27] Perioperative management of dabigatran depends on the patient's creatinine clearance and the risk of perioperative bleeding and is best guided by the consultant.[28] For patients with normal renal function, it is typically held for 2 days when no or minimal anticoagulant effect is desired at the time of the procedure and restarted 48 to 72 hours post-procedure (with prophylactic heparin or low-molecular-weight heparin in between).

Warfarin is also indicated long term for mechanical valves and in the 3 months following bioprosthetic valves. In patients with a bileaflet mechanical aortic valve replacement without atrial fibrillation, previous thromboembolism, left ventricular dysfunction, hypercoagulable condition, older generation thrombogenic valve, or more than one mechanical valve, therapeutic intravenous unfractionated heparin is usually not necessary and warfarin may be interrupted for 48 to 72 hours before, and preferably restarted within 24 hours of the surgery.[29] Mechanical valve thrombosis can be catastrophic, so for all other higher risk patients with a mechanical valve, warfarin is discontinued 5 days before surgery and subcutaneous therapeutic dose low-molecular-weight heparin is started 4 days before surgery. A prophylactic dose of low-molecular-weight heparin is started 12 to 24 hours postoperatively with the reintroduction of warfarin at 5 mg on the evening of surgery.[29, 30] High-dose vitamin K is not recommended to reverse anticoagulation because this may create a hypercoagulable state.[29]

Beta-Blockers

In the 1996 landmark randomized, double-blind, placebo-controlled trial by Mangano et al, atenolol administered intravenously preoperatively (12% to 15% were orthopaedic surgery patients) and orally up to 1 week post-operatively reduced major adverse cardiovascular events. Interestingly, however, the mortality benefit was not in the immediate perioperative period [only significantly reduced ischemia by Holter monitoring was observed (24% versus 39%; $p = .03$)] but was evident at 6 months (mortality 1% versus 10%; $p < .001$) out to 2 years.[31] After many trials since, the large, randomized, placebo-controlled POISE trial (21% were orthopaedic surgery patients) tempered the enthusiasm for initiation of perioperative beta-blockade with extended-release metoprolol started 2 to 4 hours before surgery and for 30 days afterwards. Though the risk of MI, cardiac revascularization, and atrial fibrillation was reduced, there was an increase in death, stroke, and clinically significant hypotension and bradycardia.[32] Criticisms of this trial included the high dose of extended-release metoprolol given and the absence of dose titration in these beta-blocker-naïve patients. In the subsequent DECREASE IV trial, bisoprolol that was initiated and titrated a median of 34 days before the procedure (16% were orthopaedic surgery patients) and continued for 30 days afterwards was associated with a lower incidence of cardiac death and nonfatal MI (2% versus 6%; $p = .002$).[33] Stroke risk was the same, occurring in four patients randomized to bisoprolol and in three patients to placebo. In a retrospective review of 5158 patients undergoing hip and knee arthroplasty from 2002 to 2006 in Canada, 18% were treated with beta-blockers on the day of surgery, and in 25% of these, it was discontinued. Discontinuation of beta-blockers within the week after surgery was significantly associated with MI and death.[34] Limitations of this study were not knowing whether a patient was on a beta-blocker chronically and not knowing the reason for discontinuation of the beta-blocker. In an observational cohort study of 267 consecutive total knee arthroplasties in patients who followed a perioperative beta-blocker prophylaxis institutional protocol, there were no deaths within 90 days and two nonfatal MIs (0.7%).[35] A total of 203 (76%) patients received beta-blocker prophylaxis, of whom 110 (54%) were already taking a beta-blocker and 93 (46%) were started on a beta-blocker.

According to the 2009 ACC Foundation/AHA guidelines on perioperative cardiovascular care of noncardiac surgical patients, beta-blockers should be continued perioperatively in patients already taking them.[1] Beta-blocker initiation and titration is reasonable in patients identified to have CAD or more than one Revised Cardiac Risk Index factor (Table 23-2). In the absence of CAD, the usefulness of beta-blocker initiation in patients with only one Revised Cardiac Risk Index factor is uncertain.

Statins

Postoperative cases of rhabdomyolysis have been reported with statins after noncardiac surgery.[36] However, in a prospective, case-controlled observational study of patients undergoing elective arthroplasty, there was no increase in the risk of muscular adverse effects.[37] There are data to suggest that statins with their pleotrophic and anti-inflammatory properties reduce the risk of perioperative cardiac events in high-risk surgery.[1] In addition, statin withdrawal has been associated with worse outcomes when stopped in high-risk vascular surgery.[38] Preoperative initiation of fluvastatin in intermediate-risk surgery patients (16% orthopaedic), however, showed a trend toward reduced 30-day cardiac death and MI that did not reach statistical significance in the large prospective, randomized DECREASE IV trial.[33] In patients already prescribed statins, it is reasonable to make every attempt to continue this therapy perioperatively.[1,39]

POSTOPERATIVE MANAGEMENT

Acute Myocardial Infarction

Patients with postoperative MI can be divided into those with ST segment elevation and those with non-ST segment elevation, the latter being the more common type.[3] Urgent consultation with cardiology is essential. Patients should generally be treated similarly to patients who are not postoperative, with the exception of thrombolytics, which are contraindicated in ST segment elevation MI immediately in the postoperative period.[40] Patients with the less common acute ST segment elevation MI should ideally be treated with immediate coronary artery angioplasty and possibly stenting. Medications that are required for angioplasty without stenting are aspirin (at least 162 mg) and therapeutic intravenous unfractionated heparin. Coronary artery stenting is preferred over angioplasty alone and would require additional intravenous glycoprotein IIb IIIa inhibition (eg, eptifibitide) or bivalirudin in place of heparin and a glycoprotein IIb IIIa inhibitor plus clopidogel 300 to 600 mg followed by 75 mg daily or prasugrel 60 mg followed by 10 mg daily. Although patients often do not have symptoms of non-ST segment elevation MI in the postoperative period, a troponin elevation combined with dynamic ECG changes consistent with ischemia should prompt urgent treatment including aspirin, at least 162 mg orally or 300 mg rectally, therapeutic intravenous unfractionated heparin if not contraindicated, and beta-blockade (oral preferred to intravenous). The benefit and risk of these medications in the postoperative period must be individualized. Intravenous nitroglycerin can ameliorate ischemic as well as HF symptoms that may ensue. ACE inhibitors given early after MI, particularly in patients with left ventricular dysfunction (ejection fraction

< 40%), are also recommended.[17,40] Patients who do not undergo coronary angiography should eventually have noninvasive stress testing to assess the degree of myocardium at risk. In addition, statin therapy should be initiated, with smoking cessation counseling and consideration for cardiac rehabilitation.

Arrhythmias

Perioperative atrial and ventricular tachyarrhythmias are common and can usually be controlled.[31] Sinus tachycardia is frequent and mandates consideration of an underlying cause, such as pain, hypovolemia, medication or substance withdrawal, anemia, hypoxia, fever, myocardial ischemia, or pulmonary embolus. Premature atrial complexes are ordinarily benign, but, if frequent, they may be a precursor to atrial fibrillation or other forms of supraventricular tachycardia (SVT). Treatment of an acute onset, narrow complex, regular SVT consists of vagal maneuvers (such as Valsalva or careful consideration carotid artery massage), which if unsuccessful may be followed by adenosine 6 mg intravenous rapid push, followed by 20 cc rapid flush, which will often break an AV nodal re-entrant or atrioventricular re-entrant tachycardia, or at the very least reveal the underlying atrial activity allowing further directed treatment. Treatment of SVTs, including rapid atrial fibrillation and atrial flutter, includes intravenous beta-blockade (eg, metoprolol or esmolol) or non-dihydropyridine calcium channel blockade (eg, diltiazem or verapamil) followed by oral administration. Digitalis is often least effective in the postoperative state where sympathetic tone is high, but may be considered if blood pressure is borderline. Cardioversion is not recommended unless there is urgent hemodynamic instability, because the underlying trigger is often persistent. Elective cardioversion should not be undertaken for stable atrial fibrillation or flutter in the absence of anticoagulation after 48 hours because of the risk of acute thromboembolism. Cardiology consultation with consideration of intravenous amiodarone for a brief period (days) is reasonable if the atrial arrhythmia is particularly recurrent and very symptomatic with borderline hemodynamic instability. Ideally amiodarone should not be used after 48 hours for atrial fibrillation or flutter in the absence of anticoagulation because of potential cardioversion and associated acute thromboembolic risk. Ultimately, control and treatment of the underlying cause (eg, pain, hypoxia) will often improve the tachyarrhythmias. Attention should also be placed on maintaining normal electrolytes, especially potassium and magnesium. The same goes for premature ventricular complexes that become frequent or symptomatic and/or develop into long runs of nonsustained ventricular tachycardia. Persistent ventricular tachyarrythmias necessitate cardiology consultation and an evaluation for ischemia or HF and may be treated carefully with beta-blockers, amiodarone, lidocaine, or procainamide. Cardioversion is recommended for sustained or hemodynamically compromising ventricular tachyarrhythmias. Care should also be taken when administering medications such as certain antiemetics, antipsychotics, and/or antibiotics that may prolong the QT interval, leading to iatrogenic ventricular tachyarrhythmias such as polymorphic ventricular tachycardia (torsades de pointes). Last, bradyarrhythmias may also be iatrogenically induced (eg, medications) or due to electrolyte disturbances, ischemia, or less commonly sinus node dysfunction or heart block, which should mandate an urgent cardiology consult.

Heart Failure

A history of HF is particularly common in the elderly population who often undergo reconstructive knee surgery. It is present in 2% to 3% of patients aged 65, and in more than 80% in patients over 80. HF is equally divided into systolic (reduced ejection fraction) and diastolic dysfunction (preserved ejection fraction), both of which can lead to significant morbidity.[18] Development of postoperative HF is multifactorial, resulting from hypertension, myocardial ischemia, perioperative intravenous fluids and interstitial fluid shifts, new onset atrial fibrillation, renal failure, and anemia. If acute volume overload is present with an S3 and/or S4 and pulmonary edema, intravenous diuretic therapy is initiated. If there is clinical evidence of poor perfusion, inotropic therapy may be required (be careful with dobutamine if myocardial ischemia is thought to be the instigator because this agent increases myocardial oxygen demand). Sometimes guidance by a pulmonary artery catheter in the intensive care unit setting is utilized under the guidance of a consulting cardiologist or intensivist. If acute hypertension is thought to be contributing to acute HF, then oral (ACE inhibitors, hydralazine, nitrates) or intravenous (nitroprusside, nitroglycerin, and preferably not hydralazine because of its risk for hypotension) afterload reduction is useful. Beta-blockers and non-dihydropyridine calcium channel blockers should not be given in acute HF because these may exacerbate the condition.

SUMMARY

Because of the innovations in treating cardiovascular disorders, the population over the age of 65 will continue to increase in this country. The frequency of knee replacement surgery as well as other joint arthroplasty procedures will increase. The appropriate preoperative cardiovascular risk assessment along with the perioperative management of cardiac-related medications will reduce the risk of postoperative cardiovascular complications. Orthopaedic surgeons should identify patients requiring more focused cardiovascular care and refer appropriately for specialty management.

REFERENCES

1. Fleisher LA, Beckman JA, Brown KA, et al. 2009 ACCF/AHA focused update on perioperative beta blockade incorporated into the ACC/AHA 2007 guidelines on perioperative cardiovascular evaluation and care for noncardiac surgery: a report of the American College of Cardiology Foundation/American Heart Association task force on practice guidelines. *Circulation*. 2009;120(21):e169-e276.
2. Thygesen K, Alpert JS, White HD, et al. Universal definition of myocardial infarction. *Circulation*. 2007;116(22):2634-2653.
3. Weitz HH. Noncardiac surgery in the patient with cardiovascular disease: preoperative evaluation and perioperative care. In: Merli GJ, Wietz HH, eds. *Medical Management of the Surgical Patient,* 3rd ed. Philadelphia, PA: Saunders Elsevier; 2008.
4. Rinfret S, Goldman L, Polanczyk CA, et al. Value of immediate postoperative electrocardiogram to update risk stratification after major noncardiac surgery. *Am J Cardiol*. 2004;94(8):1017-1022.
5. Lee TH, Marcantonio ER, Mangione CM, et al. Derivation and prospective validation of a simple index for prediction of cardiac risk of major noncardiac surgery. *Circulation*. 1999;100(10):1043-1049.
6. Mantilla CB, Horlocker TT, Schroeder DR, et al. Frequency of myocardial infarction, pulmonary embolism, deep venous thrombosis, and death following primary hip or knee arthroplasty. *Anesthesiology*. 2002;96(5):1140-1146.
7. Bullock DP, Sporer SM, Shirreffs TG Jr. Comparison of simultaneous bilateral with unilateral total knee arthroplasty in terms of perioperative complications. *J Bone Joint Surg Am*. 2003;85(10):1981-1986.
8. Mahomed NN, Barrett J, Katz JN, Baron JA, et al. Epidemiology of total knee replacement in the United States Medicare population. *J Bone Joint Surg Am*. 2005;87(6):1222-1228.
9. Gandhi R, Petruccelli D, Devereaux PJ, et al. Incidence and timing of myocardial infarction after total joint arthroplasty. *J Arthroplasty*. 2006;21(6):874-877.
10. Parvizi J, Mui A, Purtill JJ, et al. Total joint arthroplasty: when do fatal or near-fatal complications occur? *J Bone Joint Surg Am*. 2007;89(1):27-32.
11. Khatod M, Inacio M, Paxton EW, et al. Knee replacement: epidemiology, outcomes, and trends in southern California: 17,080 replacements from 1995 through 2004. *Acta Orthop*. 2008;79(6):812-819.
12. Pulido L, Parvizi J, Macgibeny M, et al. In-hospital complications after total joint arthroplasty. *J Arthroplasty*. 2008;23(6 suppl 1):139-145.
13. Mantilla CB, Wass CT, Goodrich KA, et al. Risk for perioperative myocardial infarction and mortality in patients undergoing hip or knee arthroplasty: the role of anemia. *Transfusion*. 2011;51(1):82-91.
14. Watson TA, Fleisher LA. Acute heart failure in the postoperative period. In: Mebazaa A, Gheorghiade M, Zannad FM, Parrillo JE, eds. *Acute Heart Failure,* 1st ed. London: Springer; 2008.
15. Poldermans D, Bax JJ, Boersma E, et al. Guidelines for pre-operative cardiac risk assessment and perioperative cardiac management in non-cardiac surgery. *Eur Heart J*. 2009;30(22):2769-2812.
16. van Diepen S, Bakal JA, McAlister FA, et al. Mortality and readmission of patients with heart failure, atrial fibrillation, or coronary artery disease undergoing noncardiac surgery: an analysis of 38,047 patients. *Circulation*. 2011;124(3):289-296.
17. Wright RS, Anderson JL, Adams CD, et al. 2011 ACCF/AHA focused update incorporated into the ACC/AHA 2007 guidelines for the management of patients with unstable angina/non-ST-elevation myocardial infarction: a report of the American College of Cardiology Foundation/American Heart Association task force on practice guidelines developed in collaboration with the American Academy of Family Physicians, Society for Cardiovascular Angiography and Interventions, and the Society of Thoracic Surgeons. *J Am Coll Cardiol*. 2011;57(19):e215-e367.
18. Hunt SA, Abraham WT, Chin MH, et al. 2009 focused update incorporated into the ACC/AHA 2005 guidelines for the diagnosis and management of heart failure in adults: a report of the American College of Cardiology Foundation/American Heart Association task force on practice guidelines developed in collaboration with the International Society for Heart and Lung Transplantation. *J Am Coll Cardiol*. 2009;53(15):e1-e90.
19. Eagle KA, Guyton RA, Davidoff R, et al. ACC/AHA 2004 guideline update for coronary artery bypass graft surgery: a report of the American College of Cardiology/American Heart Association task force on

practice guidelines (committee to update the 1999 guidelines for coronary artery bypass graft surgery). *Circulation*. 2004;110(14):e340-e437.

20. Smith SC Jr, Feldman TE, Hirshfeld JW Jr, et al. ACC/AHA/SCAI 2005 guideline update for percutaneous coronary intervention—summary article: a report of the American College of Cardiology/American Heart Association task force on practice guidelines (ACC/AHA/SCAI writing committee to update the 2001 guidelines for percutaneous coronary intervention). *J Am Coll Cardiol*. 2006;47(1):216-235.
21. Boden WE, O'Rourke RA, Teo KK, et al. Optimal medical therapy with or without PCI for stable coronary disease. *N Engl J Med*. 20072;356(15):1503-1516.
22. Chobanian AV, Bakris GL, Black HR, et al. The seventh report of the joint national committee on prevention, detection, evaluation, and treatment of high blood pressure: the JNC 7 report. *JAMA*. 2003;289 (19):2560-2572.
23. Nuttall GA, Santrach PJ, Oliver WC Jr, et al. The predictors of red cell transfusions in total hip arthroplasties. *Transfusion*. 1996;36(2):144-149.
24. Vicenzi MN, Meislitzer T, Heitzinger B, et al. Coronary artery stenting and non-cardiac surgery—a prospective outcome study. *Br J Anaesth*. 2006;96(6): 686-693.
25. Grines CL, Bonow RO, Casey DE Jr, et al. Prevention of premature discontinuation of dual antiplatelet therapy in patients with coronary artery stents: a science advisory from the American Heart Association, American College of Cardiology, Society for Cardiovascular Angiography and Interventions, American College of Surgeons, and American Dental Association, with representation from the American College of Physicians. *Circulation*. 2007;115(6):813-818.
26. Fuster V, Ryden LE, Cannom DS, et al. 2011 ACCF/AHA/HRS focused updates incorporated into the ACC/AHA/ESC 2006 guidelines for the management of patients with atrial fibrillation: a report of the American College of Cardiology Foundation/American Heart Association task force on practice guidelines developed in partnership with the European Society of Cardiology and in collaboration with the European Heart Rhythm Association and the Heart Rhythm Society. *J Am Coll Cardiol*. 2011;57(11):e101-e198.
27. Connolly SJ, Ezekowitz MD, Yusuf S, et al. Dabigatran versus warfarin in patients with atrial fibrillation. *N Engl J Med*. 2009;361(12):1139-1151.
28. Douketis JD. Pharmacologic properties of the new oral anticoagulants: a clinician-oriented review with a focus on perioperative management. *Curr Pharm Des*. 2010;16(31):3436-3441.
29. Bonow RO, Carabello BA, Chatterjee K, et al. 2008 focused update incorporated into the ACC/AHA 2006 guidelines for the management of patients with valvular heart disease: a report of the American College of Cardiology/American Heart Association task force on practice guidelines (writing committee to revise the 1998 guidelines for the management of patients with valvular heart disease). *J Am Coll Cardiol*. 2008;52(13):e1-e142.
30. Douketis JD, Berger PB, Dunn AS, et al. The perioperative management of antithrombotic therapy: American College of Chest Physicians evidence-based clinical practice guidelines (8th edition). *Chest*. 2008;133(6 suppl):299S-339S.
31. Mangano DT, Layug EL, Wallace A, et al. Effect of atenolol on mortality and cardiovascular morbidity after noncardiac surgery: multicenter study of perioperative ischemia research group. *N Engl J Med*. 1996; 335(23):1713-1720.
32. Devereaux PJ, Yang H, Yusuf S, et al. Effects of extended-release metoprolol succinate in patients undergoing non-cardiac surgery (POISE trial): a randomised controlled trial. *Lancet*. 2008;371(9627): 1839-1847.
33. Dunkelgrun M, Boersma E, Schouten O, et al. Bisoprolol and fluvastatin for the reduction of perioperative cardiac mortality and myocardial infarction in intermediate-risk patients undergoing noncardiovascular surgery: a randomized controlled trial (DECREASE-IV). *Ann Surg*. 2009;249(6):921-926.
34. van Klei WA, Bryson GL, Yang H, et al. Effect of beta-blocker prescription on the incidence of postoperative myocardial infarction after hip and knee arthroplasty. *Anesth*. 2009;111(4):717-724.
35. Heim KA, Lachiewicz MP, Soileau ES, et al. Beta-blocker prophylaxis for total knee arthroplasty patients: a case series. *J Surg Orthop Adv*. 2010;19 (3):162-165.
36. Forestier F, Breton Y, Bonnet E, et al. Severe rhabdomyolysis after laparoscopic surgery for adenocarcinoma of the rectum in two patients treated with statins. *Anesthesiology*. 2002;97(4):1019-1021.
37. Laisalmi-Kokki M, Tolonen K, Miettinen H, et al. Perioperative chronic use of statins and the risk of muscle complaints in patients undergoing knee and hip endoprosthesis surgery. *J Clin Anesth*. 2010;22 (2):81-87.
38. Skrlin S, Hou V. A review of perioperative statin therapy for noncardiac surgery. *Semin Cardiothorac Vasc Anesth*. 2010;14(4):283-290.

39. Chassot PG, Delabays A, Spahn DR. Perioperative antiplatelet therapy: the case for continuing therapy in patients at risk of myocardial infarction. *Br J Anaesth.* 2007;99(3):316-328.

40. Antman EM, Anbe DT, Armstrong PW, et al. ACC/AHA guidelines for the management of patients with ST-elevation myocardial infarction: a report of the American College of Cardiology/American Heart Association task force on practice guidelines (committee to revise the 1999 guidelines for the management of patients with acute myocardial infarction). *J Am Coll Cardiol.* 2004;44(3):E1-E211.

24 Perioperative Considerations for Total Knee Arthroplasty

Matthew C. Morrey

Total knee arthroplasty is commonly performed in a patient population that inherently carries significant medical comorbidities that can adversely affect the outcome. With a myriad of medical conditions requiring consideration, including cardiac disease, renal function, diabetes, obesity, and pulmonary status, among others, it is imperative that treating surgeons not only be familiar with such conditions, but also have an awareness of how these may affect their patients during the preoperative, intraoperative, and postoperative periods. While some of these conditions may be managed by the treating surgeon, others may warrant thorough evaluation by appropriate specialists in an effort to optimize these patients before their surgical procedure.

Although there are many medical comorbidities that affect outcomes following joint replacement arthroplasty, this chapter focuses on those that are most commonly encountered and evaluated before total knee arthroplasty. It specifically covers those that can be safely managed by the treating surgeon and those that often require subspecialty consultations (Table 24-1).

TABLE 24-1. Common Perioperative Comorbidities Associated with Total Joint Arthroplasty

Obesity
Anemia
Disease-modifying antirheumatic drugs Glucocorticosteroids
Diabetes
Renal disease
Pulmonary disease
Cardiac disease

OBESITY

The continued increase in the rate of obesity in the United States (body mass index, BMI, > 30) is an alarming trend which has worsened over the past decade. One recent study cited obesity rates in the United States as high as 32.2% among adult women and 35.5% among adult men.[1] Often, these patients present to the orthopaedic surgeon with legitimate knee pathology, many of whom would benefit from total knee arthroplasty. The relationship between obesity and total joint arthroplasty has been examined and debated, and while there is no definitive answer as to when to surgically intervene or not based on one's BMI, there is enough in the literature to arrive at some discrete conclusions that may guide the orthopaedic surgeon when caring for these patients.

While the definition of obesity is still open to some interpretation, the most commonly used criteria is that of the BMI, which is derived from an individual's body weight divided by the square of his or her height (Fig. 24-1). While this metric has been widely adopted in the medical literature, it does not differentiate between age, percentage of body fat, or distribution of muscle mass. Nonetheless, BMI has been widely utilized in the orthopaedic literature when discussing the obese patient and the implications this has on joint replacement arthroplasty.

There has been much in the literature regarding total joint arthroplasty and obesity that reflects the growing trend toward obesity in the United States. Because of the perioperative implications, associated outcomes, and complications, the specifics of total knee arthroplasty in the obese are covered fully in a later chapter. The purpose for mentioning it in the context of this chapter is that, as the treating surgeon, one must be cognizant of the issues surrounding obesity and total joint arthroplasty, because this will certainly affect operative decision making as well as one's ability to adequately counsel their patients preoperatively. As such, there are multiple specific questions that are of importance to the orthopaedic surgeon as they pertain to the obese patient (Table 24-2).

Recent literature has answered these questions and shown that total joint arthroplasty in the obese patient can be a successful procedure. Many of these patients have good satisfaction scores and improved function. It is important to note, however, that they are at risk for increased wound infection, increased likelihood of blood clot formation, and increased risk of perioperative cardiopulmonary complications, as well as other complications.[2-6] As previously mentioned, many of these specific issues are formally addressed in later chapters.

PREOPERATIVE ANEMIA

Pre- and postoperative anemia is common in patients receiving total joint arthroplasty and it has been demonstrated that anemic patients are more likely to require allogeneic blood transfusion (ABT) when compared to nonanemic patients.[7] The importance of this relationship is demonstrated by the fact that increased numbers of ABTs

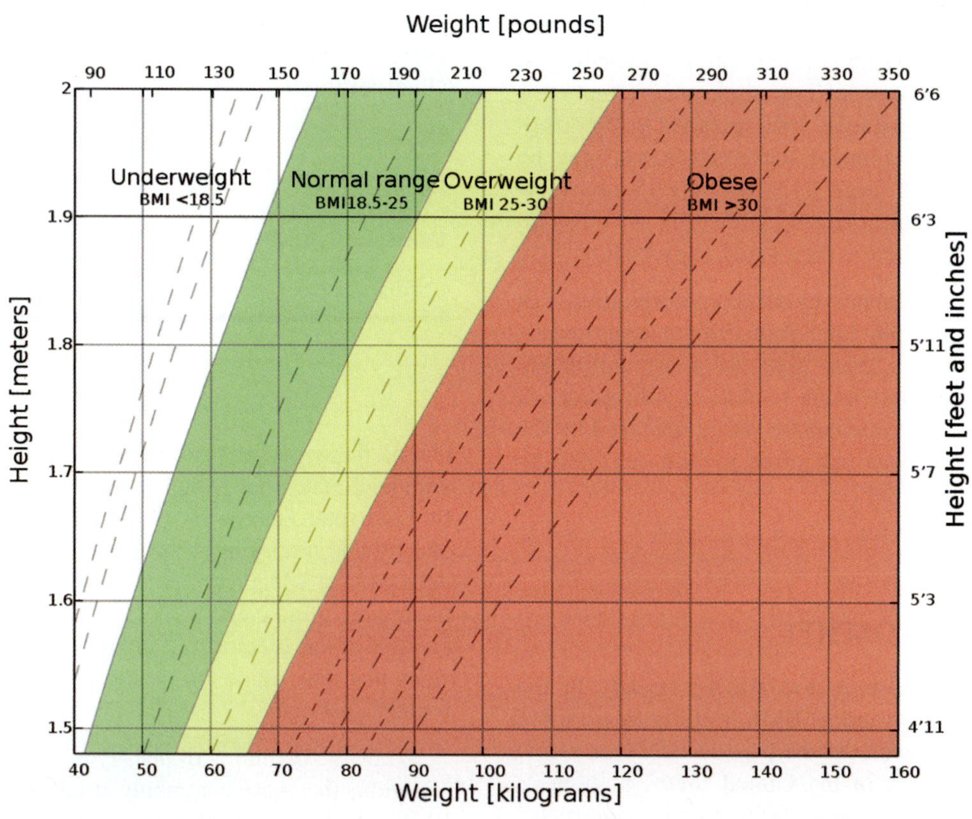

FIGURE 24-1. *Standard BMI conversion chart.*

TABLE 24-2. Questions Specific to Total Joint Arthroplasty in the Obese Patient

Does joint replacement improve the functional outcome of the obese patient?
Are there increased medical complications associated with total joint replacement in the obese?
Does joint replacement in the obese lead to higher complication and/or revision rate?
Is there a specific BMI which predisposes one to increased complications?
Are there any cost implications associated with total joint arthroplasty in the obese?

have been implicated with higher postoperative infection rates, longer hospitalizations, and increased overall mortality rates.[8-10] Allogeneic blood transfusion has also been associated with disease transmission, including HIV, hepatitis B and C, and others (Fig. 24-2). Therefore, early detection, evaluation, and optimization of preoperative anemia have become increasingly more important in an effort to reduce the need for ABT.

The reported criteria for preoperative anemia is somewhat debatable, with hemoglobin levels ranging from a more strict definition of <10 g/dL to a more liberal value of <13 g/dL.[11,12] Using this as a baseline definition, several strategies for optimizing preoperative anemia have been identified as offering significant benefit before knee arthroplasty (Table 24-3). These include preoperative oral or intravenous iron therapy, recombinant human erythropoietin (rHuEPO) therapy, and autologous transfusion techniques—mainly, preoperative autologous blood donation (PAD). In an effort to provide a better understanding of each of these strategies and how they may be effective in treating preoperative anemia before total joint arthroplasty, we offer a brief summary of each modality.

Estimated Risk of Allogenic Blood Transfusion	
Risk	Frequency per Unit Blood Transfused
Viral	
HIV	1:1,000,000
Hepatitis B	1:100,000
Hepatitis C	1:500 - 1:5,000
Cytomegalovirus (CMV)	Variable; 1:2,500
Transfusion Reaction	
Alloimmunization	Common
Allergic Reaction	1:100
Fever / Urticaria	1:100
Nonfatal hemolytic reation	1:6,000
Fatal hemolytic reaction	1:600,000

FIGURE 24-2. *Estimated risk of allogeneic blood transfusion. Modified from Keating et al.*[17]

TABLE 24-3. Strategies for Optimization of Preoperative Anemia

A.	Supplemental iron therapy
B.	Erythropoietin (rHuEPO) therapy
C.	Preoperative autologous blood donation

Supplemental Iron Therapy

The administration of preoperative iron (either orally or intravenously) has been shown to decrease the need for allogeneic blood transfusion postoperatively. A recent cohort study by Cuenca et al reported a statistically significant difference in the rate of postoperative ABT after total knee replacement (6% for patients treated via oral iron vs. 32% for the control).[13] Conventional dosing of oral iron preoperatively is 200 mg tds (180 mg of elemental iron) for a 2-week period before surgery, while intravenous (IV) dosing with the latest generation of iron (ferric carboxymaltose) can be given in larger doses (up to 1000 mg) in a single infusion (15–30 minutes).[14] Concerns of increased infection risk secondary to bacteremia associated with IV iron administration had been raised; however, in a recent prospective study of 985 patients, no significant association between IV iron administration and increased infection risk was found.[15]

Erythropoiesis-Stimulating Agents

Although several erythropoiesis-stimulating agents (ESAs) exist, only epoetin alfa is currently approved by the U.S. Food and Drug Administration (FDA) for use in patients undergoing major surgery. A 1998 systematic review of the literature demonstrated that epoetin alfa minimized perioperative blood transfusion in patients undergoing elective orthopaedic procedures.[16] The recommended dosing schedule of 300 IU/kg/day for 15 days perioperatively, or 600 IU/kg in four weekly doses beginning 3 weeks before elective surgery, has been shown to increase preoperative hemoglobin concentrations and appears to reduce the need for perioperative ABT.[17]

Concerns over increased thromboembolic risks associated with ESAs have been raised. In a 2007 study involving patients undergoing elective spinal surgery who did not receive prophylactic anticoagulation, the incidence of deep vein thrombosis (DVT) was 4.7% for those who had received epoetin alfa versus 2.1% in those patients not receiving epoetin alfa. This prompted the FDA to include boxed warnings on the packages of ESAs, recommending use of DVT prophylaxis in surgical patients receiving ESAs.[18] It is worth noting that this study focused on elective spine surgery in a patient population that often goes without formal DVT prophylaxis and may not be as applicable to total knee arthroplasty patients who, as a matter of standard of practice, receive some form of pharmacologic DVT prophylaxis.

Autologous Blood Donation

Autologous blood donation (ABD) before elective surgery has been a fairly popular option for elective total joint surgery. The utilization of ABD can decrease the risk of disease transmission and minimize the potential errors associated with blood type compatibility. There are, however, inherit concerns regarding this practice before elective surgery, such as an induced preoperative anemia, risk of ischemic events, and other complications.[19] Another issue surrounding the use of ABD, which may be contributing to a more recent decline in its use, is the concept of "overdonation." The Cleveland Clinic recently reported that upwards of 50% of blood donated for elective surgery goes unused.[20] The practice of ABD does remain a viable option, however, for those patients with multiple antibodies in whom proper blood donation may be difficult.

In summary, perioperative anemia is associated with an increased morbidity and mortality. While blood transfusion is certainly an acceptable means for dealing with this condition, it is associated with certain risks, such as postoperative infection, acute transfusion reaction, and longer hospital stays. With several pharmacological alternatives proving to be effective, as well as being advocated by the FDA and the American Red Cross, perhaps the need for ABD can be limited to select patients.

DISEASE-MODIFYING ANTIRHEUMATIC AGENTS AND GLUCOCORTICOSTEROIDS

Total knee arthroplasty in the patient population with rheumatoid disease or other inflammatory arthropathies is often a balancing act between minimizing perioperative complications while still maintaining control of the patient's underlying condition. While current pharmacologic treatments such as disease-modifying antirheumatic drugs (DMARDs) and glucocorticosteroids (GS) have been instrumental in improving patient symptoms and overall quality of life, they pose particular challenges for the treating orthopaedic surgeon. Compromised wound healing, infection, and adrenal insufficiency have all been recognized as legitimate concerns when dealing with this patient population.

Bongartz et al recently reported the risk of postoperative prosthetic joint infection to be as high as 2% in rheumatoid patients undergoing primary total joint arthroplasty and almost 6% in those undergoing revision surgery.[21] Because of the known relationship that DMARDs and GS have with increased rates of infection, the important question is how should these medications be handled in the perioperative setting in an effort to minimize their potential complications. While there is no clear consensus on how best to manage these medications, most current recommendations deal with the nonbiologic DMARDs, methotrexate being the most commonly used. Several studies have implicated methotrexate as a causative factor in the increased risk of perioperative infection and wound dehiscence,[22,23] while others have concluded that methotrexate, when conventionally dosed, has no influence on increased infection or wound dehiscence rates.[24] Table 24-4 outlines the suggested perioperative management for the most commonly used nonbiologic DMARDs as suggested by the Mayo Clinic Department of Rheumatology.

The use of biologic response modifiers (BRMs) appears to place this patient population at a higher overall infection risk when compared to traditional DMARDs. These medications, which include anti-tumor necrosis factor-alpha agents such as entanercept and infliximab, may be more dose dependent in nature and appear to be more problematic during the first 3 months of therapy.[25] Because these treatments are fairly novel, little exists in the literature in terms of recommendations for their perioperative management. Table 24-5 represents the suggested perioperative treatment of these medications as described by the Mayo Clinic Department of Rheumatology.

The use of GS has been implicated as a risk factor in increased postsurgical infection rates in a variety of surgical subspecialties, especially in those patients taking higher than normal doses. This may be attributable to a glucocorticosteroid-induced hyperglycemic state seen perioperatively in this patient population. Further, this may also be related to the common practice of using GS up to and at the time of surgery, as opposed to DMARDs, which are commonly used 1 to 2 weeks before surgery. Because the risk for adrenal suppression and its associated complications, such as circulatory shock, is very real, a balance must be reached in GS dosing during the perioperative period in an effort to prevent adrenal insufficiency. Table 24-6 summarizes the formal recommendations for perioperative GS dosing.

Interestingly, in a case control study analyzing predictors of increased infection rate in total hip and total knee arthroplasty, no association between elevated rates of infection and low-dose GS use (6 mg of prednisolone daily) was identified.[26] Nonetheless, because of the abundance of literature showing a general increased infection rate in other surgical specialties associated with GS use, as well as the devastating consequences associated with infected total joint replacement, the vast majority of orthopaedic surgeons exercise great caution when dealing with patients on chronic GS treatment.

DIABETES

The Center for Disease Control has estimated that nearly 8.3% of the United States population has been diagnosed with diabetes; the majority of these patients being older than 65 years of age.[27] It is also reported that an estimated 7 million people are diabetic but are undiagnosed. As such, the

TABLE 24-4. Recommended Perioperative Management of Common Nonbiologic DMARDs

Nonbiologic DMARD	Recommended Management
Methotrexate	Stop 2 weeks preop; Resume 10–14 days postop
Leflunomide	Stop 2 weeks preop; Resume 10–14 days postop
Azothioprine	Stop 1 week preop; Resume 5–7 days postop
Chlorambucil	Stop 1 week preop; Resume 5–7 days postop
Cyclophosphamide	Stop 1 week preop; Resume 5–7 days postop
Minocycline	Continue usual dosing
Sulfasalizine	Continue usual dosing

TABLE 24-5. Recommended Perioperative Management of Biologic Response Modifiers

Biologic Response Modifier	Recommended Management
Etanercept	Stop 1 week preop; Resume 7–14 days postop
Infiximab	Stop 2–4 weeks preop; Resume 2–4 weeks postop
Golimumab	Stop 2–4 weeks preop; Resume 7–14 days postop
Certolizumab	Stop 2–4 weeks preop; Resume 7–14 days postop
Rituximab	Stop 4 weeks preop from last dose; Resume 4 weeks preceding next dose

TABLE 24-6. Suggested Perioperative GS Dosing Guidelines

Stress to Patient	Glucocorticosteroid Dose
Minor (sedation not required)	25 mg hydrocortisone or 5 mg IV methylprednisolone on day of surgery
Moderate (sedation required)	50–75 mg hydrocortisone or 10–15 mg IV methylprednisolone on day of surgery; taper dose to baseline over 1–2 days postop
Severe (sedation required)	100–150 mg hydrocortisone or 20–30 mg IV methylprednisolone on day of surgery; taper dose to baseline over 1–3 days postop

Adapted from Cousin DB, Wood KE. Corticosteroid supplementation for adrenal insufficiency. *JAMA*. 2002;287:238-240.

orthopaedic surgeon performing total knee arthroplasty will undoubtedly be dealing with this patient population as well as their associated perioperative risks. Because diabetes is the leading cause of kidney failure in the United States, as well as a significant cause of heart disease and stroke, it is imperative that these patients be thoroughly evaluated and optimized before any surgical procedure.

It has been demonstrated that when blood glucose is properly controlled, the perioperative outcomes of patients with diabetes versus those without diabetes are similar.[28] Because of the potential perioperative complications, such as cardiovascular compromise and nephropathy, associated with the diabetic patient, elective surgery should be delayed if fasting preoperative blood glucose levels are greater than 200 mg/dL. Associated cardiac manifestations can be difficult to diagnose because the symptoms are often atypical, as is seen in the setting of silent cardiac ischemia.[29] As such, these patients often benefit from a preoperative cardiology consultation.

Diabetic nephropathy is also a common perioperative condition in the diabetic patient and is first identified by the presence of increased levels of microalbuminuria. Elevated levels of serum creatinine are routinely seen as the nephropathy progresses. Early recognition of this developing condition is important, because nephropathy is often associated with hypertension and coronary artery disease. Careful fluid management and avoidance of nephrotoxic drugs are crucial to avoiding further progression.

Postoperative management of the diabetic patient most often involves intravenous insulin infusion protocols because these have demonstrated better postoperative glycemic control.[30] However, this has been shown to increase the risk of postoperative hypoglycemia. While there does not appear to be a consensus as to what the optimal glycemic goals should be postoperatively, current infusion protocols remain the standard of care during this period. Suggested "ideal" postoperative glucose levels have been between 100 and 180 mg/dL.

RENAL DISEASE

The patient with renal disease often requires thorough evaluation by their internist in most cases and a nephrologist in advanced cases. In addition to the routine evaluation, the workup should include nutritional status (paying close attention to sodium, protein, and free fluid intake), as well as electrolyte intake monitoring. Additionally, many of these patients are on a variety of medications, most of which are renally dosed. As such, the glomerular filtration rate for these patients must be calculated and utilized to appropriately continue many of these medications (Table 24-7). The immediate preoperative assessment should also include a complete laboratory workup including chest X-ray, electrocardiogram (ECG) (especially if electrolyte imbalance is suspected), cardiac stress test, and full chemistry workup.

Certain medications should be used with great caution or avoided altogether since they may cause unnecessary stress to the patient's renal function. Many of these medications alter the electrolyte balance and ultimately the patient's volume status.

Patients with chronic renal insufficiency may require dialysis. It is recommended that these patients undergo their dialysis session 24 hours before their surgical procedure. Heparin should be avoided during this time.

Finally, a certain percentage of renal patients have likely undergone kidney transplant. In these cases, immunosuppressive medications should not be held because withholding them places the transplanted organ at risk. These patients should be carefully monitored for postoperative infection.

TABLE 24-7. Common Perioperative Medications Requiring Renal Dosing Adjustments

Vancomycin
Aminoglycosides
Digoxin
Atenolol
ACE inhibitors
Phenobarbital
Gabapentin

NOTE: Consult pharmacist for all medications in patients with renal failure.

PULMONARY DISEASE

Because the occurrence of pulmonary conditions arising after general anesthesia is fairly common, it is important to identify and optimize those patients who may be at higher risk for such perioperative issues. It is commonly accepted that many anesthetic agents used during surgery depress the respiratory drive, which can lead to hypoxemia and hypercarbia, as well as depress diaphragmatic function.[31] Other preoperative medications can dry natural, protective secretions, further compromising the patient's respiratory status. These conditions often carry over to the postoperative period and, as such, can pose a significant risk to those patients with preexisting pulmonary disease.

Ideally, the preoperative assessment should help to identify those patients at higher risk for postoperative pulmonary complications. This includes identification of risk factors such as smoking history, age (>60 years), history of congestive heart failure, chronic lung disease, and functional dependence. Patients with suspected or known lung disease should be evaluated with pulmonary function studies to evaluate their level of impairment. In patients with severe impairment, a preoperative arterial blood gas may be of use. These patients often merit formal pulmonology evaluation and clearance.

The preoperative assessment of pulmonary risk stratification is important, because early recognition may lead to decreased postoperative complications. Depending on the type of pulmonary compromise, preoperative patient education during this period can be beneficial. Smokers should be educated on the importance of cessation because quitting 6 to 8 weeks before surgery has been shown to be beneficial.[32] Those patients with chronic coughs should be encouraged to perform deep breathing exercises as well as perform incentive spirometry and periodic coughing to decrease secretions. In those patients with known pulmonary conditions who are on chronic bronchodilators or steroids, continuation of these medications should be encouraged during the perioperative period.

CARDIAC DISEASE

Evaluating and optimizing the cardiac patient before an elective orthopaedic procedure is paramount to minimizing the potential for perioperative complications. Because cardiac disease has the potential for serious perioperative complications, an entire chapter has been dedicated to this topic. However, it is worth mentioning briefly in this chapter because the preoperative evaluation regarding cardiac disease is of the utmost importance in terms of minimizing perioperative mobidity. As such, risk stratification is of great importance and can often be accomplished via detailed history and physical exam, ECG, and chest radiograph. Further diagnostic studies can be ordered as needed, depending on the patient evaluation. In general, patients with known cardiac disease should be evaluated by their internist or cardiologist, and communication between that individual and the treating surgeon is imperative to minimizing perioperative complications associated with cardiac disease.

In the preoperative setting, it is also important to establish risk factors before elective orthopaedic surgery, since these may warrant a more comprehensive evaluation by a cardiologist. These risk factors should include a history of ischemic heart disease, congestive heart failure, and cerebrovascular disease. If present, the need for noninvasive stress testing should be considered preoperatively.

As previously mentioned, because of the importance of cardiac disease as it relates to elective orthopaedic surgery, as well as the potential for a number of different perioperative manifestations and complications, an entire chapter has been devoted to detailed discussion of the topic.

SUMMARY

In summary, while it has been shown that joint replacement arthroplasty can be a tremendously successful operative intervention, various medical comorbidities become factors in the perioperative care of these patients. Often, many of these conditions can be successfully managed by the treating surgeon. However, in those patients who have severe or multiple comorbidities, referral to a subspecialist is invaluable in terms of evaluating, optimizing, and minimizing perioperative complications in these patients before their elective joint replacement arthroplasty.

REFERENCES

1. Flegal K, Carroll M, Ogden C, et al. Prevalence and trends in obesity among US adults. 1999-2008. *JAMA*. 2010;303(3):235-241.
2. Bourne R, Mukhi S, Zhu N, et al. Role of obesity on the risk for total hip or knee arthroplasty. *Clin Orthop Relat Res*. 2007;465:185-188.
3. Foran JR, Mont MA, Etienne G, et al. The outcome of total knee arthroplasty in obese patients. *J Bone Joint Surg Am*. 2004;86(8):1609-1615.
4. McQueen DA, Long MJ, Algotar AM, et al. The effect of obesity on quality-of-life improvement after total knee arthroplasty. *Am J Orthop*. 2007;36(8): E117-E120, E127.
5. Namba RS, Paxton L, Fithian DC, et al. Obesity and perioperative morbidity in total hip and total knee arthroplasty patients. *J Arthroplasty*. 2005;20(7 suppl 3):46-50.
6. Miric A, Lim M, Kahn B, et al. Perioperative morbidity following total knee arthroplasty among obese patients. *J Knee Surg*. 2002;15(2):77-83.
7. Gombotz H, Rehak PH, Shander A, et al. Blood use in elective surgery: the Austrian Benchmark Study. *Transfusion*. 2007;47:1468-1480.
8. Keating EM, Meding JB, Faris PM, et al. Predictors of transfusion risk in elective knee surgery. *Clin Orthop Relat Res*. 1998;357:50-59.
9. Beattie WS, Karkouti K, Wijeysundera DN, et al. Risk associated with preoperative anemia in noncardiac surgery: A single-center cohort study. *Anesthesiology*. 2009;110:574-581.
10. Carson JL, Duff A, Poses RM, et al. Effect of anaemia and cardiovascular disease on surgical mortality and morbidity. *Lancet*. 1996;348:1055-1060.
11. Foss NB, Kristensen MT, Kehlet H. Anaemia impedes functional mobility after hip fracture surgery. *Age Ageing*. 2008;37:173-178.
12. Rosencher N, Kerkkamp HE, Macheras G, et al. Orthopedic Surgery Transfusion Hemoglobin European Overview (OSTHEO) study: blood management in elective knee and hip arthroplasty in Europe. *Transfusion*. 2003;43:459-469.
13. Cuenca J, Garcia-Erce JA, Martinez F, et al. Preoperative haematinics and transfusion protocol reduce the need for transfusion after total knee replacement. *Int J Surg*. 2007;5:89-94.
14. Bisbe E, Garcia-Erce A, Diaz-Lobo A, et al. A multicentre comparative study on the efficacy of intravenous ferric carboxymaltose and iron sucrose for correcting preoperative anaemia in patients undergoing major elective surgery. *Br J Anaesth*. 2011; 107(3):477-478.
15. Hoen B, Paul-Dauphin A, Kessler M. Intravenous iron administration does not significantly increase the risk of bacteremia in chronic hemodialysis patients. *Clin Nephrol*. 2002;57:457-461.
16. Laupacis A, Fergusson D. Erythropoietin to minimize peri-operative blood transfusion: a systematic review of randomized trials: the International Study of Perioperative Transfusion (ISPOT) Investigators. *Transfus Med*. 1998;8:309-317.

17. Keating EM, Meding JB. Perioperative blood management practices in elective orthopaedic surgery. *J Am Acad Orthop Surg*. 2002;10(6):393-400.
18. Epogen [package insert]. Thousand Oaks, CA: Amgen Inc.; 2009.
19. Popovsky MA, Whitaker B, Arnold NL. Severe outcomes of allogeneic and autologous blood donation: frequency and characterization. *Transfusion*. 1995;35(9):734-737.
20. Kumar A. Perioperative management of anemia: limits of blood transfusion and alternatives to it. *Cleveland Clin J Med*. 2009;76(suppl 4):S112-S118.
21. Bongartz T, Halligan CS, Osmon DR, et al. Incidence and risk factors of prosthetic joint infection after total hip or knee replacement in patients with rheumatoid arthritis. *Arthritis Rheum*. 2008;59(12):1713-1720.
22. Sany J, Anaya JM, Canovas F, et al. Influence of methotrexate on the frequency of postoperative infectious complications in patients with rheumatoid arthritis. *J Rheumatol*. 1993;20(7):1129-1132.
23. Bridges S, Lopez Mendez A, Han K, et al. Should methotrexate be discontinued before elective orthopaedic surgery in patients with rheumatoid arthritis? *J Rheumatol*. 1991;18:984-988.
24. Grennan DM, Gray J, Loudon J, et al. Methotrexate and early postoperative complications in patients with rheumatoid arthritis undergoing elective orthopaedic surgery. *Ann Rheum Dis*. 2001;60:214-217.
25. Bongartz T, Sutton AJ, Sweeting MJ, et al. Anti-TNF antibody therapy in rheumatoid arthritis and the risk of serious infections and malignancies: systematic review and meta-analysis of rare harmful effects in randomized controlled trials. *JAMA*. 2006;295(19):2275-2285.
26. Berbari EF, Hanssen AD, Duffy MC, et al. Risk factors for prosthetic joint infection: case-control study. *Clin Infect Dis*. 1998;27(5):1247-1254.
27. The Expert Committee on the Diagnosis and Classification of Diabetes Mellitus. Report of the Expert Committee on the Diagnosis and Classification of Diabetes Mellitus. *Diabetes Care*. 2011;34(suppl. 1):S66-S68.
28. Gavin LA. Management of diabetes mellitus during surgery. *West J Med*. 1989;151(5):525-529.
29. Juul AB, Wetterslev J, Kofoed-Enevoldsen A, et al. The Diabetic Postoperative Mortality and Morbidity (DIPOM) Trial: rationale and design of a multicenter, randomized, placebo-controlled, clinical trial of metoprolol for patients with diabetes mellitus who are undergoing major noncardiac surgery. *Am Heart J*. 2004;147(4):677-683.
30. Gandhi GY, Murad MH, Flynn DN, et al. Effect of perioperative insulin infusion on surgical morbidity and mortality: systematic review and meta-analysis of randomized trials. *Mayo Clin Proc*. 2008;83(4):418-430.
31. Rock P, Passannante A. Preoperative assessment: pulmonary. *Anesthesiol Clin North Am*. 2004;22(1):77-91.
32. Chow, C, Devereaux, P. The optimal timing of smoking cessation before surgery. *Arch Intern Med*. 2011;171(11):989-990.

25

Sources and Controls of Microorganisms in the Operating Room During Total Joint Replacement Surgery

Merrill A. Ritter

Despite the many changes in total joint arthroplasty over the past 50 years, little has changed as it relates to the infection rates, which vary between 0.25% and 2%.[1] Sir John Charnley was one of many who offered changes that actually lowered his infection rates to where they are today by working in a so-called "greenhouse." Over a 10-year period of time, he lowered his infection rate from 10% to 1%.[2] He finally stated that he doubted if the infection rate could be lowered more than 0.5%. Attempts to determine the patients who are most likely to get an infection have resulted in a list of comorbidities, yet even with this understanding the postoperative infections persist.[1]

This chapter does not try to further this understanding but only to help with the understanding of the various sources and controls of microorganisms that exist in the operating room.

For 6 years in the early 1970s, the surgical team sampled every orthopaedic surgical procedure. We sampled the environment at the wound and back instrument table by air settle plates [colony-forming units (CFU)/ft^2/h] and volumetric Reynier air samples (CFU/ft^3). We also sampled the periphery of the room by air settle plates (CFU/ft^2/h) (Fig. 25-1). Opening and closing wound cultures and the nares of the surgical personnel and patients were obtained for each procedure. Data were continuously upgraded as to postoperative wound infections. Also during this time period, many other experiments were performed to evaluate the contamination of multiple variables, which are referred to in this chapter.

As surgeons, we have been taught to help, not add to the problems of pain and suffering. Postoperative wound infections are devastating to the patient and surgeon—physically, emotionally, and economically. Thus an old adage, "An ounce of prevention is worth a ton of cure," is appropriate here.

There are three basic principles that are worthwhile to the following information. To learn them first only helps to understand the rest:

1. Individuals shed bacteria continuously from their bodies, but the amount varies.
2. The bacteria on people are either indigenous (within the pores and cannot be eliminated) or exogenous (acquired by contact and removable with washing).
3. Bacteria have mass, attach to fomites, and settle.

SOURCE

The source of bacteria in the operating room is people.[3,4] Concerns in the past and present frequently get bogged down into passing the blame onto what we cannot see.

The operating room environment is basically "bug free" if allowed to be closed and empty overnight. The air that enters the operating room passes through a HEPA filter that

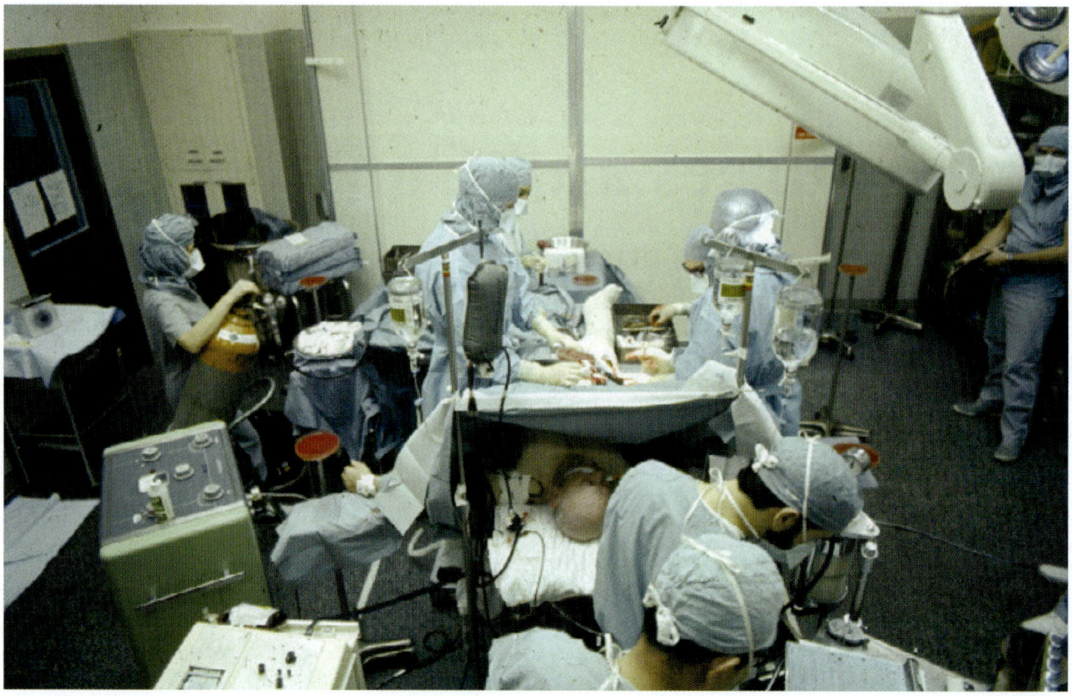

FIGURE 25-1. *A conventional operating room with a wall-less horizontal laminar airflow system. Air settle plates were positioned at the wound, back instrument table, and about the room at the wound height. Volumetric sampling was at the wound and back instrument table. All of the sampling was for every orthopaedic procedure whether or not the laminar airflow was used or not.*

removes bacteria just before it enters the room itself. It is the introduction of people that produces contamination within the operating room environment.[4]

Humans

The bacteria within the environment of an operating room are statistically increased as the number of people enter.[3,4] The colony-forming units per square foot per hour increase proportionately as do the number of people within the operating room (Fig. 25-2).[3] Humans are noted to shed normally between 1000 and 10,000 organisms per minute.[6] Those who shed in excess of 10,000 organisms per minute are referred to as "shedders" (13% of men, 1% of premenopausal women, and 5% of postmenopausal women).[5]

The major source of bacterial shedding is from the male gender. Male surgeons must look to themselves first before passing judgment on the cause of a postoperative wound infection.[5,6]

Staphylococcus aureus, a frequent isolate from postoperative wound infections, was cultured from approximately one-third of all operating room personnel.[6] *Staphylococcus epidermis* is just as frequent a source of wound infections and is cultured almost every time from all operating room personnel.

Methicillin-resistant *Staphylococcus aureus* (MRSA) has been isolated from 2.6% of our preoperative patients and methicillin-sensitive *Staphylococcus aureus* (MSSA) from 17.6%. Thus it is people who are the source of most of the operating room bacteria. The number of bacteria only increases with the number of people and whether or not an individual is a shedder. Bathing reduces this shedding only temporarily (minutes) before returning to higher levels and therefore is not a control factor.[1]

Surfaces

Surface contamination basically remains in a constant state of equilibrium.[7] Disinfecting the surfaces may help temporarily but has no lasting effect. To substantiate these data, we used compression Rodac plates to evaluate the surfaces of the operating room floor before and after surgery,

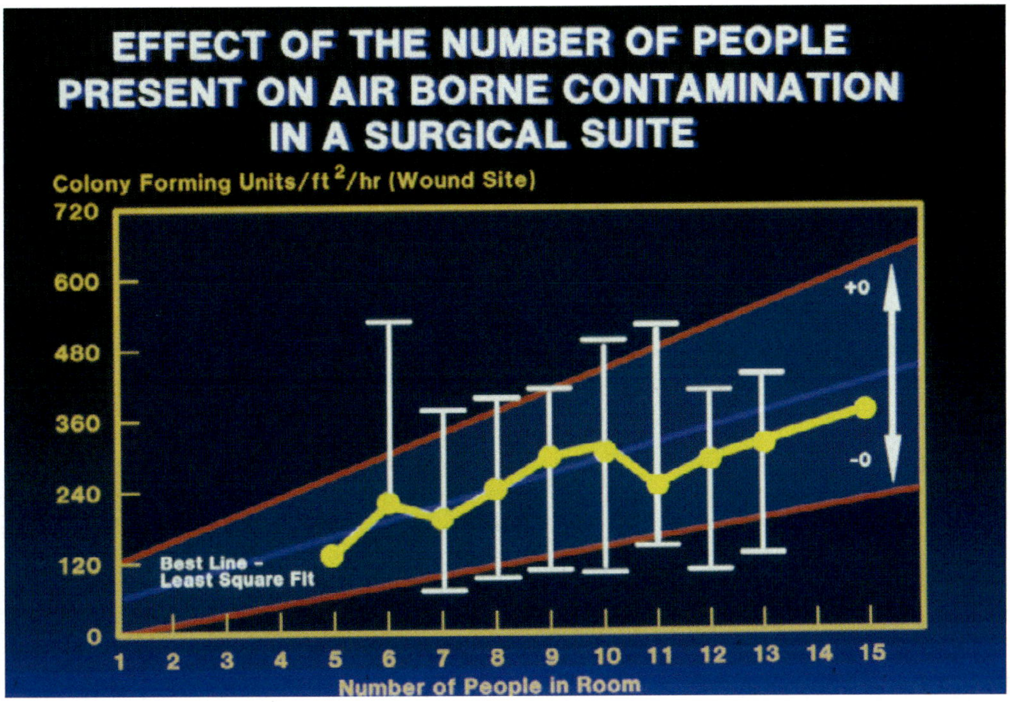

FIGURE 25-2. *A graph of the number of CFU/ft²/h versus the number of people present in the operating room.*

immediately after disinfecting and 5 minutes after disinfecting. Before surgery, there was an average of 43 colonies per plate, 51 after surgery, 27 immediately after disinfecting, and 40 after conventional use of the room. These results support the conclusion that a reduction of surface contamination returns to its previous level, rapidly making complete asepsis unobtainable.

CONTROL

Environment

During the course of our surveillance, we were able to evaluate various operating room environmental controls: a conventional operating room without any environmental control, horizontal laminar air floor without walls (Fig. 25-1), horizontal laminar airflow with walls (Fig. 25-3), and vertical laminar airflow without walls (Fig. 25-4). We have never evaluated a vertical downflow with walls (Charnley greenhouse).

It is obvious from sampling all the orthopaedic procedures (Table 25-1) that horizontal laminar airflow reduced the number of bacteria at the wound, back instrument table, and the periphery of the wound ($p < .005$); however, the periphery was not as clean as the area within the filtered air (ie, the back table and the wound).[8]

Looking at only total hip replacements (THRs) and different airflow systems (Table 25-2), horizontal laminar airflow seemed to work the best in our hands.[9] Obviously, the contamination in a vertical downflow system without walls brings the environmental bacteria from below the wound up to the wound itself because of the negative pressure that develops when surgical teams lean over the wound and the hot lamps that are in the path of the air.

Laminar airflow does not only reduce the number of bacteria at the wound site, it has also been shown statistically to reduce the number of infections as well.[10] Recently, however, Hooper et al have noted a statistically significant increase in infections with the use of space suits and laminar airflow.[11] It is speculated that the system used was downflow. This only accentuates the need for proper use of the systems. Positioning personnel within the laminar flow is critical. If one is to impede the air, then a body exhaust system is a must, especially with a horizontal unit.[12] Salvati et al found more total knee replacement infections with a horizontal laminar airflow system. This was determined to be secondary to one of the scrubbed personnel being between the airflow surface and the patient.[12]

A

B

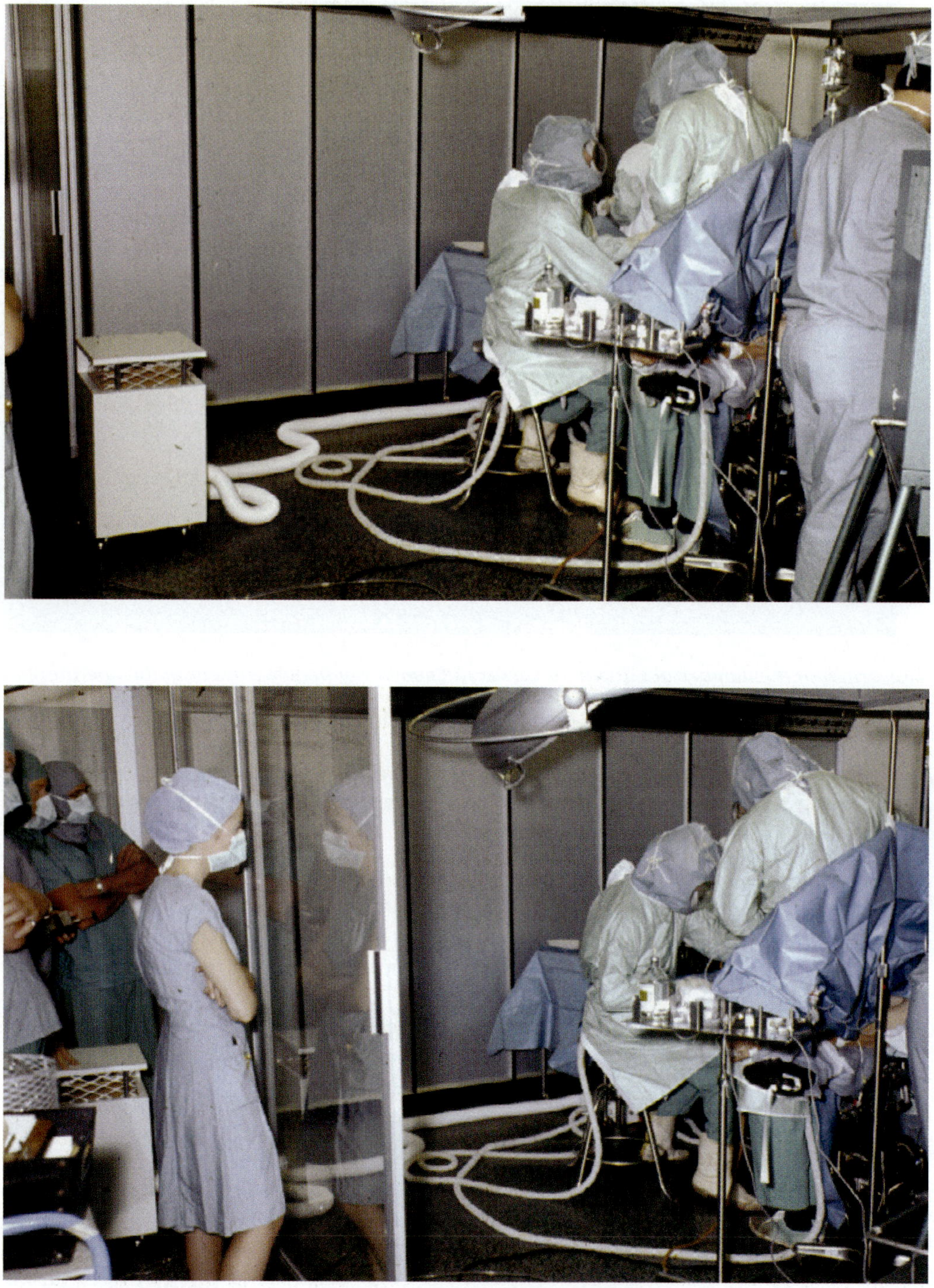

FIGURE 25-3. *A horizontal laminar airflow with the walls retracted (**A**) or with them extended (**B**).*

TABLE 25-1. Comparison of Contamination Found in Conventional vs. Laminar Airflow Operating Rooms (OR)

Air-Sampling Device	Conventional OR	Laminar Airflow OR	Reduction (%)	Probability (*p*)
Reyneir				
Wound[a]	100	7	93%	<.005
Back table[a]	74	5	93%	<.005
Air settle plates				
Wound[b]	288	23	92%	<.005
Back table[b]	332	9	97%	<.005
Periphery of room				
Operating table[b]	281	111	61%	<.005

[a]CFU/ft^3
[b]CFU/ft^2/h

TABLE 25-2. CFU/ft^2/h for Three Different Laminar Airflow Reports During Total Hip Replacement

	Horizontal Laminar Airflow		Vertical Laminar Airflow
	Wall-less	Walled	(Wall-less)
Number of THR cases	189	102	100
Wound CFU/ft^2/h	18	16	50
Back table CFU/ft^2/h	5	1	26

Ultraviolet (UV) light has many great attributes. Not only does it kill the bacteria, whereas laminar airflow tries to keep the area about the wound bacteria free, it is very inexpensive. There is a downside, however, since all operating room personnel and patients need to be protected from the ultraviolet light itself. Work by Berg-Perier supports the benefits and addresses the simplicity of its use.[13] Body exhaust is basically a requirement to avoid burns and very helpful if a member of the operating room scrub team is a shedder.[13]

In a 19-year period at our institution, there were 47 infections in 5980 joints. The infection rate for cases without UV (but with laminar airflow) was 1.77% and the infection rate of cases with UV was 0.57% ($p < .0001$). A procedure without UV has 3.1 times the odds of an infection compared to a procedure with UV ($p < .0001$). The total hip replacement infection rate dropped from 1.03% to 0.72% ($p = .5475$) and the total knee replacement infection rate dropped from 2.20% to 0.50% ($p < .0001$) by utilizing UV light. Revision surgery, previous infection, age, body mass index, cement, and diagnosis were not statistically associated with an elevated infection rate.

Although safety concerns accompany the use of UV lights in the operating room, when appropriate precautions

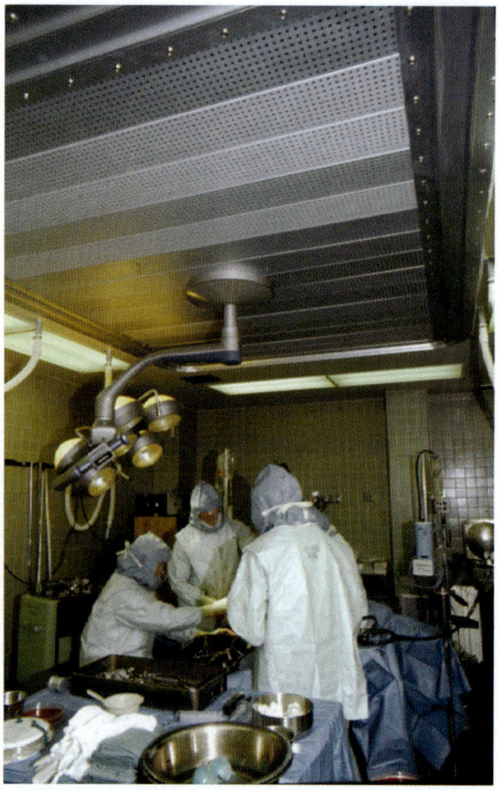

FIGURE 25-4. *A vertical wall-less laminar airflow unit.*

are taken, UV lights appear to be an effective control for lowering the infection risk in the operating room and offer a much reduced expense versus the installation of a laminar airflow system. It is obvious that there is a plethora of bacteria being forced into the operating room environment by people; thus, how well do our conventional controls work?

Clothing

As we change our normal street clothes into surgical attire, there is a certain sort of an aura that we have gone from an area that is with bacteria to an area that is without. However, the porosity of most cloth scrub clothes measures between 100 and 500 μm (bacteria measure 1 μm and fomite-carrying bacteria measure 20 to 30 μm), thus making the cloth barrier very ineffective. Looking at various aspects of scrub clothes such as dresses, pants, and shirts, as well as tucking in the shirt and enclosing the feet, there is basically no difference in the environmental contamination with any of these changes.[14] Scrubs versus street clothes do not alter the operating room environment contamination.

Gowns

We evaluated the surface contamination of three types of "sterile gowns": cloth, paper, and plastic by Rodac compression plates. At this point, we were sampling at both shoulders, the xiphoid process, and at the waist. There was a 33% reduction in surface bacteria comparing paper gowns to cloth gowns and a 71% reduction using plastic gowns verses cloth gowns ($p < .05$). There was a 57% reduction comparing plastic gowns to paper gowns ($p < .05$).[15] Remember this is surface contamination not environment contamination.

It was obvious that the more enclosure that we could offer to the surgical personnel, the better the surface reduction (the plastic gown had an attached hood). The concern was, therefore, whether this would also affect the environmental bacteria. We then looked at a plastic gown with a cloth hood, facemask, and gloves versus a hooded exhaust gown and both of these versus scrub clothes. There was a 51% reduction of environmental bacteria using the plastic gown versus scrub clothes, a 69% reduction using the body exhaust gown versus the scrub clothes, and a 38% reduction using the body exhaust gown versus the plastic wrap-around gown.[16] It is obvious that the more you can enclose the people within the operating room, the better off you are; however, remember principle number one: people continue to shed bacteria and therefore the enclosures must include everyone within the operating room, including visitors, circulation nurses, and anesthesiologists. If all are not involved, then the amount of bacteria within the operating room will still stay at the same equilibrium despite the use by the few who have scrubbed and, since people continue to shed bacteria at the same rate, clothing that does not exhaust the bacteria eventually fails as the bacteria come about the open surfaces (ie, head, neck, and below the gown). Even in an exhaust gown, the exhaust only works about the head and neck. Therefore, there are still bacteria coming out from under the base of the gown, although possibly a lesser amount.

Head covers

The length of the operating room personnel's hair and the means of enclosing the hair with various head covers were investigated.[16] Despite the head cover and the length of the hair, there was no change in the amount of environmental bacterial contamination. Remember that people shed bacteria at a continuous rate, therefore it is the person not his dress style.

Masks

The disposable mask has a filter efficiency of greater than 95%.[16] However, we need not determine the actual filter efficiency but the bacterial reduction within the environment by the operating room personnel with and without surgical masks. We have shown that there was no influence on the environmental bacteria by the use of a mask.[4] Masks allow patients and individuals to talk and thus help prevent the projection of bacteria directed toward the wound, but they do not reduce environmental bacteria.[4,17]

The next time that you wear a mask within the operating room, place your hand in front of the mask and blow as hard as you can. You will note that air does not pass through this excellent filter. Thus bacteria come from around the sides and are not filtered out.

Body exhausts

As previously noted, the body exhaust is an excellent means at reducing bacterial contamination within the environment; however, all personnel, including anesthesiologists, visitors, and circulating nurses, must use it, otherwise its effect alone is negligible.[16] To substantiate its use in laminar airflow, we evaluated wound air settle plates with and without body exhaust systems. There was absolutely no difference in the amount of colony-forming units per square foot per hour at the wound sight with or without the body exhaust[16]; however, positioning personnel within the horizontal laminar flow is critical.

Shoe covers

We evaluated various shoe covers, examining both the surface and the environment. The type of shoe or shoe cover had absolutely no effect on the surface or operating room environmental contamination.[18]

Prepping and Scrubbing

As surgeons, we have been taught from the beginning of our medical training the need for reducing the number of skin bacteria, both about the area of the wound and our hands, by prepping and scrubbing, respectively. But no matter how long we scrub or prep, or use the currently available agents, wound infection rates stay about the same. Therefore, is there a different or better way to maintain a maximum reduction of bacteria on the hands and about the wound?

Organisms

There are two microbial populations on the skin: transient and indigenous. The transient populations are acquired by touch and are easily removed with minimal washing. For this reason, hand washing should be the number one infection control policy throughout a hospital. The indigenous population inhabits the sebaceous glands and ducts of the skin. The skin, culturing through 20 cell layers deep, continues to grow demonstrable numbers of bacteria.[19]

The bacteria that inhabit the skin do so in different percentages depending on the location. For example, diphtheroids are primarily in the groin and micrococcus is on the hands. The predominate skin organisms include gram-negative rods (*Klebsiella*, *Proteus*, *Acinetobacter*, and *Enterobacter*) *Staphylococcus aureus*, *Staphylococcus epidermis*, micrococcus, and diptheroids.[20]

Time of cleaning

The statement, "More is better," does not necessarily apply to cleaning the skin. As far back as 1939, Price[21] showed by his basin technique that the number of bacteria on the skin did not change significantly from 2 to 10 minutes of scrubbing (the time allotted for the experiment). Other studies using Betadine and Phisohex show no difference in the colony counts of hands scrubbed for 5 minutes versus 10 minutes.[22] Using different compounds this time could be reduced to 2 minutes with chlorhexidine[23] or less than 1 minute with an alcohol hexachlorophene foam.[24] Since we are not killing the indigenous bacteria, which grow from the depths of the sebaceous glands, we probably need only a couple of minutes of scrubbing with the current agents supplied by the hospital (Fig. 25-5).

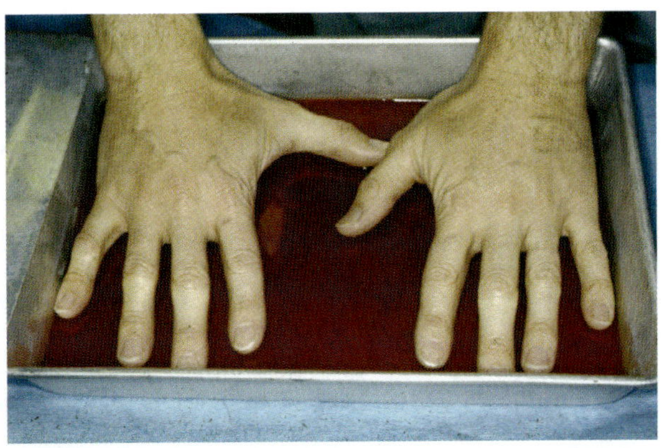

FIGURE 25-5. *Hand sampling in sterile agar cake pans before scrubbing, after scrubbing, and after the gloves were removed.*

Compounds

There are four basic compounds used: hexachlorophene, alcohol, iodine, and chlorhexidine. Hexachlorophene is bacteriostatic, whereas alcohol, iodine, and chlorhexidine are bactericidal. Alcohol has always been known to work well but loses its effectiveness rapidly.[25]

The other components have been tested alone or against one another.[22-24,26-30] All these compounds showed at least a 90% reduction in bacteria. The chlorhexidine is very good.[23,28] However, with the addition of alcohol to the hexachlorophene as a foam, it too is just as effective,[24,26,27] as is iodine in a povidone-iodine solution without a previous povidone-iodine scrubbing agent.[30] The preparation of the compound as a foam with alcohol takes away the abrasiveness of the scrub, gets to all of the areas of the skin, and is instantly effective and long lasting.[27]

Gloves

Even though we can now decrease the amount of bacteria greater than 90% on our hands (Fig. 25-5), the glove helps to reduce the remaining 10% (Fig. 25-6). Bacteria on the gloves come from the environmental contamination of the sterile field, not the hand beneath the glove.[31]

We evaluated the bacterial contamination of the surgical gloves by pressing our gloved hands directly on blood cultures immediately after their use in total hip replacement surgery (Fig. 25-6). We filled the gloves with water to check for holes, recorded the holes on a diagram, and correlated the holes with the amount of contamination on certain areas of the hand, respectively. We sampled 212 individual gloves, 68 single gloves, 72 double gloves (72 outer and 72 inner). Thirteen percent of the single gloves, 46% of the outer double gloves, and 10% of the inner double gloves had holes. No contamination was found on a finger or a palm of a hand wearing a glove with a hole in the corresponding area.

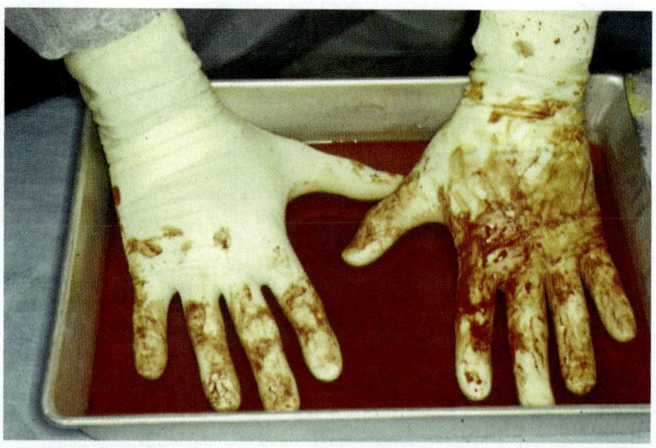

FIGURE 25-6. *Glove sampling in sterile agar cake pans after surgery.*

As noted in Table 25-3, approximately 30% of all of the gloves, whether they were single, double, inner, or outer, were contaminated. Obviously the gloves with or without holes were not the source of contamination. The contamination was from another source: the surgical field or the operating room environment.[31]

Adhesive drapes

The bacterial reduction following prepping is maintained with the use of an adhesive drape (Fig. 25-7). We have shown that adhesive drapes demonstrated no increase in bacteria multiplication, no lateral migration, no penetration of the drape, and no increase in wound contamination.[32] With antimicrobial adhesive drapes now available, there is no need for more than alcohol as a prepping agent.[33,34]

Conclusion to prepping and scrubbing

Looking realistically at what we are trying to accomplish, a sterile hand and wound, we find this is only achievable by scrubbing with a compound that kills all of the transient and superficial indigenous bacteria, then leaves an antiseptic in place to continuously suppress those bacteria migrating to the surface. This requires approximately 1 minute or less with an alcohol-antiseptic foam for the hands, without rinsing from the scrub sink and covered by an added protection of a glove. The wound needs alcohol prep for the same reason, with the addition of an antiseptic adhesive drape, to maintain a level of sterility while the drape is intact. Using these methods, the bacteria on the skin of the

TABLE 25-3. Number of Holes in Particular Gloves and the Percent Contaminated During 1½-Hour THR Cases

	Number of Holes	Contamination
Single gloves	13%	31%
Double gloves		
Outer	46%	32%
Inner	10%	39%

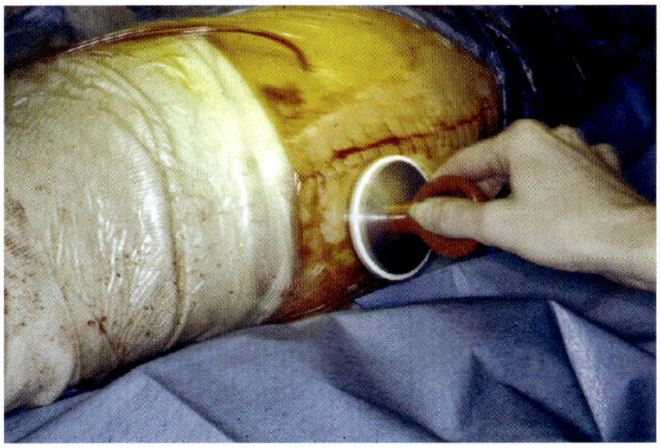

FIGURE 25-7. *Rodac sampling of a hip during surgery.*

hand and the wound are truly controlled as long as needed. There are places where an adhesive drape cannot be used (ie, face, hand, foot). These surfaces should be handled by an antiseptic spray without a detergent scrub (povidone-iodine solution or chlorhexidine).

With our present-day compounds, we should be using a 1-minute or less cleansing with alcohol foam for our hands and a 1-minute or less prep using alcohol followed by a good antiseptic adhesive drape. Times have changed, as has surgery.

The incidence of postoperative wound infections following the use of an iodophor-incorporated adhesive wound drape with a preliminary 1-minute alcohol cleanse and all operating room personnel using conventional operating room plastic gowns, hoods, masks, gloves, and a 1-minute hexachlorophene alcohol foam for the scrub was observed in 649 total hip and knee arthroplasties. Patients were followed for a minimum of 1 year for detection of an infection. An infection rate of 0.46% was noted.[34] Thus wounds need no more than an alcohol rinse and an iodophor-impregnated drape and the hands cleansed with a hexachlorophene alcohol foam before gloving.

Equipment

Knife blades are frequently disposable items. Evaluation of the bacterial contamination of these blades shows that there was no difference in contamination between the skin and deep knife blade. There was, however, less contamination of those knife blades if they were used in a laminar airflow setting versus a conventional setting (Table 25-4).[35]

Once again the environment is the source of contamination. Therefore, what effect does the environment have on the contamination of other instruments? Instruments with irregular surfaces, such as hemostats, were evaluated both in open heart and bilateral total hip replacement surgery in a conventional operating room and a horizontal laminar airflow operating room, respectively.[36]

We wanted to know what effect the scrub nurse and the environment had on the contamination of the instruments. We placed stacks of hemostats on the back instrument table and every 15 minutes for a 3-hour period of time a hemostat was placed into a jar of thioglycolate both by the scrub nurse in 10 open heart surgeries and 10 total hip surgeries (Fig. 25-8). In another series of 10 open heart surgeries and 10 total hip surgeries, sterile pickups were used to pick the instrument off the rack and place into the jar.

Tables 25-5 and 25-6 reveal that the number of contaminated hemostats were statistically reduced when laminar airflow was used (p = .001). If the scrub nurse picked the instruments up in the conventional operating room, 50% of the instruments were contaminated versus 30% if the sterile pickups were used. Spearman's correlation coefficient (0.7517) showed that the amount of contamination increased over time, especially if the scrub nurse handled the instruments.

TABLE 25-4. Microbial Contamination of Knife Blades

	Number Tested	Number Contaminated	Percentage	Probability
Skin, conventional OR	106	16	15%	
Skin, laminar airflow	102	3	3%	$p < .005$
Deep, conventional OR	165	33	20%	
Deep, laminar airflow	209	9	4%	$p < .005$

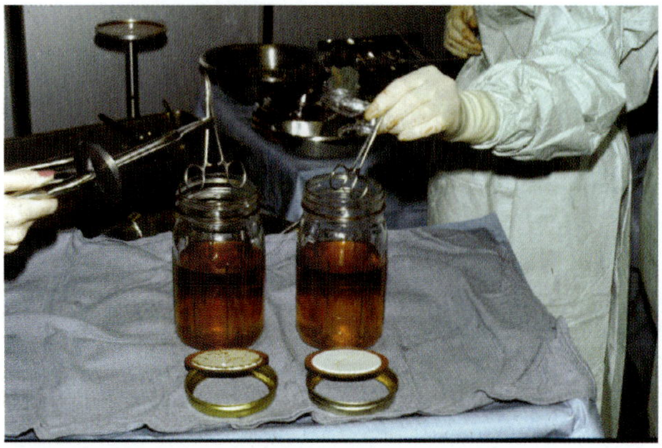

FIGURE 25-8. *Hemostat sampling in thioglycolate.*

TABLE 25-5. Average Number of Contaminated Instruments per 15 Minutes for 10 Cases (Time Tested 3 Hours)

	Conventional OR (Open Heart Surgery)	Laminar Airflow OR (Bilateral Total Hip)
Scrub nurse's gloved hands	5.33	0.92
Sterile pickups	3.58	0.49

TABLE 25-6. Average Number of Contaminated Hemostats per Case (12 Cases Sampled)

	Conventional OR (Open Heart Surgery)	Laminar Airflow OR (Bilateral Total Hip)
Scrub nurse's gloved hands	6.4	1.1
Sterile pickups	4.3	0.5

ANTIBIOTICS

An extensive discussion on the effectiveness of prophylactic antibiotics is not within the realm of this chapter. However, needless to say, it is a very important aspect of prevention of postoperative wound infections. To mention just one of many articles, Hill et al[37] showed a statistical reduction in surgical infections in a double-blinded study. Also in the ultraclean operating room evaluation by Lidwell et al,[10] there was a statistical reduction with the use of prophylactic antibiotics; however, this was not one of the variables tested.

HOST AND NUTRITION

The nutrition of the host is the most important single common denominator to the control of the onslaught of bacteria that settle into the wound. The nutritional status of the host has been evaluated[38-40] and has been shown to be a major factor.

SUMMARY

1. To prevent the problem of a postoperative wound infection, surgeons first have to evaluate the infections that their patients have developed in the past and determine the appropriate prophylactic antibiotic that will be most effective in their particular cases.
2. Some type of an environmental controlling system is needed, either laminar airflow (only if the personnel and equipment can be kept out of the path of the air), ultraviolet light, or rigid people controls. (I would be more inclined to use ultraviolet lighting.)
3. The prepping of the wound and the scrubbing of the hands are not a problem and any means of doing this is adequate. I recommend just the use of alcohol antiseptic foam for the hands and an iodophor-impregnated drape for the wounds.
4. Finally, the surgical enclosures for the scrub personnel should be some type of a plastic impermeable gown, any type of head cover, a disposable mask, and gloves; if one is a shedder, a body exhaust suit is probably necessary.

REFERENCES

1. Matar WY, Jafari SM, Restrep C, et al. Preventing infection in total joint arthroplasty. *J Bone Joint Surgery Am.* 2010:92(suppl 2):36-46.
2. Charnely J. *Low Friction Arthroplasty of the Hip: Theory and Practice.* Berlin: Springer-Verlag; 1979.

3. Eitzen HE. The effective variable human microbial shedding on the control of the contamination in surgical suites. *Proceedings of International Symposium on Contamination Control*, Sept. 1974.
4. Ritter MA, Eitzen HE, French MLV, et al. The operating room environment as affected by people and the surgical face mask. *Clin Orthop Relat Res*. 1975;111: 147-150.
5. Bethune DN. Dispersal of *Staphylococcus aureus* by patients and surgical staff. *Lancet*. 1975;1:480.
6. Mitchell NJ, Gambler DR. Clothing design for operating room personnel. *Lancet*. 1974;2(7889):1133-1136.
7. Ayliffe GA, Collins BJ, Lowbury EJ, et al. Ward floors and other surfaces as reservoirs of hospital infections. *J Hygiene (Lond)*. 1967;65(4):515-536.
8. Ritter MA, French ML. Microbiological studies in a horizontal wall-less laminar air-flow operating room during actual surgery. *Clin Orthop Relat Res*. 1973;97:16-18.
9. Ritter MA, Eitzen HE. Comparison of horizontal and vertical unidirectional (laminar) air-flow systems in orthopedic surgery. *Clin Orthop Relat Res*. 1977;129:205-208.
10. Lidwell OM, Lowbury EJ, Whyte W, et al. Effect of ultraclean air in operating rooms on deep sepsis in the joint after total hip and total knee replacement: a randomized study. *Br Med J*. 1982; 285(6334):10-14.
11. Hooper GJ, Rothwell AG, Frampton C, et al. Does the use of laminar flow and space suits reduce early deep infection after total hip and knee replacement? *J Bone Joint Surg Br*. 2011;93:85-90.
12. Salvati EA, Robinson RP, Zeno SM, et al. Infection rates after 3175 total hip and total knee replacements performed with and without a horizontal unidirectional filtered air-flow system. *J Bone Joint Surg Am*. 1982;64(4):525-535.
13. Berg-Perier M. *Ultraviolet Light in Operating Rooms*. Goteborg, Germany: Kompendietryckeriet-Kallered; 1992:1-92.
14. Ritter MA, Bradburn NC, French M. Does style make the difference? Reprinted from the *Surgical Team*, July/August 1973. Copyright 1973 by McMahon Publishing Company.
15. Alford DJ, Ritter MA, French ML, et al. The operating room gown as a barrier to bacterial shedding. *Am J Surg*. 1973;125:589-591.
16. Ritter MA, Eitzen HE, Hart JB, et al. The surgeon's garb. *Clin Orthop Relat Res*. 1980;153:204-209.
17. Letts RM, Doermer E. Conversation in the operating theater as a cause of airborne bacterial contamination. *J Bone Joint Surg Am*. 1983;65(3):357-362.
18. Ritter MA, Sieber JM, Carlson SR. Street shoes vs surgical footwear in the operating room. *Infect Surg*. 1984;3(1):81-83.
19. Ulrich JA. Microbiology of surgery suites. *Symposium on Clean Room Technology in Surgery Suites*. 1971:12-17.
20. Aly R, Maibach HI. Aerobic microbial flora of intertriginous skin. *Appl Environ Microbiol*. 1977;33(1): 97-100.
21. Price PB. The bacteriology of normal skin: a new quantitative test applied to a study of the bacterial flora and the disinfectant action of mechanical cleansing. *J Infect Dis*. 1983;62(63):301-318.
22. Tucci VJ, Stone AM, Thompson C, et al. Studies of the surgical scrub. *Surg Gynecol Obstet*. 1977;145(3): 415-416.
23. Lowbury EJ, Lilly HA. Gloved hand as applicator of antiseptic to operation sites. *Lancet*. 1975;2(7926): 153-156.
24. Eitzen HE, Ritter MA, French MLC, et al. A microbiological in-use comparison of surgical hand-washing agents. *J Bone Joint Surg Am*. 1979;61(3):403-406.
25. Price PB. Ethyl alcohol as a germicide. *Arch Surg*. 1983;38:528-542.
26. Dewar NE, Gravens DL. Effectiveness of septisol antiseptic foam as a surgical scrub agent. *Appl Microbiol*. 1973;26(4):544-549.
27. Gravens DL, Butcher HR, Ballinger WF, et al. Septisol antiseptic foam for hands of operating room personnel: an effective antibacterial agent. *Surgery*. 1973;73(3):360-367.
28. Peterson AF, Roseberg A, Alatary SD. Comparative evaluation of surgical scrub preparations. *Surg Gynecol Obstet*. 1978;146(1):63-65.
29. Ritter MA, French ML, Eitzen HE, et al. The antimicrobial effectiveness of operative-site preparative agents. *J Bone Joint Surg Am*. 1980;62:826-828.
30. Zdeblick TA, Lederman MM, Jacobs MR, et al. Preoperative use of povidone-iodine: a prospective, randomized study. *Clin Orthop Relat Res*. 1986;213:211-215.
31. Ritter MA, French ML, Eitzen HE. Evaluation of microbial contamination of surgical gloves during actual use. *Clin Orthop Relat Res*. 1976;117:103-106.
32. French MLV, Eitzen HE, Ritter MA. The plastic surgical adhesive drape: an evaluation of its efficacy as a microbial barrier. *Ann Surg*. 1976;184(1):46-50.

33. Alexander JW, Aerni S, Plettner JP. Development of a safe and effective one-minute preoperative skin preparation. *Arch Surg*. 1985;120(12):1357-1361.
34. Ritter MA, Campbell ED. Retrospective evaluation of an Iodophor-incorporated antimicrobial plastic adhesive wound drape. *Clin Orthop Relat Res*. 1988;228: 307-308.
35. Ritter MA, French ML, Eitzen HE. Bacterial contamination of the surgical knife. *Clin Orthop Relat Res*. 1975;108:158-160.
36. Ritter MA, Eitzen HE, French ML, et al. The effect that time, touch and environment have upon bacterial contamination of instruments during surgery. *Ann Surg*. 1976;184(5):642-644.
37. Doyon F, Evrard J, Mazas F, et al. Long-term results of prophylactic cefazolin versus placebo in total hip replacement. *Lancet*. 1987;1(8537):860.
38. Gherini ST, Vaughn BK, Mallory TH. Nutritional deficiencies and wound healing complications after total hip arthroplasty. *AAOS Final Program Manual*. 1990:92.
39. Jensen JE, Jensen TG, Smith TK, et al. Nutrition in orthopaedic surgery. *J Bone Joint Surg Am*. 1982;64: 1263-1272.
40. Jevsevar DS, Karlin LI. The relationship between preoperative nutritional status and complications after an operation for scoliosis in patients who have cerebral palsy. *J Bone Joint Surg Am*. 1993;75(6):880-884.

26 Screening for Methicillin-Resistant *Staphylococcus aureus* in Total Knee Arthroplasty

James C. Kudrna

Some 90 years ago, Moynihan[1] summarized the problem of surgical infections with the statement that "every operation in surgery is an experiment in bacteriology." Prevention of perioperative infection requires meticulous detail to a multitude of factors, some of which are modifiable and others that are not. In the era of evidence-based medicine, it is in the best interest of patients and physicians to follow accepted practices backed by basic science and adequate clinical data. Several articles have provided evidence-based guidelines regarding the use of perioperative antibiotics for elective and emergent orthopedic surgical procedures, preoperative skin preparation, wound closure, the use of drains and dressings, and other guidelines to assist in minimizing or preventing the risk of perioperative surgical site infections.[2] Modifiable risk factors, such as disease state, nutritional status, medications, immunosuppression, use of tobacco and alcohol, and obesity must also be optimized to minimize the infection risk. Several excellent reviews discuss these topics in detail.[3-5]

Surgical site infections following total knee arthroplasty remain devastating complications and are the most frequently reported reason for revision procedures.[6] Infection following total knee arthroplasty decreases quality of life, increases hospital length of stay, increases hospital charges, and more than doubles the risk of readmission. The percentage of patients who develop an infection following primary total knee arthroplasty remains in the range of 0.4% to 2.0%.[6-9] Medicare data reveal the rate of periprosthetic infection within the first 2 years after knee arthroplasty at 1.55%.[10,11] Infection rates in the 2- to 10-year period after knee arthroplasty are an additional 0.46%.[6] *Staphylococcus aureus* accounts for the majority of periprosthetic knee infections, with the prevalence of methicillin-resistant *Staphylococcus aureus* (MRSA) increasing and especially difficult to eradicate.[12-14] The goal of the surgical team should be to minimize the risk of these events. Prosthetic infections increase morbidity, mortality, and poor outcome for the affected patient. In the current health care environment, perioperative complications, such as infection, are being interpreted as "never-events" and are increasingly considered for nonreimbursement. Governmental and nongovernmental agencies continue to monitor these events, measure their impact on our health care system, and develop strategies to minimize their incidence.[15] The financial impact of diagnosis and treatment for these infections many times far exceeds the cost of primary knee arthroplasty, with estimates ranging from $35,000 to $90,000.[16] Any and all strategies to minimize the risk of infection should be undertaken in the preparation of patients for total knee arthroplasty procedures, with special emphasis on *Staphylococcus aureus* infection prevention.

STAPHYLOCOCCI

Staphylococci, commonly referred to as staph, are gram-positive spherical bacteria that appear microscopically in clusters resembling grapes. They are commonly cultured from the nares and skin of humans. Rosenbach in 1884 described the two pigmented types of staphylococci and proposed the nomenclature of *Staphylococcus aureus*, yellow in color, and *Staphylococcus albus,* a white species.[17] *Stapylococcus albus* is now commonly known as *Staphylococcus epidermidis*. Although in excess of 20 species of staph have been described, *S. aureus* and *S. epidermidis* are important as far as humans are concerned.[17,18] *S. aureus* colonizes primarily in the nares and on the skin, but is also found in the gastrointestinal tract and oral cavity. *S. epidermidis* is unique in colonization on the skin.

S. aureus forms large yellow colonies on rich medium, whereas *S. epidermidis* develops a relatively small white colony. *S. aureus* is often hemolytic on blood agar, whereas *S. epidermidis* is nonhemolytic. Staphylococci are facultative anaerobes that grow by aerobic respiration or by fermentation that yields primarily lactic acid. Staphylococci are catalase positive and oxidase negative.[17] *S. aureus* are capable of growing at temperatures of 15°C to 45°C and in high saline concentrations, in some species exceeding 15%. *S. epidemidis* lack the enzyme coagulase, whereas *S. aureus* strains routinely produce coagulase.[17] Most strains of *S. epidermidis* are nonpathogenic and may even play a protective role in humans, behaving as normal flora. On the contrary, *S. aureus* strains should always be considered pathogenic in humans.[19] The shape and configuration of the gram-positive cocci helps to distinguish staph species from streptococci. Streptococci are slightly oblong cells, usually appear in chains, and are catalase negative, while staphylocci are catalase producers.

Over 25% of the humans are long-term *S. aureus* nasal carriers.[20] The high incidence of *S. aureus* infections is thought to arise from the carotenoid pigment, staphyloxanthin, which is responsible for the characteristic color of the *S. aureus* colonies.[21,22] The pigment acts as a virulence factor, with an antioxidant action that helps the microbe evade death by reactive oxygen species used by the host immune system.

MRSA bacteria were once confined to health care environments, such as hospitals and extended care facilities, and patients who frequented these facilities. Since the mid-1990s, there has been a dramatic increase in the number of MRSA infections reported in humans with low exposure to the health care system. This increased incidence of MRSA infection rates has led to the recognition of new MRSA clones, which are now known as community-associated MRSA (CA-MRSA).[23-25] CA-MRSA strains differ in many ways from the older health care-associated MRSA (HA-MRSA) strains. They infect different populations, spreading among healthy younger populations, throughout the community setting, and to a lesser degree in health care environments. They have been associated with severe clinical syndromes such as necrotizing pneumonia and severe sepsis, as well as surgical site infections.[26,27] HA-MRSA has been isolated largely from an elderly population, usually with one or more comorbid health conditions and with a history of exposure to the health care environment. These strains tend to cause pneumonia, bacteremia, and invasive infections. The antimicrobial susceptibility patterns of CA-MRSA and HA-MRSA clones have resistance to all penicillins and other β-lactam and some non-β-lactam antimicrobial drugs. Statistical analysis of annual outpatient and emergency room visits between 1997 and 2005 in the United States for cellulitis or abscesses nearly doubled from 17.3 to 32.5 cases per 1000 population, with CA-MRSA isolates largely responsible for this dramatic increase.[28] The emergence of new strains of CA-MRSA has important implications, since large reservoirs of these bacteria now exist outside health care facilities. Control and containment of MRSA-related infections using currently accepted practices utilized in the health care facility setting is unlikely to be successful unless a community-based effort at eradication is developed. The emergence of some nine vancomycin-resistant strains of MRSA[29] represents a further threat to the control of these infections. Clinical reliance on vancomycin as the drug of choice against MRSA may not be possible in the near future. A program to control the spread of all MRSA clones and prevent infections in the total joint arthroplasty patient is especially important.

RISK FACTORS CONTRIBUTING TO SURGICAL SITE INFECTION

Effective prevention of surgical site infections requires consideration of preoperative, intraoperative, and postoperative factors that contribute to infection. The purpose of this discussion is to concentrate on the preoperative diagnosis and treatment of nasal contamination with staphylococci to minimize the risk of *S. aureus* and MRSA total knee infections. First, it is necessary to identify the high-risk patient undergoing knee arthroplasty. Once identified, proper strategies and patient counseling can be undertaken to develop reasonable expectations of surgical risks and to further minimize these risks with proper medical interventions.

Past history of joint infection and previous corticosteroid joint injection increase the risk of surgical site infection and cannot be eliminated.[30] Numerous other factors that increase infection risk can be modified or minimized with appropriate intervention and patient cooperation.

Included in these are obesity, smoking, alcoholism, diabetes, sickle cell disease, human immunodeficiency virus, rheumatoid or inflammatory arthritis, dental disease, chronic urinary tract infections, chemotherapeutic agents, medications, and malnutrition. Numerous literature citations document these factors as increasing surgical risk for surgical site infection.[15,31] Optimal control of these medical conditions can minimize risk of infection and enhance surgical outcomes. Identification of those patients who are known *S. aureus* nasal carriers and proper decolonization to eliminate carrier status can potentially decrease the risk of surgical site infections as well. Proper identification of risk factors and implementation of evidence-based medical interventions minimize surgical site infection risk.

MUPIROCIN

Mupirocin remains the drug of choice for nasal decolonization of contaminated patients, with very few strains of MRSA showing resistance. Also known as Bactroban or Centany, mupirocin is an antibiotic originally isolated from *Pseudomonas fluorescens* by Beecham.[32] It is bacteriostatic at low concentrations and bactericidal at high concentrations. It is used topically and remains very effective against numerous gram-positive organisms, including staphylococci. Mupirocin is a mixture of several pseudomonic acids, with pseudomonic acid A constituting greater than 90% of the mixture. Pseudomonic acids B, C, and D, each with similar chemical structure, are the other constituents.[33]

Mupirocin strongly inhibits protein and RNA synthesis in *S. aureus* and also effects DNA synthesis and cell wall formation.[33] It is used in topical form for treatment of skin infections, such as furuncles, impetigo, and open infected superficial wounds. It remains very effective against MRSA, however, it should not be used for extended periods of time, or indiscriminately, because resistance does develop and could, if it becomes widespread, destroy mupirocin's value as a treatment for MRSA. It may also contribute to the overgrowth of nonsusceptible organisms. Shortly after the clinical use of mupirocin began, some resistant strains of *S. aureus* emerged.[34]

Two distinct types were identified, one with low-level resistance and the other with high-level resistance. Other antibiotic agents such as azelaic acid, nitrofurazone, silver sulfadiazine, and ramolanin have known efficacy against the resistant strains.[35] In due time, other resistant strains will no doubt appear. Mupirocin, originally introduced by GlaxoSmithKline in 1985 under the name Bactroban, is now available in generic form. Ortho-McNeil Pharmaceutical currently markets Centany and Teva Pharmaceutical produces mupirocin ointment.

COLONIZATION WITH STAPHYLOCOCCUS

The prevalence of *S. aureus* as a cause of surgical site infections in joint arthroplasty continues to increase with it being the only cause of increasing preoperative infections between 2000 and 2005 in a recent multicenter study.[36] During this time period, MRSA incidence nearly doubled.[36] Molecular DNA analysis of *S. aureus* isolates causing surgical site infections reveals a majority of the infection strains are part of the patient's resident normal nasal flora. Perl and colleagues report this rate as high as 84.6%.[37] Thus a reasonable approach to decrease postoperative *S. aureus* surgical site infection involves eliminating *S. aureus* nasal carriage from the patient before surgical intervention. This strategy was investigated by Kalmeijer and colleagues in a group of orthopedic patients undergoing hip, knee, or spinal prosthetic implantation in the Netherlands.[38] Their study showed that decolonization with mupirocin ointment beginning 5 days before surgery decreased endogenous *S. aureus* infections 5-fold as compared to patients receiving a placebo, but the results were not statistically significant due to the small sample size of their investigation. Hacek et al,[39] in a study of 1079 hip and knee arthroplasty patients, showed a 4-fold decrease in surgical site infection with *S. aureus* for patients colonized with the bacteria and decolonized preoperatively. A prospective cohort study by Rao et al,[13] involving both hip and knee procedures, revealed a similar decreased incidence of surgical site infections. A single treatment course of intranasal mupirocin was found to be effective in reducing nasal *S. aureus* carriage for up to 1 year.[40] Hand carriage of the bacteria was also significantly decreased 6 months after therapy, further implicating the nares as the primary reservoir for hand carriage. Based on these and other reports,[13,19,41] a program to decrease the nasal carriage of *S. aureus* before surgical intervention should effectively reduce the incidence of surgical site infections.

Major questions to answer when considering a decolonization program in knee arthroplasty are: Is *S. aureus* the major cause of postoperative infection in the knee arthroplasty patient in your practice? Will a program of preoperative surveillance for *S. aureus* carriage followed by decolonization of those patients found to be positive meaningfully reduce the incidence of surgical site infection? Instituting a diagnostic and *S. aureus* decolonization program for the prospective total knee patient involves the confirmation of a molecular diagnostic assay as a rapid and reproducible test for detection, which can be performed at a reasonable cost. The real-time polymerase chain reaction (PCR)[39] procedure has been identified as a rapid, highly specific, and accurate test to determine the presence of *S. aureus* in nasal swabs. A program to reproducibly obtain nasal swabs from the preoperative patient, perform PCR testing, and treatment for those patients colonized with *S. aureus* remains a valuable and proven method to reduce surgical site infection rates. The cost of a screening program is reported to be less than $50 US.[39]

SCREENING TECHNIQUE AND TREATMENT

Patient screening for *S. aureus* carriage should be performed 2 to 4 weeks before scheduled knee arthroplasty. Nasal samples may be collected during the same visit as other scheduled preoperative tests, autologous blood donation, or educational programs. Samples are collected using premoistened, double-headed rayon-tipped swabs (Fig. 26-1). The swabs are premoistened with the Amies liquid media in the sponge at the bottom of the collection tube by simply inserting the swabs into the tube and holding for 5 seconds. During sample collection, the swabs are inserted as a pair into one nostril and then the other so that both nares are sampled with both swabs. The inside circumference of each anterior nare is rubbed for 3 to 5 seconds to obtain adequate sampling. One swab is used to perform the test using real-time PCR method for the detection of the *femA* gene unique to *S. aureus*. The second swab is used to culture the organism whenever the PCR test is positive in order to perform susceptibility testing to detect methicillin resistance and to detect the *ile*S-2 gene for demonstrating high-level mupirocin resistance. Patients with a positive nasal screen test are treated with mupirocin ointment twice daily for 5 days before surgery, with the last dose being administered the night before or the morning of surgery. Daily bathing with chlorhexidine for 5 days immediately before surgery is also recommended. At the time of hospital admission for surgery, patients are assessed for compliance and safety by whether they had complied with the decolonization program and bathing directions and whether any adverse reactions had resulted. Standard prophylactic antibiotics include 2 g of cephazolin administered within 1 hour of surgery. In cases of type 1 penicillin allergy, past history of MRSA infection, or positive MRSA nares screening, 1 g of vancomycin within 1 hour of surgery is recommended. Antibiotic prophylaxis is recommended for 24 hours postoperatively unless other circumstances require longer treatment.

Reported results with molecular diagnostic assay and decolonization have indicated a decreased incidence of *S. aureus* surgical site infections. Hacek et al[39] studied 1495 hip and knee arthroplasty patients, with screening of 912 patients, 24.5% (223) were found to be positive with *S. aureus*. In a similar study, Rao et al[19] followed 1285 hip and knee arthroplasty patients with a 25% (321) incidence of nasal carriage. Decolonization resulted in no infections in the intervention group of 321 patients over a 2-year surveillance period. From these and other studies, it can be concluded that one in four patients undergoing major total joint arthroplasty is an asymptomatic staphylococcal carrier and remains at risk for a surgical site infection.

The prevalence of *S. aureus* colonization in orthopaedic surgeons and orthopaedic surgery residents, who are in close contact with arthroplasty patients, is also of concern in the overall attempt to minimize surgical site infection. Schwarzkopf et al[42] reported on results of nasal swab cultures in 74 orthopaedic attending surgeons and 61 orthopaedic surgery residents. Of the 135 physicians, 1.5% were positive for MRSA and 35.7% were positive for methicillin-sensitive *S. aureus* (MSSA). None of the residents were MRSA positive, but 59% were MSSA positive. Of the orthopaedic attending surgeons, 2.7% were MRSA positive and 23.3% were MSSA positive. In a cohort of high-risk patients, including those undergoing joint replacement, 2.1% demonstrated nasal carriage of MRSA and 18% MSSA. The incidence of MSSA colonization in the surgeon population was greater (35.7%) than in the high-risk patient group (18%) ($p < .01$). The significance of colonization in health care providers and the impact on the incidence of surgical site infections remains unknown. Broad screening programs, including all personnel in contact with patients, at institutions performing large volumes of joint replacement may assist in determining the incidence of nasal colonization and the scope of decolonization necessary to minimize patient risk of infection. Manian[43] reported on the asymptomatic nasal carriage of mupirocin-resistant *S. aureus* and MRSA in a pet dog, which was associated with MRSA infections in household contacts. Culture of nares samples from the family dog grew mupirocin-resistant. MRSA that had a pulsed-field gel electrophoresis chromosomal pattern identical to the MRSA isolated from the patient's nares and his wife's nares. Further recurrence of MRSA infection and nasal colonization in the couple was prevented only after successful eradication of MRSA from the family dog's nares. Isolation of surgical wounds from family pets may also decrease risk of infection.

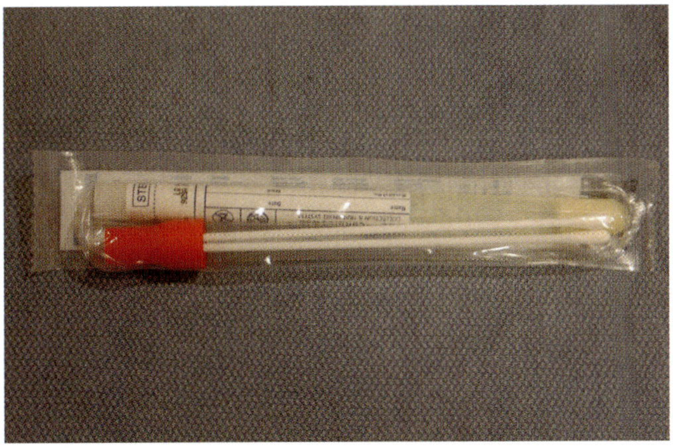

1. Open packet. Discard white cap from collection tube.

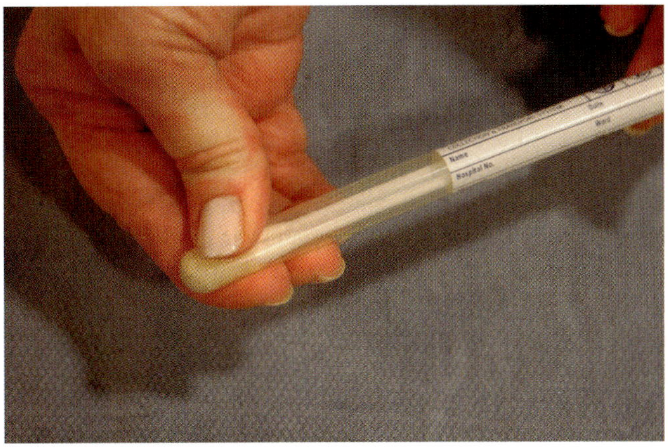

2. Moisten paired swabs before collecting sample by inserting swabs into collection tube for 5 seconds.

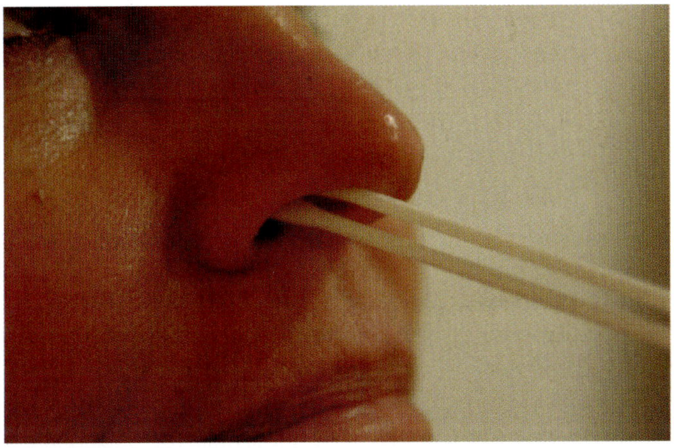

3. Insert paired swabs 1/2 inch into nostril. Rotate swabs against inside of nostril for 3 seconds. Repeat for other nostril with same paired swabs.

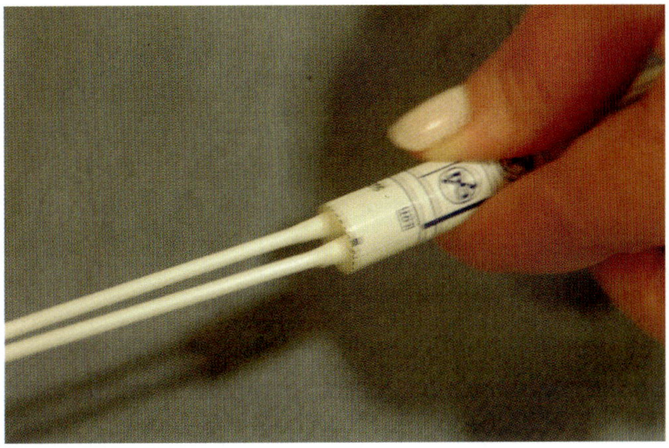

4. Return swabs in collection tube.

FIGURE 26-1. *Technique for collection of nasal specimen.*

SUMMARY

The single greatest risk factor for developing a *S. aureus* surgical site infection in hip or knee replacement surgery is a high-density nasal carriage of *S. aureus*.[20] A subsequent study[38] suggested the primary source of post-operative *S. aureus* infection is the patient's own strain of *S. aureus*, usually carried in the anterior nares. The rate of endogenous infection with *S. aureus* was 5-fold lower in a group of patients receiving recommended doses of mupirocin ointment versus a group receiving a placebo.[38] A more recent investigation reported that 9.5% of prosthetic hip or knee surgeries in a 13-month period were infected, and 89% of these infections were caused by *S. aureus*.[44] This high rate of infection resulted in the interruption of their orthopaedic surgery program until the problem could be resolved. In this group, 56% of the *S. aureus* isolates were MRSA that exhibited the community-associated phenotype (CA-MRSA) strains that are rising in prevalence across the United States.

The interest in performing *S. aureus* decolonization before major surgery has been growing during the past decade. In 1996 an unblended intervention trial using mupirocin for nasal decolonization of all patients (no surveillance for *S. aureus* was performed) undergoing major cardiothoracic surgery reported a reduction of surgical site infection in an intervention group compared to historical controls.[45] Subsequently, another study revealed similar benefit from *S. aureus* nasal decolonization in prevention of sternal wound infection for 1846 diabetic and nondiabetic patients undergoing cardiac surgery.[46] More recently, an intervention in the setting of hyperendemic MRSA colonization (point prevalence for MRSA carriage = 38%) and subsequent MRSA infection on four orthopaedic surgery wards reported a reduction in MRSA infection by using universal mupirocin decolonization and preoperative 2% triclosan bathing.[47] Other reports support the approach by suggesting preoperative surveillance for *S. aureus* to limit the unnecessary use of muporicin.[48,49] Surveillance cultures of anterior nares in those about to undergo cardiothoracic surgery were followed by mupirocin prophylaxis for all patients.[49] When the cultures were completed (at 48 hours), it was possible to discontinue muporicin therapy in 79% of their patients and limit unnecessary mupirocin treatment to 2 days. Using this strategy, a reduction of *S. aureus* surgical site infections from 1.68% to 0.37% over an 18-month period was realized.[49] Hacek et al has extended this approach by demonstrating the utility of rapid, real-time PCR molecular diagnostic testing for a preoperative surveillance purpose.[39]

A nasal screening and decolonization program for *S. aureus* before major hip and knee joint replacement surgery has resulted in a 4-fold or greater decrease in *S. aureus* surgical site infections for patients colonized with *S. aureus*.[39] This represents a very favorable outcome. A simple specimen collection technique combined with a currently available molecular microbiology test leading to focused treatment consisting of a 5-day course of nasal mupirocin preoperatively appears to prevent postsurgical infections with *S. aureus*. This protocol can be considered as a routine addition to any presurgical testing protocol and have a significant impact on infection eradication in total knee arthroplasty at a very low cost.

REFERENCES

1. Moynihan B. The ritual of a surgical operation. *Br J Surg.* 1920;8:27-35.
2. Meehan J, Jamali A, Nguyen H. Prophylactic antibiotics in hip and knee arthroplasty. *J Bone Joint Surg Am.* 2009;91(10):2480-2490.
3. Moucha C, Clyburn T, Evans R, et al. Modifiable risk factors for surgical site infection. *J Bone Joint Surg Am.* 2011;93:398-404.
4. Evans R. American Academy of Orthopaedic Surgeons Patient Safety Committee, Surgical site infection and control: an emerging paradigm. *J Bone Joint Surg Am.* 2009;91(Suppl 6):2-9.
5. Poss R, Thornhill TS, Ewald FC, et al. Factors influencing the incidence and outcome of infection following total joint arthroplasty. *Clin Orthop Relat Res.* 1984;182:117-126.
6. Garvin KL, Konigsberg B. Infection following total knee arthroplasty. *J Bone Joint Surg Am.* 2011;93: 1167-1175.
7. Mahomed N, Barrett J, Katz J, et al. Epidemiology of total knee replacement in the United States Medicare population. *J Bone Joint Surg Am.* 2005;87:1222-1228.
8. Wilson M, Kelley K, Thornhill T. Infection as a complication of total knee replacement arthroplasty. *J Bone Joint Surg Am.* 1990;72:878-883.
9. Windsor R, Bono J. Infected total knee replacements. *J Am Acad Orthop Surg.* 1994;2:44-53.
10. Bozic K, Kurtz S, Lau E, et al. The epidemiology of revision total knee arthroplasty in the United States. *Clin Orthop Relat Res.* 2010;468:45-51.
11. Kurtz S, Ong K, Lau E, et al. Prosthetic joint infection risk after TKA in the Medicare population. *Clin Orthop Relat Res.* 2010;468:52-56.
12. Ayers DC, Dennis DA, Johanson NA, et al. Instructional Course Lectures, the American Academy of Orthopaedic Surgeons–Common complications of total knee arthroplasty in the United States. *J Bone Joint Surg.* 1997;79:278-311.
13. Rao N, Cannella B, Crossett LS, et al. A preoperative decolonization protocol for *Staphylococcus aureus* prevents orthopaedic infections. *Clin Orthop Relat Res.* 2008;406(1):343-348.
14. Fulkerson E, Valle C, Wise B, et al. Antibiotic susceptibility of bacteria infection total joint arthroplasty sites. *J Bone Joint Surg Am.* 2006;88:1231-1237.
15. Boscoe JA, Slover J, Haas J. Perioperative strategies for decreasing infection. *J Bone Joint Surg Am.* 2010; 92:232-239.
16. Parvizi J, Pawasarat I, Azzam K, et al. Periprosthetic joint infection. The economic impact of methicillin-resistant infections. *J Arthroplasty.* 2010;25(6 suppl): 103-107.

17. Todar K. *Staphylococcus aureus* and staphylococcal disease. In: Todar K, ed. *Todar's Textbook of Bacteriology.* Vol 1. Madison, WI; 2009:18-22.
18. Maverakis N, Wiley B. Evidence for a multiplicity of capsular types among *Staphylococcus aureus* strains. *J Bacteriol.* 1969;99(2):472-479.
19. Rao N, Cannella B, Crosserr L, et al. Preoperative screening/decolonization for *Staphylococcus aureus* to prevent orthopedic surgical site infection. *J Arthroplasty.* 2011;26(8):1501-1507.
20. Kalmeijer M, Coertjens H, van Nieuwland-Bollen P, et al. Nasal carriage of *Staphylococcus aureus* is a major risk factor for surgical site infections in orthopedic surgery. *Infect Control Hosp Epidemiol.* 2000;21:319-323.
21. Pelz A, Wieland K, Putzbach K, et al. Structure and biosynthesis of staphyloxanthin from *Staphylococcus aureus. J Biol Chem.* 2005;280(37):32493-32498.
22. Clauditz A, Resch A, Wieland K, et al. Staphyloxanthin plays a role in the fitness of *Staphylococcus aureus* and its ability to cope with oxidative stress. *Infect Immun.* 2006;74(8):4950-4953.
23. Adcock P, Pastor P, Medley F, et al. Methicillin-resistant *Staphylococcus aureus* in two childcare centers. *J Infect Dis.* 1998;178:577-580.
24. Fridkin S, Hageman J, Morrison M, et al. Methicillin-resistant *Staphylococcus aureus* in three communities. *N Engl J Med.* 2005;352:1436-1444.
25. Dufour P, Gillet Y, Bes M, et al. Community-acquired methicillin-resistant *Staphylococcus aureus* infections in France: emergence of a single clone that produces Panton-Valentine leukocidin. *Clin Infec Dis.* 2002;35:819-824.
26. Buckingham S, McDougal L, Cathey L, et al. Emergence of community-acquired methicillin-resistant *Staphylococcus aureus* at a Memphis Tennessee children's hospital. *Pediatr Infect Dis J.* 2004;23:619-624.
27. Munckhof W, Nimmo G, Carney J, et al. Methicillin-susceptible, non-multidrug-resistant and multidrug-resistant methicillin-resistant *Staphylococcus aureus* infections: a clinical, epidemiological and microbiological comparative study. *Eur J Clin Microbiol Infect Dis.* 2008;27:355-364.
28. Hersh A, Chambers H, Maselli J, et al. National rends in ambulatory visits and antibiotic prescribing for skin and soft tissue infections. *Arch Intern Med.* 2008; 168:1585-1591.
29. Chang S, Sievert D, Hageman J, et al. Infection with vancomycin-resistant *Staphylococcus aureus* containing the vanA resistance gene. *N Engl J Med.* 2003;348:1342-1347.
30. Jerry G, Rand J, Ilstrup D. Old sepsis prior to total knee arthroplasty. *Clin Orthop Relat Res.* 1988;236: 135-140.
31. Fletcher N, Sofianos D, Berkes M, Obremskey W. Prevention of perioperative infection current concepts review. *J Bone Joint Surg Am.* 2007;89:1605-1618.
32. Fuller A, Mellows G, Woolford M, et al. Pseudomonic acid: an antibiotic produced by Pseudomonas fluorescens. *Nature.* 1971;234(5329):416-417.
33. Hughes J, Mellows G. On the mode of action of pseudomonic acid: inhibition of protein synthesis in *Staphylococcus aureus. J Antibiot.* 1978;31(4):330-335.
34. Cookson B. The emergence of mupirocin-resistance: a challenge to infection control and antibiotic prscribing practice. *J Antimicrob Chemother.* 1998;41 (1):11-18.
35. Tanaka K, Tamaki M, Watanabe S. Effect of furanomycin on the synthesis of isoleucyl-tRNA. *Biochim Biophys Acta.* 1969;195(1):244-245.
36. Anderson D, Sexton D, Kanafani Z, et al. Severe surgical site infection in community hospitals: epidemiology, key procedures, and the changing prevalence of methicillin-resistant *Staphylococcus aureus. Infect Control Hosp Epidemiol.* 2007;28: 1047-1053.
37. Perl T, Cullen J, Wenzel R, et al. Intranasal mupirocin to prevent postoperative *Staphylococcus aureus* infections. *N Engl J Med.* 2002;346:1871-1877.
38. Kalmeijer M, Coertjens H, van Nieuwland-Bollen P, et al. Surgical site infections in orthopaedic surgery: the efect of mupirocin nasal ointment in a double-blind, randomized, placebo controlled study. *Clin Infect Dis.* 2002;35:353-358.
39. Hacek D, Robb W, Paule S, et al. *Staphylococcus aureus* nasal decolonization in joint replacement surgery reduces infection. *Clin Orthop Relat Res.* 2008; 466:1349-1355.
40. Doebbeling B, Reagan D, Pfaller M, et al. Long-term efficacy of intranasal ointment. A prospective cohort study of *Staphylococcus aureus* carriage. *Arch Intern Med.* 1994;154:1505-1508.
41. Slover J, Haas J, Quirno M, et al. Cost-effectiveness of *Staphylococcus aureus* screening and decolonization program for high-risk orthopaedic patients. *J Arthroplasty.* 2011;26(3):360-366.
42. Schwarzkopf R, Richelle M, Takemoto C, et al. Prevalence of *Staphylococcus aureus* colonization in

orthopaedic surgeons and their patients. *J Bone Joint Surg Am.* 2010;92:1815-1826.

43. Manian F. Asymptomatic nasal carriage of mupirocin-resistant, methicillin-resistant *Staphylococcus aureus* (MRSA) in a pet dog associated with MRSA infection in household contacts. *Clin Infect Dis.* 2003;36:e26-e28.

44. Kourbatova E, Halvosa J, King M, et al. Emergence of community-associated methicillin-resistant *Staphylococcus aureus* USA 300 clone as a cause of health care-associated infections among patients with prosthetic joint infections. *Am J Infect Control.* 2005; 33:385-391.

45. Kluytmans J, Mouton J, VandenBergh M, et al. Reduction of surgical-site infections in cardiothoracic surgery by elimination of nasal carriage of *Staphylococcus aureus*. *Infect Control Hosp Epidemiol.* 1996; 17:780-785.

46. Cimochowski G, Harostock M, Brown B, et al. Intranasal mupirocin reduces sternal wound infection after open heart surgery in diabetics and nondiabetics. *Ann Thorac Surg.* 2001;71:1572-1579.

47. Wilcox M, Hall J, Pike H, et al. Use of peroperative mupirocin to prevent methicillin-resistant *Staphylococcus aureus* (MRSA) orthopaedic surgical site infections. *J Hosp Infect.* 2003;54:196-201.

48. Kluytmans J, Wertheim H. Nasal carriage of *Staphylococcus aureus* and prevention of nosocomial infections. *Infection.* 2005;33:3-8.

49. Nicholson M, Huseman L. Controlling the usage of intranasal mupirocin does impact the rate of *Staphylococcus aureus* deep sternal wound infections is cardiac surgery patients. *Am J Infect Control.* 2006; 34:44-48.

27

Perioperative Pain Management for Total Knee Arthroplasty

Kishor Gandhi, Jaime L. Baratta, and Eugene R. Viscusi

Postoperative pain control after total knee arthroplasty (TKA) can be challenging. A large percentage of patients consider postoperative pain control after surgery a major concern.[1-3] Inadequate control of pain in the perioperative period has been linked to adverse events, including myocardial ischemia and infarction, impaired pulmonary function, paralytic ileus, urinary retention, thromboembolism, impaired immune functions, and anxiety.[3] Aside from decreased patient satisfaction, persistent pain may impair patient rehabilitation, which is necessary for regaining muscle strength and functional status. A study examining the implications of early inpatient rehabilitation after elective joint arthroplasty in elderly patients with two or more comorbid conditions demonstrated shorter length of stay and faster attainment of functional milestones despite the comorbidities.[4] Rehabilitation is optimally achieved when an effective method of pain control is employed during the recovery process. This chapter discusses the various analgesic options for perioperative pain management after TKA.

MULTIMODAL ANALGESIA

Until the advent of neuraxial and regional anesthesia, opioids were the mainstay of treatment for moderate to severe acute pain. Opioids can cause a number of side effects, such as pruritus, nausea and vomiting, constipation, urinary retention, sedation, and respiratory depression. Opioids may not be ideal for patients requiring physical therapy since excessive sedation may impede therapy. Opioids may also inadequately control pain during movement.

The concept of multimodal pain management was introduced in the 1990s to reduce the reliance on opioid-based therapy.[5] This concept (multimodal analgesia) utilizes a combination of techniques and drugs that target different parts of the nociceptive pathway during the perioperative period (Fig. 27-1). The available modalities include neuraxial analgesia, peripheral nerve blockade, nonopioids [nonsteroidal anti-inflammatory drugs (NSAIDs), cyclooxygenase-2 (COX-2) selective inhibitors, acetaminophen, and antineuropathic drugs], and opioids. Extensive research has demonstrated the efficacy of multimodal analgesia in reducing perioperative pain.

PREEMPTIVE ANALGESIA

The success of multimodal pain management depends on preemptive administration of anti-inflammatory, antineuropathic, and analgesic regimens provided they are administered before the surgical insult. The aim of preemptive analgesia, as part of multimodal analgesia, is to limit sensitization of the peripheral and central nervous systems during

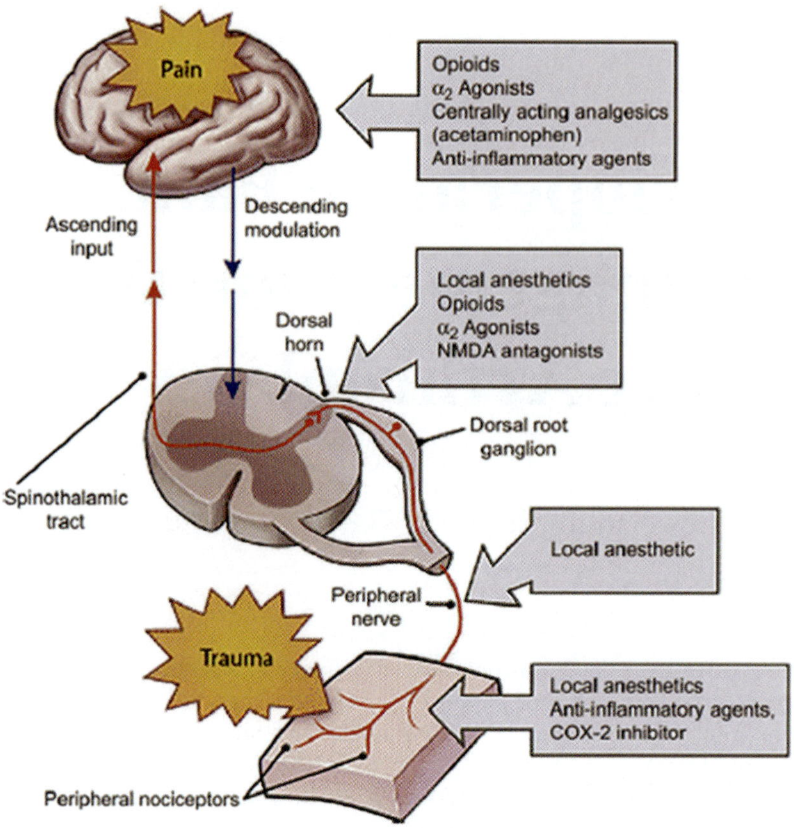

FIGURE 27-1. *Multimodal pain management pathway. (Modified with permission.[5])*

the perioperative period.[6] Sensitization or "windup" phenomenon may subsequently cause increased pain following surgery. The windup phenomenon can be reduced with initiation of pharmacological interventions before the operation. Currently, at the authors' institution, patients receive a preoperative regimen of acetaminophen, celecoxib, and pregablin, 1 to 2 hours before surgery and continued postoperatively (Table 27-1). These agents may be omitted if there are any contraindications to their use. Caution should be used with higher doses of pregabalin, which may cause excessive sedation in the elderly population.

PREOPERATIVE EVALUATION

The preoperative period is extremely important for identification of challenging patients who may not be amenable to standard modes of pain control.[7] Challenging patients include those with a history of chronic pain, the elderly population with intolerance to opioids, current substance abuse patients and those in recovery, or those with metabolic or physical limitations that limit the dosing of pain medications. Patients who should receive extensive evaluation are those who have a history of chronic opioid use. These patients are expected to have high postoperative opioid requirements. It is prudent to continue the use of all opioids (immediate and extended-release formulations) until the morning of surgery. Acute discontinuation of pain medications can risk opioid withdrawal in a tolerant patient. Identification of an ideal analgesic in such patients may be difficult and thus the use of a multimodal analgesia technique is very important. Often, the perioperative plan should involve a combination of neuraxial and regional analgesia with a targeted pharmacological approach. Opioid-tolerant patients will have the greatest benefit from a conduction block such as an epidural or regional analgesia. Discussion of an anesthetic plan should begin before the day of surgery in all patients.

TABLE 27-1. Nonopioid Analgesics and Commonly Used Dosing for TKA Patients

Drug	Preop Dose	Route of Administration	Time Before Surgery	Postop Dose
NSAIDs				
Ketorolac	15–30 mg	PO/IV	30 min - 2 h	15–30 mg Q6h
Ibuprofen	600-800 mg	PO		800 mg Q6h
COX-2 inhibitors				
Celecoxib (Celebrex)	200 mg or 400 mg	PO	30 min - 2 h	200 mg × 1
Antineuropathic				
Gabapentin (Neurontin)	600-1200 mg	PO	30 min - 2 h	600 mg BID (up to 48 h)
Pregabalin (Lyrica)	75–300 mg	PO	30 min - 2 h	75-150 mg BID
Acetaminophen				
PO (Tylenol) IV (Ofirmev)	1 g	PO/IV	30 min - 2 h	1 g Q6h (weight > 50 kg)

PO, oral; IV, intravenous; Q6h, every 6 hours; BID, twice daily.

Certain populations of patients may not benefit from neuraxial and regional anesthesia because of the presence of a neurological condition or coagulopathy. When such comorbidities exist, the clinician will need to carefully assess the risks versus the benefits. Patients with a history of severe arthritis, scoliosis, back surgery with presence of hardware, or morbid obesity may also not be candidates for neuraxial anesthesia and analgesia during TKA. Such a technique may be difficult to perform since these patients have alterations in landmarks. These patients will need to be educated on alternative modalities of pain control after the surgery (discussed later).

ANESTHESIA FOR TOTAL KNEE ARTHROPLASTY

Neuraxial Anesthesia

Like many other orthopaedic procedures, regional anesthetic techniques may be employed for total knee arthroplasty. Surgical procedures that involve the knee can be accomplished with spinal or epidural anesthesia, general anesthesia, or peripheral nerve blocks. Most commonly, a spinal anesthetic is preferred over epidural for TKA since it offers the best surgical relaxation and analgesia. Spinal anesthesia is accomplished by inserting a spinal needle (Quincke, Sprotte, or Whitacre) into the intrathecal space, typically in the L3-L4 or L4-L5 vertebral interspace, of a seated or laterally positioned patient. Upon identification of cerebrospinal fluid (CSF), a local anesthetic is then injected, resulting in a rapid onset of spinal blockade. The baricity and volume of the local anesthetic as well as the position of the patient determine the height of the blockade.

Surgical anesthesia for TKA can also be accomplished by a combined spinal-epidural anesthetic (CSE). This technique involves the insertion of an epidural needle (Hustead, Tuohy, or Crawford) into the epidural space via a loss of resistance to air or saline and then subsequent placement of a spinal needle through the epidural needle into the intrathecal space. As stated above, once CSF is identified, a local anesthetic is injected, resulting in spinal blockade. The major advantage of a CSE over a purely spinal anesthetic is the ability to place an epidural catheter into the epidural space for administration of local anesthetics and/or epidural opioids for postoperative analgesia.

Although neuraxial anesthesia offers numerous advantages over general anesthesia for TKA, it is not without its complications. These complications include postoperative backache, postdural puncture headache, local anesthetic systemic toxicity, total spinal anesthesia, neurologic injury, and spinal or epidural hematoma.

Advantages of Neuraxial Anesthesia Over General Anesthesia

Neuraxial anesthesia has been shown to decrease postoperative morbidity and mortality after major surgery when compared with general anesthesia.[8] Specifically, cardiac and pulmonary complications have been reduced when utilizing neuraxial anesthesia, which is significantly advantageous in patients with preexisting cardiac and pulmonary comorbidities.[9-11] In addition, neuraxial anesthesia has been shown to reduce the duration of surgery, the need for transfusion, postoperative nausea and vomiting, and the incidence of thromboembolic disease (deep vein thrombosis and pulmonary embolism) in patients undergoing total joint replacement.[11] Intraoperative blood loss is also reduced when comparing neuraxial to general anesthesia during total hip replacement.[10] However, this finding has not been replicated during TKA largely because of the use of a tourniquet.[11] Numerous studies have demonstrated that major orthopaedic surgery leads to a hypercoagulable state postoperatively that is prevented by the use of epidural anesthesia.[12]

Neuraxial Anesthesia and Anticoagulation

One of the most significant complications of neuraxial anesthesia is neurologic dysfunction secondary to hemorrhagic complications. The actual incidence is unknown; however, literature cites an incidence of less than 1 in 150,000 epidurals and less than 1 in 220,000 spinal anesthetics.[13] Hemorrhage during neuraxial anesthesia most commonly occurs in the epidural space secondary to a prominent venous plexus; however, needle size and catheter placement can affect the location and magnitude of bleeding.

Because of the risk of venous thromboembolism following major orthopaedic surgery, patients frequently receive anticoagulation with unfractionated heparin, low-molecular-weight heparin, or warfarin postoperatively. Refer to Table 27-2 for guidelines regarding anticoagulation in the setting of neuraxial anesthesia. In addition, many TKA patients with cardiac comorbidities receive antiplatelet therapy (Table 27-3). NSAIDs are not a contraindication to neuraxial blockade. Of note, COX-2 inhibitors do not possess antiplatelet properties and therefore can be used perioperatively. Neuraxial anesthesia should be avoided for 10 days following thrombolytics and is contraindicated for patients on thrombin inhibitors. Herbal supplements confer no added bleeding risk during neuraxial anesthesia.[13]

General Anesthesia

Although neuraxial anesthesia provides significant advantages over general anesthesia for TKA, it cannot always be utilized. General anesthesia involves induction and maintenance of anesthesia and analgesia with intravenous and inhaled anesthetics, paralysis with neuromuscular blocking drugs, and maintenance of oxygenation and normocarbia by controlled mechanical ventilation through an endotracheal tube.

Contraindications to neuraxial anesthesia include concurrent anticoagulation and/or inability to abide by the guidelines in Tables 27-2 and 27-3 as well as patient refusal. Patients with localized knee infection without sepsis may undergo neuraxial anesthesia; however, it is recommended that the risks and benefits of neuraxial anesthesia be considered for the bacteremic patient.[14] Presence of increased intracranial pressure increases the risk of brain herniation during neuraxial anesthesia and is therefore most often avoided. Spinal anesthetics have been shown to exacerbate preexisting neurological diseases including multiple sclerosis. Epidural anesthetics have been used safely in such patients.[15] Spinal anesthetic may be performed in patients with prior lumbar surgery but may present difficulty. Each patient must be assessed on a case-by-case basis to determine the risk–benefit ratio.

POSTOPERATIVE ANALGESIA FOR TOTAL KNEE ARTHROPLASTY

Postoperative pain control is paramount to the success of total knee arthroplasty. In addition to being one of the main concerns of patients presenting for surgery, postoperative pain hinders patient rehabilitation and may lead to prolonged hospitalizations.[3] Uncontrolled postoperative pain has been implicated as a risk factor for the development of chronic pain syndromes and increased incidence of postoperative morbidities.[16] Thus choosing an appropriate method of pain control for patients undergoing TKA is crucial. A variety of methods are available for pain control, including neuraxial analgesia, peripheral nerve blockade, and nonopioid and opioid analgesics. However, a multimodal approach is the current method supported by emerging evidence and most pain guidelines.

Spinal Analgesia

Although intrathecal local anesthetics do not have a duration of action long enough to provide sufficient postoperative analgesia, intrathecal opioids, including fentanyl and morphine, may be added to the mixture to improve pain control. Morphine is most commonly used for this purpose because it has a longer duration of action, approximately 12 to 18 hours dependent on dose administered, compared to fentanyl. Intrathecal morphine, either 0.2 or 0.3 mg, has demonstrated better pain control compared to 0.1 mg or no

TABLE 27-2. Guidelines for Neuraxial Anesthesia with Heparin, Low-Molecular-Weight Heparin (LMWH), and Warfarin[13]

Anticoagulant	Block Placement	Dosing After Block Placement	Catheter Removal	Special Considerations
Heparin 5000 U SQ BID	No contraindications, although risk may be reduced when heparin injection is administered after the block.	No contraindications	No contraindications	Concurrent medications affecting clotting system. Check platelet count when administered for more than 4 days.
Heparin 5000 U SQ TID	Insufficient evidence. Assess risk/benefits for each patient.	Insufficient evidence	Insufficient evidence	Assess risk/benefits for each patient.
Heparin-induced anticoagulation	Assess coagulation status. Delay placement for 6 h after heparin discontinued.	Delay until 1 h after block placement.	Assess coagulation status. Remove catheter 2–4 h after last heparin dose.	Re-heparinize 1 h after catheter removal. Assess risk/benefits in event of bloody or difficult epidural placement.
LMWH (Lovenox) thromboprophylaxis	Delay 10–12 h after last dose.	Delay until 6–8 h after block placement.	Remove catheter 10–12 h after last dose.	Administer 2 h after catheter removal. Delay 24 h for traumatic epidural placement.
Therapeutic LMWH (Lovenox) Qday dosing	Delay at least 24 h after last dose.	Delay 1st dose 6–8 h after block and 2nd dose no sooner than 24 h after 1st dose.	Remove catheter 10–12 h after last dose.	Administer 2 h after catheter removal. Delay 24 h for traumatic epidural.
Therapeutic LMWH (Lovenox) BID dosing	Delay at least 24 h after last dose.	Delay 24 h after block placement.	Remove catheter before administration.	Administer 2 h after catheter removal. Delay 24 h for traumatic epidural.
Warfarin (Coumadin)	Discontinue 4–5 days and normal INR before block placement.	No recommendations	Remove catheter when INR<1.5.	Monitor INR daily if warfarin started when epidural in place.

U, units; SQ, subcutaneous; Qday, daily; BID, twice daily; TID, three times daily.

TABLE 27-3. Neuraxial Anesthesia and Antiplatelet Agents[13]

Drug	Recommendations
NSAIDs	No contraindications
Clopidogrel (Plavix)	Discontinue 7 days before block placement
Tilclopidine (Ticlid)	Discontinue 14 days before block placement
Abciximab (Reopro)[a]	Discontinue 24–48 h until platelet aggregation normalized
Eptifibatide (Integrilin)[a] Tirofiban (Aggrastat)[a]	Discontinue 4–8 h until platelet aggregation normalized

[a] Group IIb/IIIa are contraindicated within 4 weeks of surgery.

intrathecal morphine for total hip and knee arthroplasty. The 0.2-mg dose was found to minimize side effects associated with opioids, including nausea and vomiting, pruritus, urinary retention, and respiratory depression, when compared with larger doses of intrathecal morphine. However, intrathecal morphine has been associated with a greater incidence of pruritus when compared with intravenous morphine use. Although intrathecal morphine has been found to decrease postoperative morphine use after total hip arthroplasty, it does not confer the same effect following TKA because of the higher degree of postoperative pain and greater analgesic need associated with TKA.[17]

In addition to intrathecal opioids, nonopioid analgesics can be added to the spinal local anesthetic to improve pain control. Clonidine, an α_2-adrenergic agonist, when administered intrathecally, is believed to inhibit afferent nerves at the level of the dorsal horn and thus potentiate spinal local anesthetics and opioids. When clonidine is combined with morphine intrathecally, it has been shown to reduce intravenous morphine use and improve pain scores according to visual analog scale (VAS) assessment for 24 hours postoperatively. Clonidine can lead to significant hypotension and patients must be monitored appropriately.[18]

Overall, with the addition of opioids and/or clonidine, an intrathecal analgesic can improve postoperative pain control, but it is limited by the inability to titrate the analgesic effect. It is imperative to monitor for the adverse effects of these adjuncts, including nausea, vomiting, pruritus, urinary retention, hypotension, and respiratory depression. Although uncommon with the current low doses of intrathecal opioids used for spinal analgesia, respiratory depression, which is manifested by shallow respirations, decreased ventilatory rate, obstructive apnea, and desaturations as monitored by pulse oximetry, can be a concern and thus necessitates 24 hours of monitoring postoperatively. In certain patient populations, with preexisting risk factors for respiratory depression, including the elderly, obese, and those with a history of obstructive sleep apnea, all opioids including intrathecal opioids should be used with caution.

Epidural Analgesia

It is well known that regional analgesic techniques improve early rehabilitation largely by effectively controlling pain following TKA.[19] Epidural analgesia involves either a single injection or placement of an indwelling catheter and delivery of local anesthetics and/or opioids. A recent meta-analysis demonstrated that when comparing epidural analgesia, regardless of analgesic agent, with parenteral opioids, epidural analgesia provided superior pain relief. Specifically, when examining patients who had undergone lower extremity surgery, both local anesthetic with and without opioids and opioids alone administered via a lumbar epidural resulted in better VAS scores. However, greater improvements were demonstrated when local anesthetic was administered in the epidural.[16] When comparing a 72-hour epidural infusion of 0.125% levobupivacaine with intravenous patient-controlled analgesia (PCA) with morphine to intravenous PCA morphine alone following TKA, the epidural group showed better pain relief and decreased morphine consumption without any impairment in motor function.[20]

Although local anesthetics with or without opioids and opioids alone are most commonly utilized for epidural analgesia, the addition of epinephrine has been shown to prolong epidural blockade of both local anesthetics and opioids by inducing vasoconstriction in the epidural space and decreasing systemic absorption.[21] The addition of clonidine to a local anesthetic-opioid epidural mixture has also been shown to improve pain control after TKA but with a decrease in blood pressure and heart rate.[22] Ketamine, morphine, and epinephrine added to a ropivicaine infusion of patient-controlled epidural analgesia provided patients with better pain relief, suggesting an additive effect. Ketamine is an *N*-methyl-D-aspartate (NMDA) antagonist that acts both peripherally and centrally to abolish noxious stimuli.[23]

Although epidural analgesia results in better pain control following total joint arthroplasty, especially in the early postoperative periods, significant side effects can occur. Urinary retention, pruritus, and hypotension have been found to occur more frequently with epidural analgesia as compared to parenteral analgesia, while the frequency of nausea and vomiting and respiratory depression were equal. Sedation scores were less prevalent in the epidural group.[24] Overall there are reduced incidences of postoperative complications, such as pulmonary, cardiovascular, and infections, as well as decreased length of hospital stays with the use of epidural analgesia.[25]

Despite providing improved pain control, there are several limitations to epidural analgesia that can affect effectiveness. Complications including hypotension, risk of epidural hematoma or abscess formation, and impaired motor function and interference with rehabilitation are potential limiting factors. Incompatibility with anticoagulation is of concern with epidural catheter infusions since patients are typically anticoagulated. It is important to monitor patients for these potential side effects throughout the course of epidural analgesia. Epidural analgesia is associated with a significant rate of failure related to failed or dislodged catheters, unilateral block, leaks, and catheter migration or occlusions.[25] Hence, epidural analgesia works best in a setting in which there are adequate resources for assessment of side effects and inadequate analgesia and subsequent adjustment as indicated.

Extended-Release Epidural Morphine

A recent advancement in epidural analgesia is an extended-release epidural morphine (EREM), DepoDur, which alleviates many of the concerns discussed above with regards to indwelling epidural catheters. EREM consists of microscopic multivesicular, liposomal spherical particles with internal aqueous chambers containing morphine, resulting in 48 hours of analgesia after a single epidural injection (Fig. 27-2).[26] In a study comparing EREM to intravenous PCA morphine following TKA, patients who received EREM had decreased pain and opioid consumption.[27] The advantages of EREM include decreased incidence of hypotension,[26] compatibility with anticoagulation since there is no indwelling catheter, and elimination of complications related to catheter malfunction and migration. The side-effect profile is similar between EREM and systemic opioids and includes nausea and vomiting, pruritus, urinary retention, constipation, and respiratory depression. Of note, a recent study demonstrated that the patients who experienced significant respiratory depression were all over 65 years of age.[27] Recommendations are not to exceed 15 mg of EREM for TKA since higher dosing can cause severe side effects. Due to concerns of respiratory depression, EREM should be used cautiously in patients over 65 years old and those with obstructive sleep apnea.[28] Dose reduction is advisable in at-risk patients. EREM may be less effective in patients with significant opioid tolerance. Hourly sedation and respiratory rate monitoring are recommended for 12 to 16 hours after receiving EREM. Best results with EREM are achieved when a multimodal approach is incorporated. In this fashion, EREM doses can be reduced, achieving a better balance between analgesic efficacy and side effects.

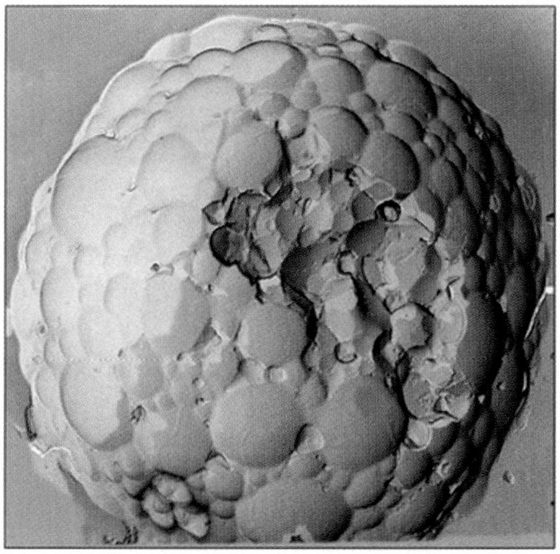

FIGURE 27-2. *Extended-release epidural morphine (DepoDur). Microscopic spherical particles with internal aqueous chambers containing morphine. After single injection of EREM in lumbar epidural space, chambers degrade to release morphine for up to 48 hours.*

Peripheral Nerve Blocks

The knee is innervated by the lumbosacral plexus. The lumbar plexus consists of the first four lumbar spinal nerves and gives rise to the lateral femoral cutaneous, femoral, and obturator nerves. The lateral femoral cutaneous nerve provides sensation to the lateral thigh, while the obturator nerve supplies motor innervation to the hip adductors and variable cutaneous innervation to the medial thigh and knee. The femoral nerve innervates the quadriceps muscle and the skin of the anteromedial thigh and continues below the knee to provide sensation to the medial leg and foot. The sciatic nerve is derived from the spinal nerves from L4 to S3 and innervates the posterior knee before branching into the peroneal and tibial nerves, which supply the majority of the lower leg and foot except that innervated by the saphenous nerve (the terminal branch of the femoral nerve).

Postoperative analgesia following TKA can be achieved by a lumbar plexus block, a femoral nerve block, or a combined femoral and sciatic nerve block. A peripheral nerve block can be achieved by injection of a local anesthetic by a single shot or a continuous catheter technique. However, a recent meta-analysis comparing lumbar epidural to peripheral nerve blockade (PNB), including single-shot femoral nerve blockade, single-shot sciatic nerve blockade, continuous femoral catheter, or continuous lumbar plexus catheter, following major knee surgery showed that there was no difference in pain scores or morphine consumption between the two groups, but the PNB group showed a better side-effect profile with a lower incidence of hypotension and urinary retention.[29] Single-injection peripheral nerve blocks are limited by the duration of the local anesthetic used; however, continuous PNB (CPNB) provides analgesia well into the postoperative period. When comparing CPNB, regardless of catheter location, the analgesia provided was superior to that of opioid analgesia with the added benefit of fewer opioid-related side effects.[30] Although recent studies have shown that CPNB catheters frequently become colonized, the rate of actual localized infection is only 0% to

3%.[31] Additional potential side effects include a risk of nerve damage, most often temporary, recently estimated to be around 1:3763,[29] and inhibition of rehabilitation secondary to persistent muscular weakness.

Lumbar plexus block

A lumbar plexus block involves blockade of the first four lumbar spinal nerves, and therefore blockade of the lateral femoral cutaneous, femoral, and obturator nerves. Blockade of these nerves will provide analgesia to the anteromedial thigh and knee as well as the lateral thigh. In patients undergoing total hip arthroplasty, a continuous lumbar plexus block was shown to substantially lower opioid requirements and provide better analgesia with less nausea and vomiting than systemic opioids.[32] Both single-injection and continuous lumbar plexus blockade have been shown to provide effective analgesia and improved mobilization following TKA; however, patients who receive a CPNB have been shown to have prolonged analgesia, reduced opioid requirements, and earlier mobilization when compared to the single-injection technique.[33] Although, lumbar plexus blocade may confer fewer side effects and the advantage of a unilateral block when compared to continuous epidural analgesia, the risk of hematoma and the compatibility with anticoagulation are similar.

Femoral nerve block

The femoral nerve supplies motor innervation to the quadriceps muscle and cutaneous innervation to the anteromedial thigh and knee as well as the medial aspect of the lower leg and foot. The femoral nerve is located lateral to the femoral artery just below the inguinal ligament (Fig. 27-3). A femoral nerve block can be accomplished by palpating the femoral artery and injecting local anesthetic 1 cm lateral and 1 cm caudal after obtaining a quadriceps twitch with the use of a stimulating needle. With increasing use of ultrasound, the femoral nerve is now commonly blocked under ultrasound guidance with or without quadriceps contraction confirmation. Because of the proximity of the femoral nerve to the femoral artery, there is a significant risk of intravascular injection during this block; however, the increasing use of ultrasound guidance may decrease this risk because the artery and needle can be visualized throughout the procedure. Local anesthetic toxicity is manifested by tinnitus, vertigo, metallic taste in the mouth, perioral numbness, restlessness, or slurred speech and can progress to seizures or cardiovascular collapse. The risk of hematoma formation and incompatibility with anticoagulation is less when compared to lumbar plexus block and neuraxial analgesia due to the easy compressibility of the femoral artery and vein.

The addition of a single-injection femoral nerve block (FNB), when added to a multimodal regimen including opioids and NSAIDs, has been shown to provide improved analgesia and decreased opioid consumption following TKA when compared to systemic opioids and NSAIDs alone.[34] It has also been shown that FNB not only improves analgesia when used adjunctively with systemic opioids but also enables early rehabilitation and decreases the length of hospital stay following TKA.[35] Continuous femoral nerve block does provide better analgesia when compared to the single-injection technique; however, it is unclear whether it shortens the length of hospital stay.[36] The obturator nerve supplies the adductors of the hip and a variable cutaneous contribution to the medial thigh and knee. Likely secondary to its variable contribution, an obturator nerve block offered no benefit when compared to placebo following TKA.[37] Both continuous epidural analgesia and continuous femoral nerve blockade result in better analgesia and faster rehabilitation when compared to systemic opioids. However, continuous FNB has been shown to have a better side-effect profile and a much lower risk of potentially irreversible nerve damage secondary to hematoma formation.[38] Nonetheless, nerve injury can occur, temporary or permanent, and is most often manifested as paresthesias, numbness, or weakness.

Sciatic nerve block

The sciatic nerve is derived from the lumbosacral plexus and provides innervation to the lateral and posterior aspect of the knee and most of the leg below the knee. A single-injection or continuous catheter can be placed with the patient in the lateral position and the nerve is most often blocked in the gluteal region when analgesia of the knee is desired. The magnitude of the contribution of the sciatic nerve to postoperative pain following TKA is unclear. At least one study demonstrated that the addition of a sciatic nerve block to a FNB did not add any analgesic benefit.[34] However, a more recent study showed that the combination of continuous femoral and sciatic nerve block provided better analgesia and decreased opioid consumption as well as the incidence of nausea and vomiting when compared to continuous FNB alone following TKA.[39] The side-effect profile and risk of hematoma formation are similar to that of the femoral nerve block. The risk of falls is increased with combined femoral and sciatic nerve blocks, and thus patient education is very important for prevention of such adverse events. The combination of FNB or lumbar plexus block and sciatic nerve block can provide total anesthesia to the knee joint. However, for analgesia, the contribution of the sciatic nerve is less certain. The clinician must evaluate the potential analgesic benefit compared to the potential loss of

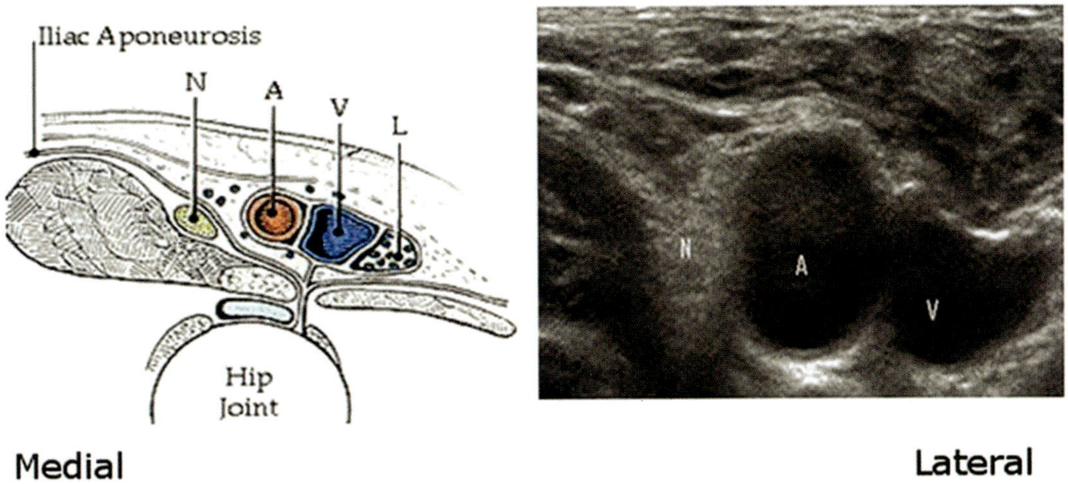

FIGURE 27-3. *Femoral nerve anatomy. N, nerve; A, artery; V, vein; L, lymphatics.*

sensation and motor function below the knee with the resulting impact on physical therapy.

Intra- and Periarticular Local Anesthetic Wound Infusion Analgesia

In recent years there has been increasing interest in high-volume local anesthetic infusion techniques for postoperative analgesia following total joint arthroplasty because of the relative simplicity and speed of placement. This technique involves infiltration of a local anesthetic directly into the tissues of the surgical field. Infusions of local anesthetic alone have been used as well as local anesthetics combined with NSAIDs and epinephrine.

A recent study showed that a local infiltration of ropivacaine, ketorolac, and epinephrine provided superior pain relief and decreased opioid consumption when compared to an epidural infusion of ropivacaine combined with intravenous ketorolac injections following TKA.[40] However, it must be noted that both infusions were administered at a rate of 4 mL/h, which is far below the typical epidural infusion rate used following TKA, so these results must be viewed with caution. A recent review of studies examining local wound infusion analgesia (LWIA) demonstrated that intraoperative LWIA administration during TKA seems to be effective for the initial 6 to 12 hours postoperatively, but the evidence to support use of a continuous catheter is unclear.[41] Still, studies have shown that continuous LWIA of local anesthetic has resulted in better pain control and decreased opioid requirements following joint replacement surgery when compared to intravenous opioids.[42] Patients who had undergone bilateral TKA with intra-articular LWIA in one knee and no injection in the other had lower VAS scores and improved range of motion in the knees that had received the injection.[43]

The use of LWIA for postoperative pain control following TKA is promising but more evidence is needed to conclude its value in the context of a multimodal analgesic regimen. It is a relatively low-risk and simple technique to perform. There has been concern over short- and long-term wound infection; however, one study documented no difference in infection rate or wound healing at 12 months following intra-articular injection after TKA.[44] There are insufficient data at this time to compare the efficacy and safety of LWIA to other current standards, such as epidural or regional anesthesia. Clearly, further studies are warranted.

Multimodal Nonopioid Analgesics

Effective pain control is imperative in the perioperative setting following TKA. Uncontrolled pain may lead to increased morbidity and mortality as well as impaired rehabilitation. The American Society of Anesthesiologists set forth guidelines regarding acute pain management in the perioperative setting. These guidelines strongly recommend the use of a multimodal regimen, including the use of around-the-clock NSAIDs, acetaminophen, and COX-2 inhibitors, whenever possible in addition to regional techniques.[45]

Acetaminophen

Acetaminophen is a well-known antipyretic and analgesic agent. It is most commonly used in the oral form but recently became available in the United States as an intravenous formulation. Acetaminophen acts as a central analgesic agent and lacks the side effects associated with NSAIDs, most notably with regard to bleeding, bone healing, renal impairment, and gastrointestinal irritation. The main mechanism of action remains uncertain. Proposed mechanisms include the inhibition of COX, and recent findings suggest it is highly selective for COX-2. Acetaminophen also has NMDA receptor antagonism and cannabinoid activity. Other proposed mechanisms include nitric oxide and 5-HT3 activity. Acetaminophen exerts weak anti-inflammatory properties. Overall, the side effects are minimal, with hepatotoxicity being the most serious side effect, but this complication is rare when total daily doses do not exceed 4 g.[28]

With relatively few side effects and the recent approval of the intravenous formulation, acetaminophen will likely have an expanded role in a multimodal analgesic regimen following TKA in the future. Following major orthopaedic surgery, patients who received intravenous acetaminophen (1 g every 6 hours for 24 hours) reported significantly better pain control and satisfaction as well as 33% less morphine consumption compared to placebo.[46] When compared to ketorolac, intravenous propacetamol (a prodrug of acetaminophen) provided similar pain relief following total joint arthroplasty as well as superior analgesia in the first 6 hours when compared to placebo.[47] Intravenous administration of acetaminophen avoids the first-pass metabolism associated with oral administration, minimizing hepatic toxicity. The recommended dose is 1 g intravenously every 6 hours, not to exceed 4 g per day in adults.

NSAIDs and COX-2 inhibitors

NSAIDs exert their antipyretic, analgesic, and anti-inflammatory effects peripherally by inhibiting prostaglandin synthesis and the stimulation of nociceptors. NSAIDs specifically act on the COX-1 and COX-2 enzymes, while COX-2 inhibitors are selective. The advantage of COX-2 selective inhibitors is that the selectivity reduces the effect on platelet aggregation and increased bleeding time that is associated with COX-1 inhibition. In addition, the use of COX-2 inhibitors may result in decreased gastric mucosal irritation associated with NSAIDs. Recently, several COX-2 inhibitors were removed from the market secondary to the association with increased cardiovascular side effects. As a class, the NSAIDs, both selective and nonselective, all have some cardiovascular risk, but this has not been observed with short-term administration such as for postoperative pain control. There are still remaining concerns of bone healing with NSAIDs and COX-2 inhibitors, but little evidence exists at this time to support or refute this concern.[48] There is now vast experience with the use of NSAIDs following total joint arthroplasty and osteointegration does not appear to be affected.

The administration of NSAIDs and COX-2 inhibitors perioperatively has resulted in decreased postoperative pain and reduced opioid consumption following total hip arthroplasty.[49] Following TKA, perioperative use of COX-2 inhibitors resulted in better pain control, improved range of motion, reduced opioid consumption, decreased incidence of nausea and vomiting, and better sleep patterns as compared to placebo, thus supporting its use in a multimodal analgesic regimen.[50] There is much emphasis placed on preoperative administration of NSAIDs and COX-2 inhibitors because preoperative use has been shown to result in further reductions in pain postoperatively.[51] Overall, there is significant evidence to support the use of NSAIDs or COX-2 inhibitors perioperatively as part of a multimodal approach to postoperative pain management following TKA.

Pregabalin and gabapentin

Pregabalin and gabapentin were originally approved as anticonvulsants. Pain clinicians recognized their utility as analgesics, particularly for neuropathic pain. More recently, studies have confirmed analgesic efficacy for major orthopaedic surgery, including spine and total joint arthroplasty. These agents decrease afferent excitatory signals in the dorsal horn of the spinal cord by acting on voltage-gated calcium channels.

Several studies have shown decreased pain and opioid consumption postoperatively with preoperative administration of gabapentin for a variety of nonorthopaedic procedures.[52] Perioperative administration of gabapentin has led to decreased pain and opioid consumption as well as improved range of motion following TKA.[53] In addition to improved knee flexion postoperatively, patients report reduced anxiety perioperatively following the preoperative administration of gabapentin.[54]

There is a risk of chronic neuropathic pain following many surgical procedures and TKA is no exception. However, perioperative administration of pregabalin has been shown to reduce the incidence of chronic neuropathic pain, decrease opioid consumption, and improve rehabilitation during the first 30 days following TKA.[55] Some studies suggest that the combination of gabapentin with other non-opioid agents, such as COX-2 inhibitors, may be synergistic.[56]

Current evidence supports the use of gabapentin or pregabalin as a part of a multimodal analgesic approach following TKA. Common side effects of pregabalin and gabapentin include sedation and dizziness.

Ketamine

Ketamine is an NMDA receptor antagonist that now has a role in perioperative analgesia. Ketamine has specifically demonstrated improved postoperative pain management in opioid-tolerant patients.[57] When combined with a FNB, perioperative ketamine infusion led to decreased opioid consumption as well as improved range of motion following TKA.[58] Reported side effects include vivid dreams, hallucinations, nausea, vomiting, and vision changes, but these are minimal with the low doses commonly used in infusions for postoperative pain control. Ketamine may prove to have a role as part of a multimodal approach following TKA.

Opioid Analgesics

Intravenous patient-controlled analgesia

Opioids remain the most commonly used agents for postoperative pain control. Intravenous patient-controlled analgesia (IV PCA) is the most popular delivery method.[59] PCA involves patient-activated opioid administration via an infusion pump with or without a basal rate where bolus doses are preset with a lockout time and maximum hourly dose. The advantage of IV PCA is that it allows the patient to titrate the opioid according to his or her pain level and eliminates the need for the patient to rely on intermittent nursing opioid boluses. With this in mind, the patient may more easily maintain a steady state of pain control.

The opioids most commonly administered via IV PCA include morphine, fentanyl, and hydromorphone. Meperidine has fallen into disfavor largely because of the potential for seizure activity. Opioids act both peripherally and centrally by binding to opioid receptors, including mu (μ), kappa (κ), and sigma (σ). Common side effects of opioids include pruritus, nausea, vomiting, ileus, constipation, and sedation. Respiratory depression is a less common but serious opioid-related side effect. The elderly are particularly sensitive to the side effects of opioids. In addition, opioids should be administered with caution in patients with obstructive sleep apnea. Special attention must be given to morphine administration in the presence of renal failure since the active metabolites are primarily excreted by the kidneys.

Oral opioids

Oral opioids are an important component of postoperative analgesia following TKA when patients are discharged to home or to a rehabilitation facility. One oral opioid combined with two or more nonopioids can be an effective multimodal regimen outside of the hospital setting. Oral opioids are commonly prescribed as combination agents with acetaminophen. Care must be exercised to avoid overdose of acetaminophen when patients may be taking multiple agents with this drug. Table 27-4 lists commonly used oral opioids following TKA.

Hydrocodone–acetaminophen combination agents are widely prescribed for postoperative pain relief, often with the mistaken assumption that these agents are safer or less addictive than other opioids. While hydrocodone is a reasonable opioid choice, it is not safer than other opioids in any known way and remains one of the most widely abused drugs.

Because opioids are associated with a number of side effects as well as abuse, there is an emphasis on opioid reduction or avoidance in the management of postoperative pain. Hence a multimodal approach is now considered standard care.

Opioid analgesics (oral and parenteral) exhibit a broad and flat dose response curve. Clinically this expresses itself as wide variability in opioid needs from one patient to another. To provide the best balance of safety and efficacy, it is critical to titrate opioids to effect individualizing the dose as needed. This follows through to discharge medications where the need for opioids both in duration and amount varies widely and is best adjusted to the patient's needs.

PERSISTENT POSTSURGICAL PAIN FOLLOWING TKA

Although the majority of patients after TKA have excellent outcomes, a small percentage continues to endure chronic pain after surgery. The International Association of the Study of Pain describes persistent postsurgical pain as one that develops after surgery and is present for at least 3 months.[60] Despite undergoing knee replacement, 44% of

TABLE 27-4. Oral Opioids and Suggested Dosing for TKA Patients in Postoperative Period

Drug	Dosage (mg)	Frequency (h)	Duration (h)
Tramadol (Ultram)	50 100	Q4–6	6–8
Tapentadol (Nucynta)	50 75 100	Q4–6	4–6
Codeine/acetaminophen (Tylenol with Codeine #3) (Tylenol with Codeine #4)	 300/30 300/60	Q4–6	4–6
Hydrocodone/acetaminophen (Vicodin, Lortab, Norco)	5/325 7.5/325 10/325	Q4–6	3–4
Oxycodone	10–20	Q4–6	4–6
Oxycodone/acetaminophen (Percocet)	5/325 7.5/325	Q6	3–4
Morphine sulfate (MS-IR)	10–30	Q3–4	2–4
Hydromorphone (Dilaudid)	4–8	Q3–4	3–4
Oxymorphone (Opana)	10–20	Q4–6	7–11

TKA patients report persistent postsurgical pain (aching, tenderness, and fatigue) and 15% report severe, extreme persistent pain 3 to 4 years after surgery.[61] A small percentage of these patients (13%) are described as having neuropathic pain in origin.[61] Neuropathic pain is characterized by allodynia, hyperalgesia, edema, and skin discoloration in the limb. Major depression, as a comorbidity, has been found to be an independent risk factor for persistent postsurgical pain. Studies have also determined that chronic pain can affect quality of life (physical, economical, and emotional well-being) after joint replacement.[62]

Chronic pain can occur with sensitization of peripheral and central nociceptors during the surgical procedure.[63-65] Recent evidence suggests that persistent postsurgical pain may be prevented with preemptive analgesia that acts to prevent peripheral and central sensitization. Patients given perioperative pregabalin continued to postoperative day 14 showed a reduction in neuropathic pain at both 3 and 6 months.[55] These patients displayed less morphine consumption and had better range of motion with rehabilitation. In a different surgical model, ketamine administered during the intraoperative course had reduced opioid consumption at 6 weeks after surgery.[66] Further studies of preemptive analgesia after TKA are necessary.

IDEAL ANESTHESIA AND ANALGESIA FOR TKA

Regional anesthetic techniques including epidural analgesia and peripheral nerve blocks (femoral, lumbar plexus, sciatic) have all demonstrated analgesic benefit for TKA. The benefits of intra- and periarticular local anesthetic wound infusions are less well understood. An ideal anesthetic and analgesic plan for TKA includes one that maximizes patient comfort, minimizes side effects, and promotes early mobilization and physical therapy. The best current evidence suggests that a perioperative plan utilizing multimodal analgesic techniques, including regional anesthesia, peripheral nerve blocks, COX-2 selective inhibitors, acetaminophen, and opioids, is recommended (Fig. 27-4). In addition, agents such as NMDA receptor antagonists (ketamine, dextromethorphan), alpha-2 agonists (clonidine, dexmedetomidine), and anticonvulsants (gabapentin, pregabalin) may have opioid-sparing effects and prevent central neurospasticity. The single best approach for TKA has not yet been defined. Careful assessment of risks and benefits must be made for each technique (Table 27-5). Further studies are needed as new analgesic agents and surgical techniques are developed.

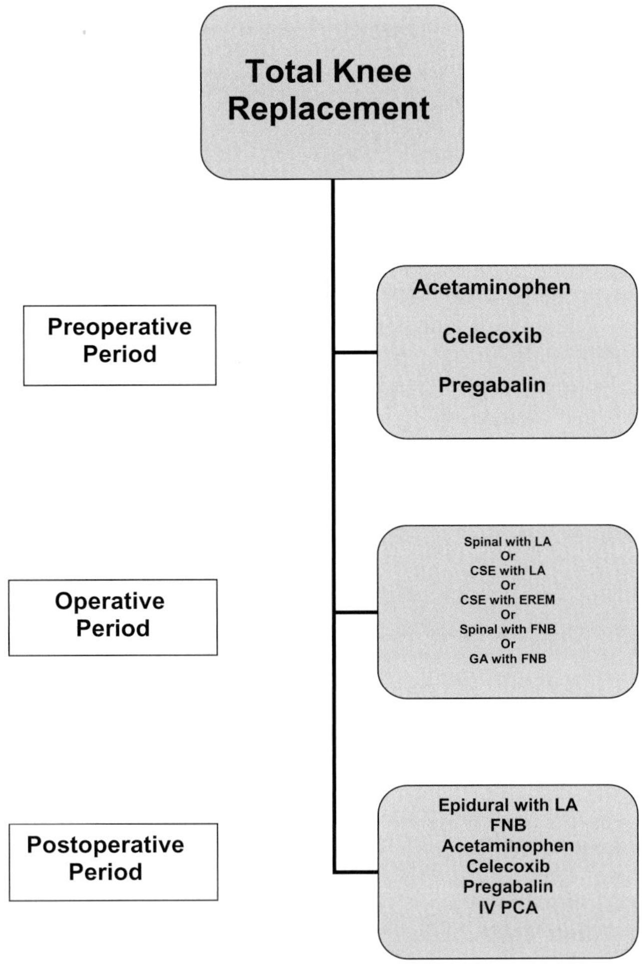

FIGURE 27-4. *Ideal anesthesia and analgesia during the perioperative course. LA, local anesthetics; GA, general anesthesia.*

TABLE 27-5. Comparison of Postoperative Analgesic Techniques for TKA

Technique	Advantages	Disadvantages
Spinal opioids	• No indwelling catheter • Compatible with postoperative anticoagulation • Reduced opioid use	• Opioid side effects • Lacks ability for titration • Limited duration
Continuous epidural	• Well-proven analgesic efficacy • Able to titrate • Reduced opioid use • Patient satisfaction • Earlier mobilization • Well-established outcome benefits	• Anticoagulation considerations • Requires infusion pump • Possible hypotension and urinary retention • Catheter malfunction/dislodgement • Labor intensive • Known side effects (opioid related or motor block)

Continued

TABLE 27-5. ***Continued***

Technique	Advantages	Disadvantages
EREM	• No indwelling catheter • Compatible with postoperative anticoagulation • Minimal associated hypotension • 48-h (prolonged) analgesia	• Opioid side effects • Caution with the elderly and obstructive sleep apnea
Single-injection lumbar plexus block	• No indwelling catheter • Compatible with postoperative anticoagulation • No concerns of hypotension and urinary retention • Reduced opioid use	• Anticoagulation considerations similar to neuraxial techniques (hematoma) • Duration of analgesia limited • Potential motor block
Continuous lumbar plexus block	• Ability to titrate • Reduced opioid use • Earlier mobilization • No concerns of hypotension and urinary retention	• Anticoagulation considerations (hematoma) • Requires infusion pump • Catheter malfunction/dislodgement • Potential motor block
Single-injection femoral nerve block	• Compatible with anticoagulation • No concerns of hypotension and urinary retention • Reduced opioid use • Analgesia of anteromedial aspect of knee	• Duration of analgesia limited • Potential motor block
Continuous femoral nerve blockade	• Ability to titrate • Reduced opioid use • Earlier mobilization • Compatible with anticoagulation • Reduced incidence of hematoma • No concerns of hypotension and urinary retention • Analgesia of anteromedial aspect of knee	• Requires infusion pump • Risk of catheter malfunction or dislodgement • Potential motor block
Sciatic nerve block	• Compatible with anticoagulation • Reduced opioid use • No concerns of hypotension and urinary retention • Analgesia of posterolateral aspect of knee	• Used in conjunction with femoral nerve block; however, controversy exists over whether addition of sciatic block improves analgesia • Duration of analgesia limited • Potential motor block
Intra/Periarticular local wound infusion analgesia (LWIA)	• Ease of placement • Compatible with anticoagulation • Few side effects • No motor block • Reduced opioid use	• Concern for wound healing/infection • Catheter malfunction/dislodgement • Efficacy not well established • Local anesthetic toxicity

Continued

TABLE 27-5. *Continued*

Technique	Advantages	Disadvantages
Nonopioids	• May reduce opioid requirements and associated side effects • Few side effects • Effective as part of multimodal analgesic regimen • May reduce chronic pain	• Side effects of individual drugs
Intravenous patient-controlled analgesia	• Effective analgesia • Gives patient ability to titrate • Safer than bolus opioids	• Opioid side effects • Technically complicated • Risk of medication and programming errors • Bulky and may impede physical therapy

REFERENCES

1. Apfelbaum JL, Chen C, Mehta SS, et al. Postoperative pain experience: results from a national survey suggest postoperative pain continues to be undermanaged. *Anesth Analg.* 2003;97:534-540.
2. Warfield CA, Kahn CH. Acute pain management: programs in U.S. hospitals and experiences and attitudes among U.S. adults. *Anesthesiology.* 1995;83: 1090-1094.
3. Joshi GP, Ogunnaike BO. Consequences of inadequate postoperative pain relief and chronic persistent postoperative pain. *Anesth Clin North Am.* 2005;23: 21-36.
4. Munin MC, Rudy TE, Glynn NW, et al. Early inpatient rehabilitation after elective hip and knee arthroplasty. *JAMA.* 1998;279(11):847-852.
5. Kehlet H, Dahl JB. The value of "multimodal" or "balanced analgesia" in postoperative pain treatment. *Anesth Analg.* 1993;77:1048-1056.
6. Gottschalk A, Smith DS. New concepts in acute pain therapy: pre-emptive analgesia. *Am Fam Physician.* 2001;63:1979-1985.
7. Gandhi K, Heitz JW, Viscusi ER. Challenges in acute pain management. *Anesth Clin.* 2011;29(2):291-309.
8. Rodgers A, Walker N, Schug S, et al. Reduction of postoperative morality and morbidity with epidural or spinal anaesthesia: results from overview of randomized trials. *BMJ.* 2000;321:1493.
9. Christopherson R, Beattie C, Frank SM, et al. Perioperative morbidity in patients randomized to epidural or general anesthesia for lower extremity vascular surgery. *Anesthesiology.* 1993;79:422-434.
10. Mauermann WJ, Shilling AM, Zuo Z. A comparison of neuraxial block versus general anesthesia for elective total hip replacement: a meta-analysis. *Anesth Analg.* 2006;103:1018-1025.
11. Hu S, Zhang ZY, Hua YQ, et al. A comparison of regional and general anaesthesia for total replacement of the hip or knee: a meta-analysis. *J Bone Joint Surg Br.* 2009;91:935-942.
12. Hollmann MW, Wieczorek KS, Smart M, et al. Epidural anesthesia prevents hypercoagulation in patients undergoing major orthopedic surgery. *Reg Anesth Pain Med.* 2001;26:215-222.
13. Horlocker TT, Wedel DJ, Rowlingson JC, et al. Regional anesthesia in the patient receiving antithrombotic or thrombolytic therapy: American Society of Regional Anesthesia and Pain Medicine evidence-based guidelines (third edition). *Reg Anesth Pain Med.* 2010;35(1):4-7.
14. Horlocker TT, Birnbach DJ, Connis RT, et al. Practice advisory for the prevention, diagnosis, and management of infectious complications associated with neuraxial techniques: a report by the American Society of Anesthesiologists Task Force on infectious complications associated with neuraxial techniques. *Anesthesiology.* 2010;112(3):530-545.
15. Barash PG, Cullen BF, Stoelting RK. *Clinical Anesthesia.* Philadelphia, PA: Lippincott Williams and Wilkins; 2006;711-714.
16. Block BM, Liu SS, Rowlingson AJ, et al. Efficacy of postoperative epidural analgesia: a meta-analysis. *JAMA.* 2003;290:2455-2463.
17. Rathmell JP, Pino CA, Taylor R, et al. Intrathecal morphine for postoperative analgesia: a randomized, controlled dose-ranging study after hip and knee arthroplasty. *Anesth Analg.* 2003;97:1452-1457.
18. Sites BD, Beach M, Biggs R, et al. Intrathecal clonidine added to a bupivacaine-morphine spinal anes-

thetic improves postoperative analgesia for a total knee arthroplasty. *Anesth Analg.* 2003;96:1083-1088.

19. Capdevila X, Barthelet Y, Biboulet P, et al. Effects of perioperative analgesic technique on the surgical outcome and duration of rehabilitation after major knee surgery. *Anesthesiology.* 1999;91:8-15.
20. Casati A, Ostroff R, Casimiro C, et al. 72-hour epidural infusion of 0.125% levobupivacaine following total knee replacement: a prospective, randomized, controlled, multicenter evaluation. *Acta Biomed.* 2008;79:28-35.
21. Huang KS, Tseng CH, Cheung KS, et al. Influence of epinephrine as an adjuvant to epidural morphine for postoperative analgesia. *Ma Zui Xue Za Zhi.* 1993; 31:245-248.
22. Forster JG, Rosenberg PH. Small dose of clonidine mixed with low-dose ropivicaine and fentanyl for epidural analgesia after total knee arthroplasty. *Br J Anaesth.* 2004;93:670-677.
23. Chia YY, Liu K, Liu YC, et al. Adding ketamine in a multimodal patient-controlled epidural regimen reduces postoperative pain and analgesic consumption. *Anesth Analg.* 1998;86:1245-1249.
24. Choi PT, Bhandari M, Scott J, et al. Epidural analgesia for pain relief following hip or knee replacement. *Cochrane Database Syst Rev.* 2003;3:CD 003071.
25. Viscusi ER. Emerging techniques in the management of acute pain: epidural analgesia. *Anesth Analg.* 2005;101:S23-29.
26. Viscusi ER, Martin G, Hartrick CT, et al. Forty-eight hours of postoperative pain relief following total hip arthroplasty with a novel, extended-release epidural morphine formulation. *Anesthesiology.* 2005;102:937-947.
27. Hartrick CT, Martin G, Kantor G, et al. Evaluation of a single-dose, extended-release epidural morphine formulation for pain after knee arthroplasty. *J Bone Joint Surg Am.* 2006;88:273-281.
28. Parvizi J, Miller AG, Gandhi K. Current concepts review: multimodal pain management after total joint arthroplasty. *J Bone Joint Surg Am.* 2011;93:1075-1084.
29. Fowler SJ, Symons J, Sabato S, et al. Epidural analgesia compared with peripheral nerve blockade after major knee surgery: a systematic review and meta-analysis of randomized trials. *Br J Anaesth.* 2008;100:154-164.
30. Richman JM, Liu SS, Courpas G, et al. Does continuous peripheral nerve block provide superior pain control to opioids? A meta-analysis. *Anesth Analg.* 2006; 102:248-257.
31. Capdevilla Z, Bringuier S, Borgeat A. Infectious risk of continuous peripheral nerve blocks. *Anesthesiology.* 2009;110:182-188.
32. Siddiqui ZI, Cepeda MS, Denman W, et al. Continuous lumbar plexus block provides improved analgesia with fewer side effects compared with systemic opioids after hip arthroplasty: a randomized controlled trial. *Reg Anesth Pain Med.* 2007;32:393-398.
33. Watson MW, Mitra D, Mclintock TC, et al. Continuous versus single-injection lumbar plexus blocks: comparison of the effects on morphine use and early recovery after total knee arthroplasty. *Reg Anesth Pain Med.* 2005;30(6):541-547.
34. Allen HW, Liu SS, Ware PD, et al. Peripheral nerve blocks improve analgesia after total knee replacement surgery. *Anesth Analg.* 1998;87:93-97.
35. Wang H, Boctor B, Verner J. The effect of single-injection femoral nerve block on rehabilitation and length of hospital stay after total knee replacement. *Reg Anesth Pain Med.* 2002;27(2):139-144.
36. Salinas FV, Liu SS, Mulroy MF. The effect of single-injection femoral nerve block versus continuous femoral nerve block after total knee arthroplasty on hospital length of stay and long-term functional recovery within an established clinical pathway. *Anesth Analg.* 2006;102:1234-1239.
37. Kardash K, Hickey D, Tessler MJ, et al. Obturator versus femoral nerve block for analgesia after total knee arthroplasty. *Anesth Analg.* 2007;105:853-858.
38. Singelyn FJ, Deyaert M, Jorist D, et al. Effects of intravenous patient-controlled analgesia with morphine, continuous epidural analgesia, and continuous three-in-one block on postoperative pain and knee rehabilitation after unilateral total knee arthroplasty. *Anesth Anal.* 1998;87:88-92.
39. Dang CP, Gautheron E, Guilley J, et al. The value of adding sciatic block to continuous femoral block for analgesia after total knee replacement. *Reg Anesth Pain Med.* 2005;30:128-133.
40. Andersen KV, Bak M, Christensen BV, et al. A randomized, controlled trial comparing local infiltration analgesia with epidural infusion for total knee arthroplasty. *Acta Orthop.* 2010;81(5):606-610.
41. Kehlet H, Andersen LO. Local infiltration analgesia in joint replacement: the evidence and recommendations for clinical practice. *Acta Anesthesiol Scand.* 2011;55:778-784.
42. Bianconi M, Ferrar L, Traina GC. Pharmacokinetics and efficacy of ropivacaine continuous wound instilla-

tion after joint replacement surgery. *Br J Anaesth.* 2003;91(6):830-835.

43. Mullaji A, Kanna R, Shetty GM. Efficacy of periarticular injection of bupivacaine, fentanyl, and methylprednisolone in total knee arthroplasty: a prospective, randomized trial. *J Arthroplasty.* 2010;25:851-857.

44. Fu P, Wu Y, Wu H, et al. Efficacy of intra-articular cocktail analgesic injection in total knee arthroplasty: a randomized controlled trial. *Knee.* 2009;16:280-284.

45. Ashburn MA, Caplan RA, Carr DB, et al. Practice guidelines for acute pain management in the perioperative setting: an updated report by the American Society of Anesthesiologists task force on acute pain management. *Anesthesiology.* 2004;100:1573-1581.

46. Sinatra RS, Jahr JS, Reynolds LW, et al. Efficacy and safety of single and repeated administration of 1 gram intravenous acetaminophen injection (paracetamol) for pain management after major orthopedic surgery. *Anesthesiology.* 2005;102:822-831.

47. Zhou TJ, Tang J, White PF. Propacetamol versus ketorolac for treatment of acute postoperative pain after total hip or knee replacement. *Anesth Analg.* 2001;92:1569-1575.

48. Abdul-Hadi O, Parvizi J, Austin MS, et al. Nonsteroidal anti-inflammatory drugs in orthopaedics. *J Bone Joint Surg Am.* 2009;91:2020-2027.

49. Fischer HB, Simanski CJ. A procedure-specific systematic review and consensus recommendations for analgesia after total hip replacement. *Anaesthesia.* 2005;60:1189-1202.

50. Buvanendran A, Kroin JS, Tuman KJ, et al. Effects of perioperative administration of a selective cyclooxygenase 2 inhibitor on pain management and recovery of function after knee replacement: a randomized controlled trial. *JAMA.* 2003;290:2411-2418.

51. Straube S, Derry S, McQuay HJ, et al. Effect of preoperative Cox-II-selective NSAIDs (coxibs) on postoperative outcomes: a systematic review of randomized studies. *Acta Anaesthesiol Scand.* 2005; 49:601-613.

52. Dierking G, Duedahl TH, Rasmussen ML, et al. Effects of gabapentin on postoperative morphine consumption and pain after abdominal hysterectomy: a randomized, double-blind trial. *Acta Anaesthesiol Scand.* 2004;48:322-327.

53. Clarke H, Pereira S, Kennedy D, et al. Gabapentin decreases morphine consumption and improves functional recovery following total knee arthroplasty. *Pain Res Manag.* 2009;14:217-222.

54. Menigaux C, Adam F, Guignard B, et al. Preoperative gabapentin decreases anxiety and improves early functional recovery from knee surgery. *Anesth Analg.* 2005;100:1394-1399.

55. Buvanendran A, Kroin JS, Della Valle CJ, et al. Perioperative oral pregabalin reduces chronic pain after total knee arthroplasty: a prospective, randomized, controlled trial. *Anesth Analg.* 2010;110:199-207.

56. Turan A, White PF, Karamanlioglu B, et al. Gabapentin: an alternative to the cyclooxygenase-2 inhibitors for perioperative pain management. *Pain Med.* 2006; 102:175-181.

57. Urban MK, Ya Deau JT, Wukovits B, et al. Ketamine as an adjunct to postoperative pain management in opioid tolerant patients after spinal fusions: a prospective randomized trial. *HSS J.* 2008;4:62-65.

58. Adam F, Chauvin M, Du Manoir B, et al. Small-dose ketamine infusion improves postoperative analgesia and rehabilitation after total knee arthroplasty. *Anesth Analg.* 2005;100:475-480.

59. Grass JA. Patient-controlled analgesia. *Anesth Analg.* 2005;101:S44-61.

60. International Association for the Study of Pain. Classification of chronic pain. Descriptions of chronic pain syndromes and definitions of pain terms. Prepared by the International Association for the Study of Pain, Subcommitte on Taxonomy. *Pain Suppl.* 1986;3:S1-226.

61. Wylde V, Hewlett S, Learmonth ID, et al. Persistent pain after joint replacement: prevalence, sensory qualities, and postoperative determinants. *Pain.* 2011;152(3):566-572.

62. Rat AC, Guillemin F, Osnowycz G, et al. Total hip or knee replacement for osteoarthritis: mid- and long-term quality of life. *Arthritis Care Res.* 2010;62:54-62.

63. Woolf C. Somatic pain—pathogenesis and prevention. *Br J Anaesth.* 1995;75:169-176.

64. Apkarian AV, Sosa Y, Sonty S, et al. Chronic back pain is associated with decreased prefrontal and thalamic gray matter density. *J Neurosci.* 2004;24(46): 10410-10415.

65. Wilder-Smith OHG, Arendt-Nielsen L. Postoperative hyperalgesia: its clinical importance and relevance. *Anesthesiology.* 2006;104(3):601-607.

66. Loftus RW, Yeager MP, Clark JA, et al. Intraoperative ketamine reduces perioperative opiate consumption in opiate-dependent patients. *Anesthesiology.* 2010;113: 639-646.

28

Anesthetic Considerations

David Kim and Sean Garvin

This chapter gives a concise and focused introduction into the specialty of anesthesia and specifically highlights the benefits of regional anesthesia for patients who undergo knee surgery. Regional anesthesia has been proven to be safe and effective and may provide a better alternative to general anesthesia. Studies have shown that regional anesthesia provides superior pain control, allowing more effective rehabilitation and shorter hospital stays. Regional anesthesia has been shown to significantly decrease blood loss, the incidence of deep vein thrombosis, surgical site infections, and respiratory complications. Even in the ambulatory setting, regional anesthesia demonstrates faster recovery from sedation, a lower incidence of postoperative nausea and vomiting, and fewer hospital admissions for pain control.

Regional anesthesia is not without its drawbacks. It requires an experienced practitioner to successfully perform these blocks. Even with the most trained professional, success is not guaranteed, and it does not carry the nearly 100% effectiveness of general anesthesia in providing surgical anesthesia.

Anesthetic care for total knee arthroplasty should take into consideration individual patient factors and be tailored to each patient's specific needs, with the goal of providing a safe intraoperative experience and postoperative analgesia that affords patients the opportunity to increase their mobility and subsequently enhance their quality of life. Neuraxial anesthesia and peripheral nerve blockade both have excellent safety profiles in experienced hands and should be included in any anesthetic plan. A thorough understanding of the applications and limitations of regional anesthesia by both anesthesiologists and surgeons is crucial for a successful perioperative experience for the patient undergoing knee surgery. Continued research efforts at optimizing the perioperative care of patients undergoing knee replacement surgery should be aimed at improving functional outcomes, while minimizing morbidity and mortality.

PREOPERATIVE EVALUATION

Before undergoing total knee arthroplasty, all patients should undergo a through preoperative anesthesia evaluation. Preoperative anesthesia evaluation is a basic element of anesthesia practice and should be performed at a time that allows for careful review of the patient's medical history, performance of necessary diagnostic investigations, a focused physical examination, and, if necessary, consultant evaluation. Studies should be ordered on a case-by-case basis in order to optimize the perioperative management of each patient.[1] Orthopaedic surgery is considered an intermediate risk procedure for cardiovascular complications, with knee arthroplasty often being performed on older patients with limited functional capacity. Specific attention should be given to cardiac, pulmonary, renal, and endocrine comorbidities because these have been associated with increased morbidity in patients undergoing major noncardiac surgery.[1,2] These patients may require more extensive workup and possibly need additional treatment, thereby delaying elective orthopaedic surgery. The American Heart Association guidelines for perioperative cardiovascular evaluation recommend further evaluation and treatment of patients with unstable coronary syndromes, recent myocardial infarction, severe mitral or aortic stenosis, decompensated heart failure, and significant arrhythmias (including atrial fibrillation with a ventricular rate of greater that 100 beats per minute).[3] Consideration should be given to administration of perioperative beta blockers in patients with greater than one clinical risk factor for coronary artery disease undergoing total knee replacement.[4]

SPECIAL POPULATIONS

Cardiac Stents

As the surgical management of the orthopaedic surgery patient has evolved, so has the care of patients with coronary artery disease. Many patients presenting for knee replacement have a history of significant coronary artery disease that has been treated with percutaneous coronary intervention with or without stenting. Patients with drug-eluting intracoronary stents have been shown to be at increased risk of cardiac events and mortality when dual antiplatelet therapy with aspirin and thienopyridine is discontinued before 1 year. Therefore, elective surgery should be delayed for at least 365 days in this patient population.[5-10] In patients with bare metal stents, elective surgery should not be performed less than 30 days after stent implantation.[3,11-13] Clopidogrel should be discontinued a minimum of 7 days before neuraxial blockade, while ticlodipine should be held for at least 10 days before spinal or epidural anesthesia.[14] Aspirin therapy in the perioperative period has been shown to be safe, without increased risk of bleeding complications, including during neuraxial anesthesia, and should be continued throughout this time in patients with coronary artery disease.[10,13,15,16]

Anticoagulated Patient

Chronic anticoagulation therapy is often prescribed for patients with atrial fibrillation, pulmonary embolism, complicated deep vein thrombosis, and cerebral thrombosis. In the past, warfarin treatment has been the mainstay of chronic anticoagulation, with patients asked to abstain for 5 days before surgery, with those as high risk for thrombosis bridged with subcutaneous low-molecular-weight heparin (LMWH).[13] Neuraxial anesthesia should not be performed if the international normalized ratio (INR) is greater than 1.4.[14] In order to decrease the risk of spinal hematoma in those patients bridged with LMWH, neuraxial anesthesia should not be performed for at least 12 hours following once daily dosing and for 24 hours following twice daily dosing.[13,14] For similar reasons, epidural catheters should be removed with INR < 1.4 for those patients on warfarin therapy and at least 2 to 4 hours before LMWH administration.[13,14]In some circumstances a patient's INR may rise unexpectedly while an epidural catheter is in place; in this instance, clinical judgment is necessary to weigh the risks of leaving the catheter in place while coagulation normalizes and the risk of bleeding on catheter removal. Fortunately, during the first few days of warfarin therapy, patients with an elevated INR have a low risk of neurologic complication on catheter removal (see section on thromboprophylaxis and epidural anesthesia).[17]

In recent years, new therapies have emerged that may supplant warfarin in its role as therapy for thrombotic complications and as chemoprophylaxis. Postoperative chemoprophylaxis for prevention of thromboembolic complications has historically included warfarin and, more recently, low-molecular-weight heparinoids, and now factor Xa inhibitors.[18-20] These include the low-molecular-weight heparinoids, direct thrombin inhibitors including dabigatran and ximelagatran (no longer available), and factor Xa inhibitors, rivaroxaban and apixaban.[21-23] Perioperative anticoagulation increases risk of bleeding complications, while insufficient anticoagulation predisposes these patients to thrombotic events. Purported benefits of these new classes of anticoagulants are good oral bioavailability, once daily dosing, and the lack of need for routine coagulation monitoring as with warfarin therapy.[24] These new medications are likely the future of perioperative anticoagulation; however, given that clinical experience is limited, caution should be used when formulating a surgical and anesthetic plan. A summary of the current recommendations of the American Society of Regional Anesthesia and the European Society of Anaesthesiology for perioperative antiplatelet and anticoagulant medications and neuraxial blockade can be found in Table 28-1.

Bilateral Total Knee Arthroplasty

Bilateral simultaneous knee arthroplasty has been demonstrated to have a decreased length of stay when compared to sequential bilateral knee arthroplasty, a decreased economic burden, and the allure to patients of only having to endure a single period of rehabilitation.[25,26] There has been an increase in the number of simultaneous bilateral total knee replacements performed over the past decade,[27] with recent research highlighting the risks specific to this population. Bilateral total knee replacements are associated with increased cardiac and pulmonary morbidity, as well as overall mortality.[28-32] Risk factors for poor outcome include

TABLE 28-1. Summary of Antithrombotic Medications with Current Recommendations from American Society of Regional Anesthesia and Pain Medicine (ASRA)[13] and European Society of Anaesthesiology (ESA)[14]

Drug Class	Medications	Neuraxial-Needle Placement	Time to Resume After Puncture/ Catheter Removal
Unfractionated heparin	Subcutaneous	No contraindication to twice daily dosing	Heparin 1 hour after block, remove 2–4 hours after last dose
	Intravenous	4–6 hours after discontinuation; check PTT before attempt	Heparin 1 hour after block, consider holding longer if traumatic placement
LMWH	Enoxaparin-Prophylaxis once daily dosing	12 hours	2 hours after catheter removal (ASRA) 4 hours after catheter removal (ESA)
	Enoxaparin-treatment twice daily dosing	24 hours	2 hours after catheter removal (ASRA) 4 hours after catheter removal (ESA)
Antiplatelet	Aspirin	No contraindication	No contraindication
	Clopidogrel	Hold for 7 days	After removal
	Ticlodipine	Hold for 10 days	After removal
	Prasugrel	Hold 7–10 days	6 hours after catheter removal
Vitamin K antagonists	Warfarin	Normal INR (ASRA) INR ≤ 1.4 (ESA)	INR <1.5(ASRA) Resume after catheter removed (ESA)
Direct thrombin inhibitors	Lepirudin/ Desirudin	ASRA suggests avoidance 8–10 hours (Check PTT) (ESA)	2–4 hours (Check PTT) (ESA)
	Argatroban	ASRA suggests avoidance 4 hours (ESA)	2 hours (ESA)
	Dabigatran	ASRA - no information Contraindicated per manufacturer	ASRA - no information 6 hours (ESA)
Anti-Xa agents	Fondaparinux	Single injection, no timeframe, avoid catheters (ASRA) 36–42 hours (ESA)	6–12 hours ESA
	Rivaroxaban	ASRA - no information 22–36 hours (ESA)	ASRA - no information 4–6 hours (ESA)
	Apixaban	ASRA- no information 26–30 hours (ESA)	ASRA - no information 4–6 hours (ESA)

PTT, partial thromboplastin time.

advanced age, male gender, history of dementia, congestive heart failure, renal disease, cerebrovascular disease, and pulmonary hypertension.[29-32] Bilateral total knee replacements should be performed only on patients who have demonstrated adequate cardiopulmonary reserve with few comorbid conditions. Figure 28-1 summarizes criteria for bilateral total knee replacement at our institution. These patients often warrant invasive hemodynamic monitoring, vigilant fluid management, and prolonged observation in a critical care environment.

Exclusion criteria for one-stage bilateral total knee replacement:

1. Age $\geq$ 80 years old
2. ASA Class $\geq$ III
3. Ischemic heart disease as evidenced by a positive stress test or a history of angina
4. Poor ventricular function; CHF within the previous year and/or LVEF $<$ 40%
5. Oxygen-dependent pulmonary disease

Patients with the following comorbidities should be considered at increased risk:

1. Insulin-dependent diabetes mellitus
2. Pulmonary hypertension
3. Steroid-dependent asthma
4. Morbid obesity (BMI > 40 kg/m^2)
5. Renal insufficiency (Cr >1.6 g/dL)
6. Chronic liver disease
7. Cerebral vascular disease

FIGURE 28-1. *Guidelines for patient selection for simultaneous bilateral total knee arthroplasty. CHF, congestive heart failure; LVEF, left ventricular ejection fraction; BMI, body mass index.*

INTRAOPERATIVE MANAGEMENT

Formulation of an anesthetic plan for total knee replacement requires careful consideration of many factors. First and foremost, patient history and individual preferences must be evaluated and the attendant risks and benefits of each anesthetic option weighed. The interplay of this information with the postoperative surgical plan for thromboembolic prophylaxis and physical therapy may significantly affect anesthetic management. Finally, an anesthesiologist's comfort with individual anesthetic techniques plays a pivotal role in this decision-making process.

ANESTHETIC TECHNIQUE

General Anesthesia

General anesthesia is probably the most common anesthetic performed for knee arthroplasty worldwide, with many centers performing one or more peripheral nerve blocks as adjuncts for intraoperative pain control, and for continued postoperative analgesia. Patients often express fear of regional anesthesia and would prefer to "be asleep" and therefore request general anesthesia. Patients are also influenced by surgeon preferences.[33] General anesthesia has the benefit of faster induction times[34,35] and near 100% success rates and may hasten time to discharge from the postanesthesia care unit. Combined with a peripheral nerve block, general anesthesia with a laryngeal mask airway is often satisfactory in the appropriately selected patient and may afford faster recovery from the general anesthetic.[35] Morbidly obese patients and those with severe gastroesophageal reflux disease should have their airways controlled with an endotracheal tube if a neuraxial technique is not feasible or is unsuccessful. Clinicians caring for patients with complex spine disease or instrumentation should weigh the risks and benefits of general versus neuraxial techniques.[36] While general anesthesia certainly has advantages, it is also associated with increased opioid use, higher early postoperative pain scores,[37] a higher incidence of nausea and vomiting,[38] and a higher risk of postoperative venous thromboembolism.[39]

Central Neuraxial Blockade

Neuraxial blockade, including epidural, spinal, and combined anesthetic techniques, provides ideal operating conditions for knee arthroplasty. Full muscle relaxation is achieved, allowing for maximal range of motion without the requirement of endotracheal intubation. Neuraxial blockade has been associated with high patient satisfaction,[33] less sedation, better pain control,[37,40] greater passive range of motion, and faster rehabilitation.[40,41] Central neuraxial blockade has been shown to decrease cardiopulmonary complications,[42,43] venous thromboemolism,[39,43] renal failure,[43] and mortality[42,43] in patients undergoing noncardiac surgery.[43]

Risks of central neuraxial blockade include a failed block,[44,45] hypotension,[46] bradycardia,[46] and urinary retention. Spinal anesthesia failure after injection of local anesthetic has been reported in as many as 17% of patients.[45] However, that incidence has been recently demonstrated to be much lower; with the use of Whitacre needles, the incidence is now on the order of 0% to 5.5%.[44,46,47] Combined spinal-epidural techniques are useful for placement at the lower lumbar levels and afford a reliable, quick onset of surgical anesthesia for knee surgery with the ability to provide supplemental anesthetic medications through the epidural catheter.

Post-dural puncture headache (PDPH) is a complication of dural puncture and is characterized by a migraine-like frontoparietal headache that has the key feature of being postural in nature and may be associated with vision changes, diplopia, light sensitivity, and vomiting.[48] Although the exact mechanism is unknown, it is likely related to leakage of cerebrospinal from the site of the durotomy.[48] When the dura is punctured with a large-bore needle such as a 17-gauge Weiss needle, PDPH occurs up to 75.3% of the time[49] in ages 20 to 40, while PDPH is much less common in the elderly and with smaller 27-gauge Whitacre-type needles (0% to 37%).[50,51] PDPH is usually benign and self-limiting and can be treated symptomatically with oral hydration, analgesics, and caffeine.[52] Larger-bore dural punctures are less likely to heal spontaneously and may require more aggressive therapy, such as epidural blood patch[53] and, in extremely rare instances, dural repair.[54] In such instances, it may be advisable to use aspirin and not warfarin for anticoagulation, to allow the option of performing a blood patch in the immediate postoperative period. Epidural abscess and hematoma are both rare complications that occur <0.12% of the time according to recent reports.[55-58] Other neurologic complications after neuraxial block are fortunately rare and have an estimated incidence in the range of 1 in 2500[59] to 30,000,[57] with a seemingly higher incidence in patients with preexisting spinal canal pathology.[36]

Peripheral Nerve Block

Over the past 30 years, a considerable amount of research has been performed examining the impact of peripheral nerve block on patient outcome in total knee arthroplasty.[60] Peripheral nerve blockade has been shown to be safe with an estimated incidence of peripheral nerve injury of 0.79%, which has not been associated with peripheral nerve blockade or type of anesthesia, but the risk was increased with longer tourniquet time and bilateral procedures.[61] Additional review of the literature indicates that peripheral nerve block for lower extremity surgery is associated with a low rate of neuropathy (0.34%), with permanent neurologic deficits being extremely rare.[59] Performance of peripheral nerve blocks for knee arthroplasty requires an anesthesiologist familiar with the innervation of the knee and detailed knowledge of anatomical landmarks in order to provide a successful block. Peripheral nerve blocks have often been used in conjunction with either neuraxial techniques[62] or general anesthesia and provide improved outcomes with opioid-sparing benefits,[60,63] fewer gastrointestinal complications,[64] fewer cases of urinary retention,[64] shorter length of stay,[64] and greater patient satisfaction,[65] without the risks of instrumentation of the neuraxis.[66] Ultrasound-guided blocks have become more routinely performed as anesthesiologists become familiar with the technical requirements and can be provided with a high success rate and possible decrement in complications with quicker block times and shorter onset.[67]

Femoral nerve block provides sensory and motor blockade to the anterior thigh via blockade of the L2-L4 ventral rami and has been shown to enhance postoperative analgesia[62,65] in patients undergoing knee replacement surgery. Both nerve stimulator and ultrasound-guided approaches have demonstrated success (85% vs. 95%, respectively),[68] with recent evidence suggesting that ultrasound-guided techniques have higher success rates, shorter onset, and better quality of motor and sensory block at lower volumes of local anesthetic.[69-71] Single-shot femoral nerve block and continuous perineural catheters have both been investigated. The combination of single-injection femoral nerve block added to epidural patient-controlled analgesia with low-concentration bupivacaine and hydromorphone has been shown to decrease visual analog pain scores for up to 2 days postoperatively, with increased passive range of motion on postoperative day 2.[62] Femoral nerve block and catheters may increase patient satisfaction,[65] decrease rescue pain medication,[71] decrease the incidence of nausea,[63] facilitate physical therapy,[62] and hasten hospital discharge.[72]

Lumbar plexus block can be performed via a posterior approach through the psoas compartment and provides sensory and motor block of L1-L4 nerve roots, providing analgesia to both obturator and femoral nerves and, when combined with sciatic nerve block, it may provide unilateral anesthesia to the operative extremity. Clinicians with significant experience in regional anesthetic techniques may combine these blocks in patients for whom general and neuraxial anesthesia could be problematic. Lumbar plexus block has been associated with rare major complications including death, cardiac arrest, high spinal anesthesia, respiratory failure, and seizure[73] and should be performed by clinicians skilled in the placement of the block with the ability to manage these possible major complications.

Sciatic nerve block has been extensively investigated as part of the anesthetic management of patients undergoing total knee arthroplasty, with the posterior approach providing motor and sensory block to the L4-S3 nerve roots. Single-injection and catheter-based techniques have been evaluated with single injections providing supplementary analgesia for up to 24 hours, with catheter techniques extending this period up to 48 hours even with dynamic motion.[74] Single-injection sciatic nerve block combined with femoral nerve block has similar pain scores, morphine consumption, and satisfaction compared to continuous epidural infusion.[75] Additionally, catheter-based techniques for sciatic nerve block when coupled with lumbar plexus block have recently been shown to provide superior analgesia, decreased morphine consumption, and improved early rehabilitation when compared to single-injection sciatic nerve block.[76] Unfortunately, few studies have been performed with epidural analgesia and sciatic nerve block, with a recent systematic review finding insufficient evidence to recommend routine sciatic nerve block for total knee replacement.[77]

Ultrasound-guided saphenous nerve block has garnered recent research interest with the increased use of ultrasound imaging for identification of sensory nerves. The saphenous nerve is a sensory branch of the femoral nerve that innervates the anteromedial aspect of the lower extremity and can provide anesthesia and analgesia to this portion of the leg without motor blockade. In a small series, block success rate has been reported as 77%,[78] 95.6%,[79] and 100%[80] with ultrasound-guided block via a subsartorial approach. In a small study,[80] saphenous block provided good analgesia in patients undergoing knee arthroscopy.[67] Continuous adductor canal blockade was found to provide adequate analgesia with low pain scores in a small preliminary study of patients undergoing total knee arthroplasty.[81] Further study is required to determine if saphenous blockade can provide adequate analgesia while maintaining motor function of the quadriceps, possibly improving early physical therapy rehabilitation.

Hypotensive Epidural Anesthesia

Hypotensive epidural anesthesia is an anesthetic technique that has been shown to decrease blood loss during hip[82-84] and knee arthroplasty.[85] Hypotensive epidural anesthesia is a safe technique that has been used without significant morbidity even in elderly patients[83] and in those with preoperative low cardiac output,[86] mild to moderate aortic stenosis,[87] and renal dysfunction.[86] Hypotensive epidural anesthesia has been shown to have a decreased blood loss when compared to the same level of hypotension induced during a general anesthetic.[82] While tourniquet application is a key component to prevention of intraoperative blood loss, there are instances in which tourniquet application is not feasible (eg, morbid obesity) or not advisable (eg, peripheral arterial disease, prosthetic vascular grafts, preexisting deep venous thrombosis) and hypotensive epidural anesthesia should be considered for these patients.

Local Anesthetic Adjuncts

The addition of opioids and alpha-2 receptor to local anesthetics delivered via the neuraxial route has been shown to not only decrease the dose of local anesthetic required to attain anesthesia but also increase the duration of analgesia.[88] Intrathecal morphine has been shown to improve pain scores when compared to single-injection femoral nerve block in patients who underwent total knee arthroplasty.[89] Caution must be used when morphine is administered via the neuraxial route because it has a long duration of action and may cause late respiratory depression; as a result, these patients may warrant an extended stay in a monitored setting.

Many different pharmacologic adjuncts have been combined with local anesthetic mixtures used for peripheral nerve blockade, including epinephrine,[90] clonidine,[91] and dexamethasone,[92] all of which have been shown to increase block duration, with various side effects including hypotension, syncope, and sedation. A recent study showed that the addition of dexamethasone to interscalene brachial plexus block was well tolerated, with a significant prolongation of analgesia duration with a concomitant decrease in narcotic consumption.[92] Prospective randomized trials of adjuncts may help delineate a dose response relationship and, if postoperative analgesia can be sufficiently prolonged, the need for perineural catheters may be diminished or altogether eliminated.

Multimodal Therapy

Collaboration between surgical and anesthesia providers allows for the establishment of perioperative multimodal analgesia regimens that include preoperative medication in an effort to provide pre-emptive analgesia using multiple classes of medications, which may improve outcomes and decrease side effects.[93] Typical regimens include preoperative long-acting oral narcotics, oral nonsteroidal anti-inflammatory drugs, and intra-articular injection of a mixture of local anesthetic, anti-inflammatory, steroid, and narcotic agents.[64,94] When combined with peripheral nerve blockade, multimodal therapy may facilitate better pain control, enhance physical therapy, shorten length of stay,[94] and decrease perioperative complications including ileus and urinary retention.[64]

Tourniquet

An intraoperative tourniquet is used widely for total knee arthroplasty. It is believed to decrease blood loss, improve the visibility of the surgical field, and provide better conditions for cementing leading to better fixation. However, several studies have demonstrated that the use of a tourniquet may be more detrimental than beneficial.[95] Besides the hemodynamic changes caused by inflation and deflation, tourniquet use may increase the risk for nerve injury, vascular injury, infection, thromboembolism, and postoperative edema.[96]

The hemodynamic shifts and metabolic insults from tourniquet use influence the anesthesiologist's decision-making process about the intraoperative monitoring needed (eg, arterial line, central venous pressure monitoring) to safely care for certain debilitated patients. Upon inflation, there is an increase in preload and afterload, which may cause patients with significant cardiac disease to decompensate leading to acute congestive heart failure. After 45 to 60 minutes, the tourniquet is known to cause significant pain and hypertension that is usually blunted using a regional technique, but is difficult to treat under general anesthesia.[97] Upon deflation, there is not only a drop in systemic vascular resistance, but also the release of ischemic metabolic factors (lactate, carbon dioxide) and emboli[98] that may significantly alter a patient's physiology. Deflation has been linked with acute pulmonary edema, emboli, and cardiac arrest.[99-101]

Through creation of a "bloodless field," the tourniquet leads to a state of increased fibrinolysis and thrombosis.[102,103] Venous stasis, endothelial damage with increased platelet adhesion, and a hypoxic hypothermic environment may contribute to this hypercoagulable state, possibly explaining the higher incidences of deep vein thrombosis and pulmonary emboli in patients with tourniquet application.[104]

Neuropraxia can occur after tourniquet use and is most likely related to both the pressure and duration of tourniquet inflation. To minimize the risk of nerve injury, it is recommended to limit the use of a tourniquet to 90 to 120 minutes.[105] Consideration must also be taken for patients with significant peripheral vascular disease. Patients with prior arterial revascularization should be excluded from the use of a tourniquet since they are at an increased risk for graft thrombosis.

Comparison studies have not shown that tourniquet use decreases total blood loss. Since the majority of blood loss occurs postoperatively, the overall total blood loss did not significantly differ whether or not a tourniquet was used.

Perioperative Bleeding

Total knee arthroplasties are known to cause significant perioperative blood loss, with reports of up to 1500 mL.[106] Blood conservation methods have been developed in preparation for the anticipated losses: preoperative autologous blood donation, iron supplementation, erythropoietin implementation, cell salvage, and the use of antifibrinolytics.

Although a tourniquet minimizes the intraoperative blood loss, most of the perioperative blood loss in total knee replacement surgery occurs after surgery. Hypotensive epidural anesthesia has shown to significantly reduce total perioperative blood loss. A study done by Juelsgaard and associates demonstrated that although intraoperative blood loss is lower with the use of a tourniquet (13 mL vs 146 mL), the overall perioperative blood loss is significantly lower among the hypotensive epidural anesthesia group (1056 mL vs 1826 mL). Nearly half of the total blood loss occurred 3 hours after surgery, and 80% occurred during the first 24 hours. In the hypotensive epidural group, 57% of the patients required no blood transfusion during their hospital stay versus 19% in the tourniquet group. Also, the overall amount of blood transfusion required was significantly lower in the epidural group (193 mL) than in the tourniquet group (775 mL).[85]

In another study comparing hypotensive epidural anesthesia and hypotensive total intravenous anesthesia in patients undergoing total hip arthroplasty, the epidural group had significantly less blood loss and transfusions than the intravenous group. The difference may be associated with nonpositive pressure ventilation, distribution of blood flow, and lower mean intraoperative central venous pressure with the epidural.[82]

POSTOPERATIVE CONSIDERATIONS

Surgical Site Infections

Surgical site infections (SSIs) are devastating complications that lead to costly and prolonged hospitalization. In 1992, a report found that each SSI led to 7.3 additional hospital days and cost $3,152.[107] A more recent review estimated the cost of a superficial surgical site infection to be $8,338.[108] In the past decade, there have been major advances in infection control practices, including operating room ventilation, sterilization methods, barrier precautions, surgical technique, hand washing, and antibiotic prophylaxis. However, despite these preventative measures, SSI remains the third most common cause of nosocomial infection, making up 14% to 16% of all nosocomial infections in hospitalized patients.[109]

Interestingly, epidural anesthesia may provide an additional preventative tool to help combat SSI. A recent retrospective study demonstrated that patients undergoing total knee and hip replacements under neuraxial anesthesia were half as likely to have an SSI versus those who had a general anesthetic. The overall risk of SSI after a total hip or knee was 2.21 times higher under a general anesthetic versus a neuraxial anesthetic (eg, epidural or spinal).[110]

It is believed that the epidural anesthesia improves tissue perfusion, maintaining normothermia and increased tissue oxygenation, thereby creating an environment that may aid in promoting host immune defenses. Postoperative pain induces a sympathetic activation causing release of endogenous catecholamines, leading to stress-induced vasoconstriction, reducing perfusion and tissue oxygenation and creating a local tissue environment that may predispose to an SSI. Superior pain control via an epidural may blunt such a stress response, leading to fewer infectious complications.

Deep Vein Thrombosis

The reported incidence of deep venous thrombosis (DVT) without prophylaxis ranges from 58% to 84% and from 17% to 57% with prophylaxis.[111,112] Studies have shown that patients who undergo total knee arthroplasty under epidural anesthesia have lower incidences of DVT. The relative risk of DVT may be reduced by up to 69% after epidural anesthesia as opposed to a general anesthetic.[113]

The proposed mechanism whereby epidural anesthesia decreases the incidence of DVT is attributed to the sympathetic blockade, which induces vasodilation and increased blood flow to the lower extremities. Also, the superior analgesia achieved with an epidural postoperatively and subsequent earlier mobilization[114] may explain the lower DVT rates. In addition, epidural anesthesia and analgesia attenuate the stress response, which decreases the release of catecholamine and cortisol, most likely leading to higher antithrombin III and lower fibrinogen levels. Epidural anesthesia and analgesia attenuate the hypercoagulable state seen after total knee arthroplasty.[115]

Though epidural anesthesia has shown to be an effective tool in lowering the incidences of DVT, there is still a high risk of developing a thrombus if no other measures are taken. Clearly a multimodal approach to DVT prophylaxis is important, which may include epidural analgesia, pneumatic compression stockings, warfarin or aspirin, and early rehabilitation. Using this approach, the rates of DVT at our institution are comparable to ones achieved with LMWH, without the risk of bleeding and epidural hematoma.[116]

Thromboprophylaxis and Epidural Analgesia

Thromboprophylaxis is essential after major knee surgery. However, since the induction of LMWH, the increased risk for epidural hematomas has often precluded the use of a neuraxial block in the perioperative setting.[117] The most recent American Society of Regional Anesthesia (ASRA) guidelines recommend that no spinal or epidural be attempted until 12 hours after the last dose of LMWH (24 hours if on a twice daily therapeutic dosing regimen).[13] See Table 28-1 for a summary of current recommendations. Most centers, including ours, do not leave an epidural catheter in place postoperatively while on LMWH because of the risk of accidental removals.

However, warfarin has been effectively used in the perioperative period, achieving significant reduction in the incidences of DVT and pulmonary embolism.[116] As mentioned earlier, a possible explanation for the reduced rates of DVT is by a sympathectomy-induced vasodilation, increasing blood flow in the lower extremities and possibly by reducing the hypercoagulability of the patient by blunting the surgical stress response. Warfarin is started on the day of surgery and an epidural patient-controlled analgesia is used until the 1st or 2nd postoperative day (POD). Despite INR levels achieved on POD 2, at our institution an epidural is often removed.[17] In a multicenter study with 4365 patients, Liu et al demonstrated the safety of removing an epidural in the setting of an INR greater than 1.4 during the initiation of warfarin therapy.[17] It is believed that the INR on POD 2 inaccurately assesses the patients "true" anticoagulated state. The therapeutic effects of warfarin are dependent on factors II and X, but the initial rise in INR is mostly due to the short half-life of factor VII. Conversely, when a patient has been off warfarin and an INR has decreased to less than 1.5, factors II and X may not have recovered sufficiently for adequate coagulation, and excessive bleeding may occur perioperatively.

Postoperative Cognitive Dysfunction, Delirium, and the Elderly

Postoperative cognitive dysfunction (POCD) and delirium are devastating conditions that reportedly affect up to 44% of the elderly after major surgery.[118] Postoperative delirium is also an extremely costly condition that can lead to increased morbidity and mortality. In 1994, the cost associated with delirium exceeded $4 billion per year.[119]

Several studies have identified multiple risk factors for POCD, with advanced age, preexisting cognitive dysfunction, electrolyte abnormalities, history of alcohol or benzodiazepine use, and impaired functional status to be the most frequently cited predictors.[118,120,121] The relative contributions of surgery and anesthesia to the development of POCD are unclear.

Anesthesia as a risk factor for POCD in the elderly has not been thoroughly investigated. The literature reveals few areas of consensus with regard to the influence of anesthesia and POCD in the elderly.[122] Studies have shown that the incidence of POCD is significantly lower in the elderly undergoing minor surgery as opposed to major surgery, especially in the ambulatory setting as opposed to a hospitalized environment.[123] It is interesting that studies have shown no difference in the incidence of POCD when an epidural is used as opposed to general anesthesia.[122,124]

The use of sedatives such as benzodiazepines in the elderly did show an increased risk of POCD, with an incidence as high as 48%.[125] Therefore, it is likely wise to limit benzodiazepine use in the elderly. However, Kadoi and colleagues demonstrated that propofol and fentanyl did not affect the cognitive performance after surgery with preservation of cerebral oxygenation.[126] Additionally, hypotensive anesthesia has not been shown to increase the incidence of POCD[83] in the elderly. Additionally, inadequate pain control has been associated with higher incidences of delirium and thus every effort should be made to ensure adequate analgesia to this group of patients.[127]

ACKNOWLEDGMENT

This chapter was written under the editorial guidance of Nigel Sharrock, MB, ChB.

REFERENCES

1. Practice advisory for preanesthesia evaluation: a report by the American Society of Anesthesiologists Task Force on Preanesthesia Evaluation. *Anesthesiology.* 2002;96:485-496.
2. Lee TH, Marcantonio ER, Mangione CM, et al. Derivation and prospective validation of a simple index for prediction of cardiac risk of major noncardiac surgery. *Circulation.* 1999;100:1043-1049.
3. Fleisher LA, Beckman JA, Brown KA, et al. ACC/AHA 2007 guidelines on perioperative cardiovascular evaluation and care for noncardiac surgery: a report of the American College of Cardiology/American Heart Association Task Force on Practice Guidelines (Writing Committee to Revise the 2002 Guidelines on Perioperative Cardiovascular Evaluation for Noncardiac Surgery): developed in collaboration with the American Society of Echocardiography, American Society of Nuclear Cardiology, Heart Rhythm Society, Society of Cardiovascular Anesthesiologists, Society for Cardiovascular Angiography and Interventions, Society for Vascular Medicine and Biology, and Society for Vascular Surgery. *Circulation.* 2007;116:e418-499.
4. Fleisher LA, Beckman JA, Brown KA, et al. 2009 ACCF/AHA focused update on perioperative beta blockade incorporated into the ACC/AHA 2007 guidelines on perioperative cardiovascular evaluation and care for noncardiac surgery: a report of the American College of Cardiology Foundation/American Heart Association Task Force on Practice Guidelines. *Circulation.* 2009;120:e169-276.
5. Grines CL, Bonow RO, Casey DE Jr, et al. Prevention of premature discontinuation of dual antiplatelet therapy in patients with coronary artery stents: a science advisory from the American Heart Association, American College of Cardiology, Society for Cardiovascular Angiography and Interventions, American College of Surgeons, and American Dental Association, with representation from the American College of Physicians. *J Am Coll Cardiol.* 2007;49:734-739.
6. Banerjee S, Varghese C, Samuel J, et al. Comparison of the impact of short (<1 year) and long-term (> or = 1 year) clopidogrel use following percutaneous coronary intervention on mortality. *Am J Cardiol.* 2008;102:1159-1162.
7. King SB III, Smith SC Jr, Hirshfeld JW Jr, et al. 2007 focused update of the ACC/AHA/SCAI 2005 guideline update for percutaneous coronary intervention: a report of the American College of Cardiology/American Heart Association Task Force on Practice Guidelines: 2007 writing group to review new evidence and update the ACC/AHA/SCAI 2005

guideline update for percutaneous coronary intervention, writing on behalf of the 2005 Writing Committee. *Circulation.* 2008;117:261-295.

8. Mehta SR, Yusuf S, Peters RJ, et al. Effects of pretreatment with clopidogrel and aspirin followed by long-term therapy in patients undergoing percutaneous coronary intervention: the PCI-CURE study. *Lancet.* 2001;358:527-533.
9. Lagerqvist B, James SK, Stenestrand U, et al. Long-term outcomes with drug-eluting stents versus bare-metal stents in Sweden. *N Engl J Med.* 2007;356: 1009-1019.
10. Douketis JD, Berger PB, Dunn AS, et al. The perioperative management of antithrombotic therapy: American College of Chest Physicians evidence-based clinical practice guidelines (8th edition). *Chest.* 2008;133:299S-339S.
11. Korte W, Cattaneo M, Chassot PG, et al. Peri-operative management of antiplatelet therapy in patients with coronary artery disease: joint position paper by members of the working group on perioperative haemostasis of the Society on Thrombosis and Haemostasis Research (GTH), the working group on perioperative coagulation of the Austrian Society for Anesthesiology, Resuscitation and Intensive Care (OGARI) and the working group thrombosis of the European Society for Cardiology (ESC). *Thromb Haemost.* 2011;105:743-749.
12. Practice alert for the perioperative management of patients with coronary artery stents: a report by the American Society of Anesthesiologists Committee on Standards and Practice Parameters. *Anesthesiology.* 2009;110:22-23.
13. Horlocker TT, Wedel DJ, Rowlingson JC, et al. Regional anesthesia in the patient receiving antithrombotic or thrombolytic therapy: American Society of Regional Anesthesia and Pain Medicine Evidence-Based Guidelines (Third Edition). *Reg Anesth Pain Med.* 2010;35:64-101.
14. Gogarten W, Vandermeulen E, Van Aken H, et al. Regional anaesthesia and antithrombotic agents: recommendations of the European Society of Anaesthesiology. *Eur J Anaesthesiol.* 2010;27:999-1015.
15. Merritt JC, Bhatt DL. The efficacy and safety of perioperative antiplatelet therapy. *J Thromb Thrombolysis.* 2004;17:21-7.
16. Horlocker TT, Wedel DJ, Schroeder DR, et al. Preoperative antiplatelet therapy does not increase the risk of spinal hematoma associated with regional anesthesia. *Anesth Analg.* 1995;80:303-309.
17. Liu SS, Buvanendran A, Viscusi ER, et al. Uncomplicated removal of epidural catheters in 4365 patients with international normalized ratio greater than 1.4 during initiation of warfarin therapy. *Reg Anesth Pain Med.* 2011;36:231-235.
18. Turpie AG, Lassen MR, Eriksson BI, et al. Rivaroxaban for the prevention of venous thromboembolism after hip or knee arthroplasty. Pooled analysis of four studies. *Thromb Haemost.* 2011;105:444-453.
19. Heit JA, Berkowitz SD, Bona R, et al. Efficacy and safety of low molecular weight heparin (ardeparin sodium) compared to warfarin for the prevention of venous thromboembolism after total knee replacement surgery: a double-blind, dose-ranging study. Ardeparin Arthroplasty Study Group. *Thromb Haemost.* 1997;77:32-38.
20. Francis CW, Berkowitz SD, Comp PC, et al. Comparison of ximelagatran with warfarin for the prevention of venous thromboembolism after total knee replacement. *N Engl J Med.* 2003;349:1703-1712.
21. Landman GW, Gans RO. Oral rivaroxaban for symptomatic venous thromboembolism. *N Engl J Med.* 2011;364:1178; author reply 1178.
22. Connolly SJ, Eikelboom J, Joyner C, et al. Apixaban in patients with atrial fibrillation. *N Engl J Med.* 2011;364:806-817.
23. Schulman S, Kearon C, Kakkar AK, et al. Dabigatran versus warfarin in the treatment of acute venous thromboembolism. *N Engl J Med.* 2009;361:2342-2352.
24. Freyburger G, Macouillard G, Labrouche S, et al. Coagulation parameters in patients receiving dabigatran etexilate or rivaroxaban: two observational studies in patients undergoing total hip or total knee replacement. *Thromb Res.* 2011;127:457-465.
25. Reuben JD, Meyers SJ, Cox DD, et al. Cost comparison between bilateral simultaneous, staged, and unilateral total joint arthroplasty. *J Arthroplasty.* 1998;13:172-179.
26. Stubbs G, Pryke SE, Tewari S, et al. Safety and cost benefits of bilateral total knee replacement in an acute hospital. *ANZ J Surg.* 2005;75:739-746.
27. Memtsoudis SG, Besculides MC, Reid S, et al. Trends in bilateral total knee arthroplasties: 153,259 discharges between 1990 and 2004. *Clin Orthop Relat Res.* 2009;467:1568-1576.
28. Restrepo C, Parvizi J, Dietrich T, et al. Safety of simultaneous bilateral total knee arthroplasty. A meta-analysis. *J Bone Joint Surg Am.* 2007;89:1220-1226.

29. Memtsoudis SG, Ma Y, Gonzalez Della Valle A, et al. Perioperative outcomes after unilateral and bilateral total knee arthroplasty. *Anesthesiology.* 2009;111: 1206-1216.
30. Memtsoudis SG, Ma Y, Chiu YL, et al. Bilateral total knee arthroplasty: risk factors for major morbidity and mortality. *Anesth Analg.* 2011;113(4):784-790.
31. Memtsoudis SG, Gonzalez Della Valle A, Besculides MC, et al. In-hospital complications and mortality of unilateral, bilateral, and revision TKA: based on an estimate of 4,159,661 discharges. *Clin Orthop Relat Res.* 2008;466:2617-2627.
32. Memtsoudis SG, Della Valle AG, Besculides MC, et al. Risk factors for perioperative mortality after lower extremity arthroplasty: a population-based study of 6,901,324 patient discharges. *J Arthroplasty.* 2010;25: 19-26.
33. Webster F, Bremner S, McCartney CJ. Patient experiences as knowledge for the evidence base: a qualitative approach to understanding patient experiences regarding the use of regional anesthesia for hip and knee arthroplasty. *Reg Anesth Pain Med.* 2011;36(5):461-465.
34. Liu SS, Strodtbeck WM, Richman JM, et al. A comparison of regional versus general anesthesia for ambulatory anesthesia: a meta-analysis of randomized controlled trials. *Anesth Analg.* 2005;101:1634-1642.
35. Williams BA, Kentor ML, Williams JP, et al. Process analysis in outpatient knee surgery: effects of regional and general anesthesia on anesthesia-controlled time. *Anesthesiology.* 2000;93:529-538.
36. Hebl JR, Horlocker TT, Kopp SL, et al. Neuraxial blockade in patients with preexisting spinal stenosis, lumbar disk disease, or prior spine surgery: efficacy and neurologic complications. *Anesth Analg.* 2010; 111:1511-1519.
37. Choi PT, Bhandari M, Scott J, et al. Epidural analgesia for pain relief following hip or knee replacement. *Cochrane Database System Rev.* 2003: CD003071.
38. Larsson S, Lundberg D. A prospective survey of postoperative nausea and vomiting with special regard to incidence and relations to patient characteristics, anesthetic routines and surgical procedures. *Acta Anaesthesiol Scand.* 1995;39:539-545.
39. Khatod M, Inacio MC, Bini SA, et al. Pulmonary embolism prophylaxis in more than 30, 000 total knee arthroplasty patients: is there a best choice? *J Arthroplasty.* 2012;27(2):167-172.
40. Capdevila X, Barthelet Y, Biboulet P, et al. Effects of perioperative analgesic technique on the surgical outcome and duration of rehabilitation after major knee surgery. *Anesthesiology.* 1999;91:8-15.
41. Williams-Russo P, Sharrock NE, Haas SB, et al. Randomized trial of epidural versus general anesthesia: outcomes after primary total knee replacement. *Clin Orthop Relat Res.* 1996:199-208.
42. van Lier F, van der Geest PJ, Hoeks SE, et al. Epidural analgesia is associated with improved health outcomes of surgical patients with chronic obstructive pulmonary disease. *Anesthesiology.* 2011;115:315-321.
43. Rodgers A, Walker N, Schug S, et al. Reduction of postoperative mortality and morbidity with epidural or spinal anaesthesia: results from overview of randomised trials. *BMJ.* 2000;321:1493.
44. Fuzier R, Bataille B, Fuzier V, et al. Spinal anesthesia failure after local anesthetic injection into cerebrospinal fluid: a multicenter prospective analysis of its incidence and related risk factors in 1214 patients. *Reg Anesth Pain Med.* 2011;36:322-326.
45. Levy JH, Islas JA, Ghia JN, et al. A retrospective study of the incidence and causes of failed spinal anesthetics in a university hospital. *Anesth Analg.* 1985;64:705-710.
46. Zayas VM, Liguori GA, Chisholm MF, et al. Dose response relationships for isobaric spinal mepivacaine using the combined spinal epidural technique. *Anesth Analg.* 1999;89:1167-1171.
47. Lynch J, Kasper SM, Strick K, et al. The use of Quincke and Whitacre 27-gauge needles in orthopedic patients: incidence of failed spinal anesthesia and postdural puncture headache. *Anesth Analg.* 1994;79:124-128.
48. Bezov D, Lipton RB, Ashina S. Post-dural puncture headache. Part I: diagnosis, epidemiology, etiology, and pathophysiology. *Headache.* 2010;50:1144-1152.
49. Lambert DH, Hurley RJ, Hertwig L, et al. Role of needle gauge and tip configuration in the production of lumbar puncture headache. *Reg Anesth.* 1997;22: 66-72.
50. Corbey MP, Bach AB, Lech K, et al. Grading of severity of postdural puncture headache after 27-gauge Quincke and Whitacre needles. *Acta Anaesthesiol Scand.* 1997;41:779-784.
51. Santanen U, Rautoma P, Luurila H, et al. Comparison of 27-gauge (0.41-mm) Whitacre and Quincke spinal needles with respect to post-dural puncture headache and non-dural puncture headache. *Acta Anaesthesiol Scand.* 2004;48:474-479.
52. Bezov D, Ashina S, Lipton R. Post-dural puncture headache. Part II: prevention, management, and prognosis. *Headache.* 2010;50:1482-1498.

53. Boonmak P, Boonmak S. Epidural blood patching for preventing and treating post-dural puncture headache. *Cochrane Database System Rev.* 2010:CD001791.
54. Harrington H, Tyler HR, Welch K. Surgical treatment of post-lumbar puncture dural CSF leak causing chronic headache. Case report. *J Neurosurg.* 1982;57:703-707.
55. Cameron CM, Scott DA, McDonald WM, et al. A review of neuraxial epidural morbidity: experience of more than 8,000 cases at a single teaching hospital. *Anesthesiology.* 2007;106:997-1002.
56. Phillips JM, Stedeford JC, Hartsilver E, et al. Epidural abscess complicating insertion of epidural catheters. *Br J Anaesth.* 2002;89:778-782.
57. Moen V, Dahlgren N, Irestedt L. Severe neurological complications after central neuraxial blockades in Sweden 1990-1999. *Anesthesiology.* 2004;101:950-959.
58. Grewal S, Hocking G, Wildsmith JA. Epidural abscesses. *Br J Anaesth.* 2006;96:292-302.
59. Brull R, McCartney CJ, Chan VW, et al. Neurological complications after regional anesthesia: contemporary estimates of risk. *Anesth Analg.* 2007;104:965-974.
60. Allen HW, Liu SS, Ware PD, et al. Peripheral nerve blocks improve analgesia after total knee replacement surgery. *Anesth Analg.* 1998;87:93-97.
61. Jacob AK, Mantilla CB, Sviggum HP, et al. Perioperative nerve injury after total knee arthroplasty: regional anesthesia risk during a 20-year cohort study. *Anesthesiology.* 2011;114:311-317.
62. YaDeau JT, Cahill JB, Zawadsky MW, et al. The effects of femoral nerve blockade in conjunction with epidural analgesia after total knee arthroplasty. *Anesth Analg.* 2005;101:891-895.
63. Paul JE, Arya A, Hurlburt L, et al. Femoral nerve block improves analgesia outcomes after total knee arthroplasty: a meta-analysis of randomized controlled trials. *Anesthesiology.* 2010;113:1144-1162.
64. Hebl JR, Dilger JA, Byer DE, et al. A pre-emptive multimodal pathway featuring peripheral nerve block improves perioperative outcomes after major orthopedic surgery. *Reg Anesth Pain Med.* 2008;33:510-517.
65. Fowler SJ, Symons J, Sabato S, et al. Epidural analgesia compared with peripheral nerve blockade after major knee surgery: a systematic review and meta-analysis of randomized trials. *Br J Anaesth.* 2008;100:154-164.
66. Fischer HB, Simanski CJ, Sharp C, et al. A procedure-specific systematic review and consensus recommendations for postoperative analgesia following total knee arthroplasty. *Anaesthesia.* 2008;63:1105-1123.
67. Walker KJ, McGrattan K, Aas-Eng K, et al. Ultrasound guidance for peripheral nerve blockade. *Cochrane Database System Rev.* 2009:CD006459.
68. Marhofer P, Schrogendorfer K, Koinig H, et al. Ultrasonographic guidance improves sensory block and onset time of three-in-one blocks. *Anesth Analg.* 1997;85:854-857.
69. Salinas FV. Ultrasound and review of evidence for lower extremity peripheral nerve blocks. *Reg Anesth Pain Med.* 2010;35:S16-25.
70. Neal JM, Brull R, Chan VW, et al. The ASRA evidence-based medicine assessment of ultrasound-guided regional anesthesia and pain medicine: Executive summary. *Reg Anesth Pain Med.* 2010;35:S1-9.
71. Aveline C, Le Roux A, Le Hetet H, et al. Postoperative efficacies of femoral nerve catheters sited using ultrasound combined with neurostimulation compared with neurostimulation alone for total knee arthroplasty. *Eur J Anaesthesiol.* 2010;27:978-984.
72. Ilfeld BM, Mariano ER, Girard PJ, et al. A multicenter, randomized, triple-masked, placebo-controlled trial of the effect of ambulatory continuous femoral nerve blocks on discharge-readiness following total knee arthroplasty in patients on general orthopaedic wards. *Pain.* 2010;150:477-484.
73. Auroy Y, Benhamou D, Bargues L, et al. Major complications of regional anesthesia in France: The SOS Regional Anesthesia Hotline Service. *Anesthesiology.* 2002;97:1274-1280.
74. Wegener JT, van Ooij B, van Dijk CN, et al. Value of single-injection or continuous sciatic nerve block in addition to a continuous femoral nerve block in patients undergoing total knee arthroplasty: a prospective, randomized, controlled trial. *Reg Anesth Pain Med.* 2011;36(5):481-488.
75. Davies AF, Segar EP, Murdoch J, et al. Epidural infusion or combined femoral and sciatic nerve blocks as perioperative analgesia for knee arthroplasty. *Br J Anaesth.* 2004;93:368-374.
76. Cappelleri G, Ghisi D, Fanelli A, et al. Does continuous sciatic nerve block improve postoperative analgesia and early rehabilitation after total knee arthroplasty?: a prospective, randomized, double-blinded study. *Reg Anesth Pain Med.* 2011;36(5):489-492.
77. Abdallah FW, Brull R. Is sciatic nerve block advantageous when combined with femoral nerve block for postoperative analgesia following total knee

arthroplasty?: a systematic review. *Reg Anesth Pain Med.* 2011;36(5):493-498.

78. Tsai PB, Karnwal A, Kakazu C, et al. Efficacy of an ultrasound-guided subsartorial approach to saphenous nerve block: a case series. *Can J Anaesth.* 2010;57: 683-688.
79. Saranteas T, Anagnostis G, Paraskeuopoulos T, et al. Anatomy and clinical implications of the ultrasound-guided subsartorial saphenous nerve block. *Reg Anesth Pain Med.* 2011;36:399-402.
80. Manickam B, Perlas A, Duggan E, et al. Feasibility and efficacy of ultrasound-guided block of the saphenous nerve in the adductor canal. *Reg Anesth Pain Med.* 2009;34:578-580.
81. Lund J, Jenstrup MT, Jaeger P, et al. Continuous adductor-canal-blockade for adjuvant post-operative analgesia after major knee surgery: preliminary results. *Acta Anaesthesiol Scand.* 2011;55:14-19.
82. Eroglu A, Uzunlar H, Erciyes N. Comparison of hypotensive epidural anesthesia and hypotensive total intravenous anesthesia on intraoperative blood loss during total hip replacement. *J Clin Anesth.* 2005;17: 420-425.
83. Williams-Russo P, Sharrock NE, Mattis S, et al. Randomized trial of hypotensive epidural anesthesia in older adults. *Anesthesiology.* 1999;91:926-935.
84. Sharrock NE. Eliminating blood transfusions: don't forget hypotensive anesthesia. *Anesthesiology.* 2002; 96:252-253.
85. Juelsgaard P, Larsen UT, Sorensen JV, et al. Hypotensive epidural anesthesia in total knee replacement without tourniquet: reduced blood loss and transfusion. *Reg Anesth Pain Med.* 2001;26:105-110.
86. Sharrock NE, Beksac B, Flynn E, et al. Hypotensive epidural anaesthesia in patients with preoperative renal dysfunction undergoing total hip replacement. *Br J Anaesth.* 2006;96:207-212.
87. Ho MC, Beathe JC, Sharrock NE. Hypotensive epidural anesthesia in patients with aortic stenosis undergoing total hip replacement. *Reg Anesth Pain Med.* 2008;33:129-133.
88. Axelsson K, Gupta A. Local anaesthetic adjuvants: neuraxial versus peripheral nerve block. *Curr Opin Anaesthesiol.* 2009;22:649-654.
89. Frassanito L, Vergari A, Zanghi F, et al. Post-operative analgesia following total knee arthroplasty: comparison of low-dose intrathecal morphine and single-shot ultrasound-guided femoral nerve block: a randomized, single blinded, controlled study. *Eur Rev Med Pharmacol Sci.* 2010;14:589-596.
90. Cuvillon P, Nouvellon E, Ripart J, et al. A comparison of the pharmacodynamics and pharmacokinetics of bupivacaine, ropivacaine (with epinephrine) and their equal volume mixtures with lidocaine used for femoral and sciatic nerve blocks: a double-blind randomized study. *Anesth Analg.* 2009; 108:641-649.
91. Popping DM, Elia N, Marret E, et al. Clonidine as an adjuvant to local anesthetics for peripheral nerve and plexus blocks: a meta-analysis of randomized trials. *Anesthesiology.* 2009;111:406-415.
92. Vieira PA, Pulai I, Tsao GC, et al. Dexamethasone with bupivacaine increases duration of analgesia in ultrasound-guided interscalene brachial plexus blockade. *Eur J Anaesthesiol.* 2010;27:285-288.
93. Duellman TJ, Gaffigan C, Milbrandt JC, et al. Multi-modal, pre-emptive analgesia decreases the length of hospital stay following total joint arthroplasty. *Orthopedics.* 2009;32:167.
94. Peters CL, Shirley B, Erickson J. The effect of a new multimodal perioperative anesthetic regimen on postoperative pain, side effects, rehabilitation, and length of hospital stay after total joint arthroplasty. *J Arthroplasty.* 2006;21:132-138.
95. Smith TO, Hing CB. Is a tourniquet beneficial in total knee replacement surgery? A meta-analysis and systematic review. *Knee.* 2010;17:141-147.
96. Wakankar HM, Nicholl JE, Koka R, et al. The tourniquet in total knee arthroplasty. a prospective, randomised study. *J Bone Joint Surg Br.* 1999;81:30-33.
97. Valli H, Rosenberg PH, Kytta J, et al. Arterial hypertension associated with the use of a tourniquet with either general or regional anaesthesia. *Acta Anaesthesiol Scand.* 1987;31:279-283.
98. Sharrock NE, Go G, Williams-Russo P, et al. Comparison of extradural and general anaesthesia on the fibrinolytic response to total knee arthroplasty. *Br J Anaesth.* 1997;79:29-34.
99. O'Leary AM, Veall G, Butler P, et al. Acute pulmonary oedema after tourniquet release. *Can J Anaesth.* 1990;37:826-827.
100. Gielen M. Cardiac arrest after tourniquet release. *Can J Anaesth.* 1991;38:541.
101. McGrath BJ, Hsia J, Epstein B. Massive pulmonary embolism following tourniquet deflation. *Anesthesiology.* 1991;74:618-620.
102. Katsumata S, Nagashima M, Kato K, et al. Changes in coagulation-fibrinolysis marker and neutrophil elastase following the use of tourniquet during total knee arthroplasty and the influence of neutrophil

elastase on thromboembolism. *Acta Anaesthesiol Scand.* 2005;49:510-516.

103. Aglietti P, Baldini A, Vena LM, et al. Effect of tourniquet use on activation of coagulation in total knee replacement. *Clin Orthop Relat Res.* 2000:169-177.

104. Harvey EJ, Leclerc J, Brooks CE, et al. Effect of tourniquet use on blood loss and incidence of deep vein thrombosis in total knee arthroplasty. *J Arthroplasty.* 1997;12:291-296.

105. Sapega AA, Heppenstall RB, Chance B, et al. Optimizing tourniquet application and release times in extremity surgery. A biochemical and ultrastructural study. *J Bone Joint Surg Am.* 1985; 67:303-314.

106. Lotke PA, Faralli VJ, Orenstein EM, et al. Blood loss after total knee replacement. Effects of tourniquet release and continuous passive motion. *J Bone Joint Surg Am.* 1991;73:1037-1040.

107. Mangram AJ, Horan TC, Pearson ML, et al. Guideline for prevention of surgical site infection, 1999. Centers for Disease Control and Prevention (CDC) Hospital Infection Control Practices Advisory Committee. *Am J Infect Control.* 1999;27:97-132; quiz 133-134; discussion 96.

108. Carey K, Stefos T, Shibei Z, et al. Excess costs attributable to postoperative complications. Medical care research and review. *MCRR.* 2011;68:490-503.

109. Emori TG, Gaynes RP. An overview of nosocomial infections, including the role of the microbiology laboratory. *Clin Microbiol Rev.* 1993;6:428-442.

110. Chang CC, Lin HC, Lin HW. Anesthetic management and surgical site infections in total hip or knee replacement: a population-based study. *Anesthesiology.* 2010;113:279-284.

111. Lieberman JR, Geerts WH. Prevention of venous thromboembolism after total hip and knee arthroplasty. *J Bone Joint Surg Am.* 1994;76:1239-1250.

112. Stulberg BN, Insall JN, Williams GW, et al. Deep-vein thrombosis following total knee replacement. An analysis of six hundred and thirty-eight arthroplasties. *J Bone Joint Surg Am.* 1984;66:194-201.

113. Sharrock NE, Haas SB, Hargett MJ, et al. Effects of epidural anesthesia on the incidence of deep-vein thrombosis after total knee arthroplasty. *J Bone Joint Surg Am.* 1991;73:502-506.

114. Farag E, Dilger J, Brooks P, et al. Epidural analgesia improves early rehabilitation after total knee replacement. *J Clin Anesth.* 2005;17:281-285.

115. Tuman KJ, McCarthy RJ, March RJ, et al. Effects of epidural anesthesia and analgesia on coagulation and outcome after major vascular surgery. *Anesth Analg.* 1991;73:696-704.

116. Miric A, Lombardi P, Sculco TP. Deep vein thrombosis prophylaxis: a comprehensive approach for total hip and total knee arthroplasty patient populations. *Am J Orthop.* 2000;29:269-274.

117. U.S. Department of Health and Human Resources. *FDA Public Heath Advisory: Reports of Epidural or Spinal Hematomas with the Concurrent Use of Low Molecular Weight Heparin and Spinal/epidural Anesthesia or Spinal Puncture.* 1997.

118. Robinson TN, Raeburn CD, Tran ZV, et al. Postoperative delirium in the elderly: risk factors and outcomes. *Ann Surg.* 2009;249:173-178.

119. Franco K, Litaker D, Locala J, et al. The cost of delirium in the surgical patient. *Psychosomatics.* 2001;42:68-73.

120. Marcantonio ER, Goldman L, Mangione CM, et al. A clinical prediction rule for delirium after elective noncardiac surgery. *JAMA.* 1994;271:134-139.

121. Williams-Russo P, Urquhart BL, Sharrock NE, et al. Post-operative delirium: predictors and prognosis in elderly orthopedic patients. *J Am Geriatr Soc.* 1992; 40:759-767.

122. Wu CL, Hsu W, Richman JM, et al. Postoperative cognitive function as an outcome of regional anesthesia and analgesia. *Reg Anesth Pain Med.* 2004;29:257-268.

123. Canet J, Raeder J, Rasmussen LS, et al. Cognitive dysfunction after minor surgery in the elderly. *Acta Anaesthesiol Scand.* 2003;47:1204-1210.

124. Williams-Russo P, Sharrock NE, Mattis S, et al. Cognitive effects after epidural vs general anesthesia in older adults. A randomized trial. *JAMA.* 1995; 274:44-50.

125. Rasmussen LS, Steentoft A, Rasmussen H, et al. Benzodiazepines and postoperative cognitive dysfunction in the elderly. ISPOCD Group. International study of postoperative cognitive dysfunction. *Br J Anaesth.* 1999;83:585-589.

126. Kadoi Y, Saito S, Kunimoto F, et al. Comparative effects of propofol versus fentanyl on cerebral oxygenation state during normothermic cardio-pulmonary bypass and postoperative cognitive dysfunction. *Ann Thoracic Surg.* 2003;75:840-846.

127. Lynch EP, Lazor MA, Gellis JE, et al. The impact of postoperative pain on the development of postoperative delirium. *Anesth Analg.* 1998;86:781-785.

29 Blood Loss in Total Knee Arthroplasty

Jonathon Salava and Ali Oliashirazi

Among the many goals of the orthopaedic surgeon in total knee arthroplasty is minimizing the risk and complications of surgery. Despite many advances in the management and prevention of blood loss and resulting anemia from total knee arthroplasty, the potential need for allogeneic blood transfusion remains. The small, but potentially devastating, risks of disease transmission, transfusion reaction, and immunosuppression or infection from allogeneic transfusions have led to the implementation of multiple blood preservation techniques. Current preservation strategies include preoperative, intraoperative, and postoperative management protocols to reduce the need for postoperative transfusion.

COMPLICATIONS OF ALLOGENEIC BLOOD TRANSFUSION

With the reported benefits of avoiding and treating postoperative anemia,[1] it is not surprising that transfusion rates in unilateral total knee arthroplasty (TKA) may be as high as 40%.[2] The orthopaedic surgeon, however, must always be cognizant of the potential complications when blood products are given. It has been estimated that as many as 20% of transfusions result in some type of adverse effect,[3] whether it is something as mild as a fever or as serious as disease transmission. Transmission of infectious diseases may be the traditional concern, but there are a number of other causes of transfusion-related morbidity and mortality as well.

Disease Transmission

Despite the dramatic decrease in risk of disease transmission from allogeneic blood transfusion (ABT), it may well remain the primary concern of both patients and surgeons alike. In 1995, Lackritz and colleagues estimated the risk of transfusion of human immunodeficiency virus (HIV) at 1 in 450,000 to 660,000 for ABT.[4] The following year Schreiber and coworkers published a similar risk of transfusion-transmitted HIV (1 in 493,000). The Schreiber study also estimated the risk for human T-cell lymphotrophic virus (HTLV) at 1 in 641,000, hepatitis C virus (HCV) at 1 in 103,000, and hepatitis B virus (HBV) at 1 in 641,000.[5] Recent data suggest that with more sensitive serologic testing and a decline in the incidence of some of these diseases, the risk of transfusion transmission is even lower. Dodd and colleagues provided an updated risk of 1 in ~2 million for HIV and HCV, 1 in ~3 million for HTLV, and 1 in 205,000-488,000 for HBV (Fig. 29-1).[6] Additional threats to the blood supply include West Nile virus,[7] babesiosis,[8] malaria, Chagas disease, hepatitis G, SEN virus, TT virus, human herpes virus 8, coronavirus, and the prion-transmitting variant Creutzfeldt-Jakob disease.[9]

Immunomodulation

Transfusion of allogeneic blood not only puts patients at risk for direct disease transmission but has also been shown to suppress the immune system and increase the overall risk of infection. Although the exact mechanisms of transfusion-related immunomodulation (TRIM) have yet to be fully elu-

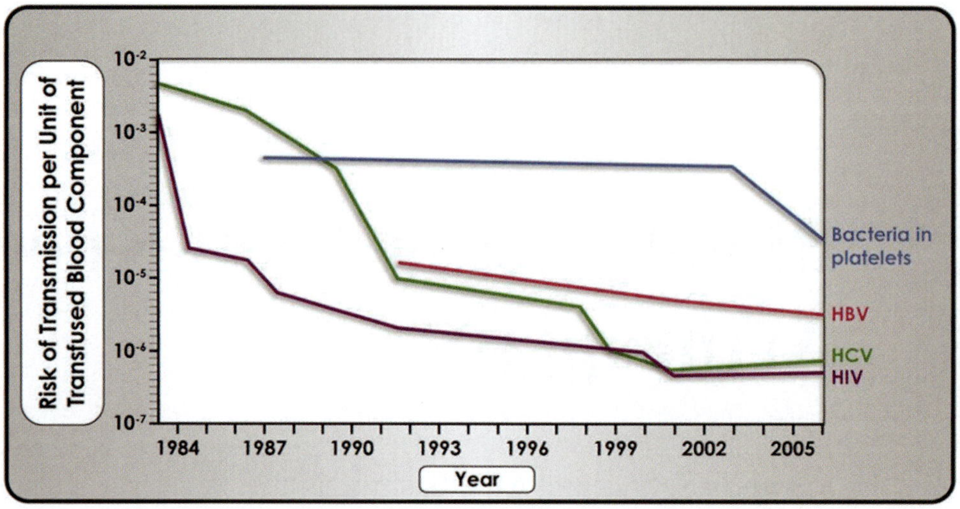

FIGURE 29-1. *This graph represents the risk of transmission of HIV, HBV, HCV, and bacterial infection in the United States. Large decreases in the 1980s and 1990s reflect decreasing incidence as well as the introduction of screening tests. (Figure by David Kendall, graphic artist, Office of Medical Education Marshall University Joan C. Edwards School of Medicine. Adapted from Dodd et al. Transfusion. 2002;42:975-979 and Stramer S. Arch Pathol Lab Med. 2007;131:702-707.)*

cidated, several classes of likely mediators have been identified. Through the actions of allogeneic mononuclear cells, white blood cell (WBC)-derived soluble mediators, and/or soluble human leukocyte antigen (HLA) peptides, a number of immune abnormalities and deficiencies are liable to occur.[10,11] In a population of hip arthroplasty patients, Kendall and coworkers demonstrated how TRIM could potentially increase the risk of infection. They found that through reductions of specific lymphocyte subgroups, when patients received allogeneic blood, cell-mediated immune response was suppressed.[12] Whether or not TRIM results in a clinically significant increase in infection rates continues to be debated. While some studies have shown transfusion of allogeneic blood to be associated with an overall increase in infection rate in orthopaedic surgery,[13-18] others have refuted this increased risk.[19,20] Some of these discrepancies may lie in the fact that some studies assess rates of wound infections alone, while others consider all infections, including in the lungs and urinary tract.

In addition to infection risk, TRIM can also have effects on cancer recurrence. Although tumors are not commonly encountered within the realm of joint arthroplasty, the risks of transfusion in the setting of tumor surgery are worthy of mention. Three separate meta-analyses of observational studies have been performed to assess any association with ABT and tumor recurrence. All of these studies demonstrated a statistically significant increase in cancer recurrence and overall mortality in transfused versus untransfused patients.[21-23] As with infection, however, there is contradictory evidence in Vamvakas' meta-analysis of randomized controlled trials that shows no TRIM effect on cancer recurrence.[24]

Transfusion-Related Mortality

Beyond these transfusion-associated morbidities, the Federal Food and Drug Administration has identified common causes of transfusion-related mortality as well. In recent years, the leading cause of transfusion-related mortality has been transfusion-related acute lung injury (TRALI). Forty-seven percent of fatalities related to transfusion from 2005 to 2010 have been attributed to TRALI.[25] This adverse effect occurs when antibodies from the donor attack the WBCs in the microcirculation of the lungs of the recipient. This reaction typically occurs within 6 hours of the transfusion with a clear temporal relationship.[16] Accounting for 24% of fatalities, hemolytic transfusion reactions (HTRs) are the second most common cause of mortality.[25] This includes both ABO and non-ABO incompatibilities, which result in an immune-mediated destruction of transfused donor red blood cells (RBCs) by recipient antibodies.[16] The third most common cause of transfusion-related death in the United States is transfusion-associated circulatory overload (TACO) (12% of fatalities).[25] TACO is defined as acute pulmonary edema secondary to congestive heart failure due to a rapid or massive transfusion of blood in patients with a decreased cardiac reserve.[16] Microbial infection, as discussed previously, is the fourth most common cause of transfusion-related mortality.[25] Other noninfectious causes of mortality related to transfusions include anaphylaxis, transfusion-associated graft-versus-host disease, and posttransfusion purpura.

With the effective blood preservation techniques available today, avoidance of transfusion is certainly the most effective means by which one can prevent these associated complications. For those settings in which transfusion may be necessary, however, Vamvakas and Blajchman have summarized five interventions available to further reduce transfusion complications.[26] One, the number of exposures to allogeneic blood could be reduced by avoiding pooled blood products and utilizing conservative transfusion guidelines. Two, reduce the number of WBC antibodies through the use of fresh-frozen plasma and platelets from male or nulliparous women. Three, utilize information systems to verify the identity of blood products and intended recipients alike. Four, use WBC-reduced RBCs if transfusion is needed. Five, utilize pathogen reduction techniques for platelets and fresh-frozen plasma.[16]

RISK FACTORS FOR TRANSFUSION

Although there are numerous blood preservation techniques available to the total joint surgeon, the cost-effectiveness of some of these methods remains unclear. To better serve the knee arthroplasty patient, as well as the health care system as a whole, it becomes important to understand which patients will benefit from these techniques. As such, numerous studies have included analysis of the risk factors associated with blood loss and the need for transfusion.

Anemia

The most significant risk factor for the need for postoperative ABT is preoperative anemia. A lower hemoglobin or hematocrit has consistently been associated with a higher rate of transfusion in total knee arthroplasty[27-30] and other major orthopaedic procedures.[31-35] Bong and colleagues found a 4-fold increase in the probability of postoperative transfusion when the preoperative hemoglobin was <10 g/dL versus >13 g/dL.[2] Salido et al found a linear relationship between preoperative hemoglobin and transfusion rate such that every 1 g/dL decrease in hemoglobin resulted in a 2.5 times increase in the probability of needing a transfusion following total hip or knee arthroplasty.[29] As one might expect, chronic diseases, such as rheumatoid arthritis, that have been associated with anemia may result in a similar increase in risk of transfusion.[36]

Age

Another potential risk factor commonly encountered in total joint arthroplasty (TJA) patients is advanced age. Unfortunately, the role that age plays in predicting who is at risk for needing a transfusion is not clear. Although some studies have not demonstrated age to be a predictor of need for transfusion,[28,29,34] there are an equal number that have found age to be a significant risk factor in TJA.[2,27,34,35,37] This discrepancy persists even after eliminating total hip studies and focusing on TKA alone.[2,28] Another difficulty in interpreting the data is deciding whether or not to include transfusion of predonated autologous blood into the analysis. Keating, for example, found age to be an insignificant factor in overall transfusion rate. While analyzing risk of ABT alone, however, age was identified as an independent risk factor in unilateral TKA.[28]

Gender and Size

The contribution that gender and body size make in assessing the risk of blood loss and transfusion is just as unclear. When looking at blood loss specifically, several studies have found males to have a higher blood loss in TJA.[30,34,36] Interestingly, females tend to have a greater risk of requiring blood transfusion.[29,38,39] This may be expla-ined by males' generally higher hematocrit and their larger blood volume reserve. Although males may lose more red blood cells than females, their reserve allows for a greater drop in hemoglobin and hematocrit. This is supported by Keating's findings that a lower weight and estimated blood volume (75 × mass in kg) resulted in a significant increase in the probability of transfusion.[28] Low body mass index (BMI) has also been shown to be a risk factor for ABT.[35,40] Similarly, stature had an effect on risk of transfusion in Salido's study, as they found an increased risk in patients of short stature.[29]

In an effort to better identify those patients who will be at greatest risk of transfusion, some investigators have combined some of these factors to guide their blood management protocol. For example, Pola and colleagues did not find age, gender, hypertension, or BMI alone to be significant risk factors. When two or more of these factors were present, however, there was a significant increase in probability of transfusion (40% vs. 19% with <2 risk factors).[34] In their series, Hatzidakis and coworkers found that patients with a hemoglobin ≥15 g/dL had zero risk of transfusion, and by utilizing age, they also found zero risk in patients <65 years old with a hemoglobin of 13 to 15 g/dL.[27] Because of these findings, some of the more costly and time-consuming preservation techniques are not recommended in these patients.

Factors of Care

Beyond patient factors, there are additional institutional and surgical factors that may increase a patient's risk of needing a transfusion. One such factor that concerns every surgeon's team is length of surgery. Although its effect on transfusion requirements is not heavily studied, there are data to suggest a significant association with length of surgery.[29] A significantly increased risk has also been seen in bilateral and revision arthroplasty.[35] In the era of evolving work duty restrictions, another hospital factor to consider is house staff turnover. During house staff turnover months, Bell and colleagues did find a greater decline in postoperative hemoglobin levels compared to nonturnover months. This did not, however, translate into a significant increase in allogeneic transfusion rates.[38]

PREOPERATIVE BLOOD MANAGEMENT

Preoperative Autologous Donation

Preoperative autologous donation (PAD) became a popular technique in reducing the risk of ABT after concerns of disease transmission arose. A steady increase in its utilization was seen from the early 1980s to its peak of 5% of transfusions in 1992.[41,42] A larger number of these PAD transfusions occur in orthopaedic patients; TKA and total hip arthroplasty (THA) together account for over half of its use.[43] While numerous studies have heralded its benefits, there are still risks and costs associated with autologous donation and transfusion that drive researchers to define the optimum patient population.

Generally, patients are only encouraged to donate blood for autologous use if the procedure realistically carries the possibility of transfusion. If the surgery has a greater than 10% likelihood of transfusion, then the patient is eligible but is subjected to additional criteria before donating. Patients should be relatively healthy, without contraindications to blood donations, and have a baseline hemoglobin of at least 11 g/dL and a hematocrit of 33%.[44,45] There should be at least a 72-hour window between PAD and surgery. Initiating donations several weeks before surgery is optimal, however, in order to allow more complete red blood cell regeneration. Autologous blood units are handled and stored separately from allogeneic units, which imparts additional costs (Fig. 29-2). Once collected, the autologous blood may be stored for 5 to 6 weeks, and if frozen, it remains viable for 24 hours once it is thawed.[44]

Numerous studies have demonstrated how PAD can reduce the risk of needing an ABT in joint arthroplasty. Keating and his coworkers found a 4-fold decrease in the rate of ABT in TKA recipients who participated in autologous predonation (3% vs. 14%). The discrepancy was even greater when evaluated in anemic unilateral TKA patients with preoperative hemoglobin levels of 10 to 13 g/dL (4% vs. 30%).[28] A 3- to 4-fold decrease has been seen in other studies as well. Bierbaum and coworkers found decreased rates of ABT in primary (6% vs. 18%), bilateral (16% vs. 57%), and revision (11% vs. 30%) arthroplasty with use of PAD.[18] Similar decreases in ABT were seen in the work from Hatzidakis et al. In their retrospective analysis of 489 total joint arthroplasties, PAD decreased the rate of ABT from 15% to 3% in primaries and from 49% to 19% in revision and bilateral arthroplasties.[27] In Walsh and colleagues' retrospective review of 1159 THAs, they found that nearly 50% of patients who did not donate autologous blood required ABT. Conversely, those who were able to predonate 1 or 2 units of blood saw a reduction in transfusion rates down to 10% and 2%, respectively.[40]

Although appealing to the patient, the surgeon must be aware of the drawbacks of PAD, including preoperative anemia with associated risk of need for transfusion (autologous or allogeneic), risk of transfusion reaction, or disease transmission due to errors, cost, and wastage. In TJA, PAD has been shown to result in phlebotomy-induced anemia [46] and an associated increase in the overall risk of transfusion (allogeneic and autologous).[47] In the THA literature, this increase has been up to 53% for a single unit and 300% if 2 units are donated.[40] The risks to the patient include a 1 in 17,000 chance of donation-related complication (typically vasovagal episode)[48] and a 1 in 16,000 to 30,000 chance of receiving incorrect autologous units due to clerical error.[49-51] In a recent cost minimization study, the cost of PAD was estimated at approximately $892 for TKA, yet this was less than relying on allogeneic blood alone for managing postoperative anemia ($1352).[52] What further compounds the cost concerns of collecting and storing the autologous donations is that so much is wasted. Due to less stringent donation criteria, unused blood meant for autologous transfusion cannot be pooled and is typically discarded. Unfortunately, the wastage rates from autologous donation can be quite high and vary widely from 30% to 76%.[2,18,27,28,53]

A

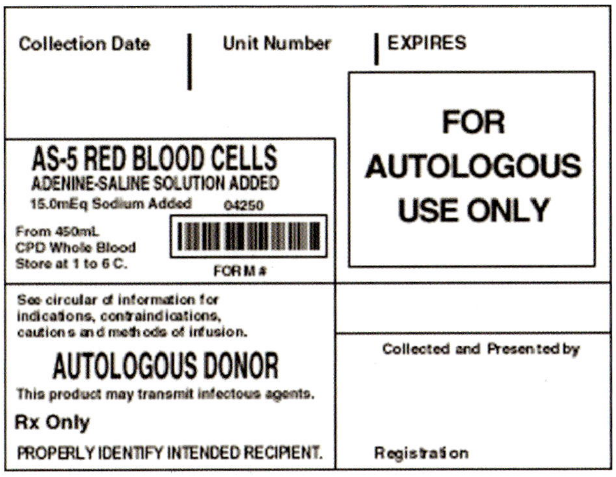

B

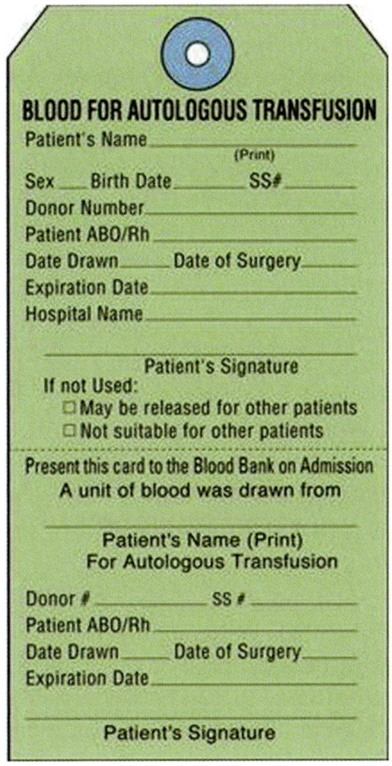

FIGURE 29-2. *Autologous blood donation deviates little from standard volunteer donation. To minimize error with autologous transfusion, the collected blood is marked as autologous (**A**) and the donor receives a tag (**B**) to ensure that, if needed, the predonated blood is used.*

Erythropoietin

As discussed above, one of the greatest predictors or factors in assessing a patient's need for allogeneic blood following TKA is his or her preoperative hemoglobin and hematocrit. Although PAD may decrease one's risk of ABT postoperatively, there are few measures available to the orthopaedic surgeon to actually maximize the patient's hemoglobin preoperatively. Erythropoietin (EPO) is a glycoprotein that is naturally excreted by the kidneys and stimulates red blood cell production in bone marrow.[54] Recombinant human EPO is a commercially available form that is produced with an identical amino acid sequence and administered before surgery to increase hemoglobin levels.

The preoperative use of EPO, alone or with additional preservation strategies, has demonstrated increased preoperative hemoglobin levels and decreased rates of ABT. Faris et al found ABT rates following perioperative administration of EPO that were one-half to one-third of a placebo group in their controlled, double-blinded, prospective study of 200 major orthopaedic surgeries.[55] Bezwada and coworkers prospectively analyzed the effects of EPO alone and in combination with PAD in 240 primary, revision, and bilateral total knee and hip arthroplasties. Even though they were able to demonstrate an increase in immediate preoperative hemoglobin levels, EPO alone did not significantly reduce the ABT rate compared to PAD. When used in combination, however, there was a significant decrease in ABTs versus either modality used alone.[56] Cushner and coworkers also compared EPO to PAD in the setting of TKA in anemic patients with hemoglobin levels of 10 to 13 g/dL and found comparable rates of ABT between these two preoperative blood conservation techniques. The EPO group, however, did have significantly higher hemoglobin levels at discharge (10.8 g/dL vs. 9.7 g/dL). They concluded that although ABT rates were similar between the two groups, these were lower compared to historical controls.[46]

The ideal dosing regimen for EPO has yet to be clearly defined. In the study by Faris, both 100 IU/kg and 300 IU/kg dosing significantly reduced ABT rates, but the higher dose was particularly more effective in the anemic population (hemoglobin between 10 and 13 g/dL).[55] This increased effect with 300 IU/kg dosing has been reproducible, as seen by de Andrade and colleagues as well.[32] A four-dose regimen described by Goldberg et al, including 600 IU/kg given subcutaneously at 21 days, 14 days, 7 days, and 1 day before surgery, has demonstrated a greater increase in hemoglobin than 300 IU/kg daily dosing. This regimen has been well tolerated and has also had similar ABT avoidance rates.[56,57] The Cushner study dose of 40,000 units given 21, 14, and 7 days before surgery was also effective and well tolerated.[46] The dose of iron supplementation used in conjunction with EPO is not well defined either. Typically patients are given 325 mg of ferrous sulfate two to three times a day.[55,56] Some variations on iron supplementation have been described as well. Feagan and his colleagues demonstrated enhanced treatment response with a standard dose of 40,000 units of EPO weekly, starting at 4 weeks before surgery. However, they eliminated the dose before the day of surgery and prescribed 450 mg of ferrous sulfate daily.[58]

As with any pharmacologic agent, EPO does have adverse effects of which the surgeon should be aware. Common reactions include local skin irritation, constipation, pyrexia, and nausea.[56] Blood pressure should be monitored closely during the dosing period because of the reports of hypertension after EPO therapy.[55,59] There have also been reports of increased incidence of deep vein thrombosis (DVT) with EPO use,[60] but this is not a consistent finding in EPO usage in TJA.

INTRAOPERATIVE BLOOD MANAGEMENT

Although EPO injections and PAD have been shown to decrease the risk of patients requiring allogeneic blood after a total knee replacement, their use in the orthopaedic world remains in flux. The true effects of these preoperative methods are not likely to be uncovered because the arthroplasty surgeon likely utilizes many of the following intraoperative techniques to further minimize blood loss and the need for ABT.

Acute Normovolemic Hemodilution

Acute normovolemic hemodilution (ANH) is a blood conservation technique initiated in the immediate preoperative setting with utilization of the collected blood products intraoperatively. The ANH process includes removal of whole blood from the patient just before surgery while administering crystalloid or colloid solution simultaneously to maintain a state of normovolemia. Collected blood is then stored in blood bags containing anticoagulant. The blood remains in the operating suite and is reinfused after any major blood loss (Fig. 29-3).[42] With regards to patient selection, published guidelines recommend ANH only be considered when the surgical blood loss is expected to exceed 20% of the blood volume in patients with a preoperative hemoglobin above 10 g/dL[42] to 11 g/dL.[61] Caution should also be exercised in patients with underlying ischemic myocardial disease.[61]

There are several advantages that ANH has over other conservation techniques like PAD. The value of ANH lies in the reduction of red blood cells lost intraoperatively. Due to the lowering of the hematocrit, there is a decrease in the cells lost per unit of volume. If it becomes necessary to transfuse the collected blood, the units are in the operating room, and the risk of clerical error and bacterial contamination is theoretically eliminated. There are also obvious advantages outside the operating room. First, patients do not have to invest additional time toward blood collection as they would with PAD.[42] Second, the units collected require no testing, which substantially lowers costs.[62] Studies that have included a cost analysis comparing ANH to PAD have shown PAD to cost between two to four times as much as ANH.[63,64] Additionally, the hemodilution process does not appear to prolong anesthesia or surgical time.[62,63]

While providing reduction in time investment, cost, risk of clerical error, and contamination, ANH appears to have similar efficacy in reducing ABT rates compared to PAD.

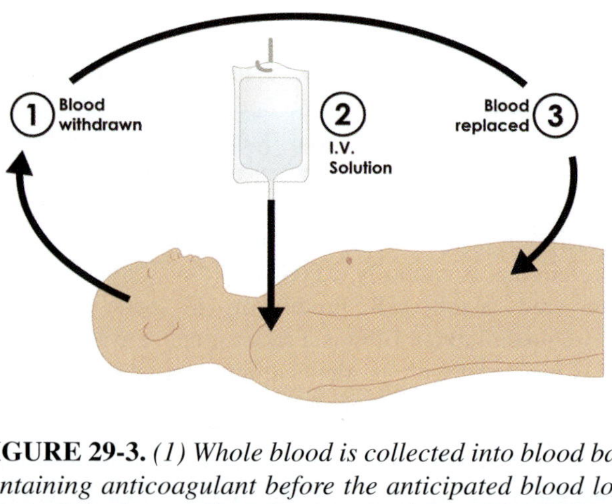

FIGURE 29-3. *(1) Whole blood is collected into blood bags containing anticoagulant before the anticipated blood loss. (2) As blood is collected, crystalloid or colloid fluid is infused to maintain a euvolemic state. (3) The sequestered blood is then reinfused after major blood loss. (Figure by David Kendall, graphic artist, Marshall University Joan C. Edwards School of Medicine.)*

Olsfanger and coworkers analyzed the effectiveness of ANH in reducing ABT rates in a prospective, randomized, controlled study of 30 TKAs. Allogeneic blood was transfused in all 10 of the controls, which was significantly more than in those who underwent ANH (11/20).[65] In Goodnough and colleagues' 32-patient TKA study, they found no statistical difference in the rate of ABT between the predonation and hemodilution group for unilateral primary TKA or revision/bilateral TKA.[63] In their separate prospective THA study comparing ANH and PAD, Goodnough et al again found no statistical difference between the two methods regarding rate of ABT.[64] Shulman et al also looked at ABT exposure rate in THA patients. When ANH was used in conjunction with autotransfusion of shed blood, they found a 75% decrease in ABT versus autotransfusion alone.[66] Because of its demonstrated effectiveness, several authors have proposed that ANH be used as an inexpensive alternative with fewer risks compared to PAD.

Hypotensive Anesthesia

Hypotensive anesthesia is an attractive option for minimizing intraoperative blood losses in TJA. Sharrock et al introduced hypotensive epidural anesthesia (HEA) in 1989[67] and further defined the acceptable degree of hypotension in 1993.[68] They demonstrated the ability to minimize intraoperative blood loss by further decreasing a patient's mean arterial pressure (MAP) down to 50 ± 5 mm Hg without adversely affecting cardiac, renal, or cerebral function. This was accomplished with epidural fentanyl and bupivacaine while administering low-dose intravenous epinephrine to maintain hemodynamic stability. While objective decreases in blood loss were measured, surgeons also noted significantly less bleeding while reaming the acetabulum and femur. The change in blood loss, however, was not significant enough to translate into fewer ABTs.[68]

The use of hypotensive anesthesia has expanded since its inception and several others have documented its benefits. Juelsgaard and coworkers specifically looked at blood loss and transfusion rates in TKA patients receiving either HEA or spinal anesthesia. Because a tourniquet was not used in the HEA group, there was significantly less intraoperative blood loss in the spinal group (13 mL vs. 146 mL). All postoperative blood loss measurements, however, demonstrated a significant increase in blood loss in the spinal group such that final blood loss averaged 1825 mL in the spinal group versus 1056 mL in the HEA group. This translated into fewer ABTs in the HEA group as well (43% vs. 81%).[69] Several studies in the THA literature have also demonstrated significant reductions in blood loss and ABT rates.[70-72]

Pharmacological Management

Pharmacological agents have been employed as another systemic method of reducing blood loss in TKA. Desmopressin is one agent that demonstrated reductions in blood loss and increased thrombogenicity in certain medical conditions and settings. Unfortunately, in the hemostatically normal patient undergoing TJA, there has been no benefit in reduction of blood loss or ABT rate,[73,74] and its mention here is purely historical. A class of medications that has shown promise is the antifibrinolytics, which function to decrease blood loss by inhibiting clot degradation. The three most commonly studied in joint replacement are aprotinin, epsilonaminocaproic acid (EACA), and tranexamic acid (TXA).

Aprotinin

Aprotinin is a bovine proteinase inhibitor that was initially used in cardiac surgery patients at increased risk of blood loss and transfusion. The exact mechanism of action of aprotinin is unknown, but there are two prevailing theories. One proposed mechanism is that aprotinin allows for platelet adhesion in the postoperative period by maintaining GPIb platelet receptors. The second mechanism involves an "antikallikrein" effect in which aprotinin causes a decrease in the production of active thrombin. This, in turn, results in less platelet aggregation during surgery, which allows for a greater number of functional platelets and less bleeding postoperatively.[75]

Use of aprotinin in joint replacement and other major orthopaedic surgeries has had, for the most part, good results. Capdevila and colleagues used aprotinin in 23 patients undergoing major orthopaedic hip or pelvis surgery. Although all patients, in both the study and control group, required blood transfusion, aprotinin reduced median blood loss from 5.3 L to 1.7 L and reduced transfusions from 7 units to 3.[76] In their randomized, double-blind, controlled study of 40 THA patients, Janssens et al demonstrated the effectiveness in the realm of TJA. Using an aprotinin bolus of 2×10^6 kallikrein inactivator units (KIU) followed by an infusion of 5×10^5 KIU/h through surgery, they demonstrated a 26% reduction in blood loss and 47% reduction in transfused units compared to a saline control.[77] Jeserchek et al also noted significant reductions in blood loss (62%) and transfusions (55%) with the use of aprotinin versus control.[78] In contrast, Langdown et al did not find any reduction in blood loss or transfusion rate with a 1.5×10^6 KIU bolus of aprotinin.[79]

ε–Aminocaproic acid

The mechanism of action of the other two antifibrinolytics, EACA and TXA, is to prevent plasmin from breaking down fibrin (Fig. 29-4). They are small lysine analogs that competitively inhibit both plasmin and plasminogen. Once bound to the lysine binding site, plasmin is not able to bind to fibrin clots, and EACA and TXA thus prevent fibrin clot degradation. Theories behind their effectiveness in TKA are based on the hypothesis that tourniquet use enhances local fibrinolytic activity in the affected limb. Typical dosing for EACA includes an intravenous loading dose of 100 to 150 mg/kg followed by a 10 to 15 mg/kg/h infusion. With TXA being more potent, its typical dosing is lower with a 10 to 15 mg/kg loading dose and a 1 mg/kg/h infusion rate or additional postoperative boluses.[80]

The efficacy of EACA in reducing blood loss and transfusion rates has been documented in several randomized, controlled studies in the orthopaedic literature, but a paucity of data exists regarding TKA alone. Harley and colleagues found that, compared to placebo, EACA significantly reduced mean postoperative (591 mL vs. 315 mL) and total blood loss (1198 mL vs. 867 mL) in primary THA. Although a reduction in transfusion rate was detected, it was not statistically significant.[81] Ray and coworkers compared EACA and aprotinin to placebo in the setting of primary THA as well and found similar results. The reduction in blood loss compared to placebo was significant for both agents. Again, though, reductions in transfusion rate did not reach statistical significance.[82] In their randomized controlled trial, Camarasa et al evaluated the efficacy of both EACA and TXA specifically in TKA. They noted significant decreases in both blood loss and transfusion rates with both agents. Although greater reductions in the rates of blood loss and transfusion were seen in the TXA group, they were not statistically significant compared to EACA.[83]

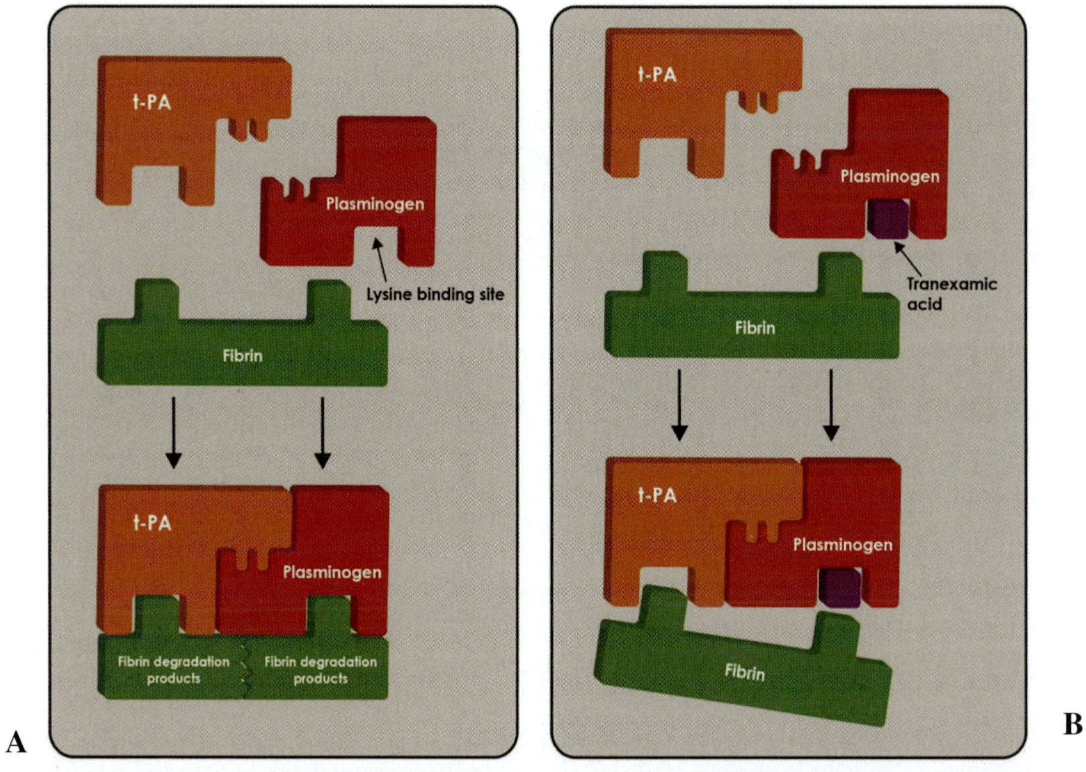

FIGURE 29-4. *Mechanism of action of tranexamic acid. The left side of the diagram depicts the activation of fibrinolysis in the absence of any fibrinolytics. On the right, the competitive inhibition of tranexamic acid at the lysine binding site prevents plasminogen from binding to fibrin for subsequent breakdown. t-PA, tissue plasminogen activator. (Figure by David Kendall, graphic artist, Marshall University Joan C. Edwards School of Medicine.)*

Tranexamic acid

Likely due to its increased potency and subsequent use, the efficacy of TXA in TKA is more extensively studied than that of EACA. In 1995, Hiippala and colleagues published some of the earliest data on use of TXA in TKA. They found a significant 45% reduction in total blood loss and a 55% reduction in number of blood units transfused with a single 15 mg/kg dose of TXA just minutes before deflating the tourniquet.[84] In a randomized, controlled follow-up study, the Hiippala group evaluated the efficacy and safety of an increased dose of TXA: 15 mg/kg just before tourniquet release with two additional 10 mg/kg doses at 3 to 4 hours and 6 to 7 hours postoperatively. Even greater reductions in total blood loss (54%) and units of blood transfused (68%) were seen with the increased dose while maintaining a low risk of DVT similar to controls.[85] Several other studies since have demonstrated similar reductions in blood loss and transfusion rates.[86-91] Cid and Lozano looked at a number of these studies in their 2005 meta-analysis. They found a 10 times reduction in the risk of being transfused when TXA is administered in TKA performed with a tourniquet.[92] Very few studies have not been able to demonstrate a reduction in blood loss or transfusion rates with use of TXA.[93,94] Engel et al found no difference with either TXA or aprotinin versus control. This was attributed to the fact that even the blood loss volumes in their control group were on a level that was only reached by administering antifibrinolytics in other studies.[93] Orpen and colleagues also found no statistical difference in total blood loss or transfusion requirements. They did, however, note a significant decrease in early postoperative blood loss and surmised that had a postoperative TXA bolus been given, as in other studies, a difference may have been detected.[94]

As with any medications, there are limitations to the utility of some of the antifibrinolytics. The application of aprotininin in current blood conservation protocols may be the most limited. First, it had the highest cost of all of the antifibrinolytics at approximately $1200 per patient, compared to approximately $1 and <$15 per patient for EACA and TXA.[95,96] The more important, and severe, limitation of aprotinin is the apparent increased risk in mortality in cardiac surgery. With the increased all-cause 30-day mortality found in the BART trial, the marketing and distribution of aprotinin has been suspended worldwide.[80] Its efficacy makes aprotinin worth mentioning should further analysis demonstrate the drug's safety. EACA and TXA each have an acceptable safety profile with few complications: nausea, vomiting, and diarrhea. Because the antifibrinolytics suppress fibrin clot breakdown, concern over the potential for increasing DVT risk has been raised. Many of the studies evaluating these pharmacologic agents, however, have demonstrated no increased risk of DVT or embolism.[76,78,81-85,93,94] Although these studies suggest no increased risk of DVT, a history of thromboembolic disease is a recommended contraindication for antifibrinolytics.

In order to try to eliminate potential systemic adverse effects and complications of intravenously administered antifibrinolytics, more recent research has focused on local application of TXA in knee arthroplasty. Because topical application of TXA had resulted in blood loss reductions in dental, cardiac, and spinal procedures, Wong and coworkers studied the novel application of topical TXA in knee arthroplasty. In their randomized, controlled, double-blinded trial, 100 patients either received 1.5 g or 3 g of TXA in 100 mL of saline or a control solution of just 100 mL of normal saline. Their results were similar to those seen with intravenous TXA. Significant reductions in blood loss were seen in both treatment groups (315 mL in the 1.5-g group and 400 mL in the 3-g group). A reduction in transfusions was also found, although it did not reach statistical significance (p = .083). There were no transfusions, however, in the 3-g treatment group. There was no increased risk of DVT detected with topical use of TXA.[97] Ishida et al also analyzed the effects of local TXA application through intra-articular injection. In this study, 2 g of TXA was administered into the knee joint via a closed suction drain followed by drain clamping. Application of TXA by this method also resulted in significant reductions in blood, but did not show a reduction in transfusions. There were no noted DVTs in the study.[98]

Tissue Hemostasis

While hypotensive anesthesia and antifibrinolytics may systemically help decrease intraoperative and early postoperative blood loss, an effective means of addressing blood loss more directly is through local tissue hemostasis. There have been several supplements added to standard surgical technique for TKA to try to control intraoperative bleeding and maintain a dry surgical field. The end goal of these techniques and devices is to coagulate and/or seal likely sources of bleeding.

Electrocautery may be the most common method of obtaining hemostasis, but newer devices claim to be just as effective while being gentler on the patient's tissues. One such device is the bipolar radiofrequency (RF) sealer, which delivers radiofrequency energy to saline for sealing and coagulating soft tissue (Fig. 29-5). It functions at cooler temperatures of 100°C or less, resulting in less charring and smoke production.[99] The temperature remains high enough, however, to seal bleeding vessels by shrinking collagen fibers in their walls. Two studies by Marulanda and coworkers demonstrated, in comparison to standard electrocautery, significant reductions in TKA in both intraoperative and total blood loss with this technology.[99,100] Weeden et al also noted significant reductions in hemoglobin decline and nearly one-third as many ABTs with use of a bipolar sealer in TKA compared to conventional electrocautery.[101,102] In comparison, use of bipolar sealers in THA have had mixed results; while some studies have demonstrated efficacy in reducing the need for ABT,[103] others have shown no difference in THA.[104,105] There have been rare reports of tibial nerve neuropathies following use of bipolar sealers in TKA. Lyons et al presented a postoperative neuropathy rate of 3.7% with use of bipolar RF compared to zero in the conventional electrocautery group. This was felt to be a consequence of generous use in the posterior compartment.[106]

Another method of improving hemostasis within the wound in TKA is with topical sealants. Topical fibrin sealants are biological adhesives that initiate the final stages of coagulation. Levy and colleagues studied the efficacy of a fibrin glue spray applied just after prosthesis cementing in TKA. There were significant decreases in both postoperative blood loss and transfusion rates.[107] Wang et al also found a significant decrease in postoperative blood loss by 55% with use of fibrin sealant. The reduction in blood transfusions in the fibrin group approached statistical significance as well.[108] Molloy and colleagues compared the effects of topical fibrin spray to intravenous tranexamic acid. Both agents resulted in significant reductions in blood loss (16% for fibrin and 13% for TXA). Although both the fibrin and the TXA treatment groups experienced reductions in transfusion rates, the drop was more substantial for TXA (53% vs. 35% reduction).[109] The main disadvantage of fibrin spray is its expense, as it can be almost 100 times as expensive as TXA.[109]

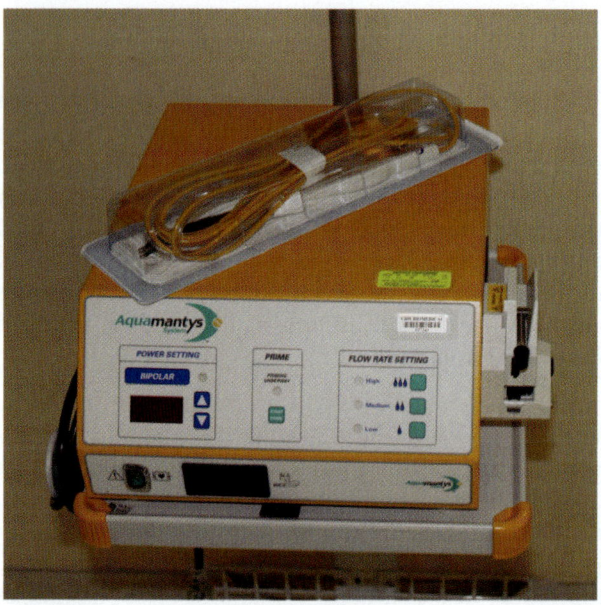

FIGURE 29-5. *The Aquamantys® system is a bipolar sealing system that delivers radiofrequency energy and saline for hemostatic control of bone and soft tissues.*

Recently, several studies have evaluated the utility of topical or intra-articular platelet-rich plasma (PRP) in TKA. PRP is obtained after centrifuging a unit of autologous whole blood with a blood separator and isolating the factor-rich buffy coat. Two prevalent growth factors in the solution are platelet-derived growth factor and transforming growth factor beta; both have been associated with improved hemostasis and wound healing.[110,111] The proposed advantage with PRP is sealing of tissues and augmentation of the healing cascade by using autologous products and theoretically eliminating infection and risks of error. Gardner et al found a statistically significant reduction in the postoperative hemoglobin drop with PRP. Additional benefits included fewer narcotics, greater functional range of motion at discharge, and shorter length of stay. Data on transfusion rates were not reported.[110] Everts and colleagues performed a similar prospective study comparing PRP plus fibrin spray to controls. Significant reductions in transfusions and drops in hemoglobin were seen in this treatment group as well. Reductions in wound leakage and wound infections were also noted.[111] In a contrasting study, Diiorio and colleagues retrospectively evaluated their series of TKA patients who had received PRP intraoperatively. Compared to controls, there were no significant differences in blood loss, passive range of motion, narcotic requirement, or length of stay.[112] Further studies will likely be needed to better identify the role that PRP will have in TKA in the future.

Much of the attention regarding hemostasis is focused on the soft tissue bleeding encountered during knee replacement. There are, however, a few options for controlling bone bleeding. The bipolar sealer device described previously is one such tool.[113] Another technique described in the literature involving osseous blood loss is plugging of the intramedullary canal. Raut et al showed that by plugging the defect left by the femoral intramedullary guide with acrylic cement blood loss could significantly be reduced by 20%.[114] Kumar et al confirmed that plugging the intramedullary femoral defect significantly reduces postoperative drainage. Rather than using cement, the plug in the Kumar study was made from autologous bone from previous cuts.[115] More recent studies continue to demonstrate the benefits of sealing the intramedullary canal and recommend that it be done regularly when utilizing an intramedullary guide (Fig. 29-6).[116]

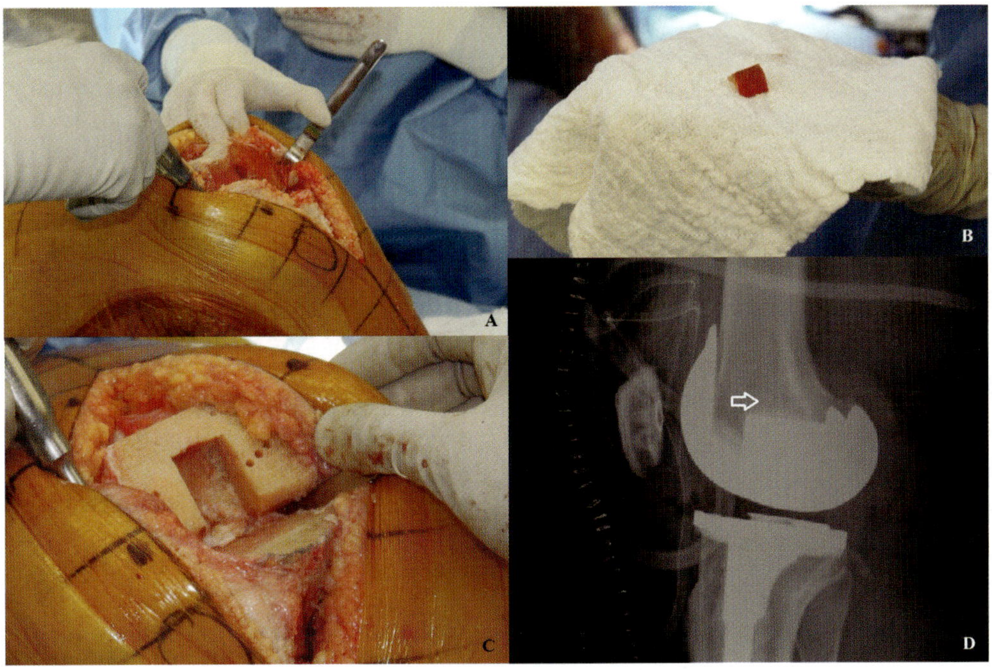

FIGURE 29-6. *(**A**) After using the opening reamer for placement of the intramedullary femoral guide, a significant defect communicating with the medullary canal remains. (**B**) Autologous bone from previous condyle or box cuts can be fashioned to plug this void. (**C**) Before cementing the posterior-stabilizing components, the autograft bone is packed into place to seal the canal. (**D**) Postoperative radiographs demonstrate the position of the plug (white arrow).*

Tourniquet Use

There is a long history of pneumatic tourniquet use in TKA. The claimed advantages include minimizing blood loss, improving the visualization of the surgical field, and improving interdigitation of cement. There are, however, plenty of reported disadvantages of tourniquet application as well: nerve or vascular injury, muscle damage, and increased incidence of venous thromboembolism.[117] Out of the 16 outcome measures in Smith and Hing's meta-analysis of tourniquet use in TKA, the only significant advantage they found was in intraoperative blood loss. Other outcomes, including postoperative blood loss, total blood loss, transfusion rate, and operative time, were similar between the tourniquet and nontourniquet groups. They identified, however, that there are a number of factors which may influence tourniquet effectiveness: location, exsanguination technique, cuff width, cuff pressure, and timing of cuff deflation.[117] Several studies have tried to clarify the optimal time of cuff deflation. Except for one study,[118] the vast majority of these investigations conclude that release of the tourniquet before skin closure and application of a compressive bandage is not effective for reducing blood loss in TKA.[119-124]

Computer-Assisted Surgery

Computer-assisted surgery (CAS) has been employed to improve the intraoperative accuracy of TKA component positioning, but some authors have found an advantage in terms of decreased blood loss as well. Because navigation pins placed in the distal femur and proximal tibia do not require conventional breaching of the medullary canals (Fig. 29-7), blood loss should theoretically be less. Kalairajah and colleagues demonstrated this expected reduction in blood loss in their prospective randomized controlled study. The CAS patients experienced a significant reduction in blood loss (15%) as well as calculated drop in hemoglobin (32%) versus conventional TKAs.[125] Conteduca and coworkers found an identical reduction in blood loss (15%) with computer navigation.[126] Miller and his coauthors evaluated the blood conservation potential of CAS TKA in the morbidly obese population. They found that blood loss was significantly greater in morbidly obese patients regardless of technique (conventional vs. CAS). Separately, there was a significant reduction in blood loss (24%) with CAS regardless of BMI.[127] These studies demonstrate that despite the increase in surgical time and placement of bicortical tracking pins, CAS can significantly reduce blood loss

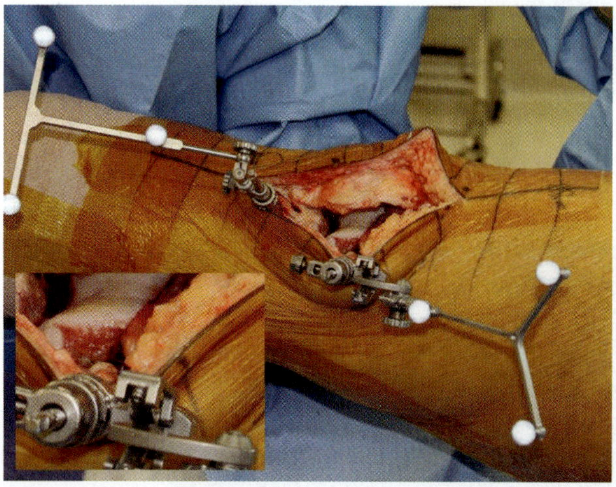

FIGURE 29-7. *Femoral and tibial pins for the computer navigation arrays are placed within the surgical wound. With their smaller diameter and minimal penetrance, they do not breach the medullary canal to the same degree as conventional intramedullary guides.*

in TKA. What has not been reliably shown in the literature, however, is a reduction in the more clinically relevant outcome: post-TKA transfusion rates.

POSTOPERATIVE BLOOD MANAGEMENT

Drain Usage and Cell Salvage

A fair amount of debate exists regarding the use of drains following TKA. They are thought to reduce hematoma formation and the incidence of deep infection, but very few studies have confirmed this effect. Early drain systems, including Penrose drains, were actually found to result in higher rates of infection,[128] but in 1961, Waugh and Stinchfield introduced a closed suction drainage that showed promise in reducing infection rates.[129] Their improved outcomes, however, were not statistically significant, and several others have since shown that closed wound drainage is not valuable for blood conservation or most other outcomes following TJA.[130-135] Some authors have attempted to improve the efficacy of closed suction drainage by limiting early blood losses with clamping. There have not, however, been any significant reductions in blood loss in doing so.[136,137]

Although the use of a closed suction drain alone has not been shown to be beneficial, the reinfusion of blood salvaged intraoperatively and drained postoperatively offers a simple and relatively inexpensive form of autologous transfusion. Blood is typically collected via a filtered closed suction drain or processed through a cell saver machine and then reinfused into the patient (Figs. 29-8 and 29-9). Numerous studies have documented significant reductions in ABT rates of up to 71% as well as reductions in volume of homologous blood transfused as high as 86% with the use of such systems.[138-147] However, there are few data regarding the efficacy and safety of blood salvage across the full spectrum of knee replacement surgery. Henderson and colleagues undertook such an investigation that evaluated reinfusion in unicompartmental, unilateral, bilateral, and revision knee replacement. They found significant reductions in the number of patients requiring ABT and the number of ABT units per patient for all four types of knee replacement. The safety of reinfusion was confirmed as well, as there were no adverse events detected.[148] There have been few contrasting studies in which cell salvage did not reduce transfusion requirements in TKA patients enough for authors to recommend cell salvage in all unilateral TKAs.[149-152] Interestingly, in three of these studies,[149-151] reinfusion was combined with PAD, which itself has demonstrated reduction in ABT requirements. As such, one might not expect to see as much benefit from cell salvage and reinfusion in this scenario.

Pain Control

There are few data in the literature that evaluate the effects of pain control regimens on blood loss and transfusion rates in TKA. In their prospective study, Chelly et al analyzed a number of outcome measures in three different pain control groups: patient-controlled analgesia (PCA), PCA plus continuous femoral infusion (CFI) block, and PCA plus epidural analgesia (EPA).[153] Significant reductions in blood loss and transfusions were found in both the CFI and EPA groups versus PCA alone. Although not statistically significant, CFI did provide an additional 8% reduction in blood loss and 18% reduction in transfusion rate beyond EPA. Coupled with the additional benefits of decreased complication rates and shorter hospital stay, the authors state that CFI represents a better alternative than PCA or EPA for postoperative pain management following TKA. There is evidence in the THA literature as well that supports the finding that supplementation of general anesthesia with EPA[154,155] or lumbar plexus block[156] can significantly reduce postoperative blood loss.

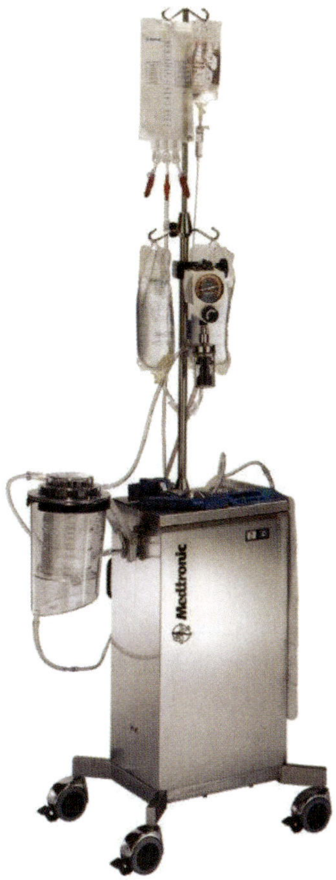

FIGURE 29-8. *The Medtronic autoLog® Autotransfusion System is an example of an intraoperative cell salvage device. Blood within the surgical field is suctioned into the device with a heparin solution. The collected blood products are filtered and processed for intraoperative transfusion. (Used with permission from Medtronic, Inc.)*

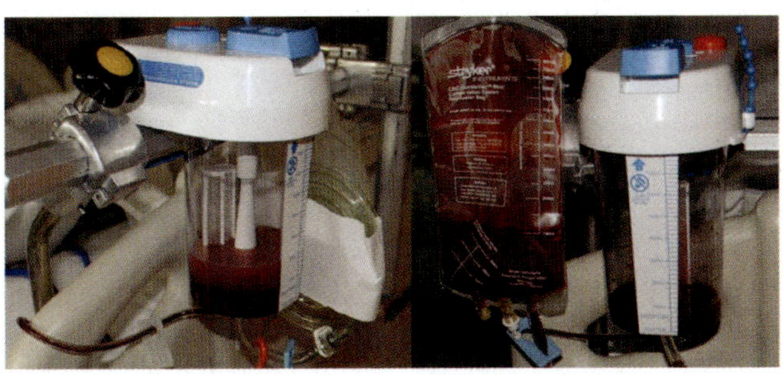

FIGURE 29-9. *The Stryker Constavac CBCII is an example of a reinfusion drain that collects blood lost in the deep portions of the surgical site postoperatively and allows for safe reinfusion of these products through a closed system.*

Rehabilitation

There have been several studies in the TKA literature that have evaluated the effect of position and timing of therapy or motion on blood loss. Speck et al randomized TKA patients into flexion or extension groups, and they reported a drainage reduction of up to 33% when patients were placed into flexion postoperatively.[157] Ong and Taylor tried to elicit whether this reduction in postoperative drain output was due to flexion or rather elevation of the knee. They found that both elevated extension and knee flexion reduced hemoglobin loss by 25% compared to level extension. As such, they recommended elevation of the leg to 35° with the knee in extension as a safe and effective method of reducing blood loss.[158] In contrast, Lotke et al analyzed two variables (timing of motion initiation and timing of tourniquet release) in four different groups of patients. The group of patients in whom the tourniquet was released intraoperatively and had continuous passive motion initiated immediately after surgery experienced a significant increase in total blood loss. When groups were combined to evaluate the effect of early motion alone, however, there was no longer any difference between early versus delayed motion postoperatively.[123] Ma and colleagues compared outcomes in TKA patients who were either splinted in full extension or held in 70° of flexion for the first 24 hours after surgery. As in the Lotke study, the authors were unable to detect any significant difference in blood loss, need for transfusion, or any other measured outcomes.[159] With conflicting results in the literature, and no significant effects on additional functional outcomes, it remains difficult to fully recommend flexion over extension positioning, or vice versa. If anything, the literature seems to favor initial elevation of the knee with early initiation of motion.

CONCLUSIONS

Blood loss and the need for transfusions will long remain an area of interest in TKA. Although improving, the risks associated with transfusion of allogeneic blood persist, and the total joint surgeon should be familiar with the techniques available to minimize the need for ABT. In planning for blood loss, the surgeon should also be aware of those patients with risk factors for needing ABT, including preoperative anemia, advanced age, female gender, bilateral TKA, and revision TKA.

Preoperative management of blood loss associated with TKA includes autologous blood donation and maximizing patients' preoperative hemoglobin levels. Use of PAD has demonstrated reductions in transfusions of allogeneic blood, but this comes at a cost. Patients are required to dedicate time for donation, and the financial burden is much greater than some of the other blood conservation techniques. Although it does significantly reduce the risk of disease transmission, there can still be complications during donation or transfusion processes. EPO, too, has been effective in blood conservation protocols by improving preoperative anemia. It may be most beneficial in those donating autologous blood or with more severe anemia.

Except for hemodilution, the focus of intraoperative blood management techniques is to reduce a patient's potential need for ABT by limiting or minimizing blood loss. ANH is essentially a form of autologous donation, but because it is performed in the operating room, the cost, complication rate, and opportunity for clerical error are much lower. The remainder of the intraoperative techniques address blood loss at a multitude of levels. Hypotensive anesthesia decreases the MAP to bleeding structures. It has been shown to be safe and effective down to 50 ± 5 mm Hg. Tourniquet use limits blood loss while also improving visualization of the surgical field and interdigitation of cemented components. Although it may comfort the surgeon to release the tourniquet to ensure adequate hemostasis before closure, the vast majority of the blood preservation literature does not support this. Of the pharmalogic agents used in TKA, TXA is the most studied, and it has demonstrated significant reductions in blood loss and ABTs while maintaining a relatively low cost and complication profile. These tools should all be used in conjuncture with good surgical technique utilizing electrocautery or a bipolar sealer for hemostasis,and using plugs or CAS to minimize blood loss from the medullary canal.

The central focus following TKA is rehabilitation, but postoperative blood loss may still play a significant role in patients' outcomes. As with timing of tourniquet release, there is a surgeon comfort level that may dictate the use of a drain postoperatively. Although hematoma and deep infection are valid concerns, the data do not support the use of closed suction drainage for improving blood loss, infection, or function outcomes in TKA. When drains are employed for the purposes of reinfusion, however, there have been significant reductions in blood loss and ABT rates documented in the literature. With regard to therapy and motion, elevation appears to be helpful in reducing blood loss, and there does not appear be any major contraindications to early motion. Effective pain control may facilitate this early return of motion while reducing blood loss as well.

With appropriate preoperative risk assessment and preparation, good surgical technique, and proper postoperative management, the total knee surgeon should be able to reduce the need for transfusion and positively affect early and long-term outcomes for all TKA patients.

PEARLS AND PITFALLS

The following are some pearls and pitfalls for the surgeon to consider:

- Although the risk of disease transmission continues to decrease with allogeneic blood transfusion, there are still other risks that make avoidance ideal.
- Preoperative anemia is the single greatest risk factor associated for needing a blood transfusion after total knee arthroplasty.
- Preoperative donation of autologous blood may be attractive to both patient and physician, but potential complications, cost burden, and wastage rates limit its use.
- Erythropoietin use is one of the most effective means of elevating a patient's hemoglobin preoperatively. It is typically supplemented with ferrous sulfate.
- Acute normovolemic hemodilution is an inexpensive alternative to PAD for the patient at increased risk of needing ABT.
- Of the pharmacologic agents available for use in TKA, tranexamic acid is the best studied, with numerous series demonstrating significant decreases in transfusion rates without any increase in DVTs or other complications.
- Tourniquet use has been shown to decrease intraoperative blood loss. Although tourniquet deflation may be performed to assess patellar tracking, deflation before closure for ensuring hemostasis has not been shown to decrease blood loss or ABT.
- Techniques used in minimizing intraoperative blood loss include electrocautery, bipolar sealer, plugging the intramedullary canal, and avoiding canal opening by using computer navigation.
- Closed suction drains are not well supported in the TKA literature, but cell salvage and reinfusion drains appear to be safe and effective methods of returning blood losses to TKA patients.
- With regard to blood loss and transfusion, there are no contraindications to early postoperative motion.

SUGGESTED READING

Brecher ME, Goodnough LT. The rise and fall of preoperative autologous blood donation. *Transfusion.* 2001; 41(12):1459-1462.

Keating EM, Meding JB. Perioperative blood management practices in elective orthopedic surgery. *J Am Acad Orthop Surg.* 2002;10(6):393-400.

Muller U, Exadaktylos A, Roeder C, et al. Effect of a flow chart on use of blood transfusions in primary total hip and knee replacement: prospective before and after study. *BMJ.* 2004;328(7445):934-938.

Sinclair KC, Clarke HD, Noble BN. Blood management in total knee arthroplasty: a comparison of techniques. *Orthopedics.* 2009;32(1):19.

Vuille-Lessard E, Boudreault D, Girard F, et al. Red blood cell transfusion practice in elective orthopedic surgery: a multicenter cohort study. *Transfusion.* 2010; 50(10):2117-2124.

REFERENCES

1. Lotke PA, Barth P, Garino JP, et al. Predonated autologous blood transfusions after total knee arthroplasty: immediate versus delayed administration. *J Arthroplasty.* 1999;14(6):647-650.
2. Bong MR, Patel V, Chang E, et al. Risks associated with blood transfusion after total knee arthroplasty. *J Arthroplasty.* 2004;19(3):281-287.
3. Walker, RH. Transfusion risks. *Am J Clin Pathol.* 1987;88(3):374-378.
4. Lackritz EM, Satten GA, Aberle-Grasse J, et al. Estimated risk of transmission of the human immunodeficiency virus by screened blood in the United States. *N Engl J Med.* 1995;333(26):1721-1725.
5. Schreiber GB, Busch MP, Kleinman SH, et al. The risk of transfusion-transmitted viral infections. *N Engl J Med.* 1996;334(26):1685-1690.
6. Dodd RY, Notari EP IV, Stramer SL. Current prevalence and incidence of infectious disease markers and estimated window-period risk in the American Red Cross blood donor population. *Transfusion.* 2002;42: 975-979.
7. Pealer LN, Marfin AA, Petersen LR, et al. Transmission of West Nile virus through blood transfusions in the United States in 2002. *N Engl J Med.* 2003;349 (13):1236-1245.
8. Gubernot DM, Lucey CT, Lee KC, et al. Babesia infection through blood transfusions: reports received by the US Food and Drug Administration, 1997-2007. *Clin Infect Dis.* 2009;48:25-30.
9. Blajchman MA, Vamvakas EC. The continuing risk of transfusion-transmitted infection. *N Engl J Med.* 2006;355(13):1303-1305.
10. Blajchman MA, Alexander JW. Mechanisms of transfusion-induced immunosuppression. *Transfusion.* 1990;30:651-658. 10.
11. Vamvakas EC, Blajchman MA. Transfusion-related immunomodulation (TRIM): an update. *Blood Rev.* 2007;21:327-348.
12. Kendall SJ, Weir J, Aspinall R. Erythrocyte transfusion causes immunosuppression after total hip repla-cement. *Clin Orthop Relat Res.* 2000;381: 145-155.
13. Innerhofer P, Klingler A, Klimmer C, et al. Risk for postoperative infection after transfusion of white blood cell-filtered allogeneic or autologous blood components in orthopedic patients undergoing primary arthroplasty. *Transfusion.* 2005;45:103-110.
14. 14. Innerhofer P, Walleczek C, Luz G, et al. Transfusion of buffy-coat-depleted blood components and risk for postoperative infection in orthopedic patients. *Transfusion.* 1999;39:625-632. 3.
15. Pulido L, Ghanem E, Joshi A, et all. Periprosthetic joint infection: the incidence, timing, and predisposing factors. *Clin Orthop Relat Res.* 2008;466(7):1710-1715.
16. Rosencher N, Kerkkamp HE, Macheras G, et al. Orthopedic surgery transfusion hemoglobin European overview (OSTHEO) study: blood management in elective knee and hip arhtroplasty in Europe. *Transfusion.* 2003;43:459-469.
17. Murphy P, Heal JM, Blumberg N. Infection or suspected infection after hip replacement surgery with autologous or homologous blood transfusions. *Transfusion.* 1991;31(3):212-217.
18. Bierbaum BE, Callaghan JJ, Galante JO, et al. An analysis of blood management in patients having a total hip or knee arthroplasty. *J Bone Joint Surg Am.* 1999;81:2-10.
19. Basora M, Pereira A, Soriano A, et al. Allogeneic blood transfusion does not increase the risk of wound infection in total knee arthroplasty. *Vox Sanguinis.* 2010;98:124-129.
20. Vamvakas EC, Moore SB, Cabanela M. Blood transfusion and septic complications after hip replacement surgery. *Transfusion.* 1995;35:150-156.

21. Brand A, Houbiers JGA. Clinical studies of blood transfusion and cancer. In: Vamvakas EC, Blajchman MA, eds. *Immunomodulatory Effects of Allogeneic Blood Transfusion.* Bethesda, MD: AABB Press; 1999:145-190.

22. Chung M, Steinmetz OK, Gordon PH. Perioperative blood transfusion and outcome after resection for colorectal carcinoma. *Br J Surg.* 1993;80:427-432.

23. Vamvakas EC. Perioperative blood transfusion and cancer recurrence: meta-analysis for explanation. *Transfusion.* 1995;35:760-768.

24. Vamvakas EC. Transfusion-associated cancer recurrence and infection: meta-analysis of the randomized controlled clincial trials. *Transfusion.* 1996;36:175-186.

25. FDA. *Fatalities Reported to FDA Following Blood Collection and Transfusion. Annual Summary for Fiscal Year 2010*; 2010.

26. Vamvakas EC, Blajchman MA. Transfusion-related mortality: the ongoing risks of allogeneic blood transfusion and the available strategies for their prevention. *Blood.* 2009;113(15):3406-3417.

27. Hatzidakis AM, Mendlick RM, McKillip T, et al. Preoperative autologous donation for total joint arthroplasty. An analysis of risk factors for allogeneic transfusion. *J Bone Joint Surg Am.* 2000;82(1):89-100.

28. Keating EM, Meding JB, Faris PM, et al. Predictors of transfusion risk in elective knee surgery. *Clin Orthop Relat Res.* 1998;347:50-59.

29. Salido JA, Marin LA, Gomez LA, et al. Preoperative hemoglobin levels and the need for transfusion after prosthetic hip and knee surgery. *J Bone Joint Surg Am.* 2002;84(2):216-220.

30. Cushner F, Friedman RJ. Blood loss in total knee arthroplasty. *Clin Orthop Relat Res.* 1991;269:98-101.

31. Faris PM, Spence RK, Larholt, et al. The predictive power of baseline hemoglobin for transfusion risk in surgery patients. *Orthopedics.* 1999;22:S135-140.

32. de Andrade JR, Jove M, Landon G, et al. Baseline hemoglobin as a predictor of risk of transfusion and response to Epoetin alfa in orthopedic surgery patients. *Am J Orthop.* 1996;25(8):533-542.

33. Sculco TP, Gallina J. Blood management experience: relationship between autologous blood donation and transfusion in orthopedic surgery. *Orthopedics.* 1999; 22(1 suppl):S129-134.

34. Pola E, Papaleo P, Santoliquido A, et al. Clinical factors associated with an increased risk of perioperative blood transfusion in nonanemic patients undergoing total hip arthroplasty. *J Bone Joint Surg Am.* 2004; 86(1):57-61.

35. Parvizi J, Chaudhry S, Rasouli MR, et al. Who needs autologous blood donation in joint replacement? *J Knee Surg.* 2011;24:25-32.

36. Prasad N, Padmanabham V, Mullaji A. Blood loss in total knee arthroplasty: an analysis of risk factors. *Int Orthop.* 2007;31:39-44.

37. Nuttall GA, Santrach PJ, Oliver WC Jr, et al. The predictors of red cell transfusions in total hip arthroplasties. *Transfusion.* 1996;36:144-149.

38. Bell TH, Berta D, Ralley F. Factors affecting perioperative blood loss and transfusion rates in primary total joint arthroplasty: a prospective analysis of 1642 patients. *Can J Surg.* 2009;52(4):295-301.

39. Churchill WH, McGurk S, Chapman RH, et al. The Collaborative Hospital Transfusion Study: variations in use of autologous blood account for hospital differences in red cell use during primary hip and knee surgery. *Transfusion.* 1998;38:530-539.

40. Walsh M, Preston C, Bong M, et al. Relative risk factors for requirement of blood transfusion after total hip arthroplasty. *J Arthroplasty.* 2007;22(8):1162-1167.

41. Goodnough LT, Brecher ME, Kanter MH, et al. Transfusion medicine. First of two parts–blood transfusion. *N Eng J Med.* 1999;340:438-447.

42. Goodnough LT, Brecher ME, Kanter MH, et al. Transfusion medicine. Second of two parts–blood conservation. *N Eng J Med.* 1999;340:525-533.

43. Segal JB, Guallar E, Powe NR. Autologous blood transfusion in the United States: clinical and nonclinical determinants of use. *Transfusion.* 2001;41:1539-1547.

44. National Heart, Lung, and Blood Institute Expert Panel on the Use of Autologous Blood. Transfusion alert: use of autologous blood. *Transfusion.* 1995;35: 703-711.

45. American Association of Blood Banks. *Standards for Blood Banks and Transfusion 241 Services.* Bethesda, MD; 2002.

46. Cushner FD, Lee GC, Scuderi GR, et al. Blood loss management in high-risk patients undergoing total knee arthroplasty. *J Knee Surg.* 2006;19:249-253.

47. Forgie MA, Wells PS, Laupacis A, et al. Preoperative autologous donation decreases allogeneic transfusion but increases exposure to all red blood cell transfusion: results of a meta-analysis. International Study of Perioperative Transfusion (ISPOT) Investigators. *Arch Intern Med.* 1998;158:616-616.

48. Popovsky MA, Whitaker B, Arnold NL. Severe outcomes of allogeneic and autologous blood donation: frequency and characterization. *Transfusion.* 1995;35: 734-737.
49. Linden JV, Paul B, Dressler KP. A report of 104 transfusion errors in New York State. *Transfusion.* 1992;32:601-606.
50. Linden JV. Autologous blood errors and incidents. *Transfusion.* 1994;34(suppl):28S.
51. Yomtovian, R. Autologous transfusion complications. In: Popovsky M, ed. *Transfusion Reactions.* Bethesda, MD: AABB Press; 1996:237-280.
52. Green WS, Toy P, Bozic KJ. Cost minimization analysis of preoperative erythropoietin vs autologous and allogeneic blood donation in total joint arthroplasty. *J Arthroplasty.* 2010;25:93-96.
53. Renner SW, Howanitz PJ, Bachner P. Preoperative autologous blood donation in 612 hospitals. A College of American Pathologists' Q-Probes study of quality issues in transfusion practice. *Arch Pathol Lab Med.* 1992;116:613-619.
54. Pazdernik TL, Kerecsen L, Mrugeshkumar KS. *Pharmacology.* Philadelphia, PA: Mosby; 2003.
55. Faris PM, Ritter MA, Abels RI. The effects of recombinant human erythropoietin on perioperative transfusion requirements in patients having a major orthopaedic operation. The American Erythropoietin Study Group. *J Bone Joint Surg Am.* 1996;78:62-72.
56. Bezwada HP, Nazarian DG, Henry DH, et al. Preoperative use of recombinant human erythropoietin before total joint arthroplasty. *J Bone Joint Surg Am.* 2003;85(9):1795-1800.
57. Goldberg MA, McCutchen JW, Jove M, et al. A safety and efficacy comparison study of two dosing regimens of epoetin alfa in patients undergoing major orthopedic surgery. *Am J Orthop.* 1996;25: 544-552.
58. Feagan BG, Wong CJ, Kirkley A, et al. Erythropoietin with iron supplementation to prevent allogeneic blood transfusion in total hip joint arthroplasty. *Ann Intern Med.* 2000;133:845-854.
59. Dunn CJ, Wagstaff AJ. Epoetin alfa. A review of its clinical efficacy in the management of anaemia associated with renal failure and chronic disease and its use in surgical patients. *Drugs Aging.* 1995;7:131-156.
60. Churchill DN, Muirhead N, Goldstein M, et al. Probability of thrombosis of vascular access among hemodialysis patientes treated with recombinant human erythropoietin. *J Am Soc Nephrol.* 1994;4: 1809-1813.
61. Napier JA, Bruce M, Chapman J, et al. Guidelines for autologous transfusion. II. Perioperative haemodilution and cell salvage. *Br J Anaesth.* 1997;78:768-771.
62. Monk TG, Goodnough LT, Birkmayer JD, et al. Acute normovolemic hemodilution is a cost-effective alternative to preoperative autologous blood donation by patients undergoing radical retro-pubic prostatectomy. *Transfusion.* 1995;35:559-565.
63. Goodnough LT, Monk TG, Despotis GJ, et al. A randomized trial of acute normovolemic hemodilution compared to preoperative autologous blood donation in total knee arthroplasty. *Vox Sanguinis.* 1999;77:11-16.
64. Goodnough LT, Despotis GJ, Merkel K, et al. A randomized trial comparing acute normovolemic hemodilution and preoperative autologous blood donation in total hip arthroplasty. *Transfusion.* 2000;40:1054-1057.
65. Olsfanger D, Fredman B, Goldstein B, et al. Acute normovolaemic haemodilution decreases postoperative allogeneic blood transfusion after total knee replacement. *Br J Anaesth.* 1997;79:317-321.
66. Shulman G, Grecula MJ, Hadjipavlou AG. Intraoperative autotransfusion in hip arthroplasty. *Clin Orthop Relat Res.* 2002;396:119-130.
67. Sharrock NE, Mineo R, Urquhar B. Hemodynamic effects of low dose epinephrine and sodium nitroprusside during epidural hypotensive anesthesia. *Reg Anesth.* 1989;14(suppl):S12.
68. Sharrock NE, Mineo R, Urquhart B, et al. The effect of two levels of hypotension on intraoperative blood loss during total hip arthroplasty performed under lumbar epidural anesthesia. *Anesth Analg.* 1993;76: 580-584.
69. Juelsgaard P, Larsen UT, Sorensen JV, et al. Hypotensive epidural anesthesia in total knee replacement without tourniquet: reduced blood loss and transfusion. *Reg Anesth Pain Med.* 2001;26:105-110.
70. Niemi TT, Pitkanen M, Syrjala M, et al. Comparison of hypotensive epidural anaesthesia and spinal anaesthesia on blood loss and coagulation during and after total hip arthroplasty. *Acta Anaesthesiol Scand.* 2000; 44:457-464.
71. An HS, Mikhail WE, Jackson WT, et al. Effects of hypotensive anesthesia, nonsteroidal antiinflammatory drugs, and polymethylmethacrylate on bleeding in total hip arthroplasty patients. *J Arthroplasty.* 1991; 6(3):245-250.
72. Sharrock NE, Salvati EA. Hypotensive epidural anesthesia for total hip arthroplasty. *Acta Orthop Scand.* 1996;67:91-107.

73. Karnezis TA, Stulberg SD, Wixson RL. The hemostatic effects of desmopressin on patients who had total joint arthroplasty: a double-blind randomized trial. *J Bone Joint Surg Am.* 1994;76:1545-1550.
74. Schott U, Sollen C, Axelsson K, et al. Desmopressin acetate does not reduce blood loss during total hip replacement in patients receiving dextran. *Acta Anaesthesiol Scand.* 1995;39:592-598.
75. Hardy JF, Desrochoes J. Natural and synthetic antifibrinolytics in cardiac surgery. *Can J Anaesth.* 1992; 39:353-365.
76. Capdevila X, Calvet Y, Biboulet P, et al. Aprotinin decreases blood loss and homologous transfusions in patients undergoing major orthopedic surgery. *Anesthesiology.* 1998;88:50-57.
77. Janssens M, Joris J, David JL, et al. High dose aprotinin reduces blood loss in patients undergoing total hip replacement surgery. *Anesthesiology.* 1994;80:23-29.
78. Jeserchek R, Clar H, Aigner C, et al. Reduction of blood loss using high-dose aprotinin in major otheopaedic surgery: a prosepective, double-blind, randomized, and placebo-controlled study. *J Bone Joint Surg Br.* 2003;85:174-177.
79. Langdown AJ, Field J, Grote J, et al. Aprotinin (Trasylol) does not reduce bleeding in primary total hip arthroplasty. *J Arthroplasty.* 2000;15:1009-1012.
80. Eubanks JD. Antifibrinolytics in major orthopaedic surgery. *J Am Acad Orthop Surg*. 2010;18:132-138.
81. Harley B, Beaupre L, Jones A, et al. The effect of epsilon aminocaproic acid on blood loss in patients who undergo primary total hip arthroplasty. *Can J Surg*. 2002;45(3):185-190.
82. Ray M, Hatcher S, Whitehouse SL, et al. Aprotinin and epsiolon aminocaproic acid are effective in reducing blood loss after primary total hip arthroplasty: a prospective, randomized double-blinded placebo controlled study. *J Thromb Haemost*. 2005;3:1421-1427.
83. Camarasa MA, Olle G, Serra-Prat M, et al. Efficacy of aminocaproic, tranexamic acids in the control of bleeding during total knee replacement: a randomized clinical trial. *Br J Anaesth*. 2006;96:576-582.
84. Hiippala S, Strid L, Wennerstrand M. Tranexamic acid (Cyklokapron) reduces perioperative blood loss associated with total knee arthroplasty. *Br J Anaesth.* 1995;74:534-537.
85. Hiippala ST, Strid LJ, Wennerstrand MI, et al. Tranexamic acid radically decreases blood loss and transfusions associated with total knee arthroplasty. *Anesth Analg*. 1997;84:839-844.
86. Veien M, Sorensen JV, Madsen F, et al. Tranexamic acid given intraoperatively reduces blood loss after total knee replacement: a randomized, controlled study. *Acta Anaesthesiol Scand*. 2002;46:1206-1211.
87. Ido K, Neo M, Asada Y, et al. Reduction of blood loss using tranexamic acid in total knee and hip arthroplasties. *Arch Orthop Trama Surg*. 2000;120:518-520.
88. Alvarez JC, Santiveri FX, Ramos I, et al. Tranexamic acid reduces blood transfusion in total knee arthroplasty even when a blood conservation program is applied. *Transfusion*. 2008;48:519-525.
89. Benoni G, Fredin H. Fibrinolytic inhibition with tranexamic acid reduces blood loss and blood transfusion after knee arthroplasty: a prospective, randomised, double-blind study of 86 patients. *J Bone Joint Surg Br.* 1996;78:434-440.
90. Jansen AJ, Andreica S, Claeys M, et al. Use of tranexamic acid for an effective blood conservation strategy after total knee arthroplasty. *Br J Anaesth.* 1999;84: 596-601.
91. Ortega-Andreu M, Pérez-Chrzanowska H, Figueredo R, et al. Blood loss control with two doses of tranexamic acid in a multimodal protocol for total knee arthroplasty. *Open Orthop J*. 2011;5:44-48.
92. Cid J, Lozano M. Tranexamic acid reduces allogeneic red cell transfusions in patients undergoing total knee arthroplasty: results of a meta-analysis or randomized controlled trials. *Transfusion.* 2005;45:1302-1307.
93. Engel JM, Hohaus T, Ruwoldt R, et al. Regional hemostatic status and blood requirements after total knee arthroplasty with and without tranexamic acid or aprotinin. *Anesth Analg.* 2001;92:775-780.
94. Orpen NM, Little C, Walker G, et al. Tranexamic acid reduces early post-operative blood loss after total knee arthroplasty: a prospective randomised controlled trial of 29 patients. *Knee*. 2006;13:106-110.
95. Florentino-Pineda I, Blakemore LC, Thompson GH, et al. The effect of epsilon-aminocaproic acid on perioperative blood less in patients with idiopathic scoliosis undergoing posterior spinal fusion: a preliminary prospective study. *Spine.* 2001;26:1147-1151.
96. Johansson T, Pettersson L, Lisander B. Tranexamic acid in total hip arthroplasty saves blood and money: a randomized, double-blind study in 100 patients. *Acta Orthop*. 2005;76(3):314-319.
97. Wong J, Abrishami A, El Beheiry H, et al. Topical application of tranexamic acid reduces postoperative blood loss in total knee arthroplasty: a randomized, controlled trial. *J Bone Joint Surg Am.* 2010;92:2503-2513.
98. Ishida K, Tsumura N, Kitagawa A, et al. Intra-articular injection of tranexamic acid reduces not only blood loss but also knee joint swelling after total knee

arthroplasty. *Int Orthop.* January 2011 [Epub ahead of print].

99. Marulanda GA, Ragland PS, Seyler TM, et al. Reductions in blood loss with use of a bipolar sealer for hemostasis in primary total knee arthroplasty. *Surg Technol Int.* 2005;14:281-286.

100. Marulanda GA, Krebs VE, Bierbaum BE, et al. Hemostasis using a bipolar sealer in primary unilateral total knee arthroplasty. *Am J Orthop.* 2009;38 (12):E179-E183.

101. Weeden SH, Schmidt RH, Isabell G. Hemostatic efficacy of a bipolar sealing device in minimally invasive total knee arthroplasty. *J Bone Joint Surg Br.* 2009;91 (suppl):45.

102. Isabell G, Weeden S. Hemodynamic efficacy of a bipolar sealing device in primary total knee arthroplasty (abstract). Paper presented at Annual Meeting of Texas Orthopaedic Association, Houston, TX; 2006.

103. Marulanda GA, Ulrich SD, Seyler TM, et al. Reductions in blood loss with a bipolar sealer in total hip arthroplasty. *Expert Rev Med Devices.* 2008;5:125-131.

104. Barsoum WK, Klika AK, Murray TG, et al. Prospective randomized evaluation of the need for blood transfusion during primary total hip arthroplasty with use of a bipolar sealer. *J Bone Joint Surg Am.* 2011; 93:513-518.

105. Zeh A, Messer J, Davis J, et al. The Aquamantys System–an alternative to reduce blood loss in primary total hip arthroplasty. *J Arthroplasty.* 2010;25:1072-1077.

106. Lyons ST, Morrison K. Sensory neuropathy associated with cauterization using bipolar radio frequency device in primary TKA. Paper presented at 2010 Annual Meeting of the American Academy of Orthopaedic Surgeons, New Orleans, LA; 2010.

107. Levy O, Martinowitz U, Oran A, et al. The use of fibrin tissue adhesive to reduce blood loss and the need for blood transfusion after total knee arthroplasty. A prospective, randomized, multicenter study. *J Bone Joint Surg Am.* 1999;81:1580-1588.

108. Wang GJ, Hungerford DS, Savory CG. Use of fibrin sealant to reduce bloody drainage and hemoglobin loss after total knee arthroplasty. *J Bone Joint Surg Am.* 2001;83:1503-1505.

109. Molloy DO, Archbold HA, Ogonda L, et al. Comparison of topical fibrin spray and tranexamic acid on blood loss after total knee replacement. *J Bone Joint Surg Br.* 2007;89:306-309.

110. Gardner MJ, Demetrakopoulos D, Klepchick PR, et al. The efficacy of autologous platelet gel in pain control and blood loss in total knee arthroplasty. *Int Orthop.* 2007;31(3):309-313.

111. Everts PA, Devilee RJ, Mahoney CB, et al. Platelet gel and fibrin sealant reduce allogeneic blood transfusions in total knee arthroplasty. *Acta Anaesthesiol Scand.* 2006;50:593-599.

112. Diiorio TM, Burkholder JD, Good RP, et al. Platelet-rich plasma does not reduce blood loss or pain or improve range of motion after TKA. *Clin Orthop Relat Res.* 2012;470(1):138-143.

113. Rosenberg AG. Reducing blood loss in total joint surgery with a saline-coupled bipolar sealing technology. *J Arthroplasty.* 2007;22(4 suppl 1):82-85.

114. Raut VV, Stone MH, Wroblewski BM. Reduction of postoperative blood loss after press fit condylar knee arthroplasty with the use of a femoral intramedullary plug. *J Bone Joint Surg Am.* 1993; 75:1356-1357.

115. Kumar N, Saleh J, Gardiner E. Plugging the intramedullary canal of the femur in total knee arthroplasty. *J Arthroplasty.* 2000;15(7):947-949.

116. Ko PS, Tio MK, Tan WL, et al. Sealing the intramedullary femoral canal with autologous bone plug in total knee arthroplasty. *J Arthroplasty.* 2003;18:6-9.

117. Smith T, Hing CB. Is a tourniquet beneficial in total knee replacement surgery? A meta-analysis and systematic review. *Knee.* 2010;17:141-147.

118. Page MH, Shepard BD, Harrison JM. Reduction of blood loss in knee arthroplasty. *Aust NZ J Surg.* 1984;54:141-144.

119. Newman JH, Jackson JP, Waugh W. Timing of tourniquet removal after knee replacement. *J R Soc Med.* 1979;72:492-494.

120. Lars PJ, Lindstrand A, Toksvig-Larsen S. Tourniquet release for hemostasis increases bleeding. *Acta Orthop Scand.* 1999;70(3):265-267.

121. Widman J, Isacson J. Surgical hemostasis after tourniquet release does not reduce blood loss in knee replacement. *Acta Orthop Scand.* 1999;70(3):268-270.

122. Christodoulou AG, Ploumis AL, Terzidis IP, et al. The role of timing of tourniquet release and cementing on perioperative blood loss in total knee replacement. *Knee.* 2004;11:313-317.

123. Lotke PA, Faralli VJ, Orenstein EM, et al. Blood loss after total knee replacement: effects of tourniquet release and continuous passive motion. *J Bone Joint Surg Am.* 1991;73:1037-1040.

124. Burkhart BC, Bourne RB, Rorabeck CH, et al. The efficacy of tourniquet release in blood conservation after total knee arthroplasty. *Clin Orthop Relat Res.* 1994;299:147-152.

125. Kalairajah Y, Simpson D, Cossey AJ, et al. Blood loss after total knee replacement: effects of computer-assisted surgery. *J Bone Joint Surg Br.* 2005;87:1480-1482.

126. Conteduca F, Massai F, Iorio R, et al. Blood loss in computer-assisted mobile bearing total knee arthroplasty. A comparison of computer-assisted surgery with a conventional technique. *Int Orthop.* 2008; 18(2):442-446.

127. Millar NL, Deakin AH, Millar LL, et al. Blood loss following total knee replacement in the morbidly obese: effects of computer navigation. *Knee.* 2011; 18:108-112.

128. Stevens DB. Postoperative orthopaedic infections. A study of etiological mechanisms. *J Bone Joint Surg Am.* 1964;46:96-102.

129. Waugh TR, Stinchfield FE. Suction drainage of orthopaedic wounds. *J Bone Joint Surg Am.* 1961;43:939-1021.

130. Ritter MA, Keating EM, Faris PM. Closed wound drainage in total hip or total knee replacement. A prospective, randomized study. *J Bone Joint Surg Am.* 1994;76(1):35-38.

131. Reilly TJ, Gradisar IA, Pakan W, et al. the use of postoperative suction drainage in total knee arthroplasty. *Clin Orthop Relat Res.* 1986;208:238-242.

132. Willett KM, Simmons CD, Bentley G. The effect of suction drains after total hip replacement. *J Bone Joint Surg Br.* 1988;70(4):607-610.

133. Beer KJ, Lombardi AV, Mallory TH, et al. The efficacy of suction drains after routine total joint arthroplasty. *J Bone Joint Surg Am.* 1991;73:584-587.

134. Li C, Nijat A, Askar M. No clear advantage to use of wound drains after unilateral total knee arthroplasty. *J Arthroplasty.* 2011;26(4):519-522.

135. Esler CN, Blakeway C, Fiddian NJ. The use of a closed-suction drain in total knee arthroplasty. *J Bone Joint Surg Br.* 2003;85(11):215-217.

136. Kiely N, Hockings M, Gambhir A. Does temporary clamping of drains following knee arthroplasty reduce blood loss? A randomised controlled trial. *Knee.* 2001;8:325-327.

137. Eum DS, Lee HK, Hwang SY, et al. Blood loss after navigation-assisted minimally invasive total knee arthroplasty. *Orthopedics.* 2006;29(10 suppl):S152-154.

138. Gannon DM, Lombardi AV, Mallory, et al. An evaluation of the efficacy of postoperative blood salvage after total joint arthroplasty. A prospective randomized trial. *J Arthroplasty.* 1991;6(2):109-114.

139. Majkowski RS, Currie I, Newman JH. Postoperative collection and reinfusion of autologous blood in total knee arthroplasty. *Ann R Coll Surg Engl.* 1991;73: 381-384.

140. Heddle NM, Brox WT, Klama LN, et al. A randomized trial on the efficacy of an autologous blood drainage and transfusion device in patients undergoing elective knee arthroplasty. *Transfusion.* 1992;32:742-746.

141. Newman JH, Bowers M, Murphy J. The clinical advantages of autologous transfusion. A randomized, controlled study after knee replacement. *J Bone Joint Surg Br.* 1997;79(4):630-632.

142. Friederichs MG, Mariani EM, Bourne MH. Perioperative blood salvage as an alternative to predonating blood for primary total knee and hip arthroplasty. *J Arthroplasty.* 2002;17(3):298-303.

143. Peter VK, Radford M, Matthews MG. Re-transfusion of autologous blood from wound drains: the means for reducing transfusion requirements in total knee arthroplasty. *Knee.* 2001;8(4):321-323.

144. Moonen AF, Knoors NT, van Os JJ, et al. Retransfusion of filtered shed blood in primary total hip and knee arthroplasty: a prospective randomized clinical trial. *Transfusion.* 2007;47(3):379-384.

145. Shenolikar A, Wareham K, Newington D, et al. Cell salvage auto transfusion in total knee replacement surgery. *Transfus Med.* 1997;7(4):277-280.

146. Sinha A, Sinha M, Burgert S. Reinfusion of drained blood as an alternative to homologous blood transfusion after total knee replacement. *Int Orthop.* 2001;25 (4):257-259.

147. Strümper D, Weber EW, Gielen-Wijffels S, et al. Clinical efficacy of postoperative autologous transfusion of filtered shed blood in hip and knee arthroplasty. *Transfusion.* 2004;44(11):1567-1571.

148. Henderson MS, Newman JH, Hand GCR. Blood loss following knee replacement surgery, use it don't lose it. *Knee.* 1999;6:125-129.

149. Mauerhan DR, Nussman D, Mokris JG, et al. Effect of postoperative reinfusion systems on hemoglobin levels in primary total hip and total knee arthroplasties: a prospective randomized study. *J Arthroplasty.* 1993;8:523-527.

150. Umlas J, Foster RR, Dalal SA, et al. Red cell loss following orthopedic surgery: the case against postoperative blood salvage. *Transfusion.* 1994;34:402-406.

151. Marks RM, Vaccaro AR, Balderston RA, et al. Postoperative blood salvage in total knee arthroplasty using the Solcotrans autotransfusion system. *J Arthroplasty.* 1995;10:433-437.
152. Slagis SV, Benjamin JB, Volz RG, et al. Postoperative blood salvage in total hip and knee arthroplasty. A randomised controlled trial. *J Bone Joint Surg Br.* 1991;73:591-594.
153. Chelly JE, Greger J, Gebhard R, et al. Continuous femoral blocks improve recovery and outcome of patients undergoing total kncc arthroplasty. *J Arthroplasty.* 2001;16(4):436-445.
154. Keith I. Anaesthesia and blood loss in total hip replacement. *Anaesthesia.* 1977;32(5):444-450.
155. Rosberg B, Fredin H, Gustafson C. Anesthetic techniques and surgical blood loss in total hip arthroplasty. *Acta Anaesthesiol Scand.* 1982;26(3):189-193.
156. Twyman R, Kirwan T, Fennelly M. Blood loss reduced during hip arthroplasty by lumbar plexus block. *J Bone Joint Surg Br.* 1990;72(5):770-771.
157. Speck M, Jakob R, Brinkmann KE. Blood loss after total knee arthroplasty in relation to positioning 70 degrees flexion vs extension. *J Bone Joint Surg Br.* 1999;81(suppl 11):245.
158. Ong SM, Taylor GJ. Can knee position save blood following total knee replacement? *Knee.* 2003;10(1):81-85.
159. Ma T, Khan RJK, Smith RC, et al. Effect of flexion/extension splintage post total knee arthroplasty on blood loss and range of motion–a randomised controlled trial. *Knee.* 2008;15:15-19.

30

Soft Tissue Coverage Following Total Knee Arthroplasty

Danielle M. Pineda and Gary A. Tuma

Soft tissue coverage of knee arthroplasty is vital to the preservation of the joint and the prosthesis. Whether it is with native or reconstructed soft tissues, the importance is related to healing and preservation of the joint and prosthesis. Complications of total knee arthroplasty include poor wound healing and skin necrosis that can lead to infection and loss of prosthesis. A simple appearing wound infection may progress to exposure of bone and hardware. These abnormalities of soft tissue healing lead to increased hospital costs, decreased quality of life, and possible loss of limb. Therefore, it is important to have a firm grasp of the management of these patients to prevent further complications and morbidity.

Previous reports have quoted a rate as high as 1% to 10% of knee arthroplasty patients who have wound complications. This chapter discusses the management of these patients starting at the physiology of wound healing, progressing from simple wound infections to reconstruction of the entire soft tissue of the knee. The reconstructive ladder, which begins with skin grafts and progresses through pedicled flaps and free flaps as options for soft tissue coverage, is discussed. It is important to understand the basis for all reconstructive procedures, lining support and coverage, as they pertain to soft tissue coverage of the knee. These hallmarks of reconstruction are crucial in achieving success in healing of the knee. Though having the experience and possibly the assistance of a plastic and reconstructive surgeon is beneficial and certainly critical in specific situations, an understanding of these principles can provide guidance to an arthroplasty surgeon who is encountering difficult situations. Adherence to some basic fundamentals can result in achievement of improved outcomes for the total knee arthroplasty patient.

PHYSIOLOGY

The goal of soft tissue reconstruction is to achieve wound healing while maintaining functionality. Therefore, any chapter dealing with soft tissue would be incomplete without a brief overview of the physiology behind wound healing. Wound healing occurs in three phases: inflammatory phase, proliferative phase, and maturational phase. During the inflammatory phase, inflammatory cells migrate to the affected area. This is vital to the removal of bacteria from the area as well as to aid in diffusion of nutrients. These inflammatory cells and nutrients reach the tissue at this stage via increased vascular permeability and diffusion. After the initial inflammation, healing begins. The proliferative phase consists of angiogenesis, fibroplasias, and epithelialization. During angiogenesis, the newly healing wound develops its own blood supply. With epithelialization, the new wound becomes incorporated into the previous tissue bed. Finally in the maturational phase, wound contraction occurs.[1]

In some minor wound infections or small areas of necrosis, local recruitment of healthy tissue may be sufficient for the healing process to occur. If the area is small enough to receive diffusion of nutrients as described above, it may start the healing process and receive the appropriate inflammatory treatment. However, for larger defects or deep infections, it is necessary to place a flap or other form of soft tissue coverage in order to provide a scaffold with a healthy blood supply. This blood supply allows the tissue to receive both the body's innate nutrients and allows for adequate delivery of antibiotics to the infected area. Additionally, by recruiting additional tissues to the region, there is a decrease in surface tension that allows for increased healing. With management of any stage of wound infection or necrosis, a healthy blood supply with minimal tension is vital to the wound healing.

PREOPERATIVE EVALUATION

The preoperative evaluation is the single most important period in which to ascertain whether the patient is at increased risk for soft tissue compromise. It is important to take a thorough history and physical to stratify the patient's risk for wound healing complications. Several patient populations are at higher risk of soft tissue complications and deficient wound healing. These patients should be counseled before proceeding with surgery. Risk factors include the following:

- Diabetes mellitus,
- Tobacco abuse,
- Malnutrition,
- Peripheral vascular disease,
- Rheumatoid arthritis,
- Chronic renal insufficiency, and
- History of prior surgery.

Before any soft tissue intervention, diabetics should have good glucose control. All tobacco abusers should be given counseling on quitting and enrolled into a tobacco cessation program. All patients should undergo a complete vascular physical exam including pulse checks and Doppler evaluations. Any patients with absent pedal pulses should have an ankle-brachial index and pulmonary vascular resistance performed and appropriate consultation with a vascular surgeon.

Any previous surgeries on the knee can lead to compromised blood flow in that region. All scars should be noted and a complete surgical history should be obtained. When making a new incision near a previous scar, care should be taken to leave a large area of healthy tissue between the previous scar and the new incision, minimizing any undermining between the scars. Any narrow skin bridges are at extremely high risk for necrosis and loss of tissue in the bridging area. This is a critical time to ask a plastic and reconstructive surgeon to evaluate the patient as well, to obviate postoperative wound healing complications.

POSTOPERATIVE EVALUATION

When a patient who is status post knee arthroplasty first presents with signs of necrosis or a soft tissue injury or infection, a complete history and physical exam should be performed. Physical exam includes special attention to the extent of involvement of the affected area and a complete neuromuscular exam. It is important to ascertain whether the soft tissue injury is superficial or a more involved injury of the deeper tissue and even the prosthesis itself. In addition, patients should have laboratory tests including complete blood cell count, erythrocyte sedimentation rate, and C-reactive protein to assess proinflammatory markers and to establish a baseline from which to work. Once the extent of the depth of injury is established, a definitive plan can be implemented using the mantra lining, support, and coverage.

MANAGEMENT

When the patient presents with signs of wound healing complications, it is important to ascertain the level of injury. More superficial injuries can be managed conservatively with local care, salves, and restriction of range of motion (ROM). Deeper injuries need to be treated more aggressively with local debridement and even operative debridement and eventual soft tissue reconstruction. The depth of injury is relative to the reconstructive tenets of lining, support, and coverage. Going from superficial to deep, the layers consist of skin, subcutaneous tissue, joint capsule and patellar tendon, prosthesis, and finally the bone. The depth of injury determines the reconstructive options based on the need for lining, support, and coverage. For all patients with signs of infection, long-term intravenous (IV) access should be obtained, such as with a peripherally inserted central catheter (PICC line), and the patient should be started on IV antibiotics immediately. These antibiotics should be tailored toward intraoperative deep tissue cultures obtained during surgery.

If patients present with serious signs of infection or sepsis, they should be taken to the operating room for extensive debridement, removal of hardware, and antibiotic spacer, and then resuscitated postoperatively before any soft tissue reconstruction. Wet-to-dry dressing changes or the use of negative-pressure sponge therapy, such as vacuum-assisted closure (VAC), can be performed while the patients are recovering from the initial infection. This may require multiple trips to the operating room before definitive coverage. However, as mentioned above, a good scaffold is necessary for healing. All necrotic and infected tissue must be removed or the wound will not heal adequately.

After complete debridement is performed, the wound can be assessed for size and depth of involvement and whether or not there is involvement of the joint space. For nonhealing wounds that only affect a small portion of the skin (less than 4 cm) and do not involve any deeper tissue, management can consist of local wound care, VAC, and possibly a skin graft. For superficial wounds greater than 4 cm in size, a local fasciocutaneous flap may be utilized. Finally, for medium and large defects that involve deeper tissue, a flap may be utilized. See Figure 30-1 for an algorithm for management. This algorithm is designed much like the tenets of reconstructive surgery using the "reconstructive ladder" to determine the options available. The reconstructive ladder is based of the principle of options moving up the ladder with the simplest treatment options first, followed by the more difficult ones.

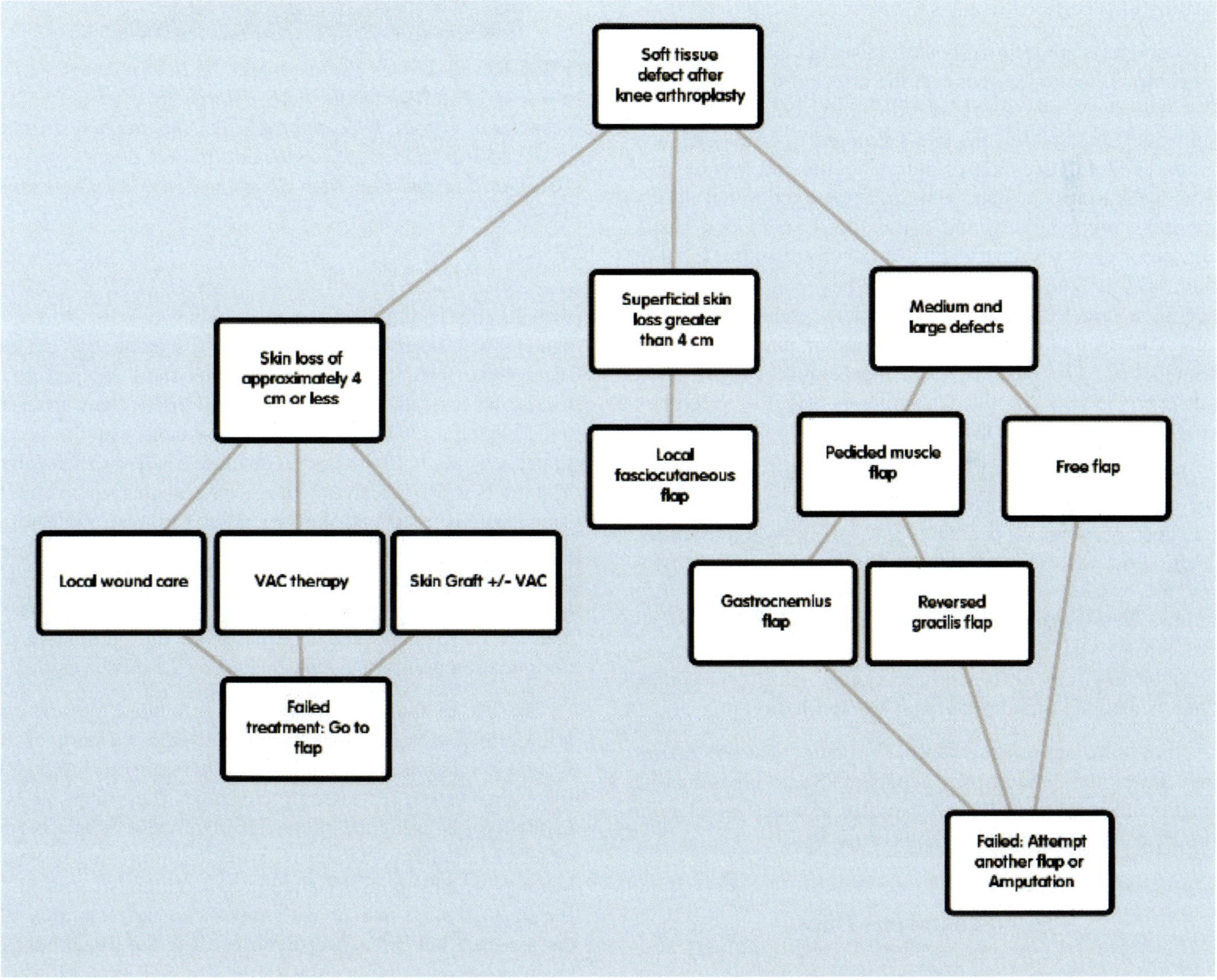

FIGURE 30-1. *Management algorithm for soft tissue defects after total knee arthroplasty. (Reprinted with permission.[1])*

Small Superficial Wounds

Smaller more superficial wounds can be managed conservatively with the addition of wound promoting devices. One such device is negative-pressure therapy such as VAC. VAC is a form of negative-pressure wound therapy that involves a contoured dressing that is sealed to the atmosphere and under continuous pressure. This allows for the removal of any fluids from the wound. It also promotes the formation of healthy granulation tissue. This device has changed the management of wounds by increasing the likelihood of salvage while limiting the morbidity. Another benefit of VAC therapy is that dressing changes only need to be performed two or three times a week, making it more tolerable for the patients. This not only improves wound healing so that a wound can undergo a skin graft, but also can be used in conjunction with skin grafts to assist in the healing of superficial wounds.

Skin grafts are frequently used in small wounds that have a healthy vascular bed beneath the affected tissue (Fig. 30-2).[2] There are two types of skin grafts commonly used: split-thickness and full-thickness skin grafts. Split-thickness grafts involve harvesting of the epidermis and less dermis. This leads to less primary skin graft contraction but allows for more secondary wound contraction. There is a better chance of graft survival with split-thickness grafts. In addition, split-thickness grafts can be meshed to allow for coverage of a larger area. The fenestrations created allow for egress of wound fluid and good contour matching of the wound bed. The final cosmetic appearance can be poor, however, because of the fenestrations and the secondary contraction limiting ROM.

Full-thickness skin grafts include both the epidermis and the complete dermal layer from the donor site. They have the best cosmetic appearance and the highest durability. They allow for the least amount of secondary wound contracture, which allows for better ROM. However, they require well-vascularized recipient beds without any bacterial colonization in order to heal. The likelihood of success is much less than with a split-thickness graft. In addition, there is a higher amount of donor site morbidity.

Skin grafts are easily performed as outpatient procedures and are well tolerated by the patient. Some complicating factors are those stated above but also include loss of graft tissue, donor site morbidity, and cosmesis.

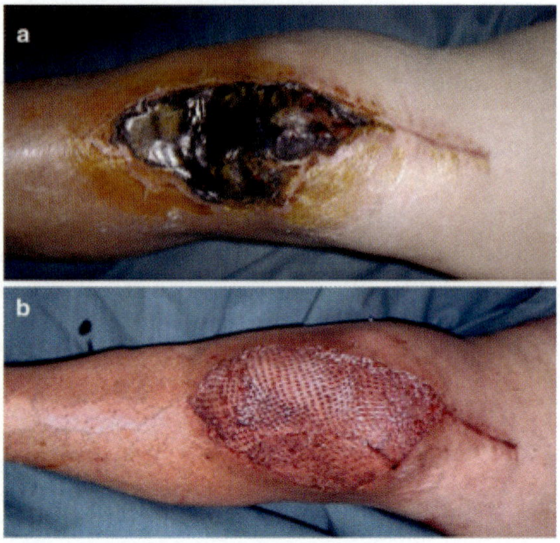

FIGURE 30-2. *This demonstrates the before and after pictures of a diabetic male with a large area of soft tissue necrosis after total knee arthroplasty. Note the fenestrations of the split-thickness skin graft and the adequate coverage. (With kind permission from Springer Science and Business Media.[2])*

Fasciocutaneous Flaps

Fasciocutaneous flaps consist of skin, fascia, and any intervening subcutaneous tissues. These flaps are useful in patients with delayed wound healing with large skin loss without joint or implant exposure. They can be utilized in patients with necrotic wounds but are discouraged in patients with active infections. Fasciocutaneous flaps are performed locally by dissecting the subcutaneous fascia away from the underlying muscle on either side of the wound. The flap is continued laterally until the fascia can close easily over the defect. The fascia is then secured with a nonabsorbable suture and the subcutaneous tissue and skin are closed in layers over the fascia. These flaps can be random in nature, meaning no discrete pedicle for their blood supply, or they can be based on perforators from underlying subcutaneous and deeper blood vessels. The arc of rotation should be based on the perforators and designed so minimal tension is placed on the rotated tissue.

The use of fasciocutaneous flaps is limited in total knee arthroplasty complications because of the location of the wound in relation to the joint. This often limits the amount of tissue than can be recruited for coverage. These flaps are best suited for use during the initial closure of the arthroplasty procedure in an attempt to recruit tissue to limit risks for wound healing complications by attempting to diminish tension. In the postoperative patient with superficial necrosis, this flap can be used but often is difficult because the tissue beneath the necrosis must be healthy so the flap will heal. However, they remain in the armamentarium for the rare patient with a superficial necrotic wound and healthy wound bed.

Pedicled Muscle Flaps

Muscle flaps are an important part of reconstruction for complications after total knee arthroplasty. These flaps are higher on the reconstructive ladder but are the workhorse of knee reconstruction. These muscle flaps can be used with and without skin to reconstruct the knee. The use of muscle flaps without skin requires a skin graft to cover; with skin, it is called a myocutaneous flap. This flap can reconstruct the knee allowing for all three mantras of reconstruction: lining, support, and coverage. These muscle flaps constitute lining by allowing for a gliding surface or replacement of the patella tendon, support in regard to the joint capsule, and coverage with soft tissue and skin. This is why these flaps are the workhorses of knee reconstruction.

Complex soft tissue defects that often have bone or hardware exposure require muscle flaps to cover the defect and provide a new blood supply for delivery of antibiotics and humoral defense factors. These flaps may be considered as local, regional, or distant depending on their anatomic region of harvest and blood supply. In addition, they are considered pedicled or free, based on whether the blood supply is left intact or anastomosed to a new blood supply. Muscle flaps are classified based on their blood supply by the Mathes and Nahai classification system (Fig. 30-3).[3]

The most commonly used flap in total knee arthroplasty reconstruction is the gastrocnemius flap. This flap is anatomically suited for knee coverage based on its origin, insertion, and arc of rotation. This flap is a type I flap with the dominant blood supply being the sural vessels with small perforators off the posterior tibial and popliteal vessels. It is also important to note that there are two muscle bellies that make up the gastrocnemius muscle: the lateral belly and medial belly. This allows for partial use of the muscle for reconstruction or the ability to use both bellies for larger defects, particularly in defects over the patellar tendon or tibial tubercle.[4] In addition, there is very little loss of function with either the use of partial or complete muscle belly harvest and rotation of the muscle. Most commonly the muscle is rotated and a skin graft is placed over the muscle belly with the donor site closed primarily. The approach to the flap is either medial, lateral, or both, depending on which muscle belly is going to be harvested. The medial muscle belly is much larger and can offer larger defect coverage. In addition, the lateral muscle belly harvest has the tibial nerve to contend with, which needs to be identified so there is no issue with postoperative foot drop. The approach is two finger breaths below the bottom edge of the tibia with an incision through skin, subcutaneous fat, and fascia exposing the muscle belly. Dissection proceeds in the subcutaneous space posteriorly until the posterior aspect of the muscle belly is encountered. Dissection then proceeds just

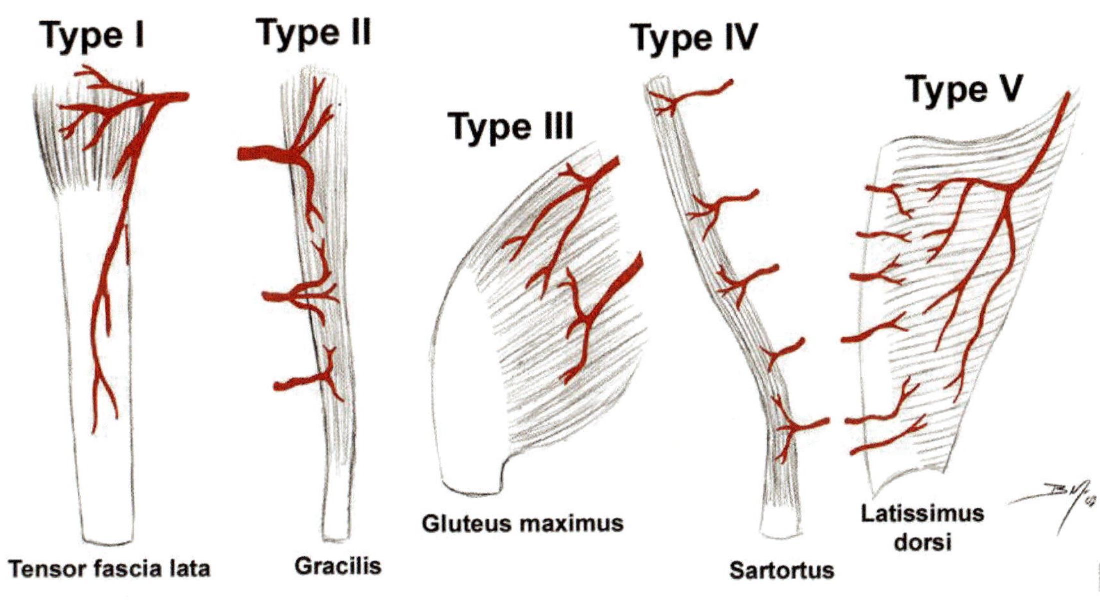

FIGURE 30-3. *Type I, one vascular pedicle; type II, dominant pedicle(s) and minor pedicle(s); type III, two dominant pedicles; type IV, segmental vascular pedicles; type V, one dominant pedicle and secondary segmental pedicles. (Reprinted with permission from Zenn MR, Jones G. Reconstructive Surgery: Anatomy, Technique, and Clinical Applications. St Louis: Quality Medical Publishing, 2012.)*

below the medial belly of the gastrocnemius muscle until the median raphe is encountered. Care is taken as not to injure the plantaris tendon or sacrifice too many perforating vessels. The muscle belly is dissected off of the insertion of the Achilles tendon. A subcutaneous tunnel is created or the overlying skin is sacrificed to allow the muscle to rotate and fill the defect. The arc of rotation is based on its origin above the knee, which is where the sural vessels, its blood supply, are located. The origin of the muscle belly can be released to gain more arc or advancement, but great care must be taken to ensure no injury to the blood supply or occlusion of the venous outflow. The muscle is inset using resorbable sutures, often over a drain. The length and total surface area of coverage can be increased by making radial incisions just through the fascia that envelops the muscle belly, allowing for the stretching of the muscle over the defect. The donor defect is closed in multiple layers over a drain and a skin graft is placed on the muscle followed by the VAC to secure the graft in place. Often it is advisable to turn the VAC setting down to 75 mm Hg when placing on a skin graft over a freshly inset muscle flap. See Figure 30-4 for an illustration of the flap. Gerwin et al performed a retrospective study of 12 patients who required soft tissue coverage of an exposed or infected total knee prosthesis. Of the 12 patients, 10 were able to retain their prosthesis after the initial event.[5] This study confirmed the efficacy of gastrocnemius flaps in defects after total knee arthroplasty.

Another useful pedicled flap is the reversed gracilis pedicle flap (Fig. 30-5).[6] This flap is also a type II flap but, when using this flap in knee reconstruction, the dominant pedicle is transected and the minor pedicles are used to perfuse this flap. This is a much less reliable flap for this reason. This flap is useful in patients who have failed a lateral or medial gastrocnemius flap. In addition, some patients have a large defect that requires both a gastrocnemius flap and a second flap for complete defect coverage.

To harvest this flap, patients are positioned in the supine position with the thigh abducted. The gracilis muscle is identified on palpation and a 10- to 15-cm sagittal skin incision is made at the anterior margin of the muscle. During the incision and dissection, care is taken to identify and protect the saphenous vein. The gracilis muscle is dissected after identifying and preserving its two major vascular pedicles. Next, the proximal tendon of the gracilis muscle is divided. Then the main vascular pedicle is clamped to ensure that the muscle remains viable. If the muscle is alive during test clamp, the main vascular pedicle is divided. The muscle then survives based on the secondary pedicle. It is flapped distally based on the secondary vascular pedicle and secured in place to cover the defect. A skin graft can be placed over the muscle flap. Subcutaneous tissue and skin are closed in layers at the donor site over a drain as well.

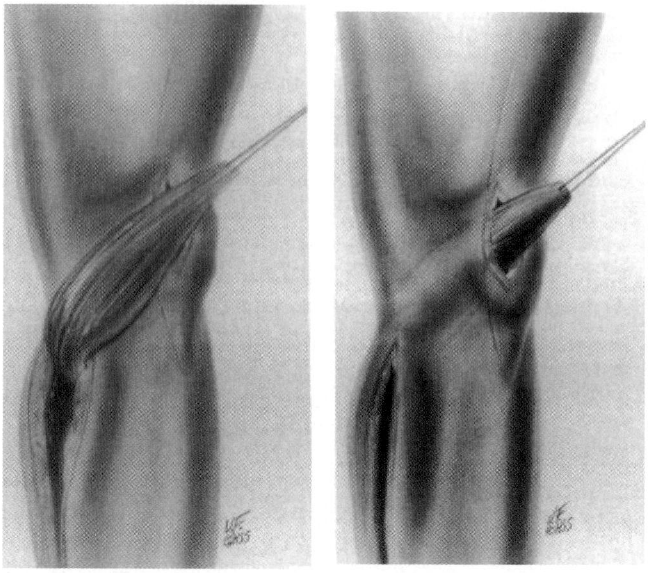

FIGURE 30-4. *Illustration of a gastrocnemius flap technique. (Reprinted with permission.[5])*

The last regional flap that can be used as muscle to reconstruct the proximal and middle third of the tibia is the soleus muscle. This is a type II muscle with proximal dominant perforators off of the posterior tibial and peroneal vessels and distal minor less reliable vessels at the distal third of the muscle belly. This anatomic configuration prevents the reliable use of the distal third of the muscle belly. The proximal portion can be rotated to cover the proximal and middle third of the tibia, skin grafted, and the donor site closed like the other harvest defects over a drain.

Free Muscle Flaps

The last rung on the ladder is reconstruction with the use of a free muscle flap. Trained plastic and reconstructive surgeons who are experienced in microvascular surgery should only attempt this reconstructive procedure. This muscle flap is the most difficult reconstructive procedure to perform. It requires the harvesting of a muscle remote from the injured knee and transplanting the muscle and anastomosing the arterial and venous supply of the muscle to recipient vessels near the defect.[7,8] The choice of muscle depends on the defect created and the size of the recipient vessels in relation to the donor vessel. There are many choices but the most common are the rectus, the latissmus, the gracilis, and the serratus muscles. There is also another tissue that is

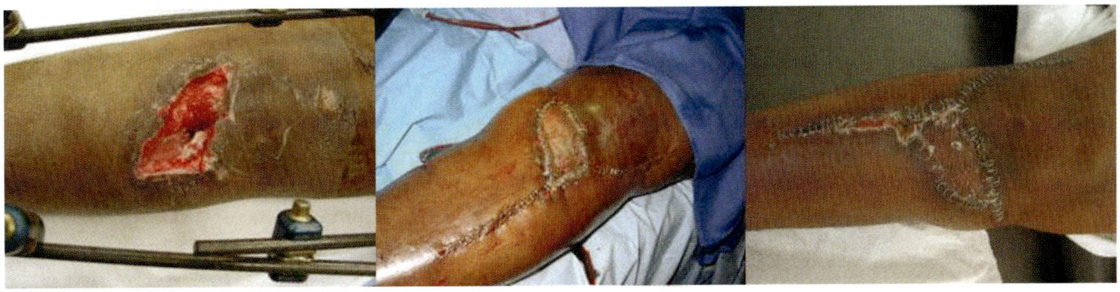

FIGURE 30-5. *Mobilization of the gracilis muscle belly as it is created into a reversed flap based on its secondary pedicle.*

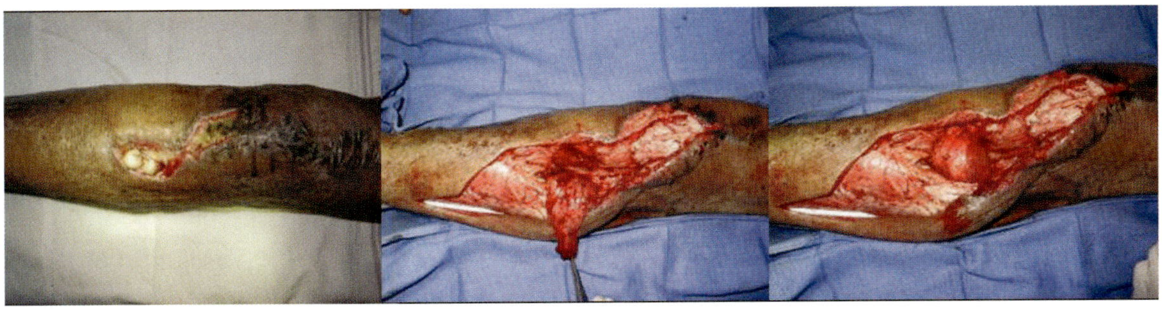

FIGURE 30-6. *Lateral gastrocnemius flap for coverage of the bone.*

quite amenable for use in healing soft tissue defects: the free omentum. All these different muscles and omentum can be used to close the soft tissue defect but require a skin graft and have donor defects that need to be closed as well. This operation requires close postoperative monitoring of the flaps in an intensive care unit setting and can require emergent return to the operating room to address changes in perfusion.

CASE EXAMPLE

A 62-year-old male was referred to the clinic 2 months after undergoing a repeat total knee arthroplasty (Fig. 30-6). He had no other pertinent medical history. On examination, the patient was noted to have a scar from the first surgery overlying his left knee and, approximately 4 cm away, a second scar from the second surgery. In between these two areas, the skin appeared necrotic with areas of dehiscence. He was scheduled for debridement in the operating room.

At the time of debridement, the necrotic skin was aggressively debrided. Underlying the necrotic skin, the soft tissue coverage appeared boggy with areas of necrosis. This tissue was sent for microbiology. The remaining tissue was debrided to a level of clean, bleeding tissue, which results in exposure of a small area of hardware. The wound was then aggressively irrigated and cleaned and a gastronemius flap was mobilized from a lateral approach. The flap was then rotated and secured achieving good coverage of the defect. A drain was left in place and a VAC dressing was placed.

The patient's knee was placed in a knee immobilizer brace for 3 to 5 days, secured over the VAC dressing. On day 5, the VAC dressing was removed and the wound was followed closely with daily dressing changes. The patient has good coverage with the flap and recovered to a full functional status without any signs of infection.

CONCLUSION

There are many options for treatment of soft tissue injury in the patient undergoing primary or revision total knee arthroplasty. Options are dependent on the level of injury and what portion of the reconstructive mantra needs to be addressed. The way in which to address these issues is to use the reconstructive ladder to approach each patient in a stepwise manner to do the least invasive treatment to address the deficit. The most important principles in dealing with complex issues in knee soft tissue reconstruction are completing adequate debridement, minimizing soft tissue tension, creating a healthy wound bed, maximizing vascularity, recruiting healthy vascularized tissue, and utilizing the assistance of a plastic and reconstructive surgeon. Last, in a high-risk patient, the assistance of a plastic and reconstructive surgeon may be sought preoperatively to plan out the reconstructive algorithm before further complications.

PEARLS AND PITFALLS

The following points should be considered for soft tissue reconstruction in total knee arthroplasty:

- A thorough history and physical exam precludes treatment of any complex knee wound with particular attention to risk factor modification and assessment of the depth of the wound.
- Before reconstruction, an aggressive debridement of all parts of the necrotic wound should be undertaken to provide a healthy scaffold for the reconstruction.
- Small superficial wounds can be treated with VAC therapy and skin grafts to cover the healthy muscle that is already present.
- Complete debridement often leaves hardware or bone exposed. In these cases, pedicled muscle flaps are often necessary to allow coverage with healthy tissue.
- Gastrocnemius flaps are the most commonly used muscle flap in knee reconstruction. Mobilization of the medial belly of the gastrocnemius muscle allows for coverage of a larger defect.

SUGGESTED READING

Markovich GD, Dorr LD, Klein NE, et al. Muscle flaps in total knee arthroplasty. *Clin Orthop Relat Res.* 1995; 321:122-130.

Menderes A, Demirdover C, Yilmaz M, et al. Reconstruction of soft tissue defects following total knee arthroplasty. *Knee.* 2002;9:215-219.

Thorne C, Beasley R, Aston S, et al., eds. *Grabb and Smith's Plastic Surgery,* 6th ed. Philadelphia, PA: Lippincott Williams & Wilkins; 2007.

REFERENCES

1. Burns J, Blackwell S. Plastic surgery. In: Townsend CM Jr, Beauchamp RD, Evers BM, Mattox KL, eds. *Sabiston Textbook of Surgery,* 18th ed. Philadelphia, PA: Elsevier; 2008.
2. Panni AS, Vasso M, Cerciello S, et al. Wound complications in total knee arthroplasty. Which flap is to be used? With or without retention of prosthesis? *Knee Surg Sports Traumatol Arthrosc.* 2011;19(7): 1060-1068.
3. Chrysopoulo MT, de la Torre JI, eds. Tissue Flap Classification. emedicine.medscape.com/article/ 1284474.
4. Ries MD, Bozic KJ. Medial gastrocnemius flap coverage for treatment of skin necrosis after total knee arthroplasty. *Clin Orthop Relat Res.* 2006;446:186-192.
5. Gerwin M, Rothaus KO, Windsor RE, et al. Gastrocnemius muscle flap coverage of exposed or infected knee prostheses. *Clin Orthop Relat Res.* 1993;286:64-70.
6. Tiengo C, Macchi V, Vigato E, et al. Reversed gracilis pedicle flap for coverage of a total knee prosthesis. *J Bone Joint Surg Am.* 2010;92:1640-1646.
7. Hierner R, Reynders-Frederix P, Bellemans J, et al. Free myocutaneous latissimus dorsi flap transfer in total knee arthroplasty. *J Plast Reconstr Aesthet Surg.* 2009;62(12):1692-1700.
8. Cetrulo CL Jr, Shiba T, Friel MT, et al. Management of exposed total knee prostheses with microvascular tissue transfer. *Microsurgery.* 2008;28(8):617-622.

31

Management of Vascular Complications Following Total Knee Arthroplasty

Sarah Fernandez, Joshua Eisenberg, Atul Rao, and Paul DiMuzio

One of the most potentially devastating complications of total knee arthroplasty (TKA) is injury to the popliteal artery, resulting in postoperative limb ischemia. Depending on the severity of the injury, sequelae can include tissue necrosis, nerve damage, and even limb loss. While arterial injury is fortunately a very rare occurrence, it is imperative that it be diagnosed and addressed promptly to minimize associated morbidity.

As the field of vascular surgery has developed over the past several decades to encompass minimally invasive techniques, the treatment for arterial injury has evolved as well. While open repair using thrombectomy and/or bypass was previously the mainstay of therapy, endovascular repair is increasingly becoming a viable option in centers equipped with the appropriate technology. Regardless of the technique used, prompt diagnosis and intervention remain the keys to minimizing the morbidity of a vascular injury following knee arthroplasty.

INCIDENCE

While large-volume single-institution studies evaluating the incidence of vascular complications in total knee arthroplasty are rare, a few studies have shown the incidence is thought to be less than 1%. The largest single-institution study reviewed 13,618 total knee arthroplasties between 1989 and 2002[1] and identified 24 arterial injuries, for an overall incidence of 0.17%. A multicenter study by Abularrage et al reviewed 26,106 total knee arthroplasties from 1996 to 2003 and determined the incidence of arterial injury to be 0.09%.[2] Several other single-institution studies have calculated similar incidences.[3,4]

MECHANISM OF INJURY

Injury to the popliteal artery during knee arthroplasty can occur through a variety of mechanisms. Overall, injuries can be classified into four major groups: direct laceration, compression of the artery after correction of a flexion deformity, arterial thrombosis, or embolization of preexisting atheromatous plaques.[5]

Direct injury of the artery can occur via multiple mechanisms. Inadvertent laceration with scalpel or cautery can be difficult to recognize in the setting of a bloodless field after tourniquet placement. Careless placement of retractors can also cause damage to the artery. Cadaver studies have demonstrated that placement of posterior retractors during TKA threaten the artery when placed laterally or more than 1 cm deep into soft tissue.[6] Additionally, anatomic distortions (ie, reoperative fields with significant scar tissue) can also increase the risk for arterial injury. Not surprisingly, prior arthroplasty has been shown in several studies to be a significant risk factor for arterial injury.[1,2,4,7]

Occasionally, when the arthroplasty corrects a significant joint deformity (particularly a flexion contracture), the artery can be placed under inadvertent traction or compressed against other structures in the knee.[5,8] Popliteal artery or superficial femoral artery thrombosis can occur either due to intimal damage and low-flow state caused by the tourniquet placement[5] or from in situ plaque rupture and intimal damage[9] due to manipulation of a diseased vessel. Plaque rupture and distal embolization can occur via the same mechanism.

RISK FACTORS FOR ARTERIAL INJURY

Clearly, patients who have preexisting atherosclerosis are at particular risk for postoperative arterial complications,[1,8] especially if a tourniquet is used.[4] In general, careful preoperative workup to elicit any history or physical findings of peripheral vascular disease is mandatory before planning elective knee arthroplasty.

A history of claudication, physical exam findings suggesting arterial insufficiency (diminished pulses, skin thinning, or ulcerations), or prior vascular surgery should prompt further preoperative workup and possibly preoperative consultation by a vascular surgeon. Lower-extremity ultrasound and determination of the ankle-brachial index (ABI) is an effective means of determining the extent of preexisting arterial disease. An ABI of less than 0.9, indicative of at least mild peripheral vascular disease, has been associated with increased risk of postoperative arterial complications[8] and consideration should be given to avoiding tourniquet use during the procedure. An ABI of less than 0.5 is indicative of severe vascular disease and preoperative evaluation by a vascular surgeon (with possible preoperative revascularization) should be considered.[9]

Several studies have attempted to identify other risk factors for arterial injury during knee arthroplasty. A multi-institution review of the National Surgical Quality Improvement Program (NSQIP) database identified African American race, reoperative procedure, dyspnea, emergency surgery status, current tobacco use, insulin-dependent diabetes mellitus, transient ischemic attack or prior stroke, impaired sensation, and recent chemotherapy as associated with increased risk of arterial injury during surgery. It is notable that most of these are also concomitant risk factors for peripheral vascular disease. However, only African American race and reoperation were found to be statistically significant risk factors.[2] Reoperative fields can be associated with scarring and distortion of normal anatomy, placing the popliteal artery at risk for damage. The African American population has a higher incidence of peripheral vascular disease,[10] which is, again, the main predisposing factor to vascular complications following arthroplasty.

DIAGNOSIS

The diagnosis (and subsequent management) of vascular complications varies depending on whether the vascular injury is detected in the intraoperative, immediate postoperative, or late postoperative period.

INTRAOPERATIVE IDENTIFICATION OF VASCULAR INJURY

Intraoperative hemorrhage can be a sign of damage to the popliteal artery, especially if the bleeding is pulsatile. Other associated signs are rapid swelling of the popliteal fossa and a change in the pulse exam.[11] Unfortunately, the presence of a tourniquet can often mask these signs. At least one recent meta-analysis regarding the timing of tourniquet release suggested that early tourniquet release (ie, before wound closure) allows the surgeon to evaluate for hemostasis and more easily detect signs of arterial bleeding.[12] Intraoperative bleeding should be managed with the basic principles of meticulous hemostasis and proximal and distal control of involved vessels. Any concern for damage to major vascular structures should prompt an intraoperative consultation by a vascular surgeon. Primary repair or patch angioplasty can be used to repair a lacerated vessel, while in the case of a completely transected vessel, a ligation with bypass (using saphenous vein from the contralateral leg) may be necessary.[1]

EARLY POSTOPERATIVE IDENTIFICATION OF VASCULAR INJURY

Both acute arterial occlusion and hemorrhage from a lacerated artery can present during the early postoperative period. A rapidly swelling joint or high drain output can be clues to postoperative hemorrhage. Immediate re-exploration and intraoperative vascular surgery consultation are indicated. The source of bleeding should be identified and controlled so that the extent of damage can be evaluated. The same repair options as for intraoperative bleeding exist, namely, primary repair or patch angioplasty of a partially transected vessel or ligation and bypass to repair a completely transected vessel.[1]

Acute arterial occlusion without concomitant hemorrhage is the most potentially catastrophic postoperative complication. The signs of acute limb ischemia—pain, pallor, parasthesias, and loss of distal pulses—are often subtle, especially in early ischemia. In the immediate postoperative arthroplasty patient, these symptoms can be masked by postoperative pain, bulky dressings, or spinal anesthesia.[1] Thus it is critical that a thorough vascular exam be conducted immediately postoperatively, with serial exams thereafter, and that any change in temperature, sensation, or pulse in the limb prompt a thorough workup for limb ischemia, with a low threshold for vascular surgery consultation.

If there is definite concern for arterial occlusion, immediate evaluation by a vascular surgeon is indicated. Early intervention and restoration of blood flow provides the highest chance for limb salvage. In patients with early signs of occlusion, arteriography before definitive surgical correction can define the anatomy of the occlusion and facilitate repair, especially in patients with preexisting vascular disease.[1] However, in patients with advanced signs of ischemia, in which any delay is undesirable, immediate exploration in the operating room is the approach of choice. Preoperatively, adequate intravenous access should be ensured, and both legs should be prepped into the field to allow for harvest of the contralateral saphenous vein.

The injury patterns resulting in acute ischemia vary, but can include the following[1]:

1. Acute occlusion of essential collateral arteries by tourniquet or joint manipulation, in the setting of a chronically occluded popliteal artery,
2. Occlusion/dissection of a patent popliteal artery by tourniquet or joint manipulation,
3. Thrombosis of popliteal artery without intimal disruption,
4. Thrombosis of preexisting popliteal artery aneurysm,
5. Superficial femoral artery occlusion/dissection by tourniquet, and
6. Distal embolization to branches of anterior tibial artery.

Figure 31-1 demonstrates occlusion of a damaged popliteal artery following total knee arthroplasty, with patency of geniculate branches.

Intraoperatively, the strategies available for repair vary based on the injury. Arterial thrombosis without arterial damage or dissection can be treated with thrombectomy; however, if intimal damage or significant arterial injury is found, ligation and bypass with saphenous vein is the preferred repair.[1]

While all arterial injuries are ideally recognized in the immediate postoperative period and revascularization

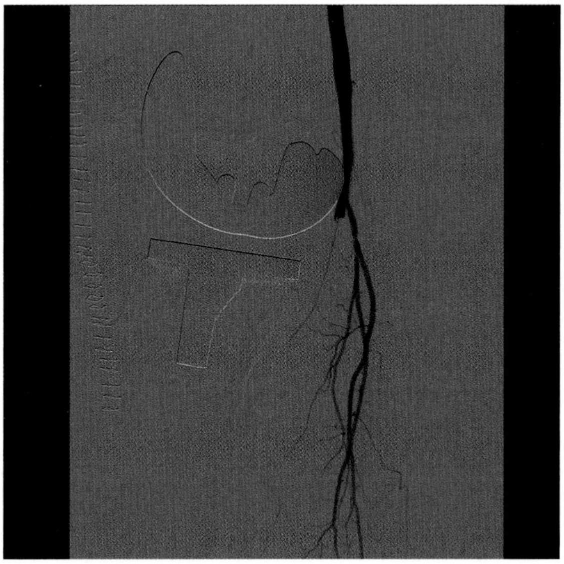

FIGURE 31-1. *Intraoperative arteriogram demonstrating popliteal artery thrombosis following total knee arthroplasty.*

occurs promptly, in reality many patients already have advanced ischemia at the time of diagnosis. Postoperative compartment syndrome after revascularization due to edema can result in secondary limb ischemia and tissue necrosis. In patients who have had ischemic symptoms for longer than 6 hours, fasciotomy is generally recommended,[1] and in all patients, a low threshold for fasciotomy should be the standard.[2]

As endovascular technology has become more popular in the vascular surgery field, the role of endovascular repair of arterial injury due to knee arthroplasty is being investigated. While the use of endovascular therapy for popliteal pseudoaneurysms in general is well described, only a few case reports discuss its use in the setting of arterial injury due to knee arthroplasty. Plagnol et al described a single case of endovascular treatment for a popliteal pseudoaneurysm following TKA in 2001.[13] In 2003 Vaidhyanath and Blanshard published a case report describing the use of a covered stent to treat a popliteal artery pseudoaneurysm after TKA.[14] More recently, Sloan et al in 2009 published a report of two cases in which an endovascular stent approach was used to successfully treat a traumatic popliteal psuedoaneurysm after TKA.[15] However, the use of endovascular techniques for acute arterial occlusion due to thrombosis has not yet been well described.

The use of an endovascular approach, consisting of an on-table arteriogram followed by appropriate intervention, has been adopted by our institution for all suspected arterial injuries after TKA. A hybrid endovascular/OR suite allows the vascular surgery team to first attempt endovascular repair while still having the full resources of an operating room in the event that conversion to an open approach is required. A variety of endovascular techniques, including angioplasty, cryoplasty, stenting, and mechanical thrombectomy have been used. Endovascular therapy avoids reoperation in the fresh postoperative field and allows simultaneous diagnosis and therapy. While large-volume studies regarding the efficacy of endovascular therapy in this patient population have not yet been published, early data suggest that endovascular therapy is at least equivalent to open surgical repair in terms of effective revascularization, hospital stay, and limb salvage.

Ultimately, regardless of the technique used for revascularization, the most critical factor in ensuring the best outcome is early diagnosis and intervention. Multiple studies have confirmed that diagnosis of acute arterial occlusion more than 24 hours postoperatively is associated with neurovascular complications, higher rate of fasciotomy, and increased risk of limb loss.[1,2,4]

LATE POSTOPERATIVE IDENTIFICATION OF VASCULAR INJURY

Pseudoaneurysms and arteriovenous fistulae can be late-presenting complications of total knee arthroplasty. Much of the literature regarding workup and management of these entities exists in the form of case reports or short case series. Thus it is difficult to determine incidence or risk factors for these complications; however, it is likely that they are similar to those for other forms of vascular injury during knee arthroplasty.

Popliteal artery pseudoaneurysms after TKA can present at any time during the postoperative period, from several days to several months following surgery.[16,17] Patients may complain of pain and/or swelling in the popliteal fossa, and physical examination may reveal a pulsatile mass in the fossa. Occasionally, popliteal artery pseudoaneurysms can present with limb ischemia due to thrombosis or distal embolization.[18] Other possible sequelae can be due to compression of surrounding structures, such as neurological symptoms or deep venous thrombosis.

Repair of popliteal artery pseudoaneurysms can be accomplished by a variety of methods. Aneurysms with a narrow neck can be treated with thrombin/acrylate injection or coil embolization.[1] Those pseudoaneurysms with a wide neck are more effectively repaired by an open ligation.[1] Endovascular stenting of the aneurysm has also been described.[13-15] Ultrasound of the pseudoaneurysm to accurately delineate the anatomy is required before planning repair.

Arteriovenous fistulae are a rare occurrence but have been reported following arthroplasty. They may present as hemarthrosis, a pulsatile mass in the popliteal fossa, or painful swelling of the lower limb.[5] Fistula formation may involve the popliteal artery or the medial or lateral geniculate arteries.[5] Operative repair of the fistula is usually required.

OUTCOMES

Vascular injury during total knee arthroplasty is a fortunately rare but potentially serious complication of surgery. Recognition of the injury and early, prompt intervention are key to avoiding tissue necrosis, long-term neurological sequelae, and limb loss. Identifying patients at risk for vascular injury (ie, reoperative patients and patients with preexisting vascular disease) is critical in minimizing their risk for vascular complications. While open repair has long been the mainstay of treatment, early results have suggested that endovascular therapy may be an effective treatment option. Postoperatively, careful neurovascular exams are critical in identifying signs and symptoms of potentially catastrophic limb ischemia. With prompt identification of the injury and appropriate therapy, the chances of preservation of neurologic function and limb salvage are maximized.

SAMPLE CASE

A 76-year-old man with a history of hypertension and hyperlipidemia underwent elective left total knee arthroplasty. The surgery was uneventful and the patient had a normal neurovascular exam postoperatively. While in the postoperative recovery unit, the patient was noted to be complaining of pain in his left leg. Additional pain medication was ordered by the housestaff; however, the patient continued to complain of worsening pain.

Examination of the leg at this time demonstrated a cool foot with no detectable dorsalis pedis or posterior tibial pulse. Capillary refill was diminished and the patient noted "numbness" when sensation was tested. An emergent vascular surgery consult was placed and the patient was started on a heparin infusion.

The patient was taken to the operating room by the vascular surgery team, and an on-table arteriogram was performed via a right femoral approach. The initial arteriogram is shown in Figure 31-2A.

The popliteal artery occlusion was first treated with balloon angioplasty, which was unsuccessful at restoring distal flow. An endovascular stent was then placed across the area of occlusion, with re-establishment of flow (Fig. 31-2B). Good runoff was noted on the poststent angiography, and palpable pulses were detectable in the left foot.

The patient's left calf was noted to be soft and, given the prompt revascularization, it was not felt that he required fasciotomy. He was transferred to the intermediate intensive care unit, with hourly neurovascular checks. The remainder of his clinical course was uncomplicated and he was discharged to a rehabilitation facility 4 days later.

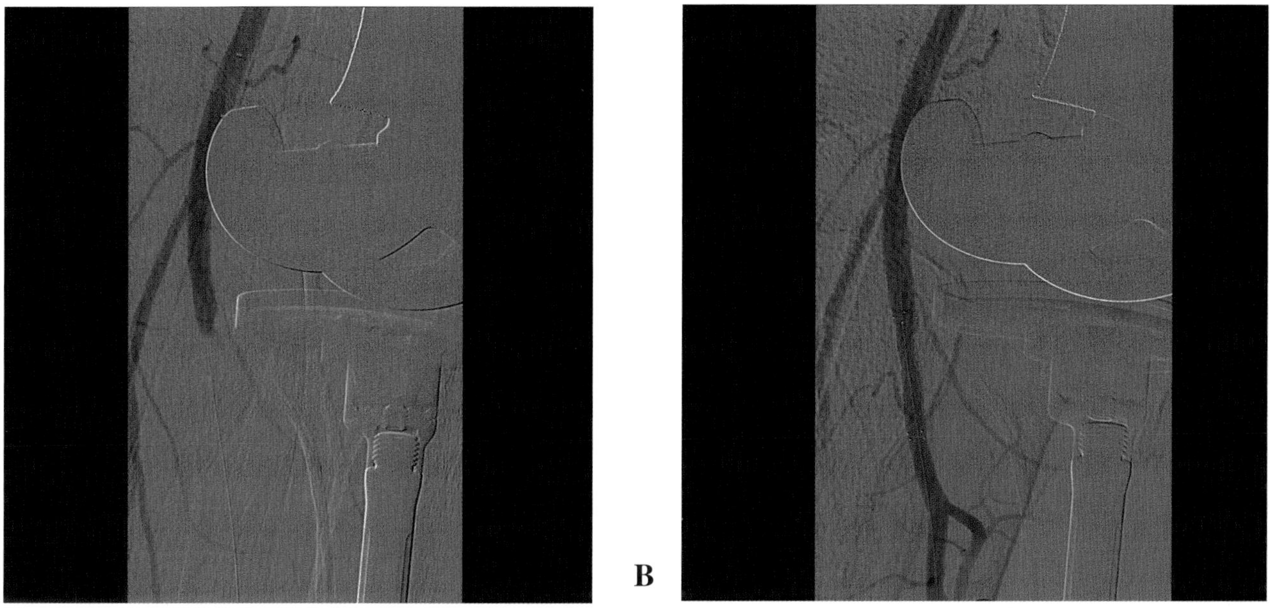

A B

FIGURE 31-2. *(A) Popliteal artery occlusion following total knee arthroplasty, before attempted endovascular repair. (**B**) Popliteal artery occlusion treated successfully with endovascular stent placement.*

REFERENCES

1. Calligaro K, Dougherty M, Ryan S, et al. Acute arterial complications associated with total knee arthroplasty. *J Vasc Surg*. 2003;38(6):1170-1177.
2. Abularrage C, Weiswasser J, Kent J, et al. Predictors of lower extremity arterial injury after total knee or hip arthroplasty. *J Vasc Surg*. 2008;47:803-807.
3. Parvizi J, Pulido L, Slenker N. Vascular injuries after total joint arthroplasty. *J Arthroplasty*. 2008;23:1115-1120.
4. Wilson J, Miranda A, Johnson B. et al. Vascular injuries associated with elective orthopaedic procedures. *Ann Vasc Surg*. 2003;17:641-644.
5. Butt U, Samuel R, Sahu A, et al. Arterial injury in total knee arthroplasty. *J Arthroplasty*. 2010;25:1311-1318.
6. Ninomiya J, Dean J, Goldberg V. Injury to the popliteal artery and its anatomic location in total knee arthroplasty. *J Arthroplasty*. 1999;14:800-807.
7. Da Silva M, Sobel M. Popliteal vascular injury during total knee arthroplasty. *J Surg Res*. 2003;109:170.
8. DeLaurentis D, Levitsky K, Booth R, et al. Arterial and ischaemic aspects of total knee arthroplasty. *Am J Surg*. 1992;164(3):237-240.
9. Smith D, McGraw R, Taylor D, et al. Arterial complications and total knee arthroplasty. *J Am Acad Orthop Surg*. 2001;9:253-257.

10. Sidaway A, Schweitzer E, Neville R, et al. Race as a risk factor in the severity of infragenicular occlusive disease: study of an urban hospital population. *J Vasc Surg*. 1990;11:536-541.

11. Saleh K, Hoeffel D, Kassim R, et al. Complications after revision total knee arthroplasty. *J Bone Joint Surg Am*. 2003;55(suppl 1):71-74.

12. Rama K, Apsingi S, Poovali S, et al. Timing of tourniquet release in knee arthroplasty. Meta-analysis of randomized controlled trials. *J Bone Joint Surg Am*. 2007;89:699-704.

13. Plagnol P, Diard N, Bruneteau P, et al. Pseudoaneurysm of popliteal artery complicating a total knee replacement: a successful percutaneous endovascular treatment. *Eur J Vasc Endovasc Surg*. 2001;21:81-83.

14. Vaidhyanath R, Blanshard K. Insertion of covered stent for treatment of a popliteal artery pseudoaneurysm following total knee arthroplasty. *Br J Radiol*. 2003;76:195-198.

15. Sloan K, Mofidi R, Nagy J, et al. Endovascular treatment for traumatic popliteal artery pseudoaneurysms after knee arthroplasty. *Vasc Endovascular Surg*. 2009;43:286-290.

16. Sandoval E, Ortega F, Garcia-Rayo M, et al. Popliteal pseudoaneurysm after total knee arthroplasty secondary to intraoperative arterial injury with a surgical pin. *J Arthroplasty*. 2008;23:1239-1241.

17. Cowell G, Boom S, Ablett M. Thrombosis of popliteal artery pseudoaneurysm by deployment of angioplasty balloon after total knee arthroplasty. *J Arthroplasty*. 2009;24(5):825.e11-e13.

18. Ibrahim M, Booth R, Clark T. Embolization of traumatic pseudoaneurysms after total knee arthroplasty. *J Arthroplasty*. 2004;19:123-125.

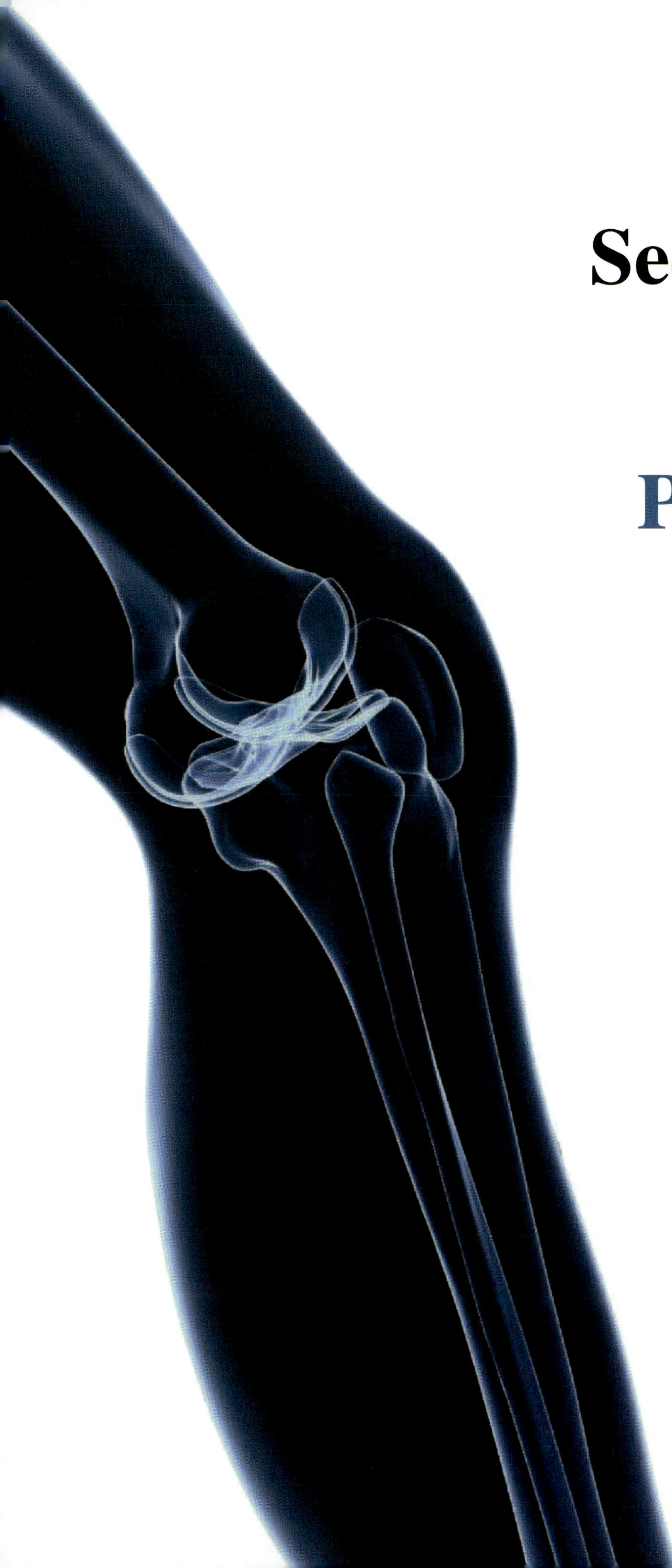

Section Three

Joint Preservation Procedures

32 Nonsurgical Evaluation and Treatment of Knee Osteoarthritis

Peter C. Vitanzo, Jr., and Barry E. Kenneally

Osteoarthritis (OA) of the knee, though extremely common in the elderly population, should not be considered an inevitable feature of aging. Unfortunately, it afflicts millions of people. Despite prevalence variations among different populations (based on age, gender, and disease definition), osteoarthritis can be a major cause of pain and disability. Furthermore, it can have a significant impact on functioning and activities of daily living in addition to imposing substantial financial costs on society. Therefore, timely recognition and evaluation of the signs and symptoms of osteoarthritis of the knee are imperative to render an appropriate treatment protocol for a patient. This includes a careful history as well as physical and radiographic examinations. Identifying and understanding risk factors can facilitate management of these patients with knee osteoarthritis and minimize health care costs. While some risk factors are consistent, others, such as physical activity, are controversial (Table 32-1).

When patients with knee OA initially present to a clinic, it is usually too early for surgical intervention (ie, total knee arthroplasty). Usually their pain intensity is not that severe, the disease process is not that advanced, they may be too young, or their functional disability is not that limiting. Frequently, patients are often not in the "right frame of mind" for surgery. They frequently want to avoid surgery as long as possible. Furthermore, since prosthetic joints have a finite life span, it is often prudent to try to delay surgery to minimize the need for multiple revision surgeries. This is particularly evident in younger patients. Therefore, it is the responsibility of the treating physician to offer suitable conservative options in order to bridge the gap before total knee arthroplasty. In patients of extreme age or with significant medical comorbidities who are poor surgical candidates, nonoperative treatment remedies may be the only appropriate alternatives. Hopefully, these conservative options can produce adequate palliative outcomes for such patients.

Fortunately, there is a myriad of effective nonsurgical treatment options that can be incorporated into the care of the patient with knee OA. These include both pharmacological and nonpharmacological treatments (Fig. 32-1). It is imperative for a physician to understand all of these available approaches in order to provide effective and comprehensive care to patients with knee OA. The unified goals of

TABLE 32-1. Knee Osteoarthritis Risk Factors

Established
Sex (female)
Obesity
Age
Prior knee injury or trauma
Osteoarthritis at other sites
Previous knee surgery
Controversial
Genetics
Physical activity
Smoking
Estrogen deficiency

treatment should be to relieve pain and improve functionality of the joint. These goals are inseparable and, taken together, they can greatly enhance the quality of life in a patient with knee OA.

When formulating a treatment plan, several factors need to be considered that include, but are not limited to, the following: risk factors (prior injury or surgery, obesity, polypharmacy, medical comorbidities), demographics (age and work requirements and environment), level of pain and disability, knee characteristics (structural damage, trauma, malalignment), level of inflammation (effusion), and the patient's desired level of functionality. It is critical to remember too that all patients are different and, as a result, treatment protocols need to be "individualized" and not "generalized" for this condition. Evidence-based, therapy algorithms would facilitate this process in different subgroups of patients with knee OA, but currently these do not exist. Therefore, the physician–patient relationship is critical to a successful outcome.

HISTORY

Before formulating an appropriate treatment protocol, it is critical for a physician to make the definitive diagnosis of knee OA. A clinician can usually achieve this diagnosis by taking a thorough history and performing a physical examination. Osteoarthritis mainly occurs in middle-aged and elderly patients. However, in select groups of people it can occur at a younger age, especially in patients with a history of surgery or trauma to the knee. African-American women also tend to develop knee OA at a younger age for reasons that are not well understood.[1]

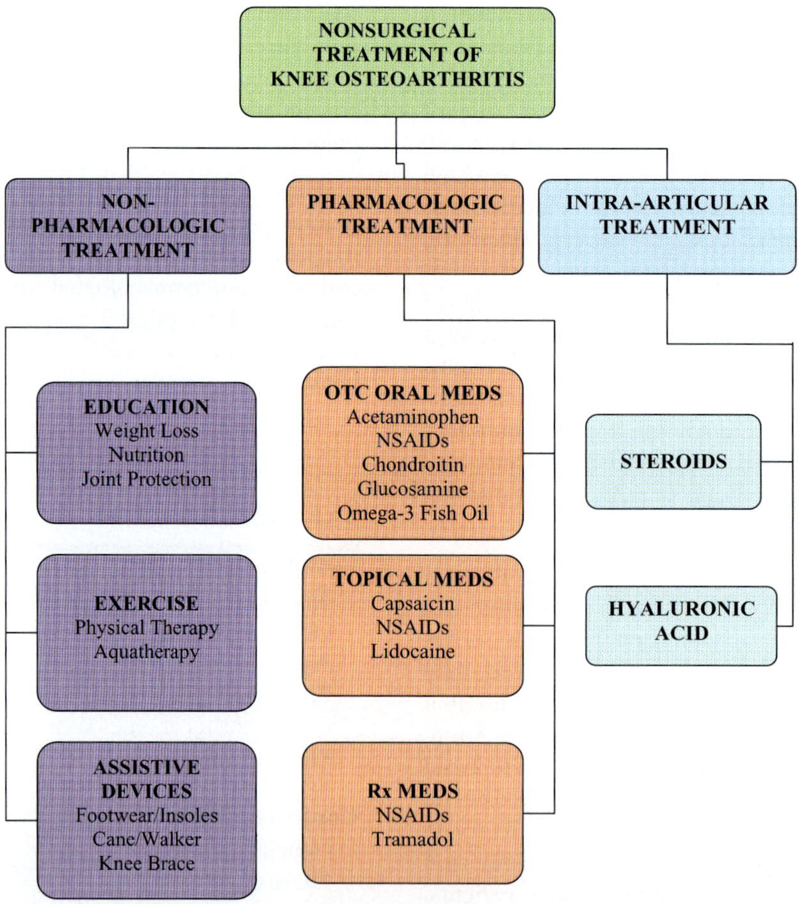

FIGURE 32-1. *Nonsurgical treatment options for knee osteoarthritis.*

An insidious onset of aching pain with gradual progression is the typical presentation of a knee OA patient. However, some patients will remain asymptomatic with the initial onset of knee OA. Pain distribution may be localized or radiating and is frequently exacerbated with increased activity and weight bearing.[2] In the early stages, pain usually improves with rest, but with disease progression, pain can occur with rest and at night. Many patients will note worsening pain with barometric pressure changes, especially cool, damp, and/or rainy weather.[3]

Joint stiffness, crepitus, and restricted range of motion of the joint are additional symptoms that may occur with worsening of knee OA. A "gelling phenomenon" (stiffness with rest and inactivity) is often described by the patient and is relieved with activity. Morning stiffness is usually only 15 to 20 minutes, far less than a patient with rheumatoid arthritis. Patients will describe pain with prolonged sitting, squatting, kneeling, and stair climbing (especially descending). Some patients will develop soft tissue swelling and/or a joint effusion as the condition progresses. Advancing knee OA can lead to a sensation of joint instability with buckling or giving out. Patients may even describe locking or catching of the knee. This is related to incongruity of the joint surface and intra-articular loose bodies from degenerative pieces of cartilage floating in the joint space.[2] Over time, patients (or more often family members) will note a deformity of the lower extremity related to advanced knee OA. This may include a varus ("bowleg") or valgus ("knock-knee") deformity. Limps and falls are common with disease progression.

PHYSICAL EXAMINATION

While the physical examination is a critical component to the diagnostic acumen of the physician, it may not yield many findings in early knee OA. Visual inspection of a patient's gait, body habitus, and joint alignment can shed light on the severity of the condition. A varus (bowleg) or valgus (knock-knee) deformity may indicate which compartment of the knee is most afflicted with OA changes, either the medial tibiofemoral or lateral tibiofemoral compartment respectively (Figs. 32-2 and 32-3). Additional signs may include soft tissue swelling, bony enlargement, or even atrophy of the quadriceps muscles, especially the vastus medialis oblique (VMO).

Palpation of the joint may yield joint line or patella facet pain, crepitus, warmth, limited range of motion, or even an effusion. Pain will often occur on extreme flexion of the joint. Compared with other joints affected with osteoarthritis, the knee has a higher tendency to develop an effusion, particularly in advanced cases.[1,2] Palpable osteophytes may be present as well as instability of the joint on specific stress testing of the ligaments.

RADIOGRAPHIC STUDIES

Radiographs can greatly complement a good physical examination of the knee joint. At least 50% to 75% of people older than 65 demonstrate some radiographic evidence

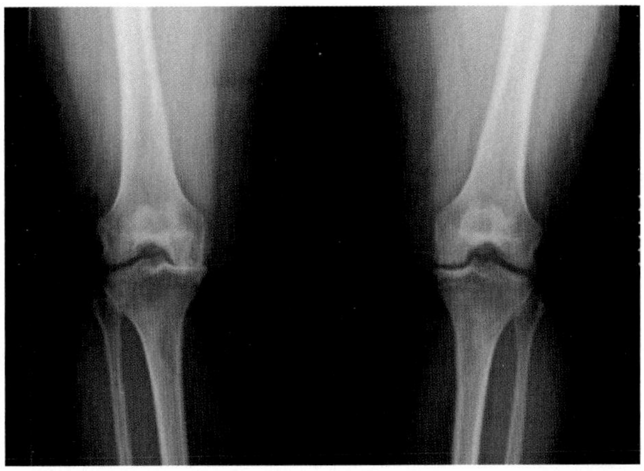

FIGURE 32-2. *Medial compartment osteoarthritis (right knee).*

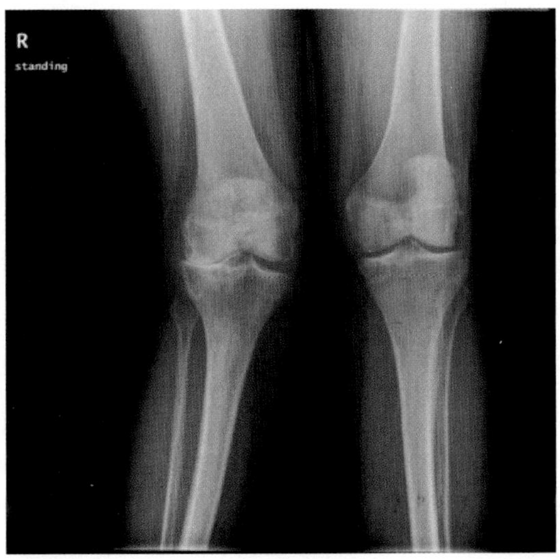

FIGURE 32-3. *Lateral compartment osteoarthritis (right knee).*

of knee osteoarthritis on plain radiographs. This number approaches 100% in patients older than 75.[4] Interestingly, only 40% to 60% of these patients may be clinically symptomatic.[4,5] This is important to note because radiographic changes do not necessarily correlate with pain intensity and visa versa. Furthermore, there is no strong correlation between the clinical outcome of osteoarthritis of the knee and its radiographic course.[6,7]

The knee joint is comprised of three compartments: the medial tibiofemoral, lateral tibiofemoral, and patellofemoral joints. Osteoarthritis may afflict any or all of these compartments, but involvement tends to be asymmetric. Unicompartmental (especially medial tibiofemoral joint) or bicompartmental (lateral tibiofemoral joint and patellofemoral joint or medial tibiofemoral joint and patellofemoral joint) involvement occurs frequently. Tricompartmental involvement is not as common.[3] If plain films are deemed necessary, it is useful to obtain an anteroposterior (AP), lateral Merchant's (patella), and posteroanterior (PA) tunnel views (Figs. 32-4 to 32-7). If possible, it is always ideal to perform these views while weight bearing to better appreciate joint space narrowing.

There are common radiographic features of knee osteoarthritis that include joint space narrowing, subchondral sclerosis, subchondral cysts, bone remodeling, and osteophytes (Table 32-2). Unlike rheumatoid arthritis, marginal bony erosions or bone demineralization are not common features of knee OA and, if present, inflammatory arthropathies should be considered in the differential.[1] The finding of osteophytes seems to be the most sensitive radiographic finding in knee OA.[5,7] Osteophytes are common at the articular margins ("marginal") of the femur and tibia as well as at the superior and inferior poles of the patella. Interior ("central") osteophytic involvement of the tibial spines and femoral condyles can also occur.

More specialized studies such as magnetic resonance imaging (MRI) and computed tomography or bone scans may be needed if the diagnosis is still unclear or if the patient is not responding appropriately to conservative treatment measures, especially if only mild OA is noted on plain radiographs.

TREATMENT

Weight Loss

Obesity has long been known to be an important risk factor for knee OA. This risk is especially strong among women.[8] Weight loss can have an important impact on symptoms, progression, and even surgical treatment of knee OA. Body mass index (BMI) is commonly used in assessing knee OA patients and is associated with OA progression.[9] In one study of women in England, it was found that for every 2-unit increase in BMI, the odds ratio for radiographic knee OA increased by 1.36.[10] This same study found no relationship between fat distribution and OA risk. The traditional theory explaining the link between OA and obesity was simply that the additional weight caused more stress on the joint. However, many patients with OA notice symptoms first in their non-weight-bearing joints such as their fingers. There is some recent evidence that the increased level of OA in the obese patient may be related to the proinflammatory effects of adipose tissue.[11-13]

Whatever the mechanism linking obesity and knee OA, weight loss has been shown to reduce pain and improve function in patients with knee OA.[14,15] The effects were even more dramatic when combined with exercise.[16] As with any patient fighting obesity, a combined program of low-impact aerobic exercise and appropriate nutrition will have the most substantial impact. Nutritionists, dieticians, personal trainers, and physical therapists can all play an important role in the treatment of knee OA. Furthermore, if despite their best efforts patients are finding weight loss difficult, it is not unreasonable to consider consultation for alternatives such as medications or even bariatric surgery.

Exercise and Activity Modification

The principles of joint protection are important in the treatment of knee OA. These principles include using proper body mechanics and posture, avoiding high-impact activities, and wearing supportive shoes and orthotic devices. Physical therapy (PT) plays a large part in teaching patients how to achieve these ideals. PT can teach patients to use proper body mechanics and help them to incorporate low-impact exercise into their health regimen.

Knee OA patients who exercise can improve strength, proprioception, and flexibility, as well as lose weight. The effect of exercise interventions on pain and function in knee OA patients have been found equivalent to nonsteroidal anti-inflammatory drugs (NSAIDs).[17] However, high-impact physical activity may actually worsen knee OA, especially among obese individuals.[18] These high-impact activities tend to be occupational, involving kneeling, squatting, stair climbing, running, and heavy lifting.[19] Some feel that these data may be skewed by workers' compensation issues. Typically, knee OA progression does not occur with regular recreational activities such as light jogging.[20]

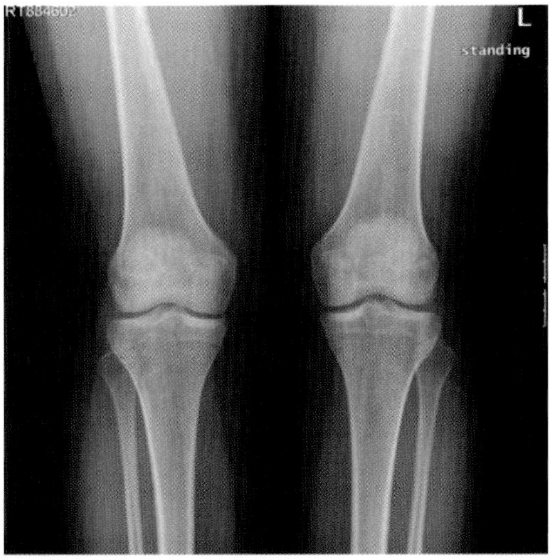

FIGURE 32-4. *AP view of normal knee.*

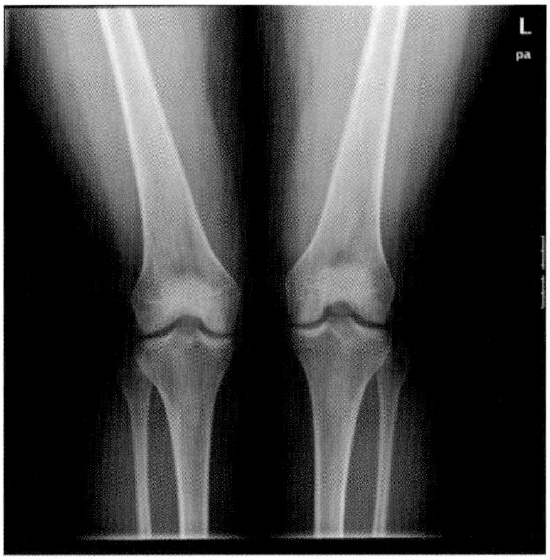

FIGURE 32-6. *Tunnel view of normal knee.*

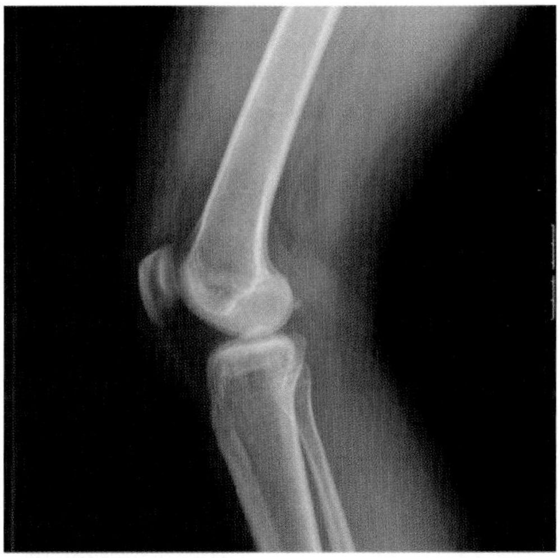

FIGURE 32-5. *Lateral view of normal knee.*

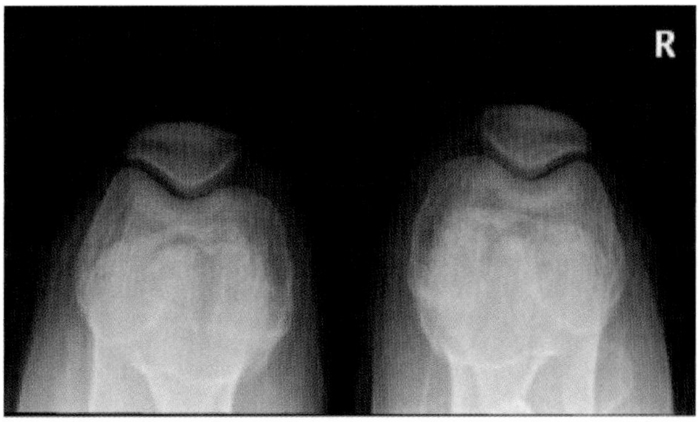

FIGURE 32-7. *Sunrise view of normal knee.*

TABLE 32-2. Knee Osteoarthritis Radiographic Features

Joint space narrowing (often medial tibiofemoral compartment)
Subchondral sclerosis
Subchondral cysts
Osteophytes ("marginal" or "central")
Bone remodeling
Varus ("bowleg") or valgus ("knock-knee") deformity
Patella subluxation
Intra-articular loose bodies

Knee OA patients should engage in exercise that is low impact and takes place in a controlled environment. Such activities include walking, aquatic exercise, cycling, yoga, Pilates, and Tai Chi. Choosing proper footwear can limit knee pain during such activities. Flexible cushioned shoes and those with heels of 1.5 inches or less can help reduce pain in knee OA.[21] Patients with isolated medial compartment OA may do better without medial arch supports. Clogs and stability shoes may create more stress at the knee than neutral or flat walking shoes.[22] Recently, there has been increasing interest on barefoot running and walking. Newer shoes provide protection for skin and soft tissues while still allowing for the natural biomechanics of barefoot motion. These shoes may reduce joint loads in patients in knee OA.[23] Patients should also be educated on finding "softer" surfaces for exercise, such as padded tracks, grass, and boardwalks, which can minimize the impact on the knees. Runners often tout wood chip trails as the softest, most comfortable surface for running. There are also various exercise machines with designs that minimize the impact on the knee, including elliptical machines, rowing machines, and stationary bicycles.

An exercise program for an OA patient should include both strengthening and aerobic activity. Although strengthening programs are more effective than aerobic in the short term, aerobic exercise has important advantages in the long term.[24] Aerobic activity also has a positive effect on mood not seen with strengthening exercises alone. This may be due to the release of endorphins. No single exercise program has been found more effective than others.[25] Since knee OA is a chronic disease, any formal rehabilitation should be structured with progression to a home program. While a structured exercise program is a great start, patients should pursue activities they enjoy, encouraging regular exercise over the long term.

Topical Therapy

There are numerous topical therapies that patients will use before presenting to a doctor. These include ice, heating pads, massage, and topical medications. Many over-the-counter (OTC) medicines will produce the sensations of cold or heat. There are also OTC pain relievers such as capsaicin, aloe (which has anti-inflammatory properties), and salicylates. Patients will frequently use ice or heat or even a combination of these two modalities for pain relief. Many patients even look toward massage therapy as an alternative approach for treating the pain of knee OA. In addition to these traditional topical therapeutic options, patients will also incorporate a variety of topical creams and ointments that are readily available over the counter.

Topical NSAIDs are effective alternatives to their systemic counterparts, but with less systemic toxicity. There are a plethora of choices for patients for these topical agents. In some studies, topical NSAIDs have been found to be as effective as oral NSAIDs in treating knee OA.[26,27] Available formulations include diclofenac, salicylates, and ibuprofen. Although systemic levels are much lower than when taking oral NSAIDs, topical NSAIDs can be absorbed systemically and can cause systemic side effects.[28]

Topical capsaicin is a safe and effective option for patients. It has been shown to be more effective than placebo at controlling pain in knee OA.[29] The chemical in this product is the active ingredient in hot peppers. Capsaicin therapy works by downregulating substance P in local tissues. No systemic side effects have been reported and capsaicin will not interact with any medications. Patients should be warned to use a glove when applying capsaicin and that there is an initial period of hypersensitivity before the substance P is downregulated.

Supplements

While there are numerous nutraceutical products on the market, the potential benefits of glucosamine and chondroitin have been studied the most extensively. Chondroitin and glucosamine are derivatives of articular glycosaminoglycans. They are thought to promote chondrocyte glycosaminioglycan production and perhaps reduce inflammation in OA while at the same time reducing pain. Measures of biomarkers in OA show that chondroitin may stimulate catabolism and inhibit proteases.[30] There have been conflicting results on studies of these supplements in OA.[31-35] Some of these trials showed that treatment may have some benefit in patients with moderate to severe disease.[33] Other studies have demonstrated a better response in milder disease.[36] A recent study of chondroitin in knee OA showed that its chondroprotective effects could be measured by MRI in as little as 6 months.[37]

Studies on supplements are limited by the many different formulations and doses that are used in studies. Some studies use glucosamine and chondroitin, while others use the agents individually. Studies on different formulations of supplements have demonstrated measurable biological differences.[30] A Cochrane review found that there was only one glucosamine formulation (Rotta) that showed consistent benefits in studies.[38] This Rotta preparation is prescribed by physicians in Europe and available OTC in the United States. This study is very important in that it demonstrated disease modification rather than just pain control.

Whether these agents are effective or not, it is very apparent that many patients are convinced that they work at least for facilitating pain control. There have been few side effects reported with either compound. The supplements may allow some patients to reduce the dose of more toxic medications. The recommended dose of chondroitin is 1200 mg per day and for glucosamine 1500 mg per day. Glucosamine should not be used in patients with seafood allergy and should be used with caution in diabetics because it may elevate blood glucose levels, although studies have not consistently found this to be the case. The side effects of chondroitin tend to be mild gastrointestinal symptoms. Liquid formulations tend to be more tolerable.

Fish oil is another supplement used to treat OA. The recommended fish oils are high in omega-3 fatty acids. Although there is limited data on the use of fish oil in OA, it has been shown to improve the lipid profile of bone marrow and joint fluid, theoretically strengthening the joints.[39] Fish oil supplements have also been shown to reduce production of proinflammatory cytokines[40] and to reduce pain in patients with OA.[41] Unfortunately, it is not clear how clinically significant these findings are in treating OA. Nevertheless, many OA patients report a favorable response. Also, many patients with OA are already taking fish oil for its cardiovascular benefits. Some clinicians express concerns over concentrated heavy metals and other pollutants in fish oil extracts. Simply increasing the amount of dietary omega-3 fatty acids may be safer. There is also prescription omega oil available but this has not been studied in OA. The best dietary sources are cold-water fish such as wild salmon, herring, mackerel, sardines, and anchovies.

Assistive Devices

Braces can serve a vital role in managing knee OA, especially in patients who cannot tolerate or have contraindications to other medical options (ie, oral medications or injections). The authors frequently incorporate unloader braces in their management of patients with knee OA. Such braces can specifically unload either the medial (majority of cases) or lateral side of the knee based on the location of the symptoms and OA findings.[42] As knee OA progresses in a particular compartment, a patient may develop alignment issues of the leg. A resultant varus (medial compartment OA) or valgus (lateral compartment OA) deformity of the lower extremity may occur. This will cause a significant shift of knee pressures to that particular compartment and likely increase pain symptoms.[43] Unloader braces can help correct this problem to more physiologic alignment.[44] These braces can reduce pain and improve functionality.[44-49] A valgus brace can "unload" the medial compartment and a varus brace can "unload" the lateral compartment. Several studies have demonstrated that medial unloader braces reduce pain and improve activity levels in patients with isolated medial compartment OA.[44-49]

Various types of canes have also been utilized for knee and hip OA pain. They can help reduce pressures on the knee, decrease pain, and, most important, assist with balance issues. It is imperative that patients be appropriately measured for and trained on how to use a cane.

Heel wedges (especially lateral wedges) can also assist in knee OA care. Since medial compartment OA is present in 80% of cases, lateral heel wedges can be very effective to lessen pain. Studies have shown that insoles of 5° to 10° can partially correct varus alignment changes.[50,51] Insoles improve pain and function and can be less cumbersome than knee braces.[44,50,52-55]

Acupuncture

In Eastern countries, acupuncture has been used to treat knee OA for thousands of years. Recently, acupuncture has seen growing popularity in the West. Unfortunately, its use has been riddled with controversy. Acupuncture studies are very difficult to interpret secondary to blinding and choosing an appropriate placebo. The most accepted design is to compare traditional acupuncture to sham acupuncture. Many studies have shown marked improvement in pain scores while few show no effect.[56-61] Recent analyses concluded that acupuncture was beneficial compared to sham acupuncture for patients with chronic knee pain.[62] While side effects are minimal, concern arises from the possibility of infection from the needles. Fortunately, the U.S. Food and Drug Administration (FDA) has now developed standards for needle sterility. Therefore, it is a reasonable complementary treatment for knee OA.

Magnets

The use of magnets in knee OA treatment is largely anecdotal. Although there is some evidence that magnets reduce knee pain in OA patients, much of the evidence is contradictory.[63] Studies involving magnet use are difficult to interpret and often lack good study design and control. A recent meta-analysis failed to provide sufficient evidence to recommend the use of magnets for pain relief.[64] Additional well-designed studies are clearly warranted and may yield promising results.

Systemic Medications

The American College of Rheumatology and the European League Against Rheumatism has established a "pyramidal" protocol for the treatment of knee OA. Acetaminophen (or paracetamol) is the first-line medication of choice for knee OA patients in conjunction with nonpharmacological means.[65,66] Its use is relatively safe compared to NSAIDs, and it is almost as effective a pain reliever. A healthy patient can usually metabolize up to 4 g/day. However, it is recommended to use the lowest effective dose that controls pain. Hepatic toxicity is a concern especially in chronic alcoholics. It is recommended that patients maintain an effective dose on a regular basis rather than take it sporadically.

The use of NSAIDs is widespread and extremely common to treat knee OA pain. They are considered second-line medication options for knee OA patients. Unfortunately, the major risks from NSAID use are gastrointestinal bleeding or perforation and renal toxicity.[67] Obviously, the lowest effective dose is preferred if needed for pain. Fortunately, in 2000, the American College of Rheumatology recommended hyaluronic acid (HA) for knee OA patients who have not responded to pharmacological therapy or patients who have a contraindication to NSAIDs. Recently, study data have shown the cardiovascular side effects of both selective and nonselective NSAIDs.[68-72] Some COX-2 inhibitors have been taken off the market because of these detrimental effects. Most experts recommend against using NSAIDs on a long-term basis. Brief periods of use for breakthrough pain or flares are tolerable.

Injectable Options

Intra-articular joint injections are frequently and successfully incorporated into the treatment regimen for knee OA. Steroid and hyaluronic acid derivatives can provide significant relief for many patients. The technique for administration of each type of injection product is the same. Various portals of injection entry can be used around the knee, including the anterolateral, anteromedial, medial midpatellar, and lateral midpatellar approaches. Evidence is conflicting as to the most accurate site for knee injection.[73,74] The authors prefer the anterolateral site for injection. However, arthrocentesis is usually performed from the lateral midpatellar site.

Intra-articular steroids

Acute inflammatory flares with effusions seem to respond particularly well to steroids. The typical steroid injection is a "cocktail" of a long-acting and/or short-acting anesthetic mixed with a steroid. A postinjection steroid flare is common and patients need to be made aware of this potential so they can recognize it and treat it accordingly. It is not uncommon to perform an arthrocentesis of an effusion at the same time as administering a steroid. Unfortunately, the benefits of intra-articular steroids tend to be short lived, but some patients do experience long-term relief of up to 6 months or longer.

Steroid injections are relatively safe and cost-effective, but there are few studies supporting their efficacy. There is a concern over the potential adverse effects of repeated injections over short intervals. Excessive steroid use can deleteriously affect cartilage and underlying bone, especially since systemic absorption does occur. This is particularly concerning for diabetics who need to monitor glucose levels closely because a transient elevation may occur after an intra-articular steroid injection.

Viscosupplementation

Fortunately, a "newer" injection treatment option is available, often referred to as "joint fluid therapy." The major roles of synovial fluid are to facilitate movement, protect the joint from trauma, and act as a transport medium for nutrients and waste products. Hyaluronic acid (HA) is critical to this function as a key component of synovial fluid and is the basis of these forms of intra-articular injections. It is the viscosity and elasticity properties of HA that allow it to facilitate lubrication (protection during slow movements) and shock absorption (protection during rapid movements).

When a person develops OA of the knee joint, the synovial fluid properties will change, particularly a decrease in HA concentration. This also includes a drop in molecular weight and charge of HA. Restoration of synovial fluid function with HA supplementation was proposed as early as the 1960s by Balasz[75] and was theorized to help with pain reduction. HA products have been used for years to treat track horses. HA use was approved by the FDA for use in humans in 1997 as a medical device and not as a drug. Currently, HA is only approved for OA of the knee. However, off-label uses for OA in other joints are common and have prompted numerous studies and investigations into use in these joints (ie, hip, shoulder, elbow, etc). There are currently six HA products available in the United States (Table 32-3).

The exact mechanism of action of HA is unclear, but theories include (1) nocioceptor analgesia, (2) restoration of the viscoelastic properties of synovial fluid, (3) suppressing inflammation, (4) stimulating HA production by synoviocytes, and (5) stimulating chondrocyte growth and collagen synthesis and decreasing chondrocyte apoptosis.[76]

Studies have looked at all these proposed theories and HA has been shown to reduce the levels of inflammatory mediators (prostaglandins, cytokines, cyclic adenosine monophosphate) in the synovial fluid of OA patients.[77-80] It also effects leukocyte activity by reducing proliferation, migration, adherence, and phagocytosis. In vitro studies have also shown that HA administration stimulates endogenous production of HA and other glycosaminoglycans.[81]

Clinical efficacy of viscosupplementation use has been questioned by some experts. This may be because patients with more severe OA of the joint on average do not tend to benefit as much as ones with milder disease, which is not unexpected. In many studies, HA was found to be at least equivalent to continuous NSAIDs use. Studies comparing intra-articular HA to steroid injections found steroids to be more effective in the short term, but HA had a longer duration of benefit for up to 6 months. The main benefit from HA injections for decreased pain seems to occur at around 6 to 13 weeks postinjection.

A recent Cochrane meta-analysis of 76 trials concluded that intra-articular HA was an effective treatment for knee OA.[82] Furthermore, intra-articular HA is part of the American College of Rheumatology's protocol for the treatment of OA.[83] There is also some evidence attesting to the cost effectiveness of intra-articular HA related to the lack of toxicity from systemic medications.[84,85]

One of the major benefits to intra-articular HA use is that adverse effects are few and tend to be local. Potential risks, although small, include hypersensitivity to local anesthetic or preservative, local pain and swelling, infection, and possibly needle breakage. Localized, pain and swelling may occur in 1% to 3% of patients, but fortunately, this responds very favorably to conservative modalities (ie, ice, NSAIDs, rest) within 1 to 3 days. Rarely, some flares can be severe enough to mimic a joint infection. These reactions are called severe acute inflammatory reactions or "pseudoseptic reactions." They seem to be more prevalent with higher-molecular-weight HA preparations (ie, hylan G-F 20). Some theorize that the reaction is a cell-mediated allergic reaction to cross-linked HA or to products used in manufacturing.[85-93] Finally, as these HA injections evolve, there is an influx of single-injection HA products (eg, Synvisc-One), which may improve health care costs and patient compliance.[94]

Hyaluronic acid injections can be used synergistically with other knee OA treatments including intra-articular steroid injections. This combination can often provide more immediate pain relief than treatment with HA alone.[87] Usually, if a patient presents with an effusion, it is best to perform an arthrocentesis with steroid injection first. A follow-up can be scheduled in 1 to 2 weeks to start HA injections to achieve a better outcome. Many feel that OA with an effusion represents a more inflammatory form of OA.

Autologous Blood Injections

Recently, there has been a rapidly growing interest in utilizing autologous blood products to treat various musculoskeletal problems. Platelet-rich plasma (a.k.a. PRP) injections are currently being studied heavily for their potential use in knee OA. The theory on the potential "healing" effects of these products stems from the growth factors that are released from these concentrated platelet-rich injec-

TABLE 32-3. Joint Fluid Therapy Products Available in the United States

Trade Name	Component	Number of Weekly Injections	Molecular Weight (in millions of Daltons)
Hyalgan (Sanofi-Aventis, Bridgewater, NJ, USA)	Sodium hyaluronate	3–5	0.50–0.73
Supartz (Orthopedics Smith & Nephew, Inc., Memphis, TN, USA)	Sodium hyaluronate	3–5	0.62–1.17
Orthovisc (DePuy Mitek, Inc., Raynham, MA, USA)	High-molecular-weight hyaluronan	3–4	1.0–2.9
Euflexxa (Bio-Technology General, Kiryat, Israel)	Sodium hyaluronate	3	2.4–3.6
Synvisc (Genzyme Biosurgery, Cambridge, MA, USA)	Hylan G-F 20	3	6.0
Synvisc One (Genzyme Biosurgery, Cambridge, MA, USA)	Hylan G-F 20	1	6.0

tions. Growth factors are actively involved in various healing processes.[95] Unfortunately, most of the clinical data on PRP use is anecdotal. Therefore, more well-designed, controlled studies need to be performed before definitive recommendations can be made for their use in knee OA.

CONCLUSION

Osteoarthritis of the knee is a complex disease of multifactorial etiology. Some risk factors are consistent while others, such as physical activity, are controversial. Additional studies are needed to further delineate these risk factors and their importance on the development and progression of knee OA. Knee OA responds best to an individualized treatment plan using various modalities. As noted previously, the physician-patient relationship is critical to the success of treatment outcome. It is imperative for the patient to be directly involved in the treatment process. Important factors to consider include the patient's biomechanics, comorbidities, physical demands, and personal preferences. A comprehensive approach to treatment often includes incorporating physical therapists, pharmacists, nutritionists, fitness trainers, prosthetic specialists, and alternative practitioners. Utilizing a team approach can maximize treatment effectiveness, minimize toxicity, and empower patients to manage their disease.

REFERENCES

1. Fife RS, Hochberg MC. Osteoarthritis. In: Klippel JH, Weyand CM, Wortmann RL, eds. *Primer on the Rheumatic Diseases.* 11th ed. Atlanta, GA: Arthritis Foundation; 1997:216-221.
2. Townes AS. Osteoarthritis. In: Barker LR, Burton JR, Zieve PD, eds. *Principles of Ambulatory Medicine.* 4th ed. Baltimore, MD: Lippincott, Williams, & Wilkins; 1995:917-929.
3. Resnick D, Niwayama G. Degenerative diseases of extraspinal locations. In: Resnick D, ed. *Diagnosis of Bone and Joint Disorders.* 3rd ed. Philadelphia, PA: W.B. Saunders; 1995:1273-1371.
4. Lane NE, Buckwalter JA. Exercise: a cause of osteoarthritis? *Rheum Dis Clin North Am.* 1993;19(3): 617-629.
5. Lanyon P, O'Reilly S, Jones A, et al. Radiographic assessment of symptomatic knee osteoarthritis in the community: definitions and normal joint space. *Ann Rheum Dis.* 1998;57(10):595-601.
6. Felson DT. The course of osteoarthritis and factors that affect it. *Rheum Dis Clin North Am.* 1993;19(3): 607-615.
7. Hart DJ, Doyle DV, Spector TD. Incidence and risk factors for radiographic knee osteoarthritis in middle-aged women: the Chingford study. *Arthritis Rheum.* 1999;42(1):17-24.
8. Felson DT, Zhang Y, Hannan MT, et al. Risk factors for incident radiographic knee osteoarthritis in the elderly: the Framingham study. *Arthritis Rheum.* 1997;40:728-733.
9. Felson DT, Goggins J, Niu J, et al. The effect of body weight on progression of knee osteoarthritis is dependent on alignment. *Arthritis Rheum.* 2004;50:3904-3909.
10. Hart DJ, Spector TD. The relationship of obesity, fat distribution and osteoarthritis in women in the general population: the Chingford Study. *J Rheumatol.* 1993;20(2):331.
11. Toussirot E, Streit G, Wendling D. The contribution of adipose tissue and adipokines to inflammation in joint diseases. *Curr Med Chem.* 2007;14:1095-1100.
12. Rojas-Rodriguez J, Escobar-Linares LE, Garcia-Carrasco M, et al. The relationship between the metabolic syndrome and energy-utilization deficit in the pathogenesis of obesity-induced osteoarthritis. *Med Hypotheses.* 2007;69:860-868.
13. Dayer JM, Chicheportiche R, Juge-Aubry C, et al. Adipose tissue has anti-inflammatory properties: focus on IL-1 receptor antagonist (IL-1Ra). *Ann N Y Acad Sci.* 2006;1069:444-453.
14. Toda Y. The effect of energy restriction, walking, and exercise on lower extremity lean body mass in obese women with osteoarthritis of the knee. *J Orthop Sci.* 2001;6:148-154.
15. Huang MH, Chen CH, Chen TW, et al. The effects of weight reduction on the rehabilitation of patients with knee osteoarthritis and obesity. *Arthritis Care Res.* 2000;13:398-405.
16. Messier SP, Loeser RF, Miller GD, et al. Exercise and dietary weight loss in overweight and obese older adults with knee osteoarthritis: the arthritis, diet, and activity promotion trial. *Arthritis Rheum.* 2004;50:1501-1510.
17. Bischoff HA, Roos EM. Effectiveness and safety of strengthening, aerobic, and coordination exercises for patients with osteoarthritis. *Curr Opin Rheumatol.* 2003;15:141-144.
18. McAlindon TE, Wilson PW, Aliabadi P, et al. Level of physical activity and the risk of radiographic and

symptomatic knee osteoarthritis in the elderly: the Framingham study. *Am J Med*. 1999;106:151-157.

19. Cooper C, Coggon D. Physical activity and knee osteoarthritis. *Lancet*. 1999;353:2177-2178.
20. Felson DT, Niu J, Clancy M, et al. Effect of recreational physical activities on the development of knee osteoarthritis in older adults of different weights: the Framingham study. *Arthritis Rheum*. 2007;57:6-12.
21. Hinman RS, Bennell KL. Advances in insoles and shoes for knee osteoarthritis. *Curr Opin Rheumatol*. 2009;21(2):164.
22. Shakoor N, Sengupta M, Foucher KC, et al. Effects of common footwear on joint loading in osteoarthritis of the knee. *Arthritis Care Res (Hoboken)*. 2010;62(7):917-23.
23. Shakoor N, Lidtke RH, Sengupta M, et al. Effects of specialized footwear on joint loads in osteoarthritis of the knee. *Arthritis Rheum*. 2008; 59(9):1214-1220.
24. Bennell K, Hinman R. Exercise as a treatment for osteoarthritis. *Curr Opin Rheumatol*. 2005;17:634-640.
25. Roddy E, Zhang W, Doherty M, et al. Evidence-based recommendations for the role of exercise in the management of osteoarthritis of the hip or knee–the MOVE consensus. *Rheumatol (Oxford)*. 2005;44:67-73.
26. Biswal S, Medhi B, Pandhi P. Long-term efficacy of topical nonsteroidal antiinflammatory drugs in knee osteoarthritis: meta-analysis of randomized placebo controlled clinical trials. *J Rheumatol*. 2006;33:1841-1844.
27. Baraf HS, Gloth FM, Barthel HR, et al. Safety and efficacy of topical diclofenac sodium gel for knee osteoarthritis in elderly and younger patients. *Drugs Aging*. 2011;28(1):27-40.
28. Makris UE, Kohler MJ, Fraenkel L. Adverse effects of topical nonsteroidal antinflammatory drugs in older adults with osteoarthritis: a systemic literature review. *J Rheumatol*. 2010;37(6):1236-1243.
29. Zhang WY, Li Wan Po A. The effectiveness of topically applied capsaicin: a meta-analysis. *Eur J Clin Pharmacol*. 1994;46:517-522.
30. Tat SK, Pelletier JP, Mineau F, et al. Variable effects of 3 different chondroitin sulfate compounds on human osteoarthritic cartilage/chondrocytes: relevance of purity and production process. *J Rheumatol*. 2010;37(3):656-664.
31. Monfort J, Pelletier JP, Garcia-Giralt N, et al. Biochemical basis of the effect of chondroitin sulfate on osteoarthritis articular tissues. *Ann Rheum Dis*. 2008;67(6):735-740.
32. Reichenbach S, Sterchi R, Scherer M, et al. Meta-analysis: chondroitin for osteoarthritis of the knee or hip. *Ann Intern Med*. 2007;146:580-590.
33. Clegg DO, Reda DJ, Harris CL, et al. Glucosamine, chondroitin sulfate, and the two in combination for painful knee osteoarthritis. *N Engl J Med*. 2006;354: 795-808.
34. Mazieres B, Hucher M, Zaim M, et al. Effect of chondroitin sulphate in symptomatic knee osteoarthritis: a multicentre, randomised, double-blind, placebo-controlled study. *Ann Rheum Dis*. 2007;66:639-645.
35. Reichenbach S, Sterchi R, Scherer M, et al. Meta-analysis: chondroitin for osteoarthritis of the knee or hip. *Ann Intern Med*. 2007;146:580-590.
36. Sawitzke AD, Shi H, Finco MF, et al. The effect of glucosamine and/or chondroitin sulfate on the progression of knee osteoarthritis: a report from the glucosamine/chondroitin arthritis intervention trial. *Arthritis Rheum*. 2008;58(10):3183-3189.
37. Wildi LM, Raynauld JP, Martel-Pelletier J. Chondroitin sulfate reduces both cartilage volume loss and bone marrow lesions in knee osteoarthritis patients starting as early as 6 months after initiation of therapy: a randomized, placebo controlled, double blind study using MRI. *Ann Rheum Dis*. 2011;70(6):982-989.
38. Towheed T, Maxwell L, Anastassiades TP, et al. Glucosamine therapy for treating osteoarthritis. *Cochrane Database Syst Rev*. 2005;2:CD002946.
39. Pritchett JW. Statins and dietary fish oils improve lipid composition in bone marrow and joints. *Clin Orthop Relat Res*. 2007;456:233-237.
40. Curtis CL, Rees SG, Cramp J, et al. Effects of n-3 fatty acids on cartilage metabolism. *Proc Nutr Soc*. 2002;61:381-389.
41. Gruenwald J, Petzold E, Busch R, et al. Effect of glucosamine sulfate with or without omega-3 fatty acids in patients with osteoarthritis. *Adv Ther*. 2009;26(9): 858-871.
42. Ahlback S. Osteoarthrosis of the knee: a radiographic investigation. *Acta Radiol Diagn (Stockh)*. 1968;suppl 277:7-72.
43. Prodromos CC, Andriacchi TP, Galante JO. A relationship between gait and clinical changes following high tibial osteotomy. *J Bone Joint Surg Am*. 1985;67:1188-1194.
44. Pollo FE, Otis JC, Backus SI, et al. Reduction of medial compartment loads with valgus bracing of the

osteoarthritic knee. *Am J Sports Med.* 2002;30:414-421.

45. Hewett TE, Noyes FR, Barber-Westin SD, et al. Decrease in knee joint pain and increase in function in patients with medial compartment arthrosis: a prospective analysis of valgus bracing. *Orthopedics.* 1998;21:131-138.
46. Matsuno H, Kadowaki KM, Tsuji H. Generation II knee bracing for severe medial compartment osteoarthritis of the knee. *Arch Phys Med Rehabil.* 1997;78:745-749.
47. Gaasbeek RD, Groen BE, Hampsink B, et al. Valgus bracing in patients with medial compartment osteoarthritis of the knee. A gait analysis study of a new brace. *Gait Posture.* 2007;26:3-10.
48. Finger S, Paulos LE. Clinical and biomechanical evaluation of the unloading brace. *J Knee Surg.* 2002;15:155-158; discussion 159.
49. Lindenfeld TN, Hewett TE, Andriacchi TP. Joint loading with valgus bracing in patients with varus gonarthrosis. *Clin Orthop Relat Res.* 1997;344:290-297.
50. Kerrigan DC, Lelas JL, Goggins J, et al. Effectiveness of a lateral-wedge insole on knee varus torque in patients with knee osteoarthritis. *Arch Phys Med Rehabil.* 2002;83:889-893.
51. Crenshaw SJ, Pollo FE, Calton EF. Effects of lateral-wedged insoles on kinetics at the knee. *Clin Orthop Relat Res.* 2000;375:185-192.
52. Sasaki T, Yasuda K. Clinical evaluation of the treatment of osteoarthritic knees using a newly designed wedged insole. *Clin Orthop Relat Res.* 1987;221:181-187.
53. Wolfe SA, Brueckmann FR. Conservative treatment of genu valgus and varum with medial/lateral heel wedges. *Indiana Med.* 1991;84:614-615.
54. Tohyama H, Yasuda K, Kaneda K. Treatment of osteoarthritis of the knee with heel wedges. *Int Orthop.* 1991;15:31-33.
55. Keating EM, Faris PM, Ritter MA, et al. Use of lateral heel and sole wedges in the treatment of medial osteoarthritis of the knee. *Orthop Rev.* 1993;22:921-924.
56. Foster NE, Thomas E, Barlas P, et al. Acupuncture as an adjunct to exercise based physiotherapy for osteoarthritis of the knee: randomised controlled trial. *BMJ.* 2007;335:436.
57. Scharf HP, Mansmann U, Streitberger K, et al. Acupuncture and knee osteoarthritis: a three-armed randomized trial. *Ann Intern Med.* 2006;145:12-20.
58. Berman BM, Singh BB, Lao L, et al. A randomized trial of acupuncture as an adjunctive therapy in osteoarthritis of the knee. *Rheumatology (Oxford).* 1999;38:346-354.
59. Williamson L, Wyatt MR, Yein K, et al. Severe knee osteoarthritis: a randomized controlled trial of acupuncture, physiotherapy (supervised exercise) and standard management for patients awaiting knee replacement. *Rheumatology (Oxford).* 2007;46:1445-1449.
60. Manheimer E, Lim B, Lao L, et al. Acupuncture for knee osteoarthritis—a randomised trial using a novel sham. *Acupunct Med.* 2006;24 suppl:S7-14.
61. Witt CM, Jena S, Brinkhaus B, et al. Acupuncture in patients with osteoarthritis of the knee or hip: a randomized, controlled trial with an additional nonrandomized arm. *Arthritis Rheum.* 2006;54:3485-3493.
62. White A, Foster NE, Cummings M, et al. Acupuncture treatment for chronic knee pain: a systematic review. *Rheum (Oxford).* 2007;46:384-390.
63. Harlow T, Greaves C, White A, et al. Randomised controlled trial of magnetic bracelets for relieving pain in osteoarthritis of the hip and knee. *BMJ.* 2004;329:1450-1454.
64. Pittler MH, Brown EM, Ernst E. Static magnets for reducing pain: systematic review and meta-analysis of randomized trials. *Can Med Assoc J.* 2007;177:736-742.
65. Hochberg MC, Altman RD, Brandt KD, et al. Guidelines for the medical management of osteoarthritis. Part II: Osteoarthritis of the knee. American College of Rheumatology. *Arthritis Rheum.* 1995;38:1541-1546.
66. Jordan KM, Arden NK, Doherty M, et al. EULAR recommendations 2003: an evidence based approach to the management of knee osteoarthritis: report of a task force of the standing committee for international clinical studies including therapeutic trials (ESCISIT). *Ann Rheum Dis.* 2003;62:1145-1155.
67. Gabriel SE, Jaakkimainen L, Bombardier C. Risk for serious gastrointestinal complications related to use of nonsteroidal anti-inflammatory drugs: a meta-analysis. *Ann Intern Med.* 1991;115:787-796.
68. Hippisley-Cox J, Coupland C. Risk of myocardial infarction in patients taking cyclo-oxygenase-2 inhibitors or conventional non-steroidal anti-inflammatory drugs: population based nested case-control analysis. *BMJ.* 2005;330:1366.
69. Graham DJ, Campen D, Hui R, et al. Risk of acute myocardial infarction and sudden cardiac death in patients treated with cyclo-oxygenase 2 selective and

non-selective non-steroidal anti-inflammatory drugs: nested case-control study. *Lancet*. 2005;365:475-481.

70. Johnsen SP, Larsson H, Tarone RE, et al. Risk of hospitalization for myocardial infarction among users of rofecoxib, celecoxib, and other NSAIDs: a population-based case-control study. *Arch Intern Med*. 2005;165:978-984.

71. Helin-Salmivaara A, Virtanen A, Vesalainen R, et al. NSAID use and the risk of hospitalization for first myocardial infarction in the general population: a nationwide case-control study from finland. *Eur Heart J*. 2006;27:1657-1663.

72. Chan AT, Manson JE, Albert CM, et al. Nonsteroidal antiinflammatory drugs, acetaminophen, and the risk of cardiovascular events. *Circulation*. 2006;113: 1578-1587.

73. Jackson DW, Evans NA, Thomas BM. Accuracy of needle placement into the intra-articular space of the knee. *J Bone Joint Surg Am*. 2002;84:1522-1527.

74. Esenyel C, Demirhan M, Esenyel M, et al. Comparison of four different intra-articular injection sites in the knee: a cadaver study. *Knee Surg Sports Traumatol Arthrosc*. 2007;15:573-577.

75. Balazs EA, Denlinger JL. Viscosupplementation: a new concept in the treatment of osteoarthritis. *J Rheumatol Suppl*. 1993;39:3-9.

76. Palacio LE, Vitanzo PC. Viscosupplementation. In: Freedman M, Morrison WB, Harwood MI, eds. *Minimally Invasive Musculoskeletal Pain Medicine*. 1st ed. New York: Informa Healthcare; 2007:53-67.

77. Caborn D, Rush J, Lanzer W, et al. A randomized, single-blind comparison of the efficacy and tolerability of hylan G-F 20 and triamcinolone hexacetonide in patients with osteoarthritis of the knee. *J Rheumatol*. 2004;31:333-343.

78. George E. Intra-articular hyaluronan treatment for osteoarthritis. *Ann Rheum Dis*. 1998;57:637-640.

79. Brandt KD, Smith GN, Jr, Simon LS. Intraarticular injection of hyaluronan as treatment for knee osteoarthritis: what is the evidence? *Arthritis Rheum*. 2000;43:1192-1203.

80. Guidolin DD, Ronchetti IP, Lini E, et al. Morphological analysis of articular cartilage biopsies from a randomized, clinical study comparing the effects of 500-730 kDa sodium hyaluronate (hyalgan) and methylprednisolone acetate on primary osteoarthritis of the knee. *Osteoarthritis Cartilage*. 2001;9:371-381.

81. Moreland LW. Intra-articular hyaluronan (hyaluronic acid) and hylans for the treatment of osteoarthritis: mechanisms of action. *Arthritis Res Ther*. 2003;5:54-67.

82. Bellamy N, Campbell J, Robinson V, et al. Viscosupplementation for the treatment of osteoarthritis of the knee. *Cochrane Database Syst Rev*. 2006;2: CD005321.

83. Recommendations for the medical management of osteoarthritis of the hip and knee: 2000 update. American College of Rheumatology Subcommittee on Osteoarthritis Guidelines. *Arthritis Rheum*. 2000;43: 1905-1915.

84. Torrance GW, Raynauld JP, Walker V, et al. A prospective, randomized, pragmatic, health outcomes trial evaluating the incorporation of hylan G-F 20 into the treatment paradigm for patients with knee osteoarthritis (part 2 of 2): economic results. *Osteoarthritis Cartilage*. 2002;10:518-527.

85. Raynauld JP, Torrance GW, Band PA, et al. A prospective, randomized, pragmatic, health outcomes trial evaluating the incorporation of hylan G-F 20 into the treatment paradigm for patients with knee osteoarthritis (part 1 of 2): clinical results. *Osteoarthritis Cartilage*. 2002;10:506-517.

86. Leopold SS, Warme WJ, Pettis PD, et al. Increased frequency of acute local reaction to intra-articular hylan GF-20 (synvisc) in patients receiving more than one course of treatment. *J Bone Joint Surg Am*. 2002; 84:1619-1623.

87. Ozturk C, Atamaz F, Hepguler S, et al. The safety and efficacy of intraarticular hyaluronan with/without corticosteroid in knee osteoarthritis: 1-year, single-blind, randomized study. *Rheumatol Int*. 2006;26:314-319.

88. Altman RD, Moskowitz R. Intraarticular sodium hyaluronate (hyalgan) in the treatment of patients with osteoarthritis of the knee: a randomized clinical trial. hyalgan study group. *J Rheum*. 1998;25:2203-2212.

89. Huskisson EC, Donnelly S. Hyaluronic acid in the treatment of osteoarthritis of the knee. *Rheumatology (Oxford)*. 1999;38:602-607.

90. Jubb RW, Piva S, Beinat L, et al. A one-year, randomised, placebo (saline) controlled clinical trial of 500-730 kDa sodium hyaluronate (hyalgan) on the radiological change in osteoarthritis of the knee. *Int J Clin Pract*. 2003;57:467-474.

91. Karlsson J, Sjogren LS, Lohmander LS. Comparison of two hyaluronan drugs and placebo in patients with knee osteoarthritis: a controlled, randomized, double-blind, parallel-design multicentre study. *Rheumatology (Oxford)*. 2002;41:1240-1248.

92. Leopold SS, Redd BB, Warme WJ, et al. Corticosteroid compared with hyaluronic acid injections for the treatment of osteoarthritis of the knee: a prospective,

randomized trial. *J Bone Joint Surg Am.* 2003;85: 1197-1203.

93. Wobig M, Bach G, Beks P, et al. The role of elasto-viscosity in the efficacy of viscosupplementation for osteoarthritis of the knee: a comparison of hylan G-F 20 and a lower-molecular-weight hyaluronan. *Clin Ther.* 1999;21:1549-1562.

94. Chevalier X, Jerosch J, Goupille P, et al. Single, intra-articular treatment with 6 ml of hylan G-F 20 in patients with symptomatic primary osteoarthritis of the knee: a randomized, multicentre, double-blind, placebo-controlled trial. *Ann Rheum Dis.* 2010;69(1): 113-119.

95. Sampson S, Reed M, Silvers H, et al. Injection of platelet-rich plasma in patients with primary and secondary knee osteroarthrities—a pilot study. *Am J Phys Med Rehabil.* 2010; 89(12):961-969.

33

NSAIDs, Weight Loss, Bracing, Lateral Heel Wedges, and Physical Therapy for the Treatment of Knee Arthritis: What Does the Evidence Show?

Justin C. Wong and Gregory K. Deirmengian

Osteoarthritis (OA) of the knee is a progressive degenerative joint disease that causes pain and leads to disability and impairment of quality of life. In the United States, the lifetime incidence of symptomatic knee osteoarthritis may be as high as 44.7%, with even higher rates among obese patients (60.5%) and those who have had prior knee injury (56.8%).[1] In its end stage, symptomatic knee osteoarthritis may be definitively treated with total joint arthroplasty. However, this intervention should be undertaken after a patient has failed an adequate trial of nonoperative management. Nonoperative treatment of knee osteoarthritis should be multifaceted and individualized to the patient, with the overarching goals of reducing pain and disability and improving quality of life.[2-5]

Nonoperative treatments for knee osteoarthritis can be categorized into pharmacologic and nonpharmacologic interventions. Pharmacologic interventions, which include acetaminophen, nonsteroidal anti-inflammatory drugs (NSAIDs), steroid injections, and viscosupplementation, should be considered an adjunct to the nonpharmacologic treatments that form the cornerstone of treatment for knee OA. Nonpharmacologic treatments include patient education regarding activity modification, weight loss, bracing, physical therapy, orthoses, and modalities such as ultrasound and transcutaneous electrical stimulation.[3] Although nonpharmacologic interventions are commonly used in clinical practice, patient and physician expectations should be aware that many of these interventions provide only mild to moderate symptomatic improvement. The purpose of this review is to explore the evidence supporting the role of these interventions in the management of knee osteoarthritis.

ACETAMINOPHEN AND NSAIDS

The American College of Rheumatology recommends pharmacologic interventions as an adjunct to nonpharmacologic therapy in patients with osteoarthritis of the knee.[2] Despite evidence demonstrating a lower effect size on pain relief, acetaminophen is often considered as first-line therapy over NSAIDs in patients with mild to moderate disease because it is considered to have less risk of serious gastrointestinal side effects.[2-4,6]

A Cochrane meta-analysis evaluating the use of acetaminophen for osteoarthritis included seven randomized controlled trials comparing acetaminophen to placebo in treatment of knee OA.[7] The median duration of trials was 6 weeks. Five studies showed improvements in pain compared with placebo, whereas two studies found no significant difference. The pooled standardized mean difference in pain between acetaminophen treatment groups and placebo was –0.13 (95% CI, –0.22 to –0.04). The Cochrane meta-analysis also included 12 randomized controlled trials comparing acetaminophen to selective or nonselective NSAIDs in the treatment of knee OA. The authors found that NSAIDs provided a modest improvement in relief of rest pain as measured by the Western Ontario and McMaster Universities Osteoarthritis Index (WOMAC) compared to acetaminophen. Of note, two studies suggested that NSAIDs offer greater pain relief in patients with higher levels of baseline pain compared to acetaminophen.

When evaluating the comparative safety of acetaminophen and NSAIDs, the Cochrane meta-analysis found no statistically significant difference in relative risk of adverse events or relative risk of withdrawing from a study due to adverse event. However, when the authors analyzed gastrointestinal (GI) adverse events and patient withdrawals due to GI events, they found that patients allocated to the nonselective NSAID treatment had a relative risk of withdrawing of 2.0 (95% CI, 1.05–3.81) and a relative risk of GI adverse event of 1.47 (95% CI, 1.08–2.00) compared to patients taking acetaminophen. Patients allocated to selective NSAID treatment had a relative risk of 0.98 (95% CI, 0.80–1.20) for GI adverse event compared to acetaminophen treatment. The authors noted that the short-term follow-up of the included studies might preclude the ability to generalize their safety results to the general population, cautioning that treating physicians should be aware of the potential GI, renal, and cardiovascular toxicities of NSAIDs.

Topical NSAIDs represent an alternate route of drug administration to minimize the potential for systemic side effects. Lin et al conducted a meta-analysis of the efficacy of topical NSAIDs in the treatment of knee osteoarthritis.[8] Thirteen randomized controlled trials, representing 1983 patients, were included. The authors found modest effect sizes on pain relief of 0.41 (95% CI, 0.16–0.66) and 0.40 (95% CI, 0.15–0.65) at weeks 1 and 2 of treatment compared to placebo. However, at weeks 3 and 4, no benefit over placebo was seen. The authors concluded that the evidence could not support long-term use of topical NSAIDs for treatment of knee osteoarthritis. A more recent meta-analysis by Biswal et al re-examined the role of topical NSAIDs and included four randomized controlled trials of topical NSAIDs versus placebo for treatment of knee osteoarthritis.[9] The studies included 709 patients, utilized either diclofenac or eltenac topical medications, and had between 4 and 12 weeks of follow-up. The authors found a pooled effect size on pain of –0.28 (95% CI, –0.42 to –0.14) and concluded that certain preparations of topical NSAIDs may provide long-term pain relief. Given that the main side effect of topical NSAIDs is self-limited skin irritation such as redness, dryness, and pruritus, their use is often considered in patients who have contraindications to use of oral NSAIDs.

WEIGHT LOSS

Modest weight reduction is recommended for overweight patients with symptomatic knee osteoarthritis.[2-5] In a meta-analysis of risk factors for the development of knee osteoarthritis, obesity was linked to the incidence of symptomatic knee osteoarthritis with a pooled odds ratio of 2.63 (95% CI, 2.28–3.05).[10] Although being overweight is correlated with an increased incidence of symptomatic knee osteoarthritis, the association with disease progression is less clear.[11-13] While longitudinal studies have failed to demonstrate altered disease progression after weight loss, gait analysis has revealed that every 1 lb of weight lost is associated with a 4-lb decrease in knee joint load during walking, potentially explaining its effect on reducing knee pain.[14]

Weight reduction may lead to modest improvements in self-reported disability as reported in a meta-analysis of four randomized controlled trials.[15] Based on 454 patients with an average weight reduction of 6 kg, the pooled effect size of weight reduction on physical disability was 0.23 (95% CI, 0.04–0.42). The pooled effect size of weight loss on pain scores was 0.20 (95% CI, 0–0.39). Using meta-regression analysis, the authors found a dose-response correlation between weight reduction and level of disability but not between weight reduction and pain scores. Although the effect of weight reduction on pain could not be reliably predicted, the authors concluded that a minimum 5% reduction in body weight over a 20-week period could lead to patients experiencing symptomatic relief.

One study that was included in the meta-analysis randomized 80 patients to either a low-energy diet or a control diet for an 8-week period. It found that a weight reduction of 10% resulted in a 28% improvement in WOMAC self-reported disability.[16] The number needed to treat to achieve an improvement of 50% or greater in WOMAC scores was 3.4. The authors did not identify a statistically significant effect on pain reduction between groups. When a similar study population was evaluated at 1-year follow-up, the low-energy diet group had maintained an 11% weight reduction and the control group had a 4% weight reduction.[17] Although neither group demonstrated a statistically significant difference from baseline in overall WOMAC scores, the low-energy diet group did experience a statistically significant decrease in pain score, which was not seen in the control group.

The Arthritis, Diet, and Activity Promotion Trial (ADAPT) was a randomized controlled trial evaluating the benefits of weight reduction and exercise, both alone and in combination, on self-reported physical function, as measured by WOMAC, pain, and other measures of mobility.[18] In this study, 316 patients were randomized to diet-only, exercise-only, diet-plus-exercise, or a healthy-lifestyle control group and were followed for 18 months. The exercise groups performed both aerobic and resistance training of the lower extremities. With regard to physical function, only the diet-plus-exercise group demonstrated a statistically significant improvement compared with the healthy-lifestyle control group. The diet-plus-exercise group also demonstrated a statistically significant reduction in pain and improvement in mobility measures, such as the stair climbing and 6-minute walk test, over the control group. The diet-only group, achieved an average 4.9% weight reduction but did not demonstrate a statistically significant improvement over the control group in WOMAC score, mobility measures, and pain. One reason cited for being unable to detect statistical significance in outcomes for the diet-only group relative to the control group is that their healthy-lifestyle control group demonstrated improvement over the course of the study. The authors attributed this finding to their use of an attention-control group as opposed to a no-treatment control. Overall, the authors concluded that a combination of exercise and diet modification provided greater improvement in symptomatic relief of knee osteoarthritis than either intervention alone.

While the evidence shows that weight loss can lead to mild to moderate improvement in physical function, the effect on pain level is less predictable. However, the other health benefits that may be realized by modest weight reduction have helped make it a common recommendation among arthritis-interest groups.[3-5]

PHYSICAL THERAPY

Patient age, pain severity, and quadriceps weakness have all been shown to be predictors of level of disability from knee osteoarthritis.[19] In order to address the role of decreased quadriceps strength on disability, the American College of Rheumatology recommends exercise in the management of osteoarthritis of the knee.[2] Regular exercise, in the form of aerobic conditioning and strength training, has been shown to provide modest improvements in patients' perceived level of disability and pain.[20-25]

Strengthening

Both isometric and dynamic resistance quadriceps-strengthening exercises may improve patients' level of disability and pain. In a randomized controlled trial evaluating the effect of both dynamic resistance and isometric resistance exercises on knee pain and functional tasks, exercise groups showed a 13% to 23% decrease in time to ascend and descend stairs after completing a 16-week training program.[20] A control group that did not undergo formal exercise therapy showed no improvement in performance of the functional tasks. Both exercise groups demonstrated similar levels of improvement in performance of mobility tests. Additionally, patients in both exercise groups had a 28% to 58% reduction in pain relative to their pretraining baseline while performing these tasks.

Supervised exercise sessions that incorporate manual therapy into a home-exercise program have been shown to provide more rapid improvement than home-based exercise alone.[26] In a randomized controlled trial, patients provided with supervised exercises as well as manual therapy twice a week for a period of 4 weeks showed a 52% improvement in WOMAC score compared to a 26% improvement observed in the home-exercise only group. This difference between groups was sustained at 1 month after supervised exercise sessions and manual therapy were completed. However, at 1 year, the WOMAC scores of both groups were equivalent, and both groups maintained a 28% to 32% improvement relative to their baseline. This lends support to the rationale of providing patients with formal physical therapy training when initiating an exercise treatment program.

Aerobic Exercise

Aerobic exercise may be used in conjunction with quadriceps strengthening or as an alternative. Roddy et al conducted a systematic review comparing the efficacy of aerobic exercise and quadriceps-strengthening programs on pain and disability.[27] The review pooled data from 13 randomized controlled trials: 2004 patients participated in a quadriceps-strengthening program and 449 patients were treated with aerobic walking. The home-based strengthening group showed a weighted pooled effect size on pain of 0.34 (95% CI, 0.23–0.42) and a weighted pooled effect size on disability of 0.32 (95% CI, 0.23–0.41). The aerobic walking group showed a weighted pooled effect size on pain of 0.52 (95% CI, 0.34–0.70) and a weighted pooled effect size on disability of 0.46 (95% CI, 0.25–0.67). The authors found no difference in efficacy between aerobic exercise and quadriceps strengthening.

The Fitness Arthritis and Seniors Trial also demonstrated equivalency between aerobic exercise and quadriceps strengthening by comparing aerobic exercise or resistance exercises with a health education control group in a randomized controlled trial.[24] Both training groups were treated with a 3-month facility-based program to ensure patients were performing exercises correctly and then were followed for an additional 15 months with periodic phone calls to encourage maintenance of exercise routine. The study found an 8% to 10% improvement in self-reported disability for both exercise groups relative to the control group. Additionally, both groups demonstrated statistically significant improvements in secondary outcome measures such as the 6-minute walk test. The added benefit for the aerobic exercise group was an improvement in their peak VO_2. An important finding from this study is that when patient outcome was analyzed by level of compliance, the authors found significant improvements in self-reported disability and functional tasks in the patients who were more compliant with their exercises. However, at 18-month follow-up, only 50% of patients were compliant with their exercise program.

Aquatic Therapy

Aquatic therapy is a form of exercise that is performed while the patient is partially immersed in water. The buoyancy of being immersed in water decreases the load observed in the knee joint and the water itself provides resistance to movement. At present, there are few studies that evaluate its effectiveness. A recent Cochrane review that focused on the role of aquatic therapy in the management of hip or knee osteoarthritis found only six randomized controlled studies addressing this issue.[28] The only study focused exclusively on patients with knee osteoarthritis found a statistically significant reduction in pain in patients assigned to 6 weeks of aquatic therapy compared to patients assigned to land-based therapy.[29] There was no functional difference between groups in terms of time for a 1-mile walking test and range of motion.

Since the Cochrane review, two additional randomized controlled trials have compared aquatic therapy and land-based therapy and found partly contradictory results. Lund et al compared aquatic therapy and land-based therapy with a control group and found that only the land-based therapy group had statistically significant improvement in pain scores and lower extremity strength at 3-month follow-up.[30] However, they noted that there was less patient dropout due to adverse effect of exercise in the aquatic therapy group and concluded that, for this reason, aquatic therapy may have a role in combination with land-based exercises. Lim et al conducted a similar study but the patient population was restricted to those with a body mass index greater than 25 kg/m^2.[31] After an 8-week intervention, these authors found significant improvement in WOMAC scores in both the aquatic and land-based therapy groups compared to controls. However, the aquatic therapy group had greater improvement in pain interference scores compared with the land-based therapy and control groups. They concluded that aquatic therapy may be helpful in obese patients, particularly if they have had difficulty with traditional land-based exercise programs.

Overall, the evidence supports the recommendation of exercise as part of the management of knee osteoarthritis. There does not appear to be a discernable difference between aerobic exercise and quadriceps-strengthening programs. The interventions may be used alone or in combination for patients suffering from knee arthritis. It should be realized that achieving long-term compliance in this patient population is difficult and physicians may have to reinforce the treatment plan for patients. It is important to note that aquatic-based therapy may play a role in the initial exercise prescription, in particular for patients who have demonstrated exacerbation of their knee pain with traditional exercise regimens.

Modalities (Transcutaneous Electrical Nerve Stimulation, Ultrasound)

Although modalities such as transcutaneous electrical nerve stimulation (TENS) and therapeutic ultrasound were not part of the clinical recommendations of the consensus guidelines of the American College of Rheumatology or American Academy of Orthopaedic Surgeons, they are commonly used in the physiotherapy setting.[2,5] TENS is believed to affect pain sensation by stimulating large fiber sensory afferent nerves that in turn activate inhibitory interneurons that modulate transmission of nociceptive neurons.[32] Although, the in vivo effects of therapeutic ultrasound are debated, it is believed that high-frequency sound waves can produce thermal and nonthermal effects in the tissue with the goal of reducing inflammation.

The authors of a recent Cochrane meta-analysis on the utility of TENS included data from 18 trials, which were considered to have low methodological quality.[32] They found a standardized mean difference (SMD) in pain intensity of –0.07 (95% CI, –0.46 to 0.32), corresponding to a difference of 0.2 cm on a 10-cm visual analog scale (VAS) scale.[32] With regard to function, they found a SMD of –0.34 (95% CI, –0.54 to –0.14), which they correlated to a 0.7-unit difference on a WOMAC disability scale ranging from 0 to 10. Overall, the authors concluded that there was a lack of quality evidence to support use of TENS.

The most recent Cochrane meta-analysis on the efficacy of therapeutic ultrasound, which included data from five small randomized controlled trials, showed that therapeutic ultrasound may improve pain and physical function in patients with knee osteoarthritis.[33] The pooled data of 320 patients and 464 knees showed a standardized mean difference in pain between ultrasound and control groups of –0.49 (95% CI, –0.76 to –0.23), which translates to 1.2 cm on a 10-cm VAS pain scale. Four of the five studies (242 patients) were pooled for the effect of ultrasound on function. The SMD of –0.64 (95% CI, –1.42 to 0.14) translated into 1.3 units on a standardized WOMAC disability scale ranging from 0 to 10. However, because of the small size and low methodological quality of the included studies, the authors felt that current data on the utility of therapeutic ultrasound for knee osteoarthritis was inconclusive.

BRACING

The aim of bracing in knee osteoarthritis is to mechanically alter the stresses that occur across the tibiofemoral or patellofemoral joint in order to improve function and decrease pain. The most common types of braces used are patellar sleeves and unloader braces. Patellar sleeves are designed to exert a medially directed force on the patella in an effort to unload the lateral femoral trochlea (Fig. 33-1).[34] Unloader braces are bulkier hinged devices that are fastened to the thigh and leg with a hinge incorporated at the knee joint (Fig. 33-2). Unloader braces are used primarily for

A

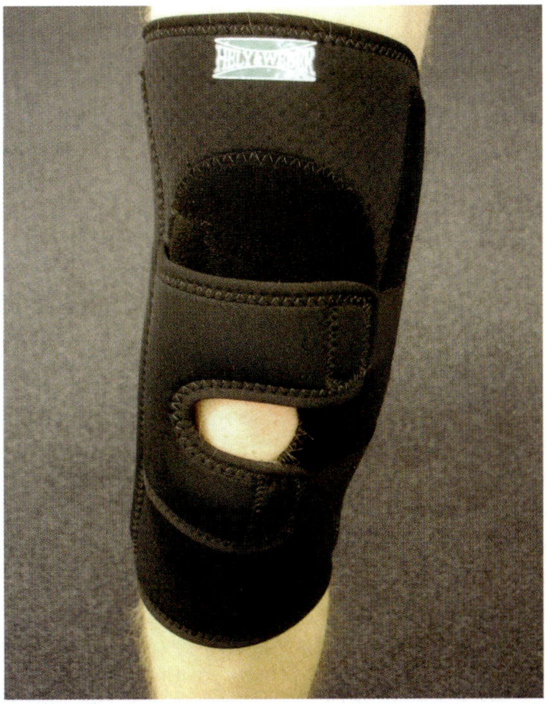

B

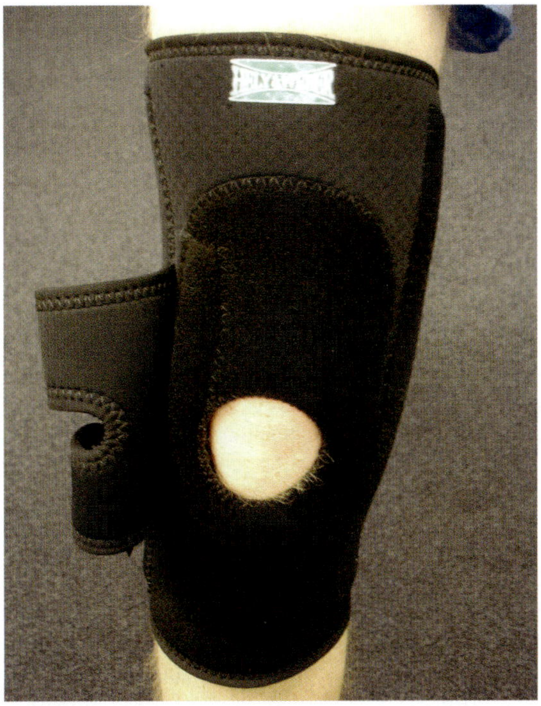

FIGURE 33-1. *Patellar sleeve. This sleeve incorporates a J-shaped buttress of padding that resists lateral patellar translation during knee range of motion: (**A**) strapped as it would be worn; (**B**) unstrapped to reveal J-shaped buttress.*

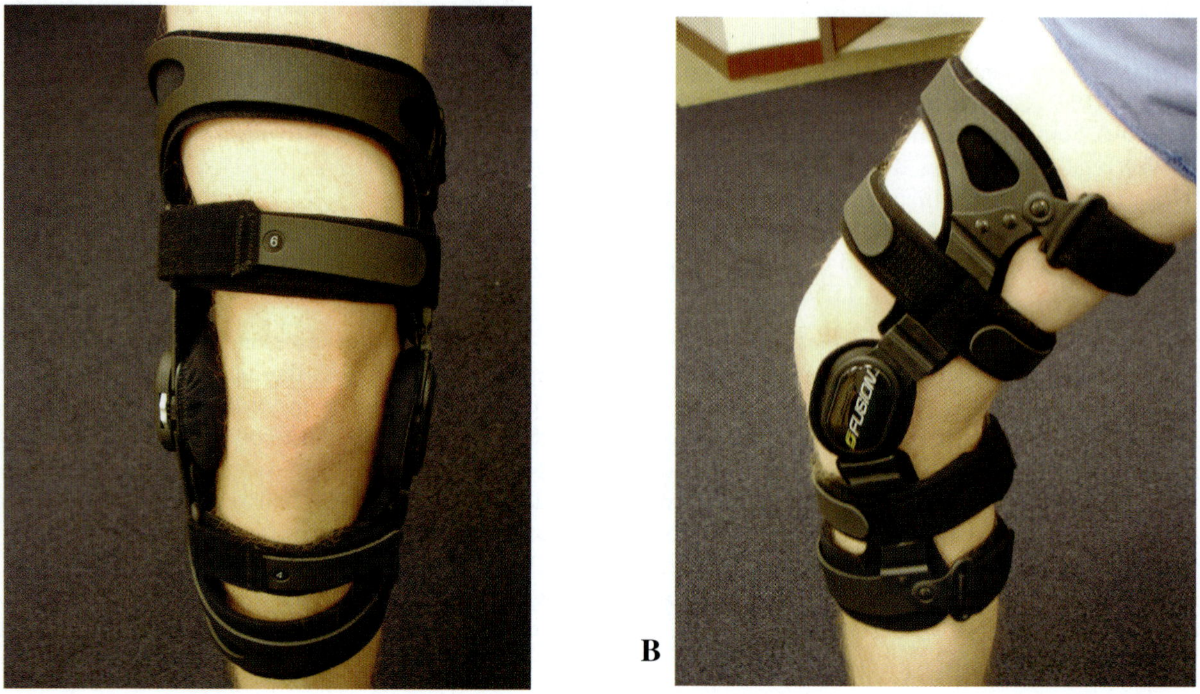

A B

FIGURE 33-2. *Valgus unloader brace. Front (**A**) and side (**B**) views. This device fits snugly to the thigh and leg with an adjustable fulcrum centered at the knee level. Through three-point fixation, the brace exerts a valgus stress on the knee.*

patients with unilateral tibiofemoral arthritis in which one proposed mechanism of action is to apply a valgus or varus stress across the knee and unload either the medial or lateral tibiofemoral compartment, respectively. Fluoroscopic analysis of patients with medial compartment joint space narrowing has shown that an average of 2 mm of condylar separation can be achieved with a properly fit brace, which also correlated with subjective improvements in knee discomfort.[35] An alternative explanation is centered on the concept that muscular contractions help to stabilize the arthritic knee but lead to higher joint reaction forces; external bracing improves the mechanical stability of the knee and allows for less muscular contractions and decreased joint reaction forces.[36]

Using gait analysis on a group of 11 patients with medial knee arthritis compared with healthy controls, Lindenfield et al demonstrated that knees with medial tibiofemoral arthritis were subjected to an increased adduction moment of the knee during the load-bearing stance phase compared with nonarthritic knees.[37] With use of a valgus-unloader brace, an average 10% reduction in the adduction moment was achieved, restoring the adduction moment to a more normal level. In this study, the use of the brace also resulted in a 48% decrease in pain and 69% increase in activity level. With gait analysis and an instrumented valgus brace, Pollo et al were able to quantify the amount of joint unloading that occurs in braced versus nonbraced conditions.[38] They found 11% and 17% decreases in the medial joint compartment load compared with no brace, when braces were set at 4° and 8° of valgus, respectively. Functionally, patients using a knee unloader brace return to a more normal pattern of walking, as determined by Draper et al with use of gait symmetry analysis.[39]

Larger, prospective, randomized controlled trials support the clinical improvements in pain and function observed in the previously mentioned biomechanical studies. Kirkley et al conducted a study of 119 patients with medial knee osteoarthritis randomized to either standard medical management without formal physical therapy, use of a neoprene sleeve, or an custom-molded unloader brace.[40] At 6-month follow-up, both the knee sleeve and unloader brace groups reported greater improvement from baseline in quality of life and function than the control group. The bracing groups also experienced a reduction in pain compared to baseline when performing mobility trials of 6-minute walk and 30-second stair climb, which was not observed in the control group. Between bracing groups, the unloader brace demonstrated statistically significant improvements in pain reduction with physical activity over the neoprene sleeve group. Additionally, the authors found a strong trend toward statistical significance that the unloader brace provided greater improvement than the neoprene sleeve in aggregate and functional WOMAC scores.

Brouwer et al performed a randomized controlled trial involving 117 patients with either medial or lateral knee osteoarthritis to determine the additive benefit of using an off-the-shelf unloader brace over other conservative measures of patient education, physical therapy, and analgesics.[41] The authors found small improvements in VAS pain score and Hospital for Special Surgery (HSS) knee scores at 3, 6, and 12-month follow-up, but these differences were not statistically significant with two-sided statistical analysis. The authors stated that the differences would have been statistically significant had one-sided statistical analysis been utilized, which would be in keeping with the belief that the use of a brace in addition to other conservative measures would confer a benefit. Analgesic use was also found to be lower in the brace group at each follow-up evaluation. Overall walking distance was also improved in the brace group compared with the control. Subgroup analysis found that bracing effects were greater for patients treated with a valgus brace for medial compartment disease compared with patients treated with a varus brace for lateral compartment disease. The authors concluded that bracing may confer some additive benefit for patients with varus knee alignment and unicompartmental disease, but they also found low patient compliance with bracing as 25 of 60 patients stopped using the brace during the study period.

One potential limitation to the study by Brouwer et al is that their bracing group utilized an off-the-shelf unloader available in only four sizes as opposed to a custom-molded brace, potentially decreasing the improvement seen with bracing. A study comparing custom-molded braces with off-the-shelf braces found that custom-molded braces provided better varus correction than an off-the-shelf brace.[42] This correlated with a statistically significant improvement in reported pain and stiffness when a custom-molded brace was utilized compared to baseline.

As mentioned previously, Kirkley et al found small improvements in quality of life and function with use of a neoprene sleeve, even though neoprene sleeves do not confer any structural stability to the knee.[40] Hunter et al conducted a randomized crossover trial to evaluate the effectiveness of a patellofemoral strap in addition to a neoprene joint sleeve for patients with lateral patellofemoral osteoarthritis.[43] The study was specifically designed to determine if the use of a patellar realigning strap, which applies a medially directed force on the patella, would provide a benefit. Despite being adequately powered, the study was unable to find a statistically significant improvement in VAS pain scores or WOMAC scores when the realigning strap was utilized.

Overall, the evidence provides some support for the use of unloader braces for unicompartmental tibiofemoral knee osteoarthritis. However, there is less evidence to support the use of neoprene sleeves in the treatment of knee osteoarthritis. Physicians should be aware that long-term compliance with brace use is low.

LATERAL HEEL WEDGE

Laterally elevated heel insoles or wedges have been designed to treat patients with predominantly medial tibiofemoral osteoarthritis. Evaluation of static lower extremity alignment when utilizing a lateral heel wedge has shown that the subtalar joint is positioned in valgus with compensatory lower extremity and postural changes that cause the mechanical axis of the leg to be more vertical, potentially causing decreased joint loading of the medial compartment.[44] A study evaluating the dynamic effect of a heel wedge during heel strike showed that it has the ability to reduce the varus thrust of the knee that is common in patients with medial compartment disease.[45]

When an elastic subtalar strap is used in conjunction with the heel wedge, subtalar motion is reduced and the heel wedge exerts its effect by altering the femoral-tibial axis and unloading the medial compartment, with greater improvements in pain relief than that observed in heel wedges without a subtalar strap.[46-48] Toda et al conducted a randomized controlled trial of patients assigned to use of a lateral heel wedge either with or without a subtalar strap. At 6-month and 2-year follow up, patients utilizing the heel wedge with subtalar strap demonstrated an improvement in their Lequesne index compared to baseline as opposed to no improvement in the patients without subtalar strapping. However, over 20% of patients withdrew from the study at the 6-month mark as a result of concerns of ineffectiveness and necessity of altered footwear when using the heel wedges.

Despite the encouraging findings of improved pain relief seen in biomechanical studies, larger randomized controlled trials have not demonstrated improvements in pain scores when lateral heel wedges were compared to a neutral wedge control group at 6-month and 2-year follow-up.[49,50] It should be noted that the lateral heel wedge utilized in these studies did not incorporate a subtalar strap, which may have affected the biomechanics of the lateral heel wedge. However, the authors did find a statistically significant decline in the reported usage of NSAIDs at 6-month and 2-year follow-up in patients in the lateral heel wedge group compared to controls. While the evidence to support the use of lateral heel wedges is limited, the possibility that patients may utilize less pain medication with orthotic use has led to the recommendation that lateral heel wedges be tried in some patients with medial knee osteoarthritis.[2,3,51]

SUMMARY

Symptomatic knee osteoarthritis may have a dramatic effect on patient quality of life. Although the disease is characterized by progressive deterioration and may ultimately require treatment by knee arthroplasty, several nonoperative treatments are available to the patient and physician. In the properly selected patient, there is a role for pharmacologic interventions such as acetaminophen and oral or topical NSAIDs. Patients should also be counseled on nonpharmacologic interventions such as modest weight reduction and exercise therapy. Some patients may benefit from use of knee sleeves, braces, and lateral heel wedges. Overall, the long-term management of knee osteoarthritis should be multimodal and requires the concerted efforts of both the patient and physician to achieve the best results.

REFERENCES

1. Murphy L, Schwartz TA, Helmick CG, et al. Lifetime risk of symptomatic knee osteoarthritis. *Arthritis Rheum.* 2008;59(9):1207-1213.
2. American College of Rheumatology Subcommittee on Osteoarthritis Guidelines. Recommendations for the medical management of osteoarthritis of the hip and knee: 2000 update. *Arthritis Rheum.* 2000;43(9): 1905-1915.
3. Zhang W, Moskowitz RW, Nuki G, et al. OARSI recommendations for the management of hip and knee osteoarthritis, Part II: OARSI evidence-based, expert consensus guidelines. *Osteoarthritis Cartilage.* 2008; 16(2):137-162.
4. Zhang W, Nuki G, Moskowitz RW, et al. OARSI recommendations for the management of hip and knee osteoarthritis, Part III: changes in evidence following systematic cumulative update research through January 2009. *Osteoarthritis Cartilage.* 2010;18(4):476-499.
5. Richmond J, Hunter D, Irrgang J. Treatment of osteoarthritis of the knee (Nonarthroplasty) *J Am Acad Orthop Surg.* 2009;17(9):591-600.
6. Zhang W, Jones A, Doherty M. Does paracetamol (acetaminophen) reduce the pain of osteoarthritis?: a meta-analysis of randomised controlled trials. *Ann Rheum Dis.* 2004;63:901-907.
7. Towheed T, Maxwell L, Judd M, et al. Acetaminophen for osteoarthritis (Review). *Cochrane Database Syst Rev.* 2006;1:CD004257.
8. Lin J, Zhang W, Jones A, et al. Efficacy of topical non-steroidal anti-inflammatory drugs in the treatment of osteoarthritis: meta-analysis of randomised controlled trials. *BMJ.* 2004:329(7461):324.
9. Biswal S, Medhi B, Pandhi P. Longterm efficacy of topical nonsteroidal antiinflammatory drugs in knee osteoarthritis: meta-analysis of randomized placebo controlled clinical trials. *J Rheumatol.* 2006;33(9): 1841-1844.
10. Blagjovec M, Jinks C, Jeffery A, et al. Risk factors for onset of osteoarthritis of the knee in older adults: a systematic review and meta-analysis. *Osteoarthritis Cartilage.* 2010;18(1):24-33.
11. Niu J, Zhang YQ, Torner J, et al. Is obesity a risk factor for progressive radiographic knee osteoarthritis? *Arthritis Rheum.* 2009;61(3):329-335.
12. Dieppe P, Cushnaghan J, Tucker M, et al. The Bristol 'OA500 study': progression and impact of the disease after 8 years. *Osteoarthritis Cartilage.* 2000;8(2):63-68.
13. Felson DT, Goggins J, Niu J, et al. The effect of body weight on progression of knee osteoarthritis is dependent on alignment. *Arthritis Rheum.* 2004;50(12): 3904-3909.
14. Messier SP, Gutenkust DJ, Davis C, et al. Weight loss reduces knee-joint loads in overweight and obese older adults with knee osteoarthritis. *Arthritis Rheum.* 2005;52(7):2026-2032.
15. Christensen R, Bartels EM, Astrup A, et al. Effect of weight reduction in obese patients diagnosed with knee osteoarthritis: a systematic review and meta-analysis. *Ann Rheum Dis.* 2007;66:433-439.
16. Christensen R, Astrup A, Bliddal H. Weight loss: the treatment of choice for knee osteoarthritis? A randomized trial. *Osteoarthritis Cartilage.* 2005;13(1): 20-27.
17. Bliddal H, Leeds AR, Stigsgaard L, et al. Weight loss as treatment for knee osteoarthritis symptoms in obese patients: 1-year results from a randomised controlled trial. *Ann Rheum Dis.* 2011;70(10):1798-1803.

18. Messier SP, Loeser RF, Miller GD, et al. Exercise and dietary weight loss in overweight and obese older adults with knee osteoarthritis: the Arthritis, Diet, and Activity Promotion Trial. *Arthritis Rheum.* 2004;50(5):1501-1510.
19. McAlindon TE, Cooper C, Kirwan JR, et al. Determinants of disability in osteoarthritis of the knee. *Ann Rheum Dis.* 1993;52(4):258-262.
20. Topp R, Woolley S, Hornyak J, et al. The effect of dynamic versus isometric resistance training on pain and functioning among adults with osteoarthritis of the knee. *Arch Phys Med Rehabil.* 2002;83(9):1187-1195.
21. Baker KR, Nelson ME, Felson DT, et al. The efficacy of home based progressive strength training in older adults with knee osteoarthritis: a randomized controlled trial. *J Rheumatol.* 2001;28(7):1655-1665.
22. Thomas KS, Muir KR, Doherty M, et al. Home based exercise programme for knee pain and osteoarthritis: a randomised controlled trial. *BMJ.* 2002;325(7367): 752.
23. O'Reilly SC, Muir KR, Doherty M. Effectiveness of home exercise on pain and disability from osteoarthritis of the knee: a randomised controlled trial. *Ann Rheum Dis.* 1999;58(1):15-19.
24. Ettinger WH Jr, Burns R, Messier SP, et al. A randomized trial comparing aerobic exercise and resistance exercise with a health education program in older adults with knee osteoarthritis: The Fitness Arthritis and Seniors Trial (FAST). *JAMA.* 1997;277(1):25-31.
25. Deyle GD, Henderson NE, Matekel RL, et al. Effectiveness of manual physical therapy and exercise in osteoarthritis of the knee: a randomized, controlled trial. *Ann Intern Med.* 2000;132(3):173-181.
26. Deyle GD, Allison SC, Matekel RL, et al. Physical therapy treatment effectiveness for osteoarthritis of the knee: a randomized comparison of supervised clinical exercise and manual therapy procedures versus a home exercise program. *Phys Ther.* 2005;85(12):1301-1317.
27. Roddy E, Zhang W, Doherty M. Aerobic walking or strengthening exercise for osteoarthritis of the knee? A systematic review. *Ann Rheum Dis.* 2005;64(4): 544-548.
28. Bartels EM, Lund H, Hagen KB, et al. Aquatic exercise for the treatment of knee and hip osteoarthritis. *Cochrane Database Syst Rev.* 2007;4:CD005523.
29. Wyatt FB, Milam S, Manske RC, et al. The effects of aquatic and traditional exercise programs on persons with knee osteoarthritis. *J Strength Cond Res.* 2001: 15(3):337-340.
30. Lund H, Weile U, Christensen R, et al. A randomized controlled trial of aquatic and land-based exercise in patients with knee osteoarthritis. *J Rehabil Med.* 2008:40(2):137-144.
31. Lim JY, Tchai E, Jang SN. Effectiveness of aquatic exercise for obese patients with knee osteoarthritis: a randomized controlled trial. *PM R.* 2010:2(8):723-731.
32. Rutjes AW, Nüesch E, Sterchi R, et al. Transcutaneous electrostimulation for osteoarthritis of the knee. *Cochrane Database Syst Rev.* 2009;4:CD002823.
33. Rutjes AW, Nüesch E, Sterchi R, et al. Therapeutic ultrasound for osteoarthritis of the knee or hip. *Cochrane Database Syst Rev.* 2010;1:CD003132.
34. McWalter EJ, Hunter DJ, Harvey WF, et al. The effect of a patellar brace on three-dimensional patellar kinematics in patients with lateral patellofemoral osteoarthritis. *Osteoarthritis Cartilage.* 2011;19(7): 801-808.
35. Komistek RD, Dennis DA, Northcut EJ, et al. An in vivo analysis of the effectiveness of the osteoarthritic knee brace during heel-strike of gait. *J Arthroplasty.* 1999;14(6):738-742.
36. Ramsey DK, Briem K, Axe MJ, et al. A mechanical theory for the effectiveness of bracing for medial compartment osteoarthritis of the knee. *J Bone Joint Surg Am.* 2007;89(11):2398-2407.
37. Lindenfield TN, Hewett TE, Andiracchi TP. Joint loading with valgus bracing in patients with varus gonarthrosis. *Clin Orthop Relat Res.* 1997;344:290-297.
38. Pollo FE, Otis JC, Backus SI, et al. Reduction of medial compartment loads with valgus bracing of the osteoarthritis knee. *Am J Sports Med.* 2002;30(3): 414-421.
39. Draper ER, Cable JM, Sanchez-Ballester J, et al. Improvement in function after valgus bracing of the knee: an analysis of gait symmetry. *J Bone Joint Surg Br.* 2000;82(7):1001-1005.
40. Kirkley A, Webster-Bogaert S, Litchfield R, et al. The effect of bracing on varus gonarthrosis. *J Bone Joint Surg Am.* 1999;81(4):539-548.
41. Brouwer RW, van Raaij TM, Verhaar JA, et al. Brace treatment for osteoarthritis of the knee: a prospective randomized multi-centre trial. *Osteoarthritis Cartilage.* 2006;14(8):777-783.
42. Draganich L, Reider B, Rimington T, et al. The effectiveness of self-adjustable custom and off-the-shelf bracing in the treatment of varus gonarthrosis. *J Bone Joint Surg Am.* 2006;88(12):2645-2652.
43. Hunter DJ, Harvey W, Gross KD, et al. A randomized trial of patellofemoral bracing for treatment of

patellofemoral osteoarthritis. *Ostearthritis Cartilage*. 2011;19(7):792-800.

44. Yasuda K, Sasaki T. The mechanics of treatment of the osteoarthritic knee with a wedged sole. *Clin Orthop Relat Res*. 1987;215:162-172.

45. Ogata K, Yasunaga M, Nomiyama H. The effect of wedged insoled on the thrust of osteoarthritis knees. *Int Orthop*. 1997;21(5):308-312.

46. Toda Y, Segal N, Kato A, et al. Effect of a novel insole on the subtalar joint of patients with medial compartment osteoarthritis of the knee. *J Rheumatol* 2001;28 (12):2705-2710.

47. Toda Y, Segal N. Usefulness of an insole with subtalar strapping for analgesia in patients with medical compartment osteoarthritis of the knee. *Arthritis Rheum*. 2002;47(5):468-473.

48. Toda Y, Tsukimura N. A 2-year follow-up of a study to compare the efficacy of lateral wedged insoles with subtalar strapping and in-shoe lateral wedged insoles in patients with varus deformity of osteoarthritis of the knee. *Osteoarthritis Cartilage*. 2006;14(3):231-237.

49. Maillefert JF, Hudry C, Baron G, et al. Laterally elevated wedged insoles in the treatment of medial knee osteoarthritis: a prospective randomized controlled trial. *Osteoarthritis Cartilage*. 2001;9(8):738-745.

50. Pham T, Maillefert JF, Hudry C, et al. Laterally elevated wedged insoles in the treatment of medial knee osteoarthritis: a two-year prospective randomized controlled study. *Osteoarthritis Cartilage*. 2004;12(1):46-55.

51. Brouwer RW, van Raaij TM, Jakma TT, et al. Bracing and orthoses for treating osteoarthritis of the knee (Review). *Cochrane Database Syst Rev*. 2005; 1:CD004020.

34 Knee Arthroscopy

Christopher C. Dodson and Michael G. Ciccotti

Knee arthroscopy is the most common procedure in orthopaedic surgery. More than 600,000 knee arthroscopies are performed annually.[1] Knee arthroscopy was originally developed as a diagnostic tool; while improvements in imaging techniques, most notably magnetic resonance imaging (MRI), has decreased the incidence of diagnostic arthroscopy, advances in arthroscopic equipment and our understanding of knee pathologies have led to an increase in the incidence and complexity of arthroscopic procedures. The most common current indications include the treatment of meniscal pathology, loose bodies, cruciate ligament reconstruction, articular cartilage procedures, patella malalignment, and assistance in intra-articular fractures.

Arthroscopic surgery demands clear visualization of all the anatomic structures and pathologic conditions with limited incisions. Adjunctive aspects to surgery, such as the use of fluids, tourniquets, leg holders, types of arthroscopes, and other instruments, must be understood before the undertaking of the actual operative procedure. Careful attention to the basic details of these aspects of arthroscopy will lead to a successful result. This chapter reviews our technique for knee arthroscopy, including basic setup, equipment, and surgical technique.

PREOPERATIVE EVALUATION

History and Physical Examination

The clinical examination of the knee begins with a thorough history that focuses on the presenting symptoms and mechanism of injury. The location and quality of pain should be ascertained as well as any previous injuries or history of surgery in the affected knee. It is important to inquire about any swelling, instability, or mechanical symptoms. Mechanical symptoms may include locking, catching, or the sensation that the knee gets "stuck" in certain positions. Also the patient should be asked about any activities that exacerbate or alleviate the symptoms. In many cases, a diagnosis can be made by history alone. For example, a young athlete who felt a "pop" in his or her knee during athletic performance almost certainly has suffered an anterior cruciate ligament (ACL) tear.

The patient's gait pattern should be inspected first. An antalgic gait is demonstrated by a shortened stance phase and is common in acute injuries of the knee. While the patient is standing, we then observe the overall alignment of the extremity for genu varus or valgus. We then begin with the least painful tests before progressing to the more painful component of the examination.

A thorough examination of the knee involves a systematic approach. In order to gain the trust and confidence of the patient, we usually begin by examining the noninjured knee first. This helps the patient relax and also serves as a baseline for what is normal for the individual patient.

Physical examination of the knee begins with inspection for any soft tissue swelling or obvious ecchymosis. Intra-articular swelling or fluid signifies an injury to the joint itself. Range of motion is then measured. Both knees should always be measured because asymmetry may be a sign of injury. A knee that cannot completely straighten (ie, a "locked knee") is usually secondary to a mechanical block from a bucket-handle tear of the meniscus or a loose body. We then begin palpation of the knee, initially focusing away from the maximal point of pain and gradually progressing toward it. All bony landmarks should be palpated for tenderness. These include the patella, medial and lateral femoral condyle, and the tibial tubercle. Additionally the medial and lateral joint line should be palpated; a tender joint line may be significant for a meniscal tear. Other common sites of tenderness include the iliotibial band, pes anserine bursa, and the patellar tendon. Once the knee is palpated, in patients who can tolerate it, we proceed with the examination of specific ligaments. The various tests for each ligament is beyond the scope of this chapter, but our routine physical examination consists of testing for varus/valgus stability at 0° and 30°, the anterior and posterior drawer, the Lachman testing, and the dial test prone at 30° and 90°. Last, we routinely axially load the knee from extension to flexion while internally and externally rotating the knee. Pain during this maneuver can be elicited secondary to a medial or lateral meniscal tear.

Imaging

We routinely obtain standing anteroposterior (AP), lateral, and Merchant view radiographs for all patients who undergo a knee evaluation. If intra-articular pathology is suspected, we obtain a noncontrast MRI. Focus points of the MRI include the medial and lateral menisci, the collateral and cruciate ligaments, and the articular cartilage in the medial, lateral, and patellofemoral compartments.

EQUIPMENT

Knee arthroscopy requires the use of basic instrumentation for all procedures. Typically a 30° arthroscope is used, but sometimes a 70° scope can be helpful during certain procedures. The remaining necessary equipment includes a light source, camera head, and video system that are connected to the arthroscope. This allows the surgeon to visualize on a monitor the intra-articular compartments of the knee. Pictures can be taken by the surgeon by often pressing a button on the arthroscope itself and can either be saved to a disk or printed to paper. A motorized shaver system and handheld instruments are the basic tools used during arthroscopy, although as technology has advanced, a variety of instruments have been designed for specific procedures. Electrothermal devices are very useful during procedures in which hemostasis is vital.

Like all arthroscopic procedures, knee arthroscopy is performed in a fluid environment. A fluid management system or "pump" is necessary to maintain joint distension, which allows for visualization of the intra-articular knee anatomy. We believe that it is paramount for the surgeon to have an intricate working knowledge of the particular pump that they use because poor "pump management" will no doubt lead to an obscured intraoperative visualization, excessive swelling, and poor outcomes. Current systems allow for the surgeon to select a desired flow rate and pump pressure.

ANESTHESIA

Arthroscopic knee surgery can be performed under general, regional, or local anesthesia. Factors to be considered include length of the surgery, the invasiveness of the procedure, and surgeon preference. We generally perform basic knee arthroscopy under general anesthesia and more invasive procedures, such as cruciate ligament reconstruction, under general anesthesia plus regional nerve block (eg, femoral nerve block). We have found this approach to be optimal since more invasive surgical procedures involve using a tourniquet for hemostasis and may involve using multiple incisions; both factors make regional anesthesia ideal for postoperative pain control. We have a limited experience performing knee arthroscopy under local anesthesia and generally limit such cases to patients who have significant medical comorbidities.[2]

SURGICAL TECHNIQUE

Preparation

Like all surgical procedures, the first step is to correctly identify the patient in the preoperative holding area and sign the surgical sight in compliance with current patient safety protocols.[3] We routinely administer broad-spectrum antibiotics covering *Staphylococcus* and *Streptococcus* organisms approximately 30 minutes before surgery. Before positioning, an examination under anesthesia is performed. This step is crucial, particularly during cases of ligamentous injuries, in order to document the degree and severity of instability.

Positioning

The patient is placed supine on the operating room table with a tourniquet placed around the thigh. The tourniquet should be placed as proximal as possible on the thigh to allow for optimal exposure of the surgical site. The decision to use or not use a tourniquet is completely surgeon's preference. Advances in pump technology that allow the surgeon to precisely control intra-articular pressure and flow rate make it possible to perform even somewhat complex arthroscopic procedures without a tourniquet raised. Some studies have shown the detrimental effects of tourniquet use[4-6] and, although rare, the surgeon would weigh these risks against the benefits, which include improved visualization, decreased blood loss, and reduced operative time. Regardless of whether or not tourniquet use is anticipated, one should always be applied in case its unexpected use is necessitated.

Some surgeons have advocated dropping the foot of the table, but we prefer to keep the table elevated and simply flex the leg off the side of the table before incision is made. To aid in the manipulation of the knee in order to help visualize the intra-articular components, either a leg holder (Fig. 34-1) or a lateral post (Fig. 34-2) can be applied. Both positioners have advantages and disadvantages and their use is almost exclusively surgeon preference and experience. The nonoperative leg is well padded and kept in extension throughout the entire procedure. It is crucial that both extremities are adequately positioned to avoid abnormal pressure that could result in neurovascular injury.

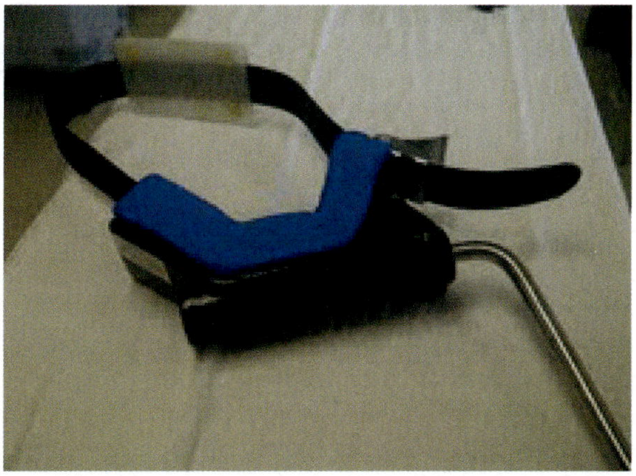

FIGURE 34-1. *An example of an arthroscopic leg holder used during knee arthroscopy. The leg holder is positioned just below the thigh and the strap can be tightened to apply extension and valgus for the medial compartment. For figure-of-four position, the strap is simply loosened.*

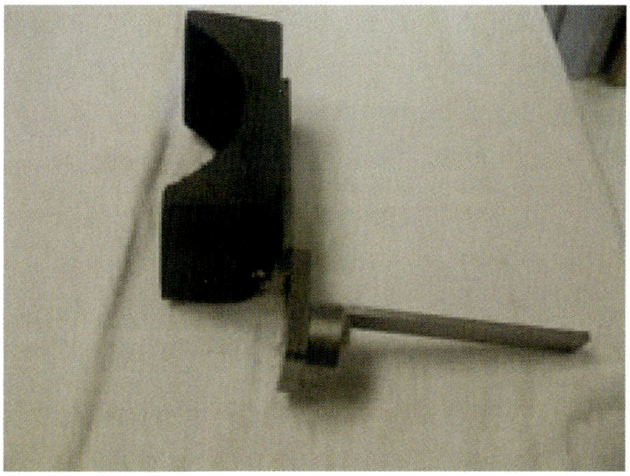

FIGURE 34-2. *Lateral post used for knee arthroscopy. The post allows for a valgus load during medial compartment evaluation. For lateral compartment evaluation, the post can be simply dropped.*

Landmarks

Anatomic landmarks and incision placement should be palpated and marked before starting the case. Using standard landmarks that can be consistently palpated and marked is helpful because after the knee is distended the anatomy is often altered and makes palpation difficult. The standard landmarks we use include the inferior pole of the patella, the medial and lateral edges of the patella tendon, and the medial and lateral joint line.

The anterolateral and anteromedial portals are then marked (Fig. 34-3). The anterolateral portal is created adjacent to the inferior pole of the patella, just lateral to the patella tendon and approximately 1 cm above the joint line. The anteromedial portal is considered the working portal of arthroscopic knee surgery and is located in a similar position medial to the patellar tendon and 5 mm above the joint line. Since this portal is so vital to the success of the surgical procedure, we will often make this portal after using a spinal needle to ensure optimal placement.

Some surgeons will add a third portal either superomedially or superolaterally to aid in arthroscopic visualization and to reduce fluid extravasation (Fig. 34-4). The portals can be created before insertion of the arthroscope, but we recommend creating them intraoperatively under direct visualization using a spinal needle for localization. Similarly, when access to the posterior compartment of the knee is necessary [eg, posterior cruciate ligament (PCL) reconstruction, loose body removal, meniscal repair], the posterior portals are created intraoperatively using previously marked landmarks and transillumination with the arthroscope.

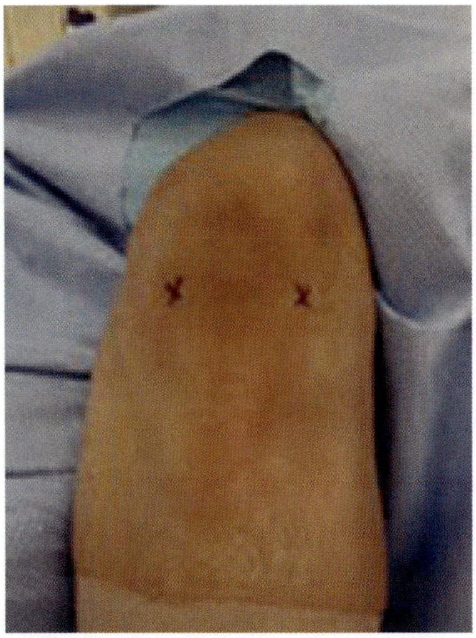

FIGURE 34-3. *Intraoperative photo of a left knee draped for the arthroscopy. The "X's" mark the anterolateral and anteromedial portal sites.*

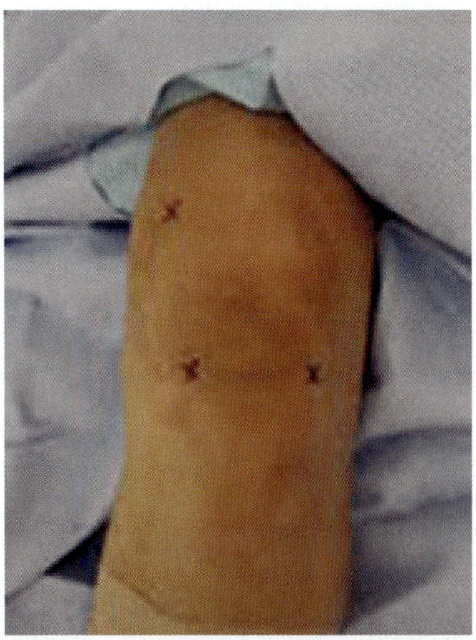

FIGURE 34-4. *Alternatively, a three-portal technique can be used. In this case, a superomedial portal is marked for outflow.*

Incision

After the patient is appropriately positioned, prepped, and draped, we begin arthroscopy with establishment of the anterolateral portal. Using a No. 11 blade, vertical or horizontal incisions can be made directed into the notch, with the knee in a flexed position. It is important that the incision is large enough to accommodate the arthroscope. We prefer to initiate the incision with the blade facing down to cut the skin and then, with the blade facing up to avoid accidentally cutting the meniscus, the incision is carried through the capsular tissue and into the notch. Although some authors have recommended lowering the handle of the blade once inside the knee joint to allow for release of the underlying fat pad, we have cautioned against teaching this technique because we have seen iatrogenic injury to the underlying articular cartilage.

Using a blunt obturator, the arthroscopic cannula is then inserted directly into the notch with the knee in a flexed position. The scope should enter easily and, if resistance is felt, the scope should be removed and the landmarks should be confirmed so that iatrogenic injury can be avoided. Once the cannula has passed easily into the notch, it is surgeon preference as to whether the cannula is advanced into the medial compartment with the knee flexed or whether the knee is brought into full extension and the arthroscope is directed under the patella into the suprapatellar pouch. When a two-portal technique is used, we advocate going directly into the medial compartment so that the anteromedial portal can be established, which aids in visualization. If a three-portal technique is used, then the cannula is advanced into the suprapatellar pouch where a superomedial or superolateral portal can be established directly under spinal needle localization.

Patellofemoral Compartment

Once in the patellofemoral compartment, the patella and trochlea should be inspected for any articular cartilage injuries (Fig. 34-5). The location and degree of articular cartilage injury should be noted for later dictation in the operative note. In cases of malalignment, the subluxation and tilt of the patella should be noted before any corrective procedures. With the knee in full extension, the arthroscope can be directed laterally into the lateral gutter to inspect for any loose bodies. The arthroscope is then directed into the medial gutter to visualize for any loose bodies as well. Regardless of whether or not the scope looks in the same direction or the opposite direction of the light source, it is important for the arthroscopist to develop a consist pattern of inspection of the knee joint that allows for maximal

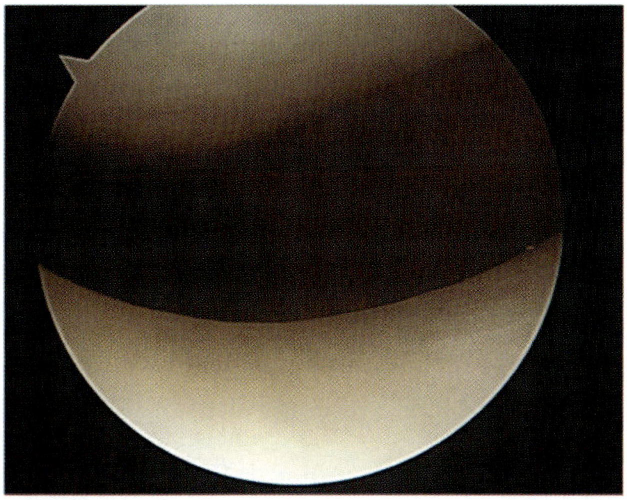

FIGURE 34-5. *The patellofemoral joint should be evaluated for any articular cartilage lesions as well as tilt or subluxation of the patella in cases of malalignment. This photo demonstrates a pristine patellofemoral joint.*

visualization at any given location in the knee. Once the scope continues medially around the curve of the condyle, a valgus stress is applied to open up the medial compartment and the arthroscope is directed into the medial compartment (Fig. 34-6).

Medial Compartment

With the arthroscope in the medial compartment, a spinal needle is used to localize the incision for the anteromedial portal. It is important to note that when meniscal pathology is expected in the medial compartment, the location of the portal should be such that arthroscopic instruments should enter the knee joint just a few millimeters above the meniscus. This will allow for ideal exposure and access of posterior medial meniscal pathology with minimal damage to the articular cartilage of the medial femoral condyle. A constant valgus force is applied to maintain exposure and minimize articular cartilage injury. Using a probe, the posterior, middle, and anterior horn is palpated and probed for injury. Any pathology is then addressed at that time, typically with a motorized shaver and a small basket biter (Figs. 34-7 and 34-8).

Intercondylar Notch

Once evaluation of the medial compartment has been completed, the scope is then placed into the intercondylar notch and the ACL is easily visible. In cases of ACL injury, the ligament may be attenuated and torn (eg, cyclops lesion) or in more chronic cases not visualized at all. Occasionally the ligamentous mucosum may prevent visualization of the ACL and can be simply debrided with a motorized shaver.

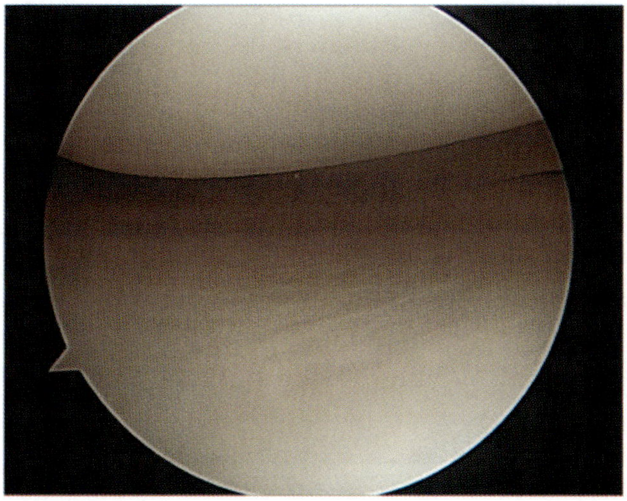

FIGURE 34-6. *Arthroscopic photo of a normal medial compartment in a left knee. The meniscus as well as surrounding articular cartilage on the medial femoral condyle and medial tibial plateau show no signs of damage.*

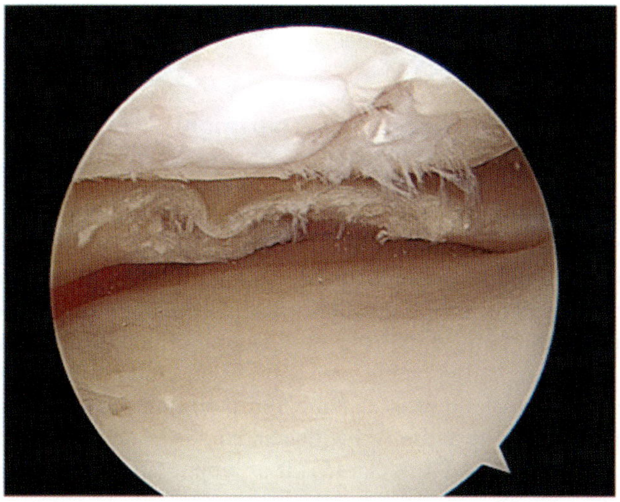

FIGURE 34-7. *Arthroscopic photo of a right knee demonstrating a degenerative medial meniscal tear and chondromalacia of the medial femoral condyle.*

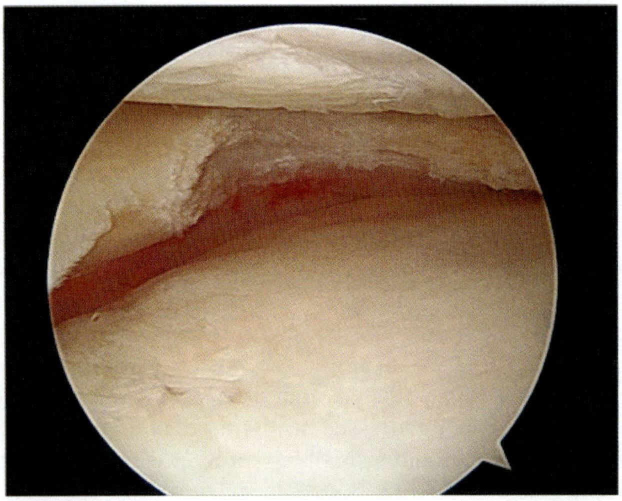

FIGURE 34-8. *Meniscectomy should remove any unstable meniscal fragments while preserving normal surrounding meniscus.*

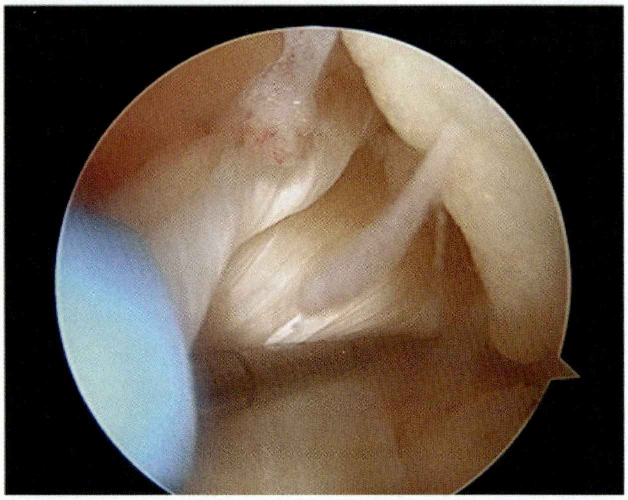

FIGURE 34-9. *The ACL is routinely probed for stability during knee arthroscopy. In cases of acute or chronic ACL injury, this may be difficult.*

After the anterior cruciate ligament is visualized, a probe should be inserted into the joint from the medial portal and the ACL, when present, should be assessed with a probe for appropriate tension (Fig. 34-9). The PCL can also be probed and assessed for tension. Once evaluation of the intercondylar notch has been completed, the probe is placed in the space between the ACL and the lateral femoral condyle and the knee is placed in the figure-of-four position. As the compartment is distracted, the arthroscope is advanced into the lateral compartment and the probe is easily manipulated in the compartment for meniscal evaluation.

Lateral Compartment

The articular cartilage and the meniscus are evaluated; the lens should be rotated in order to give a panoramic view of the compartment. Typically this is achieved with the scope looking toward the center of the knee. As the meniscus is examined, the popliteus tendon should be visible as it travels through the hiatus at the junction of middle and posterior horn of the lateral meniscus. If meniscal or articular cartilage pathology is encountered in the lateral compartment, it can be addressed with standard arthroscopic equipment (Figs. 34-10 to 34-15). It is important to note that when isolated lateral compartment pathology is expected, we establish the anteromedial portal in the figure-of-four position not in valgus. This allows for a more ideal trajectory to address the pathology in the lateral compartment. We have found that a "standard" anteromedial portal location is often too low for the lateral compartment and makes working in the compartment difficult because the tibial spines are often in the way of the instruments.

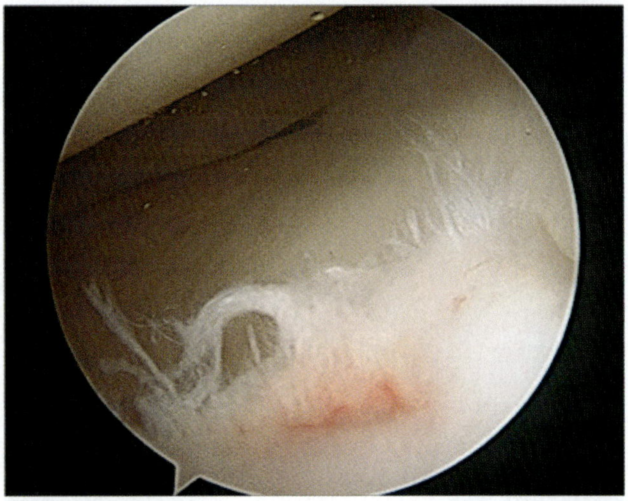

FIGURE 34-10. *Intraoperative arthroscopy photo of a 22-year-old male professional basketball player who suffered an acute injury to the anterior horn of the lateral meniscus of the right knee.*

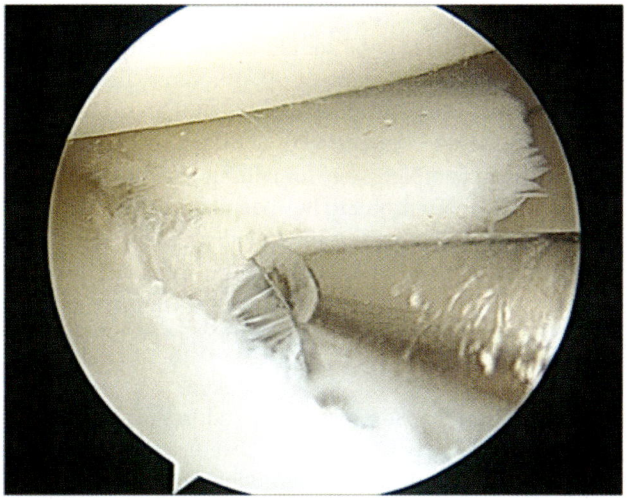

FIGURE 34-11. *Probing the anterior horn of the lateral meniscus revealed a displaced meniscal fragment from the anterior gutter of the lateral compartment.*

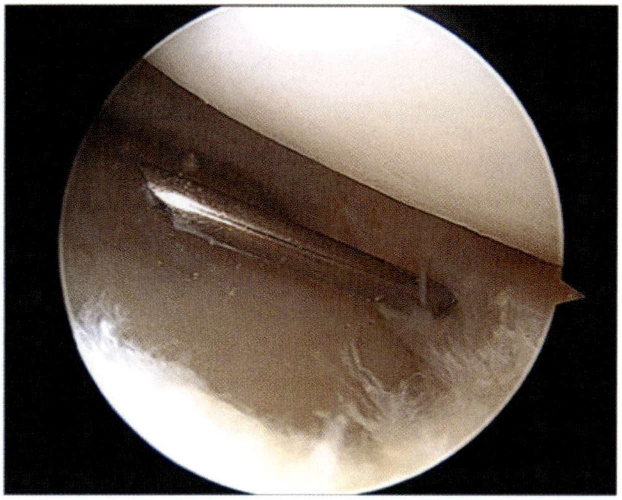

FIGURE 34-13. *Intraoperative arthroscopy photo of a left knee lateral meniscal tear with a concomitant symptomatic parameniscal cyst. The cyst is usually not visualized in arthroscopy but a spinal needle can be used to puncture the cyst.*

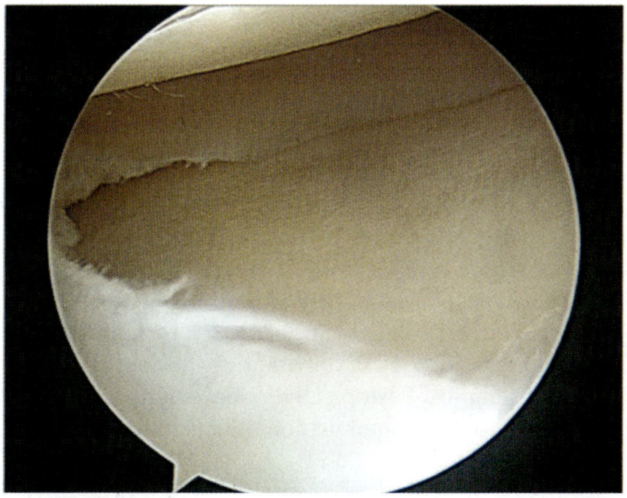

FIGURE 34-12. *Final picture demonstrating excision of the meniscal fragment and debridement of the lateral meniscal tear with minimal damage to the surrounding meniscus.*

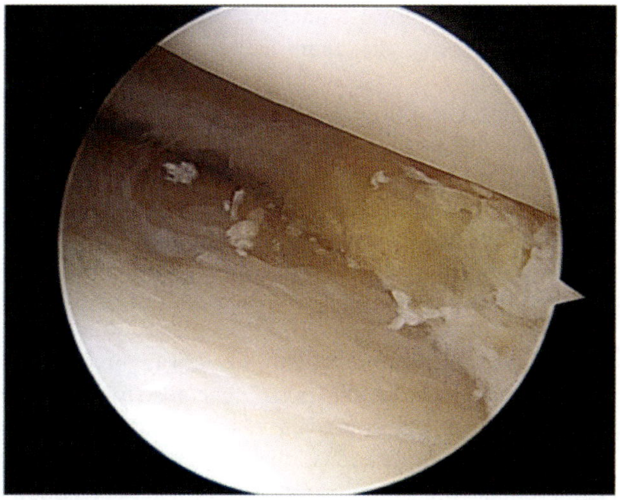

FIGURE 34-14. *Once the cyst has been punctured, the contents of the cyst can be expressed into the joint and suctioned.*

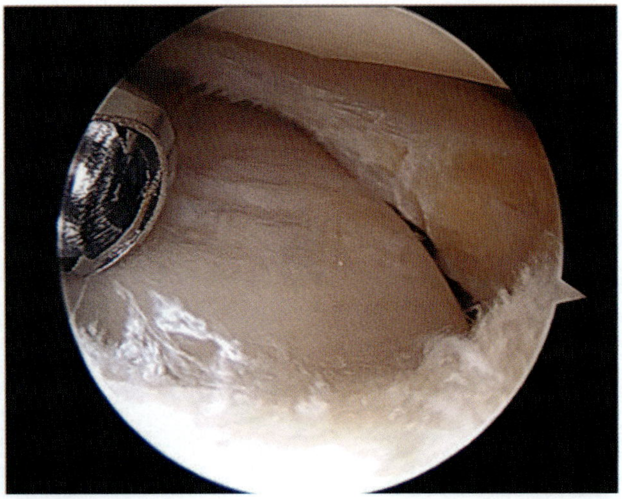

FIGURE 34-15. *After the entire contents of the cyst have been decompressed, the remaining meniscal tear itself is debrided to a stabilized rim.*

Posterior Compartment

Occasionally, inspection of the posterior compartment of the knee is necessary. This is most commonly needed during PCL reconstruction in which a posteromedial portal is necessary in order to protect the neurovascular structures during tibial tunnel drilling and to facilitate graft passage into the femoral tunnel. The scope is advanced into the posterior compartment between the PCL (if intact) and the medial femoral condyle. In order to visualize the posterior aspect of the posterior horn of the medial meniscus and the posterior joint line, a 70° arthroscope can aid in visualization. The reverse technique can be used to place the scope into the lateral posterior compartment in order to view the posterior aspect of the lateral joint.

During PCL reconstruction, we always recommend establishing a posteromedial portal. The posteromedial portal places the saphenous nerve at risk; in order to minimize neurovascular complications, the arthroscope is used to transilluminate the posterior joint line. Manual palpation is then used to verify the location and a spinal needle is inserted into the joint under direct arthroscopic visualization. A knife is used to incise the skin only and then a blunt cannula with a trocar is placed into the joint to avoid having to reestablish the portal each time an instrument is inserted or removed from the joint.

General Treatment Principles

In the majority of cases, the anteromedial portal is the working portal and a probe should be constantly used to test the stability and consistency of all structures. As pathology is encountered, it should be addressed at that time. We generally address the compartment with suspected pathology first and then complete the remaining diagnostic arthroscopy once the main problem has been addressed. For example, in cases of a medial meniscal tear, we will enter the medial compartment first, address the meniscal tear, and then enter the intercondylar notch, lateral compartment, and patellofemoral joint to confirm that there is no other pathology.

Most soft tissue pathology can be addressed using a variety of motorized shavers. In general, we use the "oscillating" function for most soft tissue work, while bony resection (eg, notchplasty during ACL reconstruction) is commonly performed with the shaver on "forward" or "reverse." The arthroscopist should be very familiar with all the different types and sizes of blades and we recommend finding a few that work well and using them consistently. In cases in which soft tissue removal may lead to bleeding, we recommend using an electrothermal device for that portion of the procedure. In order to avoid iatrogenic injury to the articular cartilage, in "tight" knees, use a curved motorized shaver. Last, but certainly not least, it is important to note that the instruments in the working portal should always be directly visualized, and we never advise using any instrument in an area where it is not clearly visible on the monitor.

CLOSURE

After the case is completed, for simple knee arthroscopy procedures the knee is irrigated and drained of fluid, and the skin incisions are closed with interrupted nylon sutures. For more complex cases, alternative sutures may be necessary for deep and superficial closure. A sterile dressing is applied only for simple cases, whereas more complex cases may require the addition of cryotherapy to reduce pain[7] and a brace for stability. Postoperative pain control can also be improved by using a combination of analgesics or narcotics as an intra-articular injection.[8]

REHABILITATION

Postoperative pain control consisting of oral narcotic medication combined with nonsteroidal anti-inflammatory medications in conjunction with ice and/or cryotherapy will help facilitate early recovery. Early rehabilitation after simple arthroscopy should focus on reducing swelling, stimulating quadriceps muscle recovery, and preventing stiffness. Weight bearing can begin immediately for simple arthroscopic cases, whereas some surgeons may protect weight bearing for more complex cases. As pain and inflammation decreases, physical therapy can be progressed as the patient tolerates in accordance with the surgeon's protocol.

COMPLICATIONS

Knee arthroscopy is generally an extremely safe procedure with rare minor complications and extremely rare major complications.[9] Intraoperatively, iatrogenic cartilage and soft tissue damage can be caused by trying to maneuver instruments in tight spaces. Using appropriately sized and shaped instruments at all times, as well as constant visualization of the instruments, is critical.

Major neurovascular injury during knee arthroscopy is extremely rare because of the relative lack of neurovascular structures in proximity to the standard portals; however, it has been described and reported.[10] Most major neurovascular injuries occur during more complex cases, such as meniscal repairs or PCL reconstruction, where multiple incisions and instruments are necessary and visualization can be more difficult. We recommend using a methodical approach during these cases, using any necessary aids (eg, second assistant during mensical repair, intraoperative fluoroscopy during PCL reconstruction) and having a thorough understanding of the surrounding anatomy to prevent these complications. Compressive neuropathy caused by positioning and tourniquet have also been reported.[11] Care should be taken to ensure that all bony prominences are well padded.

Postoperative complications after knee arthroscopy include deep venous thrombosis, compartment syndrome, and infection. The short operative time, small incisions, and use of lavage fluid make infection after knee arthroscopy extremely uncommon.[11] Since the majority of knee arthroscopy cases are done in an outpatient setting with immediate ambulation, one would suspect that the incidence of deep venous thrombosis would be low. However, it is important that the clinician have a high level of suspicion because, although the incidence is low, it is still somewhat higher than expected.[12,13] Last, compartment syndrome after knee arthroscopy is rare but reported. Compartment syndrome can occur in the operative leg with overdistension of the joint with the infusion pump[14] or in the nonoperative leg by improper positioning during a long case. It is usually in conjunction with cases in which the integrity of the joint has been disrupted (eg, posterior capsule torn in knee dislocation, or fracture treatment). During such cases, we recommend not using regional anesthesia because it can delay the diagnosis. Prompt recognition and treatment with emergent fasciotomies are essential.

CONCLUSIONS

Knee arthroscopy is a safe, effective treatment for a variety of intra-articular pathologies. Advances in technology and equipment have allowed surgeons to perform increasingly more complex procedures with a variety of arthroscopic techniques. The use of arthroscopic techniques for these procedures has led to a decrease in postoperative pain and swelling and earlier functional recovery. Although complications following knee arthroscopy are rare, the clinician must be aware of them so that, when they do occur, they can be promptly diagnosed and treated.

PEARLS AND PITFALLS

The following points should be considered when performing a knee arthroscopy:

- Create the anteromedial portal in the position in which the portal will be used—for medial compartment pathology in valgus and for lateral compartment pathology in varus.
- Avoid using the tourniquet when possible.
- For "tight" knees, use a curved motorized shaver to avoid iatrogenic injury to the articular cartilage.
- When creating a posteromedial portal, transilluminate the area to avoid iatrogenic injury to the saphenous nerve.
- Always be aware of the pump pressure and flow rate during the case—the lower, the better.

SUGGESTED READING

Petty CA, Lubowitz JH. Does arthroscopic partial meniscectomy result in knee osteoarthritis? A systematic review with a minimum of 8 years' follow-up. *Arthroscopy.* 2011;27(3):419-424.

REFERENCES

1. Rutkow IM. Surgical operations in the United States. Then (1983) and now (1994). *Arch Surg*. 1997;132: 983-990.
2. Hultin J, Hamberg P, Stenstrom A. Knee arthroscopy using local anesthesia. *Arthroscopy.* 1992;8:239-241.
3. Wong DA. Surgical site marking comes of age. *AAOS Bull*. 2004;52:30.
4. Saunders KC, Louis DL, Weingarden SI, et al. Effect of tourniquet time on postoperative quadriceps function. *Clin Orthop Relat Res.* 1979;143:194-199.
5. Reigstad O, Grimsgaard C. Complications in knee arthroscopy. *Knee Surg Sports Traumatol Arthrosc.* 2006;14(5):473-477.
6. Kieser C. A review of the complications of arthroscopic knee surgery. *Arthroscopy.* 1992;8:79-83.
7. Lessard LA, Scudds RA, Amendola A, et al. The efficacy of cryotherapy following arthroscopic knee surgery. *J Orthop Phys Ther.* 1997;26:14-22.
8. Goodwin RC, Amjadi F, Parker RD. Short-term analgesic effects of intra-articular injections after knee arthroscopy. *Arthroscopy.* 2005;21:307-312.
9. Small NC. Complications in arthroscopic surgery of the knee and shoulder. *Orthopedics.* 1993;16:985-988.
10. Kiss H, Drekonja T, Grethen C, et al. Postoperative aneurysm of the popliteal artery after arthroscopic meniscectomy. *Arthroscopy.* 2001;17:203-205.
11. Kieser C. A review of the complications of arthroscopic knee surgery. *Arthroscopy.* 1992;8:79-83.
12. Michot M, Conen D, Holtz D, et al. Prevention of deep-vein thrombosis in ambulatory arthroscopic knee surgery: a randomized trial of prophylaxis with low-molecular weight heparin. *Arthroscopy.* 2002;18: 257-263.
13. Ilahi OA, Reddy J, Ahmad I. Deep venous thrombosis after knee arthroscopy: a meta-analysis. *Arthroscopy.* 2005;21(6):727-730.
14. Bomberg BC, Hurley PE, Clark CA, et al. Complications associated with the use of an infusion pump during knee arthroscopy. *Arthroscopy.* 1992;8:224-228.

35 Closed-Wedge High Tibia Osteotomy

Hamidreza Yazdi and Reza Jamei Moayedi

Closed-wedge high tibia osteotomy (HTO) is a common effective and well-established procedure for the treatment of medial compartment knee osteoarthritis. HTO was first performed by Jackson in 1958.[1-4] In 1970, Coventry popularized this procedure and modified it.[1,3] The main indication of this procedure is unicompartmental osteoarthritis of knee[3]; however, it can be done in other conditions.[5] The goal of any HTO for varus malalignment is to shift the load to the lateral compartment.[6] Biomechanically when the mechanical axis passes through the center of the knee, about 70% of the load is borne by the medial compartment and 30% by the lateral side.[2,4] This load decreases to 50% in 4° of valgus and to 40% in 6° of valgus. For unloading the medial compartment, most authors recommend an alignment of 2° to 6° of mechanical valgus.[4,7-11]

INDICATIONS AND CONTRAINDICATIONS

Antivarus HTO is primarily indicated for pain relief and mechanical axis correction as an adjunct to other reconstructive knee procedures.[1] Medial unicompartmental osteoarthritis, posterolateral instability, varus thrust, and chronic anterior cruciate ligament deficiency are the main indications for antivarus HTO.[1]

Recently, the indications have expanded to include patients with a varus mechanical axis undergoing autogenous chondrocyte implantation, meniscal transplantation, osteochondral grafting, multiple subchondral bone microfractures, osteonecrosis, or osteochondritis dissecans of the medial side.[1,12]

Contraindications include a diagnosis of inflammatory arthritis, tricompartmental degenerative arthritis, obesity, and previous lateral meniscectomy.[1,5,13] Other principal contraindications are lateral compartment disease, fixed flexion deformity of more than 15° and less than 90° of knee flexion, symptomatic patellofemoral osteoarthritis, severe ligamentous instability, lateral translation of tibia on femur of more than 1 cm, patients' unwillingness to accept the anticipated cosmetic appearance after correction, or patients' unwillingness to be compliant with postoperative restrictions.[3,5]

This procedure should also be avoided if there is radiographic evidence of severe medial tibial bone loss or pronounced joint line obliquity due to extreme varus angulation of the proximal tibia and excessive valgus angulation of the distal femur.[1] There is no age limit for osteotomy and patients should not be excluded from consideration solely based on chronological age,[5,14-16] so physiologically young and active patients suffering unicompartmental knee osteoarithritis who are not optimal candidates for total knee replacement are ideal candidates for HTO.[5]

Mild patellofemoral degeneration is not an absolute contraindication for HTO. However, significant patellofemoral arthritis should be considered as a contraindication.[3,5]

Mild lateral compartment chondromalacia might not be an absolute contraindication to a valgus-producing osteotomy, but advanced lateral compartment degeneration is a contraindication.[5] In our experience, minimal involvement of the lateral compartment does not significantly change the results.

CLOSED-WEDGE VERSUS OPEN-WEDGE HTO

Reported advantages of closed-wedge HTO include better initial stability due to the compressive nature of the osteotomy leading to more immediate weight bearing and better healing; it requires no bone grafting or graft substitutes.[1,4] Due to the compressive force of the quadriceps tendon and good cancellous bone of the metaphysis and minimal loss of correction, the risk of nonunion is minimal.[2] Closed-wedge HTO decreases the tibial slope, which will reduce the increased anterior tibial translation in anterior cruciate ligament (ACL) deficient knees and will minimize stresses on ACL reconstruction and improve anteroposterior (AP) stability.[5]

The disadvantages of closed-wedge HTO include the necessity for either a fibular osteotomy or proximal tibiofibular joint destruction or fibular head resection,[3,4] altered proximal tibia anatomy potentially complicating future arthroplasty, and difficulty in making fine angular corrections once the bony wedge has been removed.[4] This osteotomy also shortens the leg, decreases the distance from the tibia plateau to the tibia tubercle, and increases the laxity of the lateral collateral ligament (LCL).[1]

Theoretical advantages of medial open-wedge HTO include restoring anatomy and ligamentous tension, the possibility of correction in the coronal and sagittal planes, the ability to adjust intraoperatively, the fact that only one bone cut is necessary, and the avoidance of disruption of the proximal tibiofibular joint or fibular osteotomy.[5] The disadvantages of medial open-wedge HTO include the possibility of collapse and loss of correction, the need for bone graft, a slightly higher risk of nonunion, the need for a longer period of restricted weight bearing, and increasing tibial slope.[2,5]

Due to the better healing potential of a lateral closed-wedge osteotomy, it can be advised in patients who are at risk of slower healing or nonunion, such as patients with a history of nicotine use, diabetics, patients who are steroid dependent, patients who are unwilling to have autograft or allograft, or patients on whom the osteotomy is combined with ACL reconstruction.[5] There is only one prospective randomized study comparing lateral closed-wedge HTO and medial open-wedge HTO. At 1-year follow-up, both techniques reduced pain and improved knee function and the difference was not significant, although closed-wedge HTO achieved more accurate correction.[17]

LATERAL CLOSED-WEDGE HTO VERSUS UNICOMPARTMENTAL KNEE ARTHROPLASTY

Another option for treating unicompartmental degenerative joint disease is unicompartmental knee arthroplasty (UKA). Only a few studies compare the clinical outcome of UKA versus closing-wedge HTO.[18-20] Data comparing UKA with HTO appear to support UKA over HTO.[21,22] However, Brouwer et al stated in their meta-analysis that there is prominent evidence for no significant difference in pain, knee function, and gait after HTO compared to UKA and that HTO causes more complications.[23]

PREOPERATIVE ASSESSMENT

Proper patient selection and a detailed clinical assessment are necessary when considering closed-wedge HTO.[5] This evaluation includes patients' history, including age, occupation activity level, and past medical and surgical history, and patient expectations, especially their postoperative activity level.[3,5] In the physical examination, the surgeon should focus on lower extremity range of motion, deformity, ligamentous stability, and leg length discrepancy.[5,15,24]

Essential radiographs are full-length standing alignment view, standing AP, posteroanterior flexion view (Rosenberg), and lateral as well as Merchant views of the knee.[1,2,5] Bone scan can be done to evaluate the lateral compartment in doubtful cases with normal-appearing lateral compartment in X-ray.[2,3]

PREOPERATIVE PLANNING

Preoperative planning includes the degree of correction, the wedge size, and the location of the osteotomy based on the preoperative image templating.[5] To estimate the angle of correction, the tibia plateau should be divided 0% to 100% from medial to lateral margin in full standing alignment view. Then a line needs to be drawn from the center of the femoral head and ankle to point 62% on the tibia plateau. The angle formed by these two lines equals the angle of correction.[1,4,5] The goal is to calculate the angular correction needed to produce 2° to 4° of mechanical or 8° to 10° of anatomical valgus (Fig. 35-1).[2,5,2]

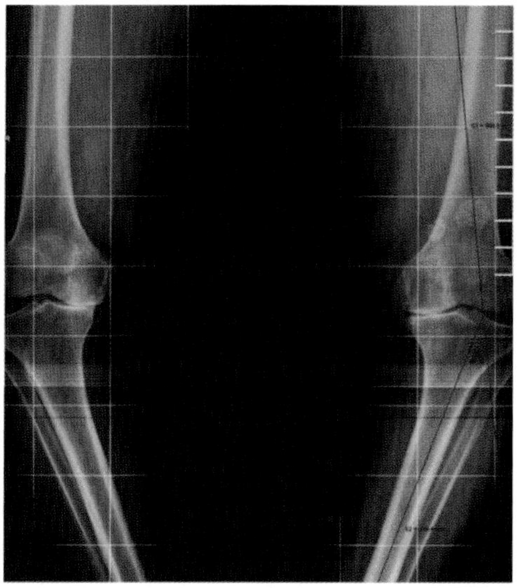

FIGURE 35-1. *The point of 62% for determination of the angle of correction.*

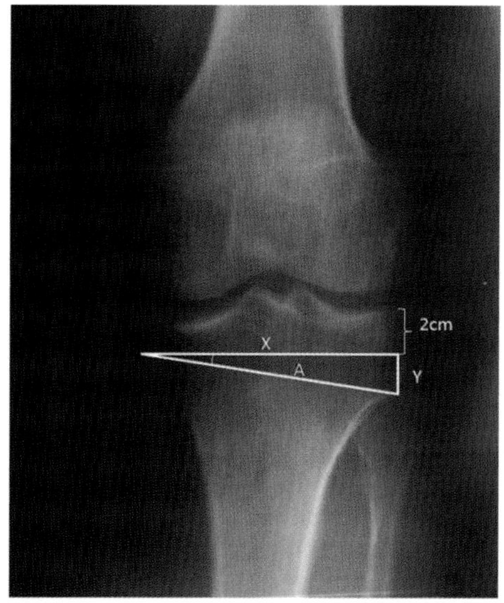

FIGURE 35-2. *The wedge height (Y) is determined by multiplying the width of the tibia (X) by the tangent of the correction angle (A).*

It should be considered that standing radiographs may overestimate the angle of correction due to osseous defects or attenuated ligaments. Each millimeter of lateral tibiofemoral joint separation causes approximately 1° of varus angulation. So comparing the amount of lateral joint space opening with the contralateral knee and subtracting the difference from the calculated angle (1°/ mm) will avoid overcorrection.[1]

Once the desired angle of correction is determined, the wedge size should be estimated on the AP X-ray of the knee. The width of tibia 2 cm distal to the joint line is measured and adjusted according to the film magnification. The tangent of correction angle (A) is obtained. The wedge height (Y) is calculated by multiplying the width of the tibia (X) by the tangent of the correction angle (A) (Fig. 35-2)[1]:

$$Y = X\,(\tan A).$$

SURGICAL TECHNIQUE

Many surgeons now perform arthroscopic examination before HTO to assess the integrity of the lateral compartment and debridement of the degenerated medial compartment.[5] Muller highly recommends arthroscopy before osteotomy,[26] but Coventry believes that if the compartment to be loaded after osteotomy appears normal on a standing X-ray and there are no symptoms of internal derangement, arthroscopy is a needless exercise.[3]

We do arthroscopic examination in most of our patients before HTO, especially when the standing X-ray is normal for the lateral compartment but the patient has some pain of this compartment or minimal increased uptake on bone scan. Surgery should be done under fluoroscopy. After preparation of the patient, a straight longitudinal incision on the anterolateral aspect of the knee is performed. Some surgeons prefer an oblique or transverse incision from the tibia tubercle to the fibular head.[1,3] We prefer to do a longitudinal incision because it seems to be better incorporated in future total knee arthroplasty (TKA) incisions, but an oblique or transverse incision also is accepted.[5]

The extensor muscles are detached from the tibia and fibula to expose the anterior fibular head and proximal tibia. The peroneal nerve is identified if needed. Coventry prefers to remove the LCL and biceps femoris tendon as a Y-conjoined structure from the head of the fibula and resect the fibular head from the head-neck junction and reattach the Y-ligament to the neck of the fibula under desired tension,[3] but fibular osteotomy, release of the proximal tibiofibular joint, or resection of the proximal medial fibular head to be able to close the osteotomy site are accepted as well.[1,2,5]

One guide wire is inserted at least 2 cm distal from the joint line and under control of image intensification, from the lateral to medial side. Another guide wire is inserted distal to the first one at a predetermined angle and according to wedge height, then the wedge of bone outlined by the wires is cut with an oscillating saw and removed. The osteotomy should end medially about 4 to 6 mm from the outer cortex of the medial tibia.

The medial cortical bridge is weakened with multiple perforations with a drill or small osteotome, and the osteotomy is closed carefully and gradually.[1-3,5]

Fixation includes cylinder cast, external fixation, staple fixation, plate fixation, or fixed angle implants.[5] We prefer to fix with two staples and applying a long leg cast for 4 weeks (Fig. 35-3), but Hofmann prefers to use rigid internal fixation and early mobilization to improve results.[27]

COMPLICATIONS

Infection

Rate of infection ranges from 0 to 10.4%.[4,5] Most are superficial and can be treated with oral antibiotics. Deep infection needs irrigation and debridement and intravenous antibiotics.[4]

Thromboembolic Disease

The incidence is 2% to 5%, but in one study using venographic examination after HTO, the incidence has been reported to be up to 41%.[28] A postoperative thromboprophylaxis regime similar to that used in TKA is recommended.[4]

Compartment Syndrome

Compartment syndrome is an uncommon complication, but Bauer et al have shown that there is an increase in compartment pressure with this operation.[4]

The risk of compartment syndrome can be increased when HTO is done in combination with an arthroscopic-assisted ligament reconstruction.[4,5] Good hemostasis and use of a drain can reduce the risk of compartment syndrome.[5,29]

Peroneal Nerve Palsy

Peroneal nerve palsy is the most common neurovascular injury after HTO.[4] The incidence ranges from 0 to 20%.[30-32] The reason may be direct trauma to nerve due to high fibular osteotomy or compartment syndrome.[4,5] In our experience, extensor hallucis longus is the most common affected muscle, and this is supported by other authors.[4]

Careful lateral dissection and avoiding excessive retraction of the nerve and prevention of compartment syndrome should be considered. Wootton et al divided the fibula into four zones and believed that no complications will be in

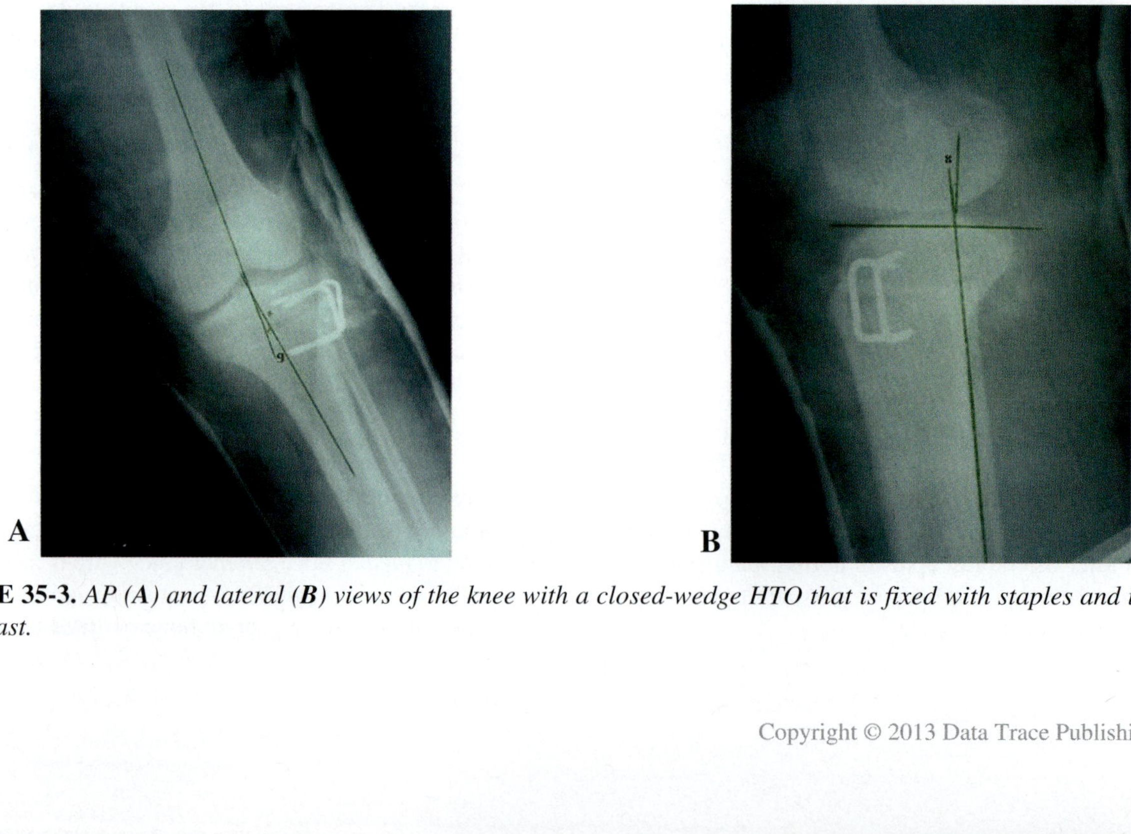

FIGURE 35-3. *AP (**A**) and lateral (**B**) views of the knee with a closed-wedge HTO that is fixed with staples and immobilized with a cast.*

zones 1 and 4, and zone 3 has the majority of complications (between 8 and 15 cm below the fibular head).[33]

Vascular Injury

The incidence of vascular injury is less than 1%.[5] Damage to the anterior tibial artery appears to be more common.[4] Proper placement of retractors posteriorly seems to protect the popliteal artery. Some authors prefer to perform osteotomy with the knee in 90° of flexion to minimize the risk of vascular damage,[15] but Zaidi et al, in their study, found that the popliteal artery is closer to the tibia in 90° of knee flexion than in full extension.[34]

Fracture

Intra-articular fractures during closing-wedge HTO have a reported incidence of 0 to 20%.[4,5] Another fracture may happen in the medial cortex of the tibia. Leaving a 6- to 10-mm bone hinge medially, stress releasing drill holes, and gradual closure of the osteotomy should be considered to minimize the risk of fracture.[4,5]

Patellar Height

Patella baja is a reported complication of closing-wedge HTO and the incidence is 7.6% to 8.8%.[35] Patella baja is caused by contracture of the patellar ligament associated with conventional cast immobilization.[4,5]

Wright et al and Coventry believe that closing-wedge HTO actually increase the patellar height in comparison with opening-wedge HTO, because of removing a wedge of bone,[3,36] so this osteotomy is preferred in patients with preoperative patellar baja over medial opening-wedge osteotomy.[5] With new methods of rigid internal fixation and early mobilization, the risk of patellar baja can be decreased.

Delayed Union and Nonunion

Nonunion is uncommon after closing-wedge HTO and the incidence is less than 1%.[4,5] These complications are more common when osteotomy is distal rather than proximal to the tibia tubercle.[3-5] Factors that have been reported to minimize the risk of nonunion or delayed union include avoidance of fracture of the medial cortex, broad and flat osteotomy cuts, avoidance of thermal necrosis with a saw blade, metaphyseal osteotomy, and rigid fixation.[4,5]

Treatment usually is a revision procedure using a more rigid fixation such as a locking plate or a compressive type of external fixator and bone graft.[4,5] Successful treatment of nonunion following HTO has been reported with conversion to TKA.[37,38]

Conversion to Total Knee Arthroplasty

Although Bae et al reported satisfactory results in TKA after HTO, Haslam et al in a study with 12.6 years follow-up found poorer results.[39,40] Most authors agree that conversion of HTO to a TKA is a much more technically demanding procedure than a primary TKA.[4] The main problems that should be considered include patella baja, wound healing problems, anatomical deformity of the proximal tibia complicating TKA, and the potential for any retained hardware.[4,40] Meticulous surgical technique considering correction of deformity, joint line height, amount of the tibia bone resection, and particular attention to skin incision and wound healing can produce better results.[40]

RESULTS

Good results have been achieved in the literature over both the medium and long term with gradual deterioration over time.[4] Most surgeons believe that, in cases of medial gonarthrosis, a slight overcorrection of 2° to 5° toward valgus can lead to better long-term results. This procedure generally provides good relief of pain and restoration of function in 80% to 90% of patients at 5 years and 50% to 65% at 10 years (Fig. 35-4).[5] The results deteriorate after 10 years,[5,41,42] but deterioration of results is most often attributed to arthritis progression rather than varus deformity recurrence.[43]

PEARLS AND PITFALLS

The following points should be considered when performing an antivarus HTO:

- This procedure is primarily indicated for pain relief and mechanical axis correction as an adjunct to other reconstructive knee procedures.
- Medial unicompartmental osteoarthritis, posterolateral instability, varus thrust, and chronic ACL deficiency are the main indications for this procedure.
- Perform an arthroscopic evaluation before the osteotomy.
- Be aware of leg shortening with this technique.

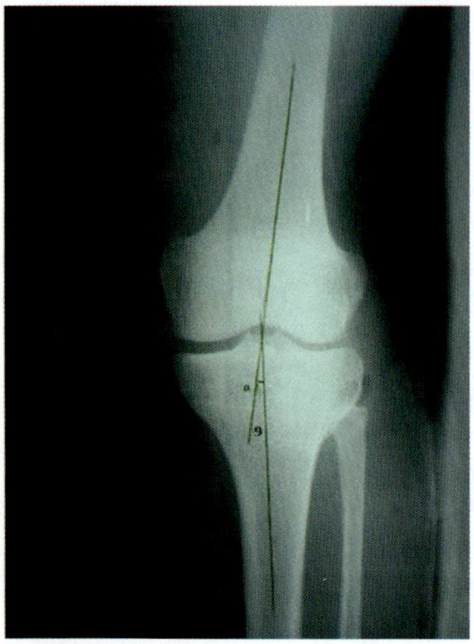

FIGURE 35-4. *AP view of the knee 7 years after a closed-wedge HTO.*

REFERENCES

1. Stuart MJ. Tibial antivarus closing wedge osteotomy. *Oper Tech Sport Med.* 2000;8(1):27-31.
2. Coventry MB. Upper tibial osteotomy for osteoarthritis. *J Bone Joint Surg.* 1985;67:1130-1140.
3. Coventry MB. Upper tibial osteotomy. *Clin Orthop Relat Res.* 1983;182:46-52.
4. Tunggal JA, Higgins GA, Waddell JP. Complications of closing wedge high tibial osteotomy. *Int Orthop.* 2010;34(2):255-261.
5. Sherman C, Canabela ME. Closing wedge osteotomy of the tibia and the femur in the treatment of gonarthrosis. *Int Orthop.* 2010;34(2):173-184.
6. Kettelkamp DB, Wegner DR, Chao EY, et al. Results of proximal tibial osteotomy. The effects of tibiofemoral angle, stance–phase, flexion–extension, and medial plateau force. *J Bone Joint Surg Am.* 1976;58:952-960.
7. Coventry MB, Listrup DM, Wallrichs SL. Proximal tibial osteotomy. A critical long-term study of eighty-seven cases. *J Bone Joint Surg Am.* 1993;75:196-201.
8. Fujisawa Y, Masuhara K, Shiomi S. The effect of high tibial osteotomy on osteoarthritis of the knee. An arthroscopic study of 54 knee joints. *Orthop Clin North Am.* 1979;10:585-608.
9. Hernigou P, Medevielle D, Debeyre J, et al. Proximal tibial osteotomy for osteoarthritis with varus deformity. A ten- to thirteen-years follow-up study. *J Bone Joint Surg Am.* 1987;69:332-354.
10. Jakob RP, Murphy SB. Tibial osteotomy for varus gonarthrosis: indication, planing and operative technique. *Instr Course Lect.* 1992;47:87-93.
11. Myrnerts R. Optimal correction in high tibial osteotomy for varus deformity. *Acta Orthop Scand.* 1980; 51:689-694.
12. Wright JM, Crockett HC, Slawski DP, et al. High tibial osteotomy. *J Am Acad Orthop Surg.* 2005;13(4): 279-289.
13. Morrey BF. Upper tibial osteotomy for secondary osteoarthritis of the knee. *J Bone Joint Surg Br.* 1989; 77:554-559.
14. Trousdale RT. Osteotomy. Patient selection, preoperative planning and results. In: Callaghan JJ, Rosenberg AG, Rubash HE, eds. *The Adult Knee.* Philadelphia, PA: Lippincott Williams and Wilkins; 2002.
15. Dowd GSE, Somayaji HS, Uthukuri M. High tibia osteotomy for medial compartment osteoarthritis. *Knee.* 2006;13:87-92.
16. Marti RK, Verhagen RA, Kerkhoffs GM, et al. Proximal tibial varus osteotomy: indications, technique and five to twenty-one years results. *J Bone Joint Surg Am.* 2001;83:164-170.
17. Brower RW, Bierma-Zeinstra SM, Van Raaij TM, et al. Osteotomy for medical compartment arthritis of the knee using a closing wedge or an opening wedge controlled by a Pudda plate. A one-year randomised controlled study. *J Bone Joint Surg Br.* 2006;88(11):1454-1459.
18. Broughton NS, Newman JH, Baily RA. Unicompartmental replacement and high tibial osteotomy for osteoarthritis of the knee. A comparative study after 5-10 years follow-up. *J Bone Joint Surg Br.* 1986;68(3):447-452.
19. Weale AE, Newman JH. Unicompartmental arthroplasty and high tibial osteotomy for osteoarthritis of the knee. A comparative study with 12 to 17 years follow up period. *Clin Orthop Relat Res.* 1994;302:134-137.
20. Varsson I, Gillquist J. Rehabilitation after high tibial osteotomy and unicompartmental arthroplasty. A comparative study. *Clin Orthop Relat Res.* 1991;266: 139-144.
21. Brojesson M, Weidenhielm L, Mattsson E, et al. Gait and clinical measurement in patients with knee osteoarthritis after surgery: a prospective 5-years follow-up study. *Knee.* 2005;12(2):121-127.

22. Stakenborg-Colsman C, Wirth CJ, Lazovic D, et al. High tibial osteotomy versus unicompartmental joint replacement in unicompartmental knee joint osteoarthritis: 7-10 years follow-up prospective randomized study. *Knee*. 2001;8(3):187-194.
23. Brouwer RW, van Raaji TM, Bierma–Zeinstra SM, et al. Osteotomy for treating knee osteoarthritis. *Cochrane Rev*. 2007;3:CD004019.
24. Noyes FR, Roberts CS. High tibial osteotomy in knees with associated chronic ligament deficiencies. In: Jackson DW, ed. *Master Technique in Orthopaedic Surgery: Reconstructive Knee Surgery*. New York: Raven Press; 1995.
25. Dugdale TW, Noys FR, Styer D. Preoperative planning for high tibial osteotomy. The effect of lateral tibiofemoral separation and tibiofemoral length. *Clin Orthop*. 2002;274:248-264.
26. Muller M, Strecker W. Arthroscopy prior to osteotomy around the knee. *Arch Orthop Trauma Surg*. 2008;128(11):1217-1221.
27. Hofmann AA, Wyatt RW, Beck SW. High tibial osteotomy: use of an osteotomy jib; rigid fixation and early motion versus conventional surgical technique and cast immobilization. *Clin Orthop Relat Res*. 1991;271:212-217.
28. Turner RS, Grifith H, Heatley FW. The incidence of deep-vein thrombosis after upper tibial osteotomy. A venographic study. *J Bone Joint Surg Br*. 1993;75:942-944.
29. Gibson MJ, Barnes MR, Allen MJ, et al. Weakness of foot dorsiflexion and changes in compartment pressures after tibial osteotomy. *J Bone Joint Surg Br*. 1986;68:471-475.
30. Bettin D, Karbowski A, Schwering L. Time-dependent clinical and roentgenographical results of Coventry high tibial valgization osteotomy. *Arch Orthop Trauma Surg*. 1998;117:53-57.
31. Naudie D, Bourne RB, Rorabeck CH, et al. The Install Award. Survivorship of the high tibial valgus osteotomy. A 10- to 22-year follow-up study. *Clin Orthop Relat Res*. 1999;18-27.
32. Wu LD, Hahne HJ, Hassenpflug T. A long-term follow-up study of high tibial osteotomy for medial compartment osteoarthrosis. *Clin J Traumatol*. 2004;7(6): 348-353.
33. Wootton JR, Ashworth MJ, MacLaren CA. Neurological complications of high tibial osteotomy. The fibular osteotomy as a causative factor: a clinical and anatomical study. *Ann R Coll Surg Engl*. 1995;77 (1):31-34.
34. Zaidi SH, Cobb AG, Bentley G. Danger to the popliteal artery in high tibial osteotomy. *J Bone Joint Surg Br*. 1995;77:384-386.
35. Scuderi GR, Windsor RE, Insall JN. Observations on patellar height after proximal tibial osteotomy. *J Bone Joint Surg Am*. 1989;71(2):245-248.
36. Wright JM, Heavrin B, Begg M, et al. Observations on patellar height following opening wedge proximal tibial osteotomy. *Am J Knee Surg*. 2001;14:163-173.
37. Sprenger TR, Doerzbacher JF. Tibial osteotomy for the treatment of varus gonarthrosis. Survival and failure analysis to twenty-two years. *J Bone Joint Surg Am*. 2003;85:469-474.
38. Yoshino N, Takai S, Watanabe L, et al. Total knee arthroplasty with long stem for treatment of nonunion after high tibial osteotomy. *J Arthroplasty*. 2004;19:528-537.
39. Bae DK, Song SJ, Ho Yoon K. Total knee arthroplasty following closed wedge high tibia osteotomy. *Int Orthop*. 2010;34:283-287.
40. Haslam P, Armstrong M, Geutjens G, et al. Total knee arthroplasty after failed high tibial osteotomy, long-term follow-up of matched groups. *J Arthroplasty*. 2007;22:245-250.
41. Virolain P, Aro HT. High tibial osteotomy for the treatment of osteoarthritis of the knee: a review of the literature and a meta-analysis of follow-up studies. *Arch Orthop Trauma Surg*. 2004;124(4):258-261.
42. Amendola A, Bonasia DE. Results of high tibial osteotomy: review of the literature. *Int Orthop*. 2010; 34(2):155-160.
43. Stuart MJ, Grace JN, Ilstrup DM, et al. Late recurrence of varus deformity after proximal tibial osteotomy. *Clin Orthop Relat Res*. 1990;260:61-65.

36 Open-Wedge High Tibial Osteotomy

Kang-Il Kim and Sang Hak Lee

High tibial osteotomy (HTO) has been an established treatment in patients with unicompartmental osteoarthritis of the knee combined with varus malalignment. However, during the past three decades, widespread application of HTO has steadily declined because of the success of total and partial knee replacement with long-term survivorship. The classic procedure of the lateral closed-wedge tibial osteotomy, popularized by Coventry, was the gold standard for correction of varus deformity with medial compartment arthritis.[1,2] However, this technique is associated with problems including peroneal nerve injury, loss of correction, shortening of the lower extremity, arthrofibrosis, and compartment syndrome.[2-4] Moreover, this method requires additional fibular procedures such as fibular osteotomy, resection of fibular head, or division of proximal tibiofibular joint. In addition, this type of correction can cause changes of tibial inclination and offset of the proximal tibia that may compromise placement of the tibial component of total knee arthroplasty in failed HTO cases. HTO with medial opening wedge has gained in popularity over recent years as a viable alternative to traditional lateral closed-wedge ostetomy.[5-8] This technique has several advantages over lateral closed-wedge osteotomy, such as freedom from peroneal nerve complications, smaller surgical exposure without any muscle detachment, more precise correction, lack of limb shortening, and easier access in case of future total knee arthroplasty.[9] Furthermore, there is no need to mobilize the fibula during the surgery. However, this procedure may need bone grafting to fill the opening gap, causing significant morbidity and increased risk of infection. Moreover, medial open-wedge HTO using internal fixation had problems that were mainly due to implant failure as well as loss of correction with small and unstable implants. Therefore, immediate weight bearing is not appropriate after this procedure and a longer rehabilitation period is required. To overcome fixation problems, Puddu and colleagues designed a special plate, which combines the roles of the buttress plate with metal block of varying height.[10] However, there is no definite consensus on optimal fixation device or surgical technique for an open-wedge HTO. Although plates are commonly used for open-wedge osteotomy, their biomechanical stability is still under investigation and longer and thicker plates have now been developed and are recommended. But bigger plates need larger incisions and cause irritation of thin medial soft tissue cover.

It is commonly recommended that a bone graft be performed if the osteotomy is 10 mm or more and delayed full weight bearing is allowed if the radiograph shows good healing at the operative site. Furthermore, healing of an osteotomy depends on the extent of surgical exposure and energy used to transect the bone besides rigid fixation. There is a need, therefore, of a surgical technique characterized by less invasive surgical methods, biological osteotomy techniques, more rigid fixation, accelerated rehabilitation, and lower risk of complications. Recently, the TomoFix system (Synthes, Solothurn, Switzerland) has been introduced based on the less invasive internal fixation principle.[6,8,11] This system design has secure fixation of locking head screws in the plate and adapts to the anatomy of the proximal tibia. The concept of angle-stable screw fixation within the plate allows stable fixation even under weight bearing without additional bone substitutes filling the osteotomy gap, although the size of the plate is much bigger than in other systems. Since the plate is securely attached with locking head screws, it permits having a minute gap (2 mm) between the tibia and the plate, which allows preservation of periosteal blood supply. With these types of new products, the open-wedge HTO has become the favored technique because it is easier to perform, and it is probably the most commonly used technique currently.

PREOPERATIVE EVALUATION

History and Examination

The predominant reason for using HTO is to obtain valgus limb alignment in patients experiencing medial joint pain and who wish to continue an active lifestyle. Although, preoperative activity level is probably more of a determinant than chronological age, an age of 60 or 65 years old is a limitation in general. History of trauma, previous surgery, professional activity, and patient's personality are of special interest. Obesity [body mass index (BMI) > 30 kg/m^2] has a negative impact on the outcome of HTO procedure.[12]

Physical examination includes evaluation of the range of motion and the instability of the ligaments. Knee motion should reveal flexion arc of over 100° and not more than 10° to 15° of flexion contracture.[13] The presence of anterior or posterior instability may require simultaneous or staged procedure with correction osteotomy and ligament reconstruction. If a patient has varus deformity and anterior cruciate ligament (ACL) insufficiency, an ACL reconstruction in addition to the open-wedge HTO can be performed simultaneously. However, performing combined procedures results in a lengthy operation with increased risk of complications, prolonged rehabilitation, and knee motion problems. Moreover, the screw-in plate for open-wedge HTO can interfere with drilling of the tibial tunnel of the ACL graft. Therefore, in these patients, valgization and extension HTO in open-wedge technique can be performed. After adequate healing of the osteotomy, a second surgery for ACL reconstruction may not be required since decrease of the slope improves sagittal stability.[14] However, tibial slope change of more than 10° is not recommended because no significant biomechanical advantages after slope alteration of more than 10° were identified in the study.[14] During gait, the torsional pattern of the limb and the presence or absence of a varus thrust should be assessed. The high adduction moment was used to describe the amount of lateral or varus thrust of the knee observed during gait. These patients are more likely to have a recurrent varus deformity following valgus HTO. When HTO is chosen for those patients in spite of a high preoperative adduction moment, overcorrection of the deformity may be helpful.[15] The soft tissue and skin as well as the vascular and neurological status of the lower extremity must also be inspected.

Imaging

Radiographic

The first goal of the radiographic examination is to confirm the indication for an osteotomy. The radiographic documentation includes a standing anteroposterior and lateral view in the extended knee position. An anteroposterior view depicts the medial and lateral joint compartment, soft tissue, and rough assessment of femorotibial alignment. A lateral view depicts the patellofemoral joint, patellar height, and posterior tibial slope. The weight-bearing posteroanterior view in 45° flexion evaluate cartilage loss with the joint space narrowing of the more posterior aspect of the femorotibial joint. The status of the patellofemoral joint, such as patellofemoral arthritis and tightening of the patella, also should be investigated with a patella axial view in 45° flexion. Although slight degenerative changes of the patellofemoral joint are not a contraindication to an HTO, the patella height and patella alignment could influence the technique of the HTO. Patella baja is a relative contraindication for open-wedge HTO since this procedure significantly lowers the patella. A weight-bearing radiograph of the entire lower limb is necessary for assessing the correct indication and the planning of any osteotomy around the knee. Varus and valgus stress views of the knee might be helpful to visualize stability of medial and lateral collateral ligaments. Joint space narrowing when stressing the presumably healthy compartment precludes osteotomy. Another goal of the radiographic assessment is to select the ideal candidate and the site of the osteotomy. The medial proximal tibial angle (MPTA) and lateral distal femoral angle (LDFA) are considered for determining the femoral or tibial cause of varus malalignment. The normal range of MPTA is 87° ± 3° and the normal range of LDFA is 87° ± 3°. If the LDFA is larger than the normal value, the cause of the varus deformity is a femoral one. Conversely, if the MPTA is markedly smaller than the normal value, the varus deformity is mainly caused by the tibia. Tibial varus slope also is important in selecting the candidates for an HTO, because the result of an HTO is better when the varus deformity is mainly due to bowing than when the deformity is essentially due to wear (Fig. 36-1).[16] Furthermore, researchers described a subgroup of patients with varus arthritic knees showing excessive valgus angulation of the femoral joint surface together with proximal tibia vara.[17] This pattern of deformity warrants special consideration because, in some extreme cases, it could require combined femoral and tibial ostetomies to restore the horizontality of the joint surface.

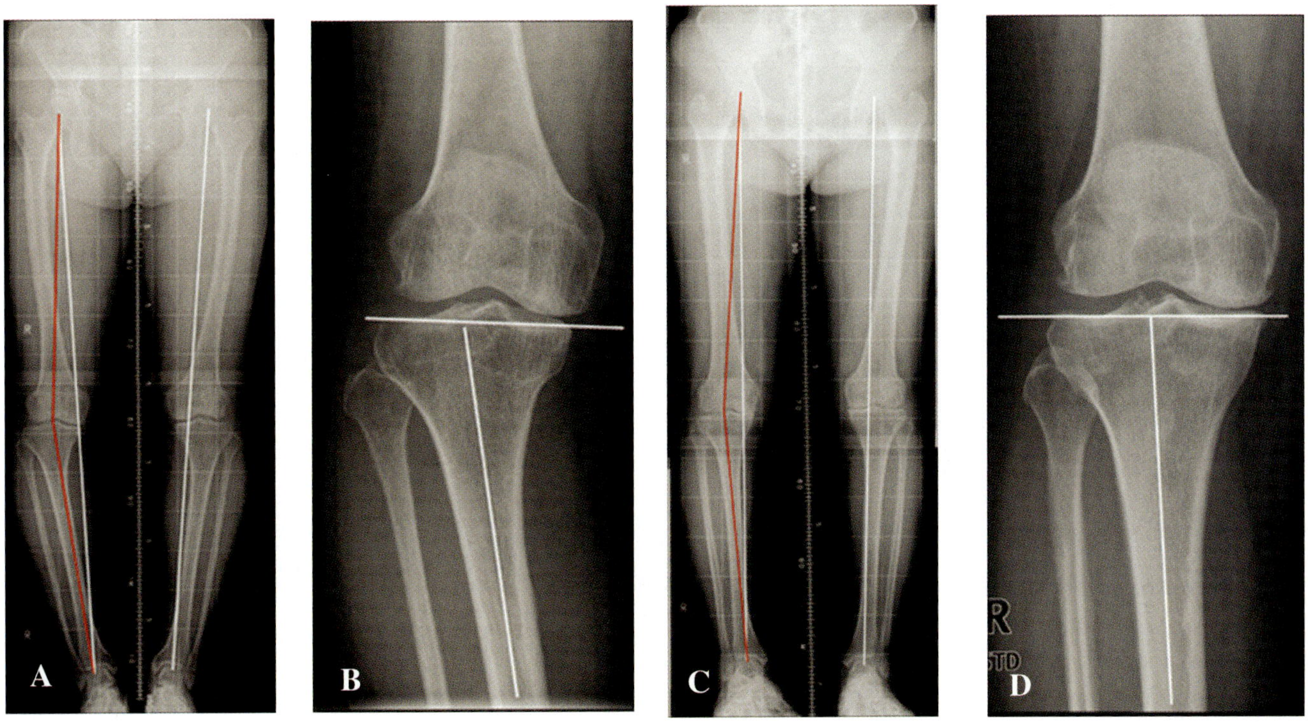

FIGURE 36-1. *The different causes of varus malalignment in two cases. (**A**) The hip-knee-ankle angle is measured as 9.5° varus malalignment. (**B**) Although medial joint space narrowing is minimal, the medial proximal tibial angle (MPTA) is significantly decreased as 77°. This patient is an ideal candidate for a high tibial osteotomy. (**C**) On the contrary, the hip-knee-ankle angle is measured as 7° varus malalignment in the other case. (**D**) The MPTA angle is in the normal range at 87°, although medial joint space is markedly narrowed. This is a borderline indication for a high tibial osteotomy and also represents an ideal candidate for partial knee replacement.*

Magnetic Resonance Imaging

Magnetic resonance imaging (MRI) is an established imaging technique for evaluation of soft tissue structures such as meniscus, ligaments, and cartilage. Although it is not mandatory, MRI offers useful information about the degree of degenerative changes and existent lesions in the affected compartment. In addition, it can assess the degenerative changes in both patellofemoral and lateral compartments. If the patients have mechanical symptoms suggesting meniscal abnormalities or loose bodies, MRI is an essential tool.

PREPARATION OF PATIENT FOR SURGERY

For the preoperative planning, templating is carried out on a weight-bearing radiograph of the entire lower limb using a cutout. The object of valgus osteotomy is to shift the weight-bearing line (WBL) 62% into the lateral tibial plateau to result in 3° to 5° of postoperative mechanical valgus.[18] In nonarthritic patients, correction is aimed at shifting the mechanical axis to 50% to 55% on the tibial plateau.[19] Transparent paper is commonly used. First, the WBL is drawn from the center of the femoral head to the center of the tibiotalar joint. The selected WBL coordinate of the tibial plateau is identified and marked at a point 62% lateral on the transverse diameter of the tibial plateau (Fig. 36-2). The new WBL is drawn from the center of the femoral head, passing the knee at the selected point, to the height of the ankle joint line. The hinge of the osteotomy is defined at the lateral cortex of the tibia and connected distally with the new and the old centers of the ankle joint. The correction angle can be measured between these two lines, A and B. The angle of correction at the proximal tibia as well as the distance to the opening of the osteotomy can be calculated.

The deformity in the sagittal plane can be accessed on the true lateral view of the knee. It is widely accepted that

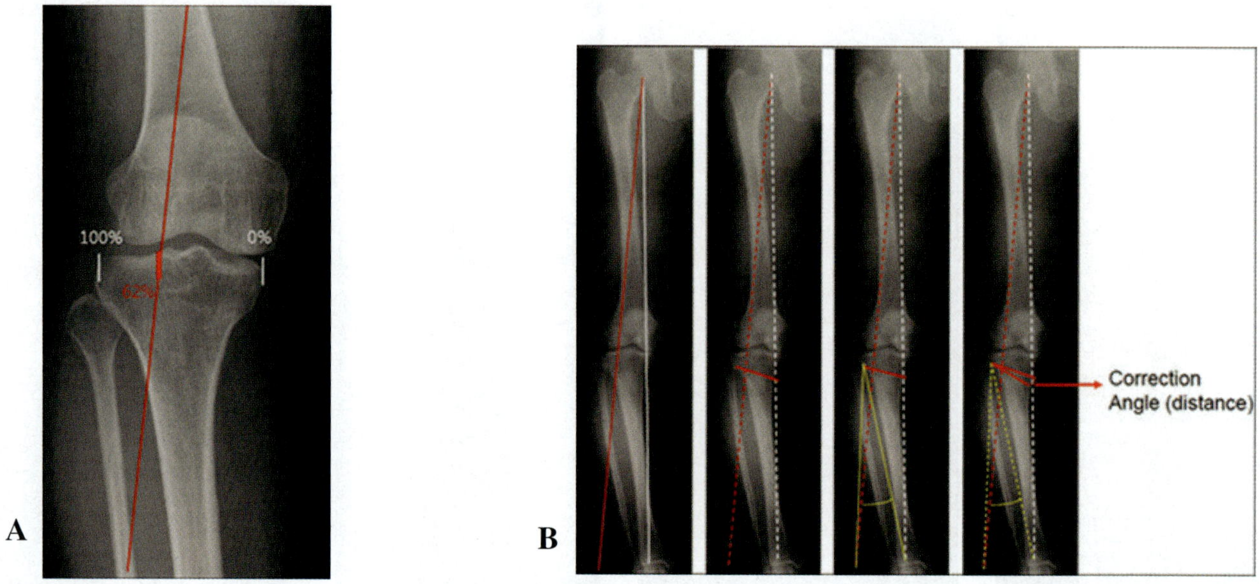

A B

FIGURE 36-2. *For the preoperative planning, templating is carried out on a weight-bearing radiograph of the entire lower limb using a cutout. The object of a valgus osteotomy is to shift the weight-bearing line 62% into the lateral tibial plateau to result in 3° to 5° of postoperative mechanical valgus.*

increasing the posterior tibial slope increases the anteroposterior component of the joint contact force and reduces the posterior subluxation of the tibia in relation to the femur, as seen in posterior cruciate ligament (PCL) deficiencies (Fig. 36-3). Alternatively, decreasing the posterior slope improves both sagittal stability by reducing anterior translation of the tibia and range of motion in knee extension deficit (Fig. 36-4). For example, in PCL insufficiency, osteotomy with an increase of the tibial inclination can be applied in patients with posterior instability to reduce posterior subluxation of the tibia. Open-wedge technique allows excellent control and manipulation of the tibial slope. Therefore, the sagittal plane deformity should be considered in cruciate ligament deficiencies.

SURGERY

Indications

The most common indication for HTO is isolated, degenerative medial compartment joint disease associated with varus tibiofemoral malalignment. Other patients who can be treated by osteotomy around the knee are those with varus malalignment of the leg and ligamentous instability of the knee. In addition, HTO should be considered in physiologically young, active adults with osteochondritis dissecans or spontaneous osteonecrosis of the medial femoral condyle, whose clinical courses are refractory to nonsurgical modalities. Fracture and other trauma, metabolic and neurological disease, and congenital and acquired deformities are also indications for HTO. The age of 65 years is cited most often, but activity level, lifestyle, and general health must be considered. Range of motion in the knee joint should be maintained from over 100° of flexion to less than 10° to 15° of flexion contracture.

Contraindications

Contraindications are medial and unicompartmental degenerative knees with (1) lateral compartment degenerative disease; (2) loss of a significant portion of the lateral meniscus; (3) concomitant symptomatic, moderate to severe patellofemoral joint disease; (4) inflammatory arthritis; (5) severe obesity, (6) poor soft tissue condition at the proximal medial tibia; and (7) systemic or local inflammation.

Positioning and Arthroscopy

For open-wedge HTO, the patient is placed in the supine position with a tourniquet under spinal or general anesthesia. The image intensifier is set up opposite the surgeon.

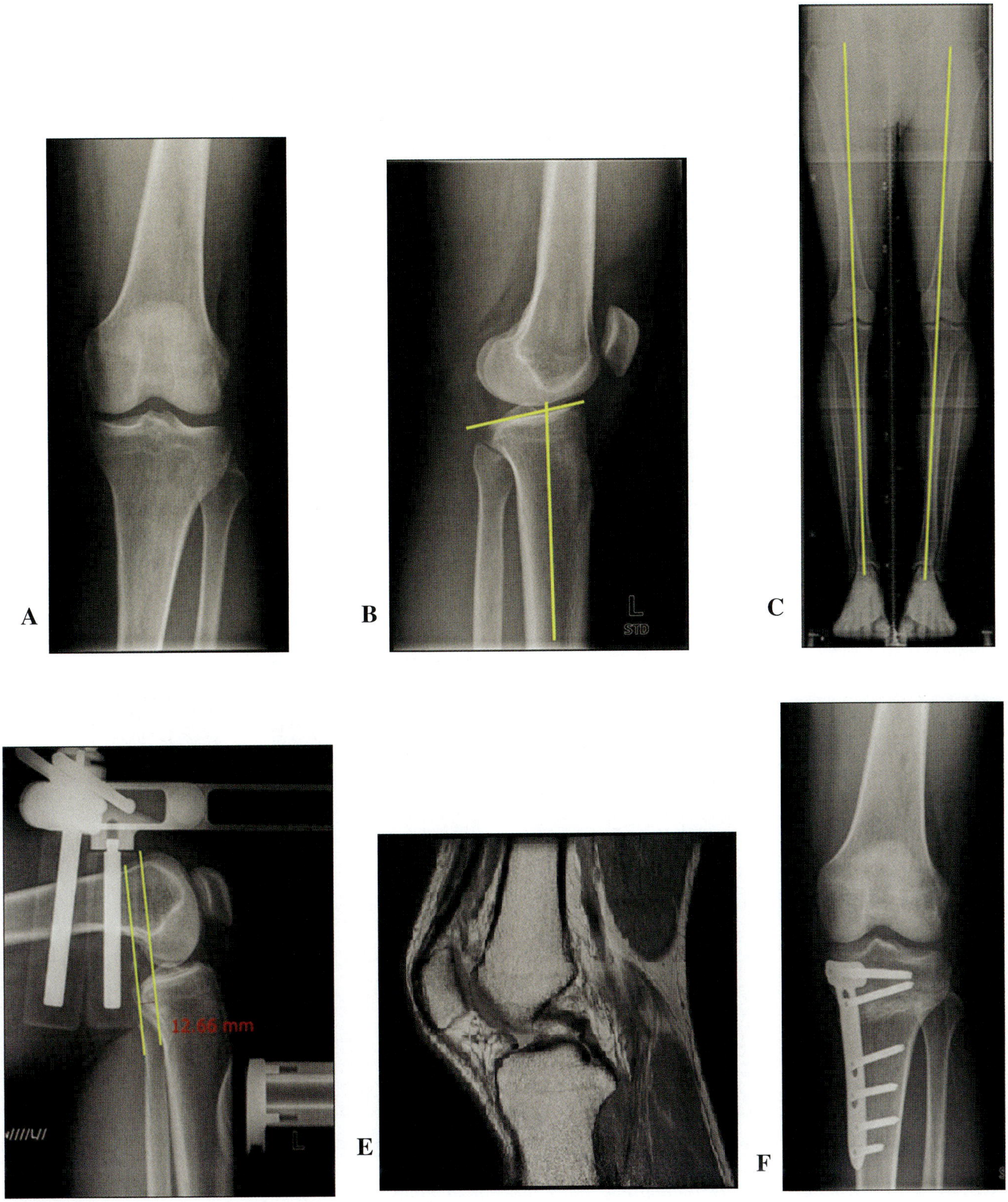

FIGURE 36-3. *See next page for figure legend.*

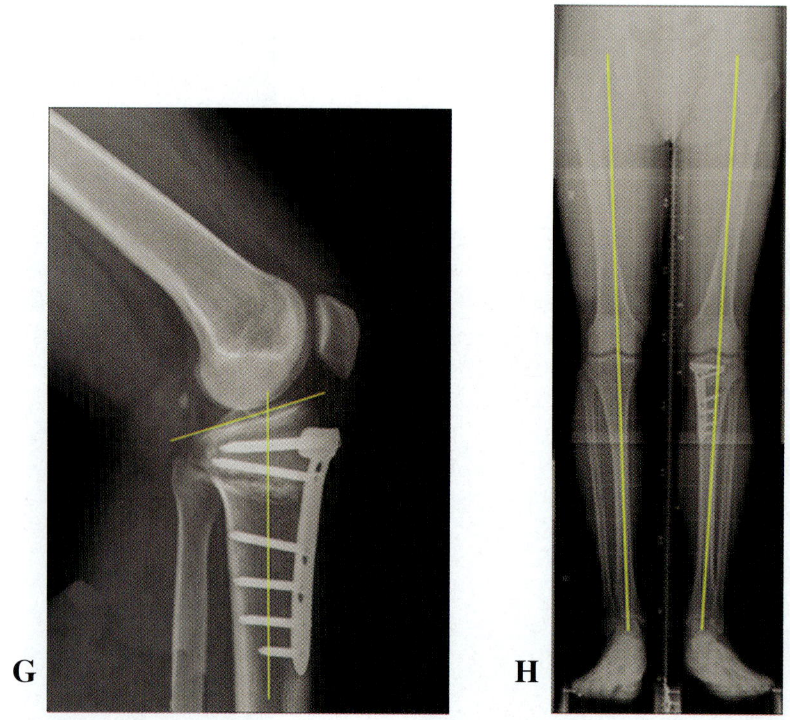

FIGURE 36-3 Continued. *(A, B) The posterior tibial slope is measured as 10° in preoperative radiographs. (C) A weight-bearing radiograph of the entire lower limb shows varus alignment in left knee joint. (D) A posterior stress radiograph using the Telos device shows 12.6-mm posterior translation of the tibia. (E) A magnetic resonance image shows continuous but deformed posterior cruciate ligament fiber, which means chronic PCL injury. (F, G, H) After open-wedge high tibial osteotomy with valgization and flexion using the TomoFix system, the posterior tibial slope is increased to 17° in postoperative radiographs.*

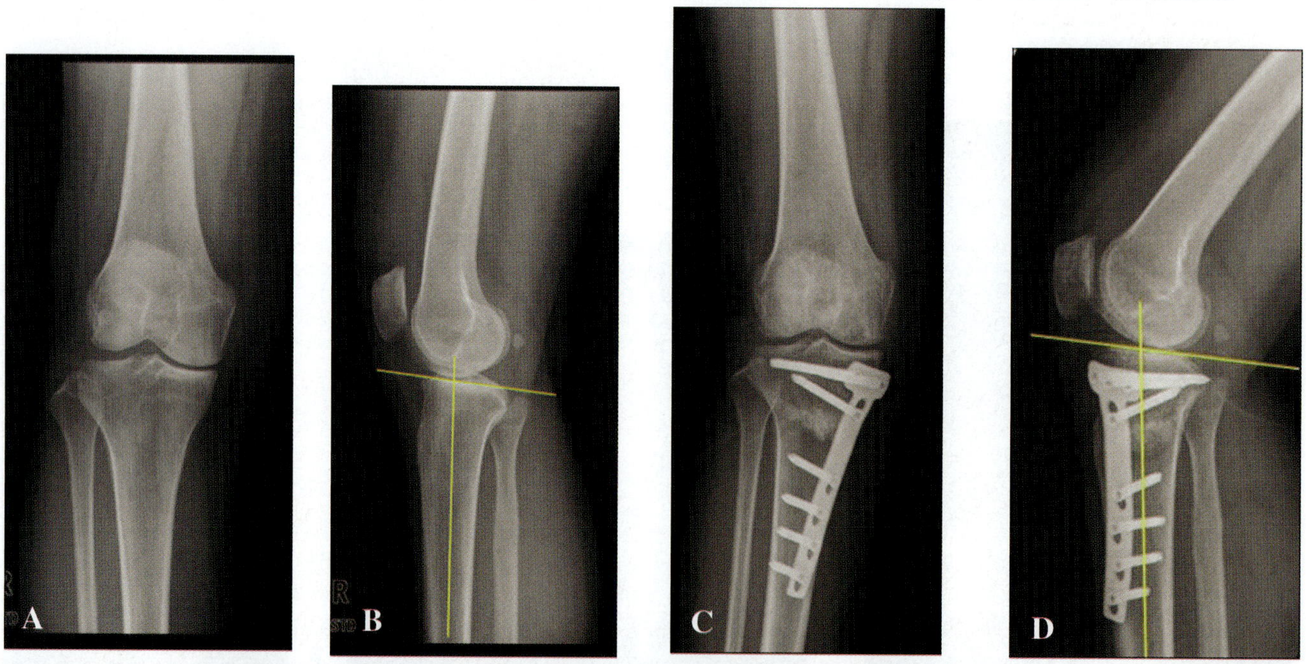

FIGURE 36-4. *(A, B) Preoperative radiographs show varus malalignment in the knee joint. The posterior tibial slope is measured as 8.5°. (C, D) After open-wedge high tibial osteotomy with valgization and extension using the TomoFix system, the posterior tibial slope is decreased to 5.5° in postoperative radiographs.*

The lower extremity is prepared and draped in the usual orthopaedic manner. Although concomitant arthroscopy is not mandatory in HTO, it may be more sophisticated care to the arthritic knee. Intra-articular pathology can be identified by arthroscopy, and excision of torn meniscus could be done with anterolateral and anteromedial portals. The lateral and patellofemoral compartments are inspected to determine if HTO is a suitable decision. Cartilage damages in the medial compartment are precisely documented, unstable cartilage flaps are debrided, and microfracturing can be performed. In cases of mechanically irritated meniscal abnormalities or loose bodies, partial meniscectomy or loose body removal is recommended.

Surgical Technique

A 4- to 5-cm incision is made horizontally on the anteromedial aspect parallel to the 1-cm superior margin of the pes anserinus (Fig. 36-5). Dissection through the sartorial fascia is performed to expose the gracilis and semitendinosus tendons, and both tendons are retracted distally and preserved (Fig. 36-6). The superficial medial collateral ligament is carefully released from the posteromedial cortex of the tibia with a Cobb elevator (Fig. 36-7). The release of the medial collateral ligament is a mandatory procedure in an open-wedge HTO. Without adequate and sufficient release of the ligament, the symptoms may not be resolved even if the varus angle is corrected because medial joint contact force is still at high stress.[14] A blunt-tip narrow radiolucent Hohm ann retractor is inserted at the posteromedial cortex to protect the neurovascular structures. The placement of the biplanar osteotomy is marked using a marking pen before the insertion of the guide pins (Fig. 36-8). Two 1.8-mm K-wires are inserted as a guide from just proximal to the insertion of the pes anserinus to the lateral cortical margin at the level of the top of the fibula and

A
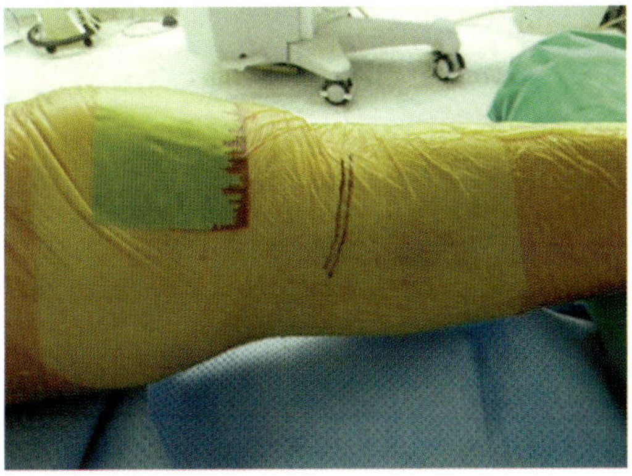

B
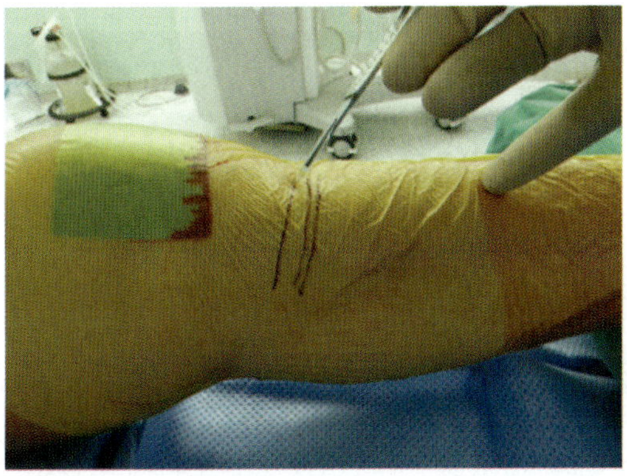

FIGURE 36-5. *(A) The gracilis and semitendinosus tendon insertions are marked for placement of skin incision on the anteromedial aspect. (**B**) A 4- to 5-cm incision is made parallel to the 1-cm superior margin of the pes anserinus.*

A
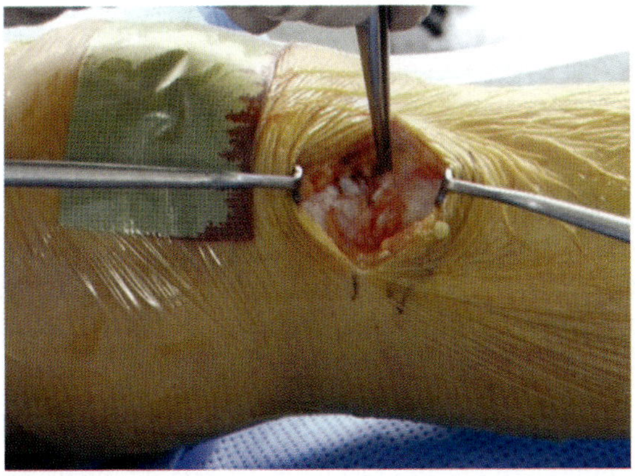

B
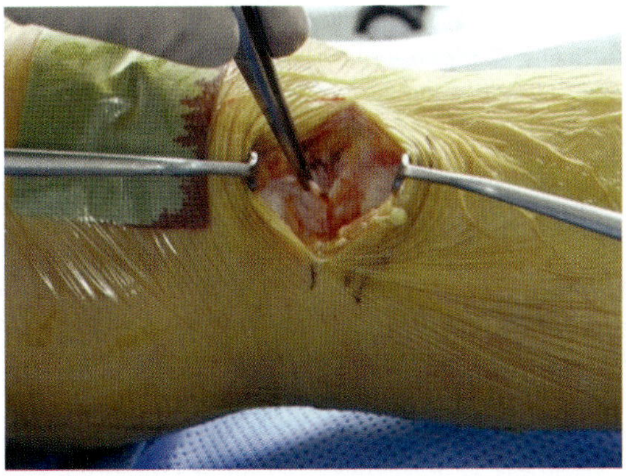

FIGURE 36-6. *After dissection through the sartorial fascia is performed, the gracilis and semitendinosus tendons (**A**) and the superficial medial collateral ligament (**B**) are identified.*

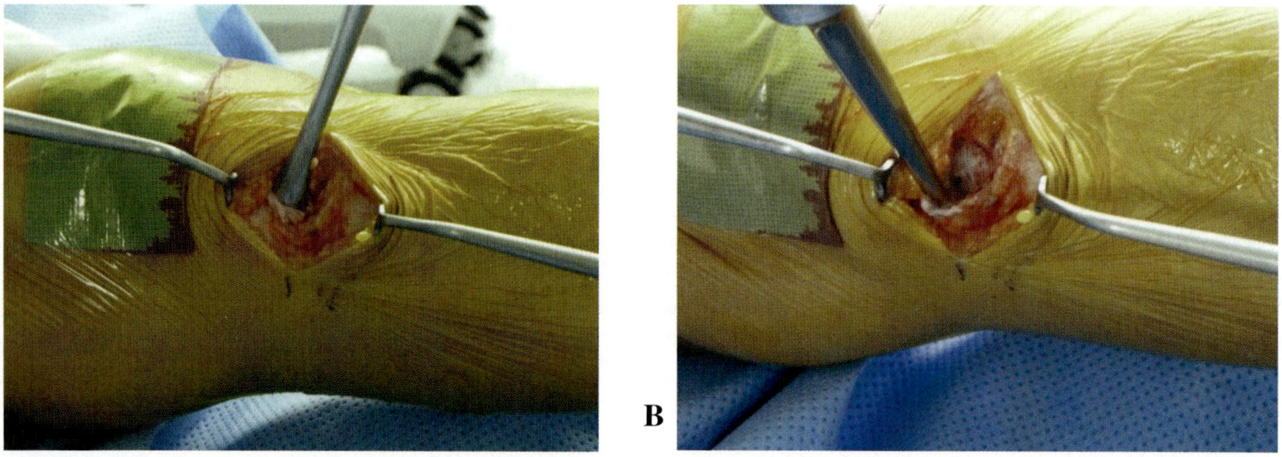

FIGURE 36-7. *The superficial medial collateral ligament is carefully subperiosteally released from the posteromedial cortex of the tibia with a Cobb elevator.*

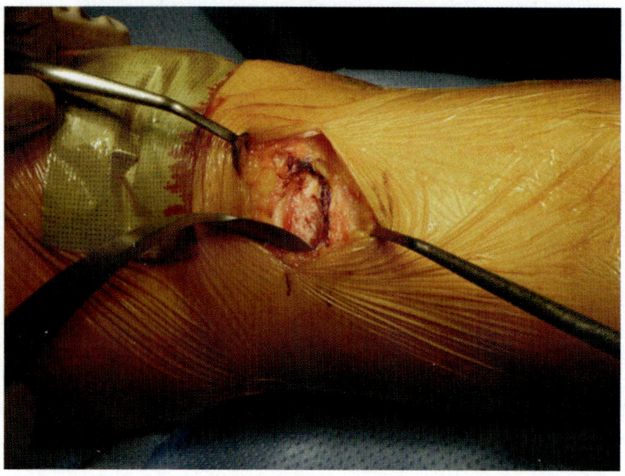

FIGURE 36-8. *The placement of the osteotomy site is marked using a marking pen before the insertion of the guide pins. These lines show the plan of the biplanar osteotomy, which is composed of horizontal and tibial tuberosity osteotomies.*

parallel to the tibial slope under image intensification (Fig. 36-9). The depth of the osteotomy can be measured from the medial cortex to the lateral hinge using the same-length K-wire. The osteotomy depth should be 10 mm shorter than the measured length (Fig. 36-10).The horizontal osteotomy is performed, parallel to the tibial slope, with the thin oscillating saw along with the two guide pins and continuous irrigation cooling of the saw blade (Fig. 36-11A). The second osteotomy at biplanar osteotomy sites starts in the anterior one-third of the proximal tibia and proximal to the insertion of the patella tendon at an angle of 130° to the first osteotomy plane (Fig. 36-11B). The broad flat chisel is inserted into the horizontal osteotomy site parallel to the two guide pins under image intensification (Fig. 36-12). Next, the narrow flat chisel is inserted into the tibial tuberosity osteotomy site. Therefore, the flat chisels are inserted into the first and second osteotomy sites (Fig. 36-13). A thick posterior cortex is especially important to note. If the posterior tibial osteotomy is not completed, it is difficult to spread in the posterior part, which can cause an increase of the posterior slope (Fig. 36-14). Therefore, a gentle and cautious posterior cortical osteotomy using an osteotome with posterior direction is sometimes needed in cases with a thicker posterior cortex in a healthy strong bone. After inserting the chisel into the transverse osteotomy, another broad flat chisel is placed between the first chisel and the guide pins. Additional flat chisels can be inserted between the ones already in place, and the gap is spread opened using chisels (Fig. 36-15). Then two osteotomies are gripped in each hand and diverted manually into valgus direction, checking valgization under image intensification. The spreader chisel is then driven into the osteotomy gap by light hammer blows and the gap is opened to the desired width by opening the spreader chisel with a large screwdriver (Fig. 36-16). The correction is now retained with a bone spreader that is inserted into the posteromedial osteotomy gap. The mechanical axis is then adjusted according to the preoperative planning under image intensification and a long straight measuring rod is placed at the center of the femoral head and at the center of the ankle joint (Fig. 36-17). To maintain posterior slope, the posterior opening gap at the most posteromedial cortex is usually 1.5 times larger than the anterior opening gap at the anteromedial cortex just behind the tibial tuberosity (Fig. 36-18). The shape of the opening gap should be trapezoidal, not rectangular, since the anterior gap is usually narrower than the posterior gap. A difference between the anterior and posterior opening of the osteotomy gap can be measured by a Vernier caliper (Fig. 36-19). While the gap is kept open with a bone spreader on the posteromedial side of the osteotomy gap, the plate is inserted into a subcutaneous tunnel and centered on the anteromedial plane of the tibia (Fig. 36-20).

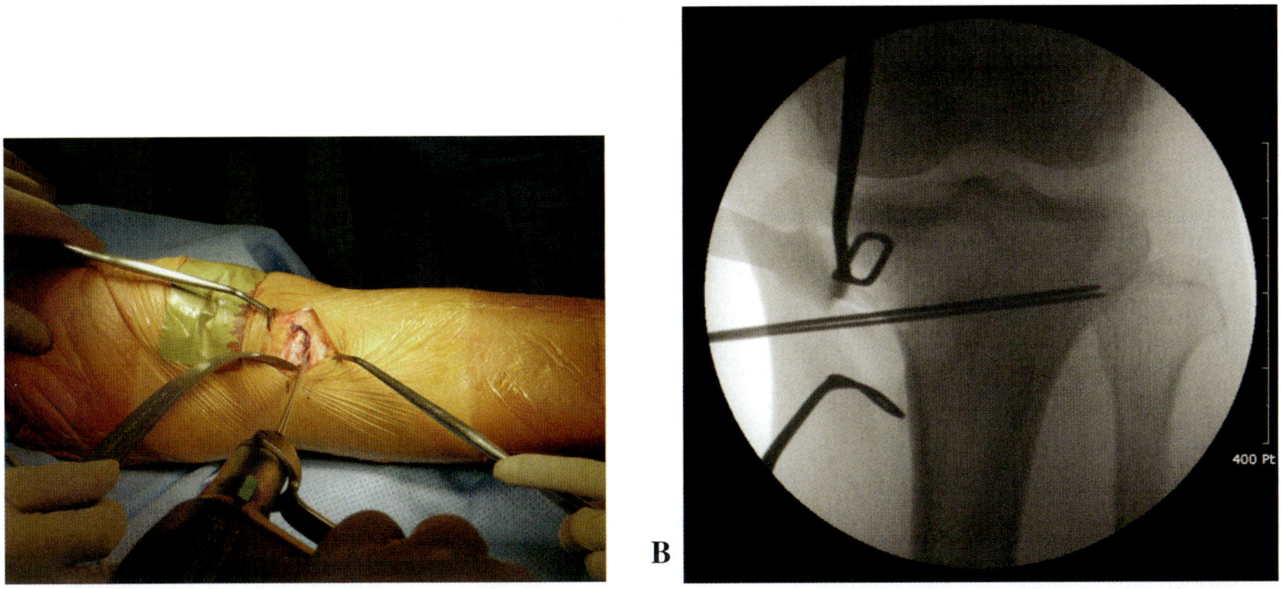

FIGURE 36-9. *(**A**) Two guide pins are inserted into the lateral cortical margin aimed at the level of the top of the fibula under the image intensifier control. (**B**) An image intensifier shows two parallel guide pins.*

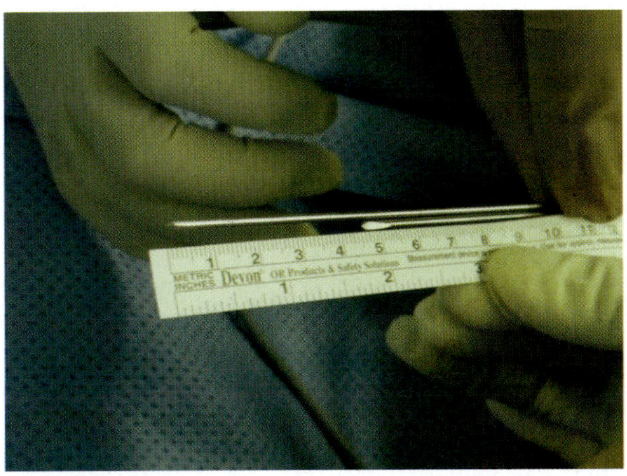

FIGURE 36-10. *The depth of osteotomy can be measured using an inserted K-wire of the same length. With this method, the osteotomy depth can be assessed from the medial cortex to the lateral hinge. To prevent breakage of the lateral cortical hinge, the osteotomy depth should be 10 mm shorter than the length of the inserted K-wire.*

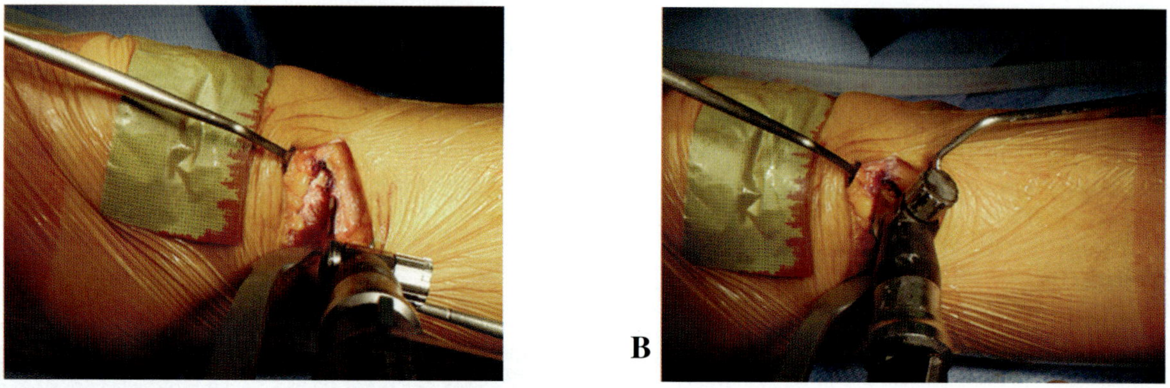

FIGURE 36-11. *(**A**) The horizontal osteotomy is performed, parallel to the tibial slope, with the thin oscillating saw. (**B**) The tibial tuberosity osteotomy is performed to an angle of 120° to 130° between the two osteotomies.*

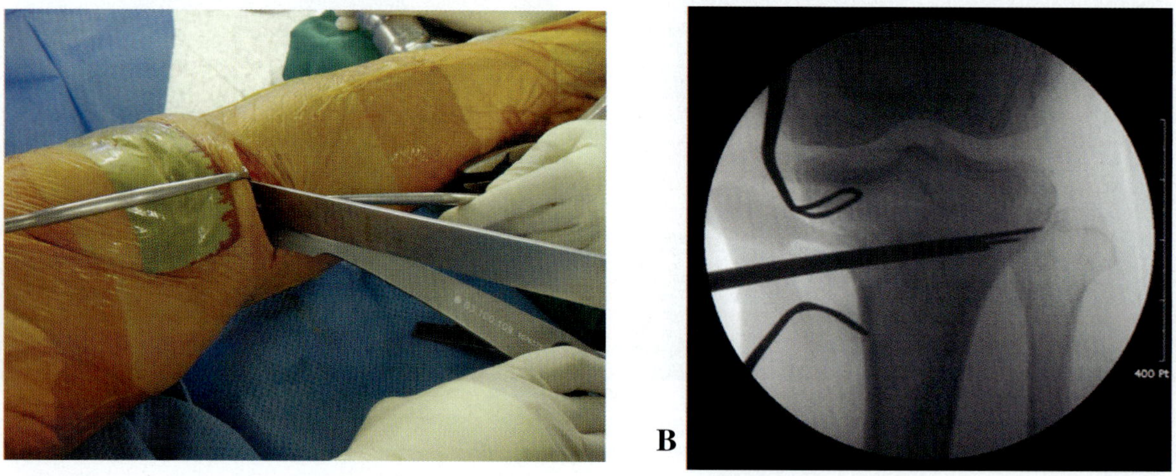

FIGURE 36-12. *(**A**) The broad flat chisel is inserted into the horizontal osteotomy site. (**B**) An image intensifier shows the flat chisel is inserted parallel to two guide pins up to 10 mm of the lateral cortex.*

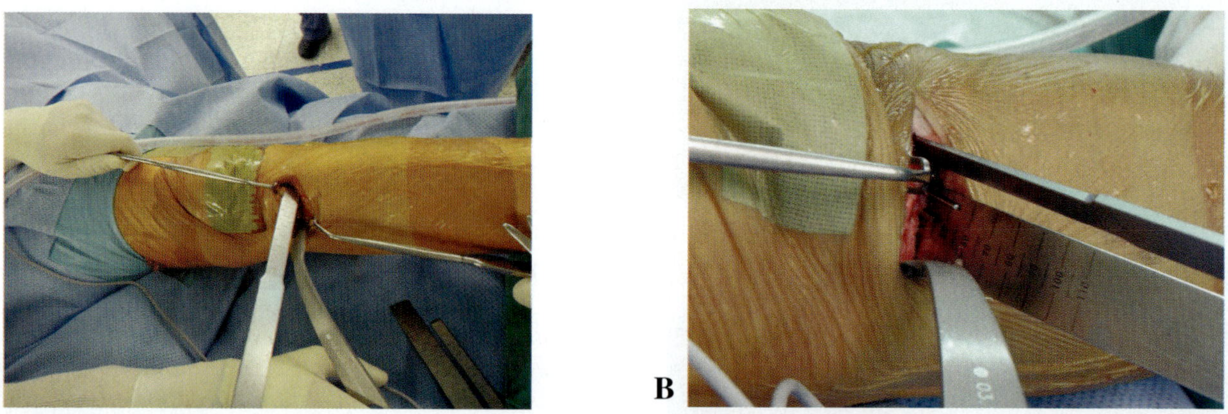

FIGURE 36-13. *(**A**) The narrow flat chisel is inserted into the tibial tuberosity osteotomy site. (**B**) Two flat chisels are positioned at the biplanar osteotomy sites.*

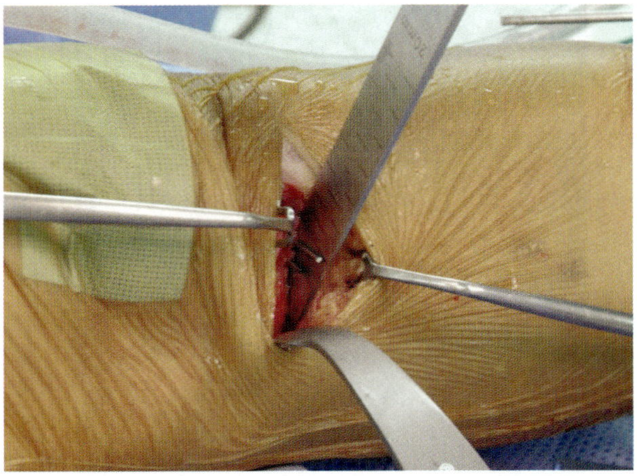

FIGURE 36-14. *Careful and complete posterior cortical osteotomy is essential.*

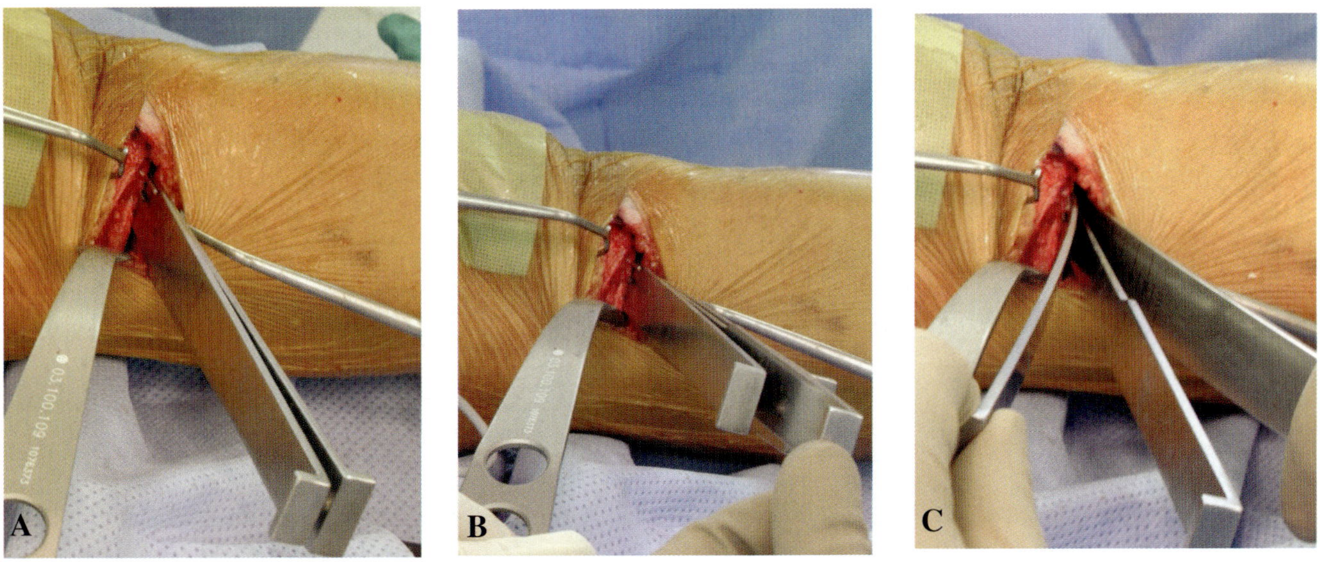

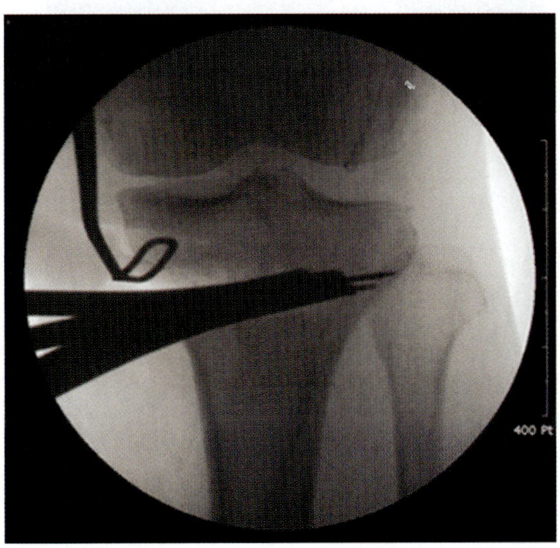

D

FIGURE 36-15. *(**A**) Additional flat chisels can be inserted between the first chisel and the guide pins. (**B**) Then additional flat chisels can be inserted between the ones already in place, and the gap is spread open using chisels. (**C**) Two osteotomies are gripped in each hand and diverted manually into a valgus direction with checking valgization in the image intensifier. (**D**) An image intensifier shows spreading of the gap using three flat chisels.*

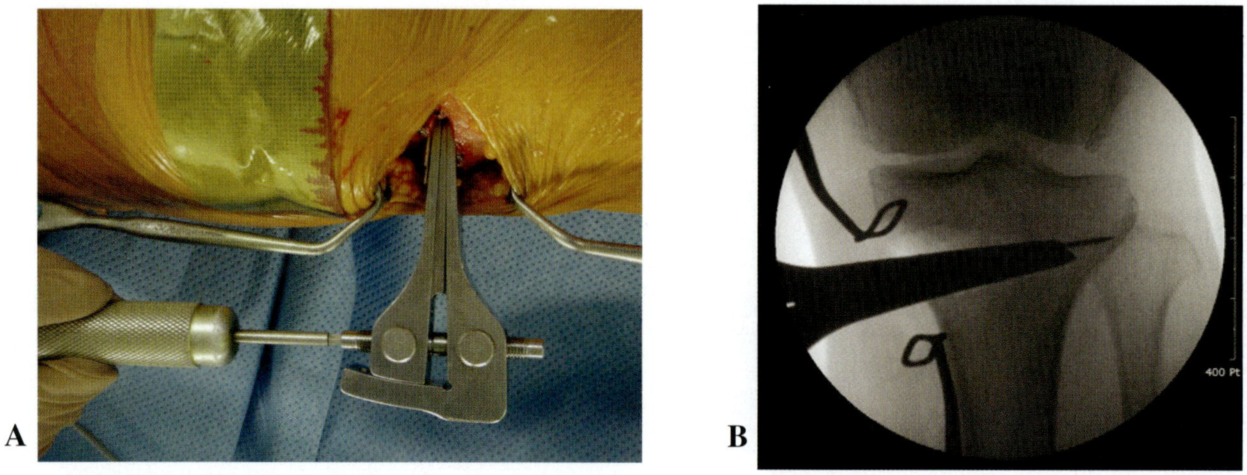

FIGURE 36-16. *(**A**) The spreader chisel is driven into the osteotomy gap and the gap is opened to the desired width by use of a driver. (**B**) An image intensifier shows opening of osteotomy gap by spreader chisel.*

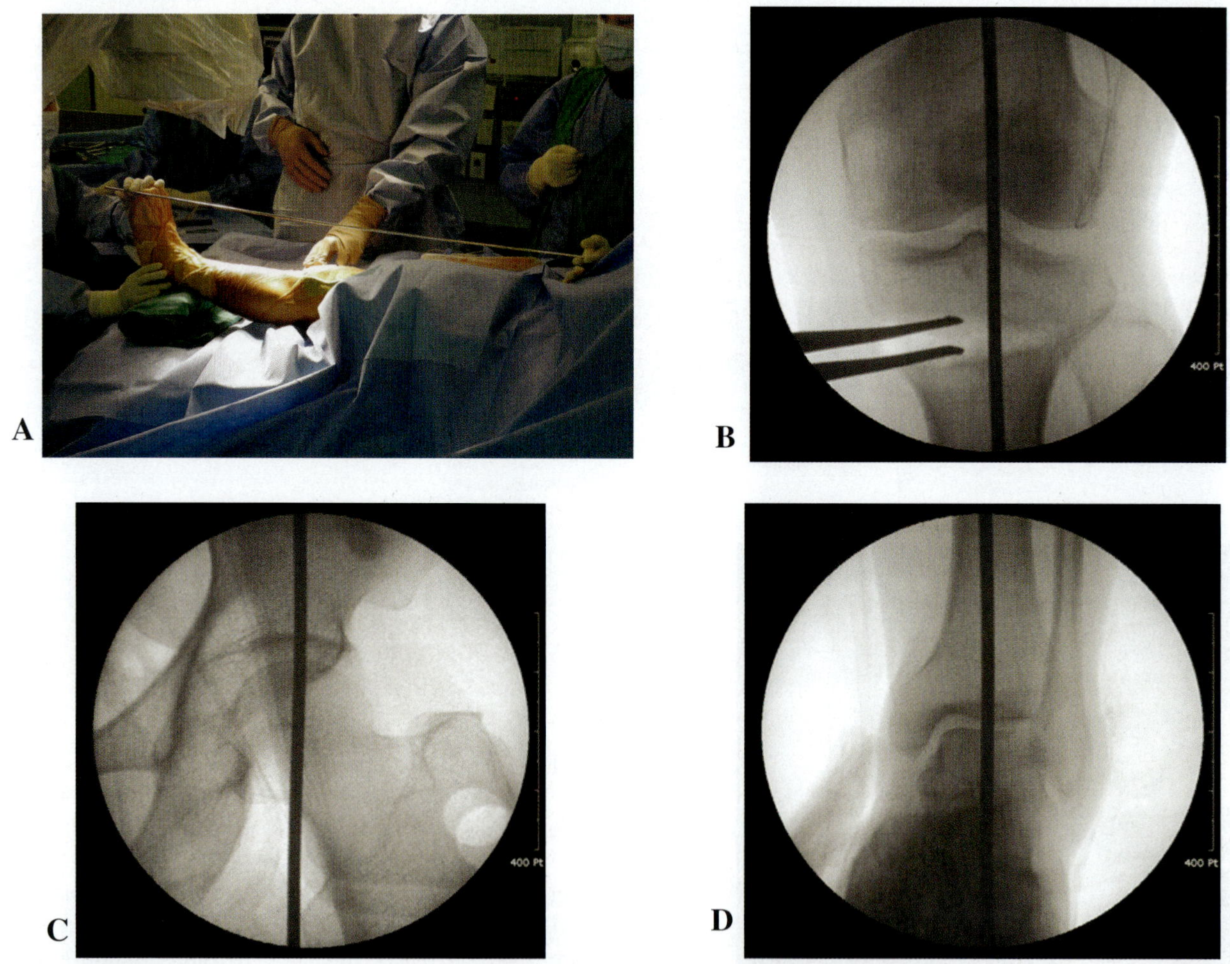

FIGURE 36-17. *A long, straight measuring rod is placed at the center of the femoral head and at the center of the upper ankle joint under image intensification.*

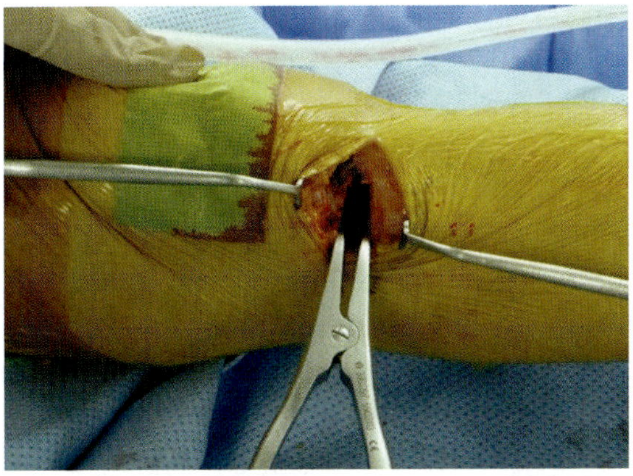

FIGURE 36-18. *The posterior opening gap is usually 1.5 times larger than the anterior opening gap after complete release of the medial collateral ligament. The shape of opening gap should be trapezoidal, not rectangular, since the anterior gap is usually narrower than the posterior gap.*

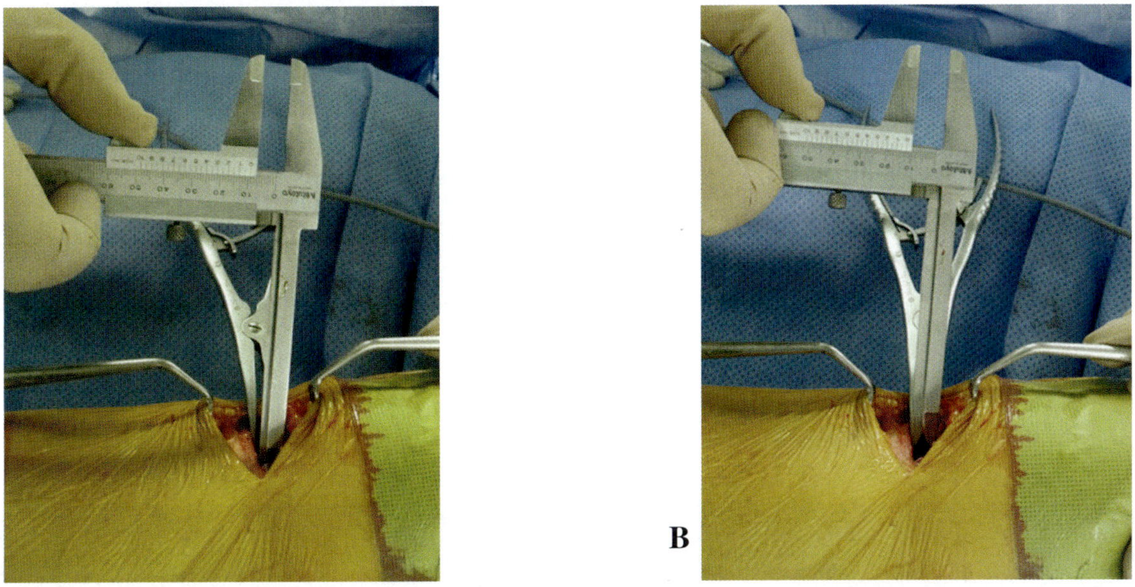

A B

FIGURE 36-19. *(**A**) An anterior ostetomy gap is measured as 8.8 mm by a Vernier caliper. (**B**) A posterior osteotomy gap (12.2 mm) is bigger than an anterior osteotomy gap.*

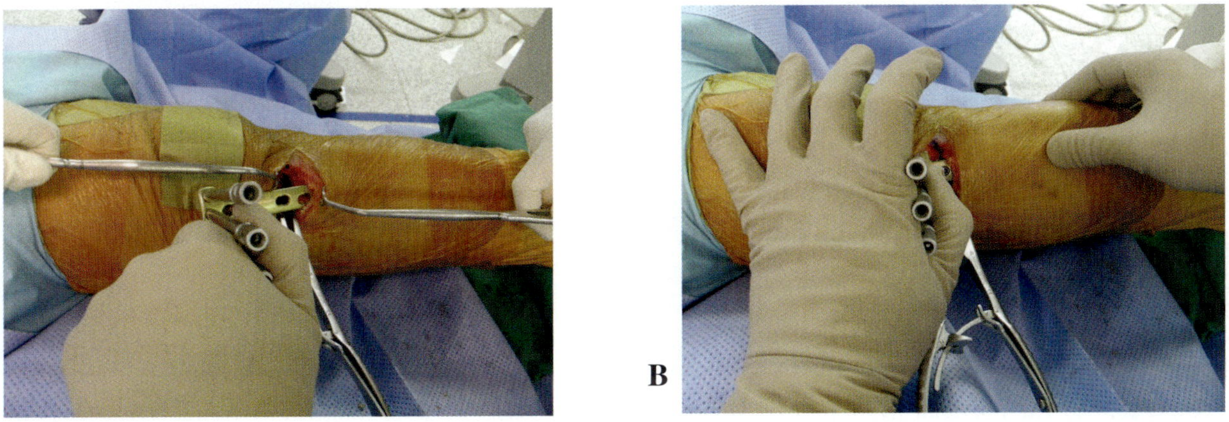

A B

FIGURE 36-20. *(**A**) While the gap is kept open with a bone spreader on the posteromedial side, the plate is inserted subcutaneously. (**B**) The plate should be positioned at the center of the anteromedial plane of the tibia.*

The K-wire is inserted into the central drill sleeve for temporarily stabilizing the plate onto the tibia. The proximal fixation of the plate is carried out with three locking head screws, which provide wide support of the tibial plateau in the subchondral area (Fig. 36-21). The temporary lag screw is then inserted just distal to the osteotomy for pretensioning (Fig. 36-22). This compresses the lateral hinge by pulling the distal osteotomy segment toward the plate fixator and

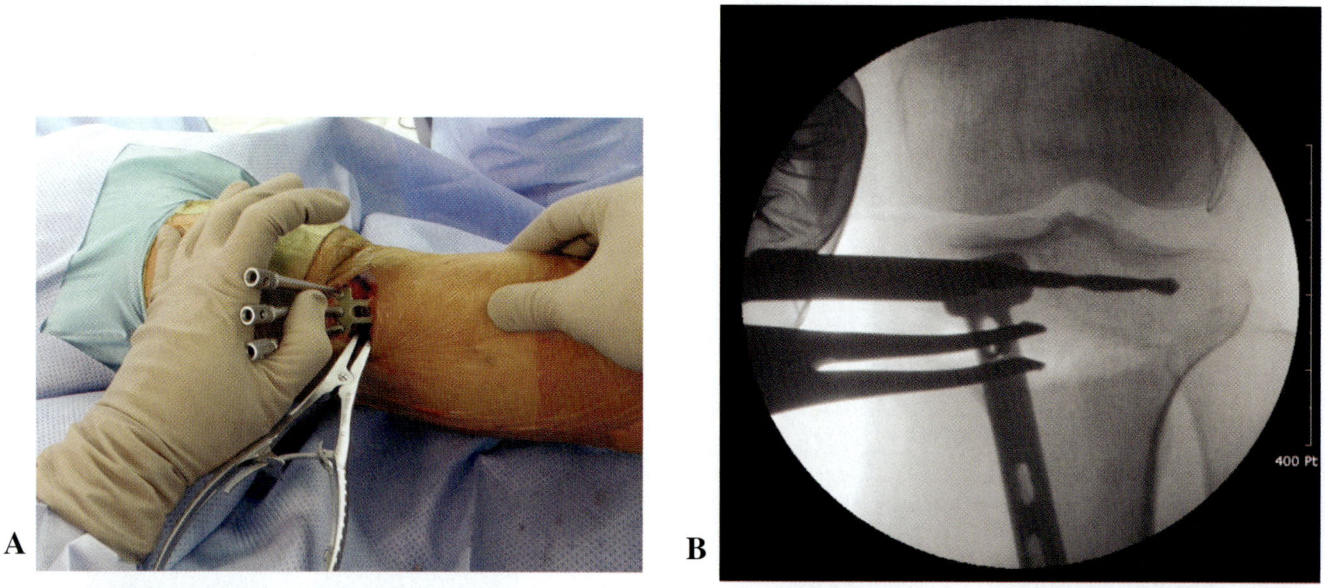

FIGURE 36-21. *(**A**) The proximal fixation of the plate is carried out with three locking head screws in the subchondral area. (**B**) An image intensifier shows the drill bit is situated in the dense subchondral area about 1 cm below the joint line.*

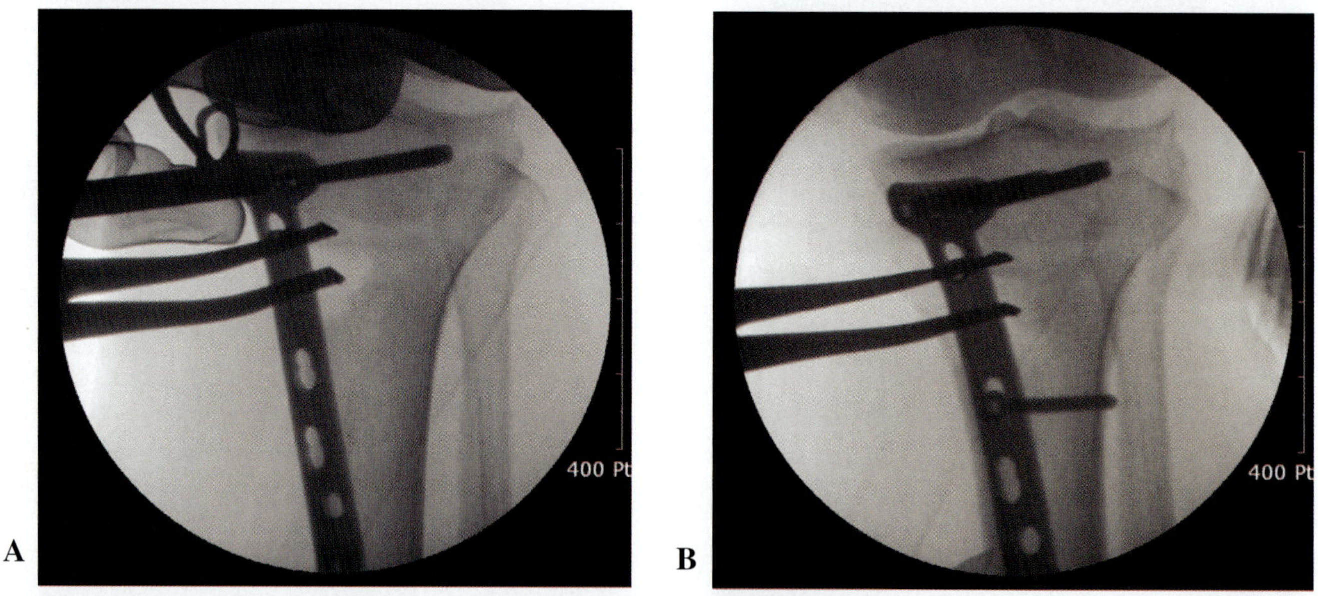

FIGURE 36-22. *(**A**) The proximal fixation of the plate is carried out with three locking head screws. (**B**) A temporary lag screw is inserted just distal to the osteotomy for compressing the lateral hinge by pulling the distal osteotomy segment toward the plate fixator and contouring the plate to the tibia.*

approximates the distal fragment to the plate. The three distal locking head screws are inserted through a small incision and a locking head screw is inserted proximal to the gap (Fig. 36-23). And then, the temporary lag screw is replaced by a bicortical locking screw. Finally, a locking head screw is inserted just proximal to the gap. Bone substitute is filled and impacted into the osteotomy gap (Fig. 36-24). It is not always necessary to transplant autogenous bone graft into the osteotomy gap. The authors recommend that autogenous cancellous bone graft from the anterior iliac crest is performed to promote rapid healing and prevent collapse, especially if the gap width exceeds 9 to 10 mm. The image intensifier is checked for documentation before the wound closure. The suction drains are inserted into both the knee joint and the wound of the proximal tibia (Fig. 36-25). The wound is closed layer by layer.

A B
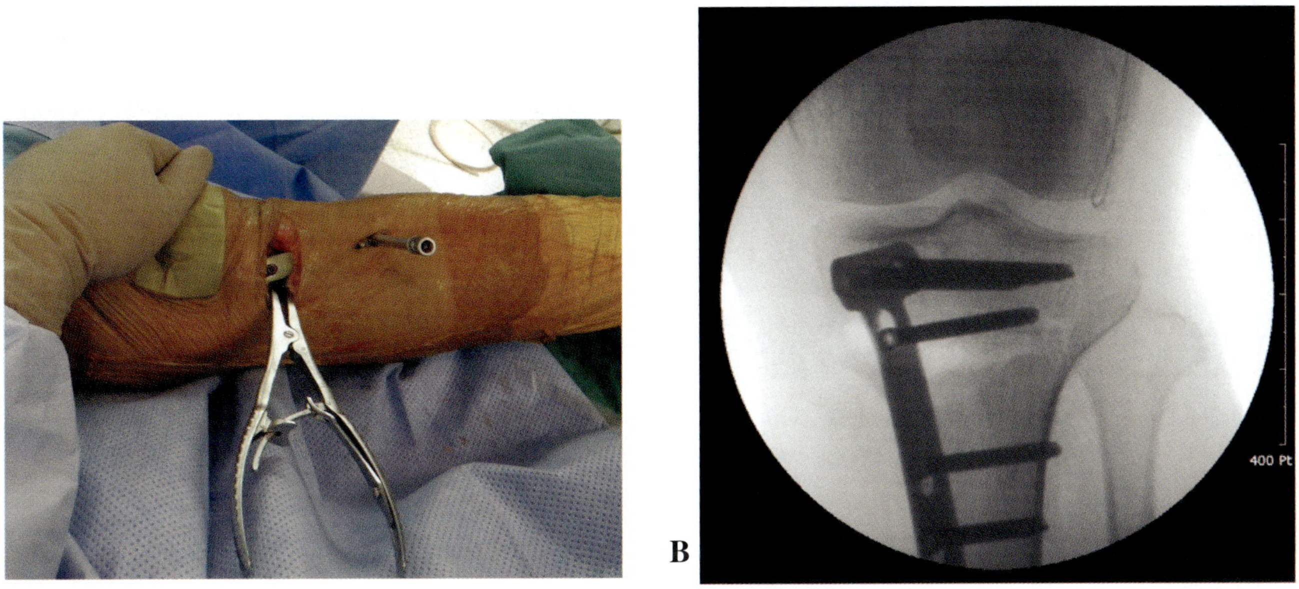

FIGURE 36-23. *(**A**) The distal three locking head screws are inserted consecutively through a small incision. (**B**) A temporary lag screw is then replaced by a bicortical locking screw and finally a locking head screw is inserted proximal of the gap.*

A B
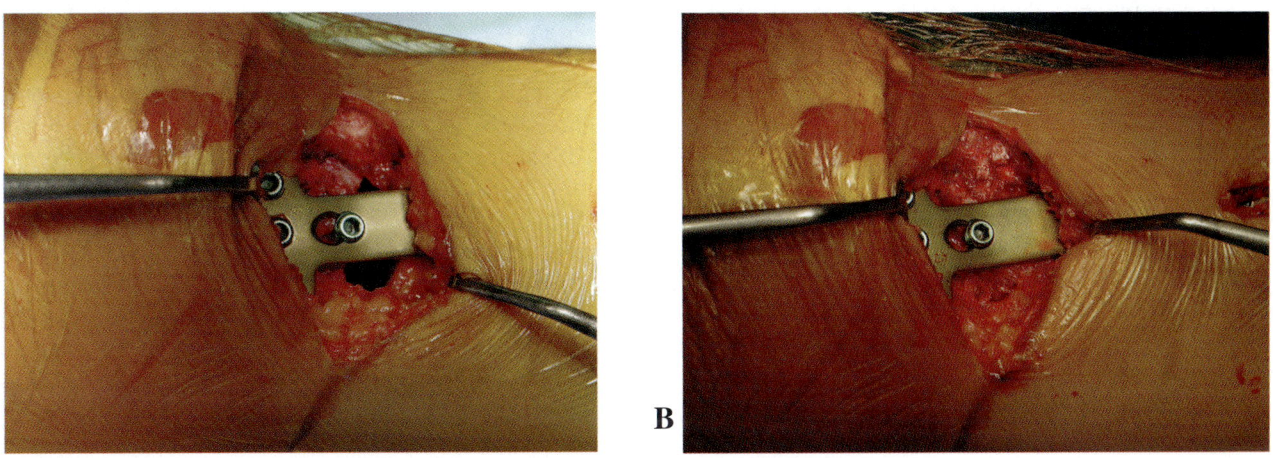

FIGURE 36-24. *(**A**) The osteotomy gap is shown beneath the plate. (**B**) If the posterior gap is measured to be larger than 10 mm, cancellous chip bone is impacted into the osteotomy gap.*

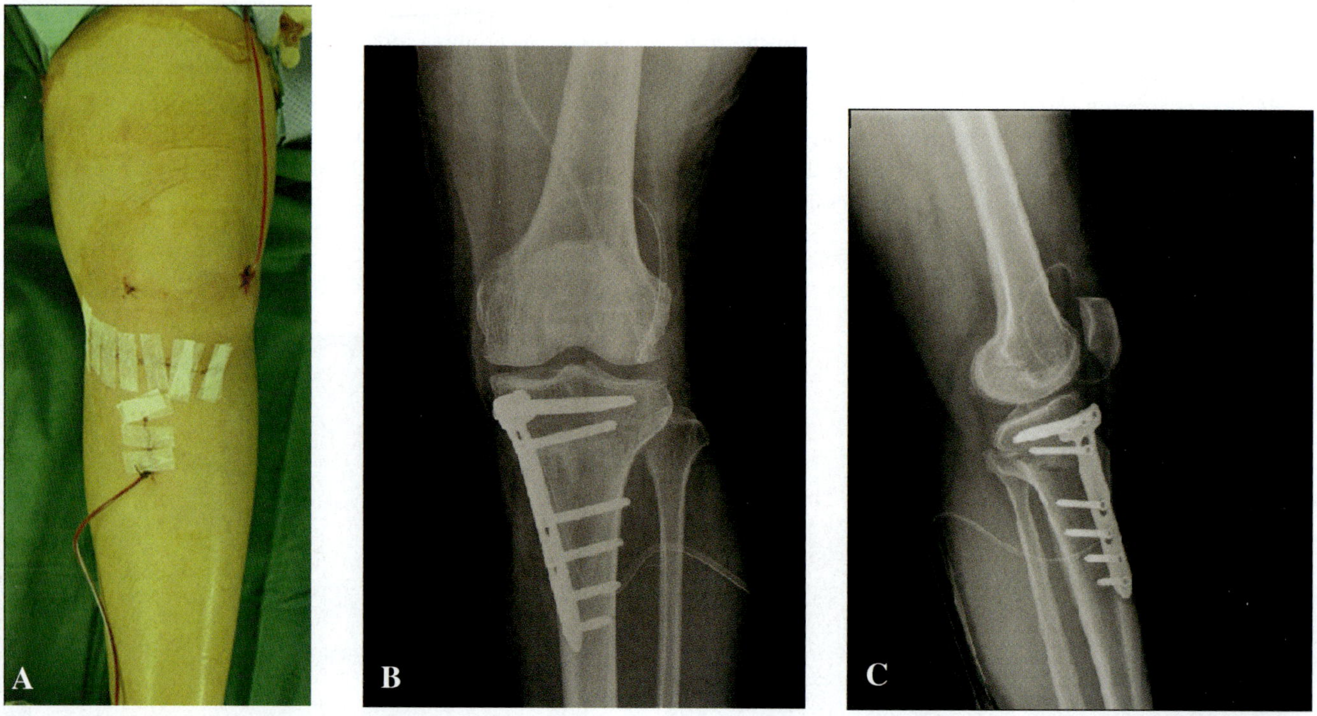

FIGURE 36-25. *(**A**) Final postoperative clinical photo showing the placement of suction drains and skin incision. (**B, C**) Immediate postoperative anteroposterior and lateral radiographs showing locking screw plated designs.*

POSTOPERATIVE MANAGEMENT

Rehabilitation

Active and passive range of motion is initiated on the 1st postoperative day. Partial weight bearing with crutch ambulation is started 3 days postoperatively. Patients are allowed to begin full weight bearing by the 6th postoperative week. Patients are also restricted for 6 months from sports that require jumping, cutting, or twisting maneuvers (Fig. 36-26). Hardware is routinely removed 2 years postoperatively.

Complications

Potential complications that may occur include delayed union, nonunion, loss of correction, overcorrection, infection, vascular injury, compartment syndrome, intra-articular fracture, limb lengthening, and thromboembolism. The rate of tibia nonunion in a medial opening-wedge HTO varies from 1.1% to 4.3%.[8,10] The delayed or nonunion may be attributed to several factors, including inadequate internal fixation, fracture of lateral cortex, and large angular correction without bone graft. Patient demographic risk factors for nonunion include tobacco use and diabetes mellitus.

Inadequate or overcorrection of lower limb alignment has been reported by many authors.[3,8,20] Careful preoperative planning is required to avoid inadequate correction. During the operation, confirmation of adequate correction should be accomplished under an image intensifier. Although an ideal position can be verified at surgery, there may be a change when postoperative full-standing radiographs are taken at 6 to 8 weeks postoperatively. Loss of the axial alignment obtained at surgery may depend closely on maintaining the initial fixation (Fig. 36-27). The gap created in a medial opening-wedge HTO facilitates instability and loss of correction. This is mainly caused by a lack of primary stability. Therefore, an opening-wedge HTO should always be supported by an internal or external fixation method. It is also important to realize that stability is largely dependent on an unharmed lateral hinge (Fig. 36-28). The osteotomy should be opened slowly in order to prevent fracturing of the lateral cortex.

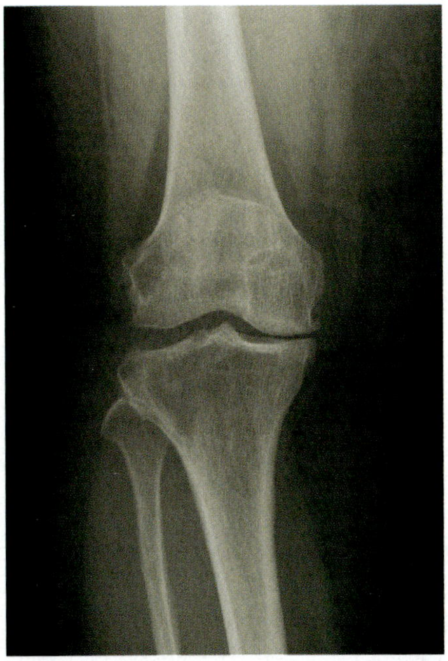

A

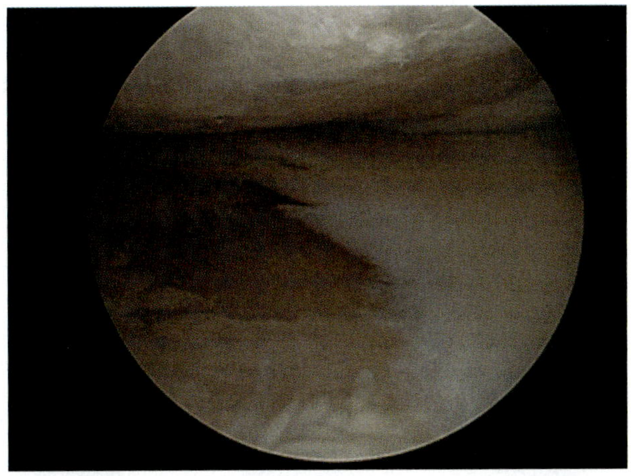

B

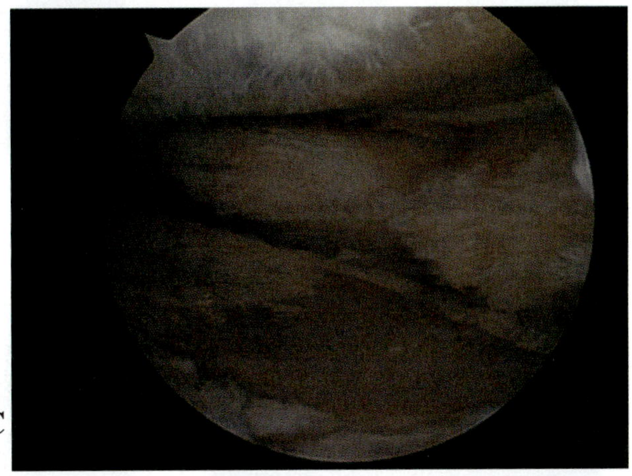

C

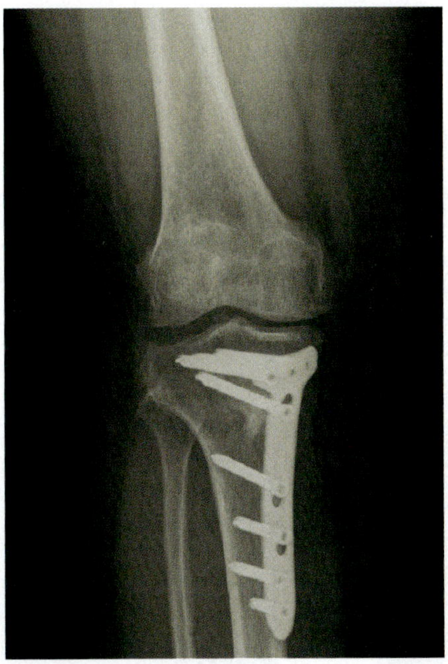

D

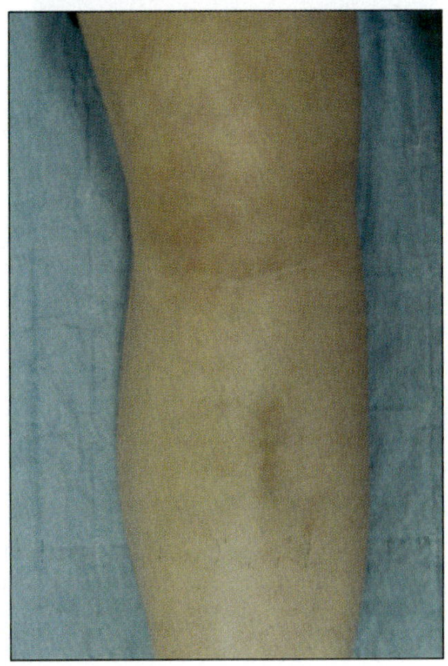

E

FIGURE 36-26. *(**A**) An anteroposterior radiograph shows varus malalignment with medial joint space narrowing. (**B**) Arthroscopic finding shows a tear of the medial meniscus and a deep chondral defect of the medial femoral condyle and medial tibial plateau. (**C**) Arthroscopic partial meniscectomy is performed. (**D**) Follow-up weight-bearing anteroposterior image shows slightly valgus alignment after open-wedge osteotomy. (**E**) Photograph shows a minimal operative scar and improved leg shape.*

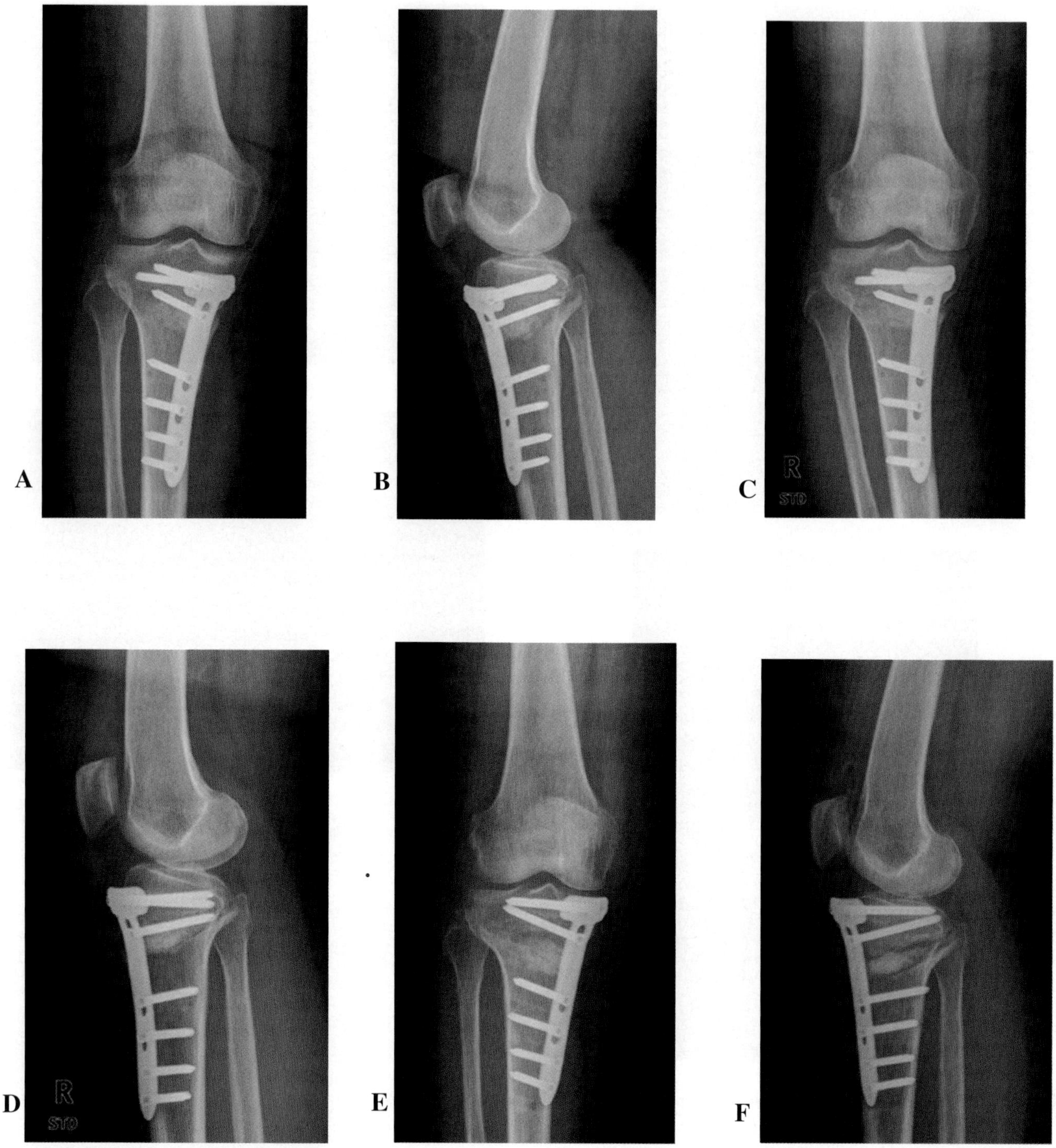

FIGURE 36-27. *(**A**, **B**) Immediate postoperative radiographs show TomoFix plate fixation after open-wedge high tibial osteotomy. (**C**, **D**) Follow-up radiographs in the 6-week postoperative period show lateral cortical breakage with loss of correction. This loss of correction was caused by early full weight bearing as well as a slightly distal plate position. (**E**, **F**) After revision open-wedge osteotomy, the proximal screw in the plate is situated in the subchondral area about 1 cm below the joint line in 6-month follow-up radiographs.*

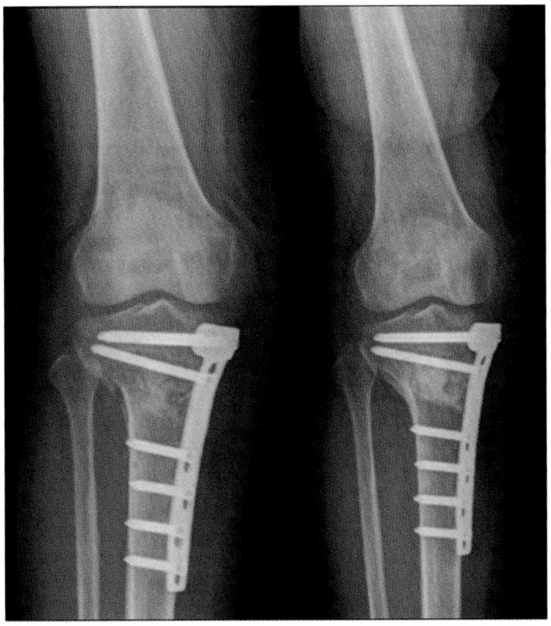

FIGURE 36-28. *Immediate postoperative radiograph shows lateral cortical breakage. Fourteen-month follow-up radiograph shows bone healing without loss of correction due to delayed weight bearing.*

Fracture of the lateral tibial plateau after open-wedge HTO is reported to be from 1% to 20%.[3,7,21] This complication can be avoided by meticulously following the described technique. The proximal osteotomy should maintain 20 mm or more thickness of tibial width proximally. Therefore, aiming the point of the guide pin to the lateral hinge area is not recommended higher than the tip of the fibular head. Fractures are also caused by the use of thick osteotomies.

Recent studies have demonstrated that a decrease in patellar height associated with medial open-wedge HTO is due to distalization of the tuberosity as a result of valgus correction and to shortening of the patellar ligament after scarring. These results caution that the high incidence of patella infera following medial opening-wedge HTO may have deleterious effects on patellofemoral biomechanics or complicate subsequent total knee arthroplasty.

In the literature, the rate of infection after a medial opening-wedge HTO varies from 2.3% to 20% (Fig. 36-29).[3,7,9,10,22] Unstable osteosynthesis causes irritation of soft tissues and may induce infection. Vascular complications are exceedingly rare following open-wedge HTO. Transection of the posterior tibial cortex risks damage to the popliteal vessels.[14] The incidence of deep vein thrombosis has been rarely reported following HTO. Turner et al[23] reported a 41% rate of deep vein thrombosis using venography after HTO in 84 patients, although only 15% of these had been diagnosed clinically.

OUTCOME

Some literature suggests that HTO provides durable and satisfactory long-term clinical results if the procedure is accurately performed in carefully selected patients, who are typically younger than 65 years and have less than 12° of angular deformity, pure unicompartmental disease, ligamentous stability, and a preoperative range of motion of at least 100°.[5,8-10,20] The two principal techniques to produce valgus realignment of the proximal tibial articular surface are lateral closing-wedge osteotomy and medial opening-wedge osteotomy. Literature comparing clinical outcome after open- versus closing-wedge HTO is very limited and long-term comparisons are completely lacking. Hoell et al[24] reported that 108 patients with varus gonarthrosis were treated with an open-wedge osteotomy by using the Puddu plate and a Coventry-type closing-wedge osteotomy. Their results showed a significant improvement of subjective and objective clinical scores in both groups. And both methods obtained safe and reproducible results for the correction considering the different operation techniques. They suggested the instability of the medial collateral ligament appeared to be an indication for open-wedge osteotomy since this can increase the stability of the medial ligament after the procedure. Recent literature has analyzed retrospectively the long-term outcome of open- and closing-wedge valgization HTO.[25] During a median follow-up of 16.5 years, 24% underwent conversion to total knee arthroplasty. Osteotomy survival was of 98% after 5 years, 92% after 10 years, and 71% after 15 years. Up to now, comparison between open- and closing-wedge HTO has shown no significant difference in survival and clinical outcomes.[3,24,25]

In medial opening-wedge osteotomy, problems are mainly due to implant failure or loss of correction. Several authors have reported successful outcome with medial open-wedge osteotomy using an internal fixator such as Puddu and TomoFix plates. DeMeo et al[26] described the midterm follow-up of opening-wedge HTO using Puddu plates. They showed that the overall survivorship at 8 years was 70%, and 57% reported subjective good to excellent results, although only 20 patients were enrolled. Total knee arthroplasty was performed in 25% at the mean 8-year follow-up. After the osteotomy, a more normal appearing weight-bearing pattern with double peaks was seen in all patients tested.

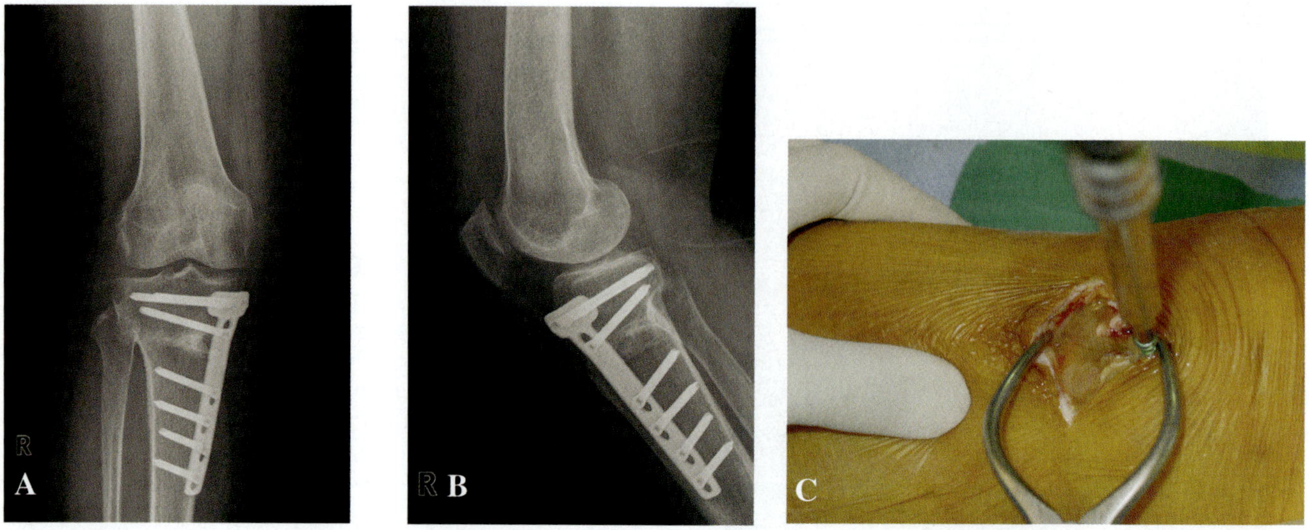

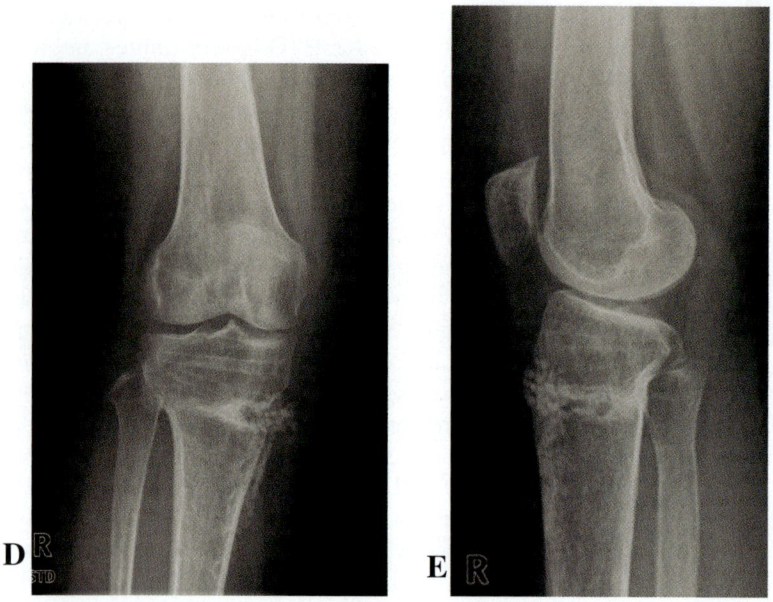

FIGURE 36-29. *(**A**, **B**) Fifteen-month follow-up radiographs show the osteotomy gap is healed with TomoFix plate fixation. (**C**) Intraoperative photograph shows pus discharge in the operative wound. (**D**, **E**) Antibiotic-impregnated cement beads are inserted into the deadspace after plate removal.*

Recent literature[20] reported 57 knees with open-wedge HTO using TomoFix and bone substitute materials. At a mean 40-month follow-up period, there were no instances of nonunion of implant failure. Niemeyer et al[27] analyzed that 69 patients treated with HTO using the TomoFix implant. A significant increase in clinical score at minimum follow-up of 36 months was found. The tibial bone varus angle was correlated significantly with greater improvement and better clinical outcome after HTO. The overall complication rate of 8.6% was mostly related to surgical causes.

PEARLS AND PITFALLS

Surgeons should keep in mind the following when performing an open-wedge osteotomy:

- To avoid over- or undercorrection of the mechanical axis, exact preoperative planning is mandatory. Potential planning errors should be recognized and corrected in time by intraoperative verification of the axis before internal fixation. Furthermore, navigation-assisted osteotomy is a helpful tool to assist in obtaining the desired intraoperative alignment (Fig. 36-30).[13,28]

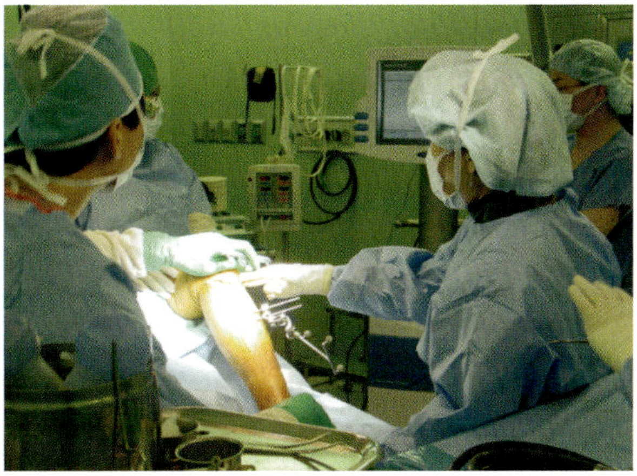

A

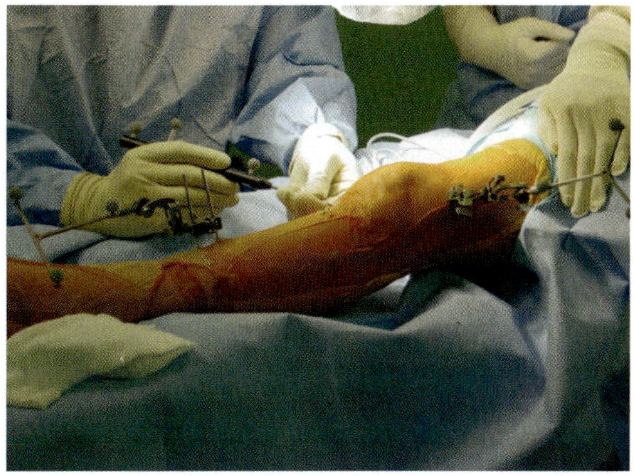

B

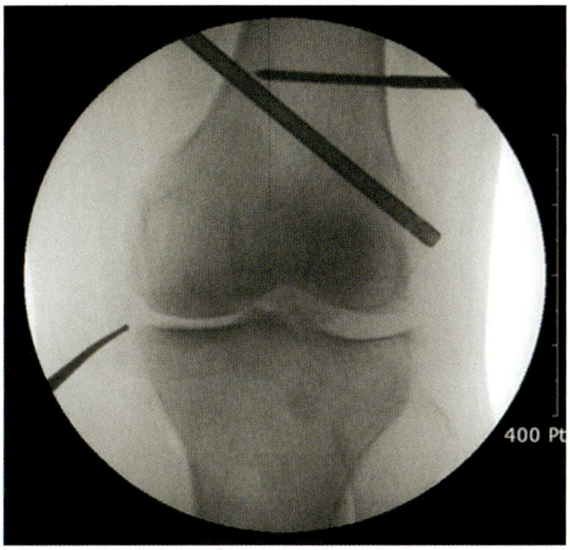

C

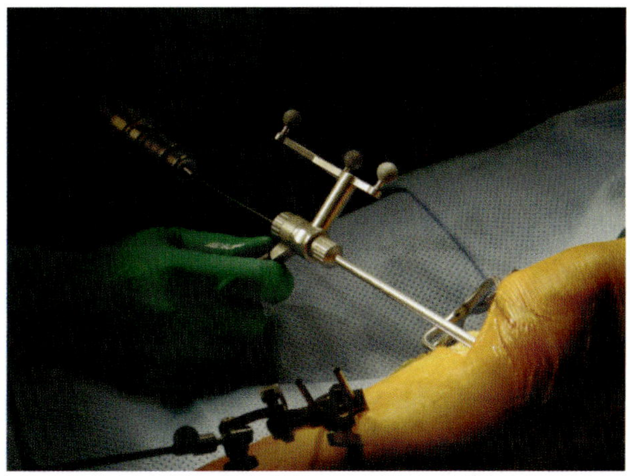

D

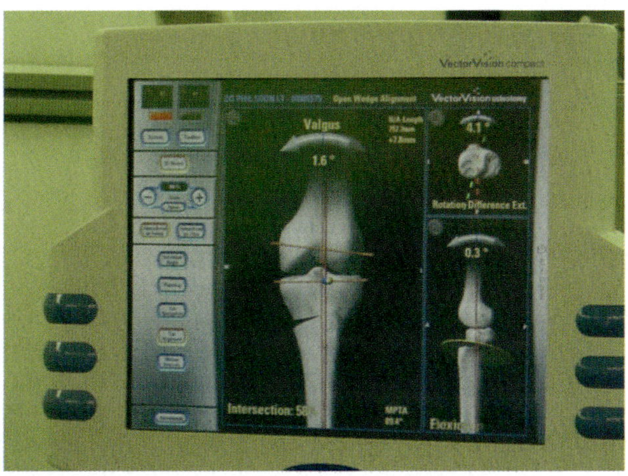

E

FIGURE 36-30. *(**A**) The femoral and tibial reference arrays are in place to find the hip joint center. (**B**, **C**) To determine the position of bony landmarks, a percutaneous pointer is being used to select the level of the medial tibial plateau under image intensification control. (**D**) Using computer-assisted navigation, the reference guide is used to select the desired slope of the osteotomy and the exact level on the tibia. The guide pins are inserted and used with the guide in making the osteotomy cut. (**E**) The computer screen gives the degree of progressive correction in real time and the point at which the mechanical axis is bisecting the tibia.* **Continued**

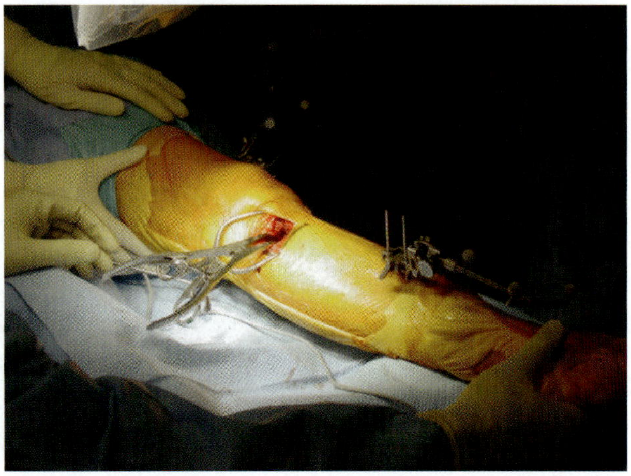

F

FIGURE 36-30 Continued. *(F) The mechanical axis is adjusted according to the preoperative planning under the navigation system during the correction retained with a bone spreader that is inserted into the posteromedial osteotomy gap.*

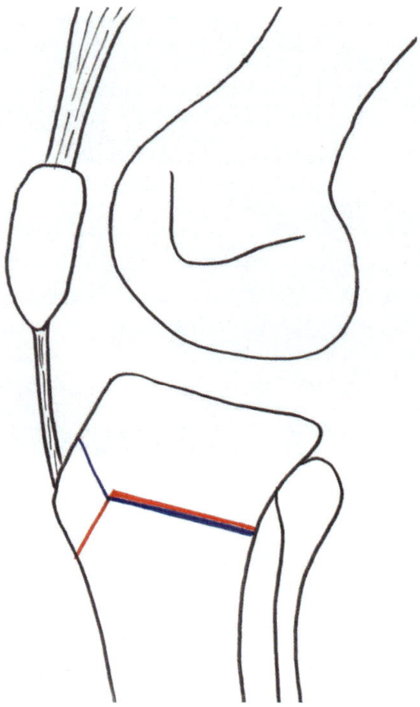

FIGURE 36-31. *Schematic drawing shows that the biplanar osteotomy (blue line) is performed proximal to the insertion of the patella tendon. In case of severe varus angulation, the biplanar osteotomy (red line) can be made distal to the insertion of patella tendon to prevent postoperative patella baja.*

- In case of severe varus angulation, the osteotomy line can be made distal to the insertion of the patella tendon to prevent postoperative patella infera (Fig. 36-31).
- Since open-wedge HTO tends to increase posterior slope, the opening of the osteotomy gap should be trapezoidal in shape (greater posteriorly than anteriorly). For this, complete posterior cortical osteotomy is essential to prevent an increase in the posterior tibial slope and to make the valgization easier.
- It is important to ensure sufficient release of the superficial medial collateral ligament to prevent stress on the medial compartment even after the valgization osteotomy. If necessary, the proximal part of the pes anserinus can also be released.

- Medial joint space should be monitored during the whole operative procedure using an image intensifier control. If the medial joint space becomes narrower after the valgization osteotomy, which means that the medial collateral ligament is still tight, it is then necessary to release the medial collateral ligament further.
- It is important to prevent breakage of the lateral cortical hinge. To preserve the thick bone as a lateral hinge, the osteotomy should not reach within 10 mm from the lateral cortex (Fig. 36-28).
- To prevent loss of correction, the proximal three locking head screws should be situated in the subchondral area about 1 cm below the joint line. The locking head screw at the D hole in the TomoFix plate should also be positioned more proximally from the osteotomy gap through the full length (Fig. 36-27).

REFERENCES

1. Coventry MB. Upper tibial osteotomy for osteoarthritis. *J Bone Joint Surg Am.* 1985;67(7):1136-1140.
2. Coventry MB, Ilstrup DM, Wallrichs SL. Proximal tibial osteotomy. A critical long-term study of eighty-seven cases. *J Bone Joint Surg Am.* 1993;75(2):196-201.
3. van den Bekerom MP, Patt TW, Kleinhout MY, et al. Early complications after high tibial osteotomy: a comparison of two techniques. *J Knee Surg.* 2008; 21(1):68-74.
4. Wildner M, Peters A, Hellich J, et al. Complications of high tibial osteotomy and internal fixation with staples. *Arch Orthop Trauma Surg.* 1992;111(4):210-212.
5. Lobenhoffer P, Agneskirchner JD. Improvements in surgical technique of valgus high tibial osteotomy. *Knee Surg Sports Traumatol Arthrosc.* 2003;11(3): 132-138.
6. Niemeyer P, Koestler W, Kaehny C, et al. Two-year results of open-wedge high tibial osteotomy with fixation by medial plate fixator for medial compartment arthritis with varus malalignment of the knee. *Arthroscopy.* 2008;24(7):796-804.
7. Song EK, Seon JK, Park SJ, et al. The complications of high tibial osteotomy: closing- versus opening-wedge methods. *J Bone Joint Surg Br.* 2010;92(9): 1245-1252.
8. Staubli AE, De Simoni C, Babst R, et al. TomoFix: a new LCP-concept for open wedge osteotomy of the medial proximal tibiaearly results in 92 cases. *Injury.* 2003;34(suppl 2):B55-62.
9. Scott WN. *Sugery of the Knee.* 4th ed. Elsevier: Philadelphia; 2006.
10. Miller BS, Downie B, McDonough EB, et al. Complications after medial opening wedge high tibial osteotomy. *Arthroscopy.* 2009;25(6):639-646.
11. Valkering KP, van den Bekerom MP, Kappelhoff FM, et al. Complications after TomoFix medial opening wedge high tibial osteotomy. *J Knee Surg.* 2009;22(3):218-225.
12. Matthews LS, Goldstein SA, Malvitz TA, et al. Proximal tibial osteotomy. Factors that influence the duration of satisfactory function. *Clin Orthop Relat Res.* 1988;229:193-200.
13. Jackson DW. *Reconstructive Knee Surgery.* 3rd ed. Philadelphia, PA: Lippincott Williams &Wilkins; 2008.
14. Lobenhoffer P. *Osteotomies Around the Knee.* Thieme: New York; 2008.
15. Wang JW, Kuo KN, Andriacchi TP, et al. The influence of walking mechanics and time on the results of proximal tibial osteotomy. *J Bone Joint Surg Am.* 1990;72(6):905-909.
16. Bonnin M, Chambat P. [Current status of valgus angle, tibial head closing wedge osteotomy in media gonarthrosis]. *Orthopade.* 2004;33(2):135-142.
17. Cooke TD, Pichora D, Siu D, et al. Surgical implications of varus deformity of the knee with obliquity of joint surfaces. *J Bone Joint Surg Br.* 1989;71(4):560-565.
18. Fujisawa Y, Masuhara K, Shiomi S. The effect of high tibial osteotomy on osteoarthritis of the knee. An arthroscopic study of 54 knee joints. *Orthop Clin North Am.* 1979;10(3):585-608.
19. Marti CB, Gautier E, Wachtl SW, et al. Accuracy of frontal and sagittal plane correction in open-wedge high tibial osteotomy. *Arthroscopy.* 2004;20(4):366-372.
20. Takeuchi R, Ishikawa H, Aratake M, et al. Medial opening wedge high tibial osteotomy with early full weight bearing. *Arthroscopy.* 2009;25(1):46-53.
21. Paccola CA, Fogagnolo F. Open-wedge high tibial osteotomy: a technical trick to avoid loss of reduction of the opposite cortex. *Knee Surg Sports Traumatol Arthrosc.* 2005;13(1):19-22.
22. Reischl N, Wahl P, Jacobi M, et al. Infections after high tibial open wedge osteotomy: a case control

study. *Arch Orthop Trauma Surg.* 2009;129(11): 1483-1487.

23. Turner RS, Griffiths H, Heatley FW. The incidence of deep-vein thrombosis after upper tibial osteotomy. A venographic study. *J Bone Joint Surg Br.* 1993;75(6): 942-944.
24. Hoell S, Suttmoeller J, Stoll V, et al. The high tibial osteotomy, open versus closed wedge, a comparison of methods in 108 patients. *Arch Orthop Trauma Surg.* 2005;125(9):638-643.
25. Schallberger A, Jacobi M, Wahl P, et al. High tibial valgus osteotomy in unicompartmental medial osteoarthritis of the knee: a retrospective follow-up study over 13-21 years. *Knee Surg Sports Traumatol Arthrosc.* 2011;19(1):122-127.
26. DeMeo PJ, Johnson EM, Chiang PP, et al. Midterm follow-up of opening-wedge high tibial osteotomy. *Am J Sports Med.* 2010;38(10):2077-2084.
27. Niemeyer P, Schmal H, Hauschild O, et al. Open-wedge osteotomy using an internal plate fixator in patients with medial-compartment gonarthritis and varus malalignment: 3-year results with regard to preoperative arthroscopic and radiographic findings. *Arthroscopy.* 2010;26(12):1607-1616.
28. Bae DK, Song SJ, Yoon KH. Closed-wedge high tibial osteotomy using computer-assisted surgery compared to the conventional technique. *J Bone Joint Surg Br.* 2009;91(9):1164-1171.

37 Alternative Proximal Tibial Osteotomy

Kang-Il Kim and Sang Hak Lee

The most common condition in patients who have a proximal tibial osteotomy (PTO) performed is isolated medial compartmental joint disease associated with varus limb alignment. Following the first report of PTO by Jackson in 1961,[1] there were several studies of osteotomy performed distal to the tibial tuberosity.[2] Over the next 10 years, the Coventry approach involving PTO proximal to the tibial tuberosity became much more widely accepted following its publication in 1965.[3,4] Up to now, the two principal techniques have been lateral closing-wedge osteotomy and medial opening-wedge osteotomy, which are performed to produce valgus realignment of the weight-bearing axis on the proximal tibial articular surface. The level of osteotomy for those two techniques is usually above tibial tuberosity and has been well described in other chapters.

In recent years, PTO above tibial tuberosity is the most popular method. This level of osteotomy has many advantages, including a high healing rate due to the increased area of metaphysis at the osteotomy site, compressive pull of the quadriceps muscle at the tibial tuberosity to aid in healing, and the ability to correct the deformity closer to the joint. Nevertheless, it has also several disadvantages, such as iatrogenic patella alta or baja, limited degree of correction, potential for tibial plateau necrosis, intra-articular fracture, and limited proximal bone stock for rigid fixation.[5,6] This technique may also have a potentially negative impact on future total knee replacement.[7] To prevent these problems, a few reports have advocated osteotomy below tibial tuberosity. This level of osteotomy has several advantages, including increased proximal bone stock for rigid fixation, ease of performing the osteotomy, and no disruption of the patellofemoral mechanism because the soft tissue stabilizers of the knee are not disrupted.[3,8] On the contrary, it also has disadvantages, such as osteotomy involving more cortical bone with its associated slower and lower healing rates and creation of a zigzag tibia.[9]

Although plates are commonly used for fixation in PTO, there is no consensus in the literature on optimal fixation device or a surgical technique for PTO. Therefore, several reports have suggested alternative PTO techniques with various implants.[3,5,8,10,11] Alternative approaches include hemicallotasis techniques with an external fixator,[12] dome-type osteotomy with a variety of devices,[3,13] and osteotomy below the tibial tuberosity with intramedullary nail or plates.[11,14] The proposed advantages of the technique with a gradual opening using a variety of external fixation devices include a controlled correction, potentially less effect on patellar height, rapid mobilization of the patients, absence of limb-length shortening, and maintenance of soft tissue tension about the knee.[12] Disadvantages of this technique include the use of an external fixation device, which can be cumbersome and poorly tolerated by the patient. With the use of an intramedullary nail, rapid rehabilitation and less invasive surgery (leaving a minimal scar) may be possible. This chapter addresses alternative PTO techniques with a literature review and introduces a novel procedure of less invasive PTO just below tibial tuberosity using an intramedullary nail, which was developed by the authors for correction of a varus knee.

SPECIAL CONSIDERATION FOR ALTERNATIVE PROXIMAL TIBIAL OSTEOTOMY

Patient selection is the most critical factor in planning and achieving a successful PTO. Even though closed-wedge and open-wedge PTOs are widespread methods to perform valgization PTO for medial varus osteoarthritis of the knee, there are still some indications for alternative PTO procedures.

The osteotomy below tibial tuberosity using an intramedullary nail or Puddu plate[11] can be used to treat young patients for varus malalignment of the leg with minimal degenerative change and less scarring. The main patient group for this procedure is young adults who are concerned about bow knee deformity with associated symptoms such as minor discomfort due to overloading of the medial compartment with no or early degenerative changes (Kellgren-Lawrence classification[15] grade 1) on radiographs. Furthermore, if main varus bony deformity is about the tibial tuberosity (correction of rotational angle is lower than usual tibial vara), it would be the best choice for correction of the deformity. Therefore, this procedure is a good option for preventing translation developed by the tibia, called zig-zag tibia, when the apex of the deformity is placed distal to the tibial tuberosity.[9] However, in cases in which there is a larger deformity correction angle and in which the bony contact after deformity correction would be smaller, acute correction with transverse osteotomy is relatively contraindicated due to the increased risk of delayed union or nonunion.

Alternatively, a dome osteotomy involves the use of a curved osteotomy that allows rotation or translation of the distal end of the tibia on the proximal fragment.[3,13,16] The dome osteotomy is typically convex superiorly and located either proximal or distal to the tibial tuberosity (Fig. 37-1). This osteotomy has indications similar to those with closed-wedge or open-wedge PTO procedures. However, this technique can be used in patients with patellofemoral problems because it avoids limb-length alteration and the potential for anterior displacement of the tibial tuberosity, which may alleviate associated patellofemoral disease. When dome osteotomy is combined with external fixation, this procedure can address large corrections of malalignment without adversely affecting the resultant joint line obliquity.[17] However, this procedure is technically demanding, with the potential difficulty of controlling alignment postoperatively and the inability to make torsional corrections.

PTO using an external fixator has several theoretical advantages: the amount of soft tissue dissection is typically less than that in internal fixation procedures; postoperative adjustment of the extent of correction can usually be accomplished without difficulty, depending on the fixation device used; axis translation to restore the mechanical axis is more easily accomplished; and angular deformity correction can be combined with lengthening, if desired.[6,12,18] Therefore, an external fixator with gradual correction technique is a good option in cases with severe genu varum deformities exceeding 15°, complex deformities in more than one plane, and an associated severe lateral collateral ligament laxity. If soft tissue problems exist, such as a previous large operation scar at the proximal tibia area, it might be wise to use an external fixator with acute or gradual correction (Fig. 37-2). Moreover, gradual correction with limb lengthening using an external fixator should be considered, when varus malalignment coexists with limb-length discrepancy (Fig. 37-3). Disadvantages include longer healing time, slower mobilization, and potentially more complex surgery with the application of the device and the need for the patient's acceptance and compliance with the postoperative management regimen.

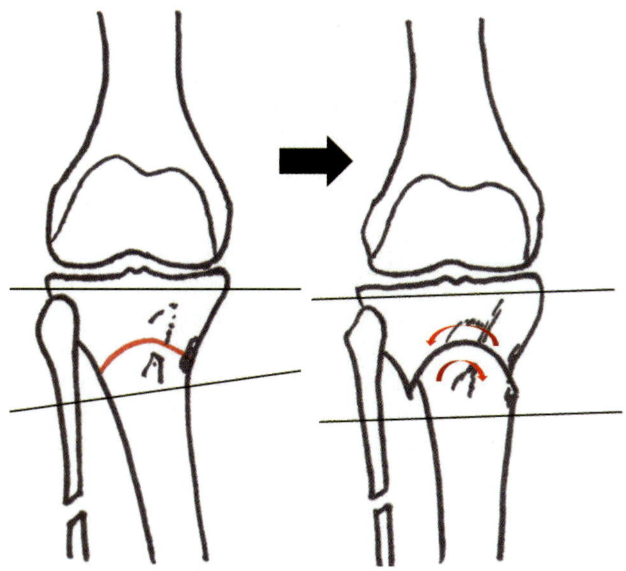

FIGURE 37-1. *Schematic drawing of the dome osteotomy above tibial tuberosity. Left, two lines on the tibia are not parallel or varus aligned preoperatively. Right, postoperatively the two tibial lines could be made parallel or even valgus aligned as desired.*

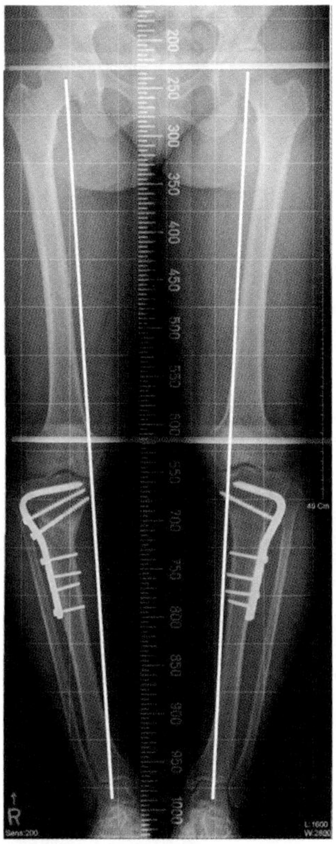

A

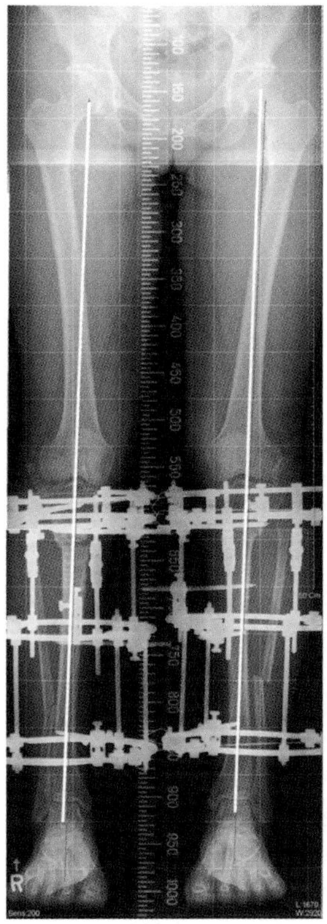

B

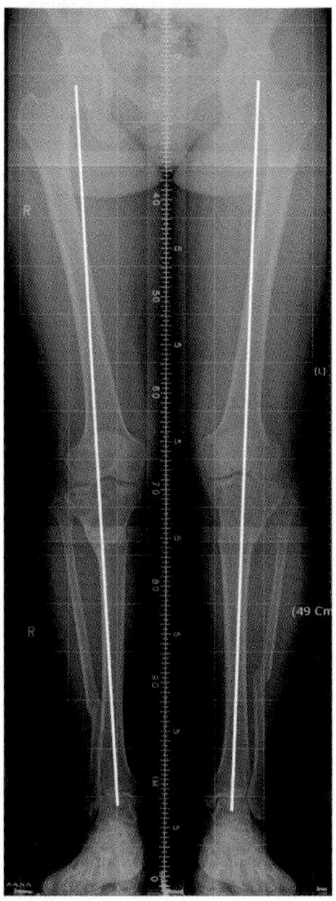

C

FIGURE 37-2. *Revision of a failed PTO case. (**A**) A 28-year-old female had bilateral PTO using a big plate in both legs but severe varus deformity exists. (**B**) Bilateral simultaneous revision PTO below tibial tuberosity was performed using a ring fixator to get earlier rehabilitation, avoid further patellar baja, and reduce soft tissue trauma to previous large scarred tissue. (**C**) The radiograph after the external fixator shows correction of varus knee in both legs.*

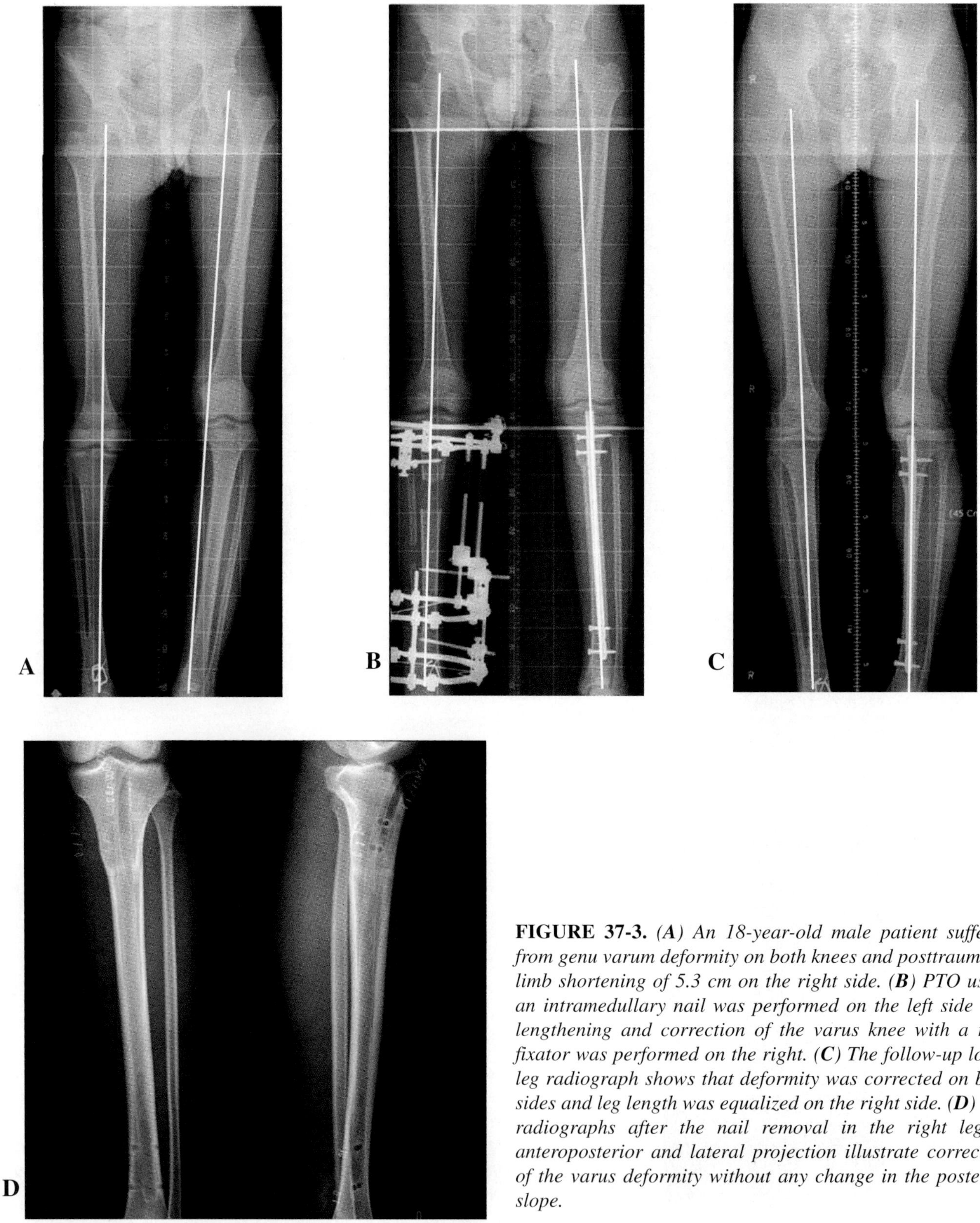

FIGURE 37-3. *(**A**) An 18-year-old male patient suffered from genu varum deformity on both knees and posttraumatic limb shortening of 5.3 cm on the right side. (**B**) PTO using an intramedullary nail was performed on the left side and lengthening and correction of the varus knee with a ring fixator was performed on the right. (**C**) The follow-up long-leg radiograph shows that deformity was corrected on both sides and leg length was equalized on the right side. (**D**) The radiographs after the nail removal in the right leg in anteroposterior and lateral projection illustrate correction of the varus deformity without any change in the posterior slope.*

ALTERNATIVE PROXIMAL TIBIAL OSTEOTOMY USING AN INTRAMEDULLARY NAIL

Preparation of Patient for Surgery

In preoperative planning, a corrected mechanical axis is drawn passing through the center of the hip and center of the knee on long-leg radiographs (Fig. 37-4). When this line was extended over the tibia, it passed from the medial aspect of tibial articular surface to the lateral aspect of the proximal tibial metaphysis. The trajectory of this line on the proximal tibia only is marked on the radiographs and a paper tracing to serve as the trajectory of the nail in the fragment of tibia proximal to the osteotomy level. The desired point of entry of the nail is obtained on the trajectory of the nail in the proximal fragment previously marked. The entry point is located more medially if the deformity to be corrected is more severe. The level of the osteotomy is influenced by the location of the most distal screw hole for proximal interlocking present on the nail; it is usually at a point 1 to 2 cm below the most distal screw hole for proximal interlocking on the nail. The level of osteotomy is also determined by the degree of correction to be achieved; the level is moved proximally or distally to respectively increase or decrease the degree of correction as required. This predetermined level of osteotomy below the tibial tuberosity is marked. The mid-diaphyseal line of the distal fragment of the tibia is marked on the paper tracing. The tibia tracing is divided at the level of osteotomy. With the proximal fragment of the tibia remaining stationary, the distal fragment is realigned to achieve desired correction such that the mid-diaphyseal line of the divided distal tibia coincides with the corrected mechanical axis (Fig. 37-5).

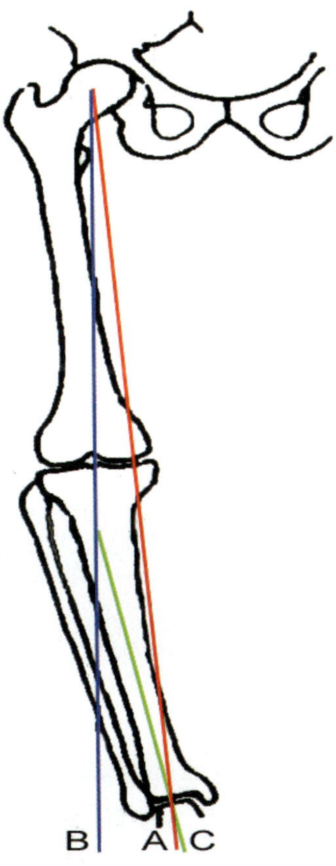

FIGURE 37-4. *In preoperative planning, three lines are marked on long-leg radiographs. The mechanical axis is marked as line A (red), the corrected mechanical axis is marked as line B (blue), and line C (green) denotes the mid-diaphyseal line of the distal fragment.*

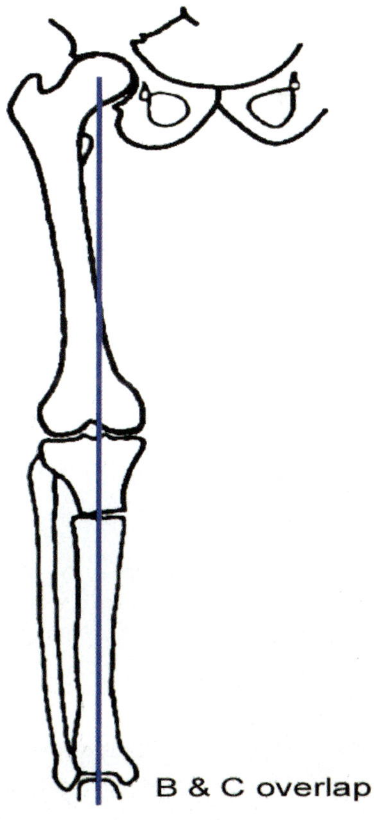

FIGURE 37-5. *A paper tracing is divided at the level of osteotomy and the distal tibia is moved to realign line C along line B. As line C overlaps the corrected mechanical axis (line B), a valgus opening is created at the osteotomy site, achieving deformity correction. The trajectory of the nail in the proximal tibia is in the valgus direction.*

Surgical Technique

With the patient in the supine position, a thigh tourniquet is applied and the leg is draped free. The entry point of the tibial intramedullary nail is made through a less than 3-cm horizontal skin incision which crosses the patellar tendon (Fig. 37-6). The level of the osteotomy and various axes are marked with a sterile marker under fluoroscopic guidance at the beginning of the procedure. Only the proximal fragment is reamed up to just short of osteotomy level under fluoroscopic guidance along the desired trajectory of entry of nail in the proximal fragment (Figs. 37-7 and 37-8). Then the osteotomy is performed percutaneously[10] through a small stab incision (<1 cm) on the anterolateral surface of tibia (Fig. 37-9).

A drill sleeve is used to protect soft tissue during drilling. Under fluoroscopic control, multiple transverse drill holes are made with a new 3.2-mm drill bit each time, at a low speed to minimize heat generation. A 0.25-inch osteotome is used to connect most of the drilled holes. The osteotomy is completed using gentle manual force because the energy used to transect the bone at the osteotomy site influences the viability of the osteotomy site and its osteogenic potential (Fig. 37-10).[10]

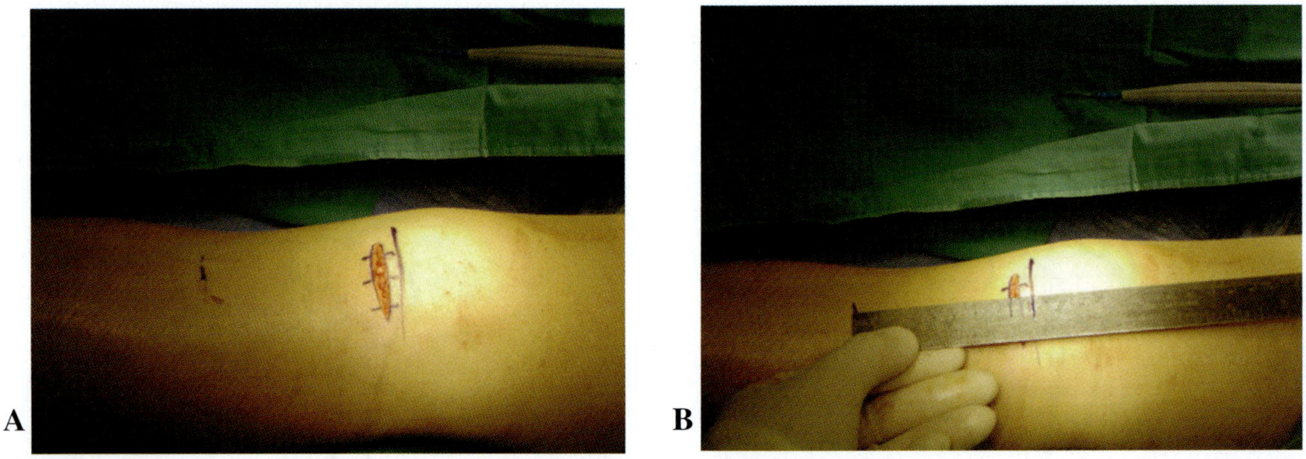

FIGURE 37-6. *(A) A less than 3-cm skin incision is made medial to the patellar tendon. (**B**) The level of osteotomy is marked under fluoroscopic guidance at the beginning of the procedure.*

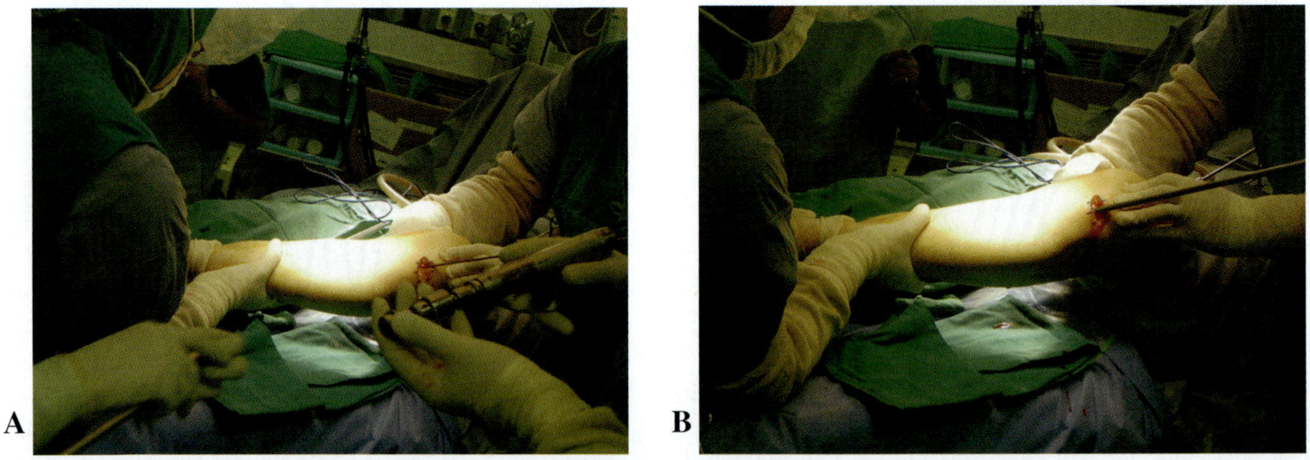

FIGURE 37-7. *(A) A guide wire is inserted through the entry point of the tibial intramedullary nail. (**B**) The reaming is performed with flexible reamers over the guide wire. Only the proximal fragment is reamed up to just short of osteotomy level under fluoroscopic guidance.*

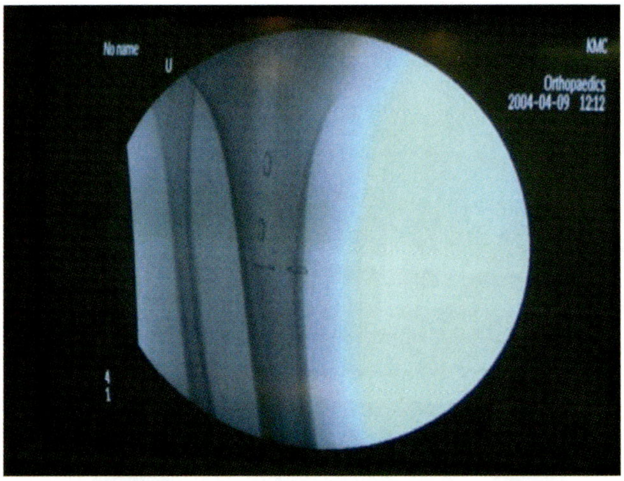

FIGURE 37-8. *The level of osteotomy is marked (transverse staples). Before the osteotomy is performed, only the proximal tibia is reamed under fluoroscopic guidance along the trajectory of the nail in the proximal fragment (valgus direction, vertical staples) obtained from the preoperative planning. Reaming is stopped just short of the osteotomy site planned.*

At this moment the fragments are still aligned with each other without any displacement due to the partially intact periosteum and soft tissue cover (Fig. 37-11). Then a guide wire is passed from the previously reamed proximal tibial entry point into the medullary canal of the distal fragment and reaming is performed with flexible reamers over the guide wire. Reaming is done by gradually increasing increments of 0.5 mm. The medullary canal is over-reamed by 0.5 mm before inserting a nail of proper size decided by standard preoperative measurement. This technique does not involve any need for reduction after completion of the osteotomy and before inserting the nail. There is no necessity to hold the reduction with the use of an external fixator[19] or any other device.[20,21] The nail is inserted through the medially located entry point with the free hand manually without the use of any blocking screws to guide the passage of the nail. The entry point of the nail and the path of the nail in the proximal fragment only were predefined by the surgeon. Beyond the osteotomy site, the path of the nail into the distal fragment of tibia is determined by the direction of the medullary canal of the distal tibia. As the nail crosses the osteotomy site and engages the medullary canal of the distal fragment at the level of the isthmus, a controlled medial opening is created naturally with the further entry of the nail down the medullary canal (Fig. 37-12). There is a change in alignment of the distal fragment due to a mismatch between the direction of the nail in the proximal fragment and the direction of the medullary canal (and the nail) in the distal fragment. When the nail engages the medullary canal and isthmus distal to the osteotomy level, the distal fragment automatically corrects into valgus alignment. This correction is achieved by a medial opening at the osteotomy site, valgus tilting of the distal fragment, and lateral translation of the distal fragment.[22] Bone graft is not needed in this procedure (Fig. 37-13). This nail is securely fixed with two or three proximal and distal interlocking screws. Suction drains are inserted into the nail insertion site.

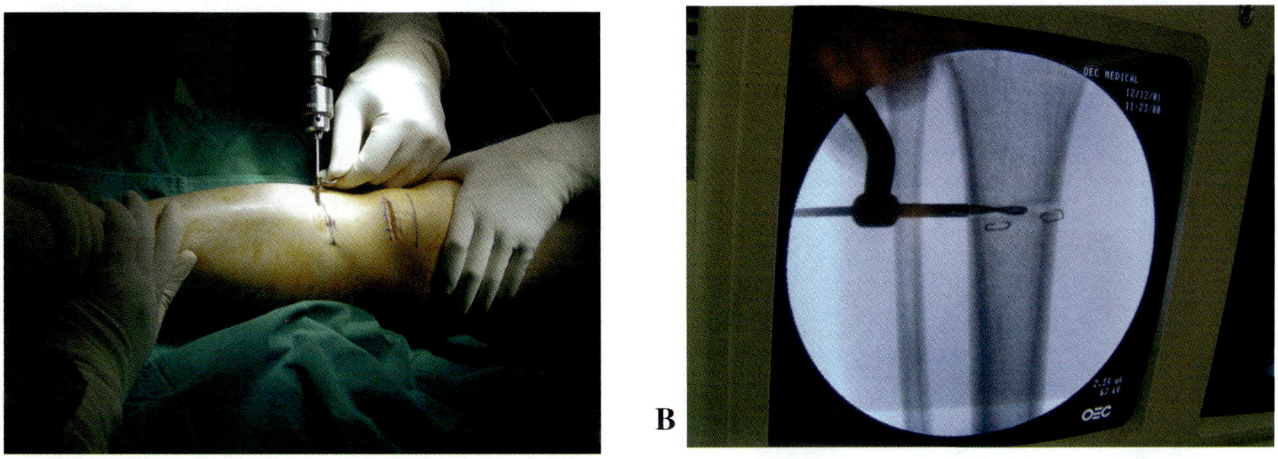

A B

FIGURE 37-9. *Osteotomy is performed through a small stab incision from the anterolateral surface of the tibia by percutaneous drilling. (**A**) A soft tissue protection drill sleeve is used. (**B**) Multiple drill holes (usually eight holes) are made in the same plane under fluoroscopic guidance at the level of osteotomy.*

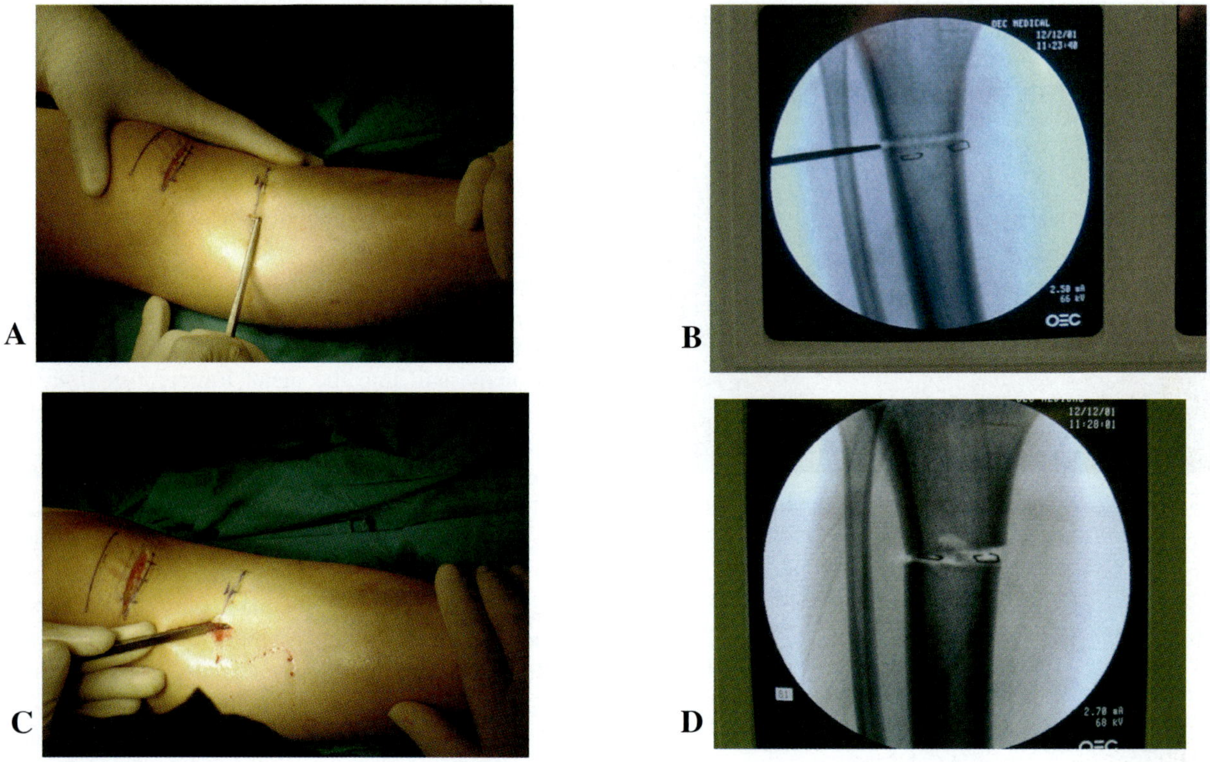

FIGURE 37-10. *(**A**) A 0.25-inch osteotome is used to connect most of the drill holes through the same skin incision. (**B**) An image intensifier shows the osteotome at the osteotomy site. (**C**, **D**) Osteotomy is completed with gentle manual force without displacement and the fragments are still aligned to each other.*

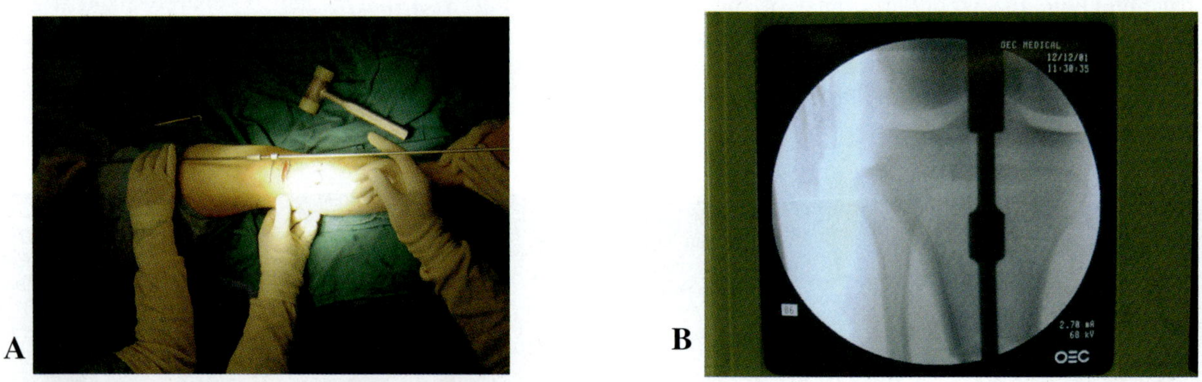

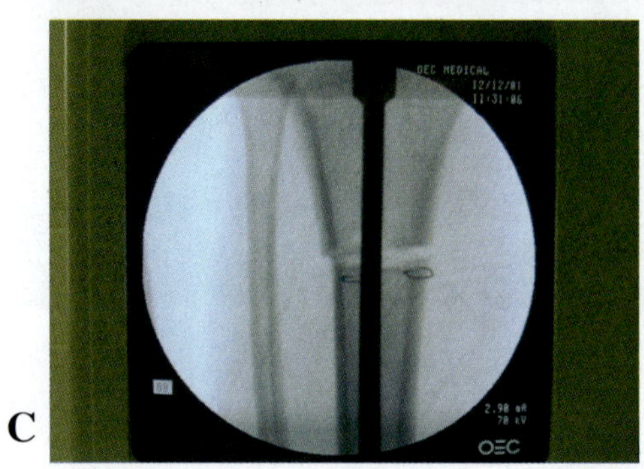

FIGURE 37-11. *The mechanical axis is then adjusted according to the preoperative planning. Under image intensification, a long, straight measuring rod is placed at the center of the femoral head and at the center of the upper ankle joint.*

A
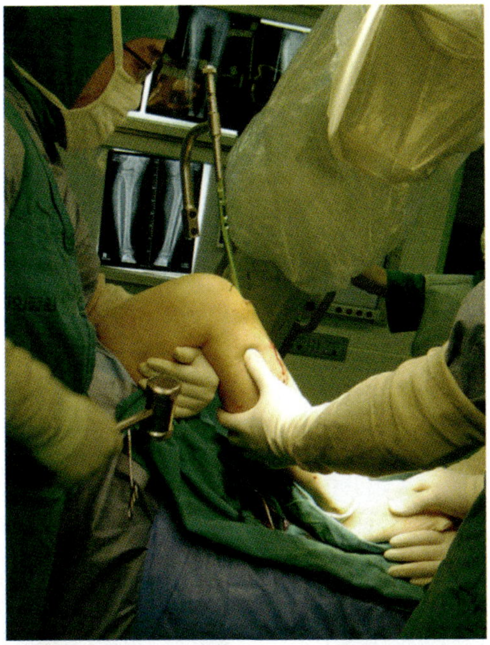

B
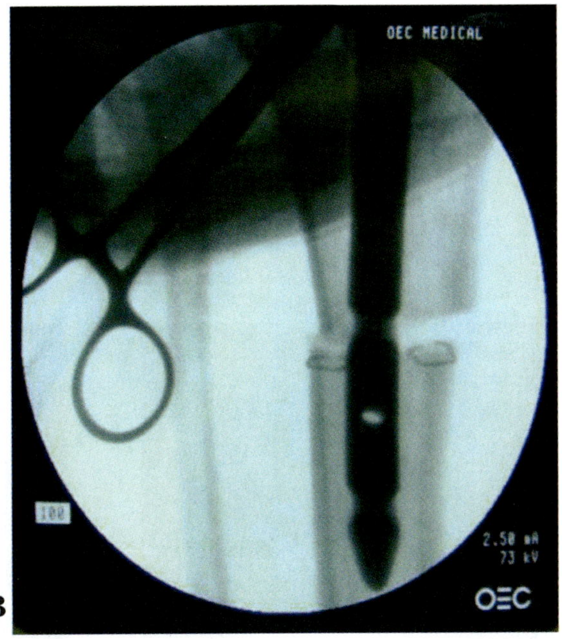

C
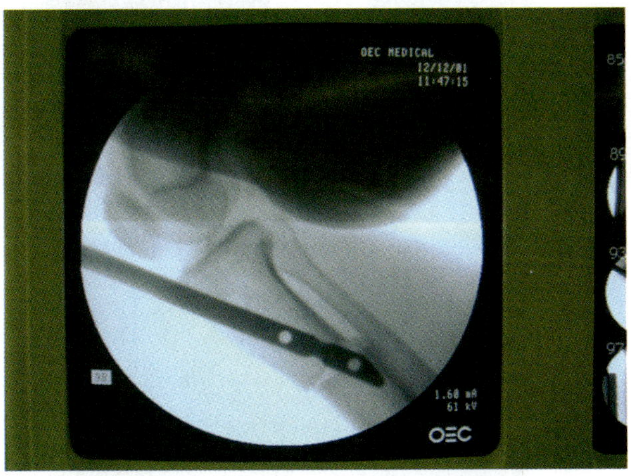

FIGURE 37-12. *A valgus correction with a medial opening was automatically created simultaneously with passing of the nail across the osteotomy site into the mid-diaphysis in the distal tibia.*

Rehabilitation

The knee is flexed to 30° with elevation and active ankle and static quadriceps exercises are started as pain permits. On the 1st postoperative day, the patient is allowed bedside leg dangling and wheelchair mobilization. On the 2nd postoperative day, the suction drain is removed. Crutch walking is started at postoperative day 3 with weight bearing allowed gradually as tolerated. Full weight bearing is normally possible after 3 or 4 weeks.

Complications

Complications prominently reported in the literature are undercorrection, overcorrection, delayed union, nonunion, delayed wound healing, loss of correction, or implant insufficiency. A frequent complication in this procedure is occasional anterior knee pain due to nail prominence. Because the entry point of nail is medial to the patellar tendon over a bare area of the medial tibial plateau, any implant prominence is easily palpable and may be symptomatic. Thus, full seating of the nail into the bone is recommended.

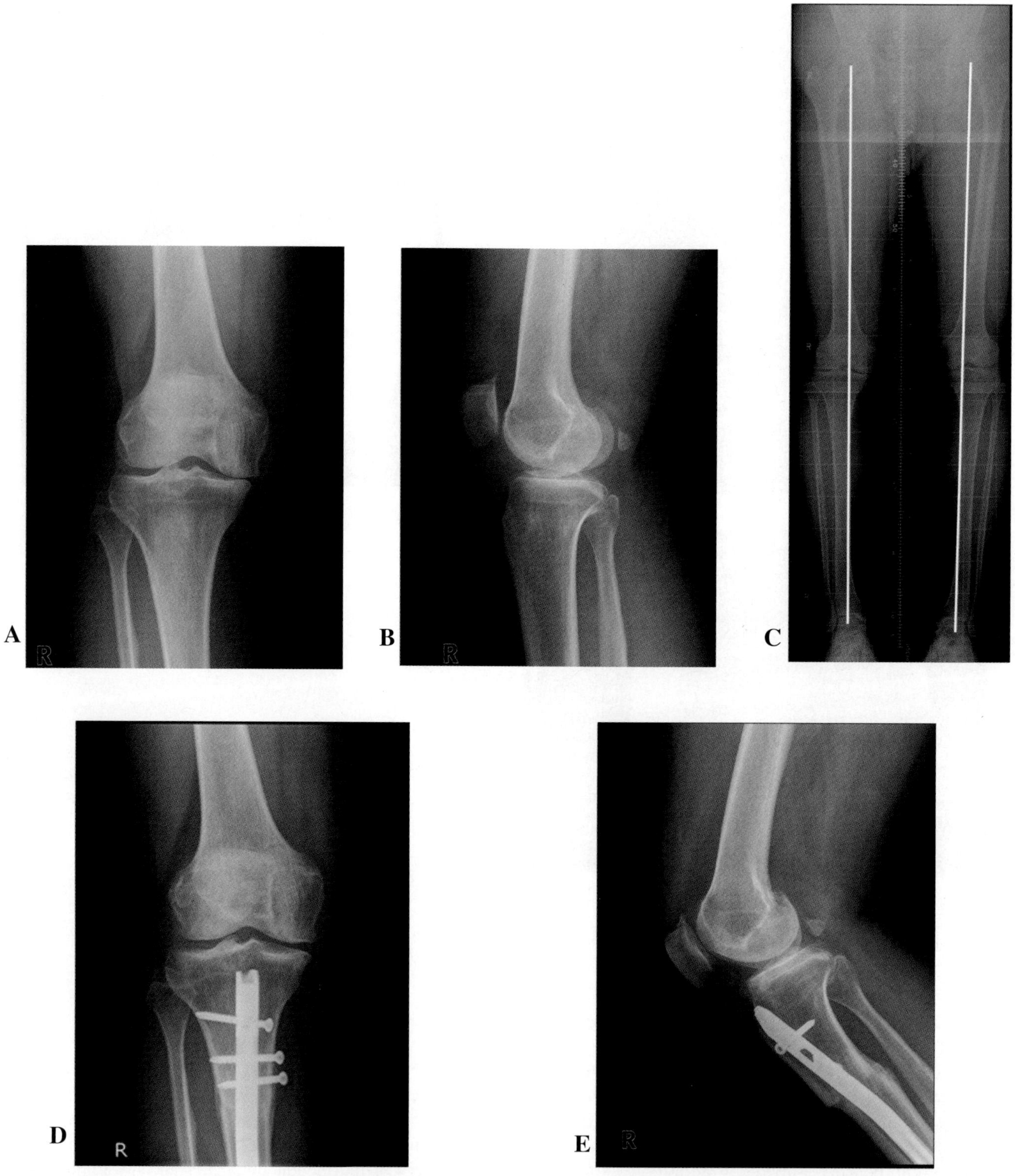

FIGURE 37-13. *(A–C) A 56-year-old male patient had bilateral genu varum deformity with a preoperative hip-knee-ankle angle of –6.1° on the right side and –5° on the left side. (**D**, **E**) The deformity was corrected using an intramedullary nail without a fibular osteotomy. A 3-year postoperative radiograph shows that the medial joint space is normalized compared with the preoperative narrowing of the space.*

OUTCOME OF ALTERNATIVE PROXIMAL TIBIAL OSTEOTOMIES

A few reports have described the advantages of PTO below tibial tuberosity, including a greater degree of correction and preservation of the proximal tibial anatomy. Sen et al reported the midterm results of PTO below tibial tuberosity using a circular external fixator in patients with medial compartment osteoarthritis.[8] They reported that the desired amount of correction can be precisely achieved without important complications, such as deletion of bone stock, patella baja, or changes of tibial slope. They concluded that the technique can be successfully applied in experienced hands for the treatment of varus gonarthrosis with a low complication rate. Gaasbeek et al reported that a new operation technique was developed to prevent patella baja in open-wedge PTO using a locking plate.[14] They performed a distal tibial tuberosity osteotomy and the tuberosity was fixed with one screw to the tibia. They evaluated radiographic results and compared them with results in open-wedge PTO with a conventional technique and concluded that the distal tuberosity osteotomy is a safe technique and that it can prevent lowering of the patella following conventional open-wedge PTO, especially in patients who need a major degree of valgus correction for medial compartment osteoarthritis of the knee.

More recent literature has reported the radiographic effects of a horizontal osteotomy made proximal to the patellar tendon insertion versus an oblique osteotomy made at the level distal to the patellar tendon insertion.[23] This literature claimed that the more distal oblique osteotomy did not statistically affect the patellar height or the sagittal tibial slope, while still allowing a similar coronal correction to the proximal horizontal osteotomy group. Additionally, it stated that the more distal osteotomy group has the advantage of a technically easier exposure, being distal to the periarticular capsule and allowing easier access to the posterior aspect to the tibia for neurovascular protection. In addition, Shim et al evaluated the results after open-wedge PTO below the tibial tuberosity for genu varum, which was treated with an autogenous tricortical iliac bone graft by using the Puddu plate.[11] They showed that PTO below the tibial tuberosity using a smaller plate in relatively young patients successfully achieved both functional and radiographic improvements without changes in patellar height or posterior tibial slope (Fig. 37-14). However, they recommended that their technique be considered in genu varum patients up to the 4th decade in life because PTO below the tibial tuberosity involves cortical bone, and it is therefore associated with slower and lower healing rates.

Dome osteotomy is less commonly used today than either the lateral closing-wedge or medial opening-wedge technique, regardless of the level of osteotomy.[5,8,24] The advantages of the dome osteotomy include no loss of leg length, plateau fracture is rare, the medial ligament is tightened without advancement, and the alignment can be manipulated postoperatively. Its disadvantages include the potential difficulty of controlling alignment postoperatively, the inability to make torsional corrections, and pin-tract problems if an external fixator is used. Gunes et al evaluated tibial slope changes after PTO below tibial tuberosity using a circular external fixator for medial compartment osteoarthritis.[17] Their results showed that there is no significant alteration in tibial slope after PTO below the tuberosity with a ring external fixation. Conversely, Cullu et al evaluated tibial slope change after a dome-type PTO above tibial tuberosity using an external fixator.[13] They hypothesized that the dome-type PTO could have more advantages over other PTO techniques since there was no removal or addition of a bone wedge, which could interfere more significantly with the geometry of the upper part of the tibia. However, their results showed a significant decrease in tibial slope after dome-type PTO. They also reported that the higher the degree of postoperative mechanical axis valgus, the higher was the degree of posterior tibial slope that resulted.

Another alternative approach is gradually opening with a variety of external fixation devices. The short-term results of this technique are comparable to those of the conventional closing-wedge osteotomy for a large correction or if tightening of the medial collateral ligament is desired.[25] Recently, Shiha et al reported a gradual correction of genu varum deformity using a ring external fixator in young patients.[12] Their results showed accurate correction at mean follow-up of 25 months and they recommended the technique as an important option in cases with severe genu varum deformities, where corrections of more than a 15° area are needed in complex deformities in more than one plane and finally in cases with an associated severe lateral collateral ligament laxity. However, they advised that their technique should be reserved for strict indications, since patient acceptance and compliance with the frame can be a problem.

The PTO is a highly effective procedure in relieving pain, correcting deformity, improving function, and preventing further progression of medial compartment osteoarthritis of the knee and can be performed using classic open- or closed-wedge techniques that are associated with good clinical results. However, since each of the alternative procedures has advantages and disadvantages depending on the type of deformity being corrected, the surgeon must weigh these in each case to select the optimal treatment plan.

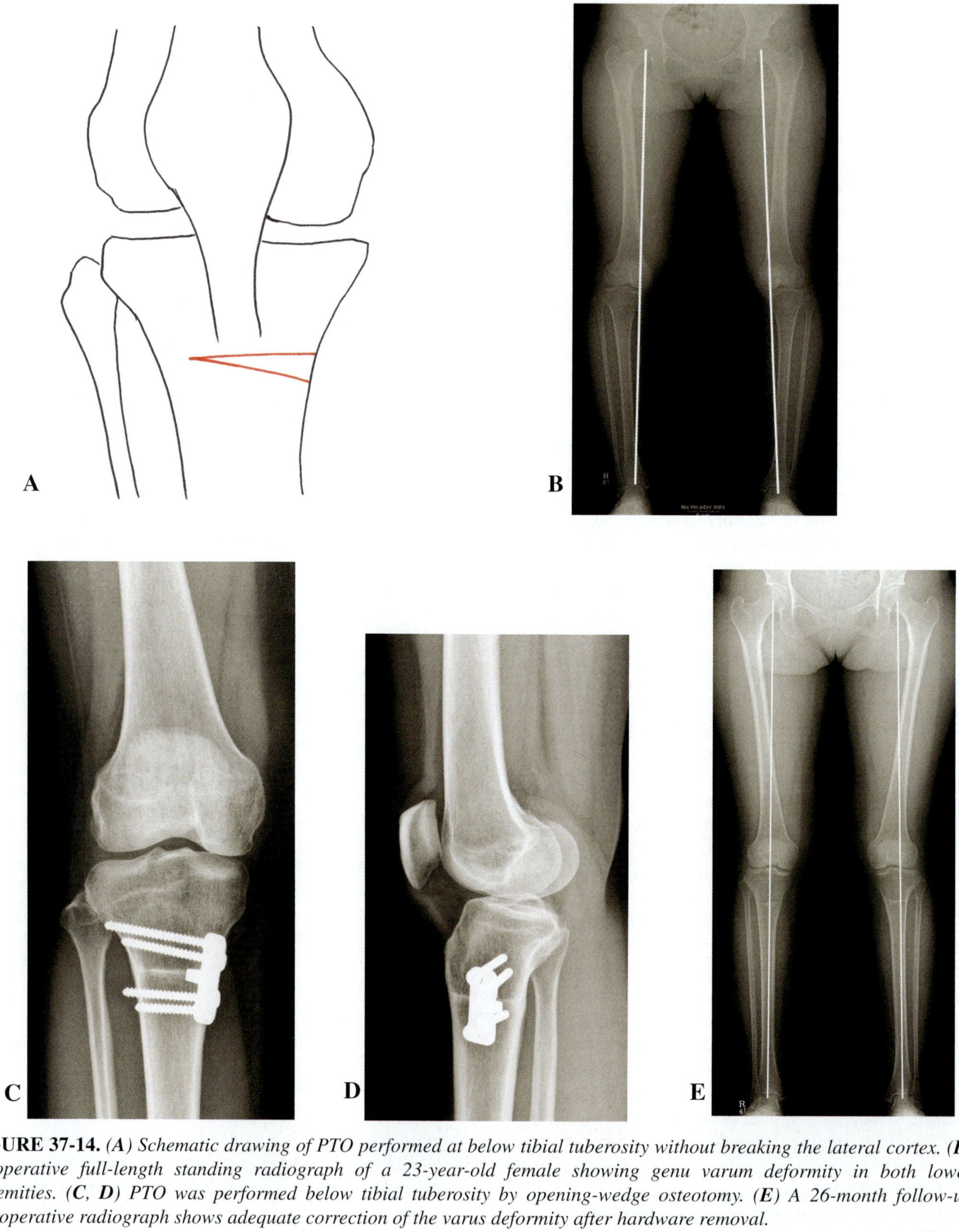

FIGURE 37-14. *(**A**) Schematic drawing of PTO performed at below tibial tuberosity without breaking the lateral cortex. (**B**) Preoperative full-length standing radiograph of a 23-year-old female showing genu varum deformity in both lower extremities. (**C**, **D**) PTO was performed below tibial tuberosity by opening-wedge osteotomy. (**E**) A 26-month follow-up postoperative radiograph shows adequate correction of the varus deformity after hardware removal.*

PEARLS AND PITFALLS

The following are some pearls and pitfall with this procedure:

- This method is technically demanding and has a steep learning curve. The degree of correction of the varus deformity at the metaphysial-diaphyseal junction is critically determined by the precise identification of the nail entry portal, the nail path, and the adequacy of the locking screws.
- The preoperative planning is extremely important to determine the exact degree of correction, entry point, and the trajectory of the nail in the proximal fragment. No such intraoperative fine tuning is possible with this technique after proximal reaming is performed and any correction different from the one preoperatively planned is not recommended.[20,26]
- Power saw and high-speed drills use in conventional techniques can cause thermal necrosis of bone ends and adjacent soft tissues.[10] Therefore, we use a new drill bit each time with a low-speed drill to minimize heat generation. Because of this less invasive surgical technique, the periosteum and soft tissue are relatively well protected, the periosteum being the most important contributor to bone healing.[10]
- Because weak fixation of the proximal fragment might lead to postoperative loss of correction, the authors recommend a nail with numerous multiplanar locking options and bicortical purchase of the proximal interlocking screws.
- If the correction in a tibial angulation case would be difficult without addressing the fibular strut, a fibular osteotomy using a similar drilling technique can be performed. With a surgeon's increase in confidence and experience with the technique, a fibular osteotomy might not be necessary (Fig. 37-15).

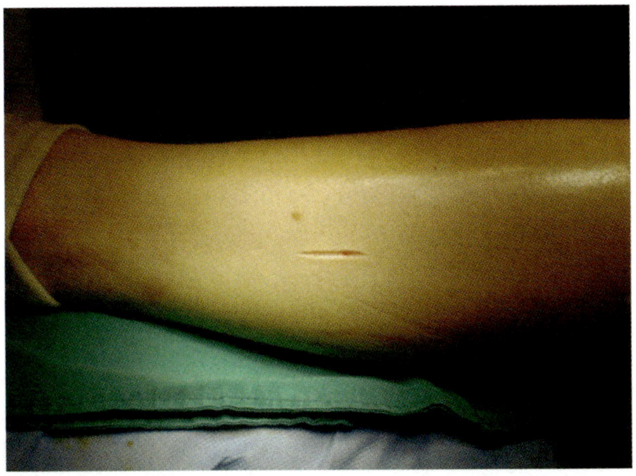

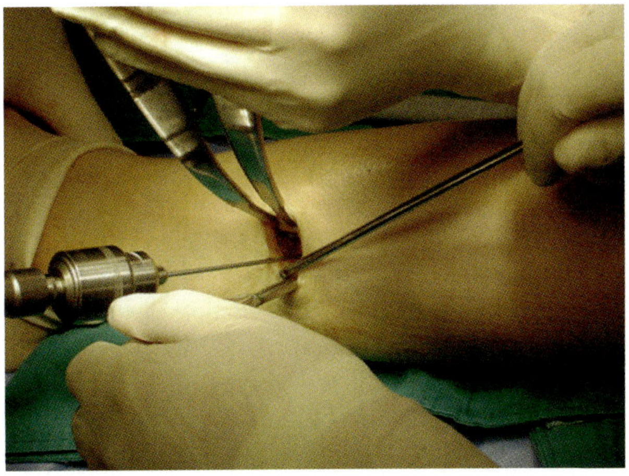

FIGURE 37-15. *The fibular osteotomy is performed with a small skin incision using a low-speed, multiple drilling technique.*

REFERENCES

1. Jackson JP, Waugh W. Tibial osteotomy for osteoarthritis of the knee. *J Bone Joint Surg Br.* 1961;43:746-751.
2. Jackson JP, Waugh W, Green JP. High tibial osteotomy for osteoarthritis of the knee. *J Bone Joint Surg Br.* 1969;51(1):88-94.
3. Adili A, Bhandari M, Giffin R, et al. Valgus high tibial osteotomy. Comparison between an Ilizarov and a Coventry wedge technique for the treatment of medial compartment osteoarthritis of the knee. *Knee Surg Sports Traumatol Arthrosc.* 2002;10(3):169-176.
4. Coventry MB. Osteotomy of the upper portion of the tibia for degenerative arthritis of the knee. A preliminary report. *J Bone Joint Surg Am.* 1965;47:984-990.
5. Paley D, Maar DC, Herzenberg JE. New concepts in high tibial osteotomy for medial compartment osteoarthritis. *Orthop Clin North Am.* 1994;25(3):483-498.

6. Schwartsman V. Circular external fixation in high tibial osteotomy. *Instr Course Lect.* 1995;44:469-474.
7. Mont MA, Alexander N, Krackow KA, et al. Total knee arthroplasty after failed high tibial osteotomy. *Orthop Clin North Am.* 1994;25(3):515-525.
8. Sen C, Kocaoglu M, Eralp L. The advantages of circular external fixation used in high tibial osteotomy (average 6 years follow-up). *Knee Surg Sports Traumatol Arthrosc.* 2003;11(3):139-144.
9. Murphy SB. Tibial osteotomy for genu varum. Indications, preoperative planning, and technique. *Orthop Clin North Am.* 1994;25(3):477-482.
10. Paley D, Tetsworth K. Percutaneous osteotomies. Osteotome and Gigli saw techniques. *Orthop Clin North Am.* 1991;22(4):613-624.
11. Shim JS, Lee SH, Jung HJ, et al. High tibial open wedge osteotomy below the tibial tubercle: clinical and radiographic results. *Knee Surg Sports Traumatol Arthrosc.* March 8, 2011 [Epub ahead of print].
12. Shiha A, El-Deen MA, Khalifa AR, et al. Ilizarov gradual correction of genu varum deformity in adults. *Acta Orthop Belg.* 2009;75(6):784-791.
13. Cullu E, Aydogdu S, Alparslan B, et al. Tibial slope changes following dome-type high tibial osteotomy. *Knee Surg Sports Traumatol Arthrosc.* 2005;13(1):38-43.
14. Gaasbeek RD, Sonneveld H, van Heerwaarden RJ, et al. Distal tuberosity osteotomy in open wedge high tibial osteotomy can prevent patella infera: a new technique. *Knee.* 2004;11(6):457-461.
15. Kellgren JH, Lawrence JS. Radiological assessment of osteo-arthrosis. *Ann Rheum Dis.* 1957;16(4):494-502.
16. Kodkani PS. Dome osteotomy of the proximal tibia for genu varum treated with a new fixation device. *J Knee Surg.* 2007;20(2):111-119.
17. Gunes T, Sen C, Erdem M. Tibial slope and high tibial osteotomy using the circular external fixator. *Knee Surg Sports Traumatol Arthrosc.* 2007;15(2):192-198.
18. Nakamura E, Mizuta H, Kudo S, et al. Open-wedge osteotomy of the proximal tibia hemicallotasis. *J Bone Joint Surg Br.* 2001;83(8):1111-1115.
19. Jung KA, Kim SJ, Lee SC, et al. "Fine-tuned" correction of tibial slope with a temporary external fixator in opening wedge high-tibial osteotomy. *Knee Surg Sports Traumatol Arthrosc.* 2008;16(3):305-310.
20. Galla MLP. High tibial open wedge valgus osteotomy stabilized with the TomoFix plate fixator. *Orthop Traumatol.* 2004;4:397-417.
21. Koshino T, Murase T, Saito T. Medial opening-wedge high tibial osteotomy with use of porous hydroxyapatite to treat medial compartment osteoarthritis of the knee. *J Bone Joint Surg Am.* 2003;85(1):78-85.
22. Paley D, Herzenberg JE, Tetsworth K, et al. Deformity planning for frontal and sagittal plane corrective osteotomies. *Orthop Clin North Am.* 1994;25(3):425-465.
23. Matar WY, Boscariol R, Dervin GF. Open wedge high tibial osteotomy: a roentgenographic comparsion of a horizontal and an oblique osteotomy on patellar height and sagittal tibial slope. *Am J Sports Med.* 2009;37(4):735-742.
24. Preston CF, Fulkerson EW, Meislin R, et al. Osteotomy about the knee: applications, techniques, and results. *J Knee Surg.* 2005;18(4):258-272.
25. Magyar G, Ahl TL, Vibe P, et al. Open-wedge osteotomy by hemicallotasis or the closed-wedge technique for osteoarthritis of the knee. A randomised study of 50 operations. *J Bone Joint Surg Br.* 1999;81(3):444-448.
26. Noyes FR, Mayfield W, Barber-Westin SD, et al. Opening wedge high tibial osteotomy: an operative technique and rehabilitation program to decrease complications and promote early union and function. *Am J Sports Med.* 2006;34(8):1262-1273.

38

Distal Femoral Varus Osteotomies for Lateral Osteoarthritis of the Knee

Yona Kosashvili, Allan E. Gross, Yaron Bar Ziv, and David Backstein

Monocompartmental knee arthritis in younger patients can present a challenge to orthopaedic surgeons. Although excellent overall results have been reported for total knee arthroplasty (TKA) at follow-up of 15 years or more,[1-3] this modality is often not preferred in younger patients. Several investigators have reported worse clinical outcomes with higher failure rates in younger patients.[4,5] A number of different procedures, including osteotomies of the proximal tibia and distal femur, have shown success in decreasing pain and increasing function, as well as delaying the need for knee arthroplasty by a decade or more in the majority of patients.[6-8]

High tibial valgus osteotomies in well-selected patients with arthritic medial compartment and varus deformity may amelerioate symptoms and delay the need for knee arthroplasty. Several studies reported good outcomes lasting more than a decade for patients with varus deformity treated by high valgus tibial osteotomy.[6,7,9-11] However, a proximal tibial varus osteotomy for correction of valgus deformity is less reliable.[12,13] When the ensuing coronal tibial slope was greater than 10°, the clinical outcomes were suboptimal, possibly due to the excessive translational forces on intra-articular structures, especially the hyaline cartilage and menisci. Thus the authors suggest that only patients with minor valgus malignment be corrected through the proximal tibia. If the resulting proximal tibial slope is expected to result in more than 10° of mediolateral slope, then a distal femoral varus osteotomy (DFVO) is preferable, either using a closing wedge on the medial side or an opening wedge of the lateral femoral cortex.

INDICATIONS AND CONTRAINDICATIONS

The indication for a DFVO is a unicompartmental, lateral arthritis with acquired or congenital valgus alignment. Prerequisites include the following:

- Active lifestyle (physical labor, high-impact sport),
- Physiologic young age,
- Minimum 90° arc of motion, and
- Capability of undergoing extensive rehabilitation.

Contraindications include the following:

- Significant osteoarthritis of the medial and/or patellofemoral compartments,
- Poor bone quality or osteoporosis (females > 60 years old, males > 65 years old),
- Knee stiffness with less than a 90° arc of motion,
- Incapability of undergoing an extensive and intensive rehabilitation process, and
- Lateral opening wedge in the context of lateral femoral condyle osteonecrosis.

PREOPERATIVE EVALUATION

Before DFVO surgery is performed, appropriate imaging is required for purposes of diagnosis and preoperative planning. This includes the following:

- Weight-bearing anteroposterior (AP) and lateral radiograph,
- Skyline (Merchant) view of patellofemoral joint,
- Full-length standing views, and
- Weight-bearing posteroanterior views at 45° of flexion (Rosenberg).

SURGICAL TECHNIQUE

Closing-Wedge DFVO

Closing-wedge DFVO has been the practice in our institution for more than three decades to correct lateral compartment gonarthritis with valgus deformity.[7,8,14] The closing-wedge osteotomy is performed by using a 90° angled blade plate. Since the blade of a 90° blade plate is placed parallel to the joint line, the distal femoral shaft–joint line angle is essentially corrected to 90° and the tibiofemoral angle to 0°. Thus, the closing-wedge DFVO technique does not require extensive preoperative measurements of angles for correction. In addition, no special instrumentation is required.

The patient is positioned supine and a tourniquet is inflated before skin incision. Image intensifier is positioned in the operating room to allow for AP and lateral fluoroscopic images throughout the procedure. A straight 15-cm midline incision is made starting just distal to the joint line and continuing proximally, which can be used in the future for TKA.

A subvastus exposure is utilized. The vastus medialis is bluntly dissected off the medial intermuscular septum and reflected and held anteriorly and laterally with a Homan retractor to expose the medial aspect of the femoral cortex and the medial femoral condyle. The knee is flexed to 90°, and a guide wire is carefully passed by hand parallel to the articular surfaces and across the joint space through a small medial arthrotomy. Under fluoroscopic control, a second wire is then drilled into the medial femoral condyle parallel to the intra-articular wire and approximately 1 cm proximal to the femoral articular surface (Fig. 38-1). Radiographic confirmation that this wire is parallel to the joint line is crucial for appropriate correction of the deformity by aligning the anatomic axis of the femur and subsequent 90° blade plate, perpendicular to femoral articular surface.

Next, three 4.5-mm drill holes are made in the medial femoral cortex at a point 2 to 2.5 cm from the articular sur-

A

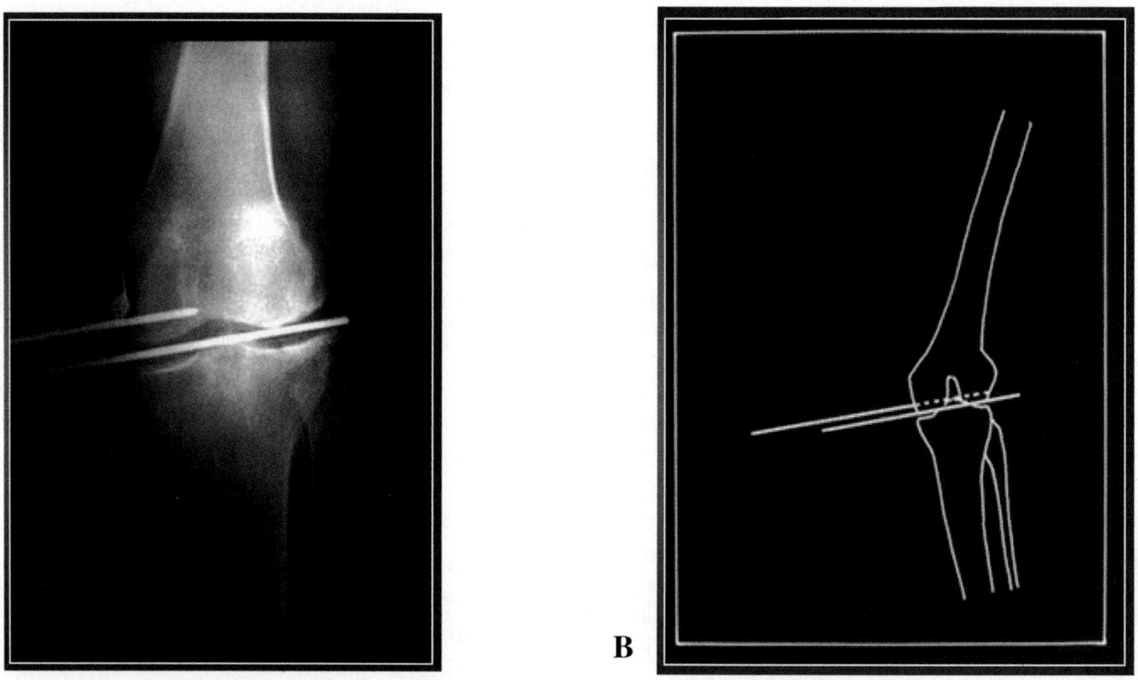

B

FIGURE 38-1. *Intraoperative radiograph (**A**) and illustration (**B**) of the parallel guides.*

face in the anterior half of the medial cortex (Fig. 38-2). These drill holes prevent uncontrolled fracture of the femur as the blade plate chisel penetrates the cortex. The chisel is then inserted parallel to the two previously inserted guide wires, to a depth of 50 to 70 mm, depending on the size of the distal femur. The plate holder is used to guide the chisel and to obtain optimal apposition of the plate to the long axis of the femur. After insertion of the chisel, AP and lateral images are obtained to confirm its alignment. The medial arthrotomy previously performed for the insertion of the intra-articular guide wire is used to visually confirm that the chisel has not penetrated the intercondylar notch.

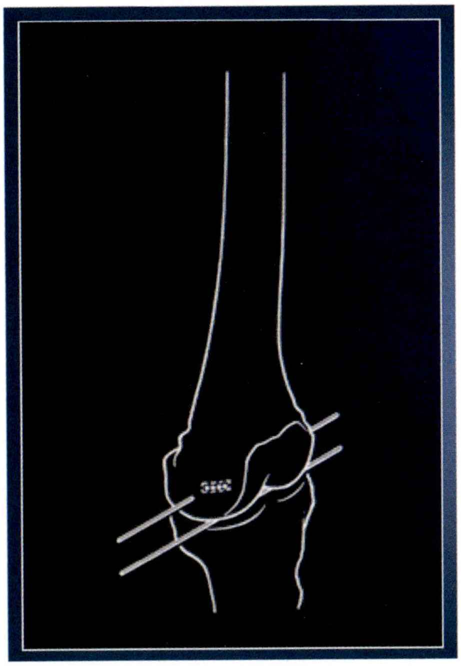

FIGURE 38-2. *Illustration of the preventive drill holes into the medial femoral cortex, placed 2.5 cm above the joint line for the insertion of the chisel (rectangle above the proximal wire).*

A longitudinal line is marked on the medial part of the femoral cortex parallel to the long axis of the femur proximal and distal to the osteotomy site to ensure that correct rotational alignment is restored after the bone resection. A closing-wedge osteotomy is made 1 cm proximal to the chisel, well above the patellofemoral joint (Fig. 38-3). The base of the osteotomy is cut with an oscillating saw while the lateral cortex is perforated with a small osteotome. This allows a correction of the deformity while preventing lateral translocation of the proximal fragment. The base of the wedge should be wide enough (5–10 mm) to allow a 90° angle between the chisel and the medial part of the femoral cortex after the wedge is removed. Since the proximal cortical fragment has a smaller diameter, it can be easily impacted into the cancellous bone of the distal fragment. This allows an increase in the magnitude of the angular correction if desired. It also provides additional stability and promotes more rapid healing of the osteotomy site.

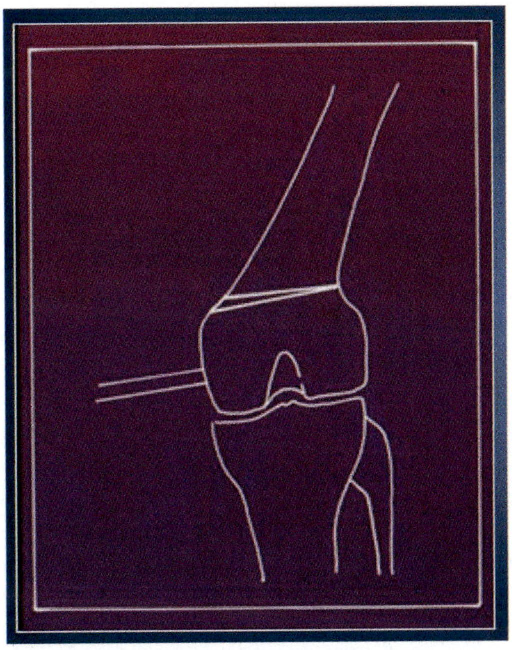

FIGURE 38-3. *Illustration of the closing-wedge osteotomy performed just above the trochlea.*

While the rotational alignment of both segments is maintained, a 90° offset dynamic compression plate is inserted. If the plate cannot be adequately brought into contact with the medial femoral diaphyseal cortex after inserting the blade, a slot can be created to better accommodate the shoulder of the blade plate until satisfactory contact is achieved. The osteotomized bony wedge is morcellized and used as an autograft along the medial aspect of the osteotomy. With the 90° blade plate positioned properly along the medial part of the femoral cortex, screws are inserted into the plate using compression techniques (Fig. 38-4). Deformity correction is achieved since the medial part of the femoral cortex and the transepycondylar femoral line are now at 90° to each other and the tibiofemoral angle is now approximately 0°. The vastus medialis is then tacked back to the medial septum using interrupted sutures, and the skin and subcutaneous tissues are closed in a routine fashion.

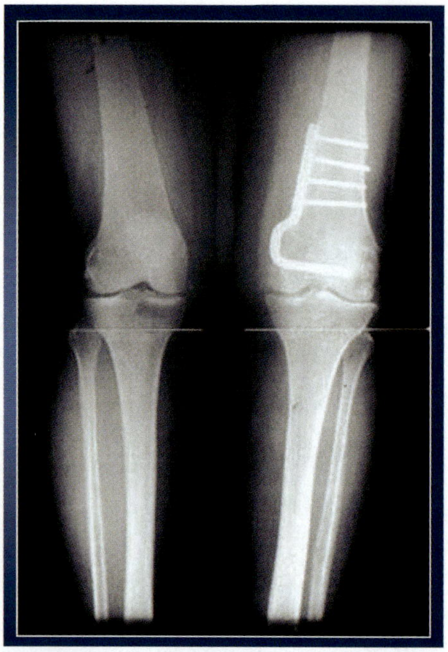

FIGURE 38-4. *Postoperative radiograph of the closing-wedge osteotomy.*

Opening-Wedge DFVO

The patient is placed in a supine position and a tourniquet is inflated before skin incision. A straight 15-cm incision on the lateral aspect of the distal femur is made starting just proximal to the joint line and continuing proximally. The vastus lateralis is carefully dissected from the lateral intermuscular septum and reflected anteriorly and medially to expose the lateral aspect of the femoral cortex. Perforating veins need to be appropriately controlled. The knee is flexed to 90° and a Homan retractor is placed posterior to the femur to protect the neurovascular structures during the osteotomy of the posterior femoral cortex.

The knee is extended to 30° of flexion over a gown pack and a guide wire is inserted from 4 to 5 cm above the lateral femoral epicondyle directed 20° obliquely in the coronal plane toward 0.5 cm above the medial femoral epicondyle under fluoroscopic control. A parallel guide wire should be temporarily positioned anterior to the femur over the first guide wire to confirm that it is above the trochlear groove. The lateral cortex is perforated by an oscillating saw, preferably by using a cutting jig placed over the guide wire in order to prevent the osteotomy from extending into the joint. The osteotomy is then completed by a sharp osteotome under fluoroscopic control severing the anterior and posterior cortices, while leaving 1 cm of a medial cortex serving as a hinge. A wedge opener is inserted to the desired degree of coronal correction, determined preoperatively, based on long-leg standing radiographs. Alternatively, the osteotomy can be opened by osteotomes inserted consecutively and stacked on each other. In both techniques the osteotomy should be gradually opened over several minutes in order prevent inadvertent fracture of the medial cortex, especially for corrections larger than 10°.

The new mechanical axis can be confirmed fluoroscopically using a long rod extending from the center of the femoral head to the center of the talus. The joint line should pass at the middle of the medial tibial plateau. The osteotomy is secured by either a femoral locking plate or by specially designed plates for this condition. Ideally, four cortical screws proximally and at least two cancellous screws distally are required. The osteotomy can be filled with shaped allogenic or tricorticocancellous grafts from the ipsilateral iliac crest. The vastus lateralis is then tacked back to the lateral septum using interrupted sutures, and the skin and subcutaneous tissues are closed in a routine fashion.

POSTOPERATIVE PROTOCOL

The postoperative protocol for both closing-wedge and opening-wedge DFVO is similar. The knee is immobilized for 24 to 48 hours in a bulky, postoperative dressing. Gentle active and active-assisted range-of-motion exercises are started 10 to 14 days postoperatively. Partial weight bearing is permitted at 6 to 8 weeks postoperatively, when radiographs indicate that the osteotomy is uniting. Gradual increase in weight-bearing status over the next 3 to 6 weeks is allowed, based on radiographic evidence of bone healing. Full activities are generally resumed 3 to 6 months after surgery.

CLINICAL OUTCOMES

Closing-Wedge DFVO

The results of closing-wedge DFVO reported in the literature are encouraging. Edgerton et al reported on 23 patients (24 knees) managed with closing-wedge DFVO and found 71% good or excellent results at a mean follow-up of 8.3 years.[15] Wang and Hsu reported good midterm success rates of DFVO even in the presence of moderate patellofemoral arthritis at a mean follow-up of 99 months.[16] Similarly, a very long-term follow-up study from our institution[8] found that knee function is expected to consistently and significantly ($p < .01$) improve following DFVO. At 1-year follow-up, 84.8% of patients had an excellent or good knee function scores, while 9.1% had fair results and 6.1% had poor results compared to the poor function encountered in 97% of these patients preoperatively. The knee function and knee scores significantly ($p < .01$) deteriorate at 10-year follow-up but remain much better ($p < .01$) than before surgery. At 10-year follow-up, 31.6% of 38 knees were either converted or planned to convert to TKA. At 15-year follow-up, 48.5% of the knees after closing-wedge DFVO were converted or planned to convert to TKA.

Despite the success of distal femoral varus osteotomies in delaying the progression of lateral compartment gonarthrosis, some of the patients are expected to require definitive treatment with TKA. Progression of osteoarthritis may be related to the patients' higher demand and the overloading of the medial compartment. To date, few reports have been made on TKA following previous DFVO, and those have either not presented objective outcomes or presented very small numbers of patients gathered from multiple centers. Nelson et al reported on 11 such patients and suggested that all TKAs need to be stemmed.[17] Moreover, constrained implants are commonly required because proper ligament balancing is difficult to achieve.

The authors recently reported on 22 DFVOs that were converted to TKAs.[18] At a 5-year average follow-up, 91% of the patients were doing well. In all cases, posterior-stabilized components were used, without a need for additional constraint. Stems (two tibial and three femoral) were required in only 23% of the cases. A potential obstacle to overcome that was noticed in that study was patella baja, which occurred in five of the patients (23%). Since a larger distal lateral femoral condyle is resected in order to restore the mechanical axis, matching the previous closing-wedge osteotomy, an overall shortening of the femur with an excessive elevation of the joint line may ensue, predisposing to patella baja.

Opening-Wedge DFVO

Puddu et al reported excellent results at 4- to 14-year follow-up in 21 patients with marked improvement in pain and knee function.[19] Similarly, Zarrouk et al reported on 80% of good to excellent outcomes in 22 patients undergoing opening-wedge DFVO with a blade plate at an average follow-up of 4.5 years.[20] However, Jacobi et al reported longer time to union and iliotibial band irritation by the lateral side plate, which encouraged them to abandon the opening-wedge osteotomy.[21] Because of the relative paucity of literature on opening-wedge osteotomy, it is difficult to establish the long-term outcomes of this procedure.

CONCLUSION

DFVO is a viable alternative for lateral compartmental knee arthritis in appropriately selected patients. This procedure may reliably improve symptoms and assist in delaying the need for TKA by more than a decade. When necessary, conversion to TKA can be performed. Care should be taken to avoid patella baja.

PEARLS AND PITFALLS

Pearls and pitfalls of this procedure include the following:

- Preoperative planning is extremely important to determine the exact degree of correction.
- This procedure is indicated for unicompartmental, lateral arthritis with acquired or congenital valgus alignment.
- Proper technique should be followed to avoid patella baja.
- Despite correct technique and ideal patient selection, some patients end up requiring TKA relatively soon.

REFERENCES

1. Buechel FF Sr. Long-term follow-up after mobile-bearing total knee replacement. *Clin Orthop Relat Res*. 2002;404:40-50.
2. Dixon MC, Brown RR, Parsch D, Scott RD. Modular fixed-bearing total knee arthroplasty with retention of the posterior cruciate ligament. A study of patients followed for a minimum of fifteen years. *J Bone Joint Surg Am*. 2005;87:598-603.
3. Font-Rodriguez DE, Scuderi GR, Insall JN. Survivorship of cemented total knee arthroplasty. *Clin Orthop Relat Res*. 1997;345:79-86.
4. Santaguida PL, Hawker GA, Hudak PL, et al. Patient characteristics affecting the prognosis of total hip and knee joint arthroplasty: a systematic review. *Can J Surg*. 2008;51:428-436.
5. Singh JA, Gabriel S, Lewallen D. The impact of gender, age, and preoperative pain severity on pain after TKA. *Clin Orthop Relat Res*. 2008;466:2717-2723.
6. Insall JN, Joseph DM, Msika C. High tibial osteotomy for varus gonarthrosis. A long-term follow-up study. *J Bone Joint Surg Am*. 1984;66:1040-1048.

7. Hutchison CR, Cho B, Wong N, et al. Proximal valgus tibial osteotomy for osteoarthritis of the knee. *Instr Course Lect.* 1999;48:131-134.
8. Kosashvili Y, Safir O, Gross A, et al. Distal femoral varus osteotomy for lateral osteoarthritis of the knee: a minimum ten-year follow-up. *Int Orthop.* 2010;34: 249-254.
9. Sprenger TR, Doerzbacher JF. Tibial osteotomy for the treatment of varus gonarthrosis. Survival and failure analysis to twenty-two years. *J Bone Joint Surg Am.* 2003;85:469-474.
10. Tjörnstrand BA, Egund N, Hagstedt BV. High tibial osteotomy: a seven-year clinical and radiographic follow-up. *Clin Orthop Relat Res.* 1981;160:124-136.
11. Vainionpää S, Läike E, Kirves P, et al. Tibial osteotomy for osteoarthritis of the knee. A five to ten-year follow-up study. *J Bone Joint Surg Am.* 1981;63:938-946.
12. Coventry MB. Proximal tibial varus osteotomy for osteoarthritis of the lateral compartment of the knee. *J Bone Joint Surg Am.* 1987;69:32-38.
13. Shoji H, Insall J. High tibial osteotomy for osteoarthritis of the knee with valgus deformity. *J Bone Joint Surg Am.* 1973;55:963-973.
14. Backstein D, Morag G, Hanna S, et al. Long-term follow-up of distal femoral varus osteotomy of the knee. *J Arthroplasty.* 2007;22:2-6.
15. Edgerton BC, Mariani EM, Morrey BF. Distal femoral varus osteotomy for painful genu valgum. A five- to 11-year follow-up study. *Clin Orthop Relat Res.* 1993;288:263-269.
16. Wang JW, Hsu CC. Distal femoral varus osteotomy for osteoarthritis of the knee. *J Bone Joint Surg Am.* 2005;87:127-133.
17. Nelson CL, Saleh KJ, Kassim RA, et al. Total knee arthroplasty after varus osteotomy of the distal part of the femur. *J Bone Joint Surg Am.* 2003;85:1062-1065.
18. Kosashvili Y, Gross AE, Zywiel MG, et al. Total knee arthroplasty after failed distal femoral varus osteotomy using selectively stemmed posterior stabilized components. *J Arthroplasty.* 2011;26:738-743.
19. Puddu G, Cipolla M, Cerullo G, et al. Osteotomies: the surgical treatment of the valgus knee. *Sports Med Arthrosc Rev.* 2007;15:15-22.
20. Zarrouk A, Bouzidi R, Karray B, et al. Distal femoral varus osteotomy outcome: is associated femoropatellar osteoarthritis consequential? *Orthop Traumatol Surg Res.* 2010;96:632-636.
21. Jacobi M, Wahl P, Bouaicha S, et al. Distal femoral varus osteotomy: problems associated with the lateral open-wedge technique. *Arch Orthop Trauma Surg.* 2011;131:725-728.

39 Osteoarticular Transfer System

Hasan M. Syed and Andreas H. Gomoll

Focal cartilage lesions in the knee represent a therapeutic challenge to the orthopaedic surgeon. Such injuries are a common cause of knee ailments with International Cartilage Repair Society (ICRS) grade III or IV defects in patients under the age of 40 accounting for more than 5% of all arthroscopies.[1,2] These cartilage defects can be secondary to trauma or be atraumatic in etiology, as is seen with osteochondritis dissecans. Patients with isolated cartilage lesions may benefit from surgical intervention both in terms of symptomatic relief and in preventing subsequent degenerative changes in the knee. Restoration of articular cartilage injuries is difficult given the lack of regenerative potential and avascularity of this tissue. Given their prevalence, different techniques have been devised to address cartilage lesions. These include chondroplasty, marrow stimulation techniques (drilling, abrasion arthroplasty, and microfracture), autologous chondrocyte implantation (ACI), fresh osteochondral allograft transplantation, and osteochondral autograft transfer (OAT). Although a viable option in the treatment of cartilage defects, fresh osteochondral allografting is limited by availability. OAT, however, involves the transfer of intact osteochondral cylinders from low-load areas of the knee to chondral defects in other, higher demand parts of the knee. The donor osteochondral plug is press fit into a recipient site. This technique has gained popularity because of its ability to transfer functional mature hyaline cartilage to areas of full-thickness cartilage loss in weight-bearing portions of the knee. Although its application is mainly limited by the amount available for harvest, it is a single-stage procedure that is relatively low cost with good outcomes in comparative studies.[3]

This technique was first demonstrated by Outerbridge in 1981, who obtained donor autograft from the lateral one-third of the patella to treat large osteochondral defects over the weight-bearing condylar surface of the knee in 10 patients. Function and symptomatology improved in these patients, although some of these patients had persistent anterior knee symptoms and loss of motion after surgery.[4] Although techniques and instrumentation have continued to evolve since then, his work laid the foundation for this procedure. Proprietary instrumentation has since been developed, allowing for both open and arthroscopic harvest and reimplantation. Animal studies have demonstrated that the donor site, if left unfilled, reconstitutes with new bone at a few millimeters from the joint surface. The remainder of the defect fills in with fibrocartilage.[5] An alternate option is to fill the donor site with allograft, recipient site tissue, or synthetic plugs.

Of the available chondral repair or reconstruction options, OAT is the only method that allows for the immediate replacement of articular lesion with mature hyaline cartilage. Multiple studies have demonstrated that the transferred plugs histologically maintain hyaline cartilage morphology. These studies have also consistently demonstrated a lack of integration of the chondral tissue between the autograft transplant and the native surrounding cartilage, even at long-term follow-up.[6-8] Although the presence of this cleft raises concern about potential graft failure of the autograft plug, Nam demonstrated that chondral defects repaired with an osteochondral autograft had significantly greater stiffness than full-thickness defects or even normal cartilage, despite the presence of these clefts.[6]

Although replacing chondral defects with hyaline cartilage is the ultimate goal of cartilage repair surgery, equally, if not more, important is biomechanical performance of the repair tissue. Studies evaluating the immediate posttransfer stiffness of the graft plugs have demonstrated that the OAT procedure does not alter the stiffness, surface integrity, or thickness of the cartilage of the donor tissue.[9] Subchondral bone remodeling is thought to be responsible for a transient decrease in stiffness seen at 6 weeks postoperatively.[6] However, at 12 weeks postoperatively, there is a return of biomechanical properties and stiffness to that of normal articular cartilage.[10]

PREOPERATIVE EVALUATION

History and Examination

A complete history, including mechanisms of injury, and physical exam should be performed for all patients complaining of knee pain. Recent acute trauma with focal pain and joint effusion is common in patients with chondral defects. Quite often, there is a history of patellar dislocation or instability. Patients generally are less than 45 years old and typically present with intermittent pain symptoms that worsen with activity. Impact-type activities generally aggravate disease in the tibiofemoral compartments, whereas patellofemoral disease is associated with use of stairs or positions of knee flexion. If the injury results in an unstable chondral or osteochondral fragment, the patient may report mechanical symptoms from a loose body.

On physical examination, patients with chondral injuries will frequently have pain at the joint line or over the femoral condyles. Exam findings are similar to those seen with meniscal disease. Depending on the acuity of the injury, an effusion may be present. Limb malalignment as well as patellar tracking must be assessed, as they may be the underlying cause of the chondral lesion. It is important to examine for concomitant injuries such as meniscal tears or ligamentous injuries. In younger patients with joint effusion and pain associated with trauma, chondral lesions must be considered in the differential.

Imaging

Radiographic

Preoperative imaging is critical in planning for OAT procedures. Standard X-rays should include standing anteroposterior and Rosenberg (45° standing posteroanterior) views to assess for osteoarthritis, osteonecrosis, and osteochondritis dissecans in the affected knee. Sunrise views are necessary to evaluate the patellofemoral compartment for degenerative changes, patellar tilt, and patellar or trochlear dysplasia. Similarly, when malalignment is suspected on clinical examination, full lower extremity bone length films help to determine the mechanical axis through the knee joint and the need for concurrent osteotomies (ie, varus or valgus neutralization osteotomies). Lateral knee views provide additional information about the joint surface as well as evaluation for possible patella alta or infera malpositioning. For suspected ostechondritis dissecans lesions, notch views are effective at visualizing the lateral aspect of the medial femoral condyle for typically located defects.[11]

Cross-sectional

In order to better assess the size and number of chondral defects, cross-sectional imaging, such as magnetic resonance (MR) and computed tomography (CT), are utilized. With advances in MR imaging, articular cartilage protocols (fast-spin-echo with or without fat suppression and/or fat-suppressed spoiled gradient-echo images that have sensitivities >95%) are available to help the surgeon determine not only the presence of full-thickness chondral defects but also the quality of the surrounding and opposing cartilage. MR imaging is also useful in assessing for any other coexisting meniscal or ligamentous pathologies. In patients in whom use of MR is contraindicated or not tolerated, as well as those with MR-incompatible hardware present near the knee joint, CT arthrogram allows for visualization of the chondral lesions by demonstrating filling of contrast fluid at the site of the defect. Although CT arthrograms are effective at determining the size and number of chondral defects, they are unable to provide a qualitative assessment of the remaining articular cartilage. As with sunrise or Merchant views with plain radiographs, CT and MR imaging allows for assessment of patellar tilt and patellar and trochlear dysplasia. However, cross-sectional imaging, particularly with CT scanning, also allows the surgeon to determine the tibial tubercle to trochlear groove distance (TT-TG). Any distance greater than 15 to 20 mm indicates patellar maltracking.

PREPARATION OF PATIENT FOR SURGERY

Once the decision for cartilage repair is made, any other pathology existing in the knee will also need to be addressed. Ligamentous reconstruction and/or meniscal repair can proceed as part of a one-stage procedure. We commonly encounter limb malalignment or patellar maltracking issues. For significant genu valgum or varum deformities, neutralization osteotomies can be performed simultaneously. Often we have found that the mechanical axis will fall directly through the affected compartment, necessitating the correction of the mechanical axis. Similarly, tibial tubercle osteotomies are performed to address patellar maltracking or instability. Any additional procedures will modify the postoperative rehabilitation protocol and usually the additional procedure will dictate the postoperative protocol. In general, patients are counseled on weight loss, smoking cessation, and maintenance of preoperative range-of-motion and knee-strengthening exercises.

SURGERY

Indications and Contraindications

Surgical candidates for OAT are generally young (<45 years) and have a symptomatic focal chondral defect without diffuse osteoarthritis. Patients with chondral defects from osteochondritis dissecans are also considered potential candidates for this procedure. The technique is limited by the size of the chondral lesion because of the availability of donor graft tissue. The typical defect size that can be addressed is between 1 and 4 cm^2.[12] Larger defects may require alternative cartilage repair techniques, including allograft osteochondral transfer. It is important to address other knee pathology such as meniscal injury, instability, or mechanical malalignment, because these issues may predispose the osteochondral autograft tissue to undue contact forces and compromise graft survival.

Contraindications include patients over the age of 55, generalized arthritis, inflammatory arthritis, obesity, and uncorrected instability, meniscal deficiency, and malalignment.

Anatomy, Approach, and Technique

OAT can be performed arthroscopically or through either a small medial or lateral parapatellar arthrotomy. This is based on the size and location of the defect as well as the surgeon's preference. Although different proprietary systems exist with variations in instrumentation, all follow the same general principles.

At the outset of the case, regardless of whether the chondral lesion will be addressed arthroscopically or through an open approach, a diagnostic knee arthroscopy is performed. Any meniscal or ligamentous injuries are addressed. The lesion itself is arthroscopically assessed (Fig. 39-1) and necessary accessory portals are established to allow for perpendicular orientation of the instrumentation to the articular surface for both the harvest and recipient sites. For arthroscopically performed OAT procedures, a transpatellar tendon portal is sometimes helpful both as a working and visualization portal. The patellar tendon is split in line with its fibers. After identifying the chondral defect(s), sizing guides are used to determine the size and number of autograft plugs needed to fill the defect (Fig. 39-2).

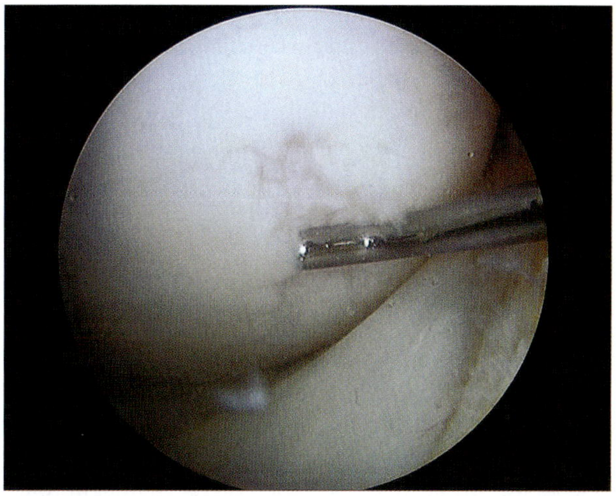

FIGURE 39-1. *Arthroscopic probe demonstrating a chondral defect of the femoral condyle.*

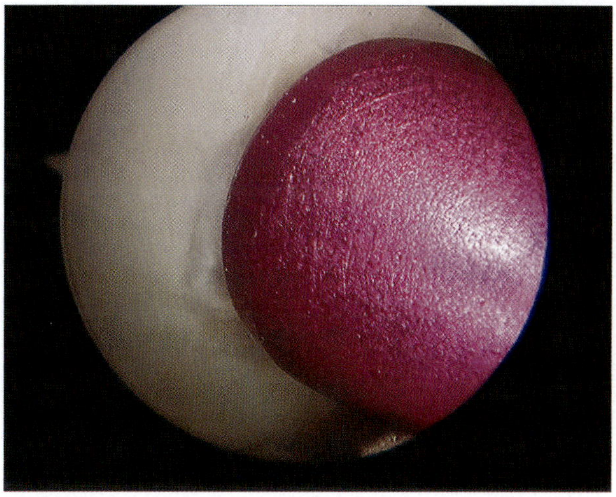

FIGURE 39-2. *The defect is measured using sizing rods to estimate the size and number of plugs required to fill the area.*

Next, an appropriately sized harvesting tube is used to obtain an osteochondral plug or plugs, generally 10 to 15 mm in length. It is critical that the harvester is introduced perpendicularly to the articular surface (Fig. 39-3). There are multiple sites recommended for autograft harvest, typically located in the lesser-weight-bearing areas of the knee. We generally prefer to obtain one to three autograft plugs from the medial trochlea, or the lateral femoral condyle from an area just proximal to the sulcus terminalis, the transition zone between the patellofemoral and tibiofemoral weight-bearing areas. After a plug has been obtained, the length is determined (Fig. 39-4).

Next, the defect site is prepared using a defect harvesting tube that is slightly undersized, to allow for press-fit fixation. The prepared defect is then checked with a depth rod to ensure that the defect is 1 mm deeper than the length of the autograft plug.

The autograft plug is then gently advanced within the harvesting tube so that a small portion of the plug is visible. The harvester is then used to gently advance the plug into the recipient site (Fig. 39-5). After the harvester is removed (Fig. 39-6), the graft is inspected to make sure it is flush with the surrounding cartilage; an oversized tamp can be used to gently seat the graft, but the use of a mallet should be avoided as much as possible (Fig. 39-7). This process is repeated for filling the remainder of the recipient site or other chondral defects.

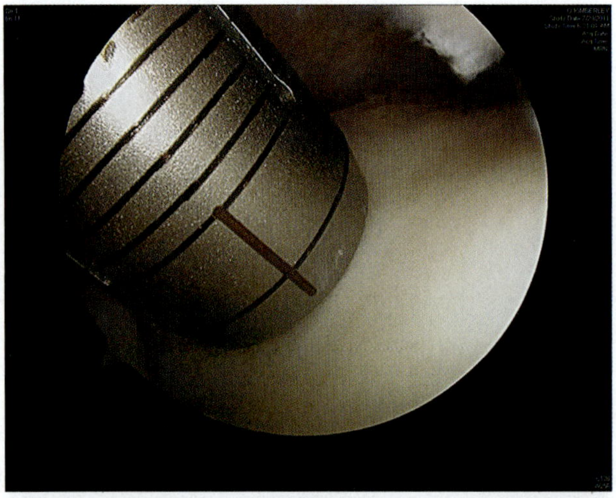

FIGURE 39-3. *An osteochondral plug is retrieved with a harvesting tube.*

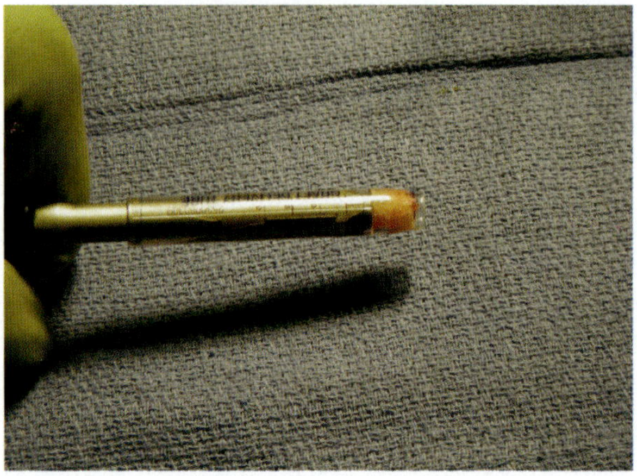

FIGURE 39-4. *The harvesting tube with the osteochondral plug ready for deployment.*

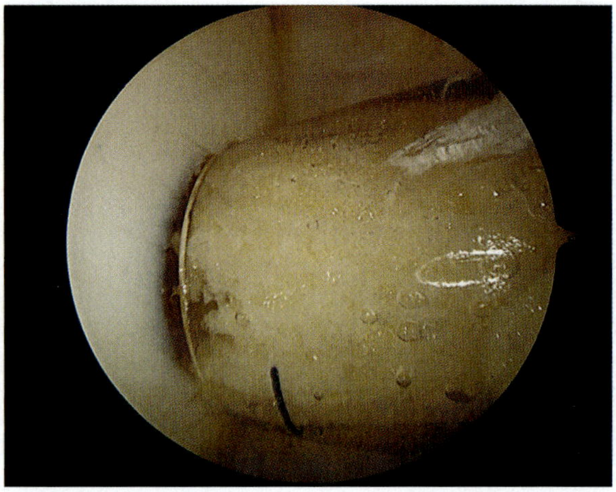

FIGURE 39-5. *Introduction of the plug into the recipient defect with gentle pressure.*

Surgical Considerations

Donor site selection

Numerous sites have been described as potential harvest sites. These include the superomedial border of the medial femoral condyle, superolateral border of the lateral femoral condyle, intercondylar notch, and proximal to the sulcus terminalis.[13] Biomechanical studies have demonstrated that contact forces are the lowest at locations just proximal to the sulcus terminalis.[14] Furthermore, cadaveric analysis has revealed that medial trochlear contact forces are less than the lateral trochlea.[15]

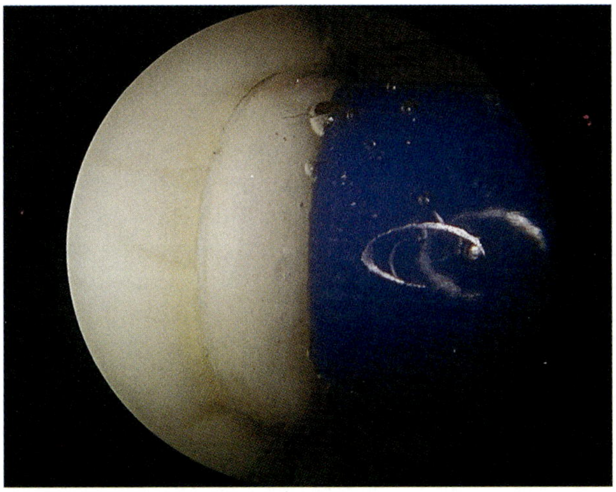

FIGURE 39-6. *Plug slightly proud before final seating.*

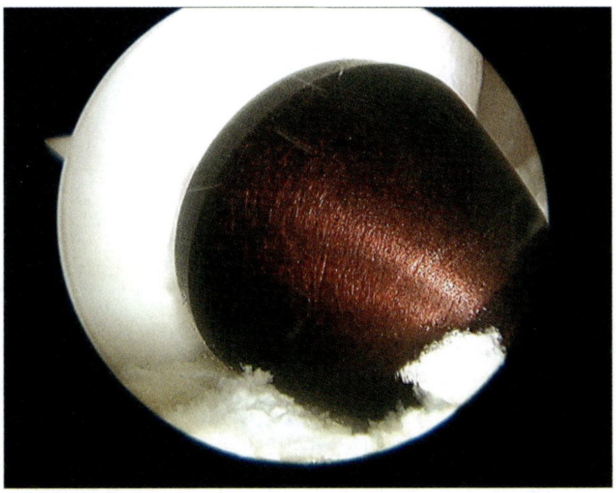

FIGURE 39-7. *Seating of the plug with the oversize tamp.*

Autograft height

The goal when placing donor plugs into chondral defects is to have them flush to the adjacent cartilage. Biomechanical studies have shown that the cartilage at the perimeter of an unfilled chondral defect experiences a significant increase in contact forces. These forces normalize when the defect is filled to the level of the surrounding tissue.[16,17] However, grafts left proud to the surrounding tissues by 0.5 mm can increase the contact forces by nearly 50% and these forces increase with increased graft elevation. Similarly, contact stress also increases when the graft is left countersunk, but much less so than seen with grafts left proud.[16] While articular congruity remains the goal, it is better to leave the graft slightly countersunk than proud.

Graft impaction

Increased forces required for graft seating with the press-fit technique have been studied and been found to be deleterious to chondrocyte viability.[18] However, typical graft impaction forces of 200 to 400 N studied in a fresh-frozen cadaver model did not reduce chondrocyte viability. However, a significant decrease in chondrocyte viability was seen when impact forces exceeded 800 N, as can be the case when donor plugs are longer than the recipient holes.[19]

Harvest site backfill

To address the residual osteochondral defect after harvest of the donor plug and decrease the risk of postoperative bleeding from the defect, backfill of the donor site has been advocated by some surgeons. Various synthetic bioabsorbable implants are commercially available for implantation. Another theoretical benefit of filling the donor site is support of the surrounding cartilage and subchondral bone, thereby preventing collapse.

POSTOPERATIVE MANAGEMENT

Rehabilitation

After OAT, patients are restricted to touch-down weight bearing on the operated extremity for 6 weeks. Active and passive range of motion is started immediately, with a continuous passive motion machine utilized if needed for 2 to 3 weeks. Return to athletic activities is individualized to the specific size and location of the chondral defect but, in general, usually it is 4 to 6 months before patients have adequate knee strength and proprioception to engage in impact activities.

Complications

Although typical postoperative issues such as infection and blood clots remain a concern as possible complications after an OAT procedure, donor site bleeding and pain are among the most common postoperative issues. When the donor site is left unfilled after harvest, painful hemarthrosis are noted in up to 8% of patients.[20] These patients will often require aspiration postoperatively for relief. Donor site morbidity and pain is often difficult to distinguish in knees in which the donor and recipient sites are in close proximity. However, studies evaluating previously asymptomatic knees in which plugs were harvested for transfer into a different joint have shown that, in the short term, 16% of such patients report knee dysfunction and pain.[12,21] Although the majority of patients report resolution of symptoms by 1 year, 3% report persistent long-term pain symptoms in the donor knee[12] and there is a wide range (9%-50%) of patients who report an incomplete return of function.[22,23]

Osteochondral autograft failure occurs in a subset of all procedures and may be related to a number of factors including technical ones. Malpositioned grafts due to inadequate sizing, angulation, or depth subject the autograft tissue to undue contact stress and may predispose it to failure. In osteochondritis dissecans, failure of incorporation of the transplanted subchondral bone to the native bone is often seen and this may be secondary to underlying osseous dysvascularity. In a prospective group of 30 patients having undergone arthroscopic autologous osteochondral grafting, although more than 75% had good to excellent results at 7-year follow-up, 10% of patients had failure of their graft tissue within 2 years postoperatively.[24]

OUTCOMES

The use of osteochondral autograft transplantation is an effective and viable option for small chondral lesions. Various studies have shown good to excellent results in over 80% of patients.[3,25,26] In a recent long-term (median follow-up 113 months) magnetic resonance imaging (MRI) evaluation of 24 patients who had undergone arthroscopic OAT procedure, MR analysis revealed good graft survival in more than 60% of patients with complete graft integration in 75% of cases.[27] Although there are few randomized controlled studies in the literature evaluating OAT versus other cartilage repair techniques, those that do exist demonstrate that the results of OAT are comparable to microfracture and autologous chondrocyte implantation in the appropriate defect size range (see Table 39-1). Osteochondral autograft transplantation, when used for the appropriate surgical indications, is a powerful technique allowing for the immediate transfer of mature hyaline cartilage to chondral lesions.

CASE EXAMPLE

A 29-year-old female, with previous right knee microfracture treatment of a medial femoral condyle chondral lesion 2 years ago, presented with nontraumatic right knee medial-sided pain, swelling, and limited activity level. Initial radiographic images were unremarkable and further workup revealed neutral mechanical alignment. After an unsuccessful trial of physical therapy and conservative measures, an MRI was performed (Fig. 39-8) and demonstrated a focal chondral defect over the medial femoral condyle without other internal pathology. A decision was made to proceed to surgery. During the diagnostic portion of the arthroscopy, the chondral defect was fully characterized and measured at 10 × 10 mm over the weight-bearing portion of the medial femoral condyle (Fig. 39-9). The chondral lesion was debrided and a donor osteochondral autograft plug obtained from an area just proximal to the lateral sulcus terminalis was harvested arthroscopically. This was then inserted into the previously prepared recipient site (Fig. 39-10). The harvest site was not backfilled. She was started on immediate active and passive range of motion and was touch-down weight bearing for the first 6 weeks postoperatively. Afterwards, the patient gradually was advanced to full weight bearing and continued therapy for strengthening and range-of-motion exercises. After 1 year postoperatively, the patient was able to return to recreational sporting activities and full range of motion without pain.

PEARLS AND PITFALLS

The following are some pearls and pitfalls for the OAT procedure:

- Assess for malalignment and patellar maltracking with appropriate imaging studies in all patients with chondral defects. If significant malalignment or patellar maltracking exists, it should be corrected at the time of surgery.
- Consider the use of filling the donor site to decrease the risk of hemarthrosis, either with the bone plug retrieved from the recipient site or a synthetic.
- Do not toggle the autograft plug harvester while introducing or retrieving the plug. This may result in distortion of the autograft plug.
- It is better to leave the graft slightly recessed as compared to leaving it proud.
- Autograft harvest and recipient site insertion must both be performed perpendicular to the articular surface.
- If the lesion site demonstrates sclerotic bone, consider drilling into the bony bed to allow for better osseous vascularization at the recipient site.

TABLE 39-1. Summary of Results of Various OAT-Related Studies in Literature

Study	Method	Type	Mean Follow-up	Results	No. of Patients	Mean Age (yrs)
Bentley et al[28] (2003)	ACI vs. mosaicplasty for OCD	Level 2 – prospective randomized	19 months	88% had good or excellent results after ACI compared with 69% after mosaicplasty	58 ACI vs. 42 mosaicplasty	31.3
Hangody & Fules[25] (2003)	Mosaicplasties grade 3–4 Outerbridge lesions or OCD	Level 4 –case series	10 years	Good to excellent results were achieved: 92% with femoral condylar mosaicplasties, 87% with tibial mosaicplasties, and 79% with patellar and/or trochlear mosaicplasties	740 (knee procedures)	NA
Chow et al[26] (2004)	Arthroscopic OAT for femoral condyle full-thickness chondral or osteochondral lesions	Level 4 –case series	45.1 months	83% good or excellent results	30	44.6
Ma et al[29] (2004)	OAT for posttraumatic OCD	Level 4 – case series	42 months	89% good or excellent results	18	29
Gudas[3] (2005)	Mosaciplasty OAT vs. MF in athletes with OCD or full-thickness cartilage defects	Level 2 – prospective randomized	37.1 months	96% good or excellent after OAT compared with 52% for the MF procedure	28 OAT vs. 29 MF	24.3
Hangody et al[30] (2010)	Mosaicplasty in competitive athletes with focal chondral or osteochondral lesions	Level 4 – case series	9.6 years	Good to excellent results were achieved: 91% with femoral condylar mosaicplasties, 86% with tibial mosaicplasties, and 74% with patellar and/or trochlear mosaicplasties	354	24.3
Muller et al[31] (2010)	OATS in athletes, grade 3 or 4 Outerbridge	Level 4 – case series	42 months	43% good or excellent results	14	41.1

MF, microfracture; OCD, osteochondral defects.

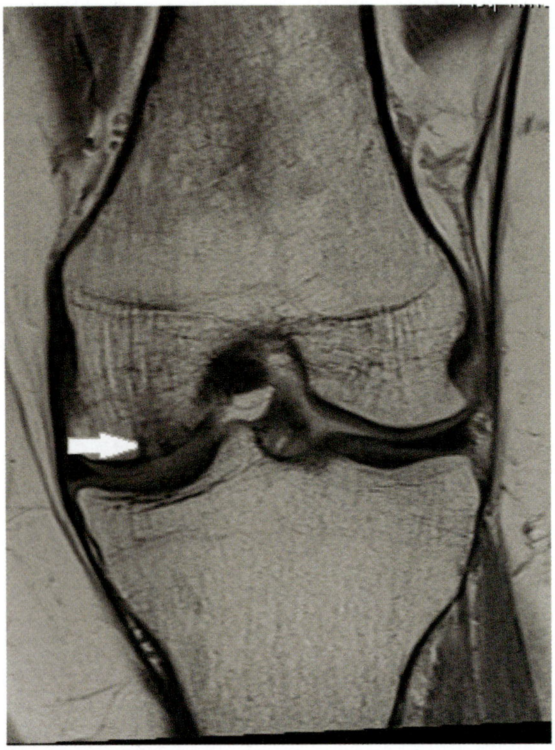

FIGURE 39-8. *MRI of right knee showing focal chondral defect (arrow) on the medial femoral condyle.*

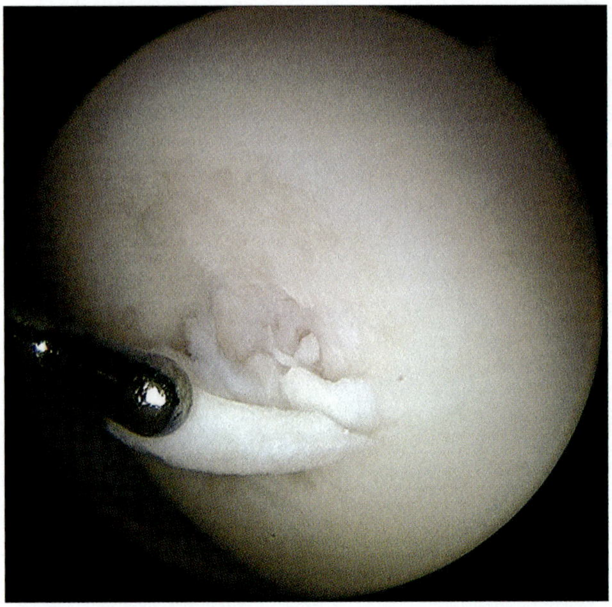

FIGURE 39-9. *Probe demonstrating full-thickness chondral defect with flap over the weight-bearing region of the medial femoral condyle.*

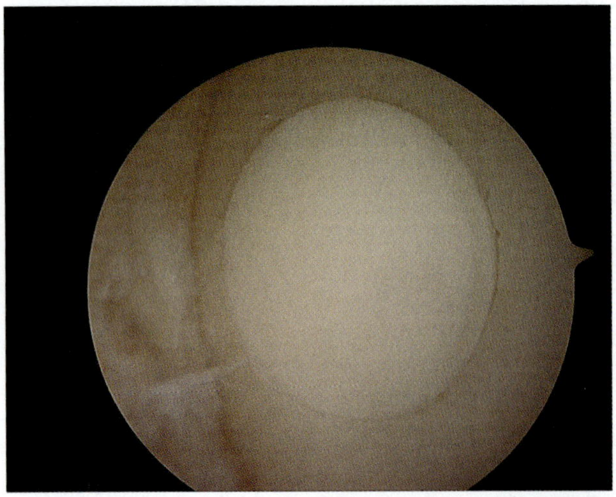

FIGURE 39-10. *Transferred autograft bone plug into the chondral defect.*

SUGGESTED READING

Gomoll AH, Farr J, Gillogly SD, et al. Surgical management of articular cartilage defects of the knee. *J Bone Joint Surg Am.* 2010;92(14):2470-2490.

REFERENCES

1. Curl WW, Krome J, Gordon ES, et al. Cartilage injuries: a review of 31, 516 knee arthroscopies. *Arthroscopy.* 1997;13:456-460.
2. Hjelle K, Solheim E, Strand T, et al. Articular carilage defects in 1,000 knee arthroscopies. *Arthroscopy.* 2002;18(7):730-734.
3. Gudas R. A prospective randomized clinical study of mosaic osteochondral autologous transplantation versus microfracture for the treatment of osteochondral defects in the knee joint in young athletes. *Arthroscopy.* 2005;21(9):1066-1075.
4. Outerbridge HK. The use of a lateral patella autograft for the repair of a large osteochondral defect in the knee. *J Bone Joint Surg Am.* 1995;77 (1):65-72.

5. Lane JG. Follow-up of osteochondral plug transfers in a goat model: a 6-month study. *Am J Sports Med.* 2004;32(6):1440-1450.
6. Nam EK. Biomechanical and histological evaluation of osteochondral transplantation in a rabbit model. *Am J Sports Med.* 2004;32(2):308-316.
7. Horas U. Autologous chondrocyte implantation and osteochondral cylinder transplantation in cartilage repair of the knee joint: a prospective, comparative trial. *J Bone Joint Surg Am.* 2003;85(2):185-192.
8. Glenn RE. Comparison of fresh osteochondral autografts and allografts: a canine model. *Am J Sports Med.* 2006;34(7):1084-1093.
9. Kuroki H. Mechanical effects of autogenous osteochondral surgical grafting procedures and instrumentation on grafts of articular cartilage. *Am J Sports Med.* 2004;32(3):612-620.
10. Nakaji N, Fujioka H, Nagura I, et al. The structural properties of an osteochondral cylinder graft-recipient construct on autologous osteochondral transplantation. *Arthroscopy.* 2006;22(4):422-427.
11. Milgram JW. Radiological and pathological manifestations of osteochondritis dissecans of the distal femur. A study of 50 cases. *Radiology.* 1978;126:305-311.
12. Hangody L, Feczko P, Bartha L, et al. Mosaicplasty for the treatment of articular defects of the knee and ankle. *Clin Orthop Relat Res.* 2001;391:S328-S336.
13. Hangody L. Autologous osteochondral mosaicplasty. Surgical technique. *J Bone Joint Surg Am.* 2004;86 (suppl):65-72.
14. Ahmad C. Biomechanical and topographical considerations for autologous osteochondral grafting in the knee. *Am J Sports Med.* 2001;29:201-206.
15. Garretson RB. Contact pressure at the osteochondral donor sites in the patellofemoral joint. *Am J Sports Med.* 2004;32(4):967-974.
16. Koh JL. The effect of graft height mismatch on contact pressure following osteochondral grafting: a biomechanical study. *Am J Sports Med.* 2004;32(2):317-320.
17. Koh JL. The effect of angled osteochondral grafting on contact pressure: a biomechanical study. *Am J Sports Med.* 2006;34(1):116-119.
18. Borazjani B. Effect of impact on chondrocyte viability during insertion of human osteochondral grafts. *J Bone Joint Surg Am.* 2006;88:1934-1943.
19. Patil S, Butcher W, D'Lima DD, Steklov N, Bugbee WD, Hoenecke HR. Effect of osteochondral graft insertion forces on chondrocyte viability. *Am J Sports Med.* 2008;36(9):1726-1732.
20. Hangody L, Vásárhelyi G, Hangody LR, et al. Autologous osteochondral grafting—technique and long-term results. *Injury.* 2008;39(suppl 1):S32-39.
21. Nishimura A, Morita A, Fukuda A, et al. Functional recovery of the donor knee after autologous osteochondral transplantation for capitellar osteochondritis dissecans. *Am J Sports Med.* 2011;39(4): 838-842.
22. Reddy S. The morbidity associated with osteochondral harvest from asymptomatic knees for the treatment of osteochondral lesions of the talus. *Am J Sports Med.* 2007;35(1):80-85.
23. Iwasaki N. Donor site evaluation after autologous osteochondral mosaicplasty for cartilaginous lesions of the elbow joint. *Am J Sports Med.* 2007;35(12): 2096-2100.
24. Marcacci M. Arthroscopic autologous osteochondral grafting for cartilage defects of the knee: prospective study results at a minimum 7-year follow-up. *Am J Sports Med.* 2007;5(12):2014-2021.
25. Hangody L, Fules P. Autologous osteochondral mosaicplasty for the treatment of full-thickness defects of weight-bearing joints: ten years of experimental and clinical experience. *J Bone Joint Surg Am.* 2003;85 (suppl 2):25-32.
26. Chow JC, Hantes ME, Houle JB, et al. Arthroscopic autogenous osteochondral transplantation for treating knee cartilage defects: a 2- to 5-year follow-up study. *Arthroscopy.* 2004;20:681-690.
27. Tetta C, Busacca M, Moio A, et al. Knee osteochondral autologous transplantation: long-term MR findings and clinical correlations. *Eur J Radiol.* 2010;76 (1):117-123.
28. Bentley G, Biant LC, Carrington RW, et al. A prospective, randomised comparison of autologous chondrocyte implantation versus mosaicplasty for osteochondral defects in the knee. *J Bone Joint Surg Br.* 2003;85(2):223-230.
29. Ma HL, Hung SC, Wang ST, et al. Osteochondral autografts transfer for post-traumatic osteochondral defect of the knee-2 to 5 years follow-up. *Injury.* 2004;35(12):1286-1292.
30. Hangody L, Dobos J, Baló E, et al. Clinical experiences with autologous osteochondral mosaicplasty in an athletic population: a 17-year prospective multicenter study. *Am J Sports Med.* 2010;38(6):1125-1133.
31. Muller S, Breederveld RS, Tuinebreijer WE. Results of osteochondral autologous transplantation in the knee. *Open Orthop J.* 2010;4:111-114.

40

Articular Cartilage Repair

Meghan Sampson, Kelsey Adair, Krushen Pillay, and Amir A. Jamali

Articular cartilage has a limited ability to heal spontaneously. Cartilage lesions in the knee are a source of significant pain, loss of function, and long-term issues such as osteoarthritis.[1] The goal of cartilage surgery is twofold: first, to address the source of pain; and second, to reduce overall joint inflammation and slow the development and progression of osteoarthritis. There are a variety of procedures to treat articular cartilage lesions with new options being developed every year. Currently mainstream techniques include microfracture, osteochondral autografting and allografting, and autologous chondrocyte implantation (ACI).

The microfracture technique is a modification of historical marrow-stimulating techniques, such as drilling and abrasion arthroplasty. The objective with marrow-stimulating techniques is to develop a well-marginated cavity surrounded by relatively healthy cartilage and to then place regularly spaced sites of penetration into the subchondral bone. Through these sites, marrow elements can enter the defect and establish the cell population and growth factors needed to form the repair tissue.[2] Unfortunately, the repair tissue formed under these circumstances may have histology characteristic of fibrocartilage, with higher amounts of collagen type I and a more disorganized cell configuration than seen in normal hyaline cartilage.

ACI was first performed in 1984 by Peterson and coworkers. They injected cultured chondrocytes into an articular defect in a rabbit knee and covered it with a periosteal flap to physically maintain the chondrocytes in place.[3] The procedure has been in clinical use in humans since the late 1980s. It is classically performed as a two-stage procedure with the first stage consisting of an arthroscopy procedure with biopsy of approximately 200 to 300 mg of mature cartilage. The chondrocytes are then recovered and expanded to approximately 12 million cells using a variety of proprietary techniques. Next an autologous periosteal or commercially available collagen patch is sewn over the defect and sealed with fibrin glue. The cells are then injected into the cavity formed by the patch.

The second broad category of cartilage repair methods involves repair of both the cartilage and the underlying bone. This osteochondral repair can be performed either with the patient's own tissue (osteochondral autograft) or tissue from a cadaver donor (osteochondral allograft). Although in some cases frozen tissue has been utilized, the gold standard for histological and clinical outcomes is a fresh osteochondral graft.

The first osteochondral autografts used large, single pieces for the graft. These grafts were obtained from the patella, the posterior femoral condyle, and the medial trochlea.[4,5] These early grafts were invasive and sometimes altered the articular biomechanics.[6] In 1993 Matsusue et al used multiple small osteochondral cylinders to compensate for the disadvantages of the single large graft.[7] Their report was one of the first cases published using osteochondral cylinders. Hangody further developed the multiple graft technique (mosaicplasty) and published his results in 1997.[8] These osteochondral cylinders are full-thickness cartilage attached to underlying bone. Once harvested from the donor site, they are transplanted to the chondral defect. The goal is to cover as much of the defect as possible with the osteochondral autograft cylinders.[6] The gaps between the cylinders usually fills in with fibrocartilage similar to that seen in microfracture.

Fresh osteochondral allografts have been in clinical use since the early 20th century.[9,10] The modern era of fresh osteochondral allografting began in the early 1970s. This procedure has become an increasingly attractive procedure in the absence of alternative methods of cartilage repair. The current indications for the procedure include the need to resurface a large portion of the knee or any resurfacing with the compromise of subchondral bone (previous trauma, avascular necrosis, or other sources of deformity).[11-24] Conceptually, fresh osteochondral allografting takes mature hyaline cartilage with living chondrocytes from a donor knee and transplants it into the damaged matching portion of the recipient knee. Hyaline cartilage is attractive for transplantation because it is avascular and aneural. Additionally, the risk of graft rejection is low, presumably due to the chondrocytes being embedded in the matrix protected from the host immune system. The osteochondral allograft also contains an osseous portion, which supports the articular cartilage. In contrast to the cells in the cartilaginous portion of the graft, the cells in the osseous portion do not survive the transplantation and are ultimately remodeled into the host bone. Both osteochondral autografts and allografts differ from the previously discussed methods of cartilage repair since the cartilage tissue is already fully mature. As a result, these grafts can exhibit identical histology to that of normal cartilage with the exception of the spaces between the grafts.

PREOPERATIVE EVALUATION

The goal of treatment of cartilage disease is to decrease pain and improve function. Thus it is critical to ascertain the location, quality, and alleviating or exacerbating factors. Some cartilage defects may become asymptomatic if given adequate healing time. It is helpful to classify the lesions as acute, subacute, or chronic. The degree of objective limitation based on alteration of sports or leisure activities is helpful in the early stages of disease. In later stages, the subjective complaints may include a limp, the need for assistive devices, instability, effusions, and difficulty with activities of daily living.

Physical examination often can identify the compartment with greatest involvement and occasionally the location of the damaged surface such as the femoral condyle. Associated injuries such as meniscal or ligamentous injuries are also identified at this time. Standard radiographs are helpful in the initial analysis of cartilage defects. However, magnetic resonance imaging (MRI), particularly with high-resolution images and cartilage-specific sequences, can be of great value. Unfortunately, many of these cartilage-specific sequences are not readily available for widespread use at this time. Deformities in the knee have traditionally been considered as either in the coronal plane or sagittal plane. However, in many cases, the deformities are complex and associated with a torsional component. We recommend full-length standing digital radiographs reconstructed on one long image. In cases of coronal deformities, the cartilage repair procedure can be combined with a tibial or femoral osteotomy based on the location and magnitude of the maximal deformity. For patellofemoral lesions, lateral retinacular lengthening or tibial tubercle osteotomy can be used as an adjunctive procedure based on the preoperative assessment.

Microfracture, Osteochondral Autografts, and Autologous Chondrocyte Implantation

Both microfracture and osteochondral autografting can be performed at the time of routine arthroscopy. Commercially available microfracture awls are available from a number of sources. Disposable autograft kits are also readily available in various graft diameter sizes and provide all necessary instrumentation needed for the procedure. Typically, the donor graft is slightly larger than the recipient to allow for press fit and immediate stabilization. When the surgeon chooses to perform ACI, he or she has the immediate option of obtaining the biopsy and placing it in sterile tissue culture medium for delivery to the processing center.

Fresh Osteochondral Allografts

The planning for fresh osteochondral allografts is slightly more complex. A key additional issue in planning these procedures is the need for a size match between the donor and recipient. Traditionally, the mediolateral dimension of the tibia has been used because it has been correlated with multiple other size measurements in the knee as demonstrated by Mensch and Amstutz.[25] More recently, we have used MRI based measurements to specifically measure the portion of the knee to be transplanted. Despite all of these techniques, the sizing of osteochondral allografts remains challenging. We anticipate that computed tomography (CT) based sizing techniques of the graft and host will provide the optimal method of size matching in the future. Currently tissue banks rarely provide CT scans of the grafts due to logistical and cost issues.

INDICATIONS AND CONTRAINDICATIONS

Microfracture

The microfracture procedure is typically performed in relatively small, full-thickness cartilage defects.[2,26] Defects that are larger are typically optimally treated with other techniques. This technique has a variety of contraindications, including patients who have axial malalignment, have partial-thickness articular cartilage defects, are unable to depend on the opposite leg for weight bearing, or are physiologically unable to follow the rehabilitation protocol.[27]

Osteochondral Autograft

Osteochondral autografts are ideal for defects between 1 and 4 cm^2, although in certain conditions they can be used for lesions up to 9 cm^2. The larger lesions can increase the rate of donor site morbidity.[28] Fifty years of age has been typically used as an age cutoff for this procedure. Other contraindications include the presence of tumors, infection, inflammatory arthropathies, osteochondritis dissecans, generalized or rheumatoid arthritis, and malalignment.[6,29] Relative contraindications are overweight patients, tobacco addiction, and patients who are noncompliant with the rehabilitation program.[6]

Fresh Osteochondral Allografts

Fresh osteochondral allografts are commonly used in salvage reconstruction of the knee. This includes posttraumatic defects of the tibial plateau, femoral condyle, and the patella.[11,17,20,24] They have also been used in the treatment of femoral or tibial epiphyseal tumors when much of the joint surface needs to be reconstructed.[30] Other defects such as patellofemoral chondrosis, osteonecrosis, osteochondritis dissecans, and some cases of unicompartmental tibiofemoral arthrosis can be treated using osteochondral allografts.[12,14,16] Allografts can also be used when other procedures such as microfracture, osteochondral autografting, or ACI have been unsuccessful.

Other contraindications include advanced multicompartment knee arthrosis, synovitis, inflammatory disease, and crystal-induced arthropathy. There have been mixed results when used in the treatment of steroid-induced osteonecrosis. The effects of other factors, such as smoking, altered bone metabolism, chronic corticosteroid use, and nonsteroidal anti-inflammatory medications (NSAIDs), on the outcome of fresh osteochondral grafts have not been fully determined.

Autologous Chondrocyte Implantation

Autologous chondrocyte implantation can be used either as a primary treatment modality or as a second line of treatment after arthroscopic debridement or microfracture has not produced adequate results.[31] As with the other techniques, patient age, body mass index, symptoms, sporting activity level, and willingness to follow the rehabilitation protocol should all be considered before performing this procedure.[32]

ACI can be used to treat larger lesions up to 16 cm^2.[2,33] Performance of ACI on opposing surfaces and in cases with more that 50% joint space narrowing is considered a contraindication.[31,34] Active inflammatory arthritis or infections are also considered contraindications. As in other treatment modalities, the cartilage treatment will most likely be unsuccessful unless biomechanical issues are addressed either concurrently or in a staged fashion.[35]

SURGICAL TECHNIQUE

Microfracture

The microfracture procedure starts with a standard arthroscopy of the knee (Fig. 40-1). A tourniquet is applied

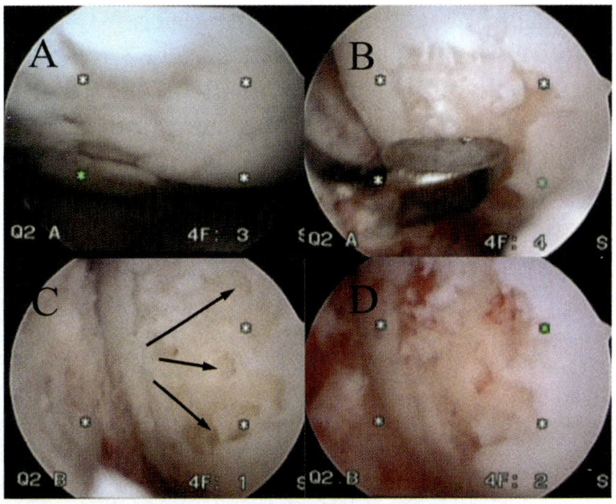

FIGURE 40-1. *Performance of microfracture of the femoral condyle. (**A**) The lesion is examined with exposed bone at the base and multiple stellate lacerations and flaps in the cartilage. (**B**) A curette is used to remove the remaining disorganized cartilage at the base of the defect and to establish clear shoulders to the defect. (**C**) The subchondral bone is penetrated with an awl forming multiple regularly spaced holes (arrows). (**D**) The water pressure in the joint is decreased, demonstrating the flow of marrow contents into the joint through the holes in the subchondral bone.*

to the knee, although it may or may not be inflated during the procedure. An examination under anesthesia is initially performed. Following the preparation and draping, a meticulous arthroscopic evaluation of all portions of the knee is performed through either a two-portal or three-portal technique. Any reparative techniques such as meniscal debridement, repair, or ligament reconstruction are performed initially since the bleeding from the microfracture site can limit visualization. Once the defect is localized, the exposed bone is debrided of all remaining unstable cartilage. Then a stable perpendicular edge of healthy cartilage around the defect is produced by debridement using a curette. This lesion helps to hold the marrow clot as it forms. The calcified cartilage cap is then removed using a curette. An arthroscopic awl is inserted into the joint and placed directly above the subchondral bone. A small mallet is then used to impact the handle of the awl and to insert the tip approximately 2 to 4 mm into the bone to create a 1- to 2-mm diameter hole in the subchondral bone plate. An awl is preferable to drilling to prevent thermal necrosis. The holes are made as close together as possible without fracturing into one another, typically 3 to 4 mm apart. The proper depth of the hole is achieved when removal of the awl leads to the egress of fat droplets entering the joint from the bone. When the arthroscopic irrigation fluid pressure is reduced, the marrow contents can be seen flowing into the joint.

Osteochondral Autograft

Osteochondral autografting can be performed as an open procedure or as an all-arthroscopic technique depending on the accessibility of the lesion (Fig. 40-2). The arthroscopic technique is performed under the same conditions as discussed above for microfracture. If a suitable lesion is identified, the lesion is sized and a donor plug is obtained from the periphery of the femoral trochlear cartilage or from the edge of the intercondylar notch, presumably from areas with minimal weight-bearing contact. It is critical to visualize the harvester (Fig. 40-3) on the donor site to be sure that the

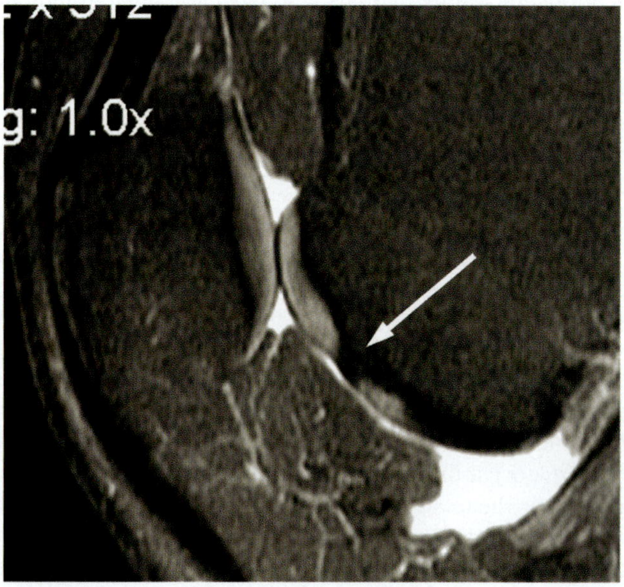

FIGURE 40-2. *One of the complications of marrow-stimulating techniques such as microfracture is filling of the defect with bone rather than cartilaginous tissue. This 36-year-old male had a microfracture of the trochlea with evidence of osseous filling of the defect (white arrow).*

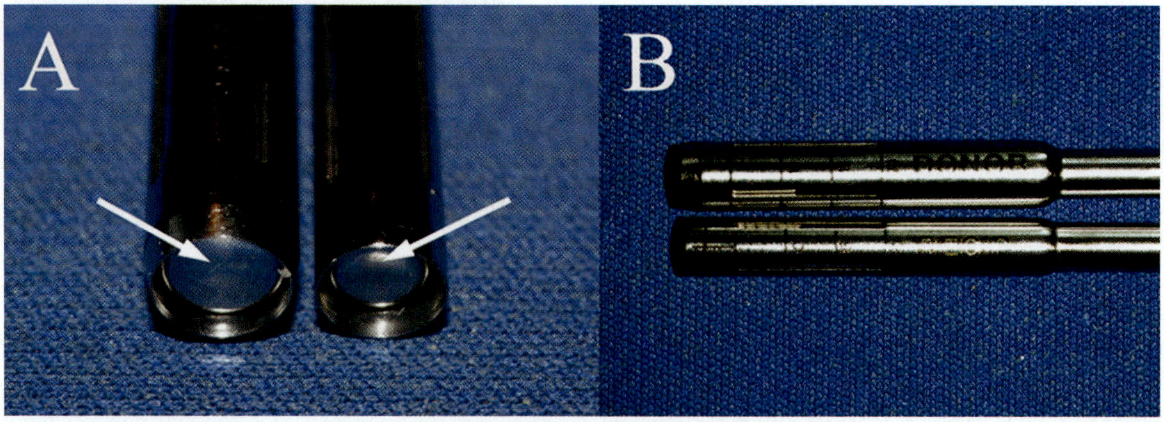

FIGURE 40-3. *Multiple kits are available for osteochondral autograft transplantation. In this set, the harvester for the donor and recipient site are shown. (**A**) The donor has a diameter of 7 mm and the recipient 6 mm to allow for press fit of the cores. The device also contains a metal plunger for controlled delivery of the cores (white arrows) (**B**) Top view of the coring devices.*

plug is harvested exactly perpendicular to its surface. Otherwise, the plug cartilage surface may be angled relative to the longitudinal dimension of the plug, leading to a proud plug with early failure. Once the plug is obtained, it is placed in normal saline until the recipient site is fully prepared. The recipient site is prepared in a similar fashion to the donor. Again, clear visualization of the entire coring device on the surface is critical in order to create a recipient site that is oriented exactly perpendicularly to the cartilage surface. The donor core can then be placed in an insertion tube and impacted into the recipient site such that it is exactly flush with the surrounding cartilage surface. In cases of multiple plugs placed together to form a mosaicplasty, we would recommend a mini-open arthrotomy for both the donor tissue harvest and the grafting itself. This can be done through one arthrotomy or through two small arthrotomies, depending on the locations of the donor and recipient sites. The optimal donor sites vary depending on the procedure. For an open procedure, the peripheries of both femoral condyles can be used as donor sites.

Resurfacing cartilage defects requires a graft length of 15 mm while osteochondral defects require a graft length of 25 mm. The grafts for osteochondral defect must be longer to account for bone loss. Once all the grafts are in place, the knee is put through a range of motion and varus and valgus stress in order to seat the grafts and to evaluate for any mechanical catching.

Fresh Osteochondral Allografts

Almost all osteochondral grafts in our practice are performed as open procedures. The areas of easiest access are the femoral condyles and patellofemoral joint. Fresh osteochondral allografting of the tibia is more challenging because of the position of the menisci. In our experience, the tibia is most efficiently resurfaced as a hybrid osteochondral hemiplateau and meniscal allograft. A tourniquet is applied to the thigh and the patient is placed supine. A leg holder device that allows stabilization of the knee between 70° and 100° of flexion is very helpful, particularly in accessing femoral condylar defects, which are often slightly posterior.

Before the first incision is made, the fresh graft is inspected to check the side and size match of the graft and the quality of the tissue. After inspection, it is chilled. Next a standard midline incision is made similar to that performed for total knee replacement. A retinacular incision is made, either medially or laterally, depending on the location of the lesion. The Hoffa's fat pad is incised, taking care to avoid disruption of the anterior horn of the meniscus. However, if needed, the meniscus can be incised anteriorly in a radial fashion at the anterior rim, leaving a 1-cm cuff for repair. This anterior horn can be repaired with nonabsorbable sutures at the end of the procedure.

The femoral condyles are a common area for cartilage lesions in the knee. Although hand-prepared and hand-sculpted grafts have been traditionally performed, current instrumentation for preparation of allograft cores has substantially improved the ease of the procedure. If a large surface needs to be covered, the grafts can be interlocked into one another in a figure-of-eight configuration. Unfortunately, this type of configuration requires a substantial amount of graft tissue and can lead to some degree of step-off at the interfaces between each graft segment (Fig. 40-4). The femoral condylar defects are often located slightly posteriorly and thus require deep flexion for perpendicular access. As the knee is flexed, the femoral condyle comes into better view. However, at the same time, the patellofemoral joint tends to tighten the space, occasionally requiring an extension of the arthrotomy into the vastus medialis muscle or lateralis muscles or quadriceps tendon. In occasional cases, the patella needs to be everted to fully access the femoral defect.

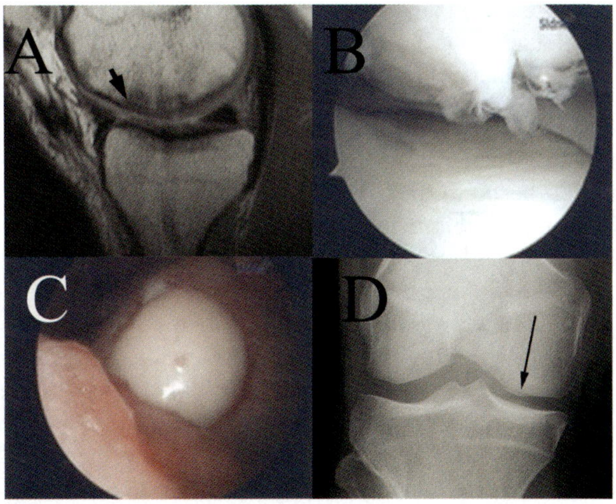

FIGURE 40-4. *Single osteochondral autograft transfer system procedure in a patient with a full-thickness defect of the medial femoral condyle noted on a sagittal MRI sequence (black arrowhead). **(B)** The lesion is noted to involve unstable flaps with extension to the subchondral bone. **(C)** One osteochondral autograft plug is inserted into the recipient site in the area of cartilage damage. **(D)** Postoperative radiograph demonstrates the osteochondral plug (black arrow).*

The specific technique for fresh osteochondral allografts using cylindrical grafts depends on the use of a cannulated system. A guide wire is driven into the center of the lesion, perpendicular to the articular surface. Next, the size of the graft is determined using sizing dowels. A reamer is used to remove the remaining articular cartilage and 5 to 15 mm of subchondral bone in the lesion. The guide pin is removed and depth measurements are made in the four quadrants of the recipient site using a ruler.

The corresponding recipient site is then located on the donor graft and either placed into a graft holder or held by hand by the surgical assistant. Next, a cylindrical coring guide is applied to the site and a coring reamer is driven in a perpendicular fashion to the surface and into the graft. At this point, the graft can be removed either by passing the coring reamer all the way through the graft or by undercutting the graft with an oscillating saw at an adequate depth. The graft is then removed and the depth measurements that were taken earlier in the recipient site at the four quadrants are used to mark along the base of the graft. An oscillating saw is used to cut a flat surface at the nonarticular end of the graft core. To remove all of the marrow elements from the graft, a high-pressure lavage system is used. The graft is inserted by hand and tamped into place so that it is flush with the adjacent cartilage. If the graft does not fit, it can be trimmed or the recipient site can be dilated. In cases of suboptimal press-fit stability or in the cases of multiple grafts, resorbable pins can be used to enhance the fixation. Next, a complete range of motion of the knee is performed to check for any catching of the articular surfaces or menisci on the graft.

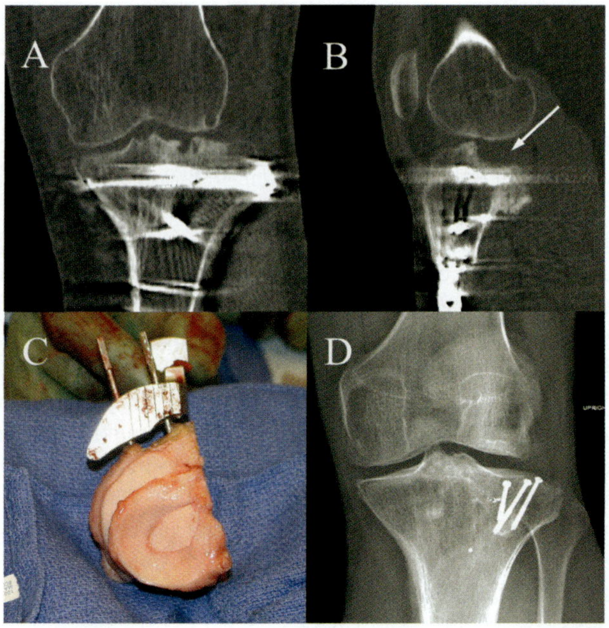

FIGURE 40-5. *A 32-year-old male sustained a bicondylar tibial plateau fracture treated with open reduction and internal fixation. The fracture healed with widening of the lateral plateau and the development of early posttraumatic arthritis. (**A**) A coronal CT scan shows the widening of the lateral tibia with formation of sclerosis and a void in the tibia. The adjacent area of the femur demonstrates some early degenerative changes including sclerosis and cyst formation. (**B**) A sagittal CT slice showing a large posterolateral defect in the tibia (white arrow). (**C**) The patient was treated with a fresh osteochondral allograft/meniscus transplant as well as a femoral allograft plug (not shown). The cutting jig from the unicompartment knee replacement set was used to cut the allograft tibial hemiplateau. (**D**) Three-year postoperative anteroposterior knee radiograph demonstrating normal joint space and a pain-free knee. The patient has returned to high-level sports including snowboarding.*

Tibial plateau allografting uses similar techniques to those used in unicompartmental knee arthroplasty (UKA) and can be performed through an arthrotomy (Fig. 40-5). The cruciate ligament attachments as well as the meniscal attachments should be protected. As stated previously, the anterior horn of the meniscus can be cut radially and secondarily repaired at the end of the procedure. A very limited horizontal cut is made using any of the commercially available UKA tibial cutting guides. Our preference is to take a cut from the tibia that matches the native tibial slope, perpendicular to the mechanical axis of the tibia, and approximately 5 to 6 mm in minimal thickness. The graft is measured and cut with a cutting jig from the UKA system after checking the cut angle with a commercially available stylus. The meniscal attachments of the graft are maintained. Once the graft is cut, its dimensions are measured and it is irrigated. The knee is flexed and the compartment is opened using rotational and coronal manipulation of the leg. The graft is gently placed under the femoral condyle with great care and the knee is brought through a range of motion. With fluoroscopy, the graft is visualized for the appropriate position, restoration of the joint line, slope, and proper orientation relative to the femoral condyle. The graft is then fixed using interfragmentary screw fixation from the submeniscal articular line at the midcoronal position to the anterior position. The meniscus is then repaired using standard suturing techniques.

Trochlear lesions are prepared as allograft cores in a similar manner to the femoral condyles. However, the trochlea is more challenging due to its concave curvature in the coronal plane and the convex curvature in the sagittal plane. This makes matching the recipient sites and donor grafts difficult. The surgeon has to be careful to match the anatomic location and the angle of approach.

The patella can be resurfaced entirely using an osteochondral allograft (Fig. 40-6). In this case, a technique similar to arthroplasty resurfacing is used. The thickness of the patella is measured and the resection of the articular surface is done leaving at least 12 to 15 mm of patellar bone. The graft is resected using a similar technique. A thickness of approximately 3 to 4 mm in the medial and lateral facets should be obtained. Next, the graft is placed in the correct position and rotation and tracking are checked. Interfragmentary cannulated screws are normally used for patellar fixation. The screws should be placed on the anterior surface of the patella into the median ridge of the graft, stopping short of the articular cartilage of the graft. Lateral retinacular lengthening or realignment procedures on the extensor mechanism can be concurrently performed. Patellar lesions that are smaller in size can be treated with cylindrical grafts like those used for the femoral condyle as discussed previously.

Autologous Chondrocyte Implantation

Autologous chondrocyte implantation is currently implemented as a two-stage procedure, with the first stage consisting of a cartilage tissue harvest. In the United States, the cartilage tissue is placed in a sterile container containing tissue culture medium and mailed to a commercial laboratory facility where the tissue is treated with a series of steps to remove the chondrocytes from the matrix and to expand their numbers. The second stage of the procedure is an open procedure analogous to the exposure needed for a fresh osteochondral allograft as stated above. The defect is prepared by removing all unhealthy cartilage down to healthy edges with stable attachment to the subchondral bone. Any remaining cartilage from the base of the defect is removed. It is also critical to avoid any bleeding bone in the base of the defect because this may compromise the chondrocyte population and introduce bone marrow-derived cells into the cavity. Once the defect is fully prepared, the tourniquet is deflated to confirm the absence of any such bleeding. In the recent past, an extension of the approach or a separate arthrotomy would be required to harvest a periosteal patch. The use of periosteal patches has fallen out of favor due to the associated need for secondary or longer primary incisions as well as the increased risk of graft hypertrophy seen with the periosteal patches. Currently, a bovine collagen membrane is commonly used. Regardless of the membrane selected, the key principle is the same. A water-tight space is created into which the mature chondrocytes are injected. A few special techniques are helpful in accurately determining the size and shape of the defect. A template can be created from the foil available in many suture packages. This template is used to achieve the correct size and shape. It is recommended to make the flap bigger than the template by 2 mm circumferentially. The membrane is then cut accordingly. If an autogenous periosteal patch is used, it can be obtained from the proximal tibia or more rarely from the edges of the femoral condyles. The overlaying fat and fibrous tissue should be removed. Next, an incision is made down to the bone and with a sharp periosteal elevator; the flap is then carefully elevated, taking care to avoid any punctures. The flap must be kept moist with normal saline at all times.[33]

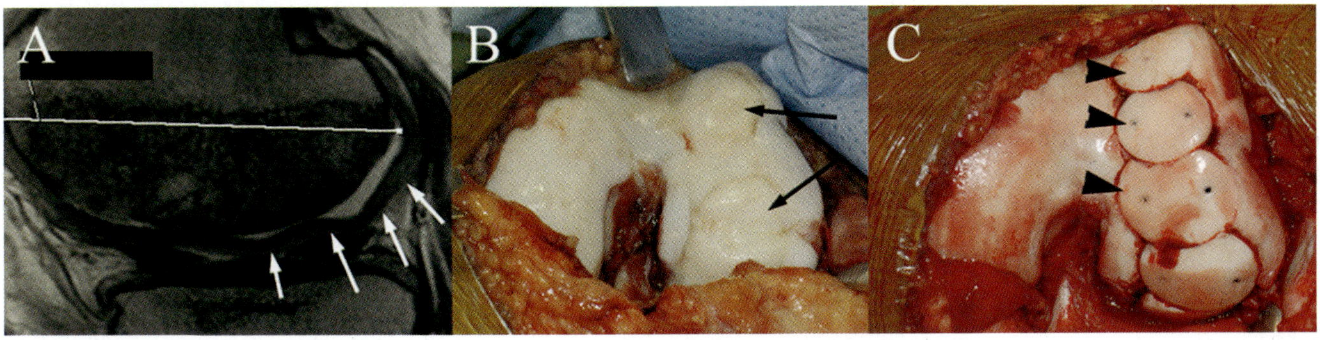

FIGURE 40-6. *A 19-year-old male, with a history of leukemia treated with chemotherapy including prednisone, developed severe bilateral knee pain and avascular necrosis. (**A**) In this case, the cartilage layer (white arrows) has completely peeled off the necrotic subchondral bone as shown in a sagittal MRI cut. (**B**) The intraoperative view shows the complete separation of the cartilage from bone (black arrows). (**C**) Multiple interlocked fresh osteochondral allografts (black arrowheads) were used to resurface the entire lateral femoral condyle.*

The defect area should be checked again and any bleeding should be controlled. A drop of fibrin glue and compression with a fingertip for 60 seconds typically is effective in controlling such bleeding. The flap is then placed over the defect and one suture is placed at each corner using 6-0 Vicryl resorbable suture. It is beneficial to mark the suture edges with a marking pen to more clearly see this small-diameter suture. Additional sutures are added at intervals of 3 to 5 mm. A superior opening should be left for the injection of the chondrocytes. Fibrin glue is then used to seal the periosteal flap between sutures.[33]

Saline solution is then injected into the pocket created over the defect using a syringe and soft catheter. It should be injected slowly, keeping an eye out for any leakage around the flap. The saline solution is suctioned away and air is injected so the pocket stays open. The chondrocytes are then implanted using a syringe and soft catheter. The injection should be performed on withdrawal, starting distally, so as to evenly distribute the chondrocytes. The opening is then closed with one to two additional sutures and sealed with fibrin glue.[33]

POSTOPERATIVE MANAGEMENT AND REHABILITATION

General Postoperative and Rehabilitation Principles

Generally, the mechanical tolerance of various types of repair tissue during their maturation is not known. As a result, our philosophy is to minimize any stresses during the first 4 to 6 weeks after cartilage repair while emphasizing the beneficial aspects of passive motion on cartilage nutrition and metabolism during this period. As such, our postoperative regimens are consistent across essentially all repair types. Microfracture and ACI are particularly at risk of damage because they depend on tissue maturation in situ. Osteochondral autograft and allografts are more durable because they represent mature tissue at the time of implantation.

Microfracture and Autologous Chondrocyte Implantation

The postoperative rehabilitation program depends on the anatomic location of the defect as well as the size. The goal is to promote the ideal environment for the mesenchymal progenitor cells from the marrow to differentiate into the chondrocyte lineage. The rehabilitation protocol for patients with lesions on weight-bearing surfaces of the femoral condyles involves using a continuous passive motion (CPM) machine starting in the recovery room.[2,36]

The beginning range of motion is 0° to 70° and is increased by 10° to 20° of flexion per day until the full range of motion is achieved. Classically, the continuous passive motion machine is utilized between 6 and 8 hours every 24 hours. Cold therapy also can be used to control both pain and inflammation for 1 to 7 days postoperatively.[27]

For 6 weeks, the patient uses crutches with no weight bearing. Immediately after the surgery, isometric exercises in a position that does not load the defect are instituted. At 6 weeks after the surgery, we initiate a gradual increase in weight bearing at 30 lb and gradually increasing by 15 lb every 2 days. The patient can use a household scale to gauge the weight that he or she is placing on the leg. We initiate stationary cycling exercises no sooner than 6 weeks, since in some cases, patients may not understand the torque setting on the bicycle and may damage the repair tissue. At 6 weeks after the surgery, gentle exercises are instituted with resistance bands. Free or machine weights on the affected joint are not permitted before 16 weeks after the surgery.

Unlike the rehabilitation for patients with lesions on the femoral condyles, patients with patellofemoral lesions must use a range-of-motion brace set at 0° to 20° for at least 8 weeks. The brace should be worn at all times except during passive motion activities. Much like patients with lesions on the femoral condyles, a CPM machine is used immediately, along with cold therapy. We typically limit weight bearing to 30 lb for 3 to 4 weeks and then to weight bearing as tolerated while wearing the range-of-motion brace locked at 0° to 20°. The brace protects the newly formed marrow clot by preventing excessive shear during its maturation. The knee brace range of motion is unlocked at 6 weeks and the patient is gradually weaned from it over the ensuing 2 to 3 weeks. We institute isometric exercises in full extension immediately along with the use of CPM. Once the brace is removed, strength training commences, initially with resistance bands and progressing to free and machine weights starting 16 weeks after the surgery. Regardless of the area treated, we do not recommend that athletes return to sports that involve quick changes in direction or jumping until at least 4 to 6 months from surgery.

Osteochondral Autografts and Allografts

For both osteochondral allografts and autografts, we prefer to protect weight bearing for a minimum of 6 weeks. Although a graft may appear stable at surgery, the host–graft interface may soften during the early healing period, potentially putting the graft at risk for subsidence during this period of time. This is particularly true for the allografts, which are at risk for an immune reaction at the bone interface and are typically larger than autografts. Our protocol is similar on the patellofemoral grafts to that used for microfracture and ACI.

Although radiographs are inexpensive and readily available, MRI is more detailed and informative about the status of the repair tissue. MRI can identify any graft anomalies, surface degradation, poor integration, synovial effusion, or bone edema.

Patients with tibial or bipolar grafts use a range-of-motion brace to control varus and valgus stress. The tibial graft with a meniscal allograft is usually limited to 90° of flexion for the first 6 weeks. Then weight bearing is increased incrementally between the 2nd and 3rd month. When the patient progresses to full weight bearing, a cane or crutch is generally used. Between the 3rd and 4th month, normal gait is typically established. Generally patients can return to sports no earlier than 6 months after the surgery and only when joint rehabilitation is complete and radiographs have been obtained showing graft–host healing.

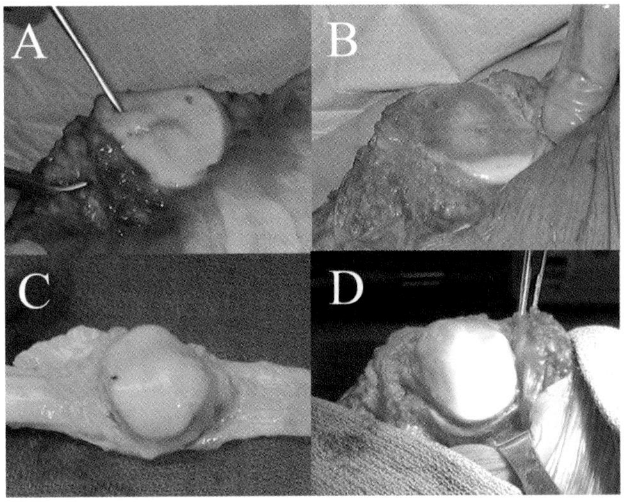

FIGURE 40-7. *A 40-year-old male with anterior knee pain and a documented patellar lesion in spite of an otherwise healthy knee. (**A**) Intraoperative view shows a full-thickness cartilage defect involving a substantial portion of the patella. (**B**) The patellar surface is cut in a fashion similar to total knee replacement (a slightly thicker cut than total knee replacement is required due to the relative thickness of the patellar allograft). (**C**) The patellar allograft is prepared in a similar fashion taking great care to control the patellar surface during the cut. (**D**) The patellar allograft is fixed to the patella using cannulated screws directed from anterior to posterior on the patella, stopping short of the subchondral bone of the patella.*

COMPLICATIONS

Microfracture

During the postoperative period, most patients progress with little difficulty, although some may have mild transient pain. Patients may also experience a grating or gritty sensation of the joint when normal weight bearing and range-of-motion activities commence. This is due to the small changes in the articular surface and it usually resolves itself in a few days or weeks.[27]

Patients may notice catching or locking in occasional cases. Steadman et al have observed that this symptom usually vanishes within 3 months. If this catching or locking is painful, one can consider limiting weight bearing and avoiding the joint angle in which the locking or catching occurs.[27] Another late complication that can occur after microfracture is recurrent effusion, which usually develops 6 to 8 weeks after the surgery, or when weight-bearing activities are starting. This effusion is usually painless and resolves itself within a couple of weeks of the onset. Sometimes this can be resolved with a second arthroscopy.[27] We have occasionally noted ossification of the microfracture defect with persistent pain (Fig. 40-7). Typically, this can best be assessed by MRI. If it does occur, other forms of cartilage restoration, such as fresh osteochondral allografting or autografting, can be considered.

Osteochondral Autografts

Complications with osteochondral autografts include fracture of the graft, implantation in an excessively prominent or deep position, hemarthrosis, and femoropatellar pain from the donor sites, and cartilage degeneration and pain from the treated defect. Graft fracture can occur from an excessively short graft or with excessively forceful impaction. Use of an oversized impactor can minimize the risk of implanting the grafts too deep. Additionally, should this occur, it is best to try to elevate the graft and bone graft beneath it and to reinsert it. If the graft will not fully seat, it is best to deepen the recipient site slightly so that it can be fully engaged to the adjacent bone and flush with the surface. Hemarthrosis can occasionally occur and would require standard treatment of knee aspiration and application of a knee wrap.[6,35]

Fresh Osteochondral Allografts

Early complications are rare and include effusion, as well as delayed or nonunion. Effusion can signify either overuse or an immune-mediated synovitis. Delayed unions or nonunions can cause discomfort and can be investigated on plain radiographs. Larger grafts are more likely to have a delayed union since the host–graft healing may take longer. Rarely, a delayed union or nonunion may require repeat surgery. Grafts that fail to integrate may lead to a sudden onset of increased pain, effusion, or crepitance. Should this occur, allograft revision or conversion to arthroplasty may be required.

Late failures of allografts can be due to lack of revascularization and gradual collapse and fragmentation of the graft. This can be diagnosed by plain radiographs, MRI, and, occasionally, arthroscopic evaluation. These failed allografts can be treated with observation if the symptoms are minimal, with the goal of avoiding global joint degeneration. Debridement can be helpful in refractory cases.[14,17] One of the most common sources of late failure is the onset of either localized or global knee osteoarthritis. In limited lesions, revision allografting appears to have an equivalent success rate as primary allografting. However, in cases in which extensive joint disease is observed, prosthetic arthroplasty is the best option.

Autologous Chondrocyte Implantation

A number of complications have been reported related to the periosteal flap used in ACI. The most common complication is hypertrophy, presumably due to friction. This is characterized by thickening and overgrowth onto the surrounding cartilage, causing catching, clicking, or crepitation in the knee. This usually occurs within the first 3 to 9 months after surgery and is initially treated by changing the rehabilitation program. If the symptoms remain, arthroscopy is performed and the flap is either shaved or removed entirely.[33]

Another potential problem with the flap is that it can delaminate in its entirety. If the flap is only partially detached, the detached piece is either debrided or excised. If the periosteal flap is completely loose, it is removed. Range-of-motion exercises, such as low resistance cycling, should be continued for the next 6 to 8 weeks to help stimulate the repair tissue to fill in the defect.[33] Graft delamination is a serious complication that occurs when the repair tissue detaches from the surrounding cartilage or underlying subchondral bone. If the graft delamination is less than 10 mm, it should be debrided. If the bone is visible, one should consider either microfracture, revision ACI, or osteochondral grafting for the uncovered portion of the defect.

Arthrofibrosis has been reported and is a particularly higher risk in cases with concurrent meniscal repair or allografting, ligament reconstruction, or inadequate rehabilitation. Standard treatments include physical therapy, dynamic bracing, and arthroscopic lysis of adhesions and knee manipulation.

OUTCOMES AND CASE EXAMPLES

Microfracture

In 2003, Steadman et al reported results from a study on patients with only traumatic chondral defects debrided and then treated with microfracture, with no associated ligament or meniscus pathology.[37] The patients were 45 years old or younger and were followed up at an average of 11 years. Significant improvement was seen on the Lysholm and Tegner scales. At the 7-year time point, 80% of patients rated themselves as "improved." The study was limited in that it was performed by the developer of the technique, a variety of defect sizes and locations were included, and, most important, there was no control group.

Knutsen et al performed a study comparing ACI to microfracture in patients with a single symptomatic cartilage defect on the femoral condyle in a stable knee. The study consisted of a total of 80 patients, with 40 undergoing ACI and 40 undergoing microfracture. At 5-year follow-up, the results of microfracture were equivalent to those of ACI, with a total of 77% survivorship for both techniques.[38] The main deficiency of the study was a small sample size and potentially inadequate power to compare the two techniques.

Osteochondral Autograft

In 2008, Hangody et al published results of a series of 789 femoral condyle defects, 31 tibial defects, and 147 patellofemoral defects.[39] Of these patients, 81% had an associated procedure (meniscal, ligamental, or bone). The follow-up was a maximum of 15 years. For femoral condyle mosaicplasty, 92% were considered good or very good, 87% for the tibia, and 74% for the patellofemoral joint. In this study, 98 second-look biopsies were performed, with 83% of the specimens demonstrating a smooth surface and hyaline or fibrocartilaginous histology.

Promising results were also obtained in a study performed by Chow et al, who reported on a series of 30 patients with an average follow-up of 45 months after arthroscopic osteochondral autografting. They had good to excellent results in 83%, with 87% reporting a normal or nearly normal knee.[40]

Fresh Osteochondral Allografts

Ghazavi et al reported on 126 knees with posttraumatic osteochondral defects treated with fresh osteochondral allografting.[17] The average follow-up was 7.5 years with a range of 2 to 20 years. There were 123 patients and in 68 an osteotomy was performed as part of the procedure. Using the Hospital for Special Surgery Knee Scoring System, 86% of the grafts were successful and 14% were failures. The survivorship was 95% at 5 years, 71% at 10 years, and 66% at 20 years. The failures in this study occurred in patients who were over 50 years old and had bipolar defects or malaligned knees and involved workers' compensation cases.

Shasha et al published a study of fresh tibial osteochondral allografts used for treating failed tibial plateau fractures.[24] The average age of the 65 patients was 42.8 years. The patients each had a defect in their proximal tibia of at least 1 cm in depth and 3 cm in diameter. With a mean average follow-up of 12 years, 44 had intact grafts and 21 had been converted to total knee replacement.

Traditionally, osteochondral allografts have been viewed as one of the optimal treatments for large, symptomatic osteochondritis dissecans lesions. Emmerson et al reported on 66 knees with this treatment.[41] The lesions were a mean 7.5 cm^2. Good to excellent results were reported in 72% at a mean follow-up of 7.7 years (minimum 2 years). Weaknesses of the study included the lack of a control group as well as the use of a nonvalidated scoring system for the analysis.

Fresh osteochondral allografts have been used in the patellofemoral joint to treat patellar and trochlear lesions, avascular necrosis, and patellofemoral arthrosis due to chronic malalignment. Jamali et al evaluated 20 knees that underwent fresh osteochondral allografting restricted to the patellofemoral joint.[42] The average follow-up was 94 months and five knees required major revision surgery such as total joint arthroplasty or revision osteochondral allografting. The authors used the nonvalidated Postel and D'Aubigné 18-point score to evaluate the results. The average score increased from 11.7 (range, 7–15) preoperatively to 16.3 (range, 12–18) at the latest follow-up. There were a total of 12 knees that were not revised and had available radiographs. Four of them had no patellofemoral osteoarthritis and six had mild patellofemoral arthritis at the latest follow-up.

Autologous Chondrocyte Implantation

Peterson et al published a report on the first 101 cases treated with ACI in their center. The best results were seen in isolated femoral condylar lesions (92% good/excellent) and the worst in the patella (67% good/excellent). Seven cases were associated with graft failure with the majority occurring at the beginning of the learning curve. Increased hyaline histological appearance was correlated with a better clinical result in a subgroup of 37 cases with an available specimen.

The durability of the technique was highlighted in a case series on 45 competitive and recreational soccer players.[43] The average follow-up was 41 months. Seventy-two percent of the players had a good to excellent result. Thirty-three percent returned to soccer, including 83% of competitive-level players and 16% of recreational players. Concomitant procedures such as osteotomies and ligament reconstruction did not affect the chance of return to soccer.

Zaslav et al performed a multicenter cohort study looking at the effectiveness of ACI in 154 knees after prior treatments had failed.[44] On average, the ACI procedure was performed 31 months after the initial cartilage treatment. The majority of the initial procedures were debridements or marrow-stimulating procedures. One hundred twenty-six patients completed the study protocol at 48-month follow-up. Of these, 76% were considered successes based on sustained improvement on a number of scales. Surprisingly, 49% of patients required subsequent surgeries, most commonly arthroscopic debridements.

PEARLS AND PITFALLS

In spite of the variety of cartilage restoration techniques currently available and many more that are being developed, the basic principles are relatively straightforward. The objectives are to decrease pain, improve function, and potentially improve the longevity of the native joint. As such, establishing a smooth surface covered with hyaline or hyaline-like cartilage tissue is vital. Each of the procedures discussed has advantages and disadvantages. Thus the surgeon can select each procedure based on practicality, the overall condition of the joint, the size and location of the lesion, and other biomechanical factors such as malalignment. Across all types of cartilage repair, protecting the repair tissue with appropriate osteotomies is critical to achieving long-term success. In some cases, correction of malalignment may be responsible for the great majority of pain relief and joint space restoration (Fig. 40-8). We are at the beginning of a new generation of less invasive cartilage repair techniques that promise to provide us with many more options for treating this challenging disease.

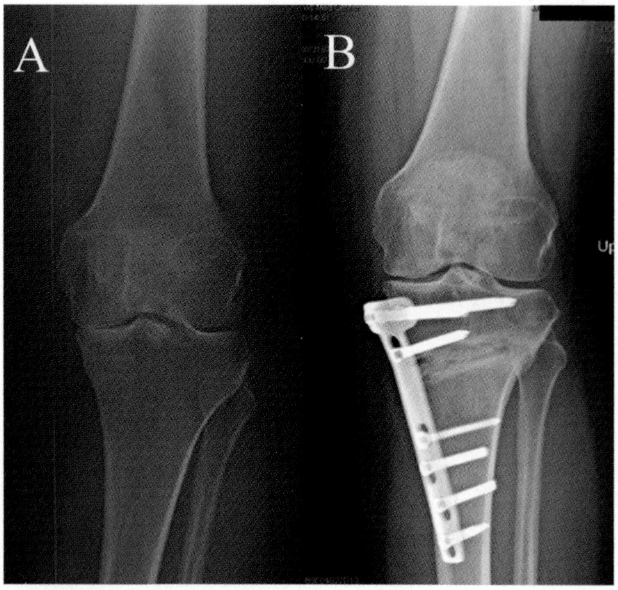

FIGURE 40-8. *The correction of malalignment is critical to establishing improved joint health and normalizing loads across the joint. (**A**) This 48-year-old female with genu varum presented with end-stage osteoarthritis involving the medial compartment of the knee. She was treated with microfracture combined with a medial tibial valgus opening-wedge osteotomy. (**B**) At 3 years, she is pain free with standing radiographs that demonstrate restoration of her medial joint space.*

REFERENCES

1. D'Anchise R, Manta N, Prospero E, et al. Autologous implantation of chondrocytes on a solid collagen scaffold: clinical and histological outcomes after two years of followup. *J Orthop Traumatol.* 2005;6:36-43.
2. Blevins FT, Steadman JR, Rodrigo JJ, et al. Treatment of articular cartilage defects in athletes: an analysis of functional outcome and lesion appearance. *Orthopedics.* 1998;21(7):761-767; discussion 767-768.
3. Grande DA, Pitman MI, Peterson L, et al. The repair of experimentally produced defects in rabbit articular cartilage by autologous chondrocyte transplantation. *J Orthop Res.* 1989;7(2):208-218.
4. Outerbridge HK, Outerbridge AR, Outerbridge RE. The use of a lateral patellar autologous graft for the repair of a large osteochondral defect in the knee. *J Bone Joint Surg Am.* 1995;77(1):65-72.
5. Yamashita F, Sakakida K, Suzu F, et al. The transplantation of an autogeneic osteochondral fragment for osteochondritis dissecans of the knee. *Clin Orthop Relat Res.* 1985;201:43-50.
6. Robert H. Chondral repair of the knee joint using mosaicplasty. *Orthop Traumatol Surg Res.* 2011; 97(4):418-429.
7. Matsusue Y, Yamamuro T, Hama H. Arthroscopic multiple osteochondral transplantation to the chondral defect in the knee associated with anterior cruciate ligament disruption. *Arthroscopy.* 1993; 9(3):318-321.
8. Hangody L, Kish G, Karpati Z, et al. Arthroscopic autogenous osteochondral mosaicplasty for the treatment of femoral condylar articular defects. A preliminary report. *Knee Surg Sports Traumatol Arthrosc.* 1997;5(4):262-267.
9. Lexer E. Substitution of whole or half joints from freshly amputated extremities by free-plastic operation. *Surg Gynecol Obstet.* 1908;6:601-607.
10. Lexer E. Joint transplantations and arthroplasty. *Surg Gynecol Obstet.* 1925;40:782-802.
11. Aubin PP, Cheah HK, Davis AM, et al. Long-term followup of fresh femoral osteochondral allografts for posttraumatic knee defects. *Clin Orthop Relat Res.* 2001;391(suppl):S318-327.
12. Bayne O, Langer F, Pritzker KP, et al. Osteochondral allografts in the treatment of osteonecrosis of the knee. *Orthop Clin North Am.* 1985;16(4):727-740.
13. Berlet GC, Mascia A, Miniaci A. Treatment of unstable osteochondritis dissecans lesions of the knee using autogenous osteochondral grafts (mosaicplasty). *Arthroscopy.* 1999;15(3):312-316.
14. Bugbee W. Fresh osteochondral allografts. *Semin Arthroplasty.* 2000;11(4):1-7.
15. Ganel A, Israeli A, Horoszowski H, et al. Osteochondral graft in the treatment of osteonecrosis of the femoral condyle. *J Am Geriatr Soc.* 1981;29(4):186-188.
16. Garrett JC. Fresh osteochondral allografts for treatment of articular defects in osteochondritis dissecans of the lateral femoral condyle in adults. *Clin Orthop Relat Res.* 1994;303:33-37.
17. Ghazavi MT, Pritzker KP, Davis AM, et al. Fresh osteochondral allografts for post-traumatic osteochondral defects of the knee. *J Bone Joint Surg Br.* 1997;79(6):1008-1013.
18. Johnson DL, Warner JJ. Osteochondritis dissecans of the humeral head: treatment with a matched osteochondral allograft. *J Shoulder Elbow Surg.* 1997;6(2): 160-163.

19. Kim CW, Jamali A, Tontz W Jr, et al. Treatment of post-traumatic ankle arthrosis with bipolar tibiotalar osteochondral shell allografts. *Foot Ankle Int.* 2002; 23(12):1091-1102.
20. Locht RC, Gross AE, Langer F. Late osteochondral allograft resurfacing for tibial plateau fractures. *J Bone Joint Surg Am.* 1984;66(3):328-335.
21. Marco F, Lopez-Oliva F, Fernandez Fernandez-Arroyo JM, et al. Osteochondral allografts for osteochondritis dissecans and osteonecrosis of the femoral condyles. *Int Orthop.* 1993;17(2):104-108.
22. Meyers MH. The treatment of osteonecrosis of the hip with fresh osteochondral allografts and with the muscle pedicle graft technique. *Clin Orthop Relat Res.* 1978;130:202-209.
23. Meyers MH, Jones RE, Bucholz RW, et al. Fresh autogenous grafts and osteochondral allografts for the treatment of segmental collapse in osteonecrosis of the hip. *Clin Orthop Relat Res.* 1983;174:107-112.
24. Shasha N, Krywulak S, Backstein D, et al. Long-term follow-up of fresh tibial osteochondral allografts for failed tibial plateau fractures. *J Bone Joint Surg Am* 2003;85(suppl 2):33-39.
25. Mensch JS, Amstutz HC. Knee morphology as a guide to knee replacement. *Clin Orthop Relat Res.* 1975;112:231-241.
26. Rodrigo JJ, Steadman JR, Silliman JF. Improvement of full-thickness chondral defect healing in the human knee after debridement and microfracture using continuous passive motion. *Am J Knee Surg.* 1994;7: 109-116.
27. Steadman JR, Rodkey WG, Rodrigo JJ. Microfracture: surgical technique and rehabilitation to treat chondral defects. *Clin Orthop Relat Res.* 2001;391 (suppl):S362-369.
28. Hangody L, Kish G, Karpati Z, et al. Mosaicplasty for the treatment of articular cartilage defects: application in clinical practice. *Orthopedics.* 1998; 21(7):751-756.
29. Hangody L, Feczko P, Bartha L, et al. Mosaicplasty for the treatment of articular defects of the knee and ankle. *Clin Orthop Relat Res.* 2001;391(suppl):S328-336.
30. Bell RS, Davis A, Allan DG, et al. Fresh osteochondral allografts for advanced giant cell tumors at the knee. *J Arthroplasty.* 1994;9(6):603-609.
31. King PJ, Bryant T, Minas T. Autologous chondrocyte implantation for chondral defects of the knee: indications and technique. *J Knee Surg.* 2002;15(3): 177-184.
32. Cole BJ, Pascual-Garrido C, Grumet RC. Surgical management of articular cartilage defects in the knee. *J Bone Joint Surg Am.* 2009;91(7):1778-1790.
33. Peterson L. Technique of autologous chondrocyte transplantation. *Tech Knee Surg.* 2002;1(1):2–12.
34. Jones DG, Peterson L. Autologous chondrocyte implantation. *J Bone Joint Surg Am.* 2006;88(11): 2502-2520.
35. Batty L, Dance S, Bajaj S, et al. Autologous chondrocyte implantation: an overview of technique and outcomes. *ANZ J Surg.* 2011;81(1-2):18-25.
36. Ohkoshi Y, Ohkoshi M, Nagasaki S, et al. The effect of cryotherapy on intraarticular temperature and postoperative care after anterior cruciate ligament reconstruction. *Am J Sports Med.* 1999;27(3):357-362.
37. Steadman JR, Briggs KK, Rodrigo JJ, et al. Outcomes of microfracture for traumatic chondral defects of the knee: average 11-year follow-up. *Arthroscopy.* 2003; 19(5):477-484.
38. Knutsen G, Drogset JO, Engebretsen L, et al. A randomized trial comparing autologous chondrocyte implantation with microfracture. Findings at five years. *J Bone Joint Surg Am.* 2007;89(10):2105-2112.
39. Hangody L, Vasarhelyi G, Hangody LR, et al. Autologous osteochondral grafting—technique and long-term results. *Injury.* 2008;39(suppl 1):S32-39.
40. Chow JC, Hantes ME, Houle JB, et al. Arthroscopic autogenous osteochondral transplantation for treating knee cartilage defects: a 2- to 5-year follow-up study. *Arthroscopy.* 2004;20(7):681-690.
41. Emmerson BC, Gortz S, Jamali AA, et al. Fresh osteochondral allografting in the treatment of osteochondritis dissecans of the femoral condyle. *Am J Sports Med.* 2007;35(6):907-914.
42. Jamali AA, Emmerson BC, Chung C, et al. Fresh osteochondral allografts: results in the patellofemoral joint. *Clin Orthop Relat Res.* 2005;437:176-185.
43. Mithofer K, Peterson L, Mandelbaum BR, et al. Articular cartilage repair in soccer players with autologous chondrocyte transplantation: functional outcome and return to competition. *Am J Sports Med.* 2005;33(11):1639-1646.
44. Zaslav K, Cole B, Brewster R, et al. A prospective study of autologous chondrocyte implantation in patients with failed prior treatment for articular cartilage defect of the knee: results of the Study of the Treatment of Articular Repair (STAR) clinical trial. *Am J Sports Med.* 2009;37(1):42-55.

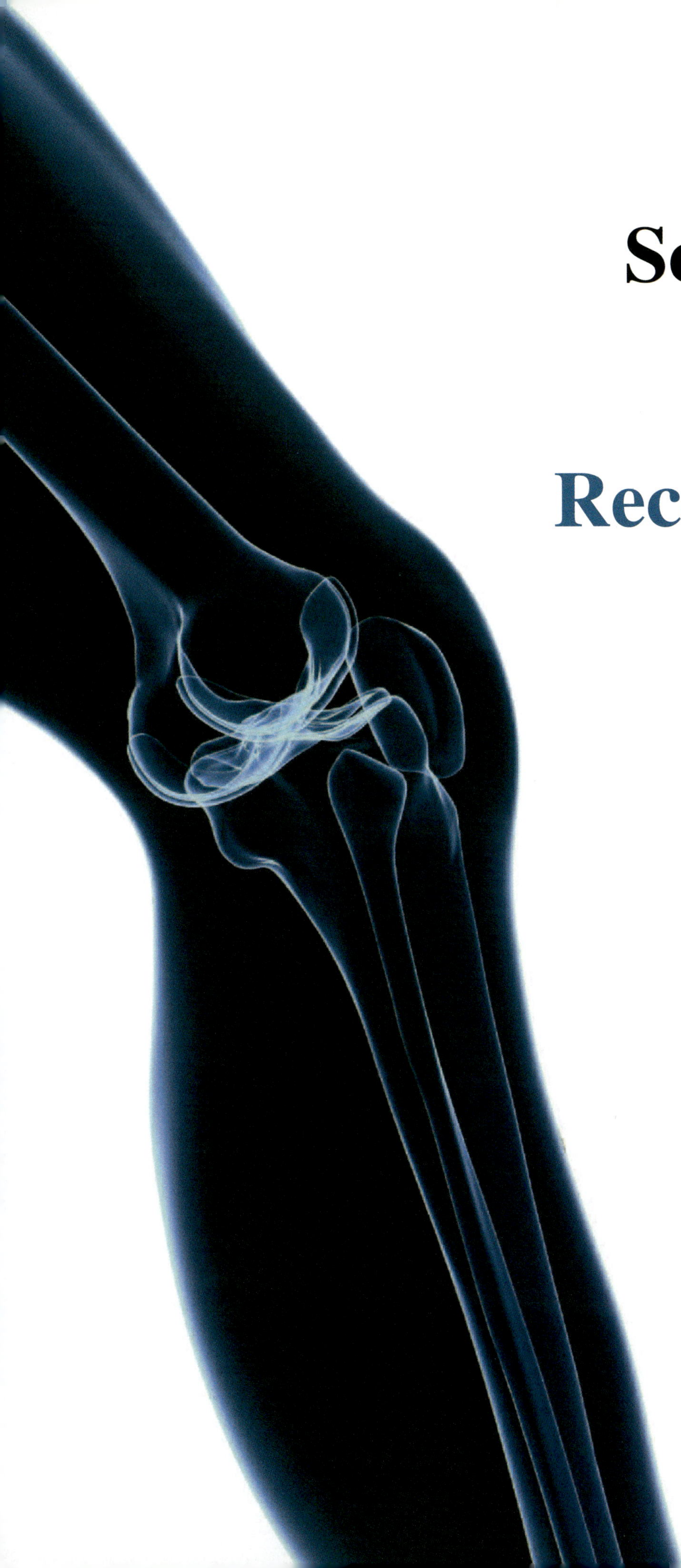

Section Four

Knee Reconstruction

41 Preoperative Clinical Evaluation

Nicholas J. Farber, Antonia F. Chen, and Brian A. Klatt

Total knee arthroplasty (TKA) is an elective procedure to replace the knee for various diseases including osteoarthritis, avascular necrosis, and posttraumatic arthritis. Outcomes following TKA are excellent and patients report substantial relief and functional improvement after surgery. A careful preoperative clinical evaluation should be performed to ensure that a TKA is clearly indicated. The clinical exam and radiographs are used by the surgeon to form a plan to correct deformities and balance the reconstructed knee. The patient should also be thoroughly screened for contraindications to TKA and assessed for risk factors that increase the risk of postoperative complications. Components of the preoperative evaluation include a history, physical examination, radiographic evaluation, and clinical testing.

HISTORY

A thorough history should be conducted to ascertain whether total knee arthroplasty is indeed indicated for the patient, identify comorbidities that would adversely affect surgery, and collect other relevant information to better prepare the clinician for the patient's surgery. Patients who are being considered for total knee replacement should be assessed for pain, stiffness, physical function, and overall disability. Certain aspects of the patient's pain should also be characterized. The onset should be described as either gradual or acute. Acute pain from a recent trauma may be indicative of a ligamentous or meniscal injury. Acute pain from activity modification suggests tendinitis or bursitis. Chronic pain is more indicative of arthritis or posttraumatic arthritis if there is a history of previous trauma.

The location of the pain should be carefully ascertained, because location is suggestive of different pathologies, each of which has different treatment plans that may or may not include TKA. Anterior knee pain is indicative of patellofemoral issues, including conditions such as patellar subluxation, prepatellar bursitis, patellar tendinitis, quad tendinitis, chondromalacia patellae, or patellofemoral arthritis. Medial pain may suggest medial meniscus tear, medial collateral ligament injury, pes bursitis, medial compartment osteonecrosis, or medial compartment arthritis. Lateral pain suggests lateral meniscus tears, lateral collateral ligament injury, iliotibial band tendinitis, or lateral compartment arthritis. Pain in the posterior portion of the knee may come from a variety of sources, including a Baker's cyst secondary to osteoarthritis, hamstring tendinitis, a gastrocnemius tear, or a meniscal root tear (Fig. 41-1).

The severity of the pain should be evaluated on a scale from 0 to 10, with 0 being no pain and 10 being the worst pain a patient has experienced. The visual analog scale (VAS) is often used to give a visual face to the amount of pain a patient is experiencing. This gives the historian an idea of how much the pain is affecting the life of the patient.

The timing of pain should be assessed, such as night pain, which wakes a patient up at night, or morning pain and stiffness. Aggravating or relieving factors of the pain should be noted, such as going up or down stairs, the number of

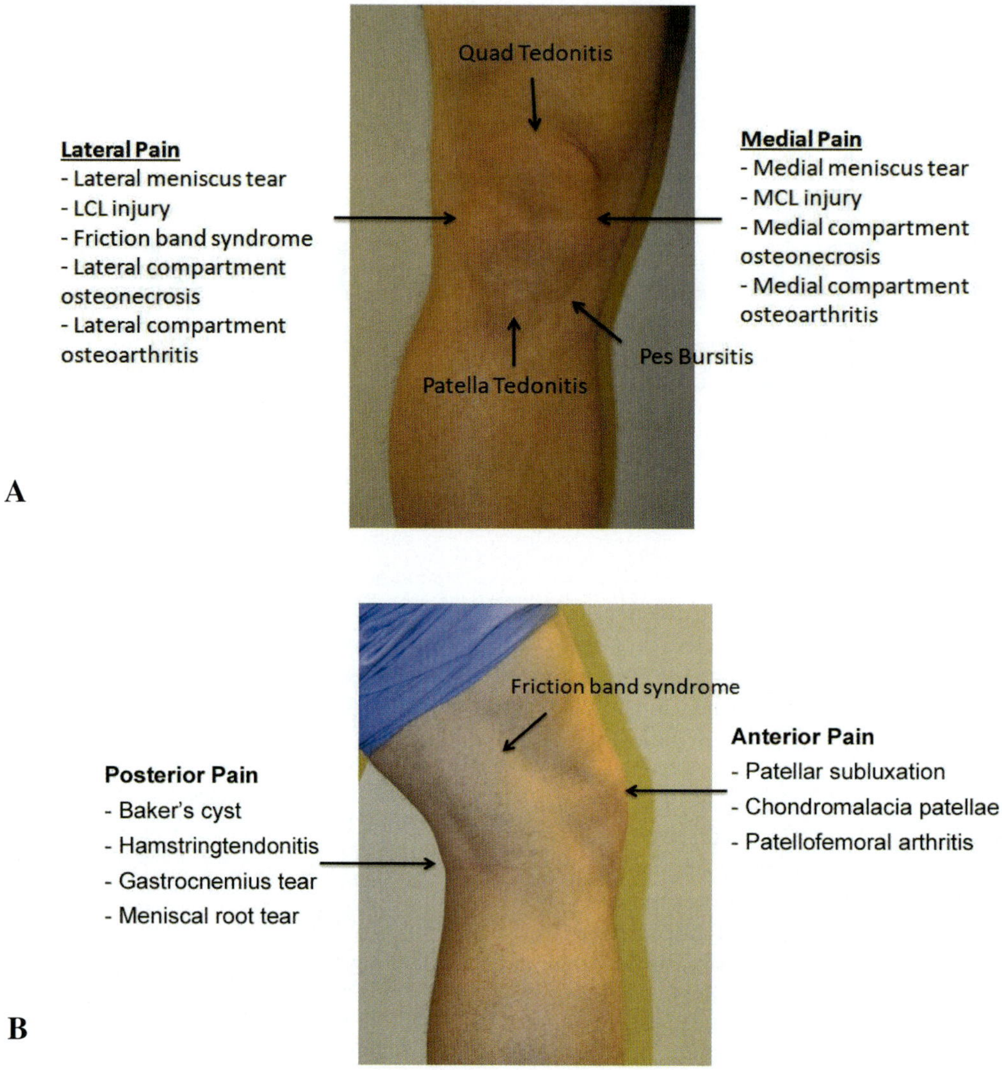

FIGURE 41-1. *Location of knee pain. Various differential diagnoses for anterior, posterior, lateral, and medial knee pain. (**A**) Anterior view of the knee. (**B**) Lateral view of the knee.*

blocks the patient can walk before he or she fatigues, and pain with activity or at rest. Pain going up and down stairs places increased force over the anterior knee, which is often due to patellofemoral disease. Pain with activity may be indicative of vascular disease, while pain at rest may be indicative of inflammatory conditions.

The etiology of the pain should be ascertained and differential sources of knee pain should be systematically excluded, most notably referred pain from hip pathology (groin pain), lumbar radiculopathy (pain down the leg over a peripheral nerve distribution), lumbar stenosis (pain relief when bending forward), vascular claudication (cramping pain with activity), and soft tissue inflammation.

Previous treatments and the patient's perceived efficacy of treatments should be noted, particularly pharmacologic, physical therapy, steroid injections, viscosupplementation, surgical procedures, and alternative treatments. If the patient did not get transient relief of pain with a steroid injection, the pathology may lie elsewhere. Usually, steroids are injected concomitantly with a local anesthetic such as lidocaine, which should give transient relief of pain for several hours. The expectations and treatment goals of the patient should be explored as TKA may not be ideal for some patients. TKA is more clearly indicated in other patients, such as those with chronic pain, joint line tenderness, morning stiffness or night pain, relief of pain from steroid injections or viscosupplementation, and pain that significantly disables activities of daily living and reduces quality of life.

Past Medical History

Identifying patients with comorbidities or other factors that increase the risk for complications is an important part of the preoperative history. The major cardiac risk factors that should be identified in the preoperative history are history of ischemic heart disease, history of congestive heart failure, history of cerebrovascular disease, preoperative treatment with insulin, and preoperative serum creatinine >2.0 mg/dL.[1] History of renal disease should also be assessed, since certain anticoagulation medications that are metabolized by the kidneys should be avoided in the postoperative period. To assess the risk of bleeding, an accurate bleeding history should be obtained and patients should complete a preoperative bleeding questionnaire. Specifically, thrombophilia has been recognized as a major risk factor for deep vein thrombosis (DVT), and so patients with clotting abnormalities that cause thrombophilia, such as protein C, protein S and antithrombin III deficiency, factor V leiden, and dysfibrinogenemia, should be identified.[2]

The increased risk of complications for obese patients following TKA is well documented. Following TKA, the odds ratio is 6.7 times higher risk for infection in obese patients compared to nonobese patients,[3] while the odds ratio is 4.8 and 9.6 for DVT in obese and morbidly obese patients, respectively, compared to nonobese patients.[4] Further, the longevity of the implants is negatively affected with increased body mass index (BMI), leading to revision TKA.[5] Although there is no specific BMI cutoff that contraindicates TKA, obese patients, especially those with BMI above 40, should attempt to lose weight before surgery and should consider bariatric surgery.[6] Diabetes mellitus is also a known risk factor for surgical complications and worse clinical outcomes, including increased incidence of infection, less range of motion, less maximal flexion, and lower Knee Society Scores compared to nondiabetic patients.[7-9] Diabetes should be under good control before proceeding with TKA.

Care should be taken to ensure the patient is in good dental health before TKA. An active oral infection should be treated, because it can lead to bacteremia and subsequent hematogenous total joint infection.[10] Examination by a dentist is not necessary for every patient, but inspection during the preoperative clinical evaluation can lead to further evaluation to reduce the risk of infection after TKA. Dental conditions that require procedures with a higher incidence of bacteremia, such as tooth extractions, root canals, or periodontal procedures, should be treated before undergoing TKA.[11]

Other important patient risk factors to identify are age, posttraumatic arthritis, extensor mechanism deficiency, neuropathic arthropathy, a history of prior infection, sleep apnea, and an inability to tolerate the procedure or comply with postoperative care.[12-14]

Past Surgical History

It is important to assess a patient's past surgical history before proceeding to surgery. Patients who have had previous reactions to anesthesia or have a family history of problems with anesthesia should be separately assessed by an anesthesiologist before undergoing a TKA. Previous orthopaedic surgeries, such as osteotomies to correct limb alignment, open reduction and internal fixation for previous fractures, and anterior cruciate ligament (ACL) reconstruction surgery, should be noted because hardware may need to be removed. Extraction devices and screw drivers must be requested and present for the procedure. These patients may also have altered anatomy and alignment from previous surgeries, and the surgeon may consider using navigation to perform the TKA. Previous surgeries, such as transplants, cardiac valve replacements, genitourinary surgery, and gastrointestinal surgery, may have specific antibiotic needs postoperatively and it may be advantageous to obtain preoperative clearance and consultation from specialists before performing a TKA.

Medications

All of the patient's current medications and allergies should be documented. A variety of drugs should be carefully monitored, supplemented, or discontinued before surgery, particularly nonsteroidal anti-inflammatory drugs (NSAIDs) and aspirin, methotrexate (MTX), antitumor necrosis factor alpha (TNF-α) drugs, glucocorticoids, anticoagulants, insulin, beta-blockers, and antibiotics. NSAIDs have been implicated in operative blood loss and increased postoperative morbidity and should be discontinued at least a week before surgery.[15,16] COX II inhibitors may be safe to continue through the period of surgery. The decision to discontinue MTX before surgery is not clear-cut, because evidence supports both continuing and discontinuing MTX preoperatively.[17-19] A prospective study on the subject suggested continuing MTX preoperatively if disease is controlled by the drug.[17] However, anti-TNF-α drugs (eg, infliximab, etanercept, adalimumab, golimumab) have been linked to infection and other studies recommend these drugs be discontinued preoperatively.[20,21] Current recommendations suggest increasing preoperative dosing of glucocorticoids therapy in patients with chronic adrenal insufficiency, although other recent evidence suggests no real benefit to additional supplementation above the patient's baseline dose.[22-24] Anticoagulants should be discontinued preoperatively in most patients; high-risk patients should be bridged with a low-molecular-weight heparin.[25] Insulin dosage should be reduced or discontinued the evening before and the day of the surgery, with the exact recommendations varying on an individual basis.[26-28] Oral hypoglycemics should be discontinued the day of the surgery.[26] Beta-blockers have been shown to confer no additional protection against postoperative cardiac morbidity in low-risk patients and should be discontinued on the day of surgery; they should, however, be used perioperatively in high-risk patients.[29]

Allergies

Allergies should be documented, with particular care given to adverse reactions to antibiotics or opioids. Some physicians recommend testing for metal allergies, but there is no test available that reliably predicts this allergy. Thus, metal allergy tests should not be routinely performed, but if a metal allergy is present, implants made of different materials may be chosen. If the patient reports a penicillin allergy, the clinician should distinguish between nonimmune-mediated drug reactions and immune-mediated reactions. If an IgE-mediated reaction is suspected, skin testing should be ordered. If the skin test is positive, penicillin, as well as other beta-lactams such as cephalosporins, should be avoided or a desensitization procedure initiated.[30] Alternatives to beta-lactams for surgical prophylaxis include clindamycin and vancomycin.[31] Reactions to opioids should be determined, and true allergies should be differentiated from drug side effects. If allergy issues become extensive, the involvement of an allergist should be considered.

Social History

A social history should be conducted, with emphasis on substance use (tobacco, ethanol, intravenous drug abuse), occupation, access to caregivers for postoperative care, hobbies that may stress the knee, and whether the domestic environment is amenable to postoperative rehabilitation. Patients who are smokers have decreased wound healing; thus it is important to counsel patients on smoking cessation preoperatively. Patients with heavy alcohol consumption are at risk of being malnourished and poor healing, as well as at increased risk of developing delirium tremens in the early postoperative period. Consideration should be given to providing medication or alcohol in the postoperative period to prevent withdrawal from occurring. Finally, a thorough review of systems should be conducted, looking for other sources of recent infection (such as sepsis, urinary tract infection, pneumonia) and neuropathy.

PHYSICAL EXAMINATION

Physical examination is a crucial part of any surgical evaluation. Observation is the first part of the physical exam and begins as soon as the clinician meets the patient. The patient's gait should be analyzed for numerous abnormalities as the patient walks in his or her usual manner and at his or her usual pace. An antalgic gait from knee pain is characterized by less time spent in the stance phase of gait, as the patient attempts to minimize weight-bearing time on the affected leg due to pain. Varus or valgus deformity of the foot is characterized by a loss of stability during the stance period, and consequently introduces varus or valgus strain, respectively, at the knee. Varus or valgus deformity of the knee is even more important for arthroplasty, so the knee should be observed for coronal malalignment as well as medial or lateral thrust during the stance phase (Fig. 41-2). Knee flexion and extension should also be measured: inadequate extension results in a shortened stance phase and requires the quadriceps to maintain stability, while inadequate flexion results in a stiff-legged gait. Measuring motion with a standard technique and recording the motion has merit, as this will be very predictive of postoperative motion.[32] An abnormal walking base may be estimated visually, with an increased walking base possibly indicating genu valgus and decreased walking base indicating genu varus. At times, gait is a result of combined disabilities. Trendelenburg gait is a result of weakened hip abductors (gluteus minimus and medius) and is manifested as a lateral lurch of the trunk toward the affected side during the stance phase. Trendelenburg gait may indicate hip pathology.

Inspection of the knee should occur, and the patient should be visually observed for prior incisions. It is important to note whether these incisions can be used for the knee replacement or will create skin necrosis if there is an inadequate skin bridge. It is recommended to use the most lateral of these incisions, because the vascularity comes from the medial side of the knee. Diffuse swelling of the knee suggests an effusion, and, while in a supine position, the

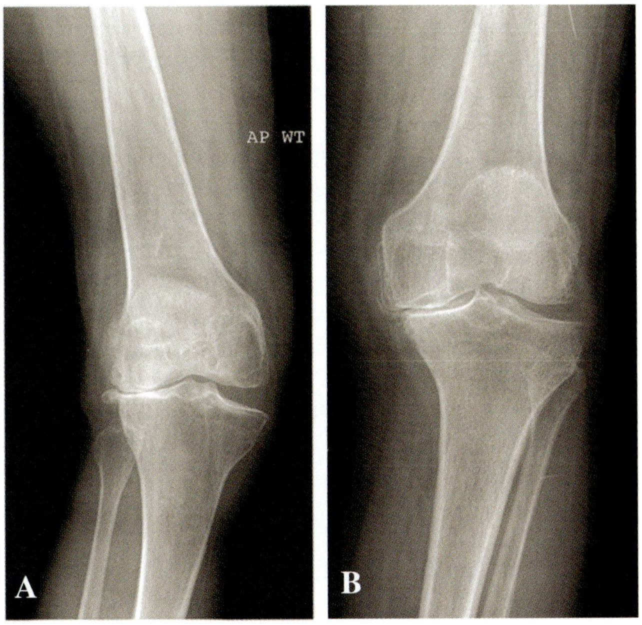

FIGURE 41-2. *Coronal malalignment of the knee. (**A**) Valgus deformity of the knee. (**B**) Varus deformity of the knee.*

patient's knee should be palpated for effusion and graded by compressing the suprapatellar pouch and observing any fluid (grade 1), slight lift-off of the patella (grade 2), a patellar ballottement (grade 3), or no ability to compress the patella against the femoral sulcus (grade 4).[33]

The degree of genu valgus or varus can be estimated by the Q angle. The Q angle should be measured in a dynamic fashion with the patient in a one-legged standing position and statically with the patient in a supine position. The knee should be completely extended, because slight flexion decreases the Q angle due to internal rotation of the tibia. While this practice is used by some, it is easier to make this measurement with the use of radiographic images. On physical exam, however, it can be determined if there is a fixed or correctable valgus or varus deformity.

The cruciate and collateral ligaments should be assessed during the exam. The integrity of the ACL is not essential, because this ligament is not preserved during TKA. Testing for the posterior cruciate ligament (PCL) can be done through the use of the posterior Lachman test and the posterior drawer test. The posterior Lachman test is performed at 30° of flexion and a posterior force is applied to the proximal end of the tibia, while the posterior drawer test is performed at 90° of flexion with a posterior force applied to the proximal end of the tibia (Fig. 41-3). PCL competency is necessary for cruciate-retaining (CR) implants. The MCL and LCL are evaluated with the leg at 30° of flexion and a varus and valgus stress applied, respectively. Similarly, if the leg is at full extension, the posteromedial and posterolateral capsules are evaluated with a valgus and varus stress, respectively.

Examination of the patellofemoral joint should begin with palpation of the medial and lateral sides of the patella looking for joint tenderness. If the patient presents mainly with locking or catching mechanical symptoms and joint line tenderness, then the problem may be meniscus related and require arthroscopic intervention, not a TKA. Apprehension should be tested for by lateral compression and indicates patellar subluxation. Patellar tracking should be evaluated in both weight-bearing and non-weight-bearing tests. For weight-bearing evaluation, the patient unilaterally stands on only the affected leg while the clinician applies an anteroposterior force on the patella. The patient slowly flexes the knee to 90°, if possible, while the clinician notes the tracking of the patella and any crepitus or locking. For non-weight-bearing evaluation, the clinician passively takes the knee through a full range of motion from full extension to flexion while observing the tracking and noting any crepitus or locking. The patellar tilt test should be performed with the knee in 20° of flexion to assess the tightness of the lateral retinaculum, while the patellar glide test performed with the knee in 20° to 30° of flexion assesses the medial and

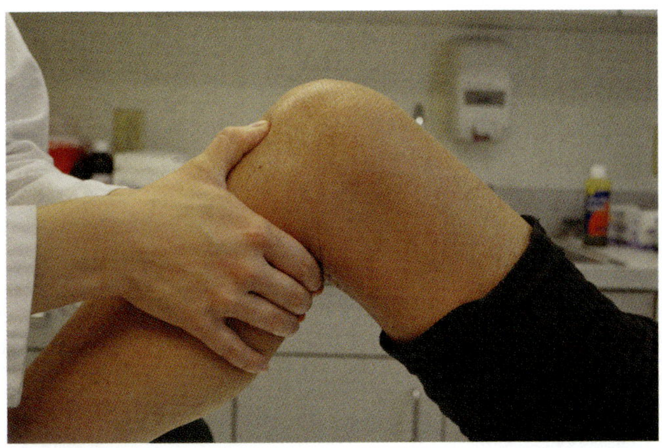

FIGURE 41-3. *Posterior drawer test. Assesses the integrity of the PCL by applying a posterior force to the proximal end of the tibia.*

lateral retinacula depending on whether lateral or medial force is applied, respectively (Fig. 41-4).

A hip examination is crucial during the preoperative clinical examination for TKA, because referred pain from the ipsilateral hip must be excluded. If an exam finds that the knee and hip on the ipsilateral side are simultaneously arthritic, the hip should be treated first; an untreated arthritic hip will lead to failure of TKA due to decreased rehabilitation.

A complete motor and sensory exam of the lower limbs should also be conducted to exclude spinal cord disease or neurologic abnormalities. The motor exam should begin with a visual inspection, looking for involuntary movements (eg, tics, tremor, chorea), muscle atrophy or hypertrophy, and muscle fasciculations. The tone of the muscles should then be examined, including a test for ankle clonus. This is followed by an assessment of the power of each muscle group, which should include testing of hip flexion, extension, adduction, and abduction; foot dorsiflexion, plantarflexion, eversion, and inversion; and toe plantarflexion and dorsiflexion. Finally, the deep (patellar and ankle) and superficial (plantar) tendon reflexes should be elicited. The sensory exam should assess each of the sensory modalities: light touch, sharp touch, temperature, vibration, and proprioception. Sensation should be examined in the peripheral nerve and dermatome distributions (Fig. 41-5).

Severe peripheral vascular disease is a relative contraindication for TKA and at-risk patients should be identified. Skin discoloration, absence of hair, dystrophic nail abnormalities, or healed vascular ulcers all signify poor circulation.[34] Dorsalis pedis and posterior tibialis pulses should be palpated bilaterally for symmetry and strength.[35] If abnormalities are found and peripheral vascular disease is suspected, ankle-brachial indexes should be obtained using Doppler ultrasound. An ankle-brachial index between 0.9 and 1.3 falls within the normal range, a value less than 0.9 requires referral to a vascular surgeon for elevated risk of arterial complications, and a value less than 0.5 indicates severe ischemia and an immediate angiogram is necessary.[33] The ankle-brachial test is unreliable if the patient presents with radiographic evidence of femoropopliteal arterial calcifications, because this falsely elevates ankle pressure and produces false negatives.[33] The popliteal fossa should also be palpated, because a mass or fullness may indicate an aneurysm, which, although rare, can lead to serious complications.[36] Finally, inspection can reveal other peripheral vascular abnormalities such as peripheral edema or venous stasis ulcers.

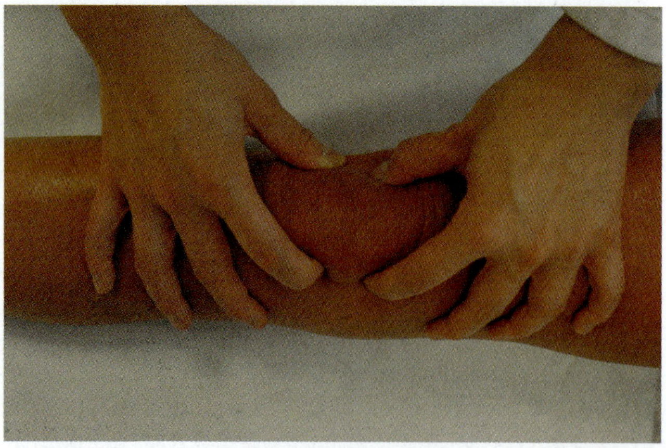

FIGURE 41-4. *Patellar tilt test. Assesses the tightness of the lateral retinaculum by tilting the lateral edge of the patella above the horizontal.*

STANDARDIZED QUESTIONNAIRES

Standardized health assessment questionnaires can help the physician assess the patient's baseline pain, functionality, and overall well-being, which can be used to determine the need for TKA. The Western Ontario and McMaster Universities Osteoarthritis Index (WOMAC) (*WOMAC Osteoarthritis Index User Guide*), Medical Outcomes Study (MOS) Short Form–36 (SF-36), MOS Short Form–12 (SF-12), and the American Knee Society score (KSS) have all been validated for such purposes.[37-40] The elements of the objective component of the KSS are a part of a good preoperative physical exam.

CLINICAL TESTING

Preoperative clinical tests are a valuable part of the preoperative evaluation and may detect abnormalities that the history, physical examination, and radiographic evaluation may miss. However, the indication for certain clinical labs should be guided by the assessment of the patient during other parts of the preoperative evaluation; extensive preoperative testing of all patients provides little to no new clinical information in the majority of cases while incurring much higher expenses.[41] The routine laboratory tests that should be performed in all patients include a complete blood count (CBC) and a basic mechanical panel (BMP).

An active local or systemic infection is an absolute contraindication for TKA. A history of prior bone or joint infection requires evaluation of the patient for an active infection through the use of laboratory tests, including a CBC with

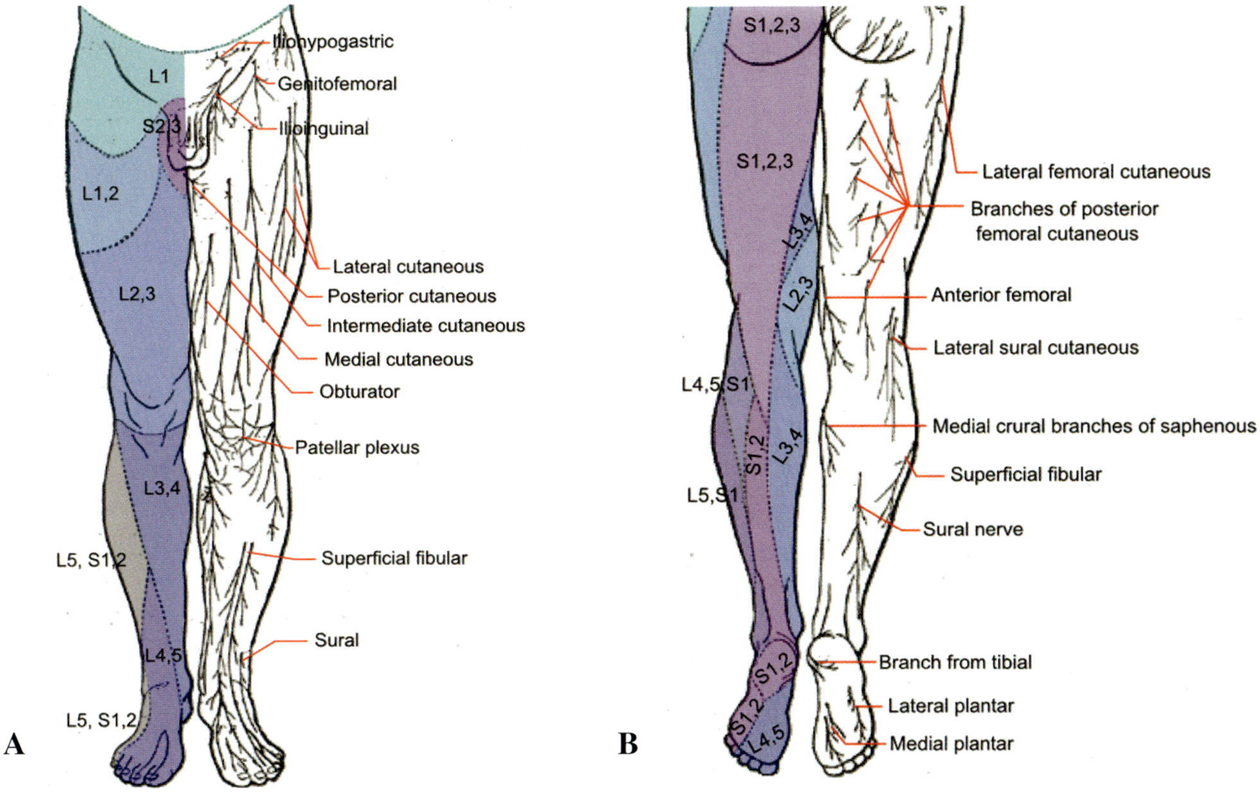

FIGURE 41-5. *Dermatomes and sensory distribution of lower extremity nerves in* **(A)** *anterior and* **(B)** *posterior views. These nerves should be routinely tested on physical exam when assessing the neurologic status of patients with lower extremity complaints. (Image courtesy of Mikael Haggstrom and the 20th U.S. edition of Gray's Anatomy of the Human Body, 1918.)*

differential, erythrocyte sedimentation rate (ESR), C-reactive protein (CRP), joint aspiration, and possibly bone and indium-labeled white blood cell scans.[42] The use of white blood cell (WBC) counts of peripheral blood, ESR, and CRP in combination provides a sensitive screening test for predicting the absence of infection and should be routinely ordered for patients with a high suspicion for infection; elevated peripheral WBC count, ESR, and CRP do not specifically confirm infection but normal values argue against infection.[43,44] If WBC counts are greater than 11,000 cells/mm^3, ESR is greater than 20, CRP is greater than 10 mg/dL, or infection is clinically suspected, then a joint aspiration with synovial fluid WBC count and differential should be performed. Normal values of these labs vary from lab to lab, and the local normal ranges should be used.

In a native knee, a synovial WBC count greater than 50,000/mm^3 or greater than 90% polymorphonuclear leukocytes is highly suggestive of joint sepsis. However, some literature suggests that this WBC count cutoff of 50,000/mm^3 lacks the sensitivity required to rule out infection, especially in more moderate infections and in potentially immunocompromised patients, because many patients with joint infection have synovial WBC count below 50,000/mm^3.[45-47] A synovial WBC count of greater than 25,000/mm^3 is a more sensitive cutoff, and patients with a WBC count below this range can more likely be ruled out for joint infection.[48] It should be noted that recent antibiotic use before joint aspiration increases the occurrence of false-negative results, and joint aspiration should be delayed 4 to 6 weeks if the patient has recently taken antibiotics.[49] The clinician should take care to exclude gout and pseudogout if synovial WBC count is elevated; gout and pseudogout are not contraindications to TKA and, if clinically suspected, synovial fluid should be analyzed for crystals to rule it in or out.[50] An alternative to synovial WBC count for assessing infection is using polymerase chain reaction to detect the presence of bacterial DNA and therefore infection; this method has greater sensitivity than the other diagnostic tests for infection.[51]

The use of gallium-67- or technetium-99m-labeled bone scans and indium-111-labeled WBC scans are not advised; they are expensive, have comparable or lesser sensitivities relative to other diagnostic tests, and overall are more appropriate for use in detecting infection before revision TKA.[48]

A urinary tract infection represents an increased risk of prosthetic infection, but is not an absolute contraindication for TKA. The testing algorithm is as follows[52]: if the patient has obstructive symptoms (ie, urine outflow problems), then the TKA should be postponed and a urologic consult arranged. If the patient instead has irritative symptoms (eg, dysuria, urgency, and frequency), then a urinalysis should be performed and analyzed for WBC count. A WBC count greater than 10,000 per mL of urine necessitates a bacterial count and culture; if the count is less than 10,000 cells per mL, the test is inconclusive and clinical judgment should be used. If the bacterial count is greater than 1000 colonies per mL, the surgery should be postponed while the patient is administered the appropriate antibiotics and then re-administered a urinalysis; if the count is less than 1000 colonies per mL, the test is inconclusive and clinical judgment should be used. If the patient presents with neither obstructive nor irritative symptoms, the patient should be cultured for microorganisms, cleared for TKA, and treated postoperatively with an 8- to 10-day regimen of antibiotics if microorganisms were found in the culture.

Preoperative coagulation studies (prothrombin time, international normalized ratio, platelet count, fibrinogen levels, and activated partial thromboplastin time) are not routine and should not be ordered unless the patient's clinical history, preoperative questionnaire, or physical examination is suggestive of a bleeding disorder.[53] If a patient is found to be anemic preoperatively, a hematology consult may be obtained to work up the cause and treatment of anemia. Preoperative electrocardiography and cardiology consult should be performed on patients identified as at risk for cardiac complications; little additional prognostic value is associated with the use of electrocardiography in patients assessed as lower risk.[54] Thoracic radiography should be performed on all patients over the age of 60, regardless of history.[55,56] Other indications for thoracic radiography include smokers of 10 cigarettes or more per day, those with cardiac or respiratory disease, and those who have had contact with tuberculosis in the past year without follow-up thoracic radiograph. This list is not all-inclusive and additional tests may be indicated based on the individual patient's physical examination or clinical history findings, as well as the clinician's judgment.

CONCLUSION

The preoperative evaluation is the time when the surgeon brings together all of the information to verify the diagnosis, identify the risk factors, and plan surgery. If the exam is thought of in this manner, all of the various components of history, physical exam, radiographic exam, and preoperative screening make sense. As when performing the surgery, each move should have purpose.

SUGGESTED READING

This recommended reading provides a revised cardiac risk index for patients undergoing orthopaedic surgeries:

Ackland GL, Harris S, Ziabari Y, et al. Revised cardiac risk index and postoperative morbidity after elective orthopaedic surgery: a prospective cohort study. *Br J Anaesth.* 2010;105(6):744-752.

This recommended reading details preoperative vascular studies and possible vascular interventions that should be performed in certain patients before total knee arthroplasty:

Garabekyan T, Oliashirazi A, Winters K. The value of immediate preoperative vascular examination in an at-risk patient for total knee arthroplasty. *Orthopedics.* 2011;34(1):52.

This recommended reading describes how preoperative motion, an important physical exam, best predicts postoperative range of motion:

Ritter MA, Stringer EA. Predictive range of motion after total knee replacement. *Clin Orthop Relat Res.* 1979;143:115-119.

REFERENCES

1. Lee TH, Marcantonio ER, Mangione CM, et al. Derivation and prospective validation of a simple index for prediction of cardiac risk of major noncardiac surgery. *Circulation.* 1999;100(10):1043-1049.
2. Chotanaphuti T, Ongnamthip P, Silpipat S, et al. The prevalence of thrombophilia and venous thromboembolism in total knee arthroplasty. *J Med Assoc Thai.* 2007;90(7):1342-1347.
3. Namba RS, Paxton L, Fithian DC, et al. Obesity and perioperative morbidity in total hip and total knee arthroplasty patients. *J Arthroplasty.* 2005;20(7 Suppl 3):46-50.

4. White RH, Henderson MC. Risk factors for venous thromboembolism after total hip and knee replacement surgery. *Curr Opin Pulm Med.* 2002;8(5):365-371.
5. Mulhall KJ, Ghomrawi HM, Mihalko W, et al. Adverse effects of increased body mass index and weight on survivorship of total knee arthroplasty and subsequent outcomes of revision TKA. *J Knee Surg.* 2007;20(3): 199-204.
6. Samson AJ, Mercer GE, Campbell DG. Total knee replacement in the morbidly obese: a literature review. *ANZ J Surg.* 2010;80(9):595-599. doi: 10.1111/j.1445-2197.2010.05396.x. Epub 2010 Aug 19.
7. England SP, Stern SH, Insall JN, et al. Total knee arthroplasty in diabetes mellitus. *Clin Orthop Relat Res.* 1990;(260):130-134.
8. Yang K, Yeo SJ, Lee BP, et al. Total knee arthroplasty in diabetic patients: a study of 109 consecutive cases. *J Arthroplasty.* 2001;16(1):102-106.
9. Papagelopoulos PJ, Idusuyi OB, Wallrichs SL, et al. Long-term outcome and survivorship analysis of primary total knee arthroplasty in patients with diabetes mellitus. *Clin Orthop Relat Res.* 1996;(330):124-132.
10. Bartzokas CA, Johnson R, Jane M, et al. Relation between mouth and haematogenous infection in total joint replacements. *BMJ.* 1994;309(6953): 506-508.
11. American Dental Association, American Academy of Orthopaedic Surgeons. Antibiotic prophylaxis for dental patients with total joint replacements. *J Am Dent Assoc.* 2003;134(7):895-899.
12. Springer BD, Della Valle CJ. Extensor mechanism allograft reconstruction after total knee arthroplasty. *J Arthroplasty.* 2008;23(7 Suppl):35-38.
13. Kim YH, Kim JS, Oh SW. Total knee arthroplasty in neuropathic arthropathy. *J Bone Joint Surg Br.* 2002; 84(2):216-219.
14. Lee GC, Pagnano MW, Hanssen AD. Total knee arthroplasty after prior bone or joint sepsis about the knee. *Clin Orthop Relat Res.* 2002;(404):226-231.
15. Robinson CM, Christie J, Malcolm-Smith N. Nonsteroidal antiinflammatory drugs, perioperative blood loss, and transfusion requirements in elective hip arthroplasty. *J Arthroplasty.* 1993;8(6):607-610.
16. Connelly CS, Panush RS. Should nonsteroidal anti-inflammatory drugs be stopped before elective surgery? *Arch Intern Med.* 1991;151(10):1963-1966.
17. Grennan DM, Gray J, Loudon J, et al. Methotrexate and early postoperative complications in patients with rheumatoid arthritis undergoing elective orthopaedic surgery. *Ann Rheum Dis.* 2001;60(3):214-217.
18. Carpenter MT, West SG, Vogelgesang SA, et al. Post-operative joint infections in rheumatoid arthritis patients on methotrexate therapy. *Orthopedics.* 1996; 19(3):207-210.
19. Perhala RS, Wilke WS, Clough JD, et al. Local infectious complications following large joint replacement in rheumatoid arthritis patients treated with methotrexate versus those not treated with methotrexate. *Arthritis Rheum.* 1991;34(2):146-152.
20. Winthrop KL, Yamashita S, Beekmann SE, et al. Mycobacterial and other serious infections in patients receiving anti-tumor necrosis factor and other newly approved biologic therapies: case finding through the Emerging Infections Network. *Clin Infect Dis.* 2008; 46(11):1738-1740.
21. Tubach F, Salmon D, Ravaud P, et al. Risk of tuberculosis is higher with anti-tumor necrosis factor monoclonal antibody therapy than with soluble tumor necrosis factor receptor therapy: the three-year prospective French Research Axed on Tolerance of Biotherapies registry. *Arthritis Rheum.* 2009;60(7):1884-1894.
22. Salem M, Tainsh RE Jr, Bromberg J, et al. Perioperative glucocorticoid coverage. A reassessment 42 years after emergence of a problem. *Ann Surg.* 1994; 219(4): 416-425.
23. Lloyd EL. A rational regimen for perioperative steroid supplements and a clinical assessment of the requirement. *Ann R Coll Surg Engl.* 1981;63(1):54-57.
24. Gröschl M, Rauh M, Dörr HG. Cortisol and 17-hydroxyprogesterone kinetics in saliva after oral administration of hydrocortisone in children and young adolescents with congenital adrenal hyperplasia due to 21-hydroxylase deficiency. *J Clin Endocrinol Metab.* 2002;87(3):1200-1204.
25. Wysokinski WE, McBane RD, Daniels PR, et al. Periprocedural anticoagulation management of patients with nonvalvular atrial fibrillation. *Mayo Clin Proc.* 2008;83(6):639-645.
26. Hoogwerf BJ. Perioperative management of diabetes mellitus: how should we act on the limited evidence? *Cleve Clin J Med.* 2006;73(Suppl 1):S95-99.
27. Pezzarossa A, Taddei F, Cimicchi MC, et al. Perioperative management of diabetic subjects. Subcutaneous versus intravenous insulin administration during glucose–potassium infusion. *Diabetes Care.* 1988; 11(1):52-58.
28. Peters A, Kerner W. Perioperative management of the diabetic patient. *Exp Clin Endocrinol Diabetes.* 1995; 103(4):213-218.
29. van Klei WA, Bryson GL, Yang H, et al. Effect of beta-blocker prescription on the incidence of postop-

erative myocardial infarction after hip and knee arthroplasty. *Anesthesiology.* 2009;111(4):717-724.

30. Gruchalla RS, Pirmohamed M. Clinical practice. Antibiotic allergy. *N Engl J Med.* 2006;354(6):601-609.

31. Li JT, Markus PJ, Osmon DR, et al. Reduction of vancomycin use in orthopedic patients with a history of antibiotic allergy. *Mayo Clin Proc.* 2000;75(9):902-906.

32. Harvey IA, Barry K, Kirby SP, et al. Factors affecting the range of movement of total knee arthroplasty. *J Bone Joint Surg Br.* 1993;75(6):950-955.

33. Tria AJ Jr. Clinical examination of the knee. In: Scott WN, ed. *Insall & Scott Surgery of the Knee.* 4th ed. Philadelphia, PA: Churchill Livingstone Elsevier; 2006:86-98.

34. Garabekyan T, Oliashirazi A, Winters K. The value of immediate preoperative vascular examination in an at-risk patient for total knee arthroplasty. *Orthopedics.* 2011;34(1):52.

35. Rush JH, Vidovich JD, Johnson MA. Arterial complications of total knee replacement. The Australian experience. *J Bone Joint Surg Br.* 1987;69(3):400-402.

36. Smith DE, McGraw RW, Taylor DC, et al. Arterial complications and total knee arthroplasty. *J Am Acad Orthop Surg.* 2001;9(4):253-257.

37. Bellamy N, Buchanan WW, Goldsmith CH, et al. Validation study of WOMAC: a health status instrument for measuring clinically important patient relevant outcomes to antirheumatic drug therapy in patients with osteoarthritis of the hip or knee. *J Rheumatol.* 1988;15(12):1833-1840.

38. Liow RY, Walker K, Wajid MA, et al. The reliability of the American Knee Society Score. *Acta Orthop Scand.* 2000;71(6):603-608.

39. McHorney CA, Ware JE Jr, Raczek AE. The MOS 36-Item Short-Form Health Survey (SF-36): II. Psychometric and clinical tests of validity in measuring physical and mental health constructs. *Med Care.* 1993;31(3):247-263.

40. Ware J Jr, Kosinski M, Keller SD. A 12-Item Short-Form Health Survey: construction of scales and preliminary tests of reliability and validity. *Med Care.* 1996;34(3):220-233.

41. Kaplan EB, Sheiner LB, Boeckmann AJ, et al. The usefulness of preoperative laboratory screening. *JAMA.* 1985;253(24):3576-3581.

42. Lee GC, Pagnano MW, Hanssen AD. Total knee arthroplasty after prior bone or joint sepsis about the knee. *Clin Orthop Relat Res.* 2002;(404):226-231.

43. Li SF, Henderson J, Dickman E, et al. Laboratory tests in adults with monoarticular arthritis: can they rule out a septic joint? *Acad Emerg Med.* 2004;11(3):276-280.

44. Li SF, Cassidy C, Chang C, et al. Diagnostic utility of laboratory tests in septic arthritis. *Emerg Med J.* 2007; 24(2):75-77.

45. Margaretten ME, Kohlwes J, Moore D, et al. Does this adult patient have septic arthritis? *JAMA.* 2007; 297(13):1478-1488.

46. McGillicuddy DC, Shah KH, Friedberg RP, et al. How sensitive is the synovial fluid white blood cell count in diagnosing septic arthritis? *Am J Emerg Med.* 2007;25(7):749-752.

47. O'Malley A, Svinos H. Towards evidence based emergency medicine: Best BETs from the Manchester Royal Infirmary. BET 3: Is the white cell count of the joint aspirate sufficiently sensitive/specific to rule in/out septic arthritis? *Emerg Med J.* 2009;26(6):435-437.

48. Love C, Tomas MB, Marwin SE, et al. Role of nuclear medicine in diagnosis of the infected joint replacement. *Radiographics.* 2001;21(5):1229-1238.

49. Gonzalez MH, Mekhail AO. The failed total knee arthroplasty: evaluation and etiology. *J Am Acad Orthop Surg.* 2004;12(6):436-446.

50. Pascual E, Batlle-Gualda E, Martínez A, et al. Synovial fluid analysis for diagnosis of intercritical gout. *Ann Intern Med.* 1999;131(10):756-759.

51. Mariani BD, Martin DS, Levine MJ, et al. The Coventry Award. Polymerase chain reaction detection of bacterial infection in total knee arthroplasty. *Clin Orthop Relat Res.* 1996;331:11-22.

52. David TS, Vrahas MS. Perioperative lower urinary tract infections and deep sepsis in patients undergoing total joint arthroplasty. *J Am Acad Orthop Surg.* 2000;8(1):66-74.

53. Rohrer MJ, Michelotti MC, Nahrwold DL. A prospective evaluation of the efficacy of preoperative coagulation testing. *Ann Surg.* 1988;208(5):554-557.

54. Noordzij PG, Boersma E, Bax JJ, et al. Prognostic value of routine preoperative electrocardiography in patients undergoing noncardiac surgery. *Am J Cardiol.* 2006;97(7):1103-1106. Epub 2006 Feb 28.

55. Nze PU, Njike C. Is routine preoperative chest X-ray indicated in elderly patients undergoing elective surgery? *Niger J Med.* 2008;17(2):150-152.

56. Ishaq M, Kamal RS, Aqil M. Value of routine preoperative chest X-ray in patients over the age of 40 years. *J Pak Med Assoc.* 1997;47(11):279-281.

42 Preoperative Imaging: Radiographic and Cross-Sectional Studies

Parag Sancheti and Ashok Shyam

For total knee replacement, it is imperative that the prosthesis implanted replicates the normal joint orientation in order to balance the weight transmission across the limb.[1,2] The main goal of preoperative planning is to define this normal joint orientation so that before surgery the surgeon can formulate a mental three-dimensional image of the joint. With this image, the surgeon can assess the severity of the disease, recognize the difficulties that will be encountered, and possibly formulate a plan to counter these difficulties. All of these things not only define the successful performance of surgery but also enhance the survival rate of the implant and reduce complication rates.[3,4] Preoperative imaging conventionally involves plain radiographs, but occasionally computed tomography (CT) scans and magnetic resonance imaging (MRI) also are required to deal with certain scenarios. Patient-specific cutting jigs and implants are now being used and require the cross-sectional studies for preoperative planning. This chapter discusses the use of plain radiographs and the indications for use of special imaging.

IMPORTANCE OF PREOPERATIVE IMAGING

As per original concepts of total knee replacement surgery, the orientation of the artificial joint should be symmetric to avoid overloading of one compartment. This is achieved by planning the surgery along the limb mechanical axis. Increased incidences of complications such as knee stiffness, patellofemoral problems, early loosening, and increased wear rates are reported in patients with a maligned knee.[5,6] In addition, the knee alignment directly affects the long-term survival of the implant.[7,8]

Preoperative imaging also helps in planning the intraoperative steps and alerts the surgeon to potential difficulties. The amount of femoral and tibia bowing helps in assessing the feasibility of the use of intramedullary rods during surgery. Knowledge of the amount and position of bone defects helps the surgeon to plan the method of dealing with the defects in advance. Other factors such as size and position of osteophytes, bone quality, and ligament integrity can be judged by preoperative imaging so that intraoperative decisions can be made more easily.

PLAIN RADIOGRAPHS

Preoperative planning depends on two factors: mechanical alignment and joint line orientation. Depending on these factors, different alignment schemes have been described, namely, classical and anatomical. In classical teaching, the aim is to create a prosthetic joint perpendicular to the tibial shaft axis to coincide with the mechanical axis. Thus a proximal tibia cut is made perpendicular to the tibia axis and the distal femoral cut is made perpendicular to the femoral mechanical axis (5°–7° valgus to the femoral anatomical axis). This creates a prosthetic joint that is perpendicular to tibia axis and has even load distribution.[9]

In anatomical teaching, the goal is to reproduce the joint line with respect to the normal mechanical alignment. This was proposed by Hungerford to recreate natural knee kinematics, especially in cruciate-retaining prostheses.[10] Thus the proximal tibial cut is taken in 3° varus, while the distal femoral cut is taken at 10° valgus to the femoral shaft axis. This results in a joint line that is parallel to the ground when the person is standing straight with feet together. The tibiofemoral axis is similarly reproduced by both methods; however, the proximal tibia cut is different and the orientation of joint line differs. The proximal tibia varus cut is difficult to reproduce technically as compared to a 90° cut and there is some evidence that this proximal tibia varus cut can cause uneven stress distribution and early clinical failure.[11,12] Although no studies have compared the two schemes, more surgeons are following the classical scheme for preoperative planning. Therefore, this chapter focuses on the classical planning scheme for total knee replacement.

Radiographs can be divided into two sets according to the requirements of the individual cases. The standard set of radiographs is required for all cases and an additional set is required when indicated. The standard set of knee radiographs includes the anteroposterior (AP) weight-bearing radiograph, single joint weight-bearing radiograph, standard lateral radiograph, varus-valgus stress view, Merchant's view, and full-length scanogram.

AP Weight-Bearing Radiograph of Both Knees

Standing radiographs are taken with the beam focused on the anterior surface of the patella (Fig.42-1). In most cases the limbs have to be rotated internally to make the patella face anteriorly. A standard distance of 100 cm between the beam and the plate is conventionally used and helps in identifying the magnification and also in standardizing the sequential radiographs. The AP weight-bearing radiographs provide a more accurate estimate of presence and degree of cartilage thinning.[13,14] The normal joint space is >3 mm in both compartments or within 50% of the contralateral knee.[15] This view also represents the position the knee acquires in functional weight bearing, and thus angular deformities in terms of varus and valgus can be better appreciated. The decrease in joint space in one compartment with an increase in joint space in the other indicates the degree of ligament stretch and instability. In severe cases, a medial or lateral translation can also be identified, which marks a more severe ligament and soft tissue pathology. Bony abnormalities, such as condylar bone defects, can be identified and classified. The severity and extent of osteophytosis can be seen on this radiograph. Depending on the size of the osteophytes, the soft tissue and capsular tenting can be judged. This will be an important aspect in intraoperative ligament balancing because removal of these osteophytes will further slacken the soft tissues. The quality of bone in cases with osteopenia can be determined. In cases with osteoporosis, uncemented fixation may be disadvantageous; however, currently no randomized trials are available to provide evidence for such an assumption. Again in cases with osteopenia, as seen in rheumatoid arthritis, a metal-backed prosthesis may be preferred compared to an all-polyethylene tibial component. The shape and size of the femoral condyle (especially the lateral femoral condyle) helps in selecting the reference line for femoral cuts. In cases with a deficiency of the lateral condyle, if posterior referencing is done with respect to the femoral condyle, the anterior femoral cut may be less laterally and might lead to internal rotation of the femoral component and anterior notching. In these scenarios with severe discrepancy between the AP diameter of the condyles, posterior referencing should be avoided.

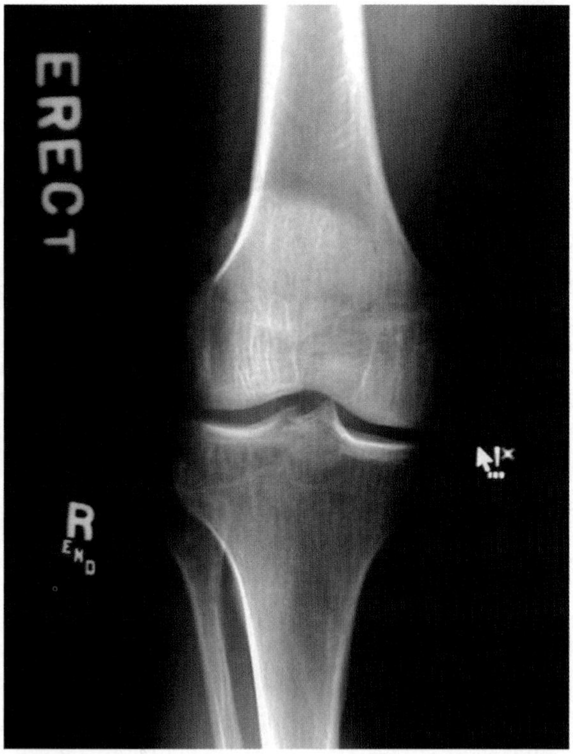

FIGURE 42-1. *Standard anteroposterior radiograph of the knee.*

Single Joint Weight-Bearing Radiographs

Single joint weight-bearing radiographs are taken with the patient standing on one leg with the patella facing forward (Fig. 42-2). The patient can use support to stand.

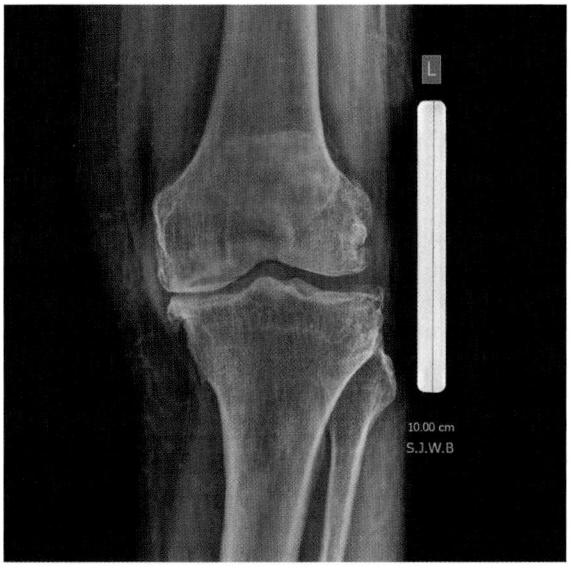

FIGURE 42-2. *Single joint weight-bearing radiograph showing mild opening of the lateral compartment.*

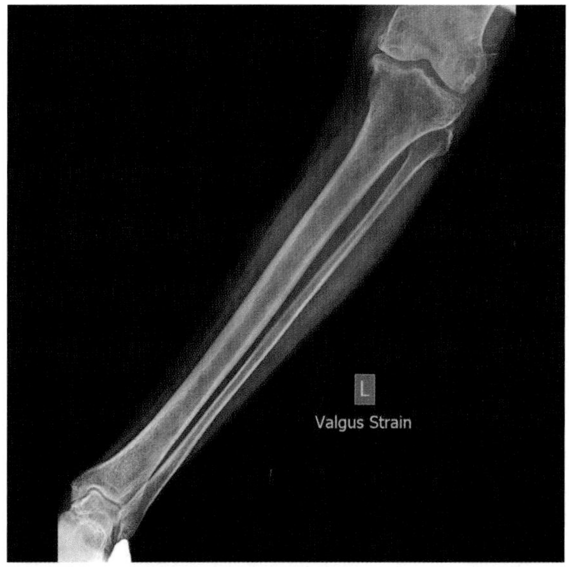

FIGURE 42-3. *Valgus stress view shows medial opening and correction of the varus deformity to almost neutral.*

These radiographs further enhance the deformity and help in judging the status of the ligaments, which are now stretched.[16] This may be especially important in cases planned for unicondylar replacement where the ligament laxity of the compartments plays a major role in deciding the planning. A significant change in the joint space orientation compared to that in AP weight-bearing radiographs indicates a greater degree of ligament laxity and may indicate use of a more constrained prosthesis.

Stress Views: Valgus and Varus

Stress views are taken in order to assess the ligament laxity and extent of correction and also to assess the amount of bone defect in cases with severe deformities (Fig. 42-3). These radiographs are taken with the patient lying supine and a varus stress applied in case of valgus deformity and a valgus stress in case of varus deformity. The amount of opening of the joint when compared to standard AP radiographs will help in assessing the amount of ligament laxity and also correctability of the deformity. In cases in which the varus deformities are fixed, more release and adjustment in the bone cuts will be required to achieve correction. Correctable varus-valgus deformities may be due to ligament laxity, bone defect, or both. Stress radiographs can help in assessing both. In cases in which the deformity is completely correctable on the stress views but has a firm end point clinically, ligaments may still be intact with the bone defect being the main reason for deformity. In cases in which overcorrection of the deformity is possible but has a definite end point clinically, the ligament may be stretched but still functionally intact. In cases in which there is overcorrection with no firm end point, ligament deficiency is assumed. Fixed deformities that are shown to be not correctable on radiograph are due to bone loss and are subsequently fixed in a deformed position due to soft tissue contracture.[17] Again the correctable deformity will require less soft tissue release intraoperatively than the fixed deformity. Stress views are also important to assess the extent of the bone defect and, according to this finding, additional inventory, such as augments and extension rods, need to be preordered.

Standard Lateral View

The standard lateral view is taken with the patient on his or her side with the selected side down and touching the film cassette (Fig. 42-4). Conventionally it is taken in 30° of flexion and a cephalad angle of 5° can be adjusted to superimpose the femoral condyles. Assessment of the knee joint with respect to severity of the degenerative process, presence of posterior osteophytes, and tibial slope can be done with this view. Assessment of sizes of the medial and lateral femoral condyles can be made with respect to the degeneration of the posterior condyle. As mentioned above, this will have bearing on the selection of the referencing

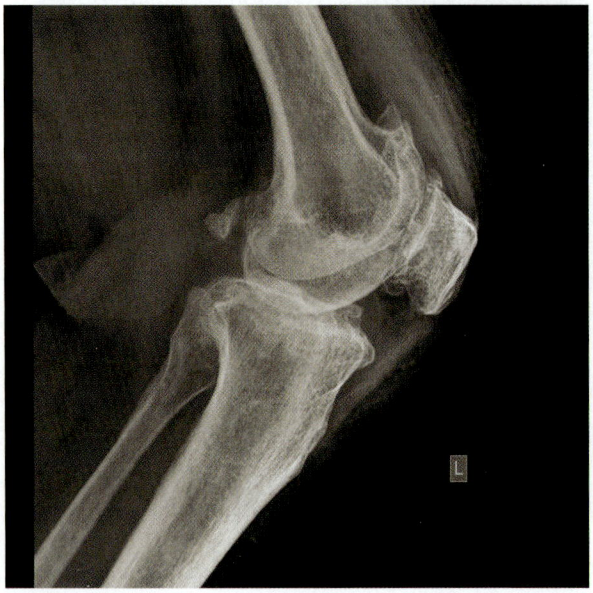

FIGURE 42-4. *Lateral radiograph of the knee showing posterior osteophytes and the status of the patellofemoral joint.*

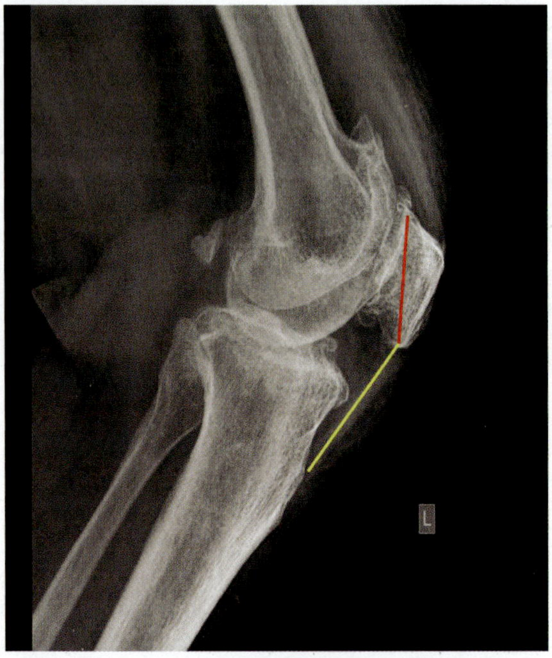

FIGURE 42-5. *The Insall-Salvati index is calculated by taking the ratio length of the patellar tendon (yellow line) to the diagonal height of the patella (red line).*

method to make femoral cuts. The patellofemoral joint can be assessed with respect to the extent of degeneration, patella height, and patella thickness. Patella height is described in terms of the Insall-Salvati index (Fig. 42-5).

The Insall-Salvati index is calculated by dividing the length of the patellar tendon by the diagonal height of the patella.[18,19] The normal values are 1.02 ± 0.2. A value above 1.2 indicates a longer patella tendon and a high-riding patella (patella alta) and a value below 0.8 indicates a short patella tendon and a low-lying patella (patella baja). Blumensaat's line is another criterion for indicating patella level and is explained in Figure 42-6. With the level of patella in mind, the difficulty in patella eversion during surgery can be judged. Also the position of the patella implant can be selected with the implant placed on the lower end of the prepared patella surface in case of patella alta and vice versa. This will help in keeping the patella level with the new joint line. Also the thickness of the patella can be assessed by this view and, in cases with a thin patella, a decision not to resurface can be made.

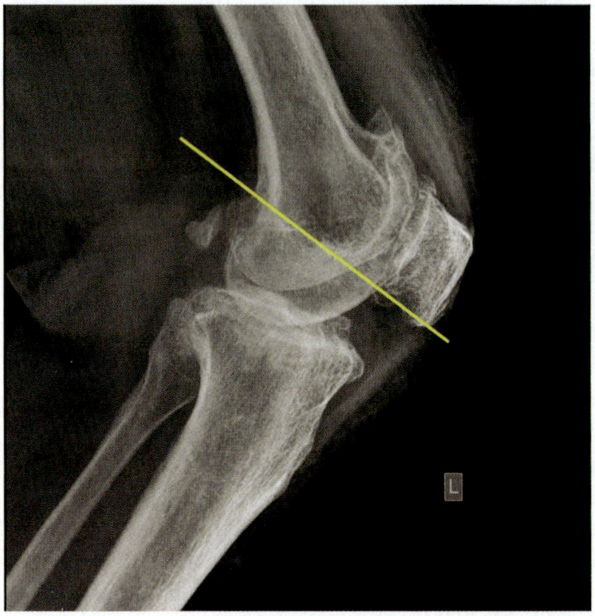

FIGURE 42-6. *The Blumensaat line is drawn on the linear radiopacity of the roof of the intercondylar notch. In this method, the patellar height is assessed according to the distance between the lower pole of the patella and the Blumensaat line in millimeters. The lower pole of the patella should normally lie on the Blumensaat line; if it is more than 10 mm above the line, it is classified as patella alta and if it is 10 mm below it is patella baja.*

Skyline (Merchant's View)

The skyline (Merchant's view) is the most commonly used axial view of the patella (Fig. 42-7).[20] The patellofemoral joint can be clearly assessed by this view and alignment and orientation of the patella in relation to the femur can be measured.[21,22] Normally, the patella is directly centered over the trochlear groove. The sulcus and congruence angles can be calculated on this view (Fig. 42-8).

The sulcus angle is calculated by drawing two lines along the trochlear groove. The sulcus angle is then bisected and another line is drawn from this bisection point to the patella ridge. The angle between these two lines is the congruence angle. Normally, the congruence angle is –6° ± 11° (minus sign when patellar apex is lateral to the bisection line). Deviation of the patella to medial or lateral side can be quantified by this angle measurement. Tightness in the retinaculum will lead to deviation of the patella to that side and a retinacular release can be planned for such cases.

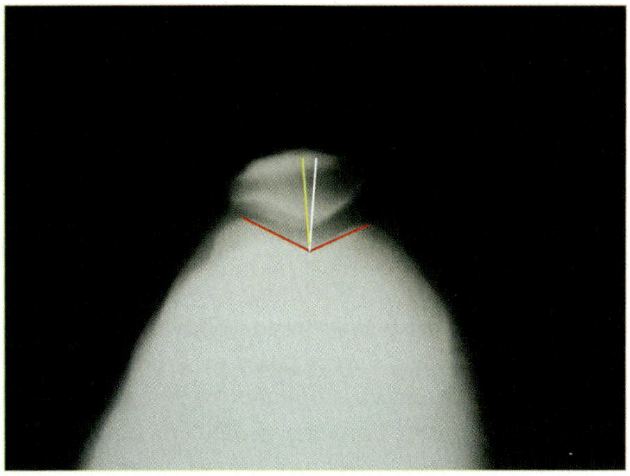

FIGURE 42-8. *Sulcus angle and the congruence angle.*

Scanogram

A scanogram is essential for assessment of alignment in all cases that are planned for total knee replacement. This helps in defining the alignment of the hip, knee, and ankle and planning of the bony cuts during surgery. A scanogram also gives an idea of relative lengths of the limbs and can detect any extra-articular deformity in the femur and tibia. An overview impression of the hip and the ankle joints can also be assessed on a scanogram (Fig. 42-9).

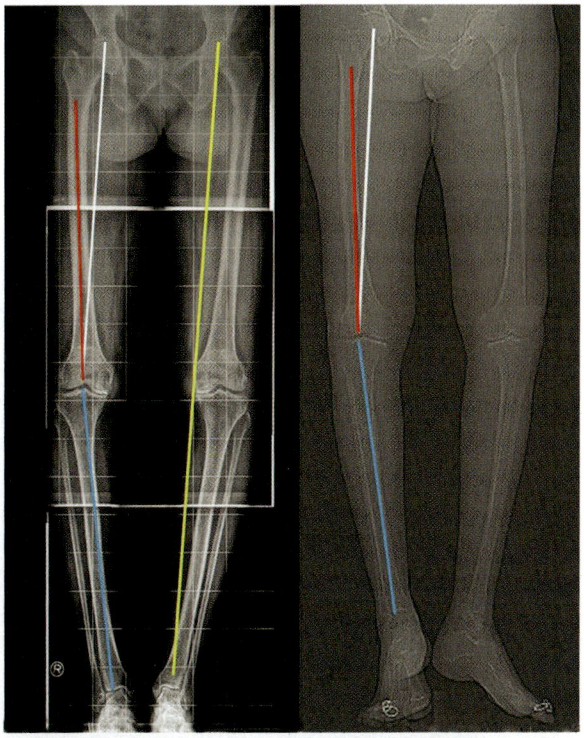

FIGURE 42-9. *Scanogram showing the mechanical femoral axis (white line), anatomic femoral axis (red line), and mechanical tibia axis (blue line). The yellow line represents the line joining the center of the hip to the center of the ankle and can be used to calculate the mechanical axis deviation. A CT scanogram can also be used for calculating the alignment axis.*

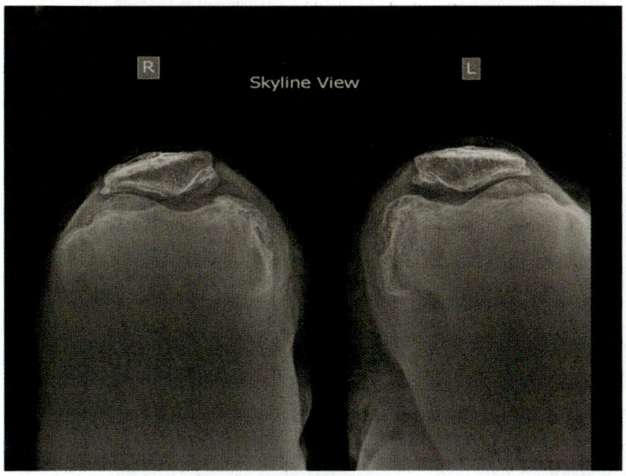

FIGURE 42-7. *Skyline (Merchant's view) showing the pathology of the patellofemoral joint.*

The mechanical axis of the leg consists of a line joining the center of the hip to the center of the knee and through the center of the ankle.[23-25] The anatomical axis of the femur is marked by joining the midpoints of two transverse lines drawn on the femoral diaphysis. The anatomical axis of the tibia is also drawn by the same methods by joining the midpoints of two transverse diaphyseal lines. There is a valgus angle of around 6° between the mechanical and anatomical axes of the femur.[26] This offset is due to developmental anatomical factors such as the length and angle of the femoral neck, width of the pelvis, femoral bowing, and femoral length. The mechanical axis is taken as a reference for correcting deformities and an alignment of 0° ± 3° is taken as the normal alignment. Thus the goal of preoperative knee arthroplasty is to bring the mechanical alignment of the limb to 0°. This helps in defining the angular deformities at the knee. If the line joining the center of the hip to the center of the knee is further extended, it will indicate the normal position of the tibia. Angular deformity can be quantified by measuring the angle between this extended line and the tibia axis. Another aspect of alignment is the knee joint line, which is normally parallel to the ground. Since the mechanical axis of the leg makes an angle of 3° with the central axis of the body, the knee joint line will be at an angle of 3° to the tibia axis and 10° to the femoral axis. Thus anatomically the distal femur is in 10° of valgus and the proximal tibia is in 3° of varus. Based on this concept, there are two different views on planning the bony cuts in total knee replacements: the classical (Fig. 42-10A) and the anatomical (Fig. 42-10B) methods.

In the anatomical method, reproduction of the anatomical joint line is the aim. Thus the distal femoral cut is made at 10° valgus and the proximal tibia cut at 3° varus. This will align the joint line perpendicular to the mechanical and weight is equally distributed across the joint. The drawback of this method is the difficulty in making accurate proximal tibia varus cuts. It is difficult for a surgeon during the learning curve to accurately cut the tibia in 3° of varus and in cases with excessive tibia varus complication such as component malalignment or subsidence. The classical method counters this problem by making the proximal tibia cut at a right angle to the tibia axis and the distal femoral cut at 5°–7° valgus. This again maintains the joint line perpendicular to the mechanical axis and parallel to the ground. The amount of the distal femoral valgus cut can be calculated from the preoperative scanogram by taking the angle between the mechanical and anatomical femoral axis.

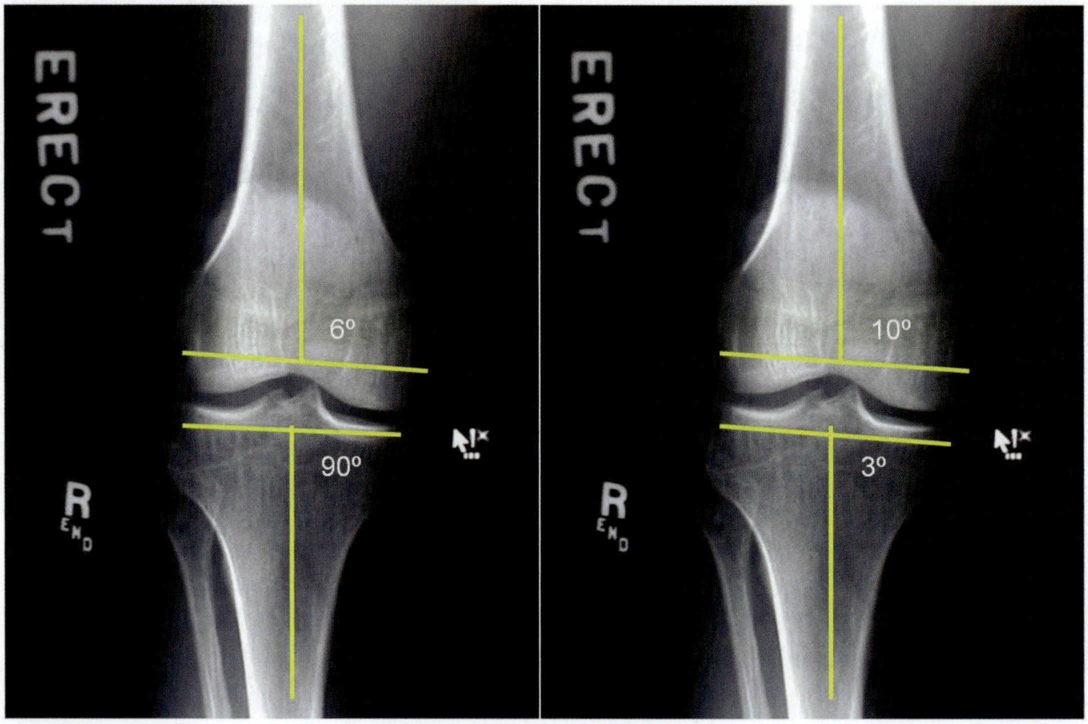

FIGURE 42-10. *Methods of deciding the distal femoral and proximal tibia cuts: (**A**) classical; (**B**) anatomical.*

The measurements of the angles and definition of the points to measure the angles need to be defined for accuracy and standardization of the process. The definition of the knee center varies. In cases in which there is no tibiofemoral subluxation, the midpoint between the medial and lateral joint line is taken as the knee center. This point defines the end point of the four axes: the femoral mechanical and anatomical axes and the tibia mechanical and anatomical axes. Further, for the femoral mechanical axis the proximal point is the center of the femoral head, whereas for the femoral anatomical axis the proximal point is the midpoint of a transverse line drawn at the upper border of the lesser trochanter. For the tibia, the distal point for both axes is the center of the ankle joint. In cases of frontal tibiofemoral subluxation, the medial and lateral boundaries of the knee joint are difficult to define and in this case the distal femoral and proximal tibial points are to be defined separately. The distal femoral point is conventionally taken as the midpoint of the intercondylar area, while the proximal medial tibial spine is taken as the proximal tibia point. After defining these points, further angular measurements can be done as described above.

The femoral neck shaft angle visible on scanograms can be a rough guide for the distal femoral cut. In cases with coxa vara, the distal femoral cut may be required to be more than the conventional 7°, while in cases with coxa valga, this cut may be required to made at a lesser angle. This is, however, an approximate measure and the actual measurement needs to be customized according to the mechanical axis in each patient.

Additional Views

Tunnel view

The tunnel view is taken with the patient in a prone position with the knee flexed by 45°. The beam is directed from posterior to anterior, oriented 45° to the horizontal.[27,28] This view can help the surgeon better visualize the intercondylar notch and its anatomy. The presence of loose bodies and osteophytes projecting from the femoral condyles can also be better visualized.

Semiflexed weight-bearing views (modified tunnel views)

This radiograph is taken with the patient standing with the knee flexed by 45° and the beam directed anterior to posterior, which helps in assessing the joint space narrowing due to degeneration of posterior femoral condyles.[29,30] The AP radiographs in these patients may appear minimally affected but semiflexed views can show definite joint space narrowing. The radiograph can also be taken at 30° of flexion to make the tibial plateau parallel to the floor to allow a better assessment of the joint space narrowing. This is indicated in cases in which the symptoms are disproportionate to the appearance on a standard AP radiograph.

Full-length tibia lateral

A full-length tibia lateral may be required to assess the posterior slope in cases with severe varus or valgus deformity or in cases with prior high tibia osteotomy. There are few methods described for measuring the posterior slope; however, the reference line of the sagittal mechanical axis is best described by joining the midpoint of the medial tibial plateau and the midpoint of the tibia plafond in the lateral view.[31] Knowledge of the angle of the posterior slope may help in deciding the amount of posterior slope required for the patient.

Kneeling view

The kneeling view is used to assess the rotational profile of the distal femur. The radiograph is taken with the patient kneeling on the radiographic plate and the beam directed at right angles to the tibia shaft. The radiograph shows the distal femur posterior condyles, and the posterior condylar axis and the trans-epicondylar axis can be measured. With these two axes the femoral condyle rotation can be judged. There is a good correlation between measurements on this view and CT scan measurements.[32] This view may be indicated in cases with posterior condylar bone loss.

Preoperative templating

Both analogue and digital templating have been found to have a high rate of anatomical variation and high inter- and intraobserver variation. More precise software with accuracy and reproducibility is desired.[33]

CROSS-SECTIONAL STUDIES

Both CT scan and MRI are indicated to better define the alignment in both the coronal and rotational planes. They are also utilized to develop three-dimensional reconstruction of the knee with the distal femur and the proximal tibia anatomy. With these details, patient-specific cutting guides and implants are now being made available for use.

Use of MRI in Preoperative Planning for Total Knee Replacement

Magnetic resonance imaging is the best tool for assessment of soft tissues and cartilage. However, the use of MRI in preoperative planning of total knee replacement (TKR) is still in the development phase. Primarily, it detects the severity of cartilage lesions and determines the integrity of the cruciate ligaments in case a cruciate-retaining prosthesis is planned. It can also be used in cases with vascular abnormality in terms of unequal distal pulses or any other arterovenous abnormalities. Delineating the anatomy of the popliteal vessels in these cases may be important to detect any anatomical variations that could become significant intraoperatively (Fig. 42-11).

Few studies have examined the use of MRI to measure coronal and rotational deformities of the limb as a part of preoperative planning. It has been found to be advantageous compared to a CT scan because no radiation is involved; however, there are problems with underestimation of deformities, especially in valgus knee deformities.[34] This may be related to the non-weight-bearing supine position in which MRI is taken. Comparison between CT scan, scanogram, and MRI scan have shown MRI to have good accuracy in determining leg axis and also rotational alignment. However, further studies will be required and cost-effectiveness needs to be studied. Underestimation of the mechanical axis deviation and leg length was also reported in a recent study.[35] MRI assessment of the condyle geometry in varus and valgus deformities showed deformed lateral femoral condyle in cases with valgus knee but no such condylar deformation in cases of varus knee.[36] Such accurate assessment of condylar geometry is also possible using MRI. However, the practical applicability of the use of MRI is still under consideration. MRI is expensive and thus should not be routinely ordered. It is contraindicated in patients with metal implants or pacemakers in situ. It is more time consuming than a standard radiograph and is difficult to do in claustrophobic patients.

Use of CT Scan in Preoperative Planning for TKR

Preoperative CT gives the surgeon an opportunity to plan preoperatively the surgical strategy for each patient individually. A customized three-dimensional surgical strategy based on the anatomical variation of the patient can be obtained.[37] It allows for accurate and precise surgical cuts and alignment[38-40] and identifies the anatomical landmarks in the knee and their relationship to each other (Fig. 42-12).

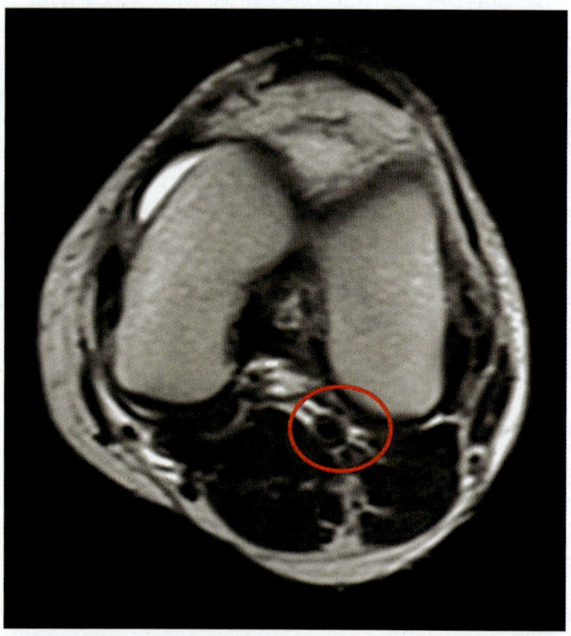

FIGURE 42-11. *Axial MRI of the distal femur can be done to assess the anatomy of the neurovascular structures.*

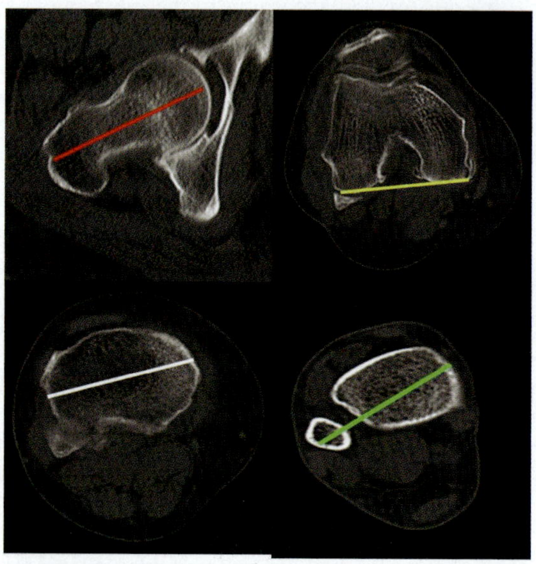

FIGURE 42-12. *Cross-sectional CT scan. Axial line through the neck of femur (red) and line tangential to the posterior femoral condyle (yellow) denote the femoral rotation. The diagonal line across the proximal tibia (white) and the distal tibiofibular axis (green) quantify the tibial torsion.*

CT scanning is an accurate imaging modality for studying the bone morphology. It is especially useful in complex cases in which there is a bone defect or when there is a patellofemoral incongruity or for distal femoral rotational alignment.[41] It helps in the anteroposterior orientation of the tibia and in determining the distal femoral resection angle in intramedullary instrumentation.[42] This is critical in avoiding patellar instability and is the recommended and most accurate method for determining the rotational profile of distal femur.[43-45] The bone–implant interface can be customized preoperatively and thus the anatomical abnormalities can also be accounted for preoperatively. CT scanograms are available (Fig. 42-9); however, most machines require the patients to lie down, thus giving a non-weight-bearing scanogram. CT scan is expensive and thus should not be routinely ordered. It is more time consuming than a standard radiograph and has a higher risk of radiation exposure.

CONCLUSION

Plain radiography is required for routine preoperative planning of total knee arthroplasty, where a good assessment of frontal plane limb alignment can be made along with an assessment of severity of the pathology. Special views and cross-sectional studies such as CT and MRI are needed in special situations. Patient-specific planning for knee arthroplasty is still in the development phase and is not widely available.

PEARLS AND PITFALLS

The following are some pearls and pitfalls of preoperative planning:

1. Preoperative planning in total knee replacement is as important as in total hip replacement and is an essential part of a successful surgery.
2. Positioning and standardization of the radiographs are a must for accurate and reproducible preoperative planning.
3. Preoperative imaging helps in planning the implant and other inventories such as augments and extension rods.
4. Stress radiographs help in assessing the amount of soft tissue release required and also in quantifying the bone defect.
5. Quality of bone may influence the choice of implant with metal-backed implants preferred in osteoporotic bones.
6. Scanograms are essential to diagnose extra-articular deformities.
7. The femoral neck shaft angle may help as a rough guide to the distal femoral cut with coxa vara requiring more distal femoral cut angulation than coxa valga.

SUGGESTED READING

Munzinger UK, Boldt JG, Keblish PA, eds. *Primary Knee Arthroplasty.* New York: Springer; 2004.

Scott WN, ed. *Insall & Scott Surgery of the Knee.* 4th ed. Philadelphia, PA: Churchill Livingstone Elsevier; 2006.

Scuderi GR, Tria AJ Jr, eds. *Surgical Techniques in Total Knee Arthroplasty.* New York: Springer; 2002.

REFERENCES

1. Hsu HP, Garg A, Walker PS, et al. Effect of knee component alignment on tibial load distribution with clinical correlation. *Clin Orthop Relat Res.* 1989; 248:135-144.
2. Sharkey PF, Hozack WJ, Rothman RH, et al. Insall Award paper. Why are total knee arthroplasties failing today? *Clin Orthop Relat Res.* 2002;404:7-13.
3. Bargren JH, Blaha JD, Freeman MAR. Alignment in total knee arthroplasty. *Clin Orthop Relat Res.* 1983; 173:178.
4. Hood RW, Vanni M, Insall JN. The correction of knee alignment in 225 consecutive total condylar knee replacements. *Clin Orthop Relat Res.* 1981; 160:94.
5. Berend ME, Ritter MA, Meding JB, et al. Tibial component failure mechanisms in total knee arthroplasty. *Clin Orthop Relat Res.* 2004;428:26-34.
6. Collier MB, Engh CA Jr, McAuley JP, et al. Factors associated with the loss of thickness of polyethylene tibial bearings after knee arthroplasty. *J Bone Joint Surg Am.* 2007;89:1306-1314.
7. Fang DM, Ritter MA, Davis KE. Coronal alignment in total knee arthroplasty: just how important is it? *J Arthroplasty.* 2009;24(6 suppl):39-43.

8. Ritter MA, Faris PM, Keating EM, et al. Postoperative alignment of total knee replacement. Its effect on survival. *Clin Orthop Relat Res.* 1994;299:153-156.
9. Hsu HP, Garg A, Walker PS, et al. Effect of knee component alignment on tibial load distribution with clinical correlation. *Clin Orthop Relat Res.* 1989;248: 135-144.
10. Hungerford DS, Kenna RV. Preliminary experience with a total knee prosthesis with porous coating used without cement. *Clin Orthop Relat Res.* 1983;176:95-107.
11. Green GV, Berend KR, Berend ME, et al. The effects of varus tibial alignment on proximal tibial surface strain in total knee arthroplasty: the posteromedial hot spot. *J Arthroplasty.* 2002;17(8):1033-1039.
12. Ritter MA, Faris PM, Keating EM, et al. Postoperative alignment of total knee replacement. Its effect on survival. *Clin Orthop Relat Res.* 1994;299:153-156.
13. Leach RE, Gregg T, Siber FJ. Weight-bearing radiography in osteoarthritis of the knee. *Radiology.* 1970;97(2):265-268.
14. Adams ME, Wallace CJ. Quantitative imaging of osteoarthritis. *Semin Arthritis Rheum.* 1991;20(6 suppl 2):26-39.
15. Ahlbäck S. Osteoarthrosis of the knee. A radiographic investigation. *Acta Radiol Diagn (Stockh).* 1968;suppl 277:7-72.
16. Rosenberg TD, Paulos LE, Parker RD, et al. The forty-five-degree posteroanterior flexion weight-bearing radiograph of the knee. *J Bone Joint Surg Am.* 1988;70(10):1479-1483.
17. Robbins GM, Masri BA, Garbuz DS, et al. Preoperative planning to prevent instability in total knee arthroplasty. *Orthop Clin North Am.* 2001;32(4):611-626, viii.
18. Insall J, Salvati E. Patella position in the normal knee joint. *Radiology.* 1971;101(1):101-104.
19. Ghelman B, Hodge JC. Imaging of the patellofemoral joint. *Orthop Clin North Am.* 1992;23(4):523-543.
20. Merchant AC, Mercer RL, Jacobsen RH, et al. Roentgenographic analysis of patellofemoral congruence. *J Bone Joint Surg Am.* 1974;56(7):1391-1396.
21. Jones AC, Ledingham J, McAlindon T, et al. Radiographic assessment of patellofemoral osteoarthritis. *Ann Rheum Dis.* 1993;52(9):655–658.
22. Fulkerson JP. Imaging of the patellofemoral joint. In: *Disorders of the Patellofemoral Joint.* 4th ed. Baltimore, MD: Williams & Wilkins; 1997:73-104.
23. Cooke TD, Li J, Scudamore RA. Radiographic assessment of bony contributions to knee deformity. *Orthop Clin North Am.* 1994;25(3):387-393.
24. Paley D, Tetsworth K. Mechanical axis deviation of the lower limbs. Preoperative planning of multiapical frontal plane angular and bowing deformities of the femur and tibia. *Clin Orthop Relat Res.* 1992;280:65-71.
25. Petersen TL, Engh GA. Radiographic assessment of knee alignment after total knee arthroplasty. *J Arthroplasty.* 1988;3(1):67-72.
26. Oguz O. Measurement and relationship of the inclination angle, Alsberg angle and the angle between the anatomical and mechanical axes of the femur in males. *Surg Radiol Anat.* 1996;18(1):29-31.
27. Camp JD, Coventry MB. Use of special views in roentgenography of the knee joint. *US Naval Med Bull.* 1944;42:56.
28. Holmblad EC. Postero-anterior x-ray view of knee in flexion. *JAMA.* 1937;9:1196-1197.
29. Buckland-Wright JC, Macfarlane DG, Jasani MK, et al. Quantitative microfocal radiographic assessment of osteoarthritis of the knee from weight bearing tunnel and semiflexed standing views. *J Rheumatol.* 1994;21(9):1734-1741.
30. Resnick D, Vint V. The "tunnel" view in assessment of cartilage loss in osteoarthritis of the knee. *Radiology.* 1980;137(2):547-548.
31. Yoo JH, Chang CB, Shin KS, et al. Anatomical references to assess the posterior tibial slope in total knee arthroplasty: a comparison of 5 anatomical axes. *J Arthroplasty.* 2008;23(4):586-592.
32. Takai S, Yoshino N, Isshiki T, et al. Kneeling view: a new roentgenographic technique to assess rotational deformity and alignment of the distal femur. *J Arthroplasty.* 2003;18(4):478-483.
33. Howcroft DW, Fehily MJ, Peck C, et al. The role of preoperative templating in total knee arthroplasty: comparison of three prostheses. *Knee.* 2006;13(6): 427-429.
34. Hinterwimmer S, Graichen H, Vogl TJ, et al. An MRI-based technique for assessment of lower extremity deformities-reproducibility, accuracy, and clinical application. *Eur Radiol.* 2008;18(7):1497-1505.
35. Liodakis E, Kenawey M, Doxastaki I, et al. Upright MRI measurement of mechanical axis and frontal plane alignment as a new technique: a comparative study with weight bearing full length radiographs. *Skeletal Radiol.* 2011;40(7):885-889.

36. Matsuda S, Miura H, Nagamine R, et al. Anatomical analysis of the femoral condyle in normal and osteoarthritic knees. *J Orthop Res.* 2004;22(1):104-109.
37. Harrysson OL, Hosni YA, Nayfeh JF. Custom-designed orthopedic implants evaluated using finite element analysis of patient-specific computed tomography data: femoral-component case study. *BMC Musculoskelet Disord.* 2007;8:91.
38. Chauhan SK, Clark GW, Lloyd S, et al. Computer-assisted total knee replacement. A controlled cadaver study using a multi-parameter quantitative CT assessment of alignment (the Perth CT Protocol). *J Bone Joint Surg Br.* 2004;86(6):818–823.
39. Chiu KY, Yau WP, Ng TP, et al. The accuracy of bextramedullary guides for tibial component placement in total knee arthroplasty. *Int Orthop.* 2008;32:467–471.
40. Jonsson B, Astrom J. Alignment and long-term clinical results of a semiconstrained knee prosthesis. *Clin Orthop Relat Res.* 1988;226:124–128.
41. Uslu MM, Ozsar B, Cirpar M, et al. Computerized tomography scout view for determining distal femoral resection angle in intramedullary instrumentation of total knee arthroplasty. *Knee Surg Sports Traumatol Arthrosc.* 2007;15(1):78-82.
42. Cates HE, Ritter MA, Keating EM, et al. Intramedullary versus extramedullary femoral alignment systems in total knee. *Clin Orthop Relat Res.* 1993;286:32–39.
43. Victor J. Rotational alignment of the distal femur: a literature review. *Orthop Traumatol Surg Res.* 2009;95(5):365-372.
44. Yau WP, Chiu KY, Tang WM. How precise is the determination of rotational alignment of the femoral prosthesis in total knee arthroplasty?: an in vivo study. *J Arthroplasty.* 2007;22(7):1042-1048.
45. Victor J, Van Doninck D, Labey L, et al. How precise can bony landmarks be determined on a CT scan of the knee? *Knee.* 2009;16(5):358-365.

43 Imaging of the Patellofemoral Joint

Ricardo Sousa and Marta Massada

The correct physiologic function of the patellofemoral (PF) joint depends on a unique coordination of static, ligamentous and osseous, and dynamic or neuromuscular elements. Many factors have been thought to contribute to abnormal pathomechanics that lead to abnormal forces across the patella. Patella alta, trochlea dysplasia, increased quadriceps or Q angle, weakened or hypoplastic vastus medialis oblique, contracted lateral retinaculum, and absent or redundant medial patellofemoral ligament have all been implicated in patellar instability and subsequent pain and even secondary degenerative changes. Patellofemoral arthritis is present, either isolated or in combination with the tibiofemoral joint, in 49% of all cases of knee osteoarthritis.[1] It is therefore important to be able to accurately choose and interpret the appropriate imaging modality that best suits each case.

PLAIN RADIOGRAPHS

Plain X-rays are always the first step when studying any painful knee. Although it does not provide information specifically on the PF joint, the anteroposterior view should always be ordered because it offers valuable information. The varus-valgus alignment is very important because it closely relates to patellar instability or progression of PF osteoarthritis.[2] Many conditions such as tibiofemoral arthritis, loose bodies, and patella bipartite can also become obvious.

Lateral View

A reliable lateral view should be taken while weight bearing with at least 30º knee flexion and perfect superimposition of the posterior femoral condyles. This much flexion is needed to tension the patellar tendon, thus allowing correct measurement of patellar height.[3] Femoral condyle superimposition is absolutely crucial for studying the trochlea.[4] The analysis of patellofemoral as well as femorotibial joint line thickness is possible and accurate but much more information can be drawn from this simple radiograph, such as anterior or posterior tibial translation, tibial slope, and so forth.[5]

Trochlea configuration is one of the major points of interest of the lateral view. The sulcus line follows the roof of the intercondylar notch or Blumensaat line and is normally posterior to the condylar line throughout the entire trochlea. Dejour et al[6] were the first to describe the "crossing sign" as the crossing of the sulcus line and the lateral condyle, meaning that the trochlea is flat. This sign is found in 96% of the population with a history of patellar dislocation and in only 3% of the control population.[4,6] Other important measurements were the deepness of the trochlea, measured as the distance between the sulcus and the lateral condyle at different angles, and the bump, which was defined as the distance between the highest point of the trochlea and a line tangent to the distal anterior femoral cortex. Accordingly, the original classification graded the dysplasia in three types, depending on the level of the crossing sign: the lower the sign, the greater the dysplasia.[6] It was demonstrated that this classification suffered from poor interobserver reproducibility[7] and a new four-type classification was proposed in 1998 that combined radiographic and computed tomography (CT) scans, features that are discussed later in the chapter.[8] Two new radiographic signs were added to the crossing sign: the supratrochlear spur and the double contour. The first represents the global prominence of the trochlea and acts as a launching ramp of the patella when it is trying to engage the trochlea. The latter is the radiographic line ending below the crossing sign and represents the subchondral condensation of the hypoplasic medial facet.

Patellar tilt can also be appreciated in the lateral view as described by Maldague and Malghem.[9,10] Position 1 or normal tilt is defined as showing the lateral facet line anterior to the patellar crest line. Mild tilt or position 2 shows both lines on the same level and position 3 or major tilt shows an inversion with the patellar crest being anterior to the lateral facet. Patellar shape is classified according to Grelsamer et al.[11] They showed that the ratio between the length of the patella and the length of its articular surface is not constant. Most patients exhibit a ratio between 1.2 and 1.5 and are classified as type I. Those exhibiting a ratio over 1.5 who have a long, not articulating inferior pole are type II and those whose inferior pole is short and have a ratio under 1.2 are type III. Interestingly, Grelsamer et al[11] found a higher prevalence of these latter two types in the group of patients with patellofemoral problems. This anatomical variant has implications in some patellar height indices.

Patella alta, an abnormally high patella, is associated with instability, whereas patella baja, an abnormally low patella, can be associated with anterior knee pain and limitation of knee flexion, essentially as a complication of knee surgery. Several radiographic techniques have been described for measuring patellar height and they can be divided into two groups: those relating the position of the patella to the femur and those that relate it to the tibia. The most commonly used indices in the literature all describe patellar height as a relation to some reference point in the tibia.

The Insall-Salvati index was first described in 1971 and measures the ratio between the length of the patellar tendon and the longest sagittal axis of the patella.[12] It is an index that is easy to measure and does not require a fixed flexion angle and the normal value interval 1.0 ± 0.2 is easily remembered. However, a patellar morphology Grelsamer type II may leave a patella alta undiagnosed. The recognition that the distal not articulating pole of the patella is not a good landmark (anatomically and physiologically the position of the articular surface is the relevant factor) led to a modification of this index by Grelsamer in 1992. As such, patellar height is calculated as the length of the patellar tendon divided by the length of the articular surface of the patella.[13] The cutoff point to define patella alta in this modified Insall-Salvati index was defined as 2.[13] Both these indices share some disadvantages. The distance of the tibial tubercle to the tibial plateau is not standard[14] and measurement is not affected by surgery, namely, tibial tubercle transfer (TTT) to a more distal or proximal position. Recognizing these limitations, Blackburne and Peel proposed a new index in 1977.[14] This index is expressed as the ratio of the length of the perpendicular line drawn from the inferior point of the patella articular surface to the tangent of the tibial plateau and the length of the entire articular surface of the patella. A normal ratio was defined as 0.8, patella baja as lower than 0.5, and patella alta as greater than 1.0. This index reflects changes after TTT but it is influenced by tibial slope. The bigger the slope the shorter the perpendicular line to the tangent of the tibial slope will be, which may leave a patella alta undetected.[13] Probably the most commonly used index in Europe was described in 1982 in France.[15] The Caton-Deschamps index is the ratio of the distance from the lower edge of the articular surface of the patella to the anterosuperior angle of the tibia outline to the length of the articular surface of the patella. A ratio smaller than 0.6 and greater than 1.2 is classified as patella baja and patella alta, respectively.[15] A major advantage of this index is that it may easily be used for determining the amount of correction needed before TTT surgery as well as for measuring changes after high tibial osteotomy. Like all other indices that use the patellar articular surface as a reference, this index may be inaccurate in certain patellae with short patellar surfaces (Fig. 43-1).[16]

Although they are less commonly used, femoral references indices are physiologically more appropriate. It

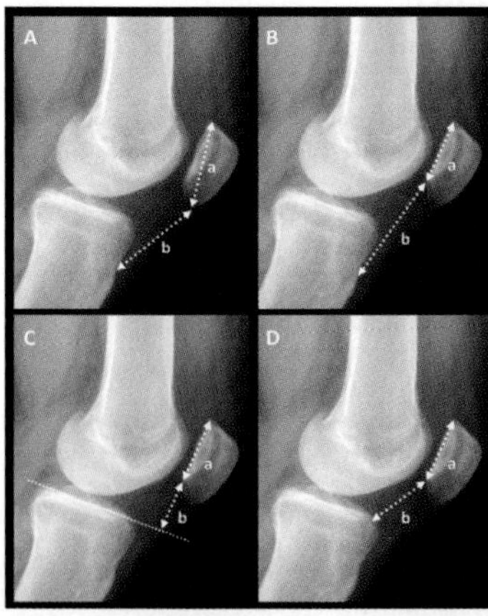

Index	Patella alta	Patella baja
Insall-Salvati	<0.8	>1.2
Modified Insall-Salvati	not defined	>2
Blackburne and Peel	<0.5	>1.0
Caton-Deschamps	<0.6	>1.2

FIGURE 43-1. *Patellar height indices (b/a): (**A**) Insall-Salvati index; (**B**) Insall-Salvati modified by Grelsamer; (**C**) Blackburne and Peel; (**D**) Caton-Deschamps.*

makes sense that the real focus should lie in the relation between the patellar articular surface and the trochlea. Bernageau[17] was one of the first to recognize it and describe patellar height as the distance between the superior line of the trochlea and the inferior edge of the articular surface of the patella with the quadriceps contracted. However, the necessary landmarks are often difficult to identify and contraction of the quadriceps is difficult to ascertain. More recently, magnetic resonance imaging (MRI) has been used to overcome these issues.[18] It provides exact articular correlation not affected by patella or trochlea osseous morphotypes. The real degree of relaxation or contraction of the quadriceps is nevertheless not possible to control because this technique is performed with the knee in extension. There are countless other techniques described in the literature indicating that a perfect index has not yet been found.[19] Some of them are but small variants of the described indices, while many others use some type of different reference. Regardless of the specific technique chosen, it is highly advisable to use an identified and reproducible index.

Axial View

Several techniques of obtaining axial radiographs of the patella have been described over the years.[20-23] They have certain major drawbacks that hamper their usefulness: some require exaggerated flexion of the knee drawing the patella into the distal femoral groove and failing to show the joint in slight to moderate flexion where most subluxation occurs, others offer distorted images as the X-ray beam strikes the film at 45° angles, and others fail to control femoral rotation.

Two major techniques gained worldwide acceptance for the amount of information they offer as well as reproducibility and reliability. In the Merchant view,[23] the patient lies supine on the table with the knees flexed over the end. The knees are slightly elevated to keep the femora horizontal and parallel with the table and the legs are strapped together at the calf to control rotation. The authors found that a 45° knee flexion was the position of least flexion which produced consistently satisfactory results, but current recommendations point toward lesser angles such as 30°.[24] The X-ray beam is directed caudally, requiring a cassette holder to place the film below the knees resting at the shins. In the Laurin view,[25] the patient is supine with a simple support or cushion under the knees to hold them in 20° flexion where the patella subluxates laterally as it enters the proximal segment of the femoral groove. The X-ray beam is directed cephalad almost parallel to the tibial crest and the proximal part of the patellofemoral joint. The patient holds the film and it is crucial that he or she is instructed to keep it perpendicular to the X-ray beam to avoid distortion. Both techniques target both knees simultaneously and require the quadriceps muscle to be relaxed.

Merchant[23] originally defined two measurements. The sulcus angle, first described by Brattström,[26] is defined by the highest points on the medial and lateral femoral condyles and the lowest point of the intercondylar sulcus. In asymptomatic knees it is approximately 138° (range 126°–150°).[23] The congruence angle is then assessed to measure patellar subluxation or lateral displacement. A line bisecting the sulcus angle is used as the reference or zero line. A second line is drawn from the apex of the sulcus angle to the lowest point on the articular ridge of the patella. The angle between these two lines is the congruence angle. If the patellar ridge is lateral to the zero line, the angle is positive; if it is medial, the angle is negative. In the original Merchant study,[23] the mean value was –6° with a standard deviation of 11°, thereby determining a congruence angle over +16° as abnormal. A few years later, Maldague and Malghem[27] compared the traditional Merchant view with another one taken at 30° flexion and passive external rotation of the foot. In a group of 27 pathologic joints, the congruence angle averaged +1.5° in the Merchant and +26.7° and +10.3° in the 30° flexion view with or without forced external rotation of the foot, respectively. Subluxation was demonstrated in 100% using this new technique versus 26% with the traditional one. Others have used direct lateral and medial stress to the patella for the measurement of force displacement relationships in the PF joint and for the demonstration of patellofemoral instability (Fig. 43- 2).[28]

In order to quantitatively measure patellar tilt, Laurin[25,29] originally proposed two methods. The lateral patellofemoral angle subtended as the angle between a line that joins the summits of both femoral condyles and a line drawn through the limits of the lateral patellar facet. In their original work, Laurin et al[25] found that 97 of 100 normal control individuals had a laterally open patellofemoral angle, while 24 of the 30 patients with patella subluxation had parallel lines and the remaining six presented with a medially open lateral patellofemoral angle. The same authors[29] also proposed measuring patellar tilt as the patellofemoral index, the ratio of thickness of the medial joint space and the lateral joint, in order to detect smaller tilts. They advocate that in a normal knee this index is under 1.6, meaning the medial joint space is slightly thicker than the lateral, and in patients with patellar instability this index is over 1.6 in 97% of the cases.[29] A different method of appreciating patellar tilt was proposed by Grelsamer et al[30] in 1993. Radiographs are taken according to Merchant except the knee is flexed 30° and not 45°. Tilt is measured by drawing a line from one corner of the patella to the other and taking the lower edge of the radiograph as a horizontal reference. It is therefore

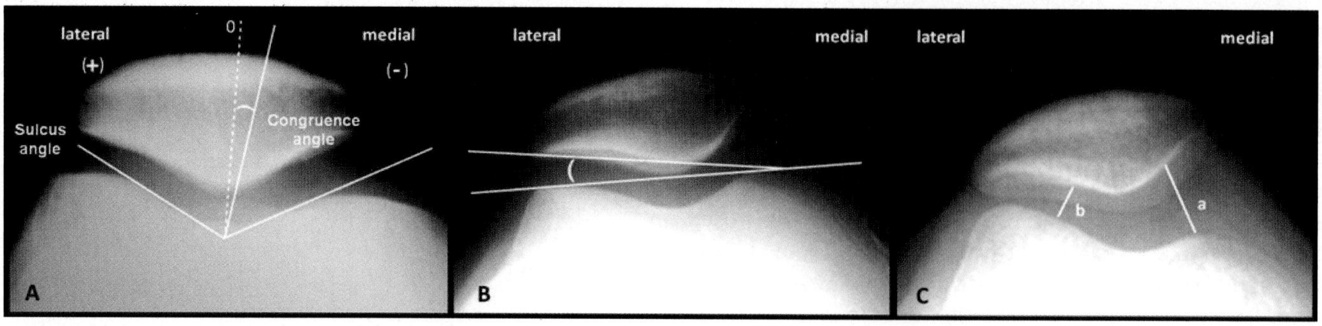

FIGURE 43-2. *Axial radiographs. (**A**) Merchant view with sulcus angle and congruence angle measurement; (**B**) Laurin view with lateral patellofemoral angle measurement; (**C**) Laurin view with patellofemoral index (a/b) measurement; normal value is <1.6.*

crucial that the cassette is held absolutely parallel to the ground and, since it is not an anatomical reference line, it is influenced by leg rotation that should therefore be neutral with the foot pointing directly upwards. Tilting of over 5° was taken to be the limit of normal being present in 85% of patients with signs and symptoms suggesting patellar malalignment but only 8% of the control patients. A significant advantage of using this technique in the total knee arthroplasty context is that it is reproducible even after patellar resurfacing. Patellofemoral osteoarthritis (OA) is best assessed in the axial view.[31,32] Ahlbäck's traditional OA grading system has been used in studies concerning the patellofemoral joint but this system was originally developed for the tibiofemoral joint.[33,34] Iwano et al[35] observed that the lateral side is usually involved and produced a simple staging system for lateral patellofemoral arthritis (Fig. 43-3). Nevertheless, it has been demonstrated that radiographic severity and apparent location of cartilage lesions in patients undergoing total knee arthroplasty for advanced osteoarthritis do not correlate well with real lesion severity and location.[36] It is important to consider this when the results of radiographic assessments alone are being considered for selecting a treatment option. More accurate cartilage diagnostic modalities (discussed later in this chapter) may be warranted if detailed information of the PF joint is required.

Other information can also be observed from the axial view, such as patellar shape, bipartite patella, or even a medial bone fragment suggestive of patellar dislocation. Wiberg[20] classified patellar shape in three types. Baumgartl[37] subsequently described a fourth type, an extreme and rare case of an inexistent medial facet. In the normal population, a type A patella is present in 16.1% of subjects, a type B in 80%, and a type C in 12.9%.[38] In a recent series of 105 patients with objective patellar instability, type A

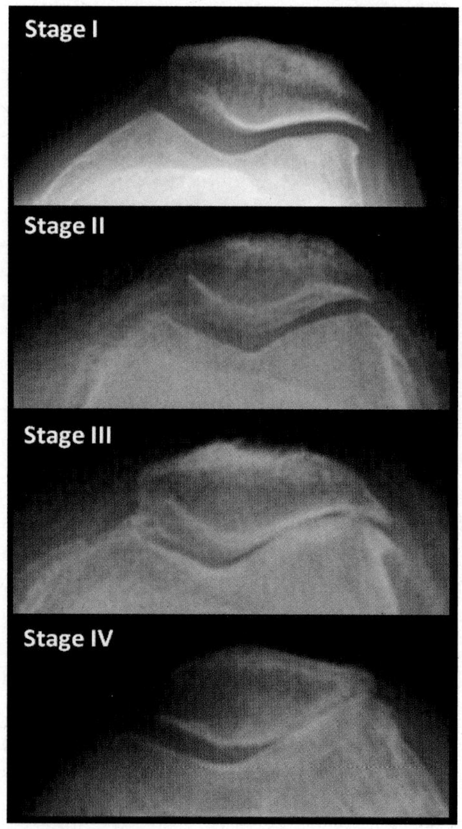

FIGURE 43-3. *Iwano's patellofemoral joint arthritis staging system. Stage I (mild OA): joint space of at least 3 mm. Stage II (moderate OA): joint space under 3 mm but no bone contact. Stage III (severe OA): bone contact less than one quarter of the surface. Stage IV (very severe OA): joint surfaces entirely touching each other.*

patella was present in 15.7% of cases, type B in 60.7%, and type C in 23.6%.[39] In this study the authors found a statistically significant association between patellar shape and patellar tilt: the more the patella is tilted, the more the patella is dysplastic (Fig. 43-4).[39] This may be due to altered biomechanics leading to increased stresses on the lateral facet and decreased stresses on the medial facet, causing insufficient development of the medial facet during growth. They also found a correlation between patellar shape type C and trochlear dysplasia grade 3.[39]

CROSS-SECTIONAL

Computed Tomograhpy

Computed tomography scanning offers the possibility of acquiring sequential axial cross-sectional images of the knee in the range of full extension to any degree of flexion using the midtransverse patella as a stable plane of reference. This has proved to be a significant advantage over axial plain radiographs of the PF joint, especially in those cases of mild patellar maltracking and alignment that can only be observed the first 20º of flexion.[40] CT additionally offers the possibility of using the posterior femoral condyles as a reference point, which has proved to be anatomically more reliable than the anterior trochlea.[41] It also allows image superimposition avoiding overlap and distortion, thus allowing the precise measurement of several different parameters. Many of the same principles used in interpreting plain radiographs, such as patellar height, sulcus, and congruence angles and even the lateral patellofemoral angle, may be extrapolated into CT scan images. There are nonetheless a few specific criteria that should be appreciated.

The tibial tubercle-trochlear groove distance (TT-TG) was first described by Goutallier and coworkers[42] using an axial radiograph at 30º flexion but gained more popularity after Henry Dejour[4] described a CT scan measurement technique in full extension. It is a measure of the coronal alignment of the extensor mechanism and has proved to be more accurate than the Q angle.[43] Two specific cuts are necessary. The first or reference cut is through the proximal trochlea and a line marking the deepest point of the trochlear groove is perpendicularly projected onto a line tangential to both posterior condyles. The second cut passes through the proximal part of the tibial tubercle and its central point is also projected onto the same line. Both cuts are then superimposed and the distance between the lines is measured. Dejour found a significant difference between a normal and unstable PF joint and defined a distance greater than 20 mm as pathological and present in 56% of patellar dislocation population and only 3% of normal knees (Fig. 43-5).[4]

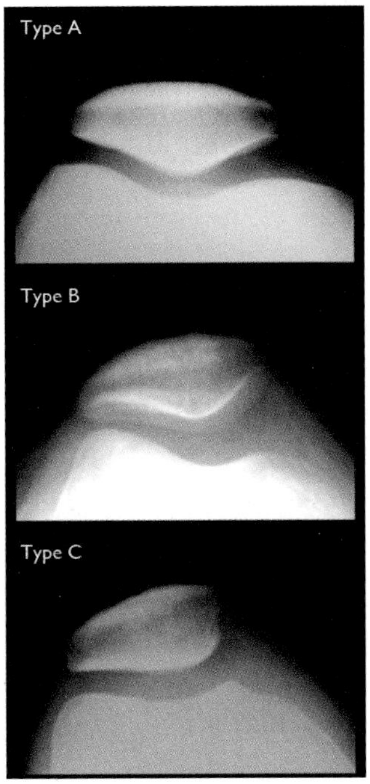

FIGURE 43-4. *Wiberg's patellar shape classification. Type A: medial and lateral facets are both concave and roughly equivalent in size. Type B: smaller medial facet with a flat or concave surface. Type C: very small, nearly inexistent medial facet describing a right angle with the lateral facet.*

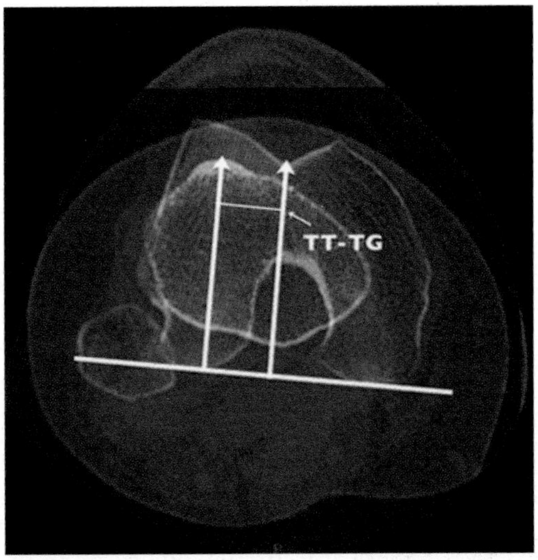

FIGURE 43-5. *CT scan with TT-TG measurement. Two cuts are superimposed in this image. The first trough of the proximal trochlea shows a line projecting from the deepest point of the trochlear groove to the posterior condylar line. The second shows a line projecting from the tibial tubercle. The distance between these lines is the value of the tibial tubercle-trochlear groove.*

Patellar tilt is also measured using the same posterior condylar line determined for TT-TG measurement as reference. A second line through the larger axis of the patella is drawn and the angle between them measures the tilt. Eighty-three percent of the patellar dislocation group has a tilt greater than 20º compared to 3% in the healthy population.[4,6] The accuracy of this measurement can be improved if one adopts the same threshold for diagnosis and uses the mean tilt of two measurements performed during relaxed and contraction of the quadriceps.[4] The relevance of measurements performed during quadriceps contraction to increase the accuracy of instability diagnosis has been extensively demonstrated.[44,45]

Trochlear analysis adds information to X-rays and helps to grade dysplasia and analyze the supratrochlear area as was proposed by David Dejour (Fig. 43-6).[8] The inclination of the lateral facet can also be measured and it shows a statistically significant difference between dysplasic and control individuals with a threshold that was determined to be 11º.[46] Although this study was performed using MRI, it has been shown that when the trochlea is flat or convex there is no mismatch between bone and cartilage.[47] The congruence angle can and should be measured in the first degrees of flexion. Schutzer et al[48] found that in a healthy PF joint the patella engages the trochlea by 10° to 20° of knee flexion. A normal congruence angle should therefore be zero or even slightly negative at this point, reflecting a centered or slightly medial patella.[49] Other secondary features, such as femoral anteversion and external tibial torsion, can also be measured if the scan is extended to the hip to determine the femoral neck axis and to the ankle to determine the bimalleolar axis, respectively.

One of the main limitations of the CT scan is its lack of ability to accurately evaluate the articular cartilage and other intra-articular soft tissue disorders. CT arthrography may be helpful in addressing this issue. In double-contrast arthrography of the knee, CT examination is performed after injection of a small amount of intra-articular contrast and air, to separate the articular cartilage from the surrounding soft tissues.[50] Though initially it was advocated that this technique had an excellent diagnostic accuracy for cartilage lesions[51] and even meniscal tears,[52] MRI (especially MR arthrography) has since been shown to be superior in detecting small cartilage lesions,[53-55] making it the imaging gold standard. Nevertheless, CT arthrography is still of real value where MRI is not available or contraindicated.

The advent of spiral scanning has made possible continuous data acquisition during active flexion and extension of the knee to give kinematic CT imaging. After obtaining and processing these images in different degrees of flexion, a cine loop of knee motion can be produced. This has been advocated as the most accurate method for evaluating patellofemoral tracking, allowing the identification of a variety of different tracking patterns that are not noted using standard radiographs.[56] However, kinetic imaging has been more extensively studied with the use of MRI.

Magnetic Resonance Imaging

Although MRI also allows measurement of several instability parameters described earlier, it has been considered more useful in evaluating the cartilage status or dynamic PF tracking abnormalities. The absence of ionizing radiation and the superior soft tissue contrast and multiplanar capabilities are other major advantages because it offers the ability to rule out associated cartilaginous and soft tissue derangements of the knee, thus helping to improve diagnostic accuracy in vague symptomatic presentations. Following acute patellar dislocation, for instance, effusion, medial patellofemoral ligament injury, and characteristic bone edema revealing lateral femoral condyle and medial patella contusions can be observed and their respective pattern may depend on trochlear dysplasia, patellar height, and TT-TG distance.[57] It can also be used to visualize the level of the distal insertion of the vastus medialis muscle that has been shown to be significantly more proximal in patients with patellar dislocations than in normal subjects.[58]

When using MRI to evaluate the aforementioned instability parameters (trochlear dysplasia, patellar tilt, TT-TG distance, etc), one must be careful in the interpretation because it has been extensively shown that the measurements taken at the cartilage level may greatly differ from those taken at the subchondral bone level as they have been originally defined in radiographs and CT scans.[47,59,60] Although this might support the claim that MRI offers more precise measurements, at this time there are no studies to define and validate these new threshold values in clinical practice.

MRI is currently the best technique to identify cartilage damage.[53-55] Degenerative disease may be identified on MRI in the early stage as slight changes on the morphology of cartilage contour or intrachondral changes in signal intensity or in the advanced stage as loss of thickness or complete cartilage loss usually seen in opposite surfaces. Traumatic injuries are also well recognized, even those as small as 0.8 mm and even without use of contrast material.[54] MR chondral injury classification is based on arthroscopic grading systems originally proposed by Outerbridge[61] and Noyes[62] and focus on recognition of defects with regions of cartilage loss and gross morphologic alteration. As in many other systems, MR classification of chondral abnormalities is from grade 0 (normal and intact cartilage) to IV (full-thickness cartilage loss).

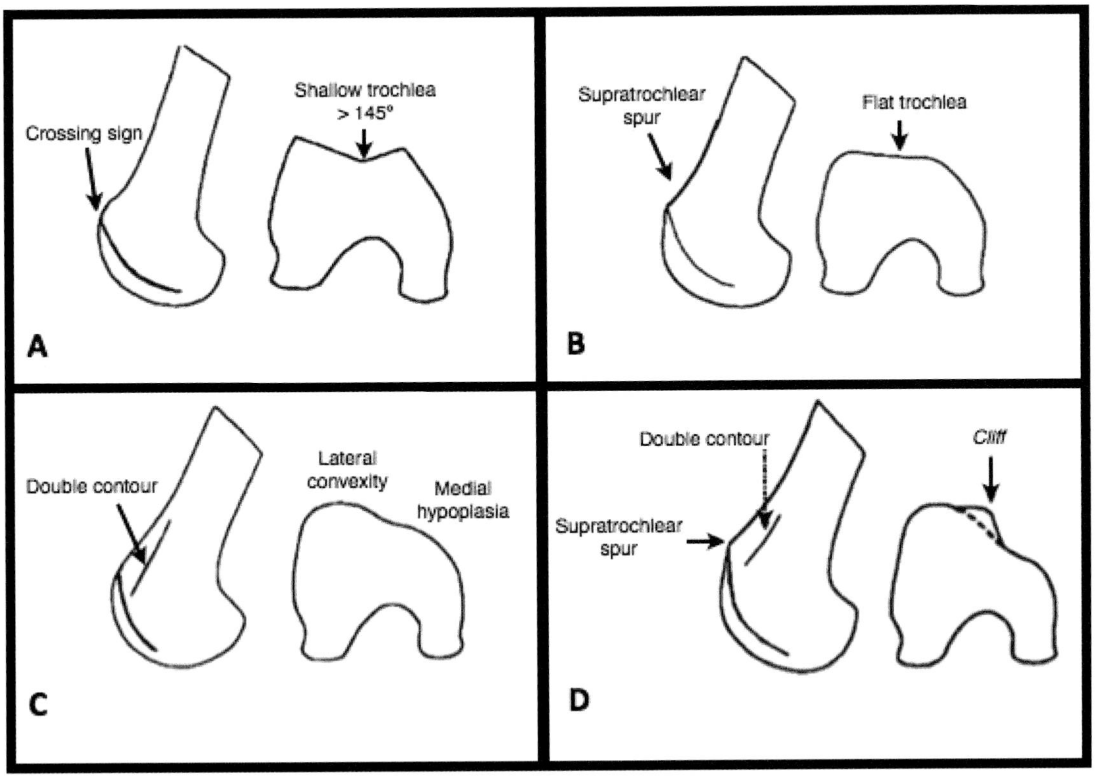

FIGURE 43-6. *Dejour trochlear dysplasia classification. (**A–D**) In each type on the left are schematics of lateral X-ray findings and on the right are schematics of the findings for the CT axial cut through the trochlea. (Adapted with permission from Dejour D, Le Coultre B. Osteotomies in patello-femoral instabilities. Sports Med Arthrosc. 2007;15(1):39-46.)*

The importance of evaluating PF tracking dynamically is widely accepted. Since Shellock et al[63] presented their initial studies in the late 1980s, kinematic MRI has become the gold standard technique. Shellock's original study[63] defined a qualitative six-type classification system for the PF tracking: normal when the apex of the patella is aligned with the femoral trochlea; lateral or medial subluxation when the apex of the patella is laterally or medially displaced relative to the femoral trochlea, respectively; excessive lateral pressure syndrome when the lateral facet of the patella is tilted toward the lateral aspect of the lateral trochlea with little or no lateral displacement (the tilting usually increases along with knee flexion); lateral to medial subluxation when the patella starts as laterally displaced and moves to a medially displaced position as the knee flexion increases; and finally patella dislocation.

Normal patellar tracking was observed in all of the asymptomatic subjects and patellar malalignment was found in 93% of the 235 patellofemoral joints with suspected abnormalities.[63] Shellock further refined the original technique by studying active versus passive motion[64] as well as loaded versus unloaded conditions.[65] These studies suggest that active movement loaded kinematic MRI enhances the diagnostic accuracy for detection of PF abnormal alignment and tracking. Another path in kinematic MRI, seemingly more objective and therefore reproducible, is the quantitative methods of which the works of Brossmann are the finest examples.[66-68] Brossmann's indices were previously described in X-rays and CT scan studies such as patellar tilt angle, lateral patellar displacement, and bisect offset defined as the percentage of patella lateral to a line passing through the deepest point of the trochlea groove perpendicular to the tangent of the posterior condyles. Outcomes revealed significant differences in the final 10° of extension compared to their values in 30° flexion of all three indices. In patients with confirmed patellar maltracking, the differences between the same parameters measured during passive and active knee extension were highly significant, thus reaffirming the crucial role of quadriceps contraction.[66] Despite all the useful information, kinematic evaluation of the PF joint still remains a promising technique but without a well-defined clinical application. Nevertheless, it has been suggested that the extra 8 to 10 minutes it takes to add a dynamic scan to a routine MRI examination of the knee may turn out to be cost-effective.[69]

OTHER IMAGING MODALITIES

Nuclear Medicine

Bone scintigraphy is a reliable imaging method to evaluate increased metabolic activity, which is usually indicative of bone remodeling or degenerative changes.[70] Scintigraphy of the knee plays a role in the detection of radiographically occult conditions such as nondisplaced fractures and early stress fractures, avascular necrosis, degenerative changes, and even evaluation of the painful knee arthroplasty.[70,71] Boegard et al[72] found good agreement between increased bone uptake and MRI-detected subchondral lesion in patients with chronic knee pain. Increased bone scintigraphic uptake has been demonstrated in patients suffering from patellofemoral pain syndrome[73] and has been reported as being higher in patients with patellar pain compared with controls.[74] Even though the conventional planar scintigraphic method for the patellofemoral joint evaluation has limits, in those patients without other objective findings, a bone scan may rule out significant patellar disease though not excluding surrounding soft tissue conditions.

To increase the accuracy of conventional scintigraphy, single photon emission computed tomography (SPECT) and especially hybrid SPECT/CT systems have been developed. This method has shown to be more specific and, to a lesser extent, more sensitive in detecting and interpreting bone and joint pathologies, providing the clinician with precise anatomical and physiological information of the patellofemoral joint.[75] SPECT/CT might be particularly helpful in the evaluation of the patellar pain patient, when patella maltracking is associated with increased load versus no change in bone metabolism.[75]

Ultrasound

Ultrasonography of the knee was traditionally limited to the evaluation of the extra-articular soft tissues of the knee. However, when careful technique is applied, it has been shown to be a reliable modality in the diagnosis of diverse knee disorders, such as injuries to the articular cartilage, menisci, tendons and ligaments, synovium, and adjacent vessels and muscles.[76] Sonography has several advantages over other cross-sectional imaging modalities. It is inexpensive, especially when compared with MRI, safe, noninvasive, and rapidly performed. In addition, sonography is not limited to standard imaging planes and its dynamic capabilities may be of value in assessing patellar tracking, measuring the sulcus angle, medial PF joint stabilizers, and so forth.[77,78] Although reports that assess the role of sonography imaging for the patellofemoral joint remain scarce, it seems apparent that with improved resolution and ultrasound imaging technology this modality can be of some use in the diagnosis of patellofemoral pathology. Nonetheless, there will always be issues relating to its operator-dependent reliability and reproducibility.

PF IMAGING AFTER TOTAL KNEE ARTHROPLASTY

Patellofemoral imaging after total knee arthroplasty (TKA) follows a lot of the same principles as the native joint. There are nonetheless a few specific criteria for imaging interpretation, especially if the patella has been resurfaced. Another major point of interest after TKA is component rotational alignment because it greatly influences patellar tracking and can be responsible for the presence of anterior knee pain, stiffness, or other serious problems such as patellar dislocation or loosening.[79]

Patellar Height

True patella baja after TKA may be a threatening complication because a shortened patellar tendon leading to distal positioning of the patella may constitute a problem difficult to address. However, this condition needs to be differentiated from pseudo-patella baja, caused by a proximal transfer of the joint line.[80] The Blackburne-Peel or the Caton-Deschamps indices are not able to differentiate between them because the tibial plateau is their tibial reference and therefore they are greatly influenced by rising of the joint line. The original or modified Insall-Salvati ratios are theoretically the best choices.[80] Nevertheless, recent work has shown that the former two methods have a better interobserver concordance than the latter two after TKA.[81]

Patellar Alignment

Specific criteria for evaluating patellar tilt and subluxation after TKA were first determined by Gomes et al[82] in 1988 and have been used ever since.[83-85] Using a classic Merchant view, tilt is measured as an angle between a line passing through the bone–patellar component interface and a line that connects the anterior border of both condyles. In asymmetric femoral components, others have suggested using a horizontal reference line instead, much as Grelsamer did for the native joint.[30,83] Subluxation or lateral displacement is measured as the distance between two parallel lines that cross the center of the patellar component and the femoral trochlea. Tilt and subluxation are considered major only when they measure >5° or >5 mm, respectively.[82,84,85]

Recently Baldini et al[85] suggested that the use of a weight-bearing axial radiographic view to evaluate total knee replacements may provide additional information over the standard radiographic view. They found it showed several tracking differences compared with the standard Merchant axial view. Specifically, lateral tilt and subluxation of the patella were significantly reduced, while the rate of uncovered patellar bone contact with the femoral trochlea was significantly increased. Probably the most important finding is that radiographic evidence of maltracking more closely correlated with clinical symptoms using the weight-bearing axial view (Fig. 43-7).

One other known source of pain and complications in knee arthroplasty is an asymmetrically thick patella.[85,86] Gomes et al[82] also defined criteria to assess the symmetry of the patellar bone resection. Two levels are measured 1.5 cm away from the medial and lateral margins of the patella, respectively. Resection is defined as asymmetrical when the difference between the two levels is ≥2 mm and a 4-mm cutoff is usually considered to define major asymmetry.[82,85,87]

Femoral Component Rotation

CT scan has long been accepted as an accurate method of measuring rotational alignment of both the femoral and tibial component, but newly developed plain radiographs are also being used. When a CT scan axial cut through both epicondyles is used, the posterior condylar line (PCL), linking the most posterior point of the medial and lateral posterior condyles, is consistently used as a reference for the rotational orientation of the femoral component. The secondary anatomical axis necessary to determine a rotational angle is not as consensual (Fig. 43-8).

Berger et al[88,89] used the surgical epicondylar axis (SEA) to determine the posterior condylar angle subtended as the angle between this axis and the PCL. The SEA is a line connecting the sulcus of the medial epicondyle and the lateral epicondylar prominence. Others have suggested that the clinical epicondylar axis (CEA), a line connecting the medial and lateral epicondylar prominences, should be used instead because the most prominent point of the medial epicondyle is much easier to identify than the sulcus in radiographic assessment.[90] More recently, Suter et al[91] confirmed earlier findings and showed that the condylar twist angle, the angle between the CEA and the PCL, is the most reliable measurement for rotational position of the

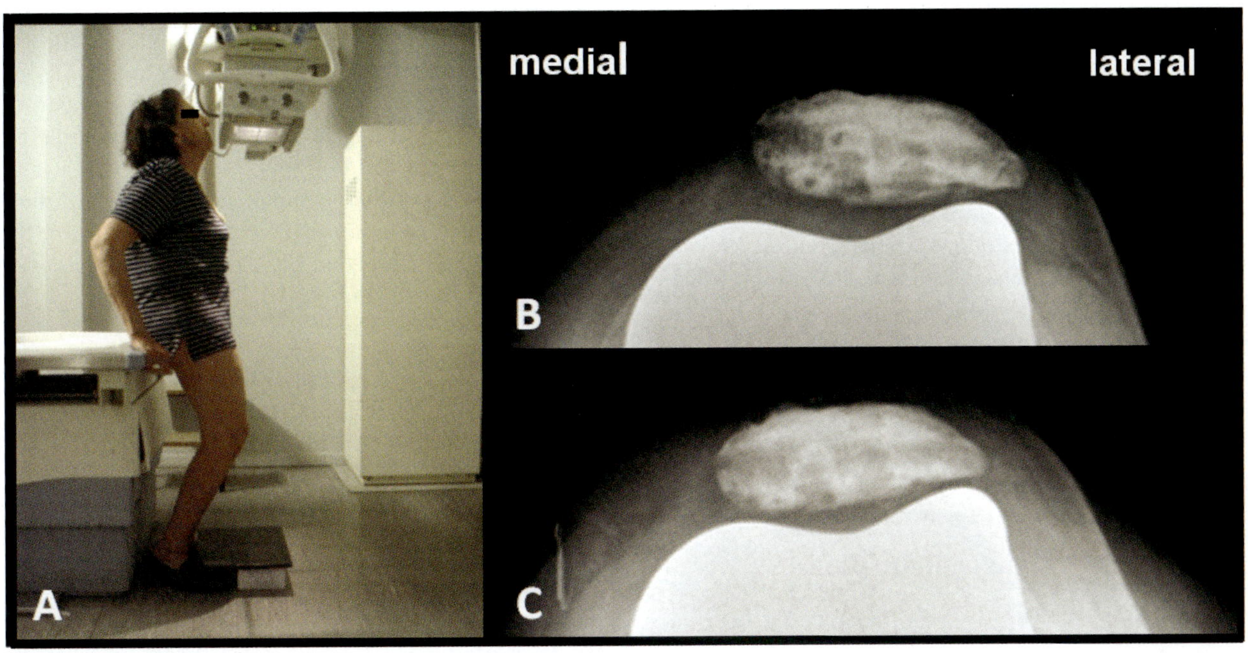

FIGURE 43-7. *Weight-bearing axial radiographic view. (**A**) Positioning of patient and X-ray beam for weight-bearing axial view; (**B**) classic Merchant view showing lateral tilt and subluxation; (**C**) weight-bearing view of the same patient showing neutralization of both tilt and subluxation.*

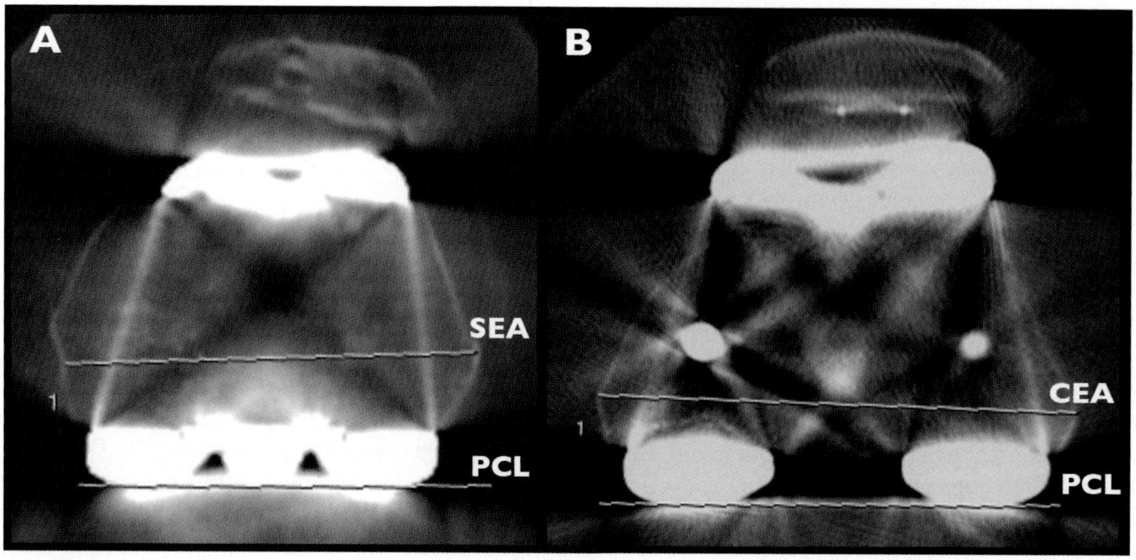

FIGURE 43-8. *Femoral component rotation measurement. Axial CT cuts through the epicondylar axis: (**A**) posterior condylar angle; (**B**) condylar twist angle. PCL, posterior condylar line, line tangent to the posterior aspect of both femoral condyles; SEA, surgical epicondylar axis, line connecting the sulcus of the medial epicondyle and the lateral epicondylar prominence; CEA, clinical epicondylar axis, line connecting the medial and lateral epicondylar prominences.*

femoral component, especially using the image cut at 30 mm above the femorotibial joint line.[91] The SEA is approximately 3° to 4° internally rotated relative to the CEA.[90,92] One should have that in mind when using this reference line because the posterior condylar angle can be estimated by subtracting 3° to 4° from the condylar twist angle.

Takai et al[93] were the first to use plain radiographs to assess the condylar twist angle, describing the so-called kneeling view. Shortly after, Kanekasu et al[94] reported their experience with a modified kneeling view using a wooden table that makes the technique more comfortable for patients with knee disorders. They compared the measurements made in 50 knees against those obtained by conventional computed tomography and found a strong correlation between them. The mean discrepancy between the two methods was 0.5° ranging from 0° to 1.9°, suggesting this radiograph is an accurate surrogate for CT scan (Fig. 43-9).[94]

Tibial Component Rotation

Three cuts of the CT scan are required to define the rotational position of the tibial component relative to the extensor mechanism, specifically the tibial tubercle. To define the tibial component axis (TCA), a cut passing through the component is made. In symmetric components it is defined as a perpendicular axis to the posterior margin of the component,[88] and in asymmetric components it is defined as a perpendicular axis to a line connecting the centers of each hemiplateau.[95] A second cut immediately below the tibial tray is used to establish the geometric center of the proximal tibia. The third and more distal cut is performed through the tibial tubercle. The latter two images are then superimposed and a line connecting the tip of the tibial tubercle and the geometric center, the tibial tubercle axis (TTA), is drawn. Rotation of the tibial component is given by the angle between the TTA and the TCA.[88] Angles up to 18° have been associated with good TKA function and are considered normal positioning (Fig. 43-10).[88,95,96]

The "Hot Patella"

A "hot patella" is a bone scintigraphy scan finding of increased tracer uptake in the patella, after total knee arthroplasty. In a recent study it was present in 51% (28/55) of patients without primary patellar resurfacing.[97] There was a positive association between a hot patella and anterior knee pain.[97] Subsequently, Ahmad et al[97] suggested that their findings appear to indicate that a hot patella in a patient with clinically defined anterior knee pain is likely to benefit from secondary patellar resurfacing (SPR). However, this hypothesis was not proved in a study of 27 SPRs where no clinical or radiological parameter was found to be related to the final outcome, including increased patellar uptake.[98] Further studies are required to clarify the real meaning of this relatively common finding after TKA. Bone scintigraphy is nevertheless useful in the assessment of the painful knee arthroplasty. A negative bone scan is reassuring and makes major complications unlikely.[99]

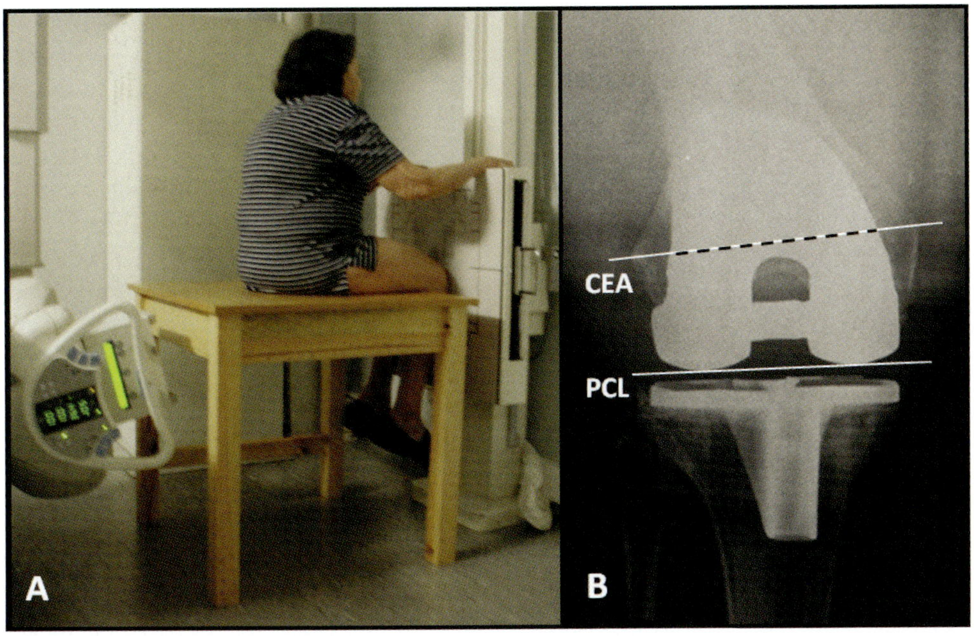

FIGURE 43-9. *Kanekasu view. (**A**) Positioning of patient, radiolucent table, and X-ray beam; (**B**) respective radiograph and condylar twist angle measurement.*

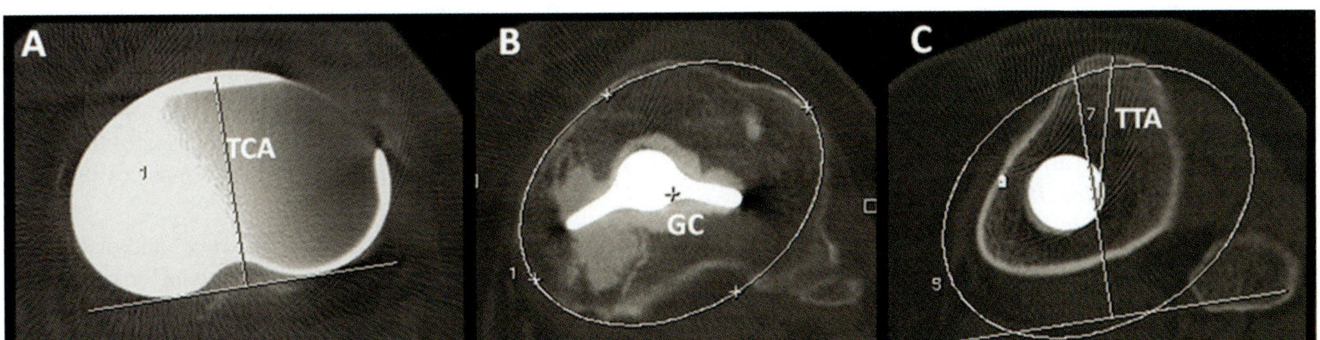

FIGURE 43-10. *Tibial component rotation measurement. (**A**) Axial CT cut through the tibial plateau to determine the tibial component axis (TCA). (**B**) Axial CT cut through the proximal tibia just below the tibial plateau to determine the geometric center (GC). (**C**) Axial CT cut through the tip of the tibial tubercle to determine the tibial tubercle axis (TTA) defined as the line connecting the geometric center of the tibia and the tip of the tibial tubercle. Rotation of the tibial component is given by the angle between the TCA and the TTA. In this example, it is 14° internally rotated.*

SUGGESTED READING

Good review and translation of the French school concepts on patellar instability:

Fithian DC, Neyret P, Servien E. Patellar instability: the Lyon experience. *Tech Knee Surg.* 2007;6(2):112-123.

A comprehensive review of many different patellar height techniques of measurement:

Phillips CL, Silver DA, Schranz PJ, et al. The measurement of patellar height: a review of the methods of imaging. *J Bone Joint Surg Br.* 2010;92:1045-1053.

A scope on the use of stress axial radiographs to enhance patellar instability diagnosis:

Teigte RA, Faerber W, Des Madryl P, et al. Stress radiographs of the patellofemoral joint. *J Bone Joint Surg Am.* 1996;78(2):193-203.

REFERENCES

1. McAlindon T, Zhang Y, Hannan M, et al. Are risk factors for patellofemoral and tibiofemoral knee osteoarthritis different? *J Rheumatol.* 1996;23:332-337.
2. Cahue S, Dunlop D, Hayes K, et al. Varus-valgus alignment in the progression of patellofemoral osteoarthritis. *Arthritis Rheum.* 2004;50:2184-2190.
3. Defrate LE, Nha KW, Papannagari R, et al. The biomechanical function of the patellar tendon during in-vivo weight-bearing flexion. *J Biomech.* 2007;40: 1716-1722.
4. Dejour H, Walch G, Nove-Josserand L, et al. Factors of patellar instability: an anatomic radiographic study. *Knee Surg Sports Traumatol Arthrosc.* 1994;2:19-26.
5. Tavernier T, Dejour D. [Knee imaging: what is the best modality]. *J Radiol.* 2001;82:387-405.
6. Dejour H, Walch G, Neyret P, et al. Dysplasia of the femoral trochlea [in French]. *Rev Chir Orthop Reparatrice Appar Mot.* 1990;76:45-54.
7. Remy F, Besson A, Migaud H, et al. Reproducibility of the radiographic analysis of dysplasia of the femoral trochlea. Intra- and interobserver analysis of 68 knees [in French]. *Rev Chir Orthop Reparatrice Appar Mot.* 1998;84:728-733.
8. Dejour D, Reynaud P, Lecoultre B. Douleurs et instabilité rotulienne. Essai de classification. *Médecine Hygiène.* 1998;56:1466-1471.
9. Maldague B, Malghem J. Significance of the radiograph of the knee profile in the detection of patellar instability. Preliminary report [in French]. *Rev Chir Orthop Reparatrice Appar Mot.* 1985;71(suppl 2):5-13.
10. Malghem J, Maldague B, Lecouvet F, et al. Plain radiography of the knee: the articular surfaces. *J Radiol.* 2008;89:692-697.
11. Grelsamer RP, Proctor CS, Bazos AN. Evaluation of patellar shape in the sagittal plane. A clinical analysis. *Am J Sports Med.* 1994;22:61-66.
12. Insall J, Salvati E. Patella position in the normal knee joint. *Radiology.* 1971;101:101-104.
13. Grelsamer RP, Meadows S. The modified Insall-Salvati ratio for assessment of patellar height. *Clin Orthop Relat Res.* 1992:170-176.
14. Blackburne JS, Peel TE. A new method of measuring patellar height. *J Bone Joint Surg Br.* 1977;59:241-242.
15. Caton J, Deschamps G, Chambat P, et al. Patella infera. Apropos of 128 cases [in French]. *Rev Chir Orthop Reparatrice Appar Mot.* 1982;68:317-325.
16. Scuderi GR. *The Patella.* New York: Springer-Verlag; 1995.
17. Bernageau J, Goutallier D, Debeyre J, et al. New exploration technic of the patellofemoral joint. Relaxed axial quadriceps and contracted quadriceps [in French]. *Rev Chir Orthop Reparatrice Appar Mot.* 1975;61(suppl 2):286-290.
18. Biedert RM, Albrecht S. The patellotrochlear index: a new index for assessing patellar height. *Knee Surg Sports Traumatol Arthrosc.* 2006;14:707-712.
19. Phillips CL, Silver DA, Schranz PJ, et al. The measurement of patellar height: a review of the methods of imaging. *J Bone Joint Surg Br.* 2010;92:1045-1053.
20. Wiberg G. Roentgenographic and anatomic studies on the femoropatellar joint. *Acta Orthop Scand.* 1941; 12:319-410.
21. Furmaier A, Breit A. Roentgenology of the femoropatellar joint with special consideration of the diagnosis chondropathia patellae [in German]. *Arch Orthop Unfallchir.* 1952;45:126-138.
22. Hughston JC, Walsh WM. Proximal and distal reconstruction of the extensor mechanism for patellar subluxation. *Clin Orthop Relat Res.* 1979;144:36-42.
23. Merchant AC, Mercer RL, Jacobsen RH, et al. Roentgenographic analysis of patellofemoral congruence. *J Bone Joint Surg Am.* 1974;56:1391-1396.
24. Davies AP, Bayer J, Owen-Johnson S, et al. The optimum knee flexion angle for skyline radiography is thirty degrees. *Clin Orthop Relat Res.* 2004:166-171.

25. Laurin CA, Levesque HP, Dussault R, et al. The abnormal lateral patellofemoral angle: a diagnostic roentgenographic sign of recurrent patellar subluxation. *J Bone Joint Surg Am.* 1978;60:55-60.
26. Brattström H. Shape of the intercondylar groove normally and in recurrent dislocation of patella. A clinical and X-ray-anatomical investigation. *Acta Orthop Scand.* 1964;suppl 68.
27. Maldague B, Malghem J. Radiology of patellar instability: contribution of the lateral radiography and the 30-degree axial view with external rotation [in French]. *Acta Orthop Belg.* 1989;55:311-329.
28. Teitge RA, Faerber WW, Des MP, et al. Stress radiographs of the patellofemoral joint. *J Bone Joint Surg Am.* 1996;78:193-203.
29. Laurin CA, Dussault R, Levesque HP. The tangential X-ray investigation of the patellofemoral joint: X-ray technique, diagnostic criteria and their interpretation. *Clin Orthop Relat Res.* 1979;144:16-26.
30. Grelsamer RP, Bazos AN, Proctor CS. Radiographic analysis of patellar tilt. *J Bone Joint Surg Br.* 1993;75: 822-824.
31. Cicuttini FM, Baker J, Hart DJ, et al. Choosing the best method for radiological assessment of patellofemoral osteoarthritis. *Ann Rheum Dis.* 1996;55: 134-136.
32. McDonnell SM, Bottomley NJ, Hollinghurst D, et al. Skyline patellofemoral radiographs can only exclude late stage degenerative changes. *Knee.* 2011;18:21-23.
33. Ahlback S. Osteoarthrosis of the knee. A radiographic investigation. *Acta Radiol Diagn (Stockh).* 1968;suppl 72.
34. Boegard T, Jonsson K. Radiography in osteoarthritis of the knee. *Skeletal Radiol.* 1999;28:605-615.
35. Iwano T, Kurosawa H, Tokuyama H, et al. Roentgenographic and clinical findings of patellofemoral osteoarthrosis. With special reference to its relationship to femorotibial osteoarthrosis and etiologic factors. *Clin Orthop Relat Res.* 1990;252: 190-197.
36. Chang CB, Seong SC, Kim TK. Evaluations of radiographic joint space—do they adequately predict cartilage conditions in the patellofemoral joint of the patients undergoing total knee arthroplasty for advanced knee osteoarthritis? *Osteoarthritis Cartilage.* 2008;16:1160-1166.
37. Baumgartl F. Anatomical and clinical importance of the femoropatellar joint [in German]. *Zentralbl Chir.* 1966;91:506-516.
38. Servien E, Ait Si ST, Neyret P. Study of the patellar apex in objective patellar dislocation [in French]. *Rev Chir Orthop Reparatrice Appar Mot.* 2003;89:605-612.
39. Panni AS, Cerciello S, Maffulli N, et al. Patellar shape can be a predisposing factor in patellar instability. *Knee Surg Sports Traumatol Arthrosc.* 2011;19: 663-670.
40. Conway WF, Hayes CW, Loughran T, et al. Cross-sectional imaging of the patellofemoral joint and surrounding structures. *Radiographics.* 1991;11:195-217.
41. Fulkerson JP, Schutzer SF, Ramsby GR, et al. Computerized tomography of the patellofemoral joint before and after lateral release or realignment. *Arthroscopy.* 1987;3:19-24.
42. Goutallier D, Bernageau J, Lecudonnec B. The measurement of the tibial tuberosity. Patella groove distanced technique and results [author's transl]. *Rev Chir Orthop Reparatrice Appar Mot.* 1978;64:423-428.
43. Redziniak DE, Diduch DR, Mihalko WM, et al. Patellar instability. *J Bone Joint Surg Am.* 2009;91:2264-2275.
44. Biedert RM, Gruhl C. Axial computed tomography of the patellofemoral joint with and without quadriceps contraction. *Arch Orthop Trauma Surg.* 1997;116:77-82.
45. Guzzanti V, Gigante A, Di LA, et al. Patellofemoral malalignment in adolescents. Computerized tomographic assessment with or without quadriceps contraction. *Am J Sports Med.* 1994;22:55-60.
46. Carrillon Y, Abidi H, Dejour D, et al. Patellar instability: assessment on MR images by measuring the lateral trochlear inclination-initial experience. *Radiology.* 2000;216:582-585.
47. Staubli HU, Durrenmatt U, Porcellini B, et al. Anatomy and surface geometry of the patellofemoral joint in the axial plane. *J Bone Joint Surg Br.* 1999;81:452-458.
48. Schutzer SF, Ramsby GR, Fulkerson JP. Computed tomographic classification of patellofemoral pain patients. *Orthop Clin North Am.* 1986;17:235-248.
49. Dupuy DE, Hangen DH, Zachazewski JE, et al. Kinematic CT of the patellofemoral joint. *AJR Am J Roentgenol.* 1997;169:211-215.
50. Vande Berg BC, Lecouvet FE, Poilvache P, et al. Spiral CT arthrography of the knee: technique and value in the assessment of internal derangement of the knee. *Eur Radiol.* 2002;12:1800-1810.
51. Ihara H. Double-contrast CT arthrography of the cartilage of the patellofemoral joint. *Clin Orthop Relat Res.* 1985:50-55.

52. Vande Berg BC, Lecouvet FE, Poilvache P, et al. Dual-detector spiral CT arthrography of the knee: accuracy for detection of meniscal abnormalities and unstable meniscal tears. *Radiology.* 2000;216:851-857.

53. Gagliardi JA, Chung EM, Chandnani VP, et al. Detection and staging of chondromalacia patellae: relative efficacies of conventional MR imaging, MR arthrography, and CT arthrography. *AJR Am J Roentgenol.* 1994;163:629-636.

54. Handelberg F, Shahabpour M, Casteleyn PP. Chondral lesions of the patella evaluated with computed tomography, magnetic resonance imaging, and arthroscopy. *Arthroscopy.* 1990;6:24-29.

55. Rand T, Brossmann J, Pedowitz R, et al. Analysis of patellar cartilage. Comparison of conventional MR imaging and MR and CT arthrography in cadavers. *Acta Radiol.* 2000;41:492-497.

56. Stanford W, Phelan J, Kathol MH, et al. Patellofemoral joint motion: evaluation by ultrafast computed tomography. *Skeletal Radiol.* 1988;17:487-492.

57. Balcarek P, Ammon J, Frosch S, et al. Magnetic resonance imaging characteristics of the medial patellofemoral ligament lesion in acute lateral patellar dislocations considering trochlear dysplasia, patella alta, and tibial tuberosity-trochlear groove distance. *Arthroscopy.* 2010;26:926-935.

58. Koskinen SK, Kujala UM. Patellofemoral relationships and distal insertion of the vastus medialis muscle: a magnetic resonance imaging study in nonsymptomatic subjects and in patients with patellar dislocation. *Arthroscopy.* 1992;8:465-468.

59. Koskinen SK, Taimela S, Nelimarkka O, et al. Magnetic resonance imaging of patellofemoral relationships. *Skeletal Radiol.* 1993;22:403-410.

60. Muellner T, Funovics M, Nikolic A, et al. Patellar alignment evaluated by MRI. *Acta Orthop Scand.* 1998;69:489-492.

61. Outerbridge RE. The etiology of chondromalacia patellae. *J Bone Joint Surg Br.* 1961;43:752-757.

62. Noyes FR, Stabler CL. A system for grading articular cartilage lesions at arthroscopy. *Am J Sports Med.* 1989;17:505-513.

63. Shellock FG, Mink JH, Deutsch AL, et al. Patellar tracking abnormalities: clinical experience with kinematic MR imaging in 130 patients. *Radiology.* 1989;172:799-804.

64. Shellock FG, Mink JH, Deutsch AL, et al. Kinematic MR imaging of the patellofemoral joint: comparison of passive positioning and active movement techniques. *Radiology.* 1992;184:574-577.

65. Shellock FG, Mink JH, Deutsch AL, et al. Patellofemoral joint: identification of abnormalities with active-movement, "unloaded" versus "loaded" kinematic MR imaging techniques. *Radiology.* 1993;188:575-578.

66. Brossmann J, Muhle C, Schroder C, et al. Patellar tracking patterns during active and passive knee extension: evaluation with motion-triggered cine MR imaging. *Radiology.* 1993;187:205-212.

67. Brossmann J, Muhle C, Bull CC, et al. Evaluation of patellar tracking in patients with suspected patellar malalignment: cine MR imaging vs arthroscopy. *AJR Am J Roentgenol.* 1994;162:361-367.

68. Brossmann J, Muhle C, Bull CC, et al. Cine MR imaging before and after realignment surgery for patellar maltracking — comparison with axial radiographs. *Skeletal Radiol.* 1995;24:191-196.

69. Witonski D. Dynamic magnetic resonance imaging. *Clin Sports Med.* 2002;21:403-415.

70. Dye SF, Chew MH. The use of scintigraphy to detect increased osseous metabolic activity about the knee. *Instr Course Lect.* 1994;43:453-469.

71. Ghelman B, Hodge JC. Imaging of the patellofemoral joint. *Orthop Clin North Am.* 1992;23:523-543.

72. Boegard T, Rudling O, Dahlstrom J, et al. Bone scintigraphy in chronic knee pain: comparison with magnetic resonance imaging. *Ann Rheum Dis.* 1999;58:20-26.

73. Naslund JE, Odenbring S, Naslund UB, et al. Diffusely increased bone scintigraphic uptake in patellofemoral pain syndrome. *Br J Sports Med.* 2005;39:162-165.

74. Dye SF, Boll DA. Radionuclide imaging of the patellofemoral joint in young adults with anterior knee pain. *Orthop Clin North Am.* 1986;17:249-262.

75. Hirschmann MT, Davda K, Iranpour F, et al. Combined single photon emission computerised tomography and conventional computerised tomography (SPECT/CT) in patellofemoral disorders: a clinical review. *Int Orthop.* 2011;35:675-680.

76. Friedman L, Finlay K, Jurriaans E. Ultrasound of the knee. *Skeletal Radiol.* 2001;30:361-377.

77. Joshi RP, Heatley FW. Imaging patellofemoral joint using ultrasound: a preliminary report. A comparison between normal subjects and patients with patellar maltracking. *Knee.* 1998;5(2):129-135.

78. Phornphutkul C, Sekiya JK, Wojtys EM, et al. Sonographic imaging of the patellofemoral medial joint stabilizing structures: findings in human cadavers. *Orthopedics.* 2007;30:472-478.

79. Rand JA. The patellofemoral joint in total knee arthroplasty. *J Bone Joint Surg Am.* 1994;76:612-620.
80. Grelsamer RP. Patella baja after total knee arthroplasty: is it really patella baja? *J Arthroplasty.* 2002;17:66-69.
81. Rogers BA, Thornton-Bott P, Cannon SR, Interobserver variation in the measurement of patellar height after total knee arthroplasty. *J Bone Joint Surg Br.* 2006;88:484-488.
82. Gomes LS, Bechtold JE, Gustilo RB. Patellar prosthesis positioning in total knee arthroplasty. A roentgenographic study. *Clin Orthop Relat Res.* 1988;236:72-81.
83. Bindelglass DF, Cohen JL, Dorr LD. Patellar tilt and subluxation in total knee arthroplasty. Relationship to pain, fixation, and design. *Clin Orthop Relat Res.* 1993;286:103-109.
84. Bindelglass DF, Vince KG. Patellar tilt and subluxation following subvastus and parapatellar approach in total knee arthroplasty. Implication for surgical technique. *J Arthroplasty.* 1996;11:507-511.
85. Baldini A, Anderson JA, Cerulli-Mariani P, et al. Patellofemoral evaluation after total knee arthroplasty. Validation of a new weight-bearing axial radiographic view. *J Bone Joint Surg Am.* 2007;89: 1810-1817.
86. Pagnano MW, Trousdale RT. Asymmetric patella resurfacing in total knee arthroplasty. *Am J Knee Surg.* 2000;13:228-233.
87. DeOrio JK, Peden JP. Accuracy of haptic assessment of patellar symmetry in total knee arthroplasty. *J Arthroplasty.* 2004;19:629-634.
88. Berger RA, Crossett LS, Jacobs JJ, et al. Malrotation causing patellofemoral complications after total knee arthroplasty. *Clin Orthop Relat Res.* 1998;356:144-153.
89. Berger RA, Rubash HE, Seel MJ, et al. Determining the rotational alignment of the femoral component in total knee arthroplasty using the epicondylar axis. *Clin Orthop Relat Res.* 1993;286:40-47.
90. Yoshino N, Takai S, Ohtsuki Y, et al. Computed tomography measurement of the surgical and clinical transepicondylar axis of the distal femur in osteoarthritic knees. *J Arthroplasty.* 2001;16:493-497.
91. Suter T, Zanetti M, Schmid M, et al. Reproducibility of measurement of femoral component rotation after total knee arthroplasty using computer tomography. *J Arthroplasty.* 2006;21:744-748.
92. Matsui Y, Kadoya Y, Uehara K, et al. Rotational deformity in varus osteoarthritis of the knee: analysis with computed tomography. *Clin Orthop Relat Res.* 2005;433:147-151.
93. Takai S, Yoshino N, Isshiki T, et al. Kneeling view: a new roentgenographic technique to assess rotational deformity and alignment of the distal femur. *J Arthroplasty.* 2003;18:478-483.
94. Kanekasu K, Kondo M, Kadoya Y. Axial radiography of the distal femur to assess rotational alignment in total knee arthroplasty. *Clin Orthop Relat Res.* 2005;434:193-197.
95. Bedard M, Vince KG, Redfern J, et al. Internal rotation of the tibial component is frequent in stiff total knee arthroplasty. *Clin Orthop Relat Res.* 2011;469: 2346-2355.
96. Barrack RL, Schrader T, Bertot AJ, et al. Component rotation and anterior knee pain after total knee arthroplasty. *Clin Orthop Relat Res.* 2001;392:46-55.
97. Ahmad R, Kumar GS, Katam K, et al. Significance of a "hot patella" in total knee replacement without primary patellar resurfacing. *Knee.* 2009;16:337-340.
98. Munoz-Mahamud E, Popescu D, Nunez E, et al. Secondary patellar resurfacing in the treatment of patellofemoral pain after total knee arthroplasty. *Knee Surg Sports Traumatol Arthrosc.* 2011;19(9):1467-1472.
99. Smith SL, Wastie ML, Forster I. Radionuclide bone scintigraphy in the detection of significant complications after total knee joint replacement. *Clin Radiol.* 2001;56:221-224.

44

Principles of Primary Total Knee Arthroplasty: Indications and Contraindications

Tad M. Mabry

Primary total knee arthroplasty (TKA) is the gold standard surgical treatment for a wide variety of conditions and patients with severe degeneration of the knee joint. The overall goals of the operation have changed little over time and include pain relief, restoration of a functional range of motion, restoration of alignment, proper stability in all planes, maintenance of a well-functioning extensor mechanism, and long-term durability.[1] The purpose of this chapter is to review some of the general principles of primary TKA, focusing on the indications and contraindications to this highly successful operation. Subsequent chapters more fully explore the complete spectrum of diagnoses and conditions about the knee requiring surgical intervention.

A recently published population-based study notes the increase in primary TKA usage over time, as well as the increasing significance of osteoarthritis as the indication for surgery.[2] The demand for primary TKA is projected to increase exponentially over the next few decades.[3] From 2005 to 2030, the number of primary TKA performed annually in the United States is expected to grow by 673%, from 450,000 cases to 3,480,000 cases.

Critical issues to consider when evaluating patients for knee replacement are noted in chapter 41, which reviews the preoperative clinical evaluation. It is mandatory to confirm that the patient's primary source of pain is the knee joint itself, rather than some distant source. Common areas to be considered as alternative sources of pain about the knee would be the spine (radiculopathy) and the hip (referred pain) (Fig. 44-1). Differential injections of the hip and the knee can be very helpful when trying to sort out the source of the patient's pain and dysfunction. Vascular claudication and

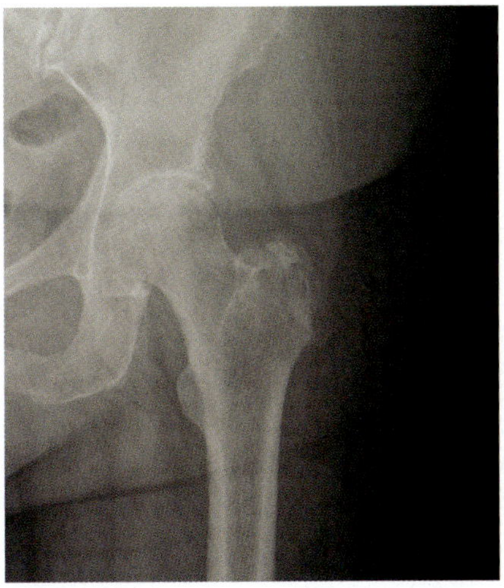

FIGURE 44-1. *Patient presenting with a chief complaint of knee pain having end-stage arthritis of the hip. Extra-articular sources of knee pain must be excluded before treating patients with TKA. Differential injections may be necessary at times.*

neuropathic pain are other potential extra-articular sources of knee pain that should be ruled out before considering TKA.

Consideration should be given to joint-preserving surgery in younger and more active patients where appropriate. Arthroplasty should always be considered as a "last resort" operation for patients with severe degenerative changes. Patients with more focal cartilage issues may be candidates for some type of cartilage repair or reconstruction.[4] Patients with meniscal pathology in the absence of severe arthritic changes may be candidates for meniscal repair or partial meniscectomy.[5] Osteotomy about the knee has been used for many years as an alternative to arthroplasty in the younger and more active patient population.[6] This is typically some type of valgus-producing tibial osteotomy in the setting of medial compartment arthritis. This can take the form of a medial opening wedge versus lateral closing wedge osteotomy and full details of these operations are noted elsewhere in this book. Patients with lateral compartment arthritis and malalignment may benefit from a varus-producing distal femoral osteotomy, which is also discussed elsewhere in greater detail. Patients with even greater malalignment may require a double osteotomy (both femoral and tibial) in order to prevent excessive obliquity of the joint line.

Unicompartmental arthroplasty is the main alternative to TKA when the option for joint-preserving surgery is no longer viable.[7] The classic indications for unicompartmental arthroplasty would include arthritis or osteonecrosis isolated to a single compartment, satisfactory range of motion, and functionally intact ligaments with passively correctable deformity.[8] These more stringent inclusion criteria have been liberalized over time;[9] however, the importance of degenerative change within the patellofemoral joint remains a point of contention. Inflammatory arthritis, as it affects the entire synovial joint, is considered a contraindication to unicompartmental arthroplasty.

Medial unicompartmental arthroplasty is by far the most common type of unicompartmental knee replacement surgery performed. Lateral unicompartmental arthroplasty, though less common, can be very effective in the appropriate patient population. Patellofemoral and bicompartmental arthroplasty have also been performed with varying degrees of success. Each of these operations is discussed elsewhere in this book in great detail.

Total knee arthroplasty remains the gold standard for the treatment of patients presenting with knee pain refractory to conservative treatment and a sufficient amount of cartilage loss to warrant total, rather than partial, joint replacement. The vast majority of TKAs are performed for the treatment of end-stage osteoarthritis. Other indications include inflammatory arthritis (eg, rheumatoid arthritis), posttraumatic arthritis, postinfectious arthritis, osteonecrosis, and neuropathic arthropathy (Table 44-1). Ideally, patients being considered for arthroplasty should have a combination of pain and disability sufficient to warrant this highly successful, but permanent and irreversible procedure.

OSTEOARTHRITIS

Osteoarthritis (OA) is the most common form of arthritis, and OA of the knee is estimated to affect 19% to 28% of adults age 45 and over.[10] Risk factors for the development of knee OA include female sex, being overweight or obese, and having a history of prior knee injury. The contribution of leg length discrepancy and malalignment to the eventual development of knee OA is still under study.[10]

As it is the most common form of arthritis, OA is also by far the predominant indication for TKA. The decision to proceed with TKA for the treatment of end-stage OA is made once nonoperative treatments have failed and other surgical options are deemed either inappropriate or less effective (Fig. 44-2). A wide variety of implant systems are available to treat patients with this condition, and many of these have demonstrated excellent results at mid- to long-term follow-up. Subsequent chapters explore in detail the wide variety of techniques and implants that have proven effective over time in allowing surgeons to reconstruct the arthritis knee.

TABLE 44-1. Indications for Primary TKA

Osteoarthritis
Inflammatory arthritis (eg, rheumatoid arthritis)
Posttraumatic arthritis
Postinfectious arthritis
Osteonecrosis
Neuropathic arthropathy

RHEUMATOID ARTHRITIS

Rheumatoid arthritis (RA) is a chronic, autoimmune inflammatory disease. While the disease process is systemic in its reach, the synovial joints are primarily affected.[11] Involvement of one or both knees in the disease process is seen in up to 90% of individuals with chronic RA. Many of these patients will eventually require TKA.[12]

There are several features unique to these patients that bear mentioning.[12] First, during the preoperative evaluation, the patient's overall medical and nutritional status should be optimized. Many of these patients may be taking a complex, multidrug regimen for disease management that should be modified perioperatively in conjunction with a rheumatologist to minimize perioperative bleeding, wound healing, or infection issues. Specific to surgical intervention, patients being considered for TKA should be evaluated for concomitant hip disease and for any cervical spine instability issues. At the time of surgery, patients with RA may present with compromised bone, soft tissue, or both. Most of these patients develop some degree of periarticular osteopenia and may be at increased risk of intraoperative fracture.[13] Cemented fixation may also be preferable in most of these cases. More significant bone loss may require the use of bone graft or metal augments. With respect to the soft tissues, RA patients may present across the entire spectrum of knee stability, from gross instability to near ankylosis. Identifying and treating these issues are essential at the time of TKA. Despite the often relatively young patient age at the time of surgery, the long-term results of TKA in RA are quite good. One long-term study of a cemented, cruciate-retaining TKA of a single design noted a 93% survivorship at 15 years free of revision for any reason and free of any revisions for aseptic loosening in patients with RA.[14] In another study of over 11,000 primary TKAs, prosthetic survivorship was greater at 15 years for patients with RA (95%) than for patients with OA (90%).[15]

POSTTRAUMATIC ARTHRITIS

Prior injury to the knee is one of the main risk factors for the development of knee arthritis.[10] Such injuries can take many forms, such as repetitive microtrauma, ligamentous disruption, cartilage injury, or intra-articular fracture on one or both sides of the joint. The severity of the injury, and the nature of any prior treatments, can have a dramatic effect on the complexity of the eventual reconstruction.[16] The potential issues subsequent to these injuries can include soft tissue defects, latent infection, retained hardware, bone loss, malunion, nonunion, and arthrofibrosis.[17]

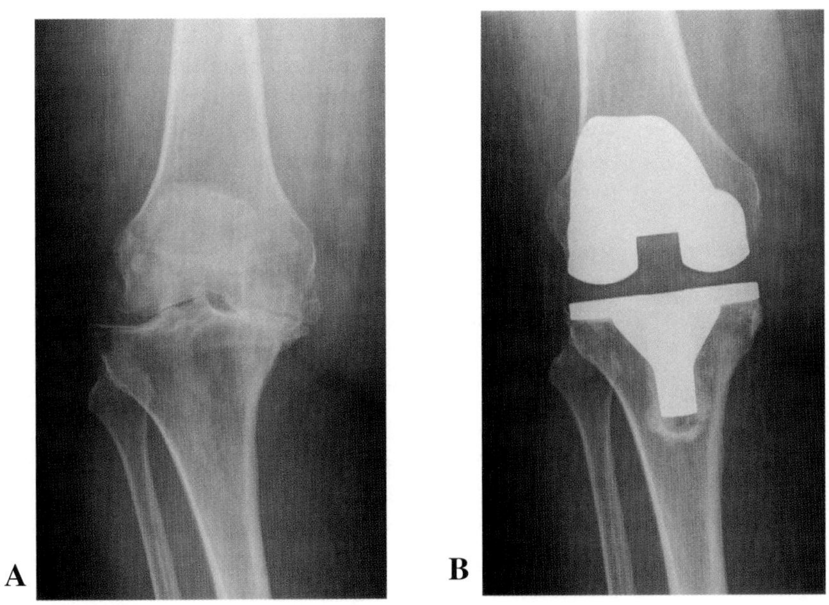

FIGURE 44-2. *Patient with severe tricompartmental OA of the knee and fixed flexion and varus deformities (**A**). Given the severity of the disease and deformity, this patient is not a candidate for joint-preserving surgery or for unicompartmental arthroplasty. After failing nonoperative treatment, this patient was treated with primary TKA (**B**).*

Preoperative planning is critical in these cases, as the surgeon must take steps to identify and plan for each of these potential pitfalls. Patients with multiple prior incisions, or patients with frank soft tissue defects, may require soft tissue coverage around the time of TKA, and plastic surgery consultation should be requested if needed. Patients must be counseled with respect to the potential increased risks of wound necrosis and infection when TKA is performed in the posttraumatic setting. It is the author's practice to assess all such patients for infection with the use of a screening ESR and CRP blood test. Aspiration, and in some cases tagged white blood cell radionuclide scanning, can be helpful in certain cases to rule out infection. Patients with ongoing infection are typically treated in a staged fashion as in the chronically infected TKA. Many patients present with retained hardware. If this hardware cannot be avoided, then specialized instruments may be required to remove the device, and the decision must be made whether to remove the hardware at the time of the TKA or to remove it in a staged manner before TKA, with or without concomitant osteotomy to treat residual deformity. Extra-articular deformity may have a significant impact on TKA and its influence is based on the location and magnitude of the malalignment. In general terms, larger-magnitude deformities and deformities closer to the joint will more often require corrective osteotomy rather than an intra-articular correction.[16] Bone loss may be addressed in the same way as one would address bone loss in the revision setting, with bone grafting, metal augmentation, and stemmed components as needed. Preoperative stiffness is one of the more common features of the posttraumatic knee, and the surgeon and patient should both be aware of the increased risk of extensor mechanism disruption complicating TKA.[17] The surgeon should be prepared to perform more extensile exposures as needed to protect the extensor mechanism, such as a quadriceps snip or tibial tubercle osteotomy.[18]

The results of TKA in the posttraumatic setting are good, but are often less favorable than the results of TKA for osteoarthritis or rheumatoid arthritis. Knee Society pain and functional scores demonstrate significant improvement, but there is a relatively high complication rate.[16,17,19,20]

POSTINFECTIOUS ARTHRITIS

Infection about the knee, whether in the form of septic arthritis or osteomyelitis, can lead to a loss of cartilage and bone and may eventually lead to severe joint destruction.[21] Many of these patients may be best treated with TKA. Keys to a successful outcome in this setting include a focused evaluation for the presence of ongoing infection, a low threshold to treat patients in a staged manner if infection remains a possibility, and the use of antibiotic-impregnated cement at the time of TKA (Fig. 44-3). The surgeon should be prepared to encounter extensive intra-articular scarring and should be prepared to perform a more extensile exposure as indicated.

One single-surgeon study of 20 knees in 19 patients yielded a 95% success rate with respect to recurrent deep infection when following the previously outlined principles.[21] Substantial improvements were noted after TKA for pain, function, and range of motion. TKA remains a viable method of reconstruction for most patients presenting with postinfectious arthritis of the knee.

OSTEONECROSIS

The knee is the next most common site for osteonecrosis of bone after the hip. Osteonecrosis of the knee is represented by three unique entities: spontaneous osteonecrosis, secondary osteonecrosis, and postarthroscopic osteonecrosis. The interested reader is referred to a recent review article that nicely outlines the pertinent features of this condition as it relates to diagnosis and surgical management.[22]

Spontaneous osteonecrosis is typically seen in older patients and is much more commonly seen in women. It is rarely bilateral and is not associated with osteonecrosis at other sites. Secondary osteonecrosis is more often seen in younger patients and is more common in men than women. Unlike spontaneous osteonecrosis, it is associated with a number of potential risk factors, including exposure to high-dose corticosteroids and alcohol abuse. In these patients, remote joint involvement (hip, shoulder) is also quite common. Postarthroscopic osteonecrosis is rare and typically affects the compartment involved with the prior arthroscopic surgical intervention. It may represent a postopera-tive subchondral fracture. There are no known risk factors beyond a history of arthroscopic surgery. Bilaterality and remote joint involvement are not seen.

Similar to the treatment of osteonecrosis about the hip, these lesions are usually treated with some form of arthroplasty if the lesion collapses. In the setting of spontaneous osteonecrosis or postarthroscopic osteonecrosis, patients may be candidates for a unicompartmental arthroplasty if the lesion is not too large (massive lesions would preclude appropriate fixation) and if the lesion is isolated to one compartment. Patients with large lesions, multicompartment involvement, or secondary osteonecrosis are typically best

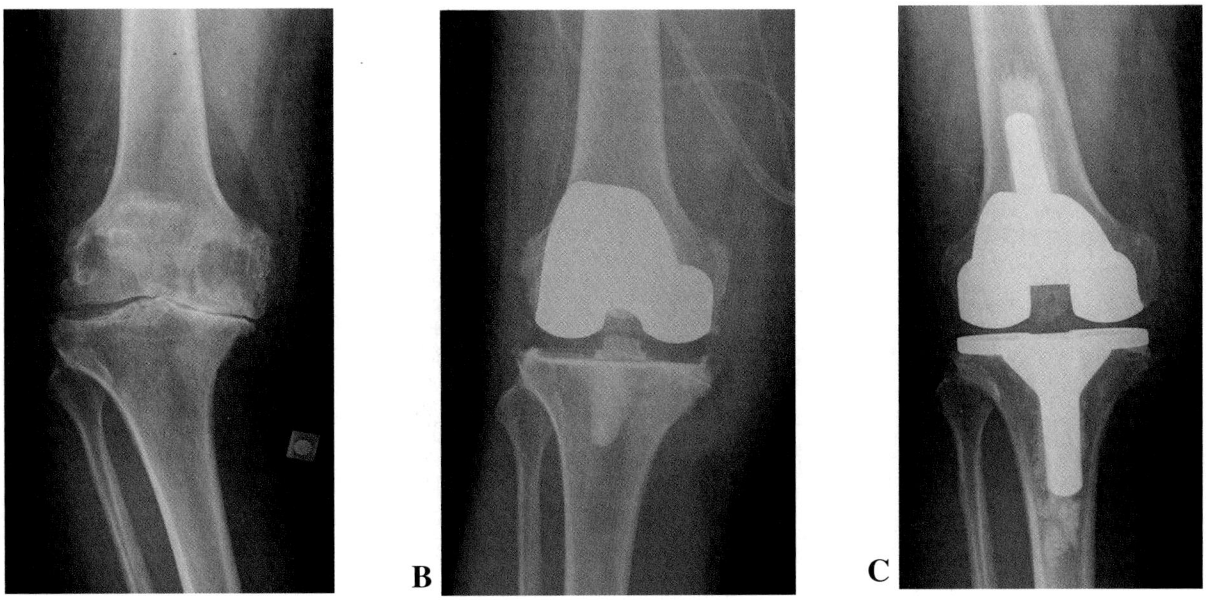

A B C

FIGURE 44-3. *This patient with postinfectious arthritis presented with persistent infection in the knee (**A**). He was treated in a staged fashion with an articulating spacer containing high-dose antibiotic-impregnated cement (**B**), followed by reimplantation 10 weeks later with a TKA containing low-dose antibiotic-impregnated cement (**C**).*

treated with TKA. Surgeons should be prepared to use bone graft or augments or both, with or without additional stem fixation, in the setting of large necrotic lesions.

NEUROPATHIC ARTHROPATHY

Neuropathic arthropathy, or Charcot joint, is a relatively rare indication for TKA. This process is believed to start with either a partial or a complete loss of nociception sense from the knee. This loss of protective sensation from the joint can lead to undetected microtrauma and eventual severe joint destruction related to bone loss and ligamentous insufficiency.[23] Although pain is not usually severe for these patients, the level of joint deformity and instability can become disabling. It is this level of disability that is the usual indication for TKA. Before considering arthroplasty, the cause of the neurologic deficit should be ascertained and, if possible, treated. Common diagnoses leading to neuropathic arthropathy of the knee include neurosyphilis, familial sensorimotor neuropathy, syringomyelia, diabetes mellitus, and stroke.

Several authors have noted reasonably successful results in this patient population.[23-25] These authors note several important principles in the treatment of this condition. First, patients with a Charcot knee joint secondary to neurosyphilis may have less successful outcomes given the frequent finding of ataxia and the relatively unstable neurologic status, which is one of the hallmarks of the condition. Second, areas of bone loss must be identified and managed appropriately. Last, ligamentous instability is often marked in these patients, and the surgeon should have a low threshold to use more constrained devices with stemmed implants if needed (Fig. 44-4).

CONTRAINDICATIONS

While there exist a number of relative contraindications to total knee replacement (Table 44-2), active infection is one of the absolute contraindications in most surgeons' hands. The infection should be cleared before implantation of a knee prosthesis.[21] This may often require a two-stage procedure with provisional bone cuts and placement of a high-dose antibiotic cement spacer (static or articulating) before conversion to definitive total knee replacement.[26] There are reports of one-stage

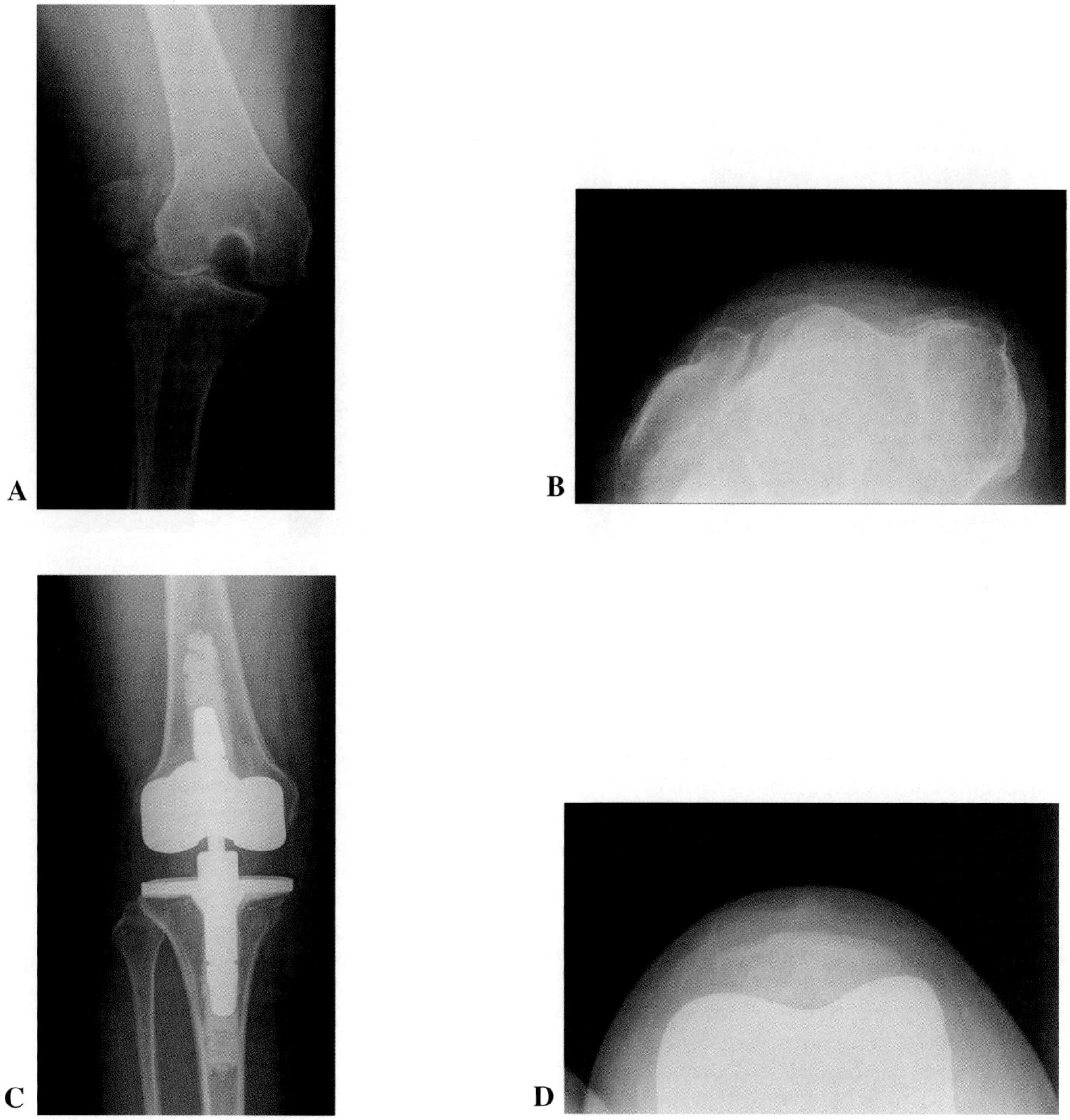

FIGURE 44-4. *This young patient with an inflammatory polyneuropathy developed bilateral Charcot knees with fixed patellar dislocations (**A**, **B**). One year following complex primary TKA with a condylar constrained knee, cemented stems, and soft tissue realignment, the patient is doing well clinically, and the patella continues to track centrally (**C**, **D**).*

TABLE 44-2. Contraindications to Primary TKA

Active infection
Nonreconstructible extensor mechanism deficiency
Severe quadriceps weakness or paralysis
Prohibitive medical risks
Cardiopulmonary disease
Immunosuppression
Nonreconstructible soft tissue envelope
Extreme morbid obesity

total knee replacement in the setting of active infection equivalent to a one-stage exchange for infected knee replacement. This has been shown to be effective functionally, although with a fairly high rate of persistent infection.[27]

Patients presenting with paralysis of the quadriceps or with a nonreconstructible extensor mechanism deficiency are not candidates for TKA. Various methods of extensor mechanism reconstruction are described later in this book. In like manner, patients with a nonreconstructible soft tissue envelope (eg, burns, skin grafts) are not appropriate for TKA. This is a very rare situation given the options for free tissue transfer, rotational flaps, and soft tissue expansion.

In order to proceed with TKA, the patient must be healthy enough to undergo major surgery. The level of medical complexity of patients presenting to the orthopaedic surgeon's office for consideration of knee replacement continues to rise over time as patients with chronic medical conditions are able to live longer with our modern medical interventions. Patients with significant medical comorbidities should be seen by a medical specialist for appropriate preoperative testing and medical optimization before surgery. Given today's anesthesia techniques and monitoring, the vast majority of patients, even with significant cardiopulmonary issues, are safe for surgical intervention. Patients who are immunocompromised should be approached carefully and should avoid surgery if the immunosuppression cannot be adequately managed. Patients on certain medications, such as prednisone or other immunomodulatory agents, may need to have these medications adjusted perioperatively to reduce the risk of infection and wound-healing complications. Patients with human immunodeficiency virus (HIV) infection should have their viral load and T-cell numbers analyzed before considering joint replacement surgery.[28,29] Special care should be taken when considering TKA for HIV-positive patients, as in all patients, who are living in difficult social circumstances given the potential for high complication rates. Patients with certain hematologic malignancies or other conditions affecting the immune system may never be safe candidates for prosthetic joint reconstruction. Patients with severe bleeding or clotting disorders must be approached with great caution around the time of any surgical intervention.

Obesity is a growing problem in the United States as well as globally. Obesity certainly can make the operation much more difficult and increase the perioperative risks of surgery.[30-34] There is also the potential for negative long-term effects on the joint with increasing patient size. There does not seem to be an absolute contraindication with respect to body weight. One of the major issues seems to be the location of the patient's extra tissue. Patients with a large pannus about the knee and particularly those patients with large skin folds about the knee may be at highest risk of perioperative wound complications. Consideration should be given to weight loss, with or without bariatric surgery, before considering total knee replacement for many of these morbidly obese patients.

CONCLUSIONS

In summary, patients with a wide variety of conditions about the knee that have failed nonoperative treatment are best treated with total knee replacement. This operation has been shown to provide durable pain relief and restoration of function to a growing number of patients. The surgeon should be aware of the potential for extra-articular sources of pain, including spine or hip pathology. Such entities should always be specifically evaluated and excluded before considering patients for knee replacement.

The goals of surgery remain the same and include pain relief, restoration of a functional range of motion, restoration of alignment, proper stability in all planes, maintenance of a well-functioning extensor mechanism, and long-term durability. The most common indications include osteoarthritis, inflammatory arthritis (eg, rheumatoid arthritis), posttraumatic arthritis, postinfectious arthritis, osteonecrosis, and neuropathic arthropathy.

Contraindications to surgery include active infection, nonreconstructible extensor mechanism dysfunction, a compromised soft tissue envelope, severe cardiopulmonary disease, immunosuppression, bleeding disorders, clotting disorders, and extreme morbid obesity.

PEARLS AND PITFALLS

Pearls

The surgeon should keep the following goals in mind when considering a TKA:

- The primary goals of surgery include pain relief, restoration of motion, restoration of a neutral mechanical axis, appropriate ligament balance, maintenance of proper extensor mechanism function, and long-term durability.
- The best surgical outcomes begin with appropriate patient selection.

Pitfalls

Avoid total knee arthroplasty in the setting of active infection, nonreconstructible extensor mechanism dysfunction, a compromised soft tissue envelope, severe cardiopulmonary disease, immunosuppression, bleeding disorders, clotting disorders, and extreme morbid obesity. Some of these issues may be modifiable and allow for surgery to proceed, albeit at a higher risk for complications.

REFERENCES

1. Insall JN, et al. Total knee arthroplasty. *Clin Orthop Relat Res.* 1985;192:13-22.
2. Singh JA, Vessely MB, Harmsen WS. A population-based study of trends in the use of total hip and total knee arthroplasty, 1969-2008. *Mayo Clin Proc.* 2010; 85(10):898-904.
3. Kurtz S, Ong K, Lau E, et al. Projections of primary and revision hip and knee arthroplasty in the United States from 2005 to 2030. *J Bone Joint Surg Am.* 2007;89(4):780-785.
4. Gomoll AH, Farr J, Gillogly SD, et al. Surgical management of articular cartilage defects of the knee. *J Bone Joint Surg Am.* 2010;92(14):2470-2490.
5. Clarke HD, Scott WN. The role of debridement: through small portals. *J Arthroplasty.* 2003;18(3 suppl 1):10-13.
6. Iorio R, Healy WL. Unicompartmental arthritis of the knee. *J Bone Joint Surg Am.* 2003;85(7):1351-1364.
7. Borus T, Thornhill T. Unicompartmental knee arthroplasty. *J Am Acad Orthop Surg.* 2008;16(1):9-18.
8. Kozinn SC, Scott R. Unicondylar knee arthroplasty. *J Bone Joint Surg Am.* 1989;71(1):145-150.
9. Pandit H, Jenkins C, Gill HS, et al. Unnecessary contraindications for mobile-bearing unicompartmental knee replacement. *J Bone Joint Surg Br.* 2011;93(5): 622-628.
10. Neogi T, Zhang Y. Osteoarthritis prevention. *Curr Opin Rheumatol.* 2011;23(2):185-191.
11. Cooles FA, Isaacs JD. Pathophysiology of rheumatoid arthritis. *Curr Opin Rheumatol.* 2011;23(3):233-240.
12. Chmell MJ, Scott RD. Total knee arthroplasty in patients with rheumatoid arthritis: an overview. *Clin Orthop Relat Res.* 1999;366:54-60.
13. Alden KJ, Duncan WH, Trousdale RT, et al. Intraoperative fracture during primary total knee arthroplasty. *Clin Orthop Relat Res.* 2009;468(1):90-95.
14. Vessely MB, et al. The Chitranjan Ranawat Award. Long-term survivorship and failure modes of 1000 cemented condylar total knee arthroplasties. *Clin Orthop Relat Res.* 2006;452:28-34.
15. Rand JA, et al. Factors affecting the durability of primary total knee prostheses. *J Bone Joint Surg Am.* 2003;85(2):259-265.
16. Ries MD. Total knee arthroplasty: posttraumatic osteoarthritis. In: Lieberman JR, Berry DJ, Azar FM, eds. *Advanced Reconstruction: Knee.* Rosemont, IL: American Academy of Orthopaedic Surgeons; 2011: 171-180.
17. Weiss NG, et al. Total knee arthroplasty in post-traumatic arthrosis of the knee. *J Arthroplasty.* 2003;18(3 suppl 1):23-26.
18. Della Valle CJ, Berger RA, Rosenberg AG. Surgical exposures in revision total knee arthroplasty. *Clin Orthop Relat Res.* 2006;446:59-68.
19. Papadopoulos EC, et al. Total knee arthroplasty following prior distal femoral fracture. *Knee.* 2002;9(4): 267-274.
20. Weiss NG, et al. Total knee arthroplasty in patients with a prior fracture of the tibial plateau. *J Bone Joint Surg Am.* 2003;85(2):218-221.
21. Lee GC, Pagnano MW, Hanssen AD. Total knee arthroplasty after prior bone or joint sepsis about the knee. *Clin Orthop Relat Res.* 2002;404:226-231.
22. Mont MA, Marker DR, Zywiel MG, et al. Osteonecrosis of the knee and related conditions. *J Am Acad Orthop Surg.* 2011;19(8):482-494.

23. Parvizi J, Marrs J, Morrey BF. Total knee arthroplasty for neuropathic (Charcot) joints. *Clin Orthop Relat Res.* 2003;416:145-150.
24. Kim YH, Kim JS, Oh SW. Total knee arthroplasty in neuropathic arthropathy. *J Bone Joint Surg Br.* 2002;84(2):216-219.
25. Soudry M, et al. Total knee arthroplasty in Charcot and Charcot-like joints. *Clin Orthop Relat Res.* 1986; 208:199-204.
26. Burnett RSJ, et al. Technique and timing of two-stage exchange for infection in TKA. *Clin Orthop Relat Res.* 2007;464:164-178.
27. Siegel A, et al. Primary arthroplasty of infected hips and knees in special cases using antibiotic-loaded bone-cement for fixation. *J Arthroplasty.* 2001;16(8 suppl 1):145-149.
28. Habermann B, Eberhardt C, Kurth AA. Total joint replacement in HIV positive patients. *J Infect.* 2008;57(1):41-46.
29. Parvizi J, et al. Total joint arthroplasty in human immunodeficiency virus-positive patients: an alarming rate of early failure. *J Arthroplasty.* 2003; 18(3):259-264.
30. Amin AK, et al. Total knee replacement in morbidly obese patients. Results of a prospective, matched study. *J Bone Joint Surg Br.* 2006;88(10):1321-1326.
31. Amin AK, et al. Does obesity influence the clinical outcome at five years following total knee replacement for osteoarthritis? *J Bone Joint Surg Br.* 2006;88 (3):335-340.
32. Dowsey MM, et al. The impact of pre-operative obesity on weight change and outcome in total knee replacement: a prospective study of 529 consecutive patients. [Erratum appears in *J Bone Joint Surg Br.* 2010;92(6):902]. *J Bone Joint Surg Br.* 2010;92 (4):513-520.
33. Foran JRH, et al. The outcome of total knee arthroplasty in obese patients. *J Bone Joint Surg Am.* 2004; 86(8):1609-1615.
34. Samson AJ, Mercer GE, Campbell DG. Total knee replacement in the morbidly obese: a literature review. *ANZ J Surg.* 2010;80(9):595-599.

45 Patella Resurfacing in Total Knee Arthroplasty

R. Stephen J. Burnett and Robert L. Barrack

Managing patellar conditions at the time of total knee arthroplasty (TKA) is an aspect of knee replacement surgery that is frequently overshadowed by other aspects of the surgical procedure and frequently is left until the end of the TKA procedure to address the patella and extensor mechanism. In addition to the many other important issues surrounding the entire TKA procedure (templating, varus-valgus soft tissue balancing, joint line restoration, mechanical axis alignment, flexion-extension gap balancing, component sizing and orientation, implant selection, component fixation, bearing surface selection, and degree of constraint) the surgeon must also consider management of the patella once a decision is made to perform a TKA. There are numerous reports of how to manage the patella at the time of primary TKA surgery; however, the decision of whether to resurface or leave the patella nonresurfaced continues to be controversial.[1] Recently, this issue has again been reported in a large randomized clinical trial of 1715 patients, reporting no difference in outcome comparing resurfacing to nonresurfacing of the patella.[2] Regardless of the decision to resurface (or not), the goals for management of the patella and extensor mechanism at the time of TKA surgery are to provide a pain-free patellofemoral articulation with long-term survival of the TKA and to avoid patellofemoral complications. To achieve these goals, the following points must be considered: (1) restore a balanced extensor mechanism with central tracking and with no tilt or subluxation of the patella, (2) restore the composite patellar and patellofemoral joint composite thickness and avoid "overstuffing" of the patellofemoral joint, (3) avoid procedures that will devascularize the patella and extensor mechanism, and (4) avoid intraoperative and postoperative extensor mechanism complications.

The controversy and indications of whether to resurface the patella or to leave the native patella unresurfaced continues to be debated by orthopaedic surgeons performing TKA.[3] The original designs of TKA did not take into consideration the patellofemoral articulation as a potential source of pain, and the results were complicated by patients with patellofemoral symptoms despite a well-performed knee arthroplasty. Subsequent designs incorporated a femoral flange for the patellofemoral articulation and provided the option for a patellar resurfacing. These early implants were not designed to accommodate the native patella in an anatomic fashion during range of motion and were used with the recommendation that the patella required resurfacing. Complications related to patellar resurfacing became a primary concern and have been associated with the variable revision rates often reported with total knee arthroplasty. Subsequent implant design modifications have been developed to offer the surgeon the option to consider leaving the patella unresurfaced. Increased awareness of component orientation and rotation has introduced yet another improvement in the results of the patellofemoral articulation in TKA.[4] Numerous clinical trials have been developed to help clarify the indications for patellar resurfacing. Unfortunately, there is little consensus, and surgeon preference remains a personal decision. Despite the numerous trials, there are three basic strategies that have evolved: always resurface, never resurface, or selectively resurface the patella. However, the debate still persists: How does a surgeon manage the patella in total knee arthroplasty? The purpose of this chapter is to review the indications, results, technique, and complications of patella resurfacing and nonresurfacing in TKA surgery.

INDICATIONS AND CONTRAINDICATIONS

The numerous and common patellar bone and soft tissue problems and conditions that may be diagnosed preoperatively are outlined in Table 45-1. The indications for resurfacing or not resurfacing the patella remain controversial. Rheumatoid and other inflammatory arthropathies have been traditional indications for resurfacing the patella. However, these inflammatory conditions frequently occur in younger age females with a host patellar bone thickness <15 to 20 mm and osteopenic and soft bone quality and may be associated with chronic corticosteroid or immunosuppressive disease-modifying medical therapy. If the native patellar thickness is thin (<15 mm), there is balanced patellar tracking during the TKA, and with controlled medical therapy the surgeon may consider leaving the patella unresurfaced in an inflammatory arthropathy, especially in a younger patient (< 50 years) who may require further revision TKA surgery in the future. The traditional indications and contraindications for resurfacing of the patella are outlined in Table 45-2. An algorithm for patella resurfacing (Fig. 45-1) has been proposed.[5]

TABLE 45-1. Preoperative Patellar Problems and Conditions Encountered Before Primary TKA

Patellofemoral OA, RA, inflammatory conditions
Previous patella fracture ± retained patella hardware
Prior extensor mechanism procedure (proximal, distal, bone, or soft tissue procedure)
Patella maltracking (lateral subluxation, tilt)
Recurrent patellar instability/dislocation
Osteonecrosis of the patella and fragmentation
Bipartite/tripartite patella
Patellectomy
Remote quadriceps tendon or patellar tendon rupture and repair
Extensor lag
Severe patella infera/baja
Knee fusion (with or without patella/extensor mechanism intact)
Arthroscopic (or open) lateral release
Thin patellar thickness (<15 mm)

TABLE 45-2. Indications for Patellar Resurfacing and Nonresurfacing

Traditional Indications for Patellar Resurfacing
Older age
Patellofemoral symptoms/anterior knee pain
Patellofemoral radiographic changes
Inflammatory arthropathy (rheumatoid arthritis)
Obesity
Intraoperative patellar maltracking
History of patellar subluxation/dislocation
Improved stair climbing
Less anterior knee pain postoperatively
Nonanatomic patellar trochlear groove on femoral component
Significant patellofemoral articular cartilage loss noted intraoperatively
Traditional Indications for Nonresurfacing of the Patella
Short, thin patient
Younger age
Osteoarthritis/noninflammatory arthritis
Well-preserved patellofemoral articular cartilage intraoperatively
Congruent patella tracking intraoperatively
Inadequate size or thickness of the patella for resurfacing
Femoral component with anatomic trochlear groove for native patella

The normal anatomy of the patella and its relation to the femur must be understood when considering management during TKA. The anteroposterior thickness of the patella is wider over the medial half of the patella and thinner on the lateral side. Thus, if the surgeon wishes to achieve a uniform patellar thickness at the time of resurfacing, the patellar osteotomy cut must be deeper on the medial side of the patella (Fig. 45-2), which is templated preoperatively. Failure to cut the patella in this fashion will result in a thicker medial composite thickness of the resurfaced patella (Fig. 45-3).

The decision to resurface the patella or not in TKA may have several biomechanical considerations. The patella acts as a dynamic fulcrum to transmit the forces generated by the extensor mechanism through the knee and may be responsible for providing up to a 50% increase in knee extension

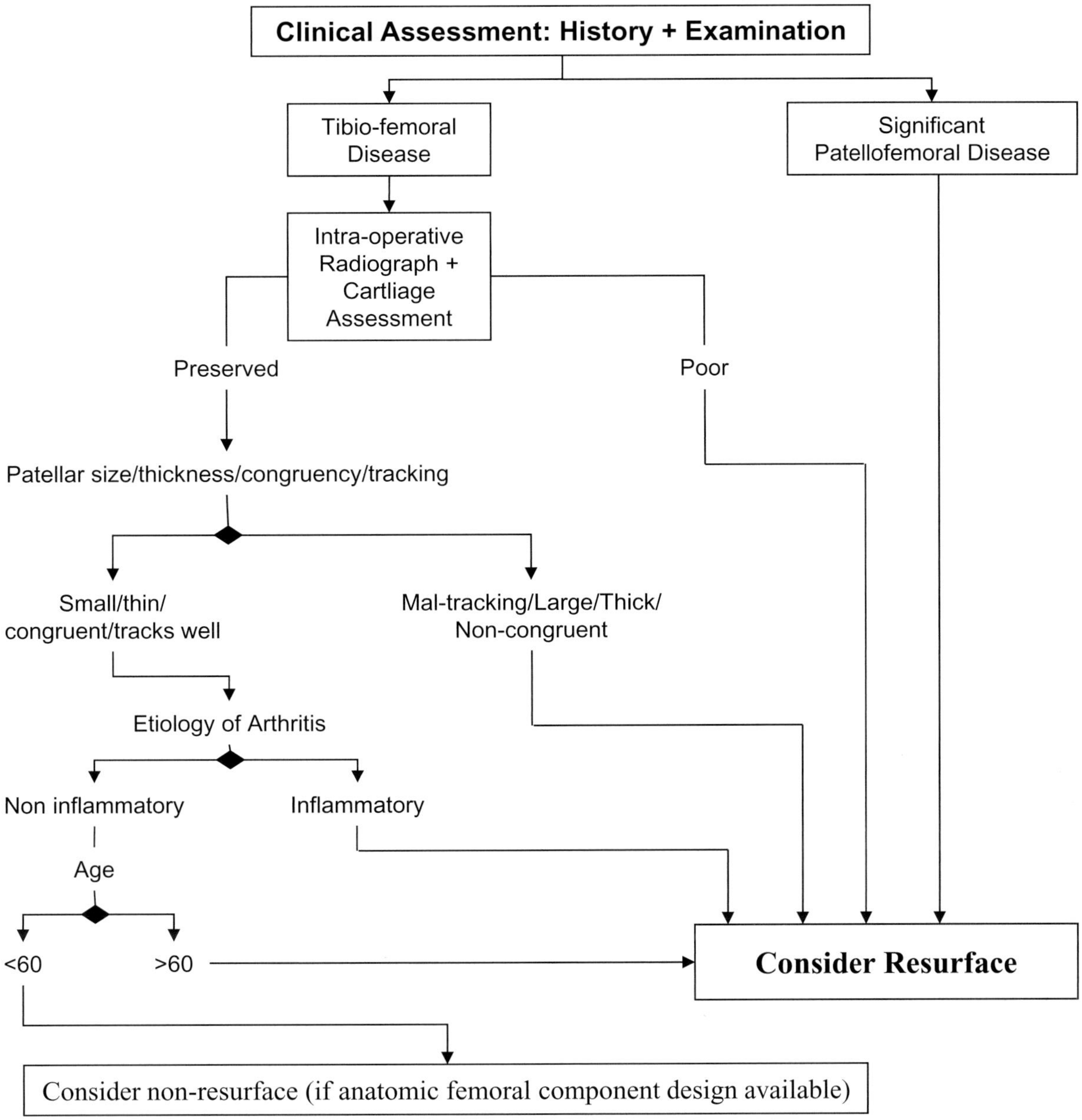

FIGURE 45-1. *A decision-making algorithm for patellar resurfacing in total knee arthroplasty. Selective resurfacing based on clinical, radiographic, and intraoperative parameters may be an option when considering how to manage the patella in TKA.*

compared with the knee without a functioning patella or patellectomy.[6] The contraction of the quadriceps mechanism has been associated with contact pressures exceeding 6.5 times body weight at the patellofemoral joint. It has been proposed that anterior knee pain following TKA may be secondary to altered biomechanics[7,8] at the patellofemoral joint. Increased patellofemoral joint forces are present with increased degrees of flexion,[9-11] which is one measure of success in TKA outcome. It has been shown that higher flexion concentrates forces onto the lateral superior and medial facets of the patella.[10] The resurfaced patella has been reported to be subjected to increased strain and

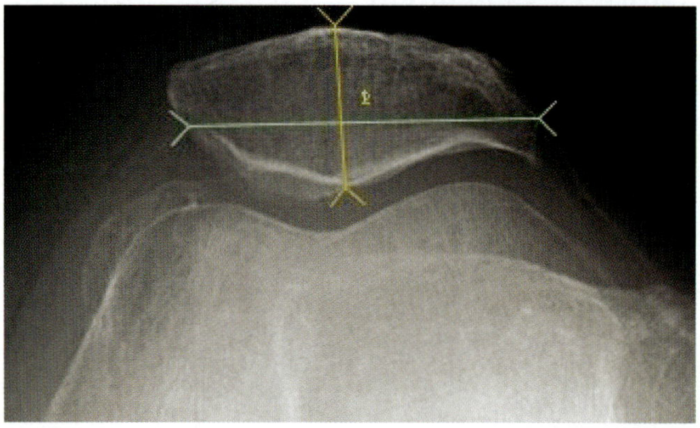

FIGURE 45-2. *The anteroposterior (AP) thickness is wider over the medial patella and thinner laterally (yellow vertical line) shown on the patellar axial view. In order to reproduce a uniform patellar thickness, the patella must be cut transversely with more resection medially than laterally (green transverse line).*

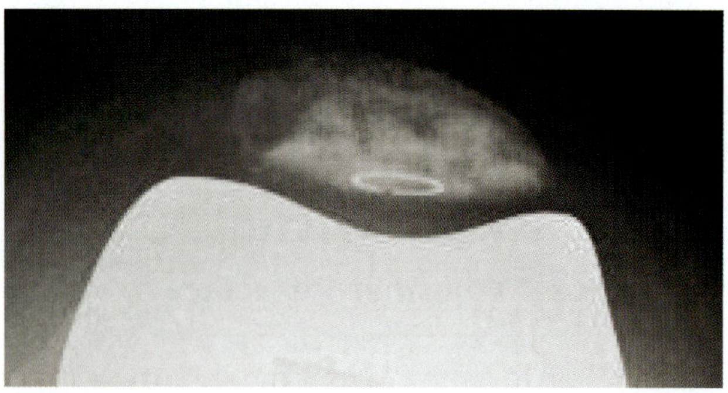

FIGURE 45-3. *The patella cut has been performed asymmetrically, shown on this patellar axial view.*

decreased tensile strength by as much as 30% to 40%.[12] The decreased thickness of bone, combined with osteopenia, may be a factor predisposing to patella fractures in the resurfaced patella. This may be worsened when combined with a lateral retinacular release, which may devascularize the extensor mechanism.[13,14] Finally, there is a question that remains to be answered: Is it logical to assume that articular cartilage is not going to wear on a metal surface?

Absolute contraindications to patella resurfacing in primary TKA include an absent patella (prior patellectomy). Patients with a prior patellectomy requiring a primary TKA for tibiofemoral arthritis have been reported with favorable results using a posterior-stabilized knee design[15]; however, TKA has a higher complication rate and inferior results if the knee has undergone prior patellectomy. Relative contraindications to patella resurfacing include a thin native patella <15 mm thickness. Despite the popularity and use of porous metal patella implants in primary and revision TKA (and their potential for soft tissue ingrowth), their use is indicated primarily when a shell of host bone remains. The use of porous metal patella components in patients with a prior patellectomy is contraindicated and will result in complications including noningrowth and subsequent erosion of the implant through the host extensor mechanism and into the subcutaneous tissues.[16]

Metal-backed patellar components have historically had a high revision rate,[17] secondary to wear through of the polyethylene and subsequent articulation of exposed titanium of the component against the patellar component. Improvements in polyethylene sterilization techniques and implant design have recently led to a renewed interest in metal-backed cementless patellar components in primary TKA, although without any published results.

PREOPERATIVE PLANNING

Preoperative patellar conditions may be identified by performing a careful preoperative history of the knee and noting any prior surgical procedures, especially remote childhood or adolescent "knee-cap" surgeries. Whenever possible, old operative reports should be sought to determine the type of extensor mechanism procedure(s) performed in the past. A directed physical exam of the knee and extensor mechanism should be performed, noting any abnormalities in the extensor mechanism function. Plain radiographs of the knee must include a patellar axial view. Adjunctive cross-sectional imaging (computed tomography, magnetic resonance imaging) may be useful in investigating patellar conditions encountered preoperatively and patellar complications associated with TKA surgery. The patellar axial radiograph (Merchant's view) is useful to assess the preoperative pathology of the patellofemoral joint, tracking within the trochlea, any degree of subluxation or lateral tilt, and thickness of host patellar bone. The lateral radiograph of the knee is useful to identify any preoperative patella infera/baja. Identifying and noting patella infera at the time of templating is useful to remind the surgeon that the exposure may be more challenging and that there may be more tension on the extensor mechanism during retraction during TKA surgery.

If the surgeon anticipates that exposure of the knee may be difficult via a standard medial parapatellar arthrotomy, then more extensile exposures should be planned. In primary TKA surgery the medial parapatellar arthrotomy is extensile and is usually sufficient. In addition, it easily allows for a more extensile quadriceps snip[18] exposure. Alternative exposures such as the mini-midvastus and subvastus exposures may also be suitable, yet less extensile. An extensive lateral release may disrupt further the superior and inferior lateral geniculate arteries and completely devascularize the extensor mechanism (Fig. 45-4), and thus should be used with caution. A tibial tubercle osteotomy may be rarely required in primary TKA exposure in cases of extreme patella infera or in rare cases such as posttraumatic proximal tibial deformity or in knee fusion takedown (and conversion to TKA). In instances of chronic patellar dislocation combined with degenerative arthritis requiring a TKA, routine management of the patella and extensor mechanism may not address the chronicity of the extensor maltracking. In such cases, proximal realignment procedures [vastus medialis obliquus (VMO) advancement] combined with tibial tubercle osteotomy realignment may be necessary to establish central extensor mechanism tracking. The surgeon should not assume that performing a TKA with patellar resurfacing and a lateral release will solve such chronic extensor mechanism maltracking and should plan preoperatively to manage this condition with realignment as required.

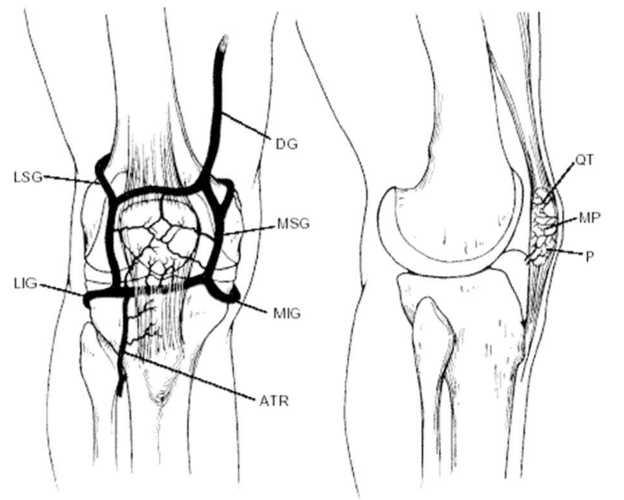

FIGURE 45-4. *Blood supply to the patella. (**Left**) The peripatellar extraosseous anastamotic ring is composed of five genicular branches [descending (DG), medial superior (MSG), medial inferior (MIG), lateral superior (LSG), lateral inferior (LIG)] and one anterior tibial recurrent (ATR) branch. (**Right**) The three intraosseous zones of patellar blood supply are the quadriceps tendon supply (QT) proximally, the midpatellar supply (MP), and the polar supply (P) distally. (Adapted from Lonner JH, Lotke PA. Aseptic complications after total knee arthroplasty. J Am Acad Orthop Surg. 1999;7(5):314.)*

TECHNIQUES: PATELLA RESURFACING AND NONRESURFACING

Exposure

Soft tissue balancing of the extensor mechanism in TKA is primarily a function of obtaining correct external rotation of the femoral and tibial components during TKA surgery, combined with joint line restoration, and ligamentous balance. If the patella is resurfaced, then optimal tracking may be achieved by medializing the patellar component and placing the implant superiorly on the patella host bone. The intraoperative extensor mechanism and patellar problems and conditions that may be encountered during primary TKA are outlined in Table 45-3. Once the surgeon completes the medial arthrotomy, it is useful to examine the tracking of the native patella and extensor mechanism before any bone or soft tissue preparation. This gives the

TABLE 45-3. Intraoperative Patellar Problems and Conditions Encountered During Primary TKA

Patella maltracking (lateral subluxation, tilt: femoral/tibial component malrotation)
Overstuffing/understuffing of the patellofemoral joint composite thickness
Tendon rupture (patellar tendon, quadriceps tendon)
Patella fracture (during preparation for resurfacing)
Devascularization of the extensor mechanism
Denervation of the vastus medialis obliquus
Asymmetric patellar bone cut during resurfacing
Patellar component malposition
Lateral patellar facet hypertrophy and impingement

surgeon a baseline for extensor tracking, patellar tilt, and subluxation before bone and soft tissue preparation. If there is extensor maltracking with trial implants, the surgeon should be alerted to a component malrotation problem and reassess femoral and tibial component external rotation.

Femoral and Tibial Component Rotation

Femoral component external rotation is crucial to extensor mechanism tracking. The femoral component should be aligned perpendicular to Whiteside's AP axis[19] and/or parallel to the transepicondylar axis (TEA), and we use both of these landmarks (Fig. 45-5) routinely during primary TKA surgery. Whether you use anterior or posterior referencing for femoral component sizing, the anterior cut on the femur should have the appearance of a "grand piano," with a resection higher on the lateral side compared to the medial. In addition, the anterior cut on the femur should be flush against the femur, without notching, and without being proud. Leaving the femoral component proud and nonflush with the femur anteriorly will overstuff the patellofemoral joint. Lateralizing the femoral component on host bone may also improve patellar tracking. [**Caution**: Excessive femoral component rotation will result in a widened medial flexion gap and a narrowed lateral flexion gap and may give the impression of false "medial laxity" in flexion.] In addition, excessive external rotation of the femoral component may result in notching of the lateral anterior femoral cortex. Elevation of the tibiofemoral joint line as a result of additional distal femoral resection may result in a relative patella baja. Proper tibial component external rotation is achieved by aligning the trial baseplate over the medial third of the tibial tubercle. An alternative is to allow the tibial baseplate to "self-align," performing a trial reduction (femoral trial and the trial polyethylene inserted into the tibial baseplate) and range of motion and then marking the rotation of the baseplate on the tibia. The surgeon should optimize tibial

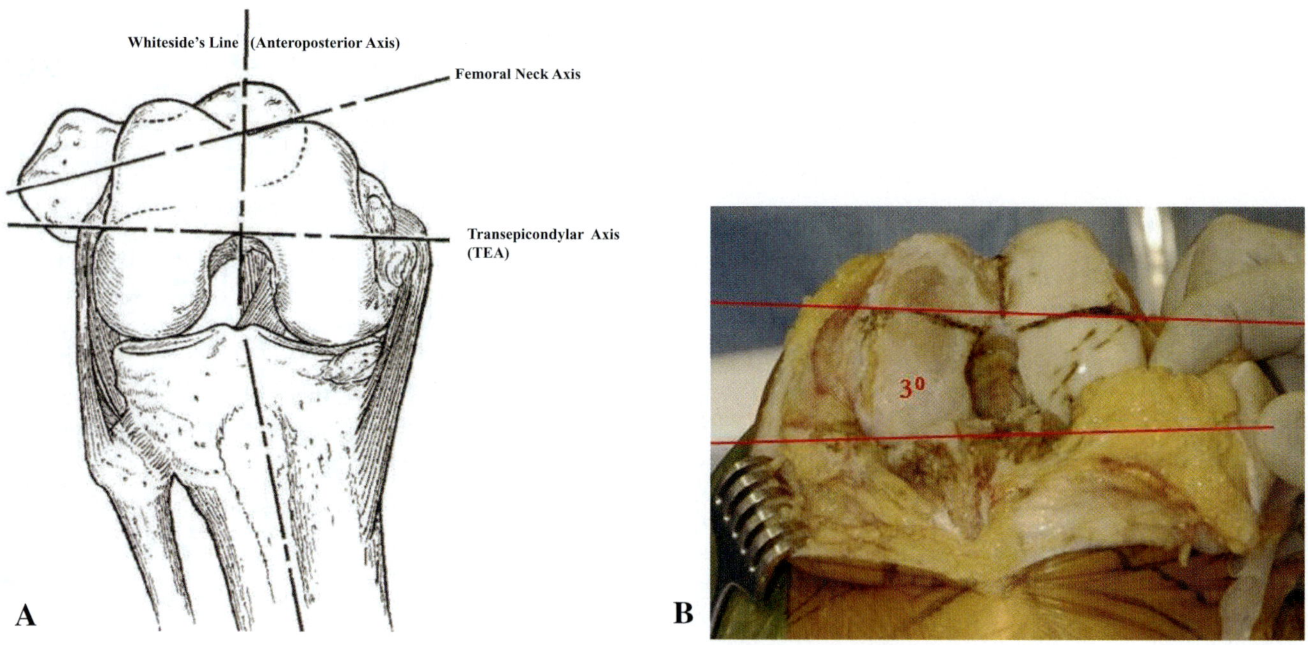

Figure 45-5. *(A) Schematic diagram demonstrating the relationship between the transepicondylar axis (TEA), "Whiteside's line" AP axis, and the femoral neck axis. Whiteside's line is drawn from the deepest portion of the trochlear groove to the most medial border of the posterior cruciate ligament origin in the intercondylar notch. (**B**) Intraoperative marking of Whiteside's line, the TEA, and the posterior femoral condylar axis (PCA), which is 3° internally rotated with respect to the TEA.*

component rotation and achieve appropriate tibial bone coverage, avoiding overhang posterolaterally on the tibia. [**Caution**: Excessive external tibial baseplate rotation will lead to excessive internal rotation of the tibia with respect to the baseplate and the patient will complain of a foot internal rotation deformity postoperatively.]

Patella Resurfacing

Frequently when we are resurfacing the patella, the patellar osteotomy cut is performed before femoral and tibial preparation in order to allow increased space for retraction once the patella is cut. Use caution when using this technique of "patella cut first" in patients with a thin patella or soft patellar bone because this may result in damage to the patella bone from retractors during femoral and tibial preparation. If the patellar bone is soft, a trial patella may be placed on the cut bone during femoral and tibial preparation. The patella may be cut using milling devices, captured saw cutting guides, and freehand saw technique and may be prepared for an inlay or onlay component. Regardless of technique, the patellar and quadriceps tendons must not be injured during the bone preparation, and the cut must produce a symmetrical patellar thickness. Asymmetric resurfacing of the patella typically involves the inadvertent preferential resurfacing of the lateral facet with underresection of bone from the medial patellar facet. Increased revision rates and symptomatic anterior knee pain have been associated with this technical error.[20] Overzealous use of patellar clamps, patellar reamer slippage, and overreaming may additionally weaken the bone. Patella resection is not a procedure to be performed multiple times, in order to avoid injury to the extensor mechanism tendons, and thus this is not a procedure for an inexperienced trainee. In addition, patellar clamps with "reamer stop" settings must be used with caution and require meticulous technique and experience. Excessive patellar resection may be associated with increased patellar strain and fracture, especially if the subchondral bone is removed. A residual bone thickness after resection of less than 15 mm may substantially increase anterior patellar strain. Preoperative templating usually dictates a thicker resection medially compared to laterally. The cut patellar thickness is then remeasured with the caliper. The implant patellar thickness of most primary patellar onlay all-polyethylene components is 9 to 10 mm. The goal of the patellar cut is to restore the composite thickness of the native patella while not underresecting the patella. The patellar sizing guide is used to establish correct positioning of the patellar component on the patella—medializing and superiorly locating the trial to enhance patellar tracking, while maintaining appropriate patellar bone coverage with the implant. We prefer to use a 3-peg onlay domed patellar component; however, inlay (or inset) patellar component designs may also be used with favorable results.[21] In one study, inset patellar fixation resistance to shear disassociation was 25% higher than that of onlay patellae.[22] Patellar reaming in preparation for a large single central peg hole may increase the anterior patellar strain greater than with smaller multiple pegged designs, predisposing to fracture. On occasion, if there is a hypertrophic lateral facet of the patella which is not covered by the implant, then we will resect this lateral facet, maintaining the integrity of the lateral retinaculum. Cemented patellar fixation is our preference in primary TKA. The patellar component is cemented in place using a pressurizing clamp that allows for adequate pressurization and removal of excess cement. Note that in patients with a thin patella composite thickness, some manufacturer's patellar pressurization clamps are inadequate for thin sizes. It is important to recognize this because unavailability of a clamp for thin patella sizes will result in inadequate pressurization. It has been reported that thermal necrosis during cementing of the patellar implant may lead to diminished local blood supply and osteonecrosis of the patellar bone,[23,24] because temperatures up to 80°C to 90°C may develop.

Lateral Release: Indications and Technique

A lateral release should rarely be necessary. The decision to perform a lateral release should be made if the femoral and tibial components have been appropriately aligned in external rotation and the patella has a tendency to sublux laterally. A significant "tilt" of the patella laterally should alert the surgeon to reassess component rotation and position of the trial implants. The technique for a lateral release begins in the lateral gutter, initially releasing longitudinally the synovium, plicae, and any soft tissue adhesions in the lateral gutter, staying lateral to the lateral collateral ligament. We avoid a full-thickness lateral release, preferring to release the synovium and inner aspect of the lateral retinaculum, followed by a staged lateral release.[25] In addition, the release is performed after the tourniquet has been deflated for two reasons. The first reason is to ensure that the quadriceps is not contracted by the tourniquet. The second reason is that the superior lateral geniculate vessels must be visualized in the superior lateral gutter; we attempt to preserve these vessels in order to minimize extensor mechanism devascularization.

Patellar Vascularity and Preservation of Blood Supply

Preservation of blood supply to the patella during standard surgical exposure has been implicated as a means of reducing the risk of avascular necrosis and subsequent fracture.[26-31] Histological evaluation of patellar specimens after patellar fracture has documented the presence of osteonecrosis.[27,32] Anatomical studies have demonstrated the extensive extraosseous and intraosseous arterial systems contributing to patellar blood supply.[14,33-35] Substantial disruption of the patellar vascular supply occurs during routine exposure in TKR.[13,14,27,28, 30,32,36-41] All of the geniculate vessels are potentially at risk during TKR surgery and subsequent patellar resurfacing. Aggressive infrapatellar fat pad resection may compromise the traversing branches supplying the inferior pole of the patella and the lateral inferior genicular artery. Standard medial parapatellar arthrotomy divides the medial superior, inferior, and descending genicular arteries. During routine lateral meniscectomy, the lateral inferior genicular branch is often cut. If a lateral retinacular release is being performed for patellar maltracking, the superior lateral genicular artery is at risk if it is not dissected out and preserved during the exposure. Nonpreservation of this artery may predispose to an increased patellar fracture risk.[42] Despite a reduced patellar vascularity noted on technetium bone scans in the early postoperative period after lateral release,[13,40,41] revascularization may occur in the patella as early as 2 months postoperatively.[13] Other studies have shown that lateral release does not lead to postoperative diminished blood flow[43]and thus the debate on this subject continues.

PREVENTION OF PATELLA FRACTURES

Operative technique, implant selection, and component alignment are controlled by the surgeon, and careful attention to these factors may reduce the risk of periprosthetic patella fracture. Proper restoration of patellar thickness and preserving the symmetry of the medial and lateral facet thickness is crucial. Achieving proper femoral and tibial component external rotation will reproduce more normal patellar tracking and reduce the subluxation and dislocation seen with malrotated implants. Avoiding a large central peg and considering designs with a smaller peripheral peg fixation system may be preferred. Repetitive patellar impingement on the polyethylene insert may result, leading to patella fatigue failure, especially at the inferior pole. It has been postulated that patellar fracture rates may be higher with the use of such posterior-stabilized implants.[44,45] Excessive patellofemoral malalignment[36,46,47] with associated patellar subluxation[48,49] leads to eccentric loading and contact forces, which may contribute to fracture risk. Attempting to maintain the patellar blood supply through limited fat pad excision, avoiding large central pegs, and maintaining the lateral superior geniculate artery during lateral retinacular release may reduce vascular compromise to the patella and reduce fracture risk.

PATELLA NONRESURFACING VERSUS RESURFACING

Randomized Trials and Meta-Analyses

Favorable results have been described for nonresurfacing of the patella at the time of TKA, with outcomes equal to patients undergoing patella resurfacing.[1,2,5,50-61] A detailed analysis of these results is beyond the scope of this chapter. However, several points are worth noting about these studies. The majority of these studies demonstrate no difference in outcomes comparing resurfacing to nonresurfacing. The higher incidence of reoperations in the nonresurfacing groups in any study may be attributed to the fact that secondary patellar resurfacing adds a surgical option for the treatment of anterior knee pain following total knee arthroplasty, thus artificially increasing the rate of reoperations in the nonresurfacing group. A knee that has undergone resurfacing of the patella and is causing significant ongoing anterior knee pain should be considered a failure, because this patient would likely be offered a revision surgery if the patella had been left nonresurfaced. Thus the results must be interpreted with caution. The existing evidence from meta-analyses indicates that patellar resurfacing may reduce the risk of reoperation with no improvement in postoperative knee function or patient satisfaction over total knee arthroplasty without patellar resurfacing. Whether it can decrease the incidence of anterior knee pain remains uncertain. Selective patellar resurfacing would be the ideal solution if sound preoperative criteria could be established. In our experience and others,[1,51] revision of a nonresurfaced patella for anterior knee pain is successful in relieving symptoms in only 50% of cases, and thus that procedure should be offered with caution. So far, a method for accurately predicting which patients can avoid patellar resurfacing has not been found. Future research looking at patellar resurfacing should focus on developing criteria for selecting those patients who would benefit from patellar resurfacing and those who would do as well without resurfacing, thereby limiting potential surgical complications.

When the patella is left unresurfaced, a "patellaplasty"[62] may be considered. This includes removal of circumferential patellar osteophyes and any fragmented articular cartilage, combined with a circumferential electrocautery of the synovium around the patella border (without causing damage to the patellar and quadriceps tendon insertions on the patella). The results[63] and technique of circumpatellar electrocautery suggest that, in the absence of patellar resurfacing, electrocautery around the margin of the patella improves the outcome of total knee replacement.

Factors to Consider in Patella Resurfacing

Isolated patellofemoral arthritis

The knee with isolated patellofemoral arthritis poses a challenging problem to the orthopaedic surgeon. Often there may be a history of previous trauma to the patella or associated patellofemoral instability in the past. Abnormal extensor mechanism biomechanics in these patients may be secondary to underlying developmental musculoskeletal abnormalities or secondary to previous reconstructive procedures. In patients with a history of proximal or distal realignment procedures of the extensor mechanism, the total knee arthroplasty may be increasingly complicated. Numerous operative procedures have been described for the treatment of isolated patellofemoral disease. The surgical options for isolated patellofemoral arthritis are diverse and include joint debridement, soft tissue, or bony extensor mechanism realignment, patellectomy, patellar resurfacing, and total knee arthroplasty. Cartilage repair and transplantation procedures may have a role in the treatment of focal cartilage defects, but this technique is not currently useful for end-stage knee arthritis.[64] Patellectomy has been advocated as an option for the treatment for severe patellofemoral arthritis.[65,66] Patellectomy decreases the strength of the quadriceps and the efficiency of the extensor mechanism while increasing the tension in the patellar tendon.[67,68] Patellofemoral maltracking and instability must be addressed even if the patella is removed to prevent extensor mechanism subluxation or dislocation. Furthermore, the results of total knee arthroplasty after previous patellectomy may be suboptimal.[69]

Recently, there has been renewed interest in patellofemoral arthroplasty because the treatment of this entity has been difficult.[70] The best results with patellofemoral arthroplasty have been obtained in patients with posttraumatic patellofemoral arthritis as compared with patients with idiopathic patellofemoral arthritis.[71] Thus, what is the best solution for isolated patellofemoral arthritis? There is a paucity of reports on the outcome of total knee arthroplasty for isolated patellofemoral arthritis. Parvizi et al[72] have reported on the results of TKA with patellar resurfacing in this population. At a minimum 2-year follow-up, 31 knees had undergone TKA for advanced patellofemoral arthritis with the use of three different TKA designs. Knee Society scores for pain and function improved, and range of motion was unchanged. Preoperative anterior knee pain was improved. Twenty-one (67%) of the knees required a lateral retinacular release and three required a formal proximal realignment procedure at the time of primary TKA with patellar resurfacing. Three patients required further intervention, including a manipulation under anesthesia, revision of the patellar implant, and an extensor mechanism realignment. Thus, resurfacing of the patella and balancing the extensor mechanism for patients with isolated patellofemoral arthritis can be demanding technically, as evidenced by the high rate of asymmetrically resurfaced patellas, the high rate of lateral retinacular release, and formal realignment procedures.

Obesity

Obesity has been studied in relation to patellar resurfacing, and routine resurfacing is often recommended.[73-75] Obese patients have been reported to experience increased rates of postoperative symptoms after TKA compared with the nonobese population.[75]. Conversely, others have noted the opposite (ie, obese patients experienced increased pain with resurfacing).[76] A weight greater than 150% of ideal body weight was associated with a two times increase in patellofemoral pain in this study. A higher rate of patellofemoral complications[74] in obese compared with nonobese patients has been reported, whereas weight, but not body mass index, was associated with postoperative anterior knee pain in nonresurfaced patellas, suggesting that total joint loading, and not obesity, may be a critical factor in the development of anterior knee pain.[3]

Rheumatoid arthritis

Inflammatory arthritis has consistently been reported as one absolute indication to resurfacing the patella in TKA. Often the patients may be sedentary, with relative osteopenia, and have stage III or IV rheumatoid disease.[77] The patella may be small in size, making resurfacing difficult or impossible to perform. Synovitis involving the extensor mechanism may be a contributing factor to peripatellar pain in patients with rheumatoid arthritis (RA). The presence of remaining articular cartilage may provide an antigenic stimulus for persistent synovial inflammation[78] and propagate the immune-mediated inflammatory response.[79,80] However, when the literature is reviewed more closely on this indication, it is interesting to note that once again it does not appear to be absolute. There are those who recommend routine resurfacing in all patients with RA[75,78,79,81-84] and others who have reported that RA is not a contraindication to leave the patella unresurfaced.[7,85,86] A lower incidence of complications from resurfacing of the patella in rheumatoid patients compared to patients with osteoarthritis (OA) has been suggested to be due to a decreased functional demand and elimination of the reaction between patellar cartilage and synovium.[84,87] In the Swedish Knee Arthroplasty Registry,[88] the satisfaction rates in patients with RA have been reported. In 1813 knees that were left unresurfaced, 15% of these were unsatisfied or unsure of the result, compared to 12% of 1208 knees that were resurfaced. Overall, rheumatoid patients were more satisfied with the results of TKA compared to OA patients, regardless of patellar resurfacing. The large number of patients in this report would indicate that the advantage of resurfacing may be in a slight increase in overall patient satisfaction.

POSTOPERATIVE MANAGEMENT

Postoperative physical therapy (PT) following primary TKA allows weight bearing as tolerated, with active range of motion of the knee permitted. Passive assisted range of motion may be performed in patients with difficulty achieving flexion, at the discretion of the treating surgeon. Outpatient physical therapy begins immediately following hospital discharge. Patients may immediately begin quadriceps strengthening isometric exercises, VMO strengthening, and light resistance exercises. We use both mechanical and pharmacological prophylaxis for venous thromboembolism postoperatively. No modification of PT is necessary for the quadriceps snip extensile exposure. If a patient has undergone a tibial tubercle osteotomy or proximal realignment procedure (rare), the PT must be modified postoperatively to limit the degree of active and passive flexion to protect the osteotomy, frequently using a hinged knee brace to lock out higher degrees of flexion. Communication between the surgeon and the physical therapist is extremely important to minimize complications and maximize patient satisfaction and recovery following primary TKA surgery.

COMPLICATIONS

Complications following primary TKA occur in approximately 1% to 3% of patients. The postoperative extensor mechanism and patellar problems and conditions that may be encountered following primary TKA are outlined in Table 45-4. While complications are rare, complications that are associated with the extensor mechanism may be problematic. Patellar tendon or quadriceps tendon ruptures are devastating complications that require early intervention, usually are not manageable with primary repair, and require advanced techniques for reconstruction.[89,90] Recognizing extensor mechanism complications requires a high index of suspicion. Similarly, isolated revision of a failed patellar resurfacing component should be undertaken with caution. The surgeon should assess for femoral or tibial component malrotation as a contributing factor to extensor mechanism problems and complications postoperatively. In patients who have undergone patella resurfacing and have ongoing anterior knee symptoms, plain X-rays may be nondiagnostic. A high index of suspicion for occult osteonecrosis of the patella must be considered. Serial radiographs may demonstrate increased sclerosis of the patella, loosening of the patellar implant, fragmentation of patellar bone, and pathological fracture of the sclerotic and osteonecrotic patella (Fig. 45-6). Management options of the osteonecrotic patella that has previously been resurfaced may include revision of the component, fracture fixation plus or minus revision of the component, or patellectomy.

TABLE 45-4. Postoperative Patellar Problems and Conditions Encountered Following Primary TKA

Patella maltracking (lateral subluxation, tilt: femoral/tibial component malrotation)
Recurrent patellar instability/dislocation
Anterior knee pain
Overstuffing/understuffing of the patellofemoral joint composite thickness
Tendon rupture (patellar tendon, quadriceps tendon)
Patella fracture (more common with patella resurfacing)
Osteonecrosis/patellar fragmentation
Patellar component malposition
Lateral patellar facet hypertrophy and impingement
Patellar component loosening
Patellar component polyethylene wear
Metal-backed patellar component complications (wear, burnishing, titanium wear debris)

PEARLS AND PITFALLS

There are numerous pearls to produce a balanced extensor mechanism tracking and optimal patellofemoral outcomes in TKA surgery. Identifying pitfalls or problems is of similar importance. These may be summarized as follows:

- Plan preoperatively for how to manage the patella (nonresurfacing versus resurfacing) and discuss this plan with the patient in advance.

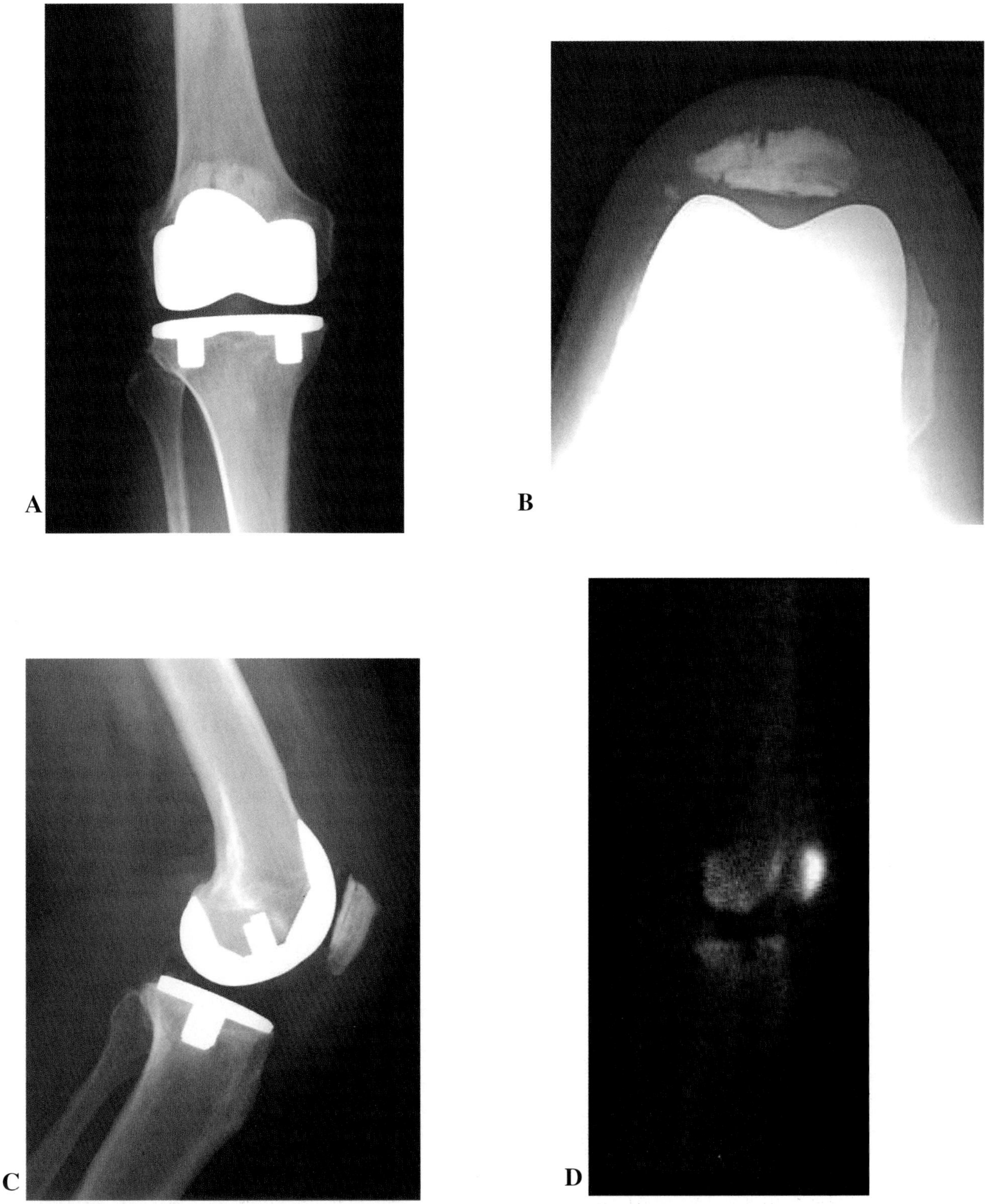

FIGURE 45-6. *See next page for figure legend.*

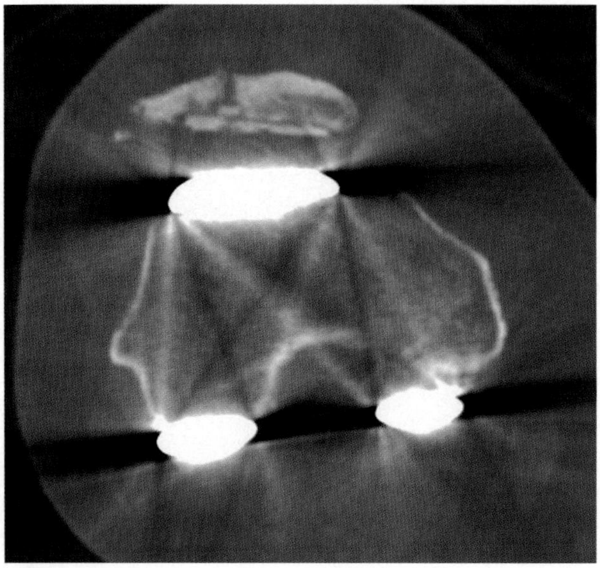

E

FIGURE 45-6. *Radiographs (**A**, **B**, **C**), bone scan (**D**), and computed tomography (**E**) in a patient referred 2 years following right TKA with patella resurfacing and severe anterior knee pain. The imaging demonstrates osteonecrosis of the patella with increased sclerosis of patellar bone, increased uptake on bone scan (diffusely), and a periprosthetic patella fracture.*

- Use an exposure that allows for intraoperative extension proximally and distally.
- Establish correct femoral and tibial component external rotation and, more important, avoid internal malrotation of components.
- Restore composite patellar thickness and do not overstuff the patellofemoral joint.
- If patellar maltracking is noted intraoperatively, reassess femoral and tibial component rotation and positioning. Avoid using a lateral release, especially if the patella tracked well preoperatively.
- Patellar component cementing should not be dismissed to the very end of the procedure when cement is doughy and unsuitable for interdigitation. Consider mixing a staged batch of cement for the patella to avoid using cement that is too doughy.
- Protect the extensor mechanism (the patellar tendon is most at risk) and ligaments carefully during bone preparation with saws, especially during the tibial cut.
- Recognize that minimally invasive TKA surgery may be fraught with complications[91] and early failure, especially with regards to the extensor mechanism, component malrotation and alignment, and soft tissue injury, and should be avoided unless the surgeon has special training and experience with these techniques.
- Recognize the potential complications that may be associated with management of the patella during TKA surgery.

SUGGESTED READING

Burnett RS. Management of patellofemoral problems in primary TKA. In: Rossi R, Bruzzone M, eds. *Soft Tissue Balancing in Primary Total Knee Arthroplasty.* Milan, Italy: Minerva Medica Spa; 2012:99-114.

REFERENCES

1. Burnett RS, Boone JL, Rosenzweig SD, et al. Patellar resurfacing compared with nonresurfacing in total knee arthroplasty. A concise follow-up of a randomized trial. *J Bone Joint Surg Am.* 2009;91(11):2562-2567.
2. Breeman S, Campbell M, Dakin H, et al. Patellar resurfacing in total knee replacement: five-year clinical and economic results of a large randomized clinical trial. *J Bone Joint Surg Am.* 2011;93(16):1473-1481.
3. Wood DJ, Smith AJ, Collopy D, et al. Patellar resurfacing in total knee arthroplasty: a prospective, ran-

domized trial. *J Bone Joint Surg Am.* 2002;84(2):187-193.

4. Barrack RL, Schrader T, Bertot AJ, et al. Component rotation and anterior knee pain after total knee arthroplasty. *Clin Orthop Relat Res.* 2001;392:36-45.
5. Burnett RS, Bourne RB. Indications for patellar resurfacing in total knee arthroplasty. *Instr Course Lect.* 2004;53:167-186.
6. Zappala FG, Taffel CB, Scuderi GR. Rehabilitation of patellofemoral joint disorders. Review. *Orthop Clin North Am.* 1992;23(4):555-566.
7. Boyd ADJ, Ewald FC, Thomas WH, et al. Long-term complications after total knee arthroplasty with or without resurfacing of the patella. *J Bone Joint Surg Am.* 1993;75(5):674-681.
8. Smith SR, Stuart P, Pinder IM. Nonresurfaced patella in total knee arthroplasty. *J Arthroplasty.* 1989;4 (suppl):S81-86.
9. Huberti HH, Hayes WC. Patellofemoral contact pressures. The influence of q-angle and tendofemoral contact. *J Bone Joint Surg Am.* 1984;66(5):715-724.
10. Hungerford DS, Barry M. Biomechanics of the patellofemoral joint. *Clin Orthop Relat Res.* 1979;144:9-15.
11. Matthews LS, Sonstegard DA, Henke JA. Load bearing characteristics of the patello-femoral joint. *Acta Orthop Scand.* 1977;48(5):511-516.
12. Reuben JD, McDonald CL, Woodard PL, Hennington LJ. Effect of patella thickness on patella strain following total knee arthroplasty. *J Arthroplasty.* 1991;6(3): 251-258.
13. Scuderi G, Scharf SC, Meltzer LP, et al. The relationship of lateral releases to patella viability in total knee arthroplasty. *J Arthroplasty.* 1987;2(3):209-214.
14. Kayler DE, Lyttle D. Surgical interruption of patellar blood supply by total knee arthroplasty. *Clin Orthop Relat Res.* 1988;229:221-227.
15. Cameron HU, Hu C, Vyamont D. Posterior stabilized knee prosthesis for total knee replacement in patients with prior patellectomy. *Can J Surg.* 1996;39(6):469-473.
16. Ries MD, Cabalo A, Bozic KJ, et al. Porous tantalum patellar augmentation: the importance of residual bone stock. *Clin Orthop Relat Res.* 2006;452:166-170.
17. Berger RA, Lyon JH, Jacobs JJ, et al. Problems with cementless total knee arthroplasty at 11 years followup. *Clin Orthop Relat Res.* 2001;392:196-207.
18. Barrack RL. Specialized surgical exposure for revision total knee: quadriceps snip and patellar turndown. *Instr Course Lect.* 1999;48:149-152.
19. Whiteside LA, Arima J. The anteroposterior axis for femoral rotational alignment in valgus total knee arthroplasty. *Clin Orthop Relat Res.* 1995;321:168-172.
20. Pagnano MW, Trousdale RT. Asymmetric patella resurfacing in total knee arthroplasty. *Am J Knee Surg.* 2000;13(4):228-233.
21. Lachiewicz PF. Implant design and techniques for patellar resurfacing in total knee arthroplasty. *Instr Course Lect.* 2004;53:187-191.
22. Rosenstein AD, Postak PD, Greenwald AS. Fixation strength comparison of onlay and inset patellar implants. *Knee.* 2007;14(3):194-197.
23. Grace JN, Sim FH. Fracture of the patella after total knee arthroplasty. *Clin Orthop Relat Res.* 1988; 230:168-175.
24. McMahon MS, Scuderi GR, Glashow JL, et al. Scintigraphic determination of patellar viability after excision of infrapatellar fat pad and/or lateral retinacular release in total knee arthroplasty. *Clin Orthop Relat Res.* 1990;260:10-16.
25. Strachan RK, Merican AM, Devadasan B, et al. A technique of staged lateral release to correct patellar tracking in total knee arthroplasty. *J Arthroplasty.* 2009;24(5):735-742.
26. Hozack WJ, Goll SR, Lotke PA, et al. The treatment of patellar fractures after total knee arthroplasty. *Clin Orthop Relat Res.* 1988;236:123-127.
27. Scott RD, Turoff N, Ewald FC. Stress fracture of the patella following duopatellar total knee arthroplasty with patellar resurfacing. *Clin Orthop Relat Res.* 1982;170:147-151.
28. Leblanc JM. Patellar complications in total knee arthroplasty. A literature review. *Orthop Rev.* 1989;18 (3):296-304.
29. Rand JA, Gustilo RB. Technique of patella resurfacing in total knee arthroplasty. *Tech Orthop.* 1988;2: 57-66.
30. Brick GW, Scott RD. The patellofemoral component of total knee arthroplasty. *Clin Orthop Relat Res.* 1988;231:163-178.
31. Lonner JH, Lotke PA. Aseptic complications after total knee arthroplasty. *J Am Acad Orthop Surg.* 1999; 7(5):311-324.
32. Insall J, Scott WN, Ranawat CS. The total condylar knee prosthesis. A report of two hundred and twenty cases. *J Bone Joint Surg Am.* 1979;61(2):173-180.

33. Bjorkstrom S, Goldie IF. A study of the arterial supply of the patella in the normal state, in chondromalacia patellae and in osteoarthrosis. *Acta Orthop Scand.* 1980;51(1):63-70.
34. Scapinelli R. Blood supply of the human patella. Its relation to ischaemic necrosis after fracture. *J Bone Joint Surg Br.* 1967;49(3):563-570.
35. Scapinelli R. Studies on the vasculature of the human knee joint. *Acta Anat (Basel).* 1968;70(3):305-331.
36. Goldberg VM, Figgie HE III, Inglis AE, et al. Patellar fracture type and prognosis in condylar total knee arthroplasty. *Clin Orthop Relat Res.* 1988(236):115-122.
37. Cameron HU, Fedorkow DM. The patella in total knee arthroplasty. *Clin Orthop Relat Res.* 1982;165: 197-199.
38. Clayton ML, Thirupathi R. Patellar complications after total condylar arthroplasty. *Clin Orthop Relat Res.* 1982;170:152-155.
39. Scott WN, Rubinstein M, Scuderi G. Results after knee replacement with a posterior cruciate-substituting prosthesis. *J Bone Joint Surg Am.* 1988;70 (8):1163-1173.
40. McMahon MS, Scuderi GR, Glashow JL, et al. Scintigraphic determination of patellar viability after excision of infrapatellar fat pad and/or lateral retinacular release in total knee arthroplasty. *Clin Orthop Relat Res.* 1990;260:10-16.
41. Wetzner SM, Bezreh JS, Scott RD, et al. Bone scanning in the assessment of patellar viability following knee replacement. *Clin Orthop Relat Res.* 1985;199: 215-219.
42. Ritter MA, Carr K, Keating EM, et al. Tibial shaft fracture following tibial tubercle osteotomy. *J Arthroplasty.* 1996;11(1):117-119.
43. Ritter MA, Campbell ED. Postoperative patellar complications with or without lateral release during total knee arthroplasty. *Clin Orthop Relat Res.* 1987; 219:163-168.
44. Aglietti P, Buzzi R, Gaudenzi A. Patellofemoral functional results and complications with the posterior stabilized total condylar knee prosthesis. *J Arthroplasty.* 1988;3(1):17-25.
45. Singerman R, Heiple KG, Davy DT, et al. Effect of tibial component position on patellar strain following total knee arthroplasty. *J Arthroplasty.* 1995;10(5): 651-656.
46. Kaufer H. Mechanical function of the patella. *J Bone Joint Surg Am.* 1971;53(8):1551-1560.
47. Figgie HE III, Goldberg VM, Figgie MP, et al. The effect of alignment of the implant on fractures of the patella after condylar total knee arthroplasty. *J Bone Joint Surg Am.* 1989;71(7):1031-1039.
48. Huberti HH, Hayes WC. Patellofemoral contact pressures. The influence of q-angle and tendofemoral contact. *J Bone Joint Surg Am.* 1984;66(5):715-724.
49. Berger RA, Crossett LS, Jacobs JJ, et al. Malrotation causing patellofemoral complications after total knee arthroplasty. *Clin Orthop Relat Res.* 1998;356:144-153.
50. Burnett RS, Boone JL, McCarthy KP, et al. A prospective randomized clinical trial of patellar resurfacing and nonresurfacing in bilateral TKA. *Clin Orthop Relat Res.* 2007;464:65-72.
51. Burnett RS, Haydon CM, Rorabeck CH, et al. Patella resurfacing versus nonresurfacing in total knee arthroplasty: results of a randomized controlled clinical trial at a minimum of 10 years' followup. *Clin Orthop Relat Res.* 2004;428:12-25.
52. Calvisi V, Camillieri G, Lupparelli S. Resurfacing versus nonresurfacing the patella in total knee arthroplasty: a critical appraisal of the available evidence. *Arch Orthop Trauma Surg.* 2009;129(9):1261-1270.
53. Fu Y, Wang G, Fu Q. Patellar resurfacing in total knee arthroplasty for osteoarthritis: a meta-analysis. *Knee Surg Sports Traumatol Arthrosc.* 2011;19(9): 1460-1466.
54. He JY, Jiang LS, Dai LY. Is patellar resurfacing superior than nonresurfacing in total knee arthroplasty? A meta-analysis of randomized trials. *Knee.* 2011;18(3): 137-144.
55. Helmy N, Anglin C, Greidanus NV, et al. To resurface or not to resurface the patella in total knee arthroplasty. *Clin Orthop Relat Res.* 2008;466(11):2775-2783.
56. Li S, Chen Y, Su W, et al. Systematic review of patellar resurfacing in total knee arthroplasty. *Int Orthop.* 2011;35(3):305-316.
57. Liu ZT, Fu PL, Wu HS, et al. Patellar reshaping versus resurfacing in total knee arthroplasty. Results of a randomized prospective trial at a minimum of 7 years' follow-up. *Knee.* April 22, 2011 [Epub ahead of print].
58. Pavlou G, Meyer C, Leonidou A, et al. Patellar resurfacing in total knee arthroplasty: does design matter? A meta-analysis of 7075 cases. *J Bone Joint Surg Am.* 2011;93(14):1301-1309.
59. Smith AJ, Wood DJ, Li MG. Total knee replacement with and without patellar resurfacing: a prospective,

randomised trial using the profix total knee system. *J Bone Joint Surg Br.* 2008;90(1):43-49.

60. Swan JD, Stoney JD, Lim K, et al. The need for patellar resurfacing in total knee arthroplasty: a literature review. *ANZ J Surg.* 2010;80(4):223-233.
61. Wood DJ, Smith AJ, Collopy D, et al. Patellar resurfacing in total knee arthroplasty: a prospective, randomized trial. *J Bone Joint Surg Am.* 2002;84(2):187-193.
62. Barrack RL, Schrader T, Bertot AJ, et al. Component rotation and anterior knee pain after total knee arthroplasty. *Clin Orthop Relat Res.* 2001;392:46-55.
63. van Jonbergen HP, Scholtes VA, van Kampen A, et al. A randomised, controlled trial of circumpatellar electrocautery in total knee replacement without patellar resurfacing. *J Bone Joint Surg Br.* 2011;93(8): 1054-1059.
64. Brittberg M, Lindahl A, Nilsson Aea. Treatment of full thickness cartilage defects in human knee with cultured autologous chondrocytes. *N Engl J Med.* 1994;331:889-895.
65. Ackroyd CE, Polyzoides AJ. Patellectomy for osteoarthritis: a study of 81 patients followed from two to twenty-two years. *J Bone Joint Surg Br.* 1970; 60:353-357.
66. Compere CL, Hill JA, Lewinnek GE, et al. A new method of patellectomy for patellofemoral arthritis. *J Bone Joint Surg Am.* 1979;61:714-719.
67. Haxton HA. The function of the patella and the effects of its excision. *Surg Gynecol Obstet.* 1945;80:389-341.
68. Sutton FS, Thompson CH, Lipke Jea. The effect of patellectomy on knee function. *J Bone Joint Surg Am.* 1976;58:537-540.
69. Laskin RS, Paletta G. Total knee replacement in the patient who has undergone a patellectomy. *J Bone Joint Surg Am.* 1995;77(1708-1712).
70. Cartier P, Sanouiller JL, Grelsamer R. Patellofemoral arthroplasty: 2-12-year follow-up study. *J Arthroplasty.* 1999;5:49-55.
71. Argensen JN, Guillame JM, Aubaniac JM. Is there a place for patellofemoral arthroplasty? *Clin Orthop Relat Res.* 1995;321:162-167.
72. Parvizi J, Stuart MJ, Pagnano MW, et al. Total knee arthroplasty in patients with isolated patellofemoral arthritis. *Clin Orthop Relat Res.* 2001;392:147-152.
73. Feller JA, Bartlett RJ, Lang DM. Patellar resurfacing versus retention in total knee arthroplasty. *J Bone Joint Surg Br.* 1996;78(2):226-228.
74. Healy WL, Wasilewski SA, Takei R, et al. Patellofemoral complications following total knee arthroplasty. Correlation with implant design and patient risk factors. *J Arthroplasty.* 1995;10(2):197-201.
75. Picetti GD, McGann WA, Welch RB. The patellofemoral joint after total knee arthroplasty without patellar resurfacing. *J Bone Joint Surg Am.* 1990;72(9):1379-1382.
76. Stern SH, Insall JN. Total knee arthroplasty in obese patients. *J Bone Joint Surg Am.* 1990;72(9):1400-1404.
77. Steinbrocker O, Traeger C, Batterman R. Theraputic criteria in rheumatoid arthritis. *JAMA.* 1949;140:659-662.
78. Scott RD. Prosthetic replacement of the patellofemoral joint. *Orthop Clin North Am.* 1979;10(1):129-137.
79. Sledge CB, Ewald FC. Total knee arthroplasty experience at the Robert Breck Brigham Hospital. *Clin Orthop Relat Res.* 1979;145:78-84.
80. Steinberg J, Sledge CB, Noble J, et al. A tissue-culture model of cartilage breakdown in rheumatoid arthritis. Quantitative aspects of proteoglycan release. *Biochem J.* 1979;180(2):403-412.
81. Barrack RL, Wolfe MW, Waldman DA, et al. Resurfacing of the patella in total knee arthroplasty. A prospective, randomized, double-blind study. *J Bone Joint Surg Am.* 1997;78(8):1121-1131.
82. Levitsky KA, Harris WJ, McManus J, et al. Total knee arthroplasty without patellar resurfacing. Clinical outcomes and long-term follow-up evaluation. *Clin Orthop Relat Res.* 1993;286:116-121.
83. Ranawat CS. The patellofemoral joint in total condylar knee arthroplasty. Pros and cons based on five- to ten-year follow-up observations. *Clin Orthop Relat Res.* 1986;205:93-99.
84. Scott RD, Reilly DT. Pros and cons of patella resurfacing in total knee replacement. *Orthop Trans.* 1980; 4:328-329.
85. Shoji H, Yoshino S, Kajino A. Patellar replacement in bilateral total knee arthroplasty. A study of patients who had rheumatoid arthritis and no gross deformity of the patella. *J Bone Joint Surg Am.* 1989;71(6):853-856.
86. Fern ED, Winson IG, Getty CJ. Anterior knee pain in rheumatoid patients after total knee replacement. Possible selection criteria for patellar resurfacing. *J Bone Joint Surg Br.* 1992;74(5):745-748.
87. Scott RD, Turoff N, Ewald FC. Stress fracture of the patella following duopatellar total knee arthroplasty with patellar resurfacing. *Clin Orthop Relat Res.* 1982;170:147-151.

88. Robertson O, Dunbar M, Pehrsson T, et al. Patient satisfaction after knee arthroplasty: a report on 27,372 knees operated on between 1981 and 1995 in Sweden. *Acta Orthop Scand.* 2000;71(3):262-267.
89. Browne JA, Hanssen AD. Reconstruction of patellar tendon disruption after total knee arthroplasty: results of a new technique utilizing synthetic mesh. *J Bone Joint Surg Am.* 2011;93(12):1137-1143.
90. Burnett RS, Butler RA, Barrack RL. Extensor mechanism allograft reconstruction in TKA at a mean of 56 months. *Clin Orthop Relat Res.* 2006;452:159-165.
91. Barrack RL, Barnes CL, Burnett RS, et al. Minimal incision surgery as a risk factor for early failure of total knee arthroplasty. *J Arthroplasty.* 2009;24(4):489-498.

46 Unicompartmental Knee Arthroplasty

Peter M. Bonutti, Bhaveen H. Kapadia, Qais Naziri, Aaron J. Johnson, and Michael A. Mont

Unicompartmental knee arthroplasty (UKA), also called a partial knee arthroplasty, has been used to treat unicompartmental arthritis of either the medial or lateral knee compartment. In 80% to 90% of patients it is used for the medial compartment.[1,2] However, controversy exists regarding the present use of these procedures: surgical approach, bearing design, and appropriate patient selection. This chapter describes the historic and current indications for UKA, reviews the proper surgical technique, explains the preoperative and postoperative evaluation, and reports on the outcomes of various studies.

HISTORY

The introduction of monocompartmental arthritis treatment began with the use of a metallic hemiarthroplasty for tibial plateau resurfacing in the late 1950s by McKeever and in the early 1960s by MacIntosh. Both of these devices had reportedly good short-term clinical outcomes for 72 of 103 knees at a mean follow-up of 8 years (range, 5–13 years) and 39 of 40 knees at a mean follow-up of 3 years (range, 1–10 years), respectively.[3,4] In the 1970s the designs evolved to employ metallic femoral components articulating with polyethylene inserts cemented into the tibial plateau. Although these early designs were not always successful, they led to a better understanding for the evolution of designs for UKA.

First-generation implants, the Marmor (Smith & Nephew, Memphis, TN) and the St. Georg Sled (Waldemar Link, Hamburg, Germany), were fixed-bearing implants with a polyethylene tibial insert that relied on native ligaments for stability. Although these implants successfully improved range of motion and provided symptomatic relief, they had a host of problems, including progression of adjacent compartment arthritis, loosening, subsidence on both the femoral condyle and the tibial plateau, and high rates of component wear.[5-9] Some of the contributing factors that resulted in these suboptimal outcomes were improper prosthesis designs, a poor understanding of appropriate patient selection criteria, and a steep procedure learning curve.[10] Fortunately, analysis of these issues allowed for improvements in the second-generation of implants. The Marmor implant was redesigned to lower the load off of cancellous bone to redistribute much of it onto cortical bone.[8] This was because prior failures were mostly attributed to the implant's placement on cancellous bone and the consequent subsidence of the medial tibial plateau.[11]

Metal-backed components were introduced in an attempt to resolve some of these issues by allowing for a more even distribution of forces through the increased rigidity of the baseplate, easier polyethylene exchange to account for spacer wear, and increased resistance to subsidence through improved force distribution. One particularly negative aspect of the metal-backed implant, however, was that it required greater amounts of bone resection.[12] An example of a metal-backed, fixed-bearing implant was the Porous Coated Anatomic (PCA; Howmedica, Mahwah, NJ). The most common causes of failure of this prosthesis were component loosening and polyethylene wear.[13] One specific area of the PCA component that was problematic was the constrained range of motion that led to increased stresses on the bearing surface, which led to high rates of polyethylene wear. This prompted the design of unicompartmental components with less constraint.

These third-generation implants sought to address the issues of these early metal-backed components by implementing designs with reduced constraint and consequently reduced wear rates. This was affected by changing the thickness of the insert, the contact area between the insert and the femoral component, and the bearing congruency between the two.[14] The concept of full congruency was implemented in mobile-bearing implants by having three separate components. These were a metal femoral component that articulated with a polyethylene meniscal component, which translated in the sagittal plane on a flat metal tibial surface. Although the advent of the mobile-bearing prostheses addressed the problem of polyethylene wear, it also introduced a new mode of failure: dislocation of the mobile insert from the tibial base.[9,15-17]

Currently, both mobile-bearing designs and fixed-bearing designs are used when performing UKA. Advantages and disadvantages of each, along with survivorship and clinical outcomes, are discussed in this chapter.

TABLE 46-1. Indications and Contraindications for UKA

Indications	
	Degenerative osteoarthritis limited to a single tibiofemoral compartment
	Older patients with moderate activity
	Ligamentous stability
Contraindications	
	Rheumatic disease
	Absence of the anterior cruciate ligament
	Patellofemoral disease
	Younger age
	Obesity

PREOPERATIVE EVALUATION

As necessary with any patient evaluation, it is important to conduct a thorough history and physical examination and obtain radiographs of the affected joint. For UKA, in particular, it is critical to evaluate patients for appropriate selection criteria, because these can determine the success or failure of the implant. Initially, UKA was indicated for elderly patients who had osteoarthritis of only one tibiofemoral compartment and no ligamentous injuries (Table 46-1).[18] Patients who were young, obese, or had patellofemoral disease were not indicated for UKA.[19-21] Rheumatic disease was also considered a contraindication, because it tends to involve all knee compartments.[22,23]

Indications

The indication for UKA has historically been in patients who are sedentary. Naal et al surveyed 83 patients following UKA to assess sports participation postoperatively.[24] At a mean follow-up of 18 months (range, 12–28 months), the patients reported a return to activity of 95% with a decrease in the minimum time engaged in activities from 66 minutes before surgery to 55 minutes after surgery. The frequency of activities was 2.9 (sessions per week) preoperatively and remained similar at 2.8 at a later follow-up. Although the frequency of activity was maintained, there was a decline in high-impact activities. They concluded that the indications for UKA should include those individuals who are moderately active, since there is a reasonable chance of maintaining activity postoperatively.

Unicompartmental arthroplasty was historically indicated for patients over 60 years of age. Recently, this has been re-evaluated.[25,26] Pennington et al reported a 92% survivorship in 41 patients (45 knees) who had a mean age of 58 years (range, 37–60 years) at a mean 11 years (range not given) follow-up.[25] In a comparison study at 10-year follow-up in patients below (512 knees) and above (52 knees) 60 years of age, Price et al showed a survivorship of 91% and 96%, respectively, with mean Hospital for Special Surgery scores of 94 points for the younger patients and 86 points for the older group.[27] In another large study of 1173 UKAs, Cartier et al found a mean survivorship of 95% in patients who had a mean age of 53 years (range, 30–60 years) at 10-year follow-up.[28] Based on these reported survivorships, some surgeons will consider younger patients (50–60 years of age) for UKA.

Contraindications

Assessment of a patient requires attention to knee pathology as well as to comorbidities. Although conflicting reports exist in the literature about the effect of increased body mass index (BMI) on success rates, it appears that patients who have a BMI greater than 32 to 35 kg/m^2 may have an increased risk for component failure.[29] Bonutti and Dethmers conducted a review of 34 patients (40 knees) with a BMI of 35 kg/m^2 or greater and 33 patients (40 knees) with a BMI below 35 kg/m^2.[12] At a 2-year follow-up, there was a significant difference in implant survivorship of 90% and 100%, respectively ($p = .05$). The mean time to failure was 33 months (range, 9–54 months) following surgery. Furthermore, the mean Knee Society pain scores were 96 points (range, 80–100 points) in the higher BMI group compared to 98 points (range, 84–100 points) in the lower BMI group ($p = .017$). The mean Knee Society function scores were 95 points (range, 50–100 points) in the higher BMI group, in comparison to 97 points (range, 80– 100 points) in the lower BMI group ($p = .127$). These results suggest that patients with a BMI of 35 kg/m^2 or greater have a higher risk of early failures and poorer clinical outcomes.

Berend et al evaluated the association between obesity and survivorship of 79 medial UKAs (69 patients). At a mean follow-up of 40 months (range, 24–69 months), there were 16 failures (78% survivorship). In these patients, the mean BMI was higher (35 kg/m^2) than in patients who had surviving implants (31 kg/m^2; $p = .04$). It was found that a BMI of greater than 32 kg/m^2 was predictive of failure ($p = .04$).[29]

In a contrasting retrospective review, Naal et al found no correlation between BMI and failures or survivorship.[30] Clinical outcome 2 years after surgery was reviewed for 83 consecutive UKAs. Three knees failed (survivorship of 96.4%) and were converted to total knee arthroplasty; however, there was no significant association with increased BMI and failures ($p = .387$).

On physical examination, it is critical to assess the integrity of the anterior cruciate ligament (ACL). One of the typical contraindications for UKA was an absence or deficiency of the ACL. It has been postulated that a deficient ACL contributes to an increased failure rate of a UKA, because the absence of this ligament allows for more sliding between the tibia and femur and consequently polyethylene wear.[31,32] The high failure rate has been attributed to the instability of the knee joint after UKA with a deficient or absent ACL. However, some studies have reported on concomitant UKA and ACL reconstruction and suggest that at early- and mid-term follow-up these patients have good survivorship and clinical outcomes. Pandit et al compared the knee kinematics of 10 patients after ACL reconstruction and UKA to those of 10 UKA patients with an intact ACL and found that relatively normal knee kinematics is restored after a combined UKA and ACL reconstruction.[33] At an approximate mean follow-up of 3.4 years (range, 3–5 years), all clinical scores were improved postoperatively with no statistically significant differences between the two groups. A mean Oxford Knee score of 45 points (range, 42–48 points) and 43 points (range, 42–45 points) was reported for the reconstruction and intact groups, respectively. Supporting results were reported by Tinius et al, who reviewed 27 knees (27 patients) with combined ACL reconstruction and medial UKA.[34] The study showed that at a mean clinical follow-up of 50 months (range, 9–71 months), a combined ACL reconstruction and UKA restored native knee stability, improved clinical outcomes, and prevented UKA failure. Since there was no comparative group in this study, the results were compared to recent literature reporting UKA clinical outcomes and failure rates.

Imaging Evaluation

Routine radiographic evaluation consists of anteroposterior, lateral, and tangential axial views of the affected knee. Weight-bearing anteroposterior radiographs of the lower extremity provide a more accurate assessment of joint space width and the extent of the degenerative disease in the lateral and medial joint compartments (Fig. 46-1).

There is some difference in opinion as to whether or not patellofemoral disease is an absolute contraindication.[9,35-38] Because it has been reported in the literature that any disease in the patellofemoral compartment may worsen after UKA, Merchant views of the knee are best for visualization to ensure there is no disease (patella centered directly over the femoral trochlear articular surface).

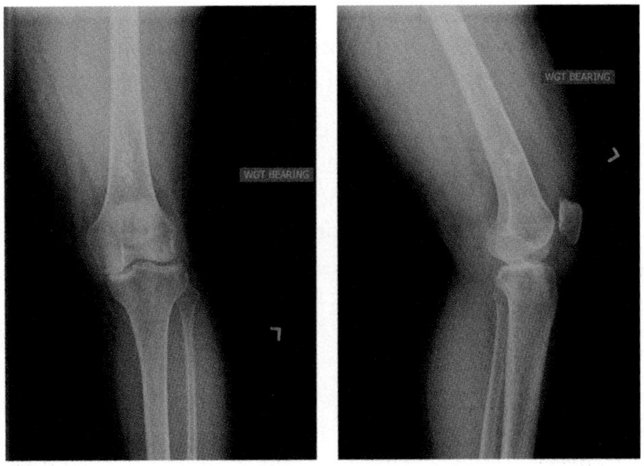

FIGURE 46-1. *Standing anteroposterior and lateral radiographs of a symptomatic knee showing medial compartment arthritis. (Reprinted with permission from Sinai Hospital of Baltimore, Inc.)*

Although single photon emission computed tomography (SPECT) scans have been shown to be accurate in detecting subclinical disease in the other compartments, it is not routinely recommended.[15] Additionally, if there is concern for soft tissue disease, such as an acute meniscal tear, ACL deficiency, or focal chondral lesions, magnetic resonance imaging (MRI) may be considered, although this is also not routinely recommended.

SURGERY

The typical approach to the UKA is through an anterior incision and a medial parapatellar arthrotomy, with reflection and dislocation of the patella.[39] One of the advantages of this procedure is that the cruciate ligaments are spared, potentially preserving the native structural stability and kinematics of the knee. With normal kinematics present, UKAs may provide a more natural gait and improved function over a standard total knee arthroplasty (TKA). Consequently, it is critical that care be taken to preserve these structures during the surgical approach during UKA.

Tibial resection is typically conservative (typically 2 mm below the arthritic surface), with the goal of preserving as much bone as possible if later conversion to TKA is necessary. Particular care should be taken to avoid breaching the posterior cortex during this resection to reduce the risk of compromising structural stability and tibial plateau fractures. Furthermore, careful sizing of the tibial component is essential, because improper sizing has led to stress fractures of the tibial plateau.[40-44] Placement of the femoral component should be as centered as possible on the condyle (Fig. 46-2). However, a lateral direction error is preferable because it affords more congruency with the tibial component in extension.[39] Deformity overcorrection may also lead to increased stresses on the adjacent compartment, thus promoting arthritic changes.[35]

All efforts should be made to eliminate cement in the posterior joint space. The use of two-stage cementing, nerve hooks, intraoperative fluoroscopy, and dental mirrors for visualization has been suggested to reduce this problem.[45]

POSTOPERATIVE MANAGEMENT AND REHABILITATION

The postoperative management following UKA is similar to that following total knee arthroplasty. Thromboembolic prevention is important to prevent developing deep vein thrombosis and potential pulmonary embolism.[46,47]

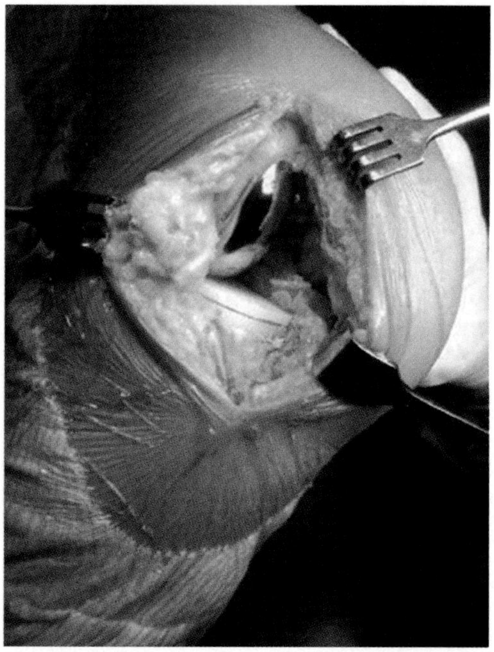

FIGURE 46-2. *Femoral and tibial components. (Reprinted from Servien E, Aitsiselmi T, Neyret P, et al. How to select candidates for lateral unicompartmental prosthesis. Curr Orthop Pract. 2008;19(4):451-458, with permission from Lippincott Williams & Wilkins.)*

Passive motion is begun as tolerated in the immediate postoperative period. Patients are also encouraged to ambulate on the day of surgery with weight bearing as tolerated with aids. Continuous passive motion devices may be used, with a knee immobilizer placed at night to reduce the risk of developing a flexion contracture. On postoperative day 1 or 2, quadriceps muscle exercises, straight leg raises, and bed to chair transfers are initiated as tolerated. A knee immobilizer may be used during ambulation until achieving stable straight leg raises. Most patients are able to walk within 1 week with a cane and discontinue it at 2 weeks. The use of a cane is often recommended for at least 2 to 4 weeks for safety, however.[48]

OUTCOMES

Results of UKA have improved in recent years with numerous reports of survivorship greater than 90% at 5- to 10-year follow-up (Table 46-2). Figure 46-3 shows postoperative standing anteroposterior and lateral radiographs. The Australian National Joint Registry reported a survival rate of 86.7% at 9 years in 31,884 UKAs.[49] In a prospective study of 50,493 medial UKAs, Koskinen et al reported an 87% survivorship at 7-year follow-up.[50]

Springer et al reported a mean time to conversion to TKA of 100 months (range, 6–207 months) in 22 failed UKAs (20 medial and 2 lateral) in 18 patients.[51] The most common reasons for revision were polyethylene wear (12 patients, 54%) and component loosening (7 patients, 31%), occurring at a mean of 101 months (range, 28–182 months) and 71 months (range, 6–125 months), respectively. Another revision study reported a mean time to revision of 60 months (range, 2–228 months) for 36 medial UKAs, with the most common reasons for revision being loosening (39%) and progression to arthritis (36%).[52] More recently, Aly et al reported that of 45 knees (43 patients) only 2 knees (4.4%) required revision at a mean follow-up of 105 months (range, 45–134 months).[53] One revision occurred because of a medial tibial plateau fracture after a fall 3 years postoperatively and the other occurred 2 years postoperatively due to aseptic component loosening.

TABLE 46-2. Survivorship and Clinical Outcomes of UKA

Study	Year	No. of Knees (Patients)	Prosthesis	Follow-up Duration in Months (Range)	Findings	Ref.
Argenson et al	2002	160 (147)	Miller-Galante	66 (36–112)	• 10-year survival rate of 94% • HSS mean was 96 points	35
Ashraf et al	2002	88 (79)	St Georg (lateral)	108 (24–252)	• 10-year survival rate was 83% • 15-year survival rate was 74% • OKS mean was 34 points	65
Berger et al	2005	62 (51)	Miller-Galante	144 (120–156)	• 10-year survival rate was 98 • 13-year survival rate was 96% • HSS mean was 92 points	66
O'Rourke et al	2005	136 (103)	Marmor	288 (204–337)	• 20-year survival rate of 84% • 25-year survival rate of 72% • KSS clinical mean was 72 • KSS functional mean was 53 • HSS mean was 74 points	67
Verdonk et al	2005	97 (86)	Oxford	81 (24–168)	• 90% satisfactory (HSS)	60
Pennington et al	2006	29 (24)	Miller-Galante	149 (37–187)	• 12.4-year survival rate of 100% • HSS mean was 93 points	68
Vorlat et al	2006	149 (140)	Oxford	126 (63–174)	• 10-year survival rate of 82%	61
Kim et al	2007	95 (68)	Oxford III	36	• 100% satisfactory (KSS) • 85% of patients satisfied with result • KSS clinical mean was 90 points • KSS functional mean was 87 points	69

Continued

TABLE 46-2. ***Continued***

Study	Year	No. of Knees (Patients)	Prosthesis	Follow-up Duration in Months (Range)	Findings	Ref.
Emerson and Higgins	2008	55 (51)	Oxford	142 (106–172)	• 10-year survival rate of 85% • KSS clinical mean was 75 points • KSS functional mean was 90 points	70
Koskinen et al	2009	46 (46)	Miller-Galante II	84 (32–157)	• 7-year survival rate of 87% • KSS clinical mean was 76 points • KSS functional mean was 93 points	50
Aly et al	2010	45 (43)	Oxford	105 (45–134)	• 8-year survival rate of 95.6% • Average HSS of 117.6 (78–198) at 117 months • 80% had an excellent mean score of 170 (173–198), 10% had a good score of 155 (140–165), 5% had a fair score 130 (120–140), and 5% had a poor score 106 (77–118)	53

HSS, Hospital for Special Surgery; KSS, Knee Society score; OKS, Oxford Knee score.

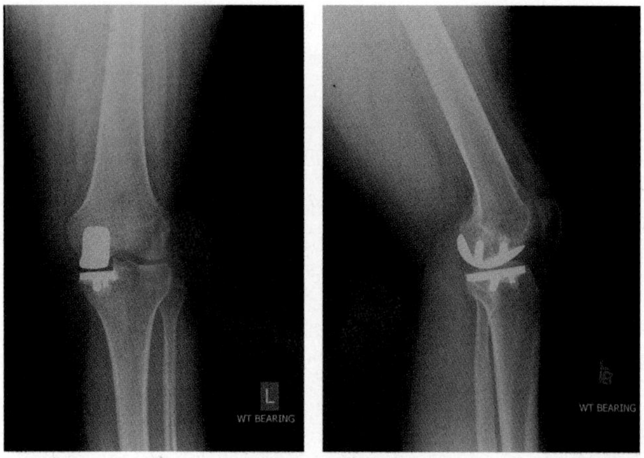

FIGURE 46-3. *Postoperative standing anteroposterior and lateral radiographs. (Reprinted with permission from Sinai Hospital of Baltimore, Inc.)*

Debate exists over whether mobile- or fixed-bearing UKA provides better outcomes (Fig. 46-4). In a study of 20 patients at 11 years by Emerson et al, mobile-bearing and fixed-bearing prosthetics were compared with reported survivorships of 99% and 93%, respectively.[54] Although there were no significant differences in clinical outcomes, as measured by Knee Society scores (p = .7), the most common mechanism of failure was different in both groups. In the fixed-bearing group, four out of eight revised knees had polyethylene wear, whereas, in the mobile-bearing device, four out of seven revised knees suffered from contralateral compartment arthritis. Other studies have reported similar results regarding clinical outcomes in both prosthetic designs.[55,56] There has been no reported evidence suggesting that one design is superior to the other, although proponents of the mobile-bearing prosthesis argue that it is more resistant to wear than the fixed-bearing prosthesis. The most prominent difference is the mechanism of failure: contralateral arthritis and dislocations in mobile-bearing designs versus polyethylene wear in fixed-bearing designs.

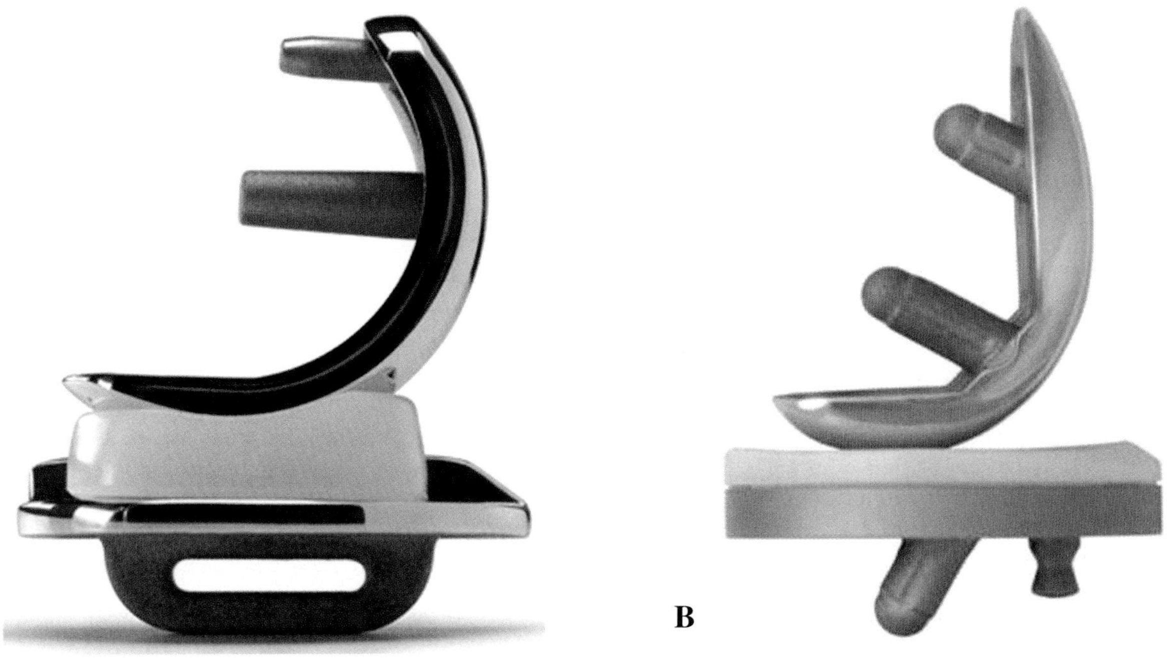

FIGURE 46-4. *(**A**) Mobile-bearing implant; (**B**) fixed-bearing implant. (Reprinted with permission from Biomet and Stryker.)*

COMPLICATIONS

Even when all possible precautions and measures are taken to ensure optimal clinical outcomes, complications are possible (Table 46-3). The most common complications are component dislocation, progression to arthritis to the contralateral compartment, component loosening, subsidence of the tibial component, and polyethylene wear. Other less common complications include pseudomeniscal synovial impingement,[57] metallosis,[58] and contralateral meniscal injury.[59]

Dislocation of the polyethylene insert is a complication more typically found in the mobile-bearing prosthesis. Verdonk et al reported a total of four dislocations out of 97 knees at a mean follow-up of 7 years (range, 2–14 years).[60] Two of the four revisions reported by Vorlat et al were caused by bearing dislocation at a mean follow-up of 126 months.[61] Dislocations of mobile-bearing implants can be identified radiographically by displacement of radio-opaque markers.[62]

Polyethylene wear is a complication of all prostheses; however, the wear rate is lower for mobile-bearing devices than with fixed-bearing devices. Kendrick et al measured the wear rate of 13 mobile-bearing medial UKAs (14 patients) using radiostereometric analysis at a mean of 21 years (range, 17–26 years).[63] A mean annual wear rate of 0.045 mm/year (range, 0.016–0.099 mm/year) was reported. A retrieval study of 47 fixed-bearing medial UKAs (47 patients) by Kendrick et al estimated a wear rate of 0.07 mm/year (range, 0.06–0.09 mm/year) at a mean follow-up

TABLE 46-3. Complications of UKA

Major	
	Dislocation
	Progression to arthritis
	Component loosening
	Subsidence of tibial component
	Polyethylene wear
	Periprosthetic fracture
Minor	
	Pseudomeniscal synovial impingement
	Metallosis
	Meniscal injury

of 8 years (range, 4–12 years).[64] Based on these studies, it appears that fixed-bearing devices are more susceptible to wear than mobile-bearing devices.

Another complication is progression to arthritis of the contralateral compartment, which is typically due to overcorrection of the varus deformity. Emerson et al found an increased postoperative valgus alignment in the prosthesis in mobile-bearing devices when compared to fixed-bearing devices. Although this resulted in reduced load on the medial side, it consequently resulted in an increase in stresses on the lateral compartment.[54] This mechanism has been postulated to be the principal cause of contralateral compartment arthritis in mobile-bearing devices.

Proximal tibia fractures are a rare but serious complication of UKA. Van Loon et al demonstrated three cases of periprosthetic facture of the tibial plateau; two occurred intraoperatively and one occurred 6 days postoperatively.[44] In one of the cases, which presented 6 days postoperatively, it was determined based on postoperative radiographs that there were fissures present in the medial tibial plateau. It was thought that these complications occurred due to surgical technique and has been supported by additional literature reporting similar cases.[41-43] Therefore, it is important during the procedure to maintain tibial cortical integrity with proper tibial component sizing, as well as careful malleting during component fixation.

CONCLUSION

Recent long-term follow-up studies (at 10 years) of UKA have survivorship rates reported between 82% and 98%, with survivorships of greater than 90% in certain populations given appropriate patient selection. Consequently, patient selection is critical for good clinical outcomes. The procedure has a high learning curve and it has been well documented that failures may be due to either improper patient selection or poor surgical technique.[53] Historically, UKA has been most successful in older, less active patients who have intact cruciate ligaments. However, recent reports suggest that this may be appropriate in some patients who are as young as 50 to 60 years of age, have moderate activity levels, and, if necessary, who undergo ACL reconstruction at the time of UKA.

PEARLS AND PITFALLS

The following are things to consider for a successful UKA:

1. A successful UKA depends on proper patient selection criteria, with attention to adjacent ligamentous stability, age, activity level, and body mass index.
2. UKA has a steep procedure learning curve and it is therefore recommended that surgeons seeking experience use conventional techniques before attempting minimally invasive surgery.
3. UKA survivorship depends on proper surgical technique, with attention to correct component sizing and careful tibial resection to avoid periprosthetic fractures of the tibial plateau.
4. Avoid varus tibial cut.
5. Avoid overstuffing the joint. Most surgeons will leave 1 to 2 mm of laxity in extension and flexion.
6. Avoid patella impingement on the femoral component.
7. Posterior slope of the tibia should be less than 7°.
8. Do not overcorrect alignment. Maintain slight varus of 1° to 2° for varus knees to avoid overloading the lateral compartment.
9. Total knee arthroplasty and osteotomies are alternatives to UKA in the correct patients.

REFERENCES

1. Ahlback S. Osteoarthrosis of the knee. A radiographic investigation. *Acta Radiol Diagn.* 1968:suppl 277:7-72.
2. Hernborg JS, Nilsson BE. The natural course of untreated osteoarthritis of the knee. *Clin Orthop Relat Res.* 1977;123:130-137.
3. Scott RD, Joyce MJ, Ewald FC, et al. McKeever metallic hemiarthroplasty of the knee in unicompartmental degenerative arthritis. Long-term clinical follow-up and current indications. *J Bone Joint Surg Am.* 1985;67:203-207.
4. MacIntosh DL, Hunter GA. The use of the hemiarthroplasty prosthesis for advanced osteoarthritis and rheumatoid arthritis of the knee. *J Bone Joint Surg Br.* 1972;54:244-255.
5. Inglis GS. Unicompartmental arthroplasty of the knee. A follow-up of 3 to 9 years. *J Bone Joint Surg Br.* 1984;66:682-684.
6. Laskin RS. Unicompartmental tibiofemoral resurfacing arthroplasty. *J Bone Joint Surg Am.* 1978;60: 182-185.

7. Mallory TH, Danyi J. Unicompartmental total knee arthroplasty. A five- to nine-year follow-up study of 42 procedures. *Clin Orthop Relat Res*. 1983;175:135-138.
8. Marmor L. Unicompartmental knee arthroplasty. Ten- to 13-year follow-up study. *Clin Orthop Relat Res*. 1988;226:14-20.
9. Maduekwe UI, Zywiel MG, Bonutti PM, et al. Scientific evidence for the use of modern unicompartmental knee arthroplasty. *Expert Rev Med Devices*. 2010;7:219-239.
10. Robertsson O, Lidgren L. The short-term results of 3 common UKA implants during different periods in Sweden. *J Arthroplasty*. 2008;23:801-807.
11. Squire MW, Callaghan JJ, Goetz DD, et al. Unicompartmental knee replacement. A minimum 15 year followup study. *Clin Orthop Relat Res*. 1999; 367:61-72.
12. Bonutti PM, Dethmers DA. Contemporary unicompartmental knee arthroplasty: fixed vs mobile bearing. *J Arthroplasty*. 2008;23:24-27.
13. Skyrme AD, Mencia MM, Skinner PW. Early failure of the porous-coated anatomic cemented unicompartmental knee arthroplasty: a 5- to 9-year follow-up study. *J Arthroplasty*. 2002;17:201-205.
14. Simpson DJ, Gray H, D'Lima D, et al. The effect of bearing congruency, thickness and alignment on the stresses in unicompartmental knee replacements. *Clin Biomech*. 2008;23:1148-1157.
15. Hart R, Konvicka M, Filan P, et al. SPECT scan is a reliable tool for selection of patients undergoing unicompartmental knee arthroplasty. *Arch Orthop Trauma Surg*. 2008;128:679-682.
16. Ashraf T, Newman JH, Desai VV, et al. Polyethylene wear in a non-congruous unicompartmental knee replacement: a retrieval analysis. *Knee*. 2004;11:177-181.
17. Price AJ, Short A, Kellett C, et al. Ten-year in vivo wear measurement of a fully congruent mobile bearing unicompartmental knee arthroplasty. *J Bone Joint Surg Br*. 2005;87:1493-1497.
18. White SH, Ludkowski PF, Goodfellow JW. Anteromedial osteoarthritis of the knee. *J Bone Joint Surg Br*. 1991;73:582-586.
19. Ashraf ST, Ackroyd CE, Newman JH. Compartmental knee arthroplasty. *Curr Orthop*. 2003;17:134-143.
20. Mont MA, Stuchin SA, Paley D, et al. Different surgical options for monocompartmental osteoarthritis of the knee: high tibial osteotomy versus unicompartmental knee arthroplasty versus total knee arthroplasty: indications, techniques, results, and controversies. *Instr Course Lect*. 2004;53:265-83.
21. Scott RD. Unicondylar arthroplasty: redefining itself. *Orthopedics*. 2003;26:951-952.
22. Goodfellow JW, Kershaw CJ, Benson MK, et al. The Oxford knee for unicompartmental osteoarthritis. The first 103 cases. *J Bone Joint Surg Br*. 1988;70:692-701.
23. Kennedy WR, White RP. Unicompartmental arthroplasty of the knee. Postoperative alignment and its influence on overall results. *Clin Orthop Relat Res*. 1987;221:278-285.
24. Naal FD, Fischer M, Preuss A, et al. Return to sports and recreational activity after unicompartmental knee arthroplasty. *Am J Sports Med*. 2007;35:1688-1695.
25. Pennington DW, Swienckowski JJ, Lutes WB, et al. Unicompartmental knee arthroplasty in patients sixty years of age or younger. *J Bone Joint Surg Am*. 2003; 85:1968-1973.
26. Parratte S, Argenson JN, Pearce O, et al. Medial unicompartmental knee replacement in the under-50s. *J Bone Joint Surg Br*. 2009;91:351-356.
27. Price AJ, Dodd CA, Svard UG, et al. Oxford medial unicompartmental knee arthroplasty in patients younger and older than 60 years of age. *J Bone Joint Surg Br*. 2005;87:1488-1492.
28. Cartier P, Khefacha A, Sanouiller JL, et al. Unicondylar knee arthroplasty in middle-aged patients: a minimum 5-year follow-up. *Orthopedics*. 2007;30:62-65.
29. Berend KR, Lombardi AV Jr, Mallory TH, et al. Early failure of minimally invasive unicompartmental knee arthroplasty is associated with obesity. *Clin Orthop Relat Res*. 2005;440:60-66.
30. Naal FD, Neuerburg C, Salzmann GM, et al. Association of body mass index and clinical outcome 2 years after unicompartmental knee arthroplasty. *Arch Orthop Trauma Surg*. 2009;129:463-468.
31. Engh GA, Ammeen D. Is an intact anterior cruciate ligament needed in order to have a well-functioning unicondylar knee replacement? *Clin Orthop Relat Res*. 2004;428:170-173.
32. Suggs JF, Li G, Park SE, et al. Function of the anterior cruciate ligament after unicompartmental knee arthroplasty: an in vitro robotic study. *J Arthroplasty*. 2004;19:224-229.
33. Pandit H, Van Duren BH, Gallagher JA, et al. Combined anterior cruciate reconstruction and Oxford unicompartmental knee arthroplasty: in vivo kinematics. *Knee*. 2008;15:101-106.

34. Tinius M, Hepp P, Becker R. Combined unicompartmental knee arthroplasty and anterior cruciate ligament reconstruction. *Knee Surg Sports Traumatol Arthrosc*. 2012;20(1):81-87.

35. Argenson JN, Chevrol-Benkeddache Y, Aubaniac JM. Modern unicompartmental knee arthroplasty with cement: a three to ten-year follow-up study. *J Bone Joint Surg Am*. 2002;84:2235-2239.

36. Buchholz HW, Heinert K. Long-term results of cemented arthroplasty. Analysis of complications fifteen years after operation. *Orthop Clin North Am*. 1988;19:531-540.

37. Berger RA, Meneghini RM, Sheinkop MB, et al. The progression of patellofemoral arthrosis after medial unicompartmental replacement: results at 11 to 15 years. *Clin Orthop Relat Res*. 2004;428:92-99.

38. Beard DJ, Pandit H, Ostlere S, et al. Pre-operative clinical and radiological assessment of the patellofemoral joint in unicompartmental knee replacement and its influence on outcome. *J Bone Joint Surg Br*. 2007;89:1602-1607.

39. Scott RD. Three decades of experience with unicompartmental knee arthroplasty: mistakes made and lessons learned. *Orthopedics*. 2006;29: 829-831.

40. Clarius M, Haas D, Aldinger PR, et al. Periprosthetic tibial fractures in unicompartmental knee arthroplasty as a function of extended sagittal saw cuts: an experimental study. *Knee*. 2010;17(1):57-60.

41. Kumar A, Chambers I, Wong P. Periprosthetic fracture of the proximal tibia after lateral unicompartmental knee arthroplasty. *J Arthroplasty*. 2008;23: 615-618.

42. Pandit H, Murray DW, Dodd CA, et al. Medial tibial plateau fracture and the Oxford unicompartmental knee. *Orthopedics*. 2007;30:28-31.

43. Rudol G, Jackson MP, James SE. Medial tibial plateau fracture complicating unicompartmental knee arthro-plasty. *J Arthroplasty*. 2007;22:148-150.

44. Van Loon P, de Munnynck B, Bellemans J. Periprosthetic fracture of the tibial plateau after unicompartmental knee arthroplasty. *Acta Orthop Belg*. 2006;72:369-374.

45. Hauptmann SM, Weber P, Glaser C, et al. Free bone cement fragments after minimally invasive unicompartmental knee arthroplasty: an underappreciated problem. *Knee Surg Sports Traumatol Arthrosc*. 2008; 16:770-775.

46. Colwell CW Jr, Froimson MI, Mont MA, et al. Thrombosis prevention after total hip arthroplasty: a prospective, randomized trial comparing a mobile compression device with low-molecular-weight heparin. *J Bone Joint Surg Am*. 2010;92:527-535.

47. Haas SB, Barrack RL, Westrich G, et al. Venous thromboembolic disease after total hip and knee arthroplasty. *J Bone Joint Surg Am*. 2008;90:2764-2780.

48. Fitz WS, Richard D. Unicompartmental total knee arthroplasty. In: Scott WN, ed. *Surgery of the Knee*. 4th ed. Philadelphia, PA: Churchill Livingstone Elsevier; 2006:1408-1420.

49. Graves SE, Davidson D, de Steiger R. *National Joint Replacement Registry Annual Report*. Australian Orthopaedic Association National Joint Replacement Registry, Adelaide, Austrailia; 2010.

50. Koskinen E, Paavolainen P, Eskelinen A, et al. Medial unicompartmental knee arthroplasty with Miller-Galante II prosthesis: mid-term clinical and radiographic results. *Arch Orthop Trauma Surg*. 2009; 129:617-624.

51. Springer BD, Scott RD, Thornhill TS. Conversion of failed unicompartmental knee arthroplasty to TKA. *Clin Orthop Relat Res*. 2006;446:214-220.

52. Saldanha KA, Keys GW, Svard UC, et al. Revision of Oxford medial unicompartmental knee arthroplasty to total knee arthroplasty–results of a multicentre study. *Knee*. 2007;14:275-279.

53. Aly T, Weam M, El-Sallakh S. The Oxford unicompartmental knee prosthesis: midterm follow-up. *Curr Orthop Pract*. 2010;21:187-89.

54. Emerson RH Jr, Hansborough T, Reitman RD, et al. Comparison of a mobile with a fixed-bearing unicompartmental knee implant. *Clin Orthop Relat Res*. 2002;404:62-70.

55. Confalonieri N, Manzotti A, Pullen C. Comparison of a mobile with a fixed tibial bearing unicompartimental knee prosthesis: a prospective randomized trial using a dedicated outcome score. *Knee*. 2004; 11:357-362.

56. Li MG, Yao F, Joss B, et al. Mobile vs. fixed bearing unicondylar knee arthroplasty: a randomized study on short term clinical outcomes and knee kinematics. *Knee*. 2006;13:365-370.

57. Jung KA, Lee SC, Hwang SH. Pseudomeniscal synovial impingement after unicondylar knee arthroplasty. *Orthopedics*. 2009;32:361.

58. Sanchis-Alfonso V. Severe metallosis after unicompartmental knee arthroplasty. *Knee Surg Sports Traumatol Arthrosc*. 2007;15:361-364.

59. Mencia MM, Ashworth MJ. Lateral meniscal injury after a successful medial unicompartmental knee arthroplasty. *J Arthroplasty.* 2010;25(2):333.e7-e8.

60. Verdonk R, Cottenie D, Almqvist KF, et al. The Oxford unicompartmental knee prosthesis: a 2-14 year follow-up. *Knee Surg Sports Traumatol Arthrosc.* 2005;13:163-166.

61. Vorlat P, Putzeys G, Cottenie D, et al. The Oxford unicompartmental knee prosthesis: an independent 10-year survival analysis. *Knee Surg Sports Traumatol Arthrosc.* 2006;14:40-45.

62. Mukherjee K, Pandit H, Dodd CA, et al. The Oxford unicompartmental knee arthroplasty: a radiological perspective. *Clin Radiol.* 2008;63:1169-1176.

63. Kendrick BJ, Simpson DJ, Kaptein BL, et al. Polyethylene wear of mobile-bearing unicompartmental knee replacement at 20 years. *J Bone Joint Surg Br.* 2011;93:470-475.

64. Kendrick BJ, Longino D, Pandit H, et al. Polyethylene wear in Oxford unicompartmental knee replacement: a retrieval study of 47 bearings. *J Bone Joint Surg Br.* 2010;92:367-373.

65. Ashraf T, Newman JH, Evans RL, et al. Lateral unicompartmental knee replacement survivorship and clinical experience over 21 years. *J Bone Joint Surg Br.* 2002;84:1126-1130.

66. Berger RA, Meneghini RM, Jacobs JJ, et al. Results of unicompartmental knee arthroplasty at a minimum of ten years of follow-up. *J Bone Joint Surg Am.* 2005;87:999-1006.

67. O'Rourke MR, Gardner JJ, Callaghan JJ, et al. The John Insall Award: unicompartmental knee replacement: a minimum twenty-one-year followup, end-result study. *Clin Orthop Relat Res.* 2005;440:27-37.

68. Pennington DW, Swienckowski JJ, Lutes WB, et al. Lateral unicompartmental knee arthroplasty: survivorship and technical considerations at an average follow-up of 12.4 years. *J Arthroplasty.* 2006; 21:13-17.

69. Kim KT, Lee S, Park HS, et al. A prospective analysis of Oxford phase 3 unicompartmental knee arthroplasty. *Orthopedics.* 2007;30:15-18.

70. Emerson RH Jr, Higgins LL. Unicompartmental knee arthroplasty with the Oxford prosthesis in patients with medial compartment arthritis. *J Bone Joint Surg Am.* 2008;90:118-122.

47 Lateral Unicompartmental Knee Arthroplasty

Jean-Noel Argenson and Sebastien Parratte

Unicompartmental femorotibial osteoarthritis usually affects the medial compartment of the knee and, more rarely, the lateral compartment.[1] The lateral compartment is considered to be involved in 5% to 10% of unicompartmental femorotibial arthroplasty cases; therefore, isolated lateral unicompartmental knee arthritis remains a challenging problem.[2,3] Surgical management of unicompartmental knee arthritis includes conservative treatment, such as external bracing, arthroscopic debridement, or femoral osteotomy, and nonconservative treatment, such as unicompartmental arthroplasty or total knee arthroplasty.[2,3] These procedures, however, have a finite life span in young and active patients and some concerns, such as functional recovery, and the possibility of return to sports should be considered.[2-6] It has been demonstrated that femoral osteotomy remains an attractive conservative procedure to avoid knee arthroplasty in younger patients with a valgus deformation and low-grade unicompartmental osteoarthritis.[7] Valgus osteotomy is challenging, however, with a high rate of complications and limited functional results for patients with Ahlback[1] grade 2 or more osteoarthritis.[8] Furthermore, total knee arthroplasty (TKA) after femoral osteotomy remains a more complex procedure because of previous skin incisions, hardware removal, and potential femoral deformity.[9] Thus for patients with symptomatic unicompartmental arthritis greater than Ahlback grade 1, nonconservative treatment should be considered even in younger patients.[2] Unicompartmental knee arthroplasty (UKA), which has been performed since the 1970s, in a patient in whom only one compartment of the knee is affected, may provide better physiological function and quicker recovery compared to total knee arthroplasty and preserves bone stock.[3-6] Furthermore, patient satisfaction is greater because the knee feels more natural.[3-6] With proper patient selection and more reliable surgical technique, 10-year results of modern UKA are now available and show survivorship greater than 90% at 10 years' follow-up.[4,5] UKA in the lateral compartment has been described, however, as technically more challenging and 10 times less performed than medial UKA, thus representing less than 1% of all knee arthroplasty procedures.[10] Both the anatomical and the biomechanical characteristics are different in the lateral compartment[2,11]; therefore, this chapter presents the specificities related to UKA in the lateral compartment for patient selection, surgical technique, and outcomes.

PREOPERATIVE EVALUATION

History and Examination

During the clinical examination of the knee, the surgeon must focus on the range of motion, with a minimum range of knee flexion of 100°, before choosing UKA as a treatment option. A contracture may be improved by only a few degrees after UKA, and this should be recognized preoperatively. A lack of extension of less than 10° is acceptable. The clinical evaluation of the patellofemoral joint is also mandatory to seek out any type of anterior knee pain described by the patient during stair climbing and descending or during squatting. The stability of the joint must be evaluated carefully in the sagittal plane for the anterior cruciate ligament (ACL) and in the frontal plane using the dedicated tests. The unicompartmental implant fills the gap left by the worn cartilage, bringing the collateral ligament back to normal tension after the procedure. During the varus stress test of the knee, the valgus deformation should be correctible and the tension of the lateral collateral ligament should be normal. The clinical results of UKA using a mobile or a fixed bearing and the in vivo kinematics have highlighted the importance of a functional ACL for unicondylar knee replacement specifically to restore the rollback, which is a crucial point for the lateral compartment.[11] Then during the clinical evaluation, the testing of the ACL should be performed with caution, especially when using the Lachman test since the pivot shift may be limited due to the pain and swelling on this arthritic knee.[12]

Imaging

Radiographic imaging

The radiological analysis systematically includes anteroposterior (AP) and lateral views of the knee, full-length X-rays in bipedal and single leg stance, varus and valgus stress radiographs, and skyline views at 30°, 60°, and 90° of knee flexion.[13] On full-length X-rays, the angle between the mechanical axis of the femur and the anatomical axis of the femur can be calculated and reproduced during the procedure at the time of the distal femoral cut. The analysis also evaluates any extra-articular bony deformity that cannot be corrected by the unicompartmental implant and searches for any femoral long hip stem that might require the use of a shorter intramedullary rod or the use of an extramedullary rod. As described first by Kozinn and Scott and later by various authors, UKA should be limited to preoperative valgus deformity of the lower limb lower than 15° degrees and greater deformities may represent a contraindication for UKA. Correction of such deformities may require soft tissue release, which should not be performed when doing UKA because that may lead to frontal femorotibial subluxation.[14]

Varus and valgus stress X-rays, performed with the patient supine using a dedicated knee stress system, are very important first to assess the presence of full-thickness articular cartilage in the uninvolved compartment and second to confirm that the deformity can be fully corrected to neutral.[13] In cases in which a UKA cannot correct the deformity or will result in overcorrection, this view indicates the need for soft tissue management and therefore the use of TKA. The lateral view of the joint confirms the absence of anterior tibial translation greater than 10 mm referencing the posterior edge of the tibial plateau and shows that tibial erosion is limited to anterior and midportions of the tibial plateau, confirming that the ACL is competent.[14] The height of the patella should also be analyzed since a patella baja will limit the exposure during minimally invasive procedures.[15]

The radiographic analysis should ensure that there is no patellofemoral loss of joint space on skyline views at 30°, 60° and 90° of flexion. The presence of periarticular osteophytes may not be a contraindication for unicondylar replacement, and these osteophytes can be removed even through a minimally invasive incision.[15] Although the status of the patellofemoral joint is not a criterion of suitability for some authors, a painful patellofemoral joint or the full loss of patellofemoral cartilage is now for us a contraindication for performing an isolated unicondylar remplacement.[16] In cases of associated wear in the lateral and in the patellofemoral compartment, bicompartmental arthroplasty combining lateral UKA and patellofemoral arthroplasty can be considered during the same procedure.[16]

Cross-sectional imaging

When there is a question regarding the status of the ACL following the clinical examination, magnetic resonance imaging may be useful to confirm that the ACL is intact.

PREPARATION OF PATIENT FOR SURGERY

Patient preparation includes physical and psychological preparation. The physical preparation includes training to maintain the range of motion and to limit the risk of knee flexion deformity, as well as muscular training to optimize the quadriceps and the hamstrings strength at the time of surgery.

The psychological preparation includes "à la carte" training concerning the hospitalization and the rehabilitation program. The patient can also meet with patients who have had recent surgery if they want to share fears and thoughts concerning the procedure. The goals for each postoperative day are presented to patients to prepare them for rehabilitation and to improve their involvement and motivation. If excessive stress related to surgery is detected, a specific program of neurolinguistic preparation is proposed to the patient.

SURGERY

Indications

The indications for lateral UKA are painful osteoarthritis (OA) or osteonecrosis limited to the lateral compartment of the knee associated with significant loss of joint space on the radiographs.[2-4,6] Lateral UKA can also be performed in case of posttraumatic arthritis limited to the lateral compartment as recently reported.[17] Age and weight may still represent debatable issues for the indication of UKA because the procedure is often presented as an alternative to either osteotomy or TKA.[2,3] As previously mentioned and according to the results of a previously published series, we consider distal femoral osteotomy as an attractive and efficient conservative procedure for the young patient with no osteoarthritis and a valgus knee.[2,3] Based on the comparative results from 10 years of follow-up studies on UKAs and TKAs, Scott and colleagues considered that UKA might assume a role in two groups of patients: middle-aged osteoarthritic patients (especially women undergoing a "first" arthroplasty) and osteoarthritic octogenarians having their "first and last" arthroplasty.[18] With survivorship studies of modern UKA comparable to TKA after the first decade, the selection process must be reconsidered and patients in their 60s and 70s would seem to have a greater chance of living out their life with either a TKA or a UKA, which in any case would be easier to revise.[3,19]

Early reports of UKA considered obesity as a relative contraindication for UKA, but recent studies found no correlation between weight and outcomes and we concur with the idea that wear is more related to activity than to weight.[20] Obesity itself is consequently not a contraindication.

Contraindications

Any type of inflammatory arthritis, such as rheumatoid arthritis, is recognized as a formal contraindication for UKA because this can be a cause of rapid degeneration of the unreplaced compartments. Mild chondrocalcinosis, which is mostly a radiographic finding, may be accepted as an indication to perform UKA, in contrast to the productive chondrocalcinosis often associated with cyclic effusion of the knee.

Anatomy

In our practice, lateral UKA corresponds to 10% of the indication for UKA and long-term results confirm those previously published, demonstrating that lateral osteoarthritis can be treated successfully by unicondylar replacement.[2] The in vivo kinematic evaluation of patients implanted with lateral UKA showed a greater posterior displacement of the femorotibial contact point during flexion as compared with patients implanted with medial UKA.[11] The technique using a fixed-bearing cemented metal-backed implant through a minimally invasive lateral parapatellar approach is described in this chapter. Due to the anatomy of the lateral compartment, some specific points of the surgical technique should be outlined, including a limited tibial resection (because the disease is most of the time located on the femoral side), a perpendicular tibial cut in the sagittal and the frontal plane (as there is no slope on the lateral compartment and limited frontal deformation of the tibia), a vertical tibial cut done close to the border of the medial part of the patellar tendon (due to the natural orientation of the lateral tibial plateau), a more proximal distal femoral cut (if there is a femoral condyle dysplasia), and an adapted femoral rotation (relative to the divergence of the femoral condyle).[21, 22] The divergence of the femoral condyle leading to the screw-home mechanism represents the most challenging point of the surgical technique for a lateral UKA, because a good position in flexion may lead to a malposition in extension.[21,22]

Approach

The procedure can be performed under general or epidural anesthesia on a routine operating table using two leg holders: one at the lateral aspect of the thigh and the second one below the foot. The knee is flexed at 90° for the skin incision; a thigh tourniquet can be used but its use is limited in our practice. The length of the skin incision varies from 8 to 10 cm depending on skin elasticity and patient morphotype. It is important to maintain proper visualization throughout the procedure and this, in part, depends on the variation in tissue elasticity. Sufficient visualization is required during the procedure and can be achieved by frequent extension-flexion manipulations to preferentially visualize either the femoral side or the tibial side. When proper visualization of the anatomical structure or the component is not obtained by shifting the position of the knee, it might be necessary to extend the size of the incision proximally. One of the classic pitfalls of the procedure is related to the length of the incision, which should not be too small, particularly at the beginning of the learning curve. An insufficient exposure may lead to skin damage by excessive tension, to implant malpositioning, or to inadequate knee balancing. The skin incision, using a minimal approach of the lateral compartment, needs to be lateral, especially at the distal portion, owing to the frequent divergence of the lateral femoral condyle. The upper limit of the incision is the superior pole of the patella extending distally toward the lateral side of the tibial tuberosity but ending 2 cm under the joint line previously located (Fig. 47-1). The proximal part of the incision is more essential for the procedure and two-

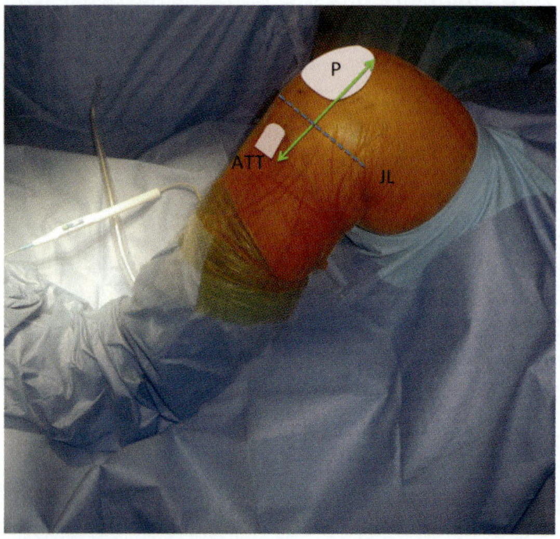

FIGURE 47-1. *The upper limit of the incision is the superior pole of the patella (P) extending distally toward the lateral side of the anterior tibial tuberosity (ATT) but ending 2 cm under the joint line previously located. The proximal part of the incision is more essential for the procedure and two-thirds of the incision should be located above the joint line (JL).*

thirds of the incision should be located above the joint line. When the lateral arthrotomy is performed and the synovial cavity opened, visualization of the joint is often easier than on the medial side due to the natural mobility of the lateral tibiofemoral joint. The lateral part of the fat pad in the way of the condyle is excised to properly visualize the condyle, the ACL, and the corresponding tibial side of the tibial plateau. It is important to note that the principles of ligament balancing existing in TKA cannot be applied to UKA because the collateral ligaments should not be released in UKA. To protect the collateral ligament and safely perform the cuts, a dedicated curved, thin Homan retractor is placed on the lateral side of the incision.

Technique

Before proceeding to the bone cuts, first bring the knee to 60° of flexion to evaluate the joint by checking the resistance of the ACL with an appropriate hook and noting the state of both the medial tibiofemoral joint and the patellofemoral joint. The osteophytes should be removed in the intercondylar notch to avoid late impingement with the ACL on the notch. This point is very important to preserve the ACL and avoid the so-called "Marie-Antoinette effect," which is famous in Europe. When osteophytes develop in the intercondylar notch, they can have a "guillotine effect" on the ACL. The osteophytes are also removed from around the lateral aspect of the patella. When performing a lateral UKA, the osteophytes on the lateral condyle should not be removed, because these osteophytes will be helpful for the positioning of the femoral compartment.[21,22] Before the vertical cut, searching and marking the anterior contact point between the tibial native tibial plateau and the anterior part of the femoral condyle can be helpful to optimize the positioning of the implant.

Tibial cut

Once the status of the patella, the ACL, and the opposite compartment has been checked, the next step is to progress to the bone cuts. In lateral UKA, the tibial resection should stay minimal, because the disease is more often on the femoral side. The tibial cut is made using an extramedullary road. The guide is placed distally around the ankle with the axis of the guide lying slightly medial to the center of the ankle joint. The proximal part of the guide rests on the anterior tibia pointing toward the axis of the tibial spines and the cutting part of the guide rests only on the upper lateral tibia to be resected. The diaphyseal part of the guide is parallel to the anterior tibial crest, and the anteroposterior position of the guide is adjusted distally to reproduce the natural upper tibial slope of the lateral compartment, usually around 0°. The amount of resection is decided after using a 4-mm probe located on the deepest part of the affected plateau, and particular care should be taken to properly define the level of the cut. To do so, it is important to control the level of resection using an "angel-wing" probe to mimic the cut, not only on the anterior part of the plateau, but also on the posterior aspect. To complete the tibial cut, the sagittal tibial cut should be done. This step is more challenging for the lateral compartment than for the medial one because of the position of the anterior aspect of the lateral tibial plateau, which is usually posterior to the lateral aspect of the patellar tendon (Fig. 47-2). Because of this anatomical consideration for the Oxford team, this cut should be done through the patellar tendon. To preserve the patellar tendon and avoid any tendonosis, we prefer using a small retractor to retract the tendon and protect it during the cut. The medial border of the plateau should be determined in flexion and extension (following the alignment of the edge of the femoral condyle on the tibial plateau when the knee is brought from flexion close to full extension), marked with the Bovie while respecting the tibial spine eminence. Once the line has been made with the Bovie, the cut can be done freehand and, of course, particular care should be taken to protect the ACL.

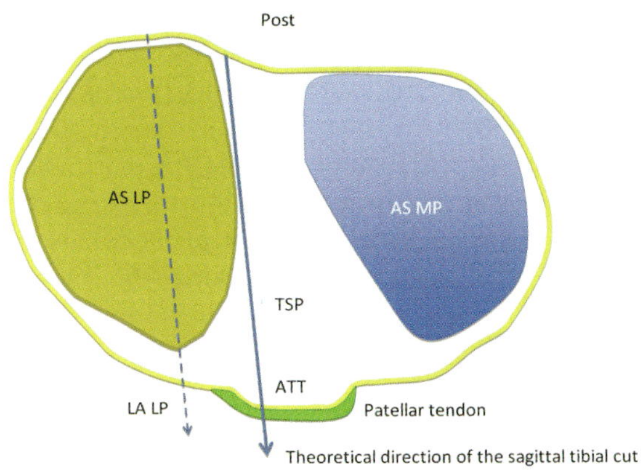

FIGURE 47-2. *To complete the tibial cut, the sagittal tibial cut should be made, which is more challenging for the lateral compartment than for the medial one because of the position of the anterior aspect of the lateral tibial plateau, which is usually posterior to the lateral aspect of the patellar tendon. AS LP, articular surface lateral plateau; AS MP, articular surface medial plateau; TSP, tibial spine prominence; LA LP, longitudinal axis of the lateral plateau; ATT, anterior tibial tubercule.*

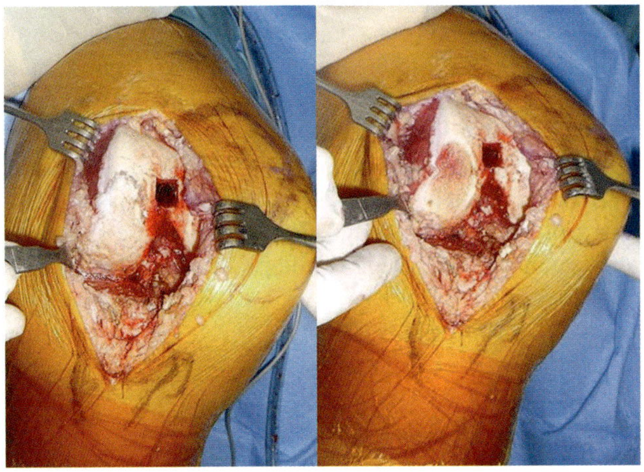

FIGURE 47-3. *The amount of bone resected from the distal femur corresponds exactly, millimeter for millimeter, to the femoral prosthesis. However, because of the potential dysplasia of the lateral femoral condyle, the amount of cut can be lower than expected.*

Femoral cut

The entrance hole of the distal femur for the intramedullary technique is centered above the roof of the intercondylar notch and prepared using an osteotome to conserve the cartilage. The drilling of the femoral medullary canal through a short incision often requires bringing the knee to 60° of flexion. In flexion, the tension from the patella on the intramedullary guide might induce incorrect alignment. Once the guide has been properly introduced, the distal femoral cut can be made by reporting the angle between the anatomic and mechanical axis previously calculated on the full weight-bearing view. This angle is usually 3° to 5°. It is critical to carefully protect the skin at the proximal part of the incision while performing this cut to avoid any skin damage. The amount of bone resected from the distal femur corresponds exactly, millimeter for millimeter, to the femoral prosthesis; however, due to the potential dysplasia of the lateral femoral condyle, the amount of cut can be lower than expected (Fig. 47-3). Therefore, once the distal femoral cut has been performed, it is crucial to check the extension space using a dedicated spacer block (Fig. 47-4). Full extension should be obtained without excessive tension. If the full extension can not be obtained, the distal femoral cut should be considered and a 2-mm recut might be required. The next challenge concerns the remainder of the femoral cuts (posterior cut and chamfers), which will then be completed using the appropriate cutting block. The rotation setup of the cutting block is the crucial point of the procedure. The size of the femoral implant should be determined using the cutting block. The size is determined once this femoral finishing guide is positioned on the distal femoral cut, searching for the best compromise between an anatomically centered position on the femoral condyle and a long axis perpendicular to the resected tibial plateau. The top of

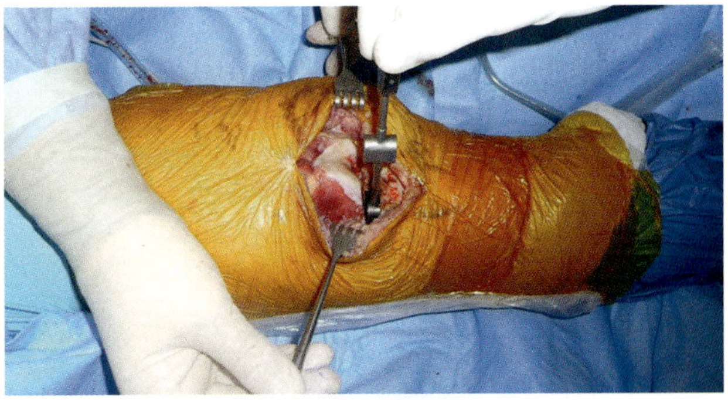

FIGURE 47-4. *Once the distal femoral cut has been performed, it is crucial to check the extension space using a dedicated spacer block.*

this finishing guide should be localized 1 to 2 mm above the deepest layer of the cartilage to avoid a potential notch between the femoral implant and the patella. In other words, ideally the femoral block should be slightly smaller anteriorly than the original femoral condyle. The control of the mediolateral position of the femoral cutting guide, which determines the position of the final implant, as previously mentioned, is crucial (Fig. 47-4). The upper position of the guide can be determined by using the landmark made with the Bovie at the beginning of the procedure corresponding to the anterior contact point in extension between the tibia and the femur. This landmark is also located at the most anterior part of the distal femoral cut. The guide is placed anteriorly and a first screw pin is used to secure the anterior position of the guide. Then, the lateral aspect of the femoral guide should follow the lateral aspect of the condyle to avoid any excessive internal rotation in extension due to the screw-home mechanism. This principle is illustrated in Figure 47-5. Because the divergence of the lateral condyle is different from one knee to another, checking the mediolateral

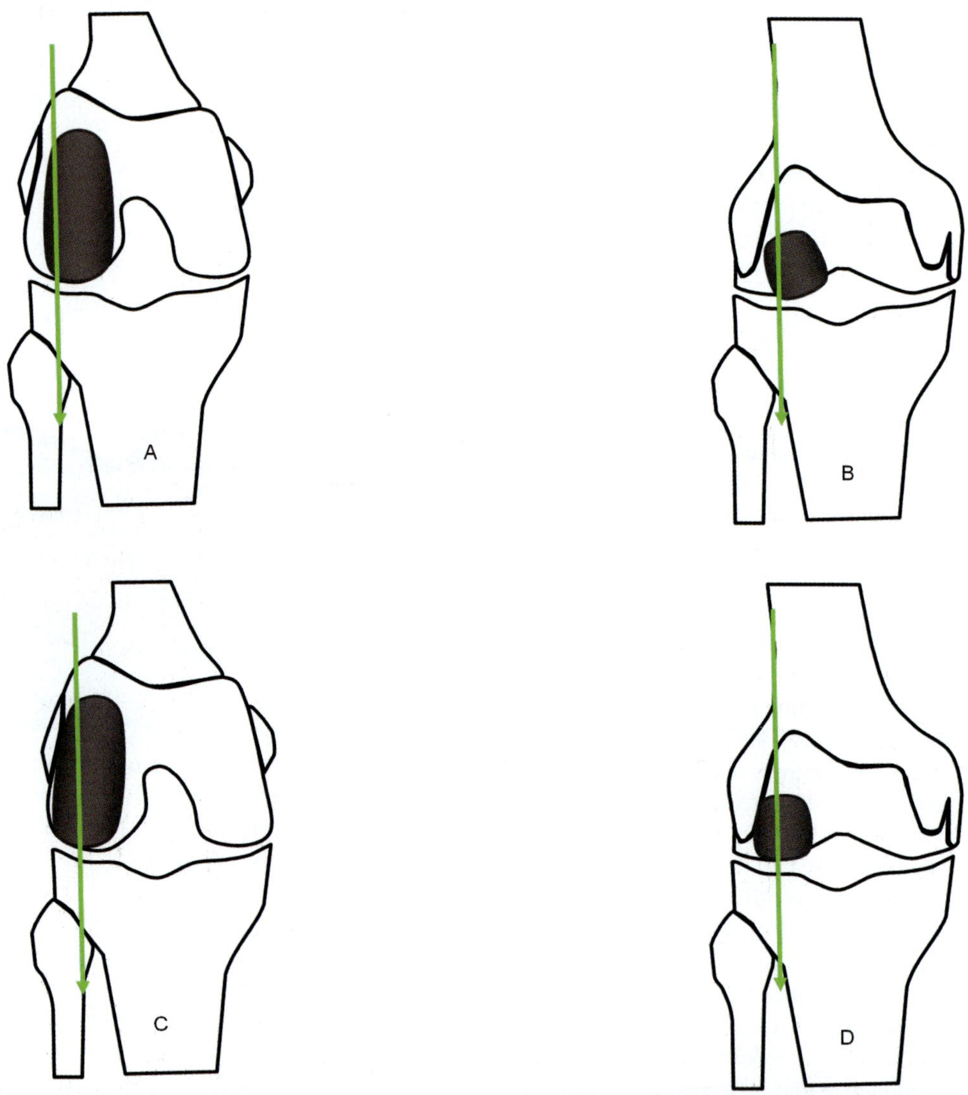

FIGURE 47-5. *Due to the screw-home mechanism consecutive to the divergence of the femoral condyle, a good positioning in flexion (**A**) may lead to an excessive internal rotation in extension and an impingement into the tibial spine eminence (**B**). Therefore, the positioning in flexion should exaggerate the lateral rotation (**C**) to obtain a satisfying position in extension (**D**).*

position of the guide on the femoral condyle is also recommended, and finally the second screw pin is used to secure the femoral guide. Once the posterior cut and the chamfrains have been made and the cutting guide removed, removal of any posterior osteophytes is necessary using a curved osteotome to increase the range of flexion and avoid any posterior impingement with the polyethylene in high flexion.

Tibial finishing and trials

The size of the tibial tray should now be determined, resulting in the best compromise between maximal tibial coverage and overhang, which might induce pain. The anteroposterior size of the tibial plateau sometimes differs from the mediolateral one, especially for female knees, thus different sizing trials are necessary to find the best compromise. It is important to keep the depth of the tibial cut as conservative as possible to take advantage of the strength of the tibial cortex and the increased area of contact proximally. The knee is then brought into maximal flexion and internally rotated. The final preparation of the tibia is completed with the appropriate guide with the underlying keel impacted in the subchondral bone. Using a minimal incision, it is important to locate carefully the posterior margin of the tibial plateau to position the keel correctly in the anteroposterior direction. It is useful to precut the future location of the keel using a reciprocating saw blade or an osteotome.

The flexion-extension gaps should be then tested with the trial components in place and inserting a trial polyethylene liner. At that step, it is important to search for any impingement of the femur against the spine eminence in extension due to a lack of external rotation in flexion. Once this has been verified, it is important to look for a 2-mm protective laxity checked close to full extension to avoid any overcorrection of the deformity leading to progression of osteoarthritis in the medial compartment. The polyethylene insert is often thicker than for the medial side in case of femoral dysplasia, even if the principle of undercorrection of the deformity for all cases of lateral UKA remains the basis for successful long-term results. All components should be cemented for better fixation because long-term results suggest that loosening is not a common mode of failure with modern cemented, metal-backed components. The tibial component is cemented first with the knee in full flexion and internally rotated to improve the exposure of the lateral compartment. When cementing the components, it is important to remove the excess cement at the posterior aspect of the knee, and the use of a 90° curved probe is useful to remove any posterior cement when using a minimal incision. Once the femoral implant has been cemented, bringing the knee close to extension helps to remove any posterior cement. Finally, the polyethylene can be inserted in flexion after the cleaning and the drying of the tibial implant. A final testing of the knee from flexion to extension (Fig. 47-6) and patellar tracking should be checked before closing. If a tourniquet has been used, it should be released before closure to adequately perform hemostasis.

POSTOPERATIVE TREATMENT AND COMPLICATIONS

Rehabilitation

In our practice, one intra-articular drain is left in for 36 hours. Postoperatively, immediate weight bearing is recommended after removal of the femoral nerve block catheter (left in for 12 hours postoperatively) protected by two crutches for 1 or 2 weeks. Manual range-of-motion physiotherapy is performed the day after surgery. Deep venous thrombosis prevention is managed using mechanical devices and low-weight heparin for 3 weeks postoperatively.

Complications

Specific complications of a lateral UKA may be related to poor patient selection, inappropriate implant design, or a surgical error. Complications related to poor patient selection include early arthritis progression and instability.[2] Arthritis progression within the 2 first years after surgery can be related to an overcorrection of the valgus deformation or to a misdiagnosed arthritis at the time of surgery. To limit the risk of misdiagnosed arthritis, it is recommended that the previously described patient selection process should be carefully followed.[2] Instability is rare and may be related either to an insufficient ACL or to excessive tibial resection, so once again preoperative patient selection and carefully followed surgical technique may limit those risks.[2]

Complications related to the implant design have been described with the early generation of mobile-bearing implants in the lateral compartment with a high rate of dislocation, and therefore fixed-bearing implants or mobile-bearing implants adapted to the lateral compartment are recommended.[2,3]

Complications related to surgical technique include fracture, in case of an excessively low tibial cut. Problems of rotation can be due to the surgical difficulty of using the screw-home mechanism and this can lead to an impingement on the tibial spine eminence with pain in extension and a lack of extension. Lack of extension can also result from a femoral cut that is too thin.[2,3]

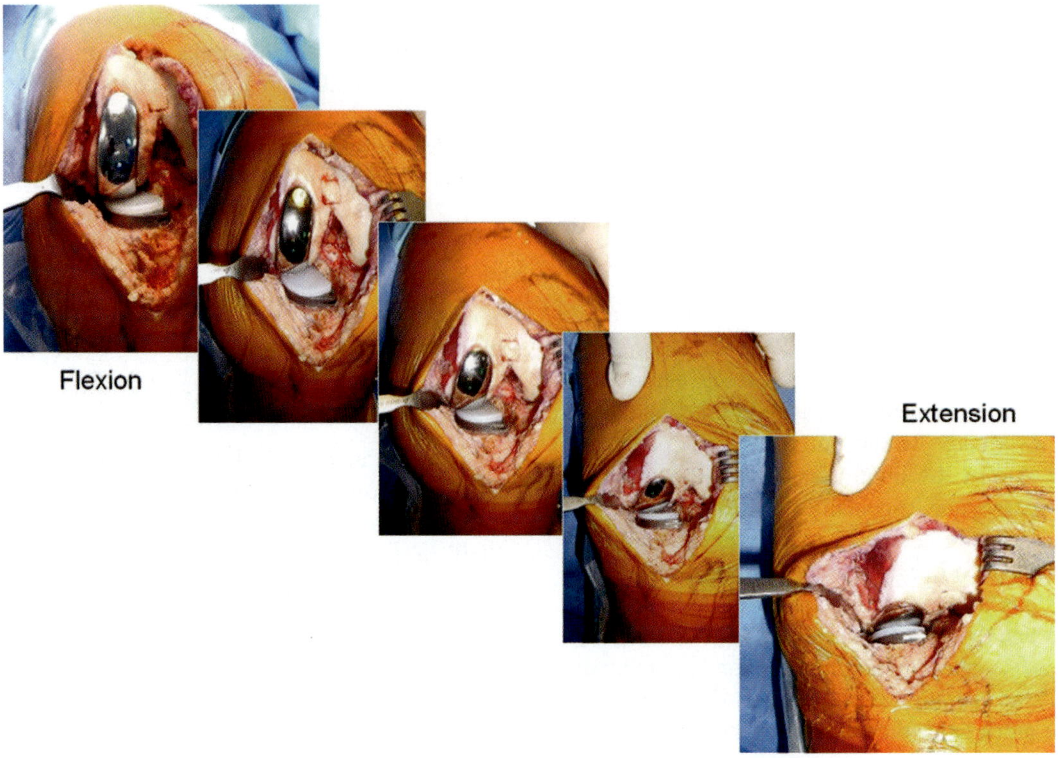

FIGURE 47-6. *Final testing of the knee shows a good adaptation from flexion to extension with no impingement in the tibial spine eminence in extension, demonstrating a good integration of the screw-home mechanism.*

OUTCOMES

Survivorship studies generated from early unicompartmental series showed that survivorship rates at 10 years were decreasing into the 85% range.[2-5] With better patient selection and reproducible instrumentation, more recent series show 10-year survivorship regularly at 90% or greater.[2] Many authors now also support the view that revision of a modern UKA is a relatively common and simple procedure.[19] Patients from the Swedish registry are more satisfied after revision of a failed UKA than after revision of a TKA.[23] Unicompartmental femorotibial osteoarthritis usually affects the medial compartment of the knee and, more rarely, the lateral compartment; therefore, there are fewer series in the literature concerning the results of lateral UKA. The results of this study have shown that lateral UKA can provide satisfying long-term clinical and radiological results and the survivorship at 10, 16, and 22 years is comparable to the survivorship obtained for medial UKA in the literature.[2] We retrospectively reported the long-term results of a series including all patients treated with an isolated lateral UKA in our institution for a confirmed diagnosis of lateral unicompartmental osteoarthritis of the knee or idiopathic osteonecrosis between February 1982 and December 2004. Forty consecutive UKAs in 39 patients performed using a cemented prosthesis have been included. There were 24 women and 15 men in the series, with 22 right knees and 18 left knees. The mean age of the patients at the time of surgery was 61 ± 7 years (range, 34–79 years). The mean body mass index of the patients was 26 ± 5 kg/m^2 (range, 18–43). According to the Ahlback classification, 2 knees (5%) were grade 2, 7 (17%) were grade 3, and 31 (78%) were grade 4. The etiologies of the lateral osteoarthritis were primary osteoarthritis in 24 knees (60%), post-traumatic (following a tibial plateau fracture) in 12 cases (30%), and secondary to an osteonecrosis in 4 cases (10%). In the series, 31 (77%) patients were engaged in labor or sports. The Knee Society knee and function scores improved significantly after lateral UKA between the preoperative and the final evaluation at a mean follow-up of 12.6 ± 4.2 years (range, 3–23 years) in this series. Preoperatively the mean active knee flexion was 115° ± 8 ° (range, 100°– 135°) and 134° ± 7° (range, 122°–153°) at final follow-up. All but 10 patients returned to their preoperative activity level (63%). At the time of the final follow-up, 23 patients (62.3%) were enthusiastic about the procedure, 9 patients (24.3%) were satisfied, 1 patient (2.7%) reported no change, and 4 patients (10.7%) were not satisfied.

The mean preoperative mechanical axis of the lower limb was 6° ± 3° of valgus (range, 0°–15° of valgus) and the mean postoperative alignment was 3° ± 2° of valgus (range, 1°–6°). Four knees (10%) showed radiolucencies (<1 mm) at the tibial bone–cement interface without any sign of progression after 5 years of follow-up. No femoral radiolucencies were observed. Concerning osteoarthritis (OA) progression, four knees required a revision for symptomatic progression at 1, 2.8, 9.8, and 13.7 years, respectively. At final follow-up 6 knees presented with isolated asymptomatic OA progression in the medial compartment and 5 knees presented an isolated asymptomatic OA progression in both medial and patellofemoral compartments. Two knees were revised without implant removal. One had a traumatic patellar fracture at 10 years in a well-functioning knee treated with an open reduction and an internal fixation with a poor result and a remaining painful patella. One knee had limited motion after 2 years due to arthrofibrosis and was arthroscopically treated with a good result. Four knees were revised for significant and painful progression of the osteoarthritis in the medial compartment in three cases and in the patellofemoral compartment in one case. For 2 of these 4 knees, a bicompartmental arthroplasty was performed in one case at 1 year by adding a medial UKA and in the other case by adding a patellofemoral arthroplasty at 2.4 years. Clinical and radiological results were satisfying for these two patients at final follow-up. The two remaining knees presenting with a painful osteoarthritis progression were revised using a TKA at 9.8 years and 13.7 years, respectively. Finally, one knee was revised with a standard posterostabilized TKA for a tibial loosening at 11 months secondary to a tibial plateau fracture with a good result at final follow-up. Considering revision for any reason, the 10-year survivorship was 92%, the 16-year survivorship was 81%, and the 22-year survivorship was 74% (95% confidence interval: 0.52–0.96).

Our results at a maximum follow-up of 23 years ranged between the results of the old and recent studies of lateral UKA reported in the literature.[2,24,25] Recent studies reported a low failure rate while the results of older series were more controversial.[2,24,25] As previously mentioned, we observed a significant improvement of the results over time, which is probably linked first to an improvement in patient selection. A 21% failure rate has been reported using the mobile-bearing Oxford unicompartmental prosthesis in the lateral compartment, with 10% rate of bearing dislocation.[26] This difference with the commonly reported excellent long-term results using the same implant for the medial compartment may be explained by the amount of femoral translation of the lateral condyle while the medial one remains fairly stationary.[2] According to these results and because of the biomechanical properties of the lateral compartment, fixed-bearing implants seem more appropriate.[2] Thus, two recent studies have shown more favorable results using fixed-bearing UKA at mid- or long-term follow-up.[2,25] As mentioned in our series, osteonecrosis limited to the lateral compartment can also be a good indication for a lateral UKA.[27]

UKA can also be used in case of posttraumatic arthritis in the lateral compartment. Sah and Scott studied the results of lateral compartment UKA for this indication (with average 5 years' follow-up).[25] They reported 10 posttraumatic cases in this series of 49 lateral UKAs placed through an anterior midline incision.[25] They compared the results of these patients with those in whom UKA was performed for "conventional" indications.[25] They found it necessary to utilize, on average, a 2-mm thicker tibial component to compensate for depression of the lateral plateau in the posttraumatic group.[25] We recently reported a series including 13 cases of posttraumatic lateral UKA performed with modern instrumentation with a mean follow-up of 10.2 years (range, 3–22.1 years) with good results.[17] In this series, we have preferred to use screws to reinforce the bone of the lateral tibial plateau and utilize an identical tibial component to that used in standard degenerative cases. Sah and Scott reported worse objective knee scores (International Knee Society knee and function) in the posttraumatic group, with 50% of patients reporting dissatisfaction with their results.[25] The survivorship in their series was 100% at 5 years, which is comparable with our results. In our series, the functional results were also inferior to those that we have previously reported for degenerative cases, but the proportion of patients who were dissatisfied (23%) was lower than that reported by Sah and Scott.[17,25]

CASE EXAMPLES

The radiographs in Figure 47-7 show the preoperative radiological analysis of a 55-year-old man with a painful lateral arthritis of the knee post menisectomy that is resistant to the medical treatment. A fixed-bearing UKA was performed in January 2001. Figure 47-8 shows the 10-year follow-up radiographs with a good functional result.

PEARLS AND PITFALLS

Some pearls and pitfalls with the use of a UKA are as follows:

- Isolated arthritis of the lateral compartment
- Limited valgus deformation

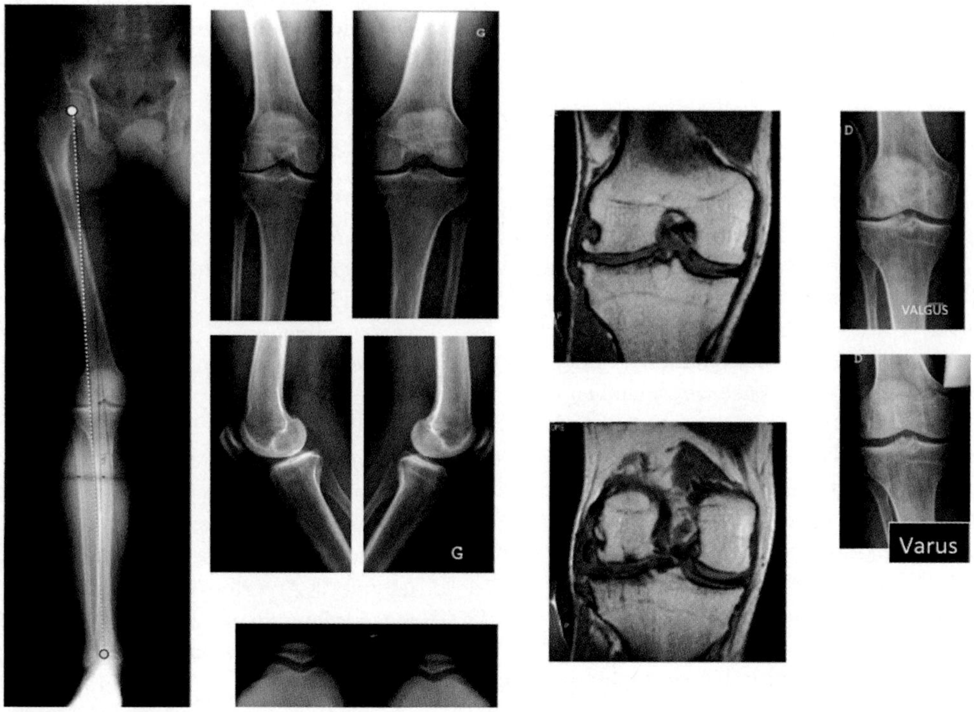

FIGURE 47-7. *Preoperative radiological analysis of a 55-year-old man with a painful lateral arthritis of the knee post menisectomy that is resistant to medical treatment. A fixed-bearing UKA was performed in January 2001.*

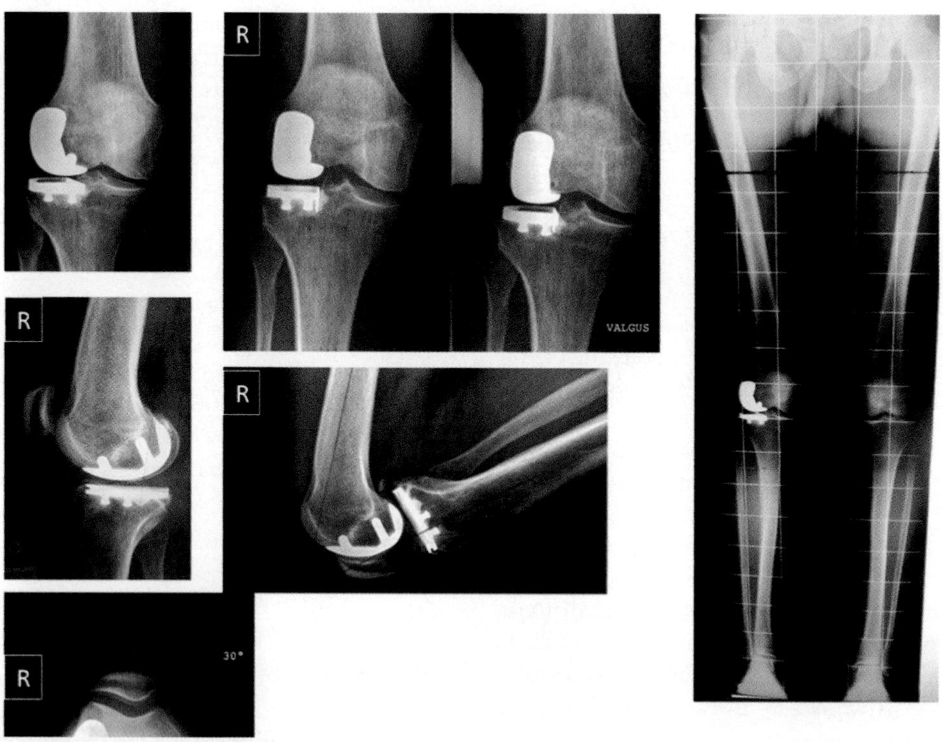

FIGURE 47-8. *Ten-year follow-up radiographs showing a good functional result, with no sign of wear or loosening.*

- Functional ACL
- Limited lateral parapatellar approach
- Fixed-bearing is recommended
- Limited tibial cut
- Control the axis of the sagittal cut for the tibia
- Conservation of the lateral osteophytes
- Check the extension space using dedicated spacer blocks
- Control of the femoral rotation considering the screw-home mechanism
- Survival comparable to TKA at 15 years

REFERENCES

1. Ahlback S. Osteoarthrosis of the knee. A radiographic investigation. *Acta Radiol Diagn (Stockh).* 1968;Suppl 277:7-72.
2. Argenson JN, Parratte S, Bertani A, et al. Long-term results with a lateral unicondylar replacement. *Clin Orthop Relat Res.* 2008;466(11):2686-2693.
3. Argenson JN, Parratte S, Bertani S, et al. The new arthritic patient and arthroplasty treatment options. *J Bone Joint Surg Am.* 2009;91(suppl 5):43-48.
4. Argenson JN, Chevrol-Benkeddache Y, Aubaniac JM. Modern unicompartmental knee arthroplasty with cement: a three- to ten-year follow-up study. *J Bone Joint Surg Am.* 2002;84(12):2235-2239.
5. Berger RA, Meneghini RM, Jacobs JJ, et al. Results of unicompartmental knee arthroplasty at a minimum of ten years of follow-up. *J Bone Joint Surg Am.* 2005; 87(5):999-1006.
6. Pagnano MW, Clarke HD, Jacofsky DJ, et al. Surgical treatment of the middle-aged patient with arthritic knees. *Instr Course Lect.* 2005;54:251-259.
7. Puddu G, Cipolla M, Cerullo G, et al. Which osteotomy for a valgus knee? *Int Orthop.* 2010;34(2):239-247.
8. Wang JW, Hsu CC. Distal femoral varus osteotomy for osteoarthritis of the knee. *J Bone Joint Surg Am.* 2005;87(1):127-133.
9. Kosashvili Y, Gross AE, Zywiel MG, et al. Total knee arthroplasty after failed distal femoral varus osteotomy using selectively stemmed posterior stabilized components. *J Arthroplasty.* 2011;26(5):738-743.
10. Scott RD. Lateral unicompartmental replacement: a road less traveled. *Orthopedics.* 2005;28:983-984.
11. Argenson JN, Komistek RD, Aubaniac JM, et al. In vivo determination of knee kinematics for subjects implanted with a unicompartmental arthroplasty. *J Arthroplasty.* 2002;17(8):1049-1054.
12. Tria AJ. Clinical examination of the knee. In: *Insall & Scott Surgery of the Knee.* Vol. 1. 4th ed. Philadelphia, PA: Churchill Livingstone Elsevier; 2006:86-98.
13. Gibson PH, Goodfellow JW. Stress radiography in degenerative arthritis of the knee. *J Bone Joint Surg Br.* 1986;68(4):608-609.
14. Kozinn SC, Scott R. Unicondylar knee arthroplasty. *J Bone Joint Surg Am.* 1989;71(1):145-150.
15. Argenson JN, Parratte S, Flecher X, et al. Unicompartmental knee arthroplasty: technique through a mini-incision. *Clin Orthop Relat Res.* 2007;464:32-36.
16. Parratte S, Pauly V, Aubaniac JM, et al. Survival of bicompartmental knee arthroplasty at 5 to 23 years. *Clin Orthop Relat Res.* 2010;468:747-755.
17. Lustig S, Parratte S, Magnussen RA, et al. Lateral unicompartmental knee arthroplasty relieves pain and improves function in posttraumatic osteoarthritis. *Clin Orthop Relat Res.* Epub 2011 Jul 12.
18. Scott RD, Cobb AG, McQueary FG, et al. Unicompartmental knee arthroplasty. Eight- to 12-year follow-up evaluation with survivorship analysis. *Clin Orthop Relat Res.* 1991;271:96-100.
19. Dudley TE, Gioe TJ, Sinner P, et al. Registry outcomes of unicompartmental knee arthroplasty revisions. *Clin Orthop Relat Res.* 2008;466(7):1666-1670.
20. Argenson JN, Parratte S. The unicompartmental knee: design and technical considerations in minimizing wear. *Clin Orthop Relat Res.* 2006;452:137-142.
21. Cartier P. Is the unicondylar prosthesis reliable? *Acta Orthop Belg.* 1985;51(4):563-571.
22. Cartier P, Cheaib S. Unicondylar knee arthroplasty: 2-10 years of follow-up evaluation. *J Arthroplasty.* 1987;2(2):157-162.
23. Robertsson O, Dunbar M, Pehrsson T, et al. Patient satisfaction after knee arthroplasty: a report on 27,372 knees operated on between 1981 and 1995 in Sweden. *Acta Orthop Scand.* 2000;71(3):262-267.
24. Goodfellow J, O'Connor J, Murray DW. The Oxford meniscal unicompartmental knee. *J Knee Surg.* 2002; 15(4):240-246.

25. Sah AP, Scott RD. Lateral unicompartmental knee arthroplasty through a medial approach. Study with an average five-year follow-up. *J Bone Joint Surg Am.* 2007;89:1948-1954.

26. Gunther T, Murray D, Miller R. Lateral unicompartmental knee arthroplasty with Oxford meniscal knee. *Knee.* 1996;3:33-39.

27. Parratte S, Argenson JN, Dumas J, et al. Unicompartmental knee arthroplasty for avascular osteonecrosis. *Clin Orthop Relat Res.* 2007;464:37-42.

48

Patellofemoral Arthroplasty

Jess H. Lonner and Eric B. Smith

Isolated patellofemoral arthritis is a common source of pain and disability. Generally, it can be treated effectively with nonsurgical interventions, such as weight reduction, physical therapy, and judicious use of injectable or oral medications. However, when the pain is refractory to these efforts, surgery may be considered. A number of surgical options have been used, with variable success, for patellofemoral arthritis, including arthroscopic debridement and lavage, patellar unloading procedures, patellectomy, cartilage grafting and bone marrow stimulation techniques, patellar resurfacing, patellofemoral arthroplasty, and total knee arthroplasty. This chapter discusses the role of patellofemoral arthroplasty (PFA) for the treatment of patellofemoral arthritis; however, this treatment may not be appropriate for all patients. Selecting appropriate patients and adhering to strict surgical indications will optimize results.

EPIDEMIOLOGY

Chondromalacia patella has been observed in 40% to 60% of patients at autopsy and in 20% to 50% of patients at the time of arthrotomy for other diagnoses.[1] The clinical prevalence of isolated patellofemoral arthritis is high, occurring in as many as 11% of men and 24% of women over the age of 55 with symptomatic osteoarthritis of the knee in one study.[2] This gender predilection is undoubtedly related to the often subtle patellar malalignment and dysplasia that is common in women. The patellofemoral cartilage is also vulnerable to direct traumatic injury, considering its unprotected location in the body.

PREOPERATIVE EVALUATION

History and Physical Examination

Evaluation of the patient under consideration should be thorough, to confirm that the pain is localized to the anterior compartment of the knee and that it emanates from the patellofemoral chondral surfaces and not soft tissues. This can usually be done by taking a detailed history of the problem and by performing a meticulous physical examination.

Patellofemoral arthritis causes anterior knee pain; therefore, the location of the patient's complaint should be anterior. The discomfort is typically exacerbated by activities such as stair climbing and descent, ambulating on hills, standing from a seated position, sitting with the knee flexed, and squatting. Walking on level ground should not be as painful. A description of anterior crepitus is common. A clear description of the location of the pain is important; discomfort anywhere but directly retropatellar, or just lateral or medial to the patella, will not be relieved with a PFA. Additional important history should include previous trauma to the knee, patellar dislocation, or any prior issues with the patellofemoral joint. A history of recurrent atraumatic patellar dislocations may suggest considerable malalignment, which may need to be corrected. These patients may have dysplasia of the distal femur, such as severe trochlear flattening or convexity. After establishing the location and quality of pain, it is important to ascertain whether there were previous interventions, such as physical therapy, weight reduction, medications, injections, or surgery.

With respect to the physical examination, pain on patella inhibition testing, patellofemoral crepitus, and retropatellar knee pain with squatting are typical. Any associated medial or lateral tibiofemoral joint line tenderness should raise one's suspicion of more diffuse chondral disease (even in the presence of relatively normal radiographs) and may be a contraindication to isolated PFA. It is also essential to rule out other potential sources of anterior knee pain, such as pes anserinus bursitis, patellar or quadriceps tendinitis, prepatellar bursitis, instability, or pain referred from the ipsilateral hip or back. Careful assessment of patellar tracking and the Q angle also are important. Patients with high Q angles frequently require a tibial tubercle realignment procedure (anteromedialization) performed before or concurrent with PFA. It is also important to assess anterior cruciate ligament (ACL) and posterior cruciate ligament (PCL) integrity (Lachman, anterior/posterior drawer, pivot shift maneuvers) because reconstruction of these ligaments may be advisable. ACL or PCL insufficiency is not an absolute contraindication for PFA; however, reconstruction may be advisable to reduce the risk of knee pain and instability and to potentially preserve the tibiofemoral articular cartilage.

Imaging

Weight-bearing radiographs, including anteroposterior, posteroanterior midflexion, lateral, and axial views, are the gold standard for addressing arthritis of the knee. Axial radiographs will demonstrate the position of the patella within the trochlear groove and the extent of arthritis. Typically loss of joint space is seen, but on occasion there will be relative radiographic patellofemoral joint space preservation with minimal or no osteophytes, despite significant cartilage loss. Lateral X-rays will occasionally demonstrate patellofemoral joint space loss and osteophytes, but are often more useful in identifying whether there is patella alta or baja. Standing anteroposterior and midflexion posteroanterior radiographs are critical to determine the presence of tibiofemoral arthritis (Fig. 48-1). Mild squaring-off of the femoral condyles and even small marginal osteophytes may be accepted, provided the patient is devoid of tibiofemoral pain with functional activities and on physical exam and that there is minimal chondral degeneration during arthroscopy or arthrotomy. Newer magnetic resonance imaging (MRI) sequences may be useful for evaluating patellofemoral arthrosis, but more importantly MRI can be used to evaluate the medial and lateral compartments for evidence of chondral wear or bone marrow edema in the femoral condyles or tibial plateau. Photographs from prior arthroscopic treatment will provide valuable information regarding the extent of anterior compartment arthrosis and the status of the tibiofemoral articular cartilage and menisci.

Indications for Patellofemoral Arthroplasty

Surgery for patients with isolated patellofemoral arthritis is indicated when anterior knee pain has become intolerable to the patient, after nonoperative treatments have failed. The outcome of patellofemoral arthroplasty can be optimized by limiting its application to patients with isolated patellofemoral osteoarthrosis, posttraumatic arthrosis, or severe chondrosis (Outerbridge grade IV). Many of these patients have undergone arthroscopy and their photos can be valuable in determining the extent of patellofemoral and tibiofemoral arthritis. This option is best reserved for patients with subjective complaints of isolated retropatellar and/or peripatellar pain and functional limitations.

Contraindications

PFA should not be performed in patients with inflammatory arthritis or chondrocalcinosis involving the menisci or tibiofemoral chondral surfaces, nor should it be offered to patients with inappropriate expectations.[3-6] The presence of medial or lateral joint line pain suggest more diffuse chondral disease and should be considered contraindications to isolated patellofemoral resurfacing. Additionally, the presence of tibiofemoral arthrosis should discourage isolated PFA. The presence of even focal grade III tibiofemoral chondromalacia can compromise the outcome after PFA, although these patients will often acknowledge resolution of the most prominent component of pain. Combining PFA with medial or lateral unicompartmental knee arthroplasty or autologous osteochondral grafting are sound considerations in these situations.[7,8] Patients who consent for partial knee arthroplasty may also be consented for possible total knee arthroplasty, in case more pronounced tibiofemoral cartilage wear is seen at the time of surgery.

Although it can be most effective for treating patellofemoral dysplasia,[9] PFA should be avoided in patients with considerable patellar maltracking or malalignment, unless they are corrected. This is not to say, however, that moderate patellar tilt, observed on preoperative tangential radiographs or at the time of arthrotomy, or trochlear dysplasia should be considered contraindications for this procedure. In such cases, a lateral retinacular recession or release may be necessary at the time of arthroplasty.[4-6] Persistent patellar subluxation may cause pain and snapping and potentially polyethylene wear of the prosthesis. Patients with excessive Q angles should undergo tibial tubercle realignment before or during PFA (although some trochlear prosthesis shapes may accommodate a slightly increased Q angle).

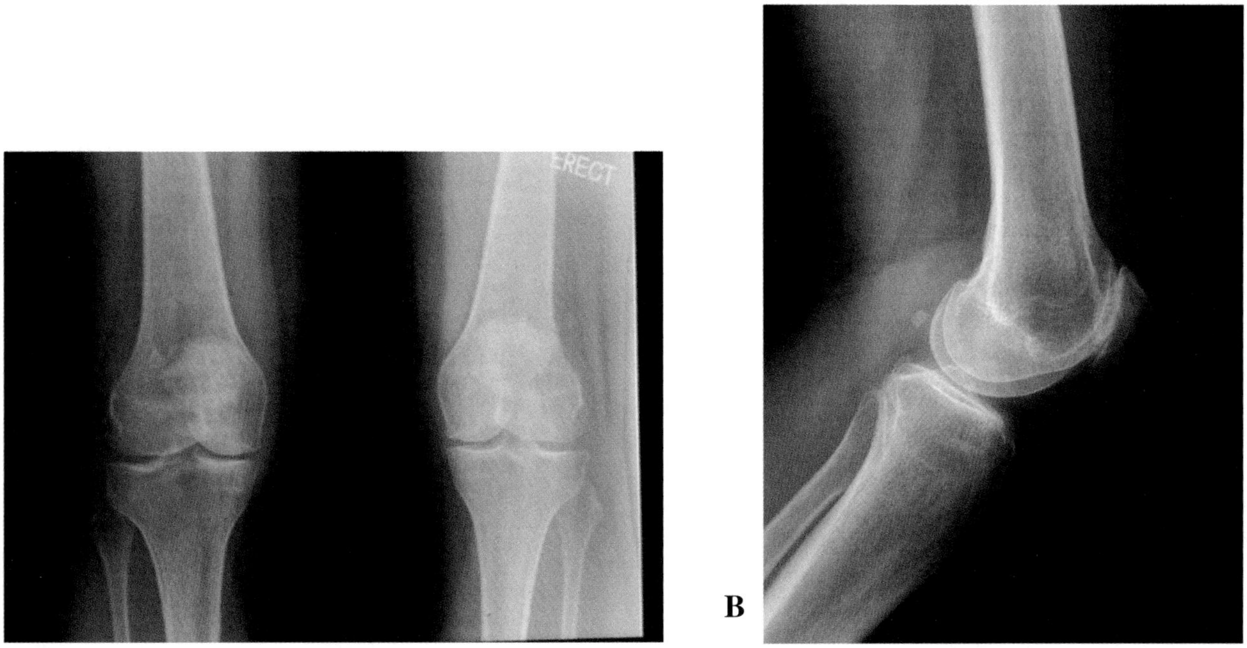

A B

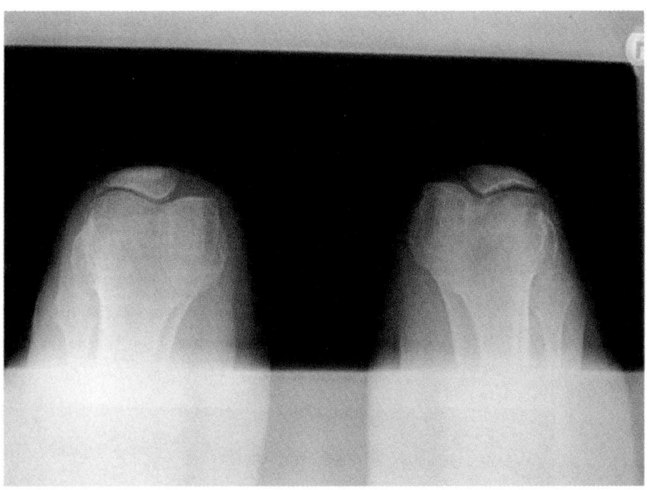

C

FIGURE 48-1. *Weight-bearing anteroposterior (**A**), lateral (**B**), and axial (**C**) radiographs demonstrating advanced patellofemoral arthrosis with sparing of the tibiofemoral compartments.*

While there are intuitive concerns, there are no data available on whether obesity or cruciate ligament insufficiency put the PFA at risk for failure. There are no age criteria for PFA provided the other criteria are met.

SURGICAL TECHNIQUE

During arthrotomy, it is essential to avoid cutting normal articular cartilage or the menisci. Before proceeding with PFA, carefully inspect the entire joint to make sure the tibiofemoral compartments are free of disease. As mentioned above, if the weight-bearing condylar surfaces have a focal full-thickness cartilage defect, consider an autologous osteoarticular graft. If there is more diffuse medial or lateral compartment wear, consider a bicompartmental arthroplasty or a total knee arthroplasty.

In addition to the design features of some contemporary components that have substantially improved patella tracking, instrumentation has been developed that is low profile, accurate, and conducive to less invasive surgical techniques. Early-generation implants required freehand preparation of all of the bony surfaces, which contributed to inaccurate trochlear component alignment. Second-generation implants typically neither offered a means for preparing the distal femur for the intercondylar tail of the implant nor were they amenable to more contemporary, less invasive surgical techniques, since they tended to be quite bulky. Newer systems have simplified the procedure and improve the anatomic mating of the implant to the articular surfaces of the transition zones.

The trochlear component should be externally rotated perpendicular to the anteroposterior axis of the femur (Whiteside axis) or parallel to the epicondylar axis to enhance patellar tracking.[5,6] This is difficult with inlay style trochlear components, which tend to be internally rotated due to the normal trochlear inclination. It is predictably accomplishable with onlay style trochlear components (Fig. 48-2).[10] Osteophytes bordering the intercondylar notch should be removed. The trochlear component should maximize coverage of the trochlea, without extending beyond the medial-lateral femoral margins anteriorly, encroaching on the weight-bearing surfaces of the tibiofemoral articulations distally, or overhanging into the intercondylar notch. The medial and lateral transitional edges of the prosthesis should be flush with or recessed approximately 1 mm from the adjacent condylar articular cartilage.[5] The proximal edge should be flush with the anterior femoral cortex, and the distal tip should be flush with the articular cartilage and not extend into the intercondylar notch. The patella is resurfaced by the same principles observed in total knee arthroplasty, restoring the original patella thickness and medializing the component. The exposed cut surface of the lateral patella that is not covered by the patellar prosthesis is removed or beveled to avoid potentially painful articulation on the trochlear prosthesis.[11] This may also enhance patella tracking by releasing tension on the lateral retinaculum.

Assessment of patellar tracking is performed with the trial components in place. Attention is paid to identify patellar tilt, subluxation, or catching of the components. Patellar tilt and mild subluxation usually can be addressed successfully by performing a lateral retinacular recession or release. As stated earlier, more severe extensor mechanism malalignment may require proximal or distal realignment.

POSTOPERATIVE MANAGEMENT

Isometrics and range-of-motion exercises are started immediately. Use of a continuous passive motion machine during hospitalization (1 to 3 days) may accelerate flexion recovery, but it is probably not necessary for most patients. Full weight bearing is permitted immediately, with support of crutches and a cane until there is adequate recovery of quadriceps strength. Thromboembolism prophylaxis is utilized for 4 to 6 weeks. Twenty-four hours of perioperative antibiotics is advisable, and appropriate precautions regarding antibiotic prophylaxis for dental procedures or other interventions should follow standard recommendations of the American Academy of Orthopaedic Surgeons.[9]

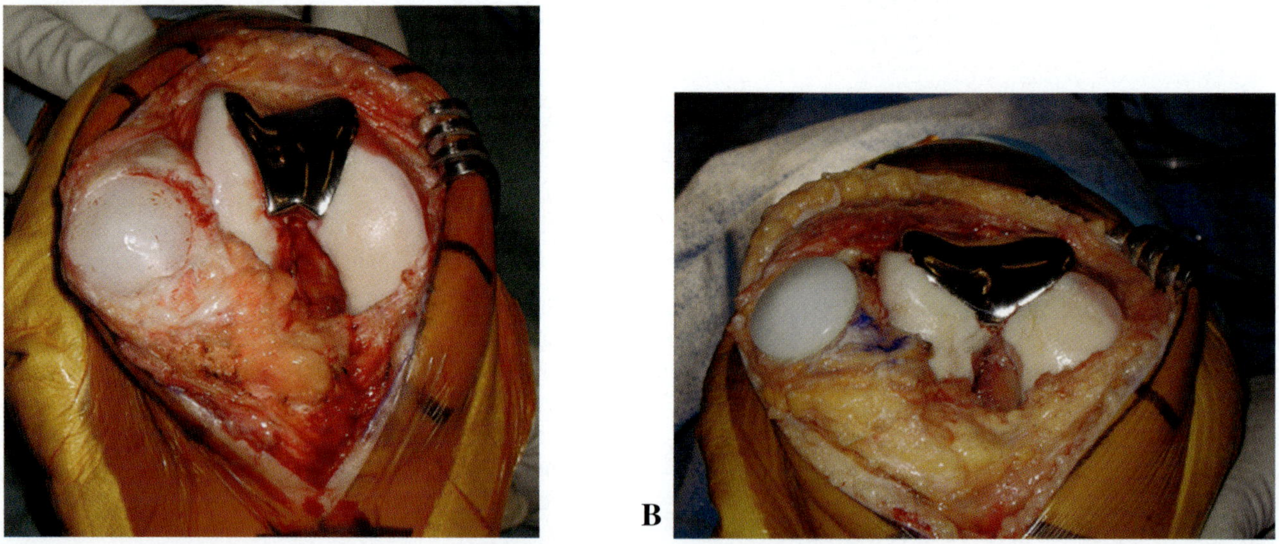

A B

FIGURE 48-2. *Intraoperative photos showing components positioned after inlay (**A**) and onlay (**B**) methods of bone preparation.*

REHABILITATION

After discharge from the hospital, patients should enter outpatient physical therapy within 1 to 2 weeks of surgery. Initial focus of therapy is on passive and active range of motion, followed by strengthening, proprioception, and endurance. In some circumstances, full recovery of quadriceps strength can take 6 months or longer, considering the severe preoperative quadriceps atrophy that is encountered in some patients with patellofemoral arthritis.

COMPLICATIONS

Complications are relatively rare after PFA. Anterior knee pain and patellar instability were a major reported reason for failure of early PFA designs and were often attributed to soft tissue imbalance or component malalignment (Table 48-1). However, many of these were likely related to trochlear component design.[6,27,28] Early-generation and contemporary inlay style trochlear designs have had a higher incidence of patellar snapping and lateral instability than onlay style designs, accounting for a higher need for secondary surgery to realign the soft tissues or revise the trochlear prosthesis in the former group. This is because many inlay style designs are internally rotated as a result of a need to be implanted flush with the surrounding articular cartilage of the trochlear peaks, whereas onlay designs can be positioned perpendicular to the anteroposterior axis of the femur.[10,28,29] A study by Hendrix et al found that revising an inlay trochlear component to an onlay prosthesis for patellar instability eliminated the problem.[29] With all design styles, a small percentage of patients will have mild anterior knee pain from soft tissue impingement or peripatellar scarring, but this occurs with a similar frequency that we see in total knee arthroplasty.[15,25]

TABLE 48-1. Clinical Results of Multiple Patellofemoral Arthroplasty Series

Series	Implant	No. of PFAs	Age	Diagnosis	Duration of Follow-up (yrs)	% of Good/ Excellent Results
Blazina[12]	Richards types I & II	57	39 (range, 19-81)	NA	2 (range, 8-42 mos)	NA
Arciero[13]	Richards type II (14); CFS-Wright (11)	25	62 (range, 33-86)	OA (25); malalignment or instability (14)	5.3 (range, 3-9 yrs)	85
Cartier[14]	Richards types II & III	72	65 (range, 23-89)	Dysplasia/grade IV chondromalacia (29); PTA (3); chondrocalcinosis (5)	4 (range, 2-12 yrs)	85
Argenson[15]	Autocentric	66	57 (range, 19-82)	Dysplasia or dislocation (22); PTA (20); OA (24)	5.5 (range, 2-10 yrs)	84
Krajca-Radcliffe[16]	Richards types I & II	16	64 (range, 42-84)	Primary OA (10) PTA (2) Recurrent dislocation (1)	5.8 (range, 2-18 yrs)	88
Tauro[17]	Lubinus	62	66 (range, 50-87)	PTA (2); primary OA (74)	7.5 (range 5-10 yrs)	45
de Winter[18]	Richards type II	26	59 (range, 22-90)	Primary OA (17); malalignment (8); PTA (1)	11 (range, 1-20 yrs)	76
Ackroyd[19]	Avon	95	NA	NA	2-5 yrs	83
Smith[20]	Lubinus	45	72 (range, 42-86)	Primary OA (44); PTA (1)	4 (range, 6 mos-7.5 yrs)	69

Continued

TABLE 48-1. *Continued*

Series	Implant	No. of PFAs	Age	Diagnosis	Duration of Follow-up (yrs)	% of Good/ Excellent Results
Kooijman[21]	Richards type II	45	50 (range, 20-77)	OA (45)	17 (range, 15 – 21 yrs)	86
Lonner[6]	Lubinus	30	38 (range, 34-51)	Primary OA (26); PTA (4) [s/p tibial tubercle realignment (10)]	4 (range, 2-6 yrs)	84
Lonner[6]	Avon trochlea; Nexgen patella	25	44 (range, 28-59)	Primary OA (25) [s/p realignment (2)]	6 mos (range, 1 mos – 1 yr)	96
Merchant[22]	LCS	15	49 (range, 30-81)	Chronic sublux or recurrent dislocation with secondary DJD (13); chondrosis (2)	3.8 yrs (range, 2.3-5.5 yrs)	93
Sisto[23]	Kinematch PFR	25	45 (range, 23-51)	OA (25) [s/p tibial tubercle elevation (6); s/p arthroscopic lateral release and debridement (13)]	73 mos (range, 32-119 mos)	100
Cartier[24]	Richards types II & III	79	60 (range, 36-81)	Dysplasia and patellar subluxation (70%); primary OA (12%); grade IV chondromalacia (7%); isolated chondrocalcinosis (6%); post patella fracture (5%)	10 yrs (range, 6-16 yrs)	77
Argenson[25]	Autocentric	66	57 (range, 21-82)	Dysplasia or dislocation (21); PTA (18); OA (18)	16 yrs (range, 12-20 yrs)	NA
Ackroyd[26]	Avon	109	68 (range, 46-86)	OA (106); Dislocation (2); PTA (1)	5.2 yrs (range, 5-8 yrs)	80%

NA, not available; OA, osteoarthritis; PTA, posttraumatic arthritis; DJD, degenerative joint disease.

Infection and thromboembolic disease are also risks after PFA; therefore, standard prophylactic strategies should be utilized to avoid these complications. An unpublished study by Lonner et al reported less than a 1% incidence of symptomatic venous thromboembolism using a multimodal approach to venous thromboembolism prophylaxis after PFA, which included aspirin or Coumadin and pneumatic calf pumps. Late failures from component subsidence, polyethylene wear, or loosening may eventually develop in the long term, but these problems occur in less than 1% of published cases combined (Table 48-1). Trochlear component loosening may be more common in cementless designs.[15,25] Arthrofibrosis is uncommon after patellofemoral arthroplasty. While it has been reported with an incidence of 7.6% to 12% in two series, both series included a number of patients who had undergone concomitant unicompartmental tibiofemoral arthroplasty, but did not mention whether the tendency for arthrofibrosis was increased in those with bicompartmental arthroplasty.[13,15]

If early patellar instability is avoided, the development of tibiofemoral arthritis is the most common "failure mechanism," occurring in approximately 20% of knees at 15 years.[21,24,25] This is more common when the underlying diagnosis is primary osteoarthritis and less common in patellofemoral dysplasia or posttraumatic arthritis.[25] In the event that revision to total knee arthroplasty is necessary to treat progressive arthritis, typically the all-polyethylene patellar component can be retained if not worn or loose, and standard total knee components can be used without the need for stems, augments, or bone graft, and without compromising the results.[30,31]

CLINICAL RESULTS

Most series have reported good and excellent results in roughly 80% to 90% of cases at short- and midterm follow-up (Table 48-1). However, clinical results of PFA are affected by trochlear component design features, as well as patient selection and surgical technique.[6,27,28,32] Outcomes and patellofemoral performance have improved, and the need for secondary soft tissue surgery to enhance patellar tracking after PFA has decreased, due to trochlear design improvements that have occurred as we have moved from first- to second-generation and now to third-generation implants, and particularly from inlay to onlay style trochlear components. The radius of curvature, width, thickness, tracking angle, and extent of constraint of the trochlear component affect patellar tracking and outcomes. Contemporary onlay designs, because of their optimized rotational alignment, have substantially reduced the incidence of patellofemoral complications, leaving tibiofemoral arthritis the major source of failure of PFAs.[6,27,28,32] Implant design, whether onlay or inlay, is likely the most critical issue affecting patellar tracking.[6,27,28] The inlay design is inset into the trochlea and tends to be more bone conserving; the onlay design is implanted flush with the anterior surface of the femoral cortex and removes the entire anterior trochlear surface. At first glance, the inlay design appears to be more appealing; however, given the variability in distal anterior femoral morphology, inlayed trochlear components often do not accurately mate with the articular geometry of the trochlear region of the femur, resulting in an offset along any of its edges. This typically results in patella catching on the trochlear component, either proximally as the knee proceeds from extension to flexion or distally as the knee proceeds from deep flexion to extension. The onlay device is more suitable for a larger variation in trochlear geometries. Unlike the inlay designs, it can be applied in patients with trochlear dysplasia without risk of having the component sit proud relative to the surrounding articular cartilage. Trying to inset a trochlear component into the bone is analogous to implanting a potato chip onto the anterior aspect of the knee: if the two surfaces are geometrically mated, then the outcome will be absolutely perfect, but if there is a mismatch, then there is an increased risk for relative component malalignment and malposition relative to the articular surfaces. This is why patella maltracking is more common with inlay-style implants. Additionally, the inlay trochlear design may also display greater variability in rotational alignment. By design, the component is rotated so that its medial and lateral edges are flush with the surrounding articular cartilage. Since most patients have a more prominent anterior lateral trochlear flange compared to the medial flange, these inlay components are often implanted in internal rotation relative to the transepicondylar and anteroposterior axes of the distal femur. This predisposes to lateral patellar subluxation that has been common with these prostheses (Fig. 48-3). Poor patellar tracking will manifest early. If related to component malposition in internal rotation with an inlay style trochlear prosthesis, revision to an onlay design with repositioning perpendicular to the anteroposterior axis of the femur can remedy the problem.[10,29]

The Australian Orthopaedic Association, National Joint Replacement Registry, has provided insight into the experience with and outcomes after PFA performed between 1999 and 2008. In that registry, 75.6% of the 977 PFAs performed in Australia were in women, usually in patients under the age of 55 (37.5%) or between the ages of 55 and 64 (29.1%). The tendency for revision after PFA varied between component types. For instance in that series, the cumulative 5-year revision rate was 18.1% with the Lubinus and 21.8% with the LCS (both inlay-style trochlear components with obtuse radii of curvatures), compared to 9.9% with the Avon (an onlay-style component that can be more accurately rotated perpendicular to the anteroposterior femoral axis). Data on some newer systems are not yet available in that registry.[32] The registry does not clearly elucidate the mechanisms of failure and reasons for revision with each individual implant, but the data corroborate other studies that show a higher incidence of patellofemoral-related (maltracking) problems with inlay-style trochlear implants compared to others (onlay style).[6,10,27-29]

Cartier et al had 85% good or excellent results in 72 first-generation PFAs followed for an average of 4 years.[14] There were numerous concomitant surgical procedures performed to enhance patellar tracking, including soft tissue realignment or tibial tubercle transfer. Longer-term follow-up of those patients, at a mean of 10 years (range, 6–16 years) after surgery, found that results deteriorated over time, primarily due to the development of tibiofemoral arthritis. That is not surprising, given the average patient age of 60 at the time of the initial PFA in that series. At most recent follow-up, 80% of those who retained their patellofemoral prostheses were pain-free and 20% had moderate or severe pain, primarily from

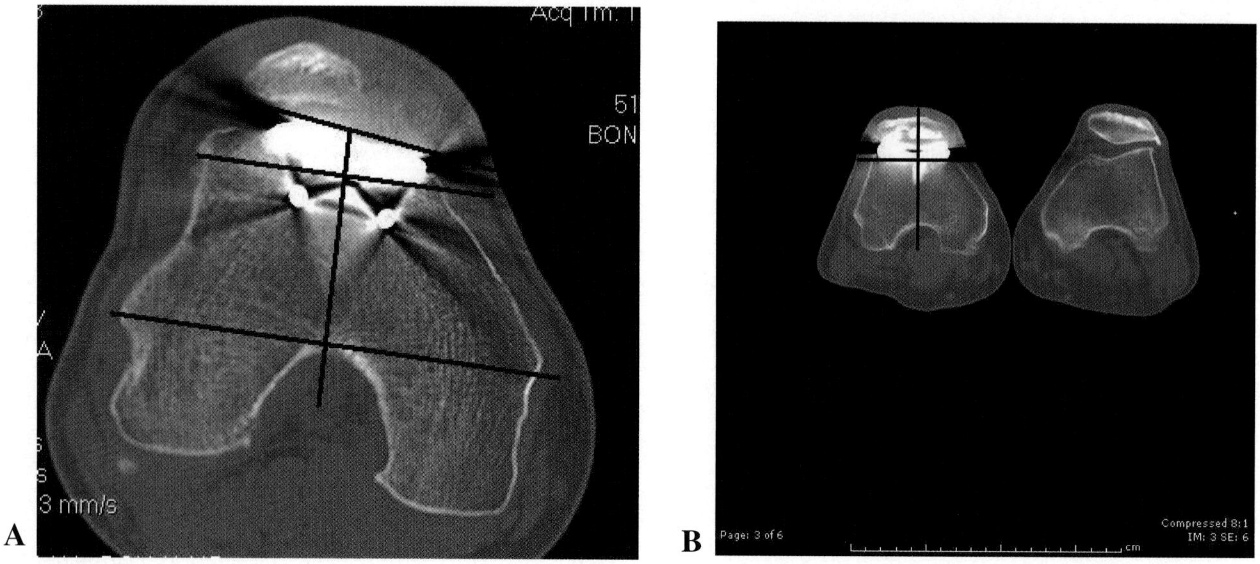

FIGURE 48-3. *(A) Axial computed tomography (CT) scan of an inlay-style implant demonstrating internal rotation relative to the anteroposterior axis of the distal femur, resulting in lateral patellar catching and subluxation. (**B**) Axial CT scan of an onlay-style trochlear prosthesis showing rotation perpendicular to the anteroposterior axis of the femur.*

tibiofemoral arthritis. Stair ambulation was considered normal in 91% of patients. No cases of patellar or trochlear loosening were identified. The authors noted that early failures peaked at 3 years and were related to inappropriate indications for the surgery and presumably to patellar maltracking problems that could likely be traced to implant design quirks. They identified a later peak in failures in the 9th and 10th years that corresponded to the development of symptomatic tibiofemoral osteoarthritis. The authors reported a survivorship of 75% at 11 years.[24] Kooijman et al reported an 86% long-term success rate with the same first-generation PFA, even though early secondary soft tissue surgery was necessary in 18% of patients and revision of the PFA was necessary for catching, imbalance, or malposition in only 16%.[21]

In a consecutive series of 30 first-generation implants and 25 second-generation implants, Lonner found that results varied depending on which trochlear design was used.[6] The incidence of patellofemoral dysfunction, subluxation, catching, and substantial pain was reduced from 17% with the earlier design to less than 4% with the more contemporary product. In another series, 14 of the same first-generation patellofemoral implants were revised to a second-generation implant that had a more favorable topography for patellar tracking. The etiologies of failure of the primary procedures were component malposition, subluxation, polyethylene wear, or overstuffing. After revision there was statistically significant improvement in knee scores for patellar tracking at a mean 5-year follow-up. Mild femorotibial arthritis (Ahlbach stage I) was predictive of a poorer clinical outcome. At most recent follow-up, there was no evidence of wear, loosening, or subluxation. This study showed that significant improvement can be obtained when revising the failed PFA with a more accommodating implant design, provided there is no femorotibial arthritis.[33]

Ackroyd et al reported on 306 second-generation PFAs and found that patellar tracking was substantially improved compared to a first-generation implant. In that series, patellar subluxation occurred in 3% and residual anterior knee pain was noted in 4%. Four percent required revision to total knee arthroplasty, mostly for tibiofemoral arthritis and none for mechanical loosening or wear.[19]

Argenson et al reported on 66 second-generation PFAs in patients with a mean age of 57 and with a mean follow-up of 16 years.[25] While most patients had substantial and sustained pain relief, 25% were revised to total knee arthroplasty for tibiofemoral arthritis (at a mean of 7.3 years after PFA) and 14% for aseptic trochlear component loosening, many of which were uncemented (at a mean of 4.5 years after PFA). The authors reported the best results when the procedure was performed for posttraumatic patellofemoral arthritis or patellar subluxation and the least favorable in those with primary degenerative arthritis. The development of tibiofemoral arthritis was the most frequent cause of failure; however, at the time of initial PFA, 14% had concomitant tibiofemoral osteotomies for early arthritis, which confounds the results. In those who retained their implants at most recent follow-up, there were significant improvements in Knee Society scores. The authors continue to advocate for the procedure as an intermediate stage before total knee arthroplasty in the absence of tibiofemoral arthritis or coronal plane malalignment.[25]

Lonner's personal experience with over 150 PFAs has demonstrated substantial improvement in anterior knee pain and stair ambulation capabilities, using a third-generation prosthesis (Gender Solutions PFJ, Zimmer, Warsaw, IN) with enhanced design features to optimize patellar tracking and with fully instrumented bone preparation,[28] and there has been a statistically significant improvement in Knee Society scores and average postoperative knee range of motion in excess of 130° (Fig. 48-4). There have been no failures from patellar catching, instability, or clinically apparent subluxation. There have been no mechanical failures at short-term follow-up. There has been one case of slight patellar subluxation noted on routine postoperative radiographs, due to chronic weakness of the vastus medialis (this improved by 6 months postoperatively with an appropriate strengthening program), one iliotibial band snapping, and one recurrent hemarthrosis. Three knees in two patients required manipulation under anesthesia 6 weeks after surgery and have maintained 115° of flexion.

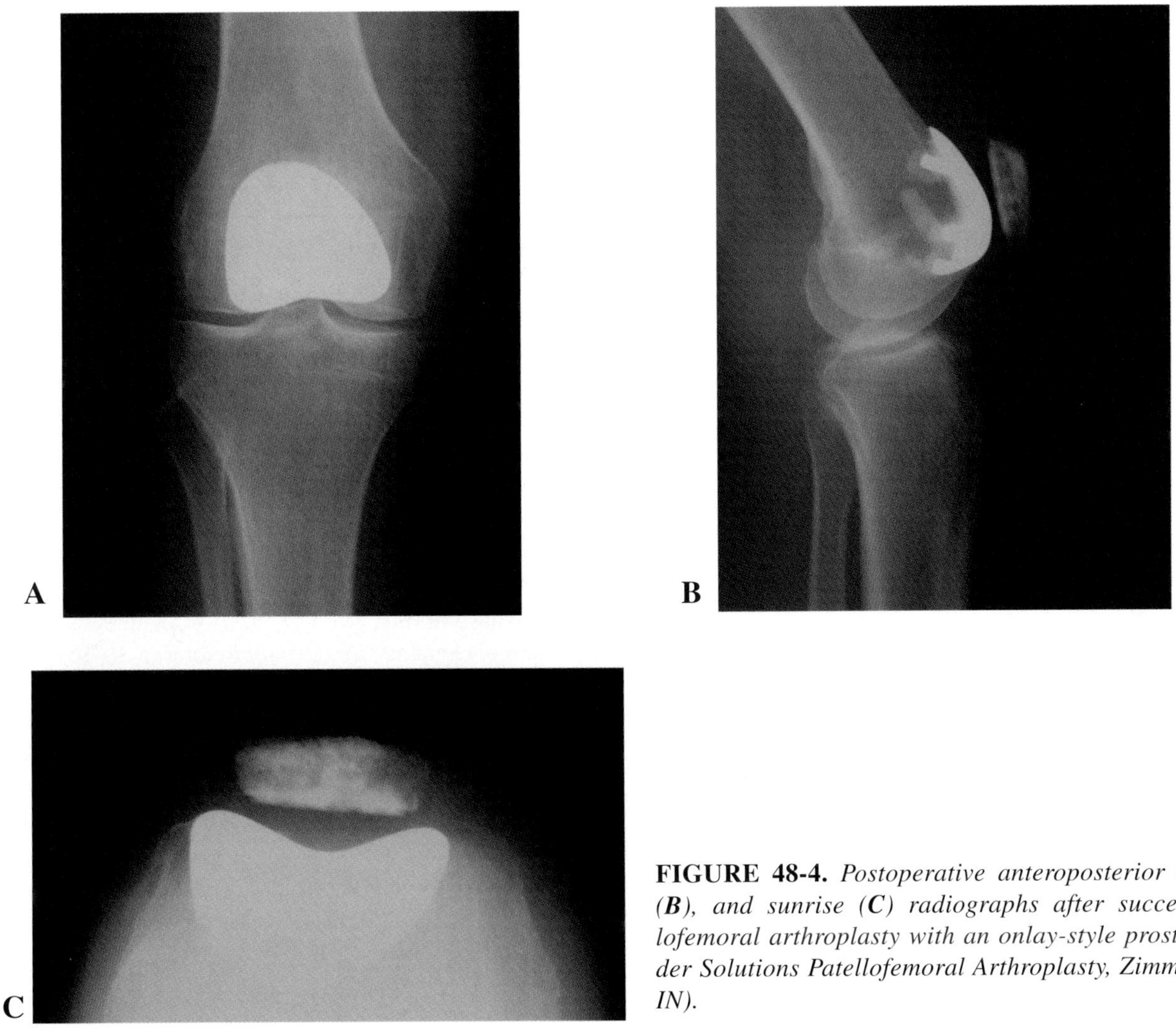

FIGURE 48-4. *Postoperative anteroposterior (**A**), lateral (**B**), and sunrise (**C**) radiographs after successful patellofemoral arthroplasty with an onlay-style prosthesis (Gender Solutions Patellofemoral Arthroplasty, Zimmer, Warsaw, IN).*

SUMMARY

Patellofemoral arthroplasty can be an effective treatment alternative for patellofemoral arthritis resulting from primary osteoarthrosis, dysplasia, or posttraumatic arthrosis in patients with normal or correctable patella alignment and tracking. PFA may provide patients with substantial pain relief of isolated patellofemoral arthrosis; however, the results can be affected by the geometric features of the trochlear component and technical issues. Residual instability may result in early failure, highlighting the importance of excluding those patients with uncorrectable patellar instability or malalignment. Implant malposition, potentially hastened by particular designs, may also contribute to failures from maltracking and mechanical catching of the patella.[4,6,17] Sparing of the tibiofemoral compartments, menisci, and cruciate ligaments allows preservation of a more kinematically sound knee joint than total knee arthroplasty.

Although sparse, long-term data suggest that loosening of cemented trochlear and all-polyethylene patellar components is uncommon and that the need for additional surgery for progressive tibiofemoral arthritis may be only approximately 25% at a mean of 15 years after PFA.[21] With emerging designs, the incidence of anterior knee pain after PFA should be comparable to that after total knee replacement surgery, namely approximately 4% to 7%.[34,35] Finally, even small amounts of tibiofemoral cartilage loss may compromise the results enough to warrant restricting this procedure to ideal candidate patients, although combining PFA with autologous osteochondral grafting for focal condylar defects or unicompartmental knee arthroplasty for associated medial or lateral arthritis may expand the application of the procedure.

PEARLS AND PITFALLS

As with many orthopaedic procedures, patient selection is critically important in obtaining excellent results with PFA. Correlating subjective complaints of anterior knee pain with objective findings of isolated patellofemoral arthrosis will optimize results. Patellar maltracking must be corrected with realignment procedures either before or concomitantly with PFA. Finally, results are maximized by utilizing newer onlay implant designs that engage the patella within the trochlear groove, have limited constraint, and a sagittal radius of curvature that mates well with the native distal femur.

REFERENCES

1. Vuorinen O, Paakkala T, Tuuturii T, et al. Chondromalacia patellae: results of operative treatments. *Arch Orthop Trauma Surg*. 1985;104:175.
2. McAlindon RE, Snow S, Cooper C, et al. Radiographic patterns of osteoarthritis of the knee joint in the community: the importance of the patellofemoral joint. *Ann Rheum Dis*. 1992;51:844-849.
3. Leadbetter WB, Seyler TM, Ragland PS, et al. Indications, contraindications, and pitfalls of patellofemoral arthroplasty. *J Bone Joint Surg Am*. 2006;88(suppl 4):122-137.
4. Lonner JH. Patellofemoral arthroplasty. *Semin Arthroplasty*. 2000;11:234-240.
5. Lonner JH. Patellofemoral arthroplasty. In: Lotke PA, Lonner JH, eds. *Master Techniques in Orthopaedic Surgery: Knee Arthroplasty*. 3rd ed. Philadelphia, PA: Wolters Kluwer Lippincott Williams & Wilkins; 2008.
6. Lonner JH. Patellofemoral arthroplasty: pros, cons, design considerations. *Clin Orthop Relat Res*. 2004; 428:158-165.
7. Lonner JH, Mehta S, Booth RE. Ipsilateral patellofemoral arthroplasty and autogenous osteochondral femoral condylar transplantation. *J Arthroplasty*. 2007;22:1130-1136.
8. Argenson JN, Parratte S, Bertani A, et al. The new arthritic patient and arthroplasty treatment options. *J Bone Joint Surg Am*. 2009;91(suppl 5):43-48.
9. Hanssen AD, Osmon DR, Nelson CL. Prevention of deep periprosthetic joint infection. *J Bone Joint Surg Am*. 1996;78:458-471.
10. Lonner JH. Patellofemoral arthroplasty. *Orthopedics*. 2010;33:1-4.
11. Lonner JH. Lateral patellar chamfer in total knee arthroplasty. *Am J Orthop*. 2001;30:713-714.
12. Blazina ME, Fox JM, Del Pizzo W, et al. Patellofemoral replacement. *Clin Orthop Relat Res*. 1979;144: 98-102.
13. Arciero R, Toomey H. Patellofemoral arthroplasty. A three- to nine-year follow-up study. *Clin Orthop Relat Res*. 1988;236:60-71.
14. Cartier P, Sanouiller JL, Grelsamer R. Patellofemoral arthroplasty. *J Arthroplasty*. 1990;5:49-55.
15. Argenson JN, Guillaume JM, Aubaniac JM. Is there a place for patellofemoral arthroplasty? *Clin Orthop Relat Res*. 1995;321:162-167.

16. Krajca-Radcliffe JB, Coker TP. Patellofemoral arthroplasty. A 2- to 18-year follow-up study. *Clin Orthop Relat Res.* 1996;330:143-151.
17. Tauro B, Ackroyd CE, Newman JH, et al. The Lubinus patellofemoral arthroplasty: a five- to ten-year prospective study. *J Bone Joint Surg Br.* 2001;83:696-701.
18. de Winter WE, Feith R, van Loon CJ. The Richards type II patellofemoral arthroplasty: 26 cases followed for 1-20 years. *Acta Orthop Scand.* 2001;72:487-490.
19. Ackroyd CE, Newman JH, Evans R, et al. The Avon patellofemoral arthroplasty. Five-year survivorship and functional results. *J Bone Joint Surg Br.* 2007;89:310-315.
20. Smith AM, Peckett WRC, Butler-Manuel PA, et al. Treatment of patellofemoral arthritis using the Lubinus patellofemoral arthroplasty. A retrospective review. *Knee.* 2002;9:27-30.
21. Kooijman HJ, Driessen APPM, van Horn JR. Long-term results of patellofemoral arthroplasty. *J Bone Joint Surg Br.* 2003;85:836-840.
22. Merchant AC. Early results with a total patellofemoral joint replacement arthroplasty prosthesis. *J Arthroplasty.* 2004;19:829-836.
23. Sisto DJ, Sarin VK. Custom patellofemoral arthroplasty of the knee. *J Bone Joint Surg Am.* 2006;88:1475-1480.
24. Cartier P, Sanouiller JL, Khefacha A. Long-term results with the first patellofemoral prosthesis. *Clin Orthop Relat Res.* 2005;436:47-54.
25. Argenson JNA, Flecher X, Parratte S, et al. Patellofemoral arthroplasty: an update. *Clin Orthop Relat Res.* 2005;440:50-53.
26. Ackroyd CE, Newman JH, Evans R, et al. The Avon patellofemoral arthroplasty. Five-year survivorship and functional results. *J Bone Joint Surg Br.* 2007;89:310-315.
27. Lonner JH. Patellofemoral arthroplasty. *J Am Acad Orthop Surg.* 2007;15:495-506.
28. Lonner JH. Patellofemoral arthroplasty: the impact of design on outcomes. *Orthop Clin N Am.* 2008;39:347-354.
29. Hendrix MRG, Ackroyd CE, Lonner JH. Revision patellofemoral arthroplasty: three- to seven-year follow-up. *J Arthroplasty.* 2008;23:977-983.
30. Lonner JH, Mont MA, Sharkey P, et al. Fate of the unrevised all-polyethylene patellar component in revision total knee arthroplasty. *J Bone Joint Surg Am.* 2003;85:56-59.
31. Lonner JH, Jasko JG, Booth RE. Revision of a failed patellofemoral arthroplasty to a total knee arthroplasty. *J Bone Joint Surg Am.* 2006;88:2337-2342.
32. Australian Orthopaedic Association National Joint Replacement Registry. Available at: http://dmac.adelaide.edu.au/aoanjrr/publications.jsp.
33. Federico DJ, Reider B. Results of isolated patellar debridement for patellofemoral pain in patients with normal patellar alignment. *Am J Sports Med.* 1997;25:663-669.
34. Laskin RS, Van Steijn M. Total knee replacement for patients with patellofemoral arthritis. *Clin Orthop Relat Res.* 1999;367:89-95.
35. Mont MA, Haas S, Mullick T, et al. Total knee arthroplasty for patellofemoral arthritis. *J Bone Joint Surg Am.* 2002;84:1977-1981.

49 Bicompartmental Arthroplasty

Gerard A. Engh

The use of unicompartmental implants to replace more than one compartment of the knee has been an option for over three decades. In fact, the earliest nonlinked implants were separate unicompartmental femoral and tibial components that replaced both tibiofemoral compartments of the knee. The earliest results with both fixed- and mobile-bearing unicompartmental implants used for bicompartmental tibiofemoral arthritis were inconsistent and often led to early revision for a variety of reasons. Instruments were not available for preparing the bone and placing the implants correctly while preserving both cruciate ligaments. Achieving proper tension on the ligaments was a daunting task. At that time, instrumentation had not been developed that integrated the placement and orientation of components to each other. Implant manufacturers and surgeons came to recognize that proper instrumentation was far easier to develop for monoblock components that replaced all three compartments of the knee. Restoring knee alignment and achieving stability was far more predictable with total knee arthroplasty instrumentation. There has not been renewed interest in this approach to tibiofemoral arthritis. The focus of this chapter is limited to bicompartmental arthroplasty for advanced arthritis involving the medial tibiofemoral and the adjacent patellofemoral joint.

WHY BICOMPARTMENTAL ARTHROPLASTY?

Roughly 85% of patients with degenerative arthritis in the knee present with advanced changes in the medial tibiofemoral compartment of the knee and some degree of arthritic change in the patellofemoral joint. Often, the anterior cruciate ligament is intact. Historically, these knees have been treated with a primary total knee replacement arthroplasty and have excellent long-term clinical results. As confidence in knee arthroplasty surgery has grown, younger and more active patients are choosing to undergo joint replacement surgery. The concept of a knee arthroplasty in which both cruciate ligaments are retained and the intact, nondiseased lateral compartment is preserved appeals to surgeons as a more conservative treatment option as well as to patients as an implant option that will accommodate their more active lifestyle. Younger patients with arthritis are particularly interested in an operative procedure that allows them to return to work in a timely fashion and in an implant that will function reliably with more rigorous physical activity.

The preservation of bone and ligaments and the potential for better knee kinematics has created a renewed interest in bicondylar arthroplasty procedures as an option for the patient who has patellofemoral changes and medial compartment arthritis. An implant that bridges the gap between a unicondylar and total knee replacement is appealing to surgeons who believe that changes in the patellofemoral compartment cannot be ignored. A bicompartmental implant offers the same potential benefits as a bicruciate-sparing unicondylar implant in terms of better function and relatively normal knee kinematics. The potential advantages in contrast to total knee arthroplasty also include less operative trauma, a quicker patient recovery, less blood loss with the surgical procedure, a more normal pattern of kinematics (femoral rollback and tibial rotation when both cruciate ligaments are preserved), and the potential for full knee flexion by preserving the lateral compartment of the knee.[1-3] In addition, if revision surgery becomes necessary, it is an easier procedure than revising a failed total knee implant. The outcome of revising a failed unicondylar implant is equivalent to the outcome of primary total knee replacement surgery as reported in the Swedish Knee Registry.[4] Such benefits most likely would be realized when revising a bicompartmental implant.

PATELLOFEMORAL COMPARTMENT

Advocates of mobile-bearing unicondylar replacements question the need for resurfacing the patellofemoral joint, despite the presence of grade 4 articular cartilage changes in either the trochlea, the underside of the patella, or both. Short-term results were excellent with the Oxford mobile-bearing device in knees that had full-thickness cartilage loss in the trochlea or articular surface of the patella (Fig. 49-1).[5] The authors cautioned using the mobile-bearing device only when eburnated bone was present in the lateral patellofemoral joint. However, most surgeons are reluctant to ignore the patellofemoral joint, anticipating that this could be the source of residual pain in the short term and may lead to progression of patellofemoral arthritis over time. Progression of arthritis in the patellofemoral joint following unicondylar arthroplasty has been reported in a study of 99 medial unicondylar replacements with follow-up of 14 years.[6] Twenty-nine patients developed patellofemoral arthritis; 23 of whom reported pain. The incidence of patellofemoral arthritis was 34% in patients with medial unicondylar arthroplasty. An interesting finding from the study was that the arthritis always occurred in the patellofemoral joint opposite the side with the unicondylar implant. Essentially, this rules out impingement between the femoral implant and the patella as the underlying cause for patellofemoral degeneration, an inference of users of mobile-bearing unicondylar implants.

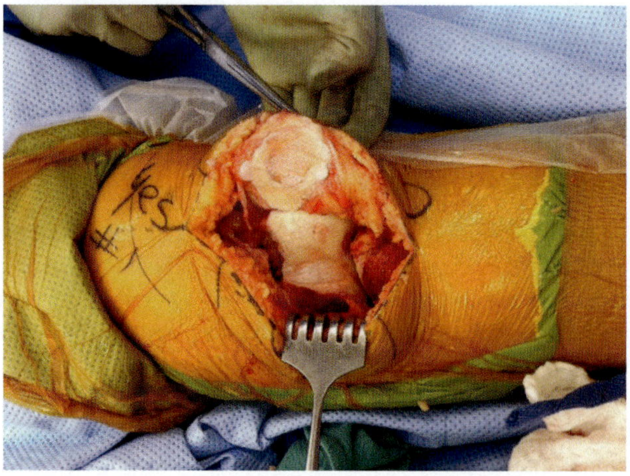

FIGURE 49-1. *An intraoperative photograph of the patellofemoral joint with eburnated bone in the medial facet and trochlea. The lateral facet and trochlea have relatively healthy articular cartilage. Advocates of the Oxford unicompartmental knee arthroplasty would consider such changes acceptable for a mobile-bearing unicondylar implant.*

HISTORICAL USE OF UNICOMPARTMENTAL IMPLANTS FOR BICOMPARTMENTAL ARTHROPLASTY

Implants for patellofemoral arthroplasty were not available until the mid-1980s. The use of custom implants was an option that was rarely used and only to resurface the underside of the patella, not the trochlear groove. Isolated patellofemoral knee arthroplasty that resurfaced both the trochlea and underside of the patella was rarely performed even after the introduction of implants specific for resurfacing both sides of the patellofemoral joint. The clinical results of isolated patellofemoral arthroplasty were marginal with the different implant systems available and were not reported until this past decade.[7,8]

Bicompartmental replacement of the medial tibiofemoral and patellofemoral compartments has only recently been reported and only in a small number of cases. The procedures were performed with first-generation implants combining separate medial unicompartmental implants with a patellofemoral replacement. Instrumentation was not available to facilitate these surgical procedures. Recently, a monoblock femoral implant that replaces one side of the tibiofemoral compartment and the patellofemoral compartment was introduced (Journey Deuce, Smith & Nephew, Memphis, TN). With this implant, there is instrumentation to align and orient the femoral and tibial components to one another. The early clinical results with this implant are largely unreported.

UNICOMPARTMENTAL VERSUS MONOBLOCK IMPLANTS FOR BICOMPARTMENTAL ARTHROPLASTY: PROS AND CONS

There are two options for resurfacing the medial tibiofemoral compartment and the patellofemoral compartment. The first is to use separate implants to replace each compartment. The second is to use a monoblock femoral component that replaces the medial femoral condyle and adjacent trochlear groove. There are advantages and disadvantages with both options.

The first option, using modular parts for separate compartments, allows positioning of the implants relative to the patient's anatomy. The surgeon can place the trochlear groove at its most advantageous location and is able to properly size and position the medial unicondylar implant for flexion and extension stability without compromising the location of the trochlear groove. Historically, bicompartmental arthroplasties were performed in this fashion without instruments designed to orient the implants in relationship to one another.

The second option, a nonmodular, monoblock femoral component, is easier to implant with conventional instrumentation. The lesser number of positioning options may be an advantage with such an implant. A monoblock femoral component eliminates the transition zone that is present between separate trochlear and femoral components. This transition zone may be a source of catching or pain if the patellar component does not articulate smoothly across this interface. The monoblock femoral component, however, must be the correct size that will maintain knee stability with proper flexion-extension bone resections from the medial compartment, yet will be wide enough to cover the distal end of the femur and place the trochlear groove in its anatomically correct position. Figure 49-2 is a postoperative radiograph showing an undersized femoral component. This femoral component is positioned in a valgus orientation and the trochlear groove is translated medially. The patella cannot track normally because of the location of the trochlear groove. A properly sized femoral component is shown in Figure 49-3. The femoral component is wide enough to cover the femoral condyles with the trochlea centered over the intercondylar eminence of the tibia.

Radiographic examples of bicompartmental arthroplasty in which independent components were used for each compartment of the knee are shown in Figures 49-4 and 49-5. A number of disadvantages are apparent with this type of surgery. First, unicondylar arthroplasty in combination with patellofemoral arthroplasty is a technically demanding procedure. Instrumentation is not available to properly orient the trochlear and femoral condylar components in relationship to each other. Second, the positioning and orientation of the unicondylar femoral implant to the trochlear component is critical. The patellar component articulates from the trochlear implant onto the femoral condylar component and simultaneously onto the lateral femoral condyle as the knee flexes. Therefore, the patellar component must cross two

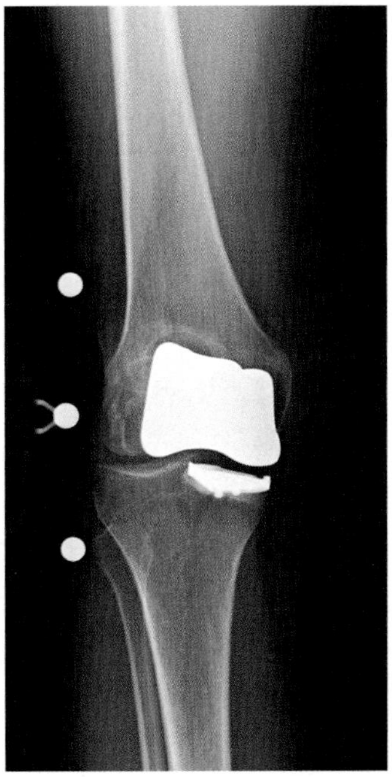

FIGURE 49-2. *An undersized bicompartmental femoral component that does not adequately cover the distal femur. The trochlear groove is displaced medially and could cause patellofemoral tracking problems.*

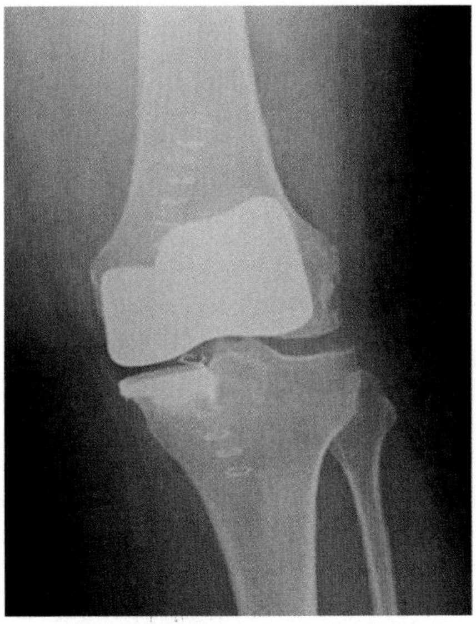

FIGURE 49-3. *A bicompartmental, monoblock femoral component that fully covers the distal femur. The trochlear groove is directly above the intercondylar eminence.*

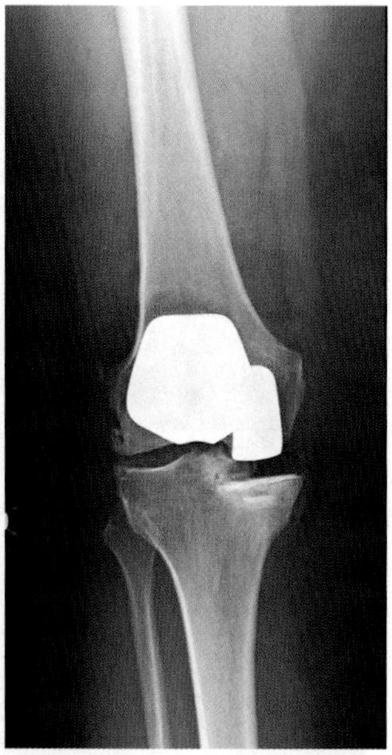

FIGURE 49-4. *Independent implants for each compartment permit the surgeon the freedom to place the components relative to the patient's anatomy. The transition zones created by separate components for the medial femoral condyle and the trochlea create a second transition zone for the patella. Impingement or tracking problems may occur with improperly placed components.*

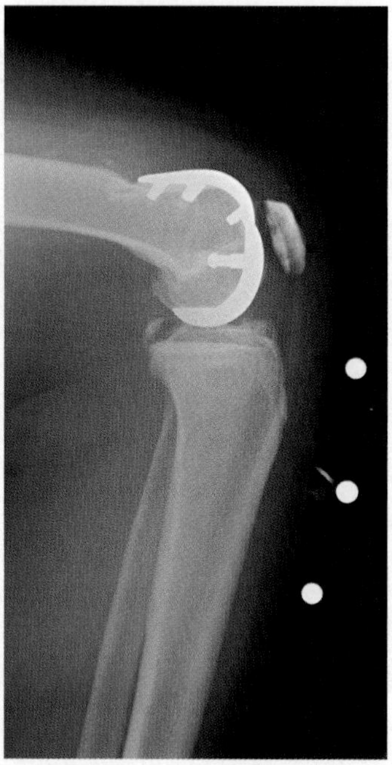

FIGURE 49-5. *Independent implants are also shown on this lateral radiograph.*

zones that are potential sites for impingement or wear of the patellar component. During stair climbing, this transition across zones occurs around 70° to 90° of flexion, when stresses across the patellofemoral joint are several times the patient's body weight. The third disadvantage may prove to be prohibitive from a practical standpoint. This is the cost of using separate unicondylar and patellofemoral components and the additional operative time required to prepare and insert separate and independent components.

RESULTS WITH UNICOMPARTMENTAL IMPLANTS FOR BICOMPARTMENTAL ARTHROPLASTY

In 1990, Cartier et al published the first clinical results of arthroplasty combining unicondylar and patellofemoral procedures.[9] These procedures were performed between 1975 and 1986. A Blazina Patella II or Patella III (Richards) patellofemoral implant with a deep trochlear design was inserted along with a medial unicondylar implant in 30 knees and a lateral unicondylar implant in six knees. The authors did not report the type of unicondylar implant that was used. The follow-up in this study was an average of 4 years (range, 2–12 years) and good or excellent results were reported for 86% of the knees.

The results of combining the implantation of a larger number of independent patellofemoral components with unicondylar implants were reported recently.[10] The authors hoped to determine if such an approach is durable without progression of arthritis in the unresurfaced lateral tibiofemoral compartment. This retrospective review of 71 patients (77 knees) with a combined medial unicondylar and patellofemoral arthroplasties was published at a mean follow-up of 11.7 years (range, 5–23 years). Thirty-five of the 77 knees (45%) had a history of patellar dislocation or trochlear dysplasia before surgery. All patients in this review had an Autocentric polyethylene patellofemoral prosthesis (DePuy, Warsaw, IN) that was cemented in place. The cobalt-chrome femoral component was cemented in only 40% of the cases. In terms of revision for radiographic loosening or disease progression in the lateral compartment, survivorship in this study was 54% at a mean 17 years. Six knees had isolated, but asymptomatic, progression of osteoarthritis in the lateral compartment. Twenty of the 27 cases with aseptic loosening were revised for loosening of the patellar component. Fifteen of these were uncemented patellofemoral implants performed before 1989.

Considerable questions remain as to how results should be interpreted from this study when this patellofemoral prosthesis was used in combination with a unicondylar implant. The Autocentric patellofemoral implant had an almost identically poor outcome when used as an isolated patellofemoral replacement.[11] The authors reported the outcome of 66 isolated patellofemoral arthroplasties performed in patients with an average age of 57 years. The survivorship was only 58% at a mean 16.2 years.

The authors of one other retrospective review reported the results of nine cases in which the Modular III (Richards/Smith & Nephew) patellofemoral implant was combined with either a Modular III (Richards/Smith & Nephew) or Genesis (Smith & Nephew, Memphis, TN) unicondylar implant.[12] The average follow-up for this small number of cases was 11.8 years (range, 4–17 years). No revisions occurred in this series. Three patients were satisfied and six patients were very satisfied with the outcome. The patellofemoral implant used in this case report study had excellent and durable results when used as an isolated patellofemoral arthroplasty. This may explain the far better outcomes with this small cohort of patients as compared to the larger cohort with the Autocentric patellofemoral implant.

RESULTS WITH MONOBLOCK IMPLANTS FOR BICOMPARTMENTAL ARTHROPLASTY

The results of the initial clinical experience with a monoblock trochlear/femoral condylar implant used for bicompartmental arthroplasty have been marginal. The early experience with a monoblock bicompartmental femur and a relatively small number of cases were recently reported in two studies.[13,14] In one study, a single surgeon performed 36 Journey-Deuce (Smith & Nephew, Memphis, TN) bicondylar arthroplasties that were followed for a mean 21 months.[13] The survival rate was 86% and 31% of the patients were unsatisfied with the outcome. The five early revisions were for anterior knee pain in the region of the proximal tibia. Aseptic loosening of the tibial tray was identified at surgery and one of the trays was broken. Another cohort comparison study with assignment determined at the patient's discretion compared 21 bicondylar implants to 33 standard total knee replacements.[14] Patients in the bicondylar arthroplasty group had improvement in Western Ontario and McMaster Universities Osteoarthritis Index (WOMAC) stiffness by 3 months, whereas patients in the total knee replacement group did not have substantial improvement until 1 year after the arthroplasty. The complication rate, however, was higher in the bicondylar group, with three revisions for persistent pain beyond 1 year postoperatively.

The two aforementioned studies[13,14] were the earliest clinical experience reported with a new implant system, unique instrumentation, and surgeons who were learning a new surgical procedure that retained both cruciate ligaments and the lateral compartment of the knee. As may have been expected, the results were not as good as with traditional total knee arthroplasty in which instrumentation, implants, and surgical technique have evolved over almost 40 years. The early benefit of this less invasive surgical procedure, the quicker recovery of knee function evident in both studies, warrants further follow-up with a second generation of bicondylar implants and instruments.

ANDERSON ORTHOPAEDIC CLINICAL EXPERIENCE

One hundred fifty-five Journey Deuce bicompartmental implants were performed at the Anderson Clinic by a single surgeon (the author of this chapter) from August 2006 through December 2010. In terms of Knee Society scores and Oxford scores, the outcome was similar to the scores of patients with Genesis II (Smith & Nephew, Memphis, TN) cruciate-retaining knees done over the same time interval (Figs. 49-6 and 49-7). Patient improvement in both Oxford and Knee Society scores was evident as experience was gained with the instrumentation and implantation for the bicompartmental procedure. This improvement is demonstrated by the slope of a line that best fits the Oxford scores to the time interval when the procedures were performed (Fig. 49-6). Over the same time interval, the Oxford scores remained constant with Genesis II cruciate-retaining knee replacements (Fig. 49-7).

Nine of the 155 patients (5.5%) who underwent bicompartmental arthroplasty at the Anderson Clinic using the Journey Deuce implant were revised to total knee implants at an average of 18 months. The reason for revision was tibial subsidence in four knees, a failed patella in two knees, progression of lateral compartment arthritis (Fig. 49-8) in two knees, and infection in one knee. The revision surgery was performed with primary total knee implants in eight knees and a unicondylar implant was implanted in the unresurfaced lateral compartment of one knee (Fig. 49-9). In the four knees revised for tibial subsidence, the medial tibial bone defect was repaired with autogenous bone from the resected lateral tibial plateau.

An ongoing, prospective clinical study was approved by the Institutional Review Board at the Inova Mount Vernon Hospital to evaluate the clinical outcomes and knee function of 50 knees randomized to either a Journey Deuce bicompartmental knee replacement or a Genesis II cruciate-retain-

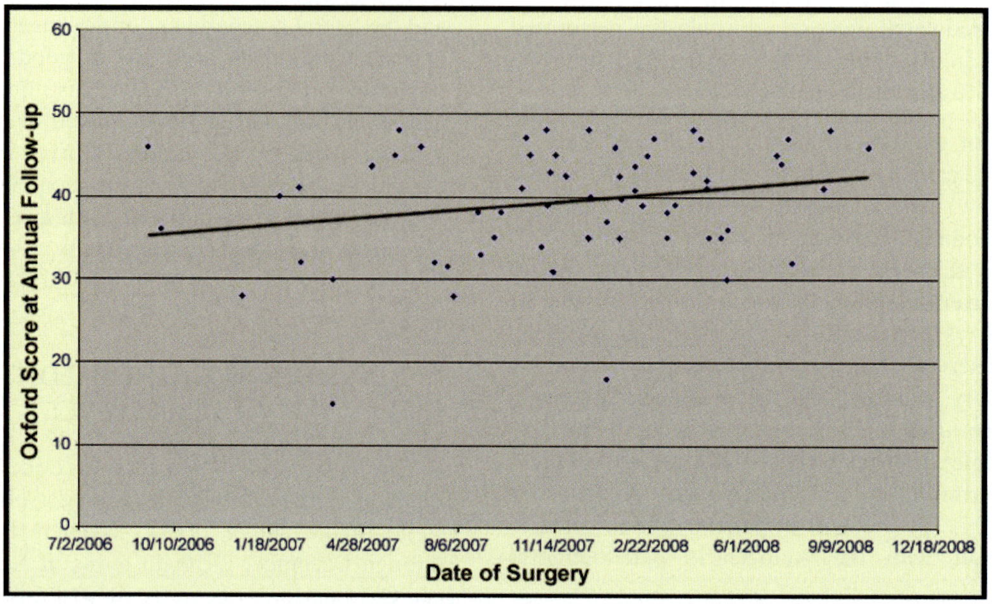

FIGURE 49-6. *Oxford Knee scores at annual follow-up for Journey Deuce (Smith & Nephew, Memphis, TN) knee replacements performed at the Anderson Orthopaedic Clinic.*

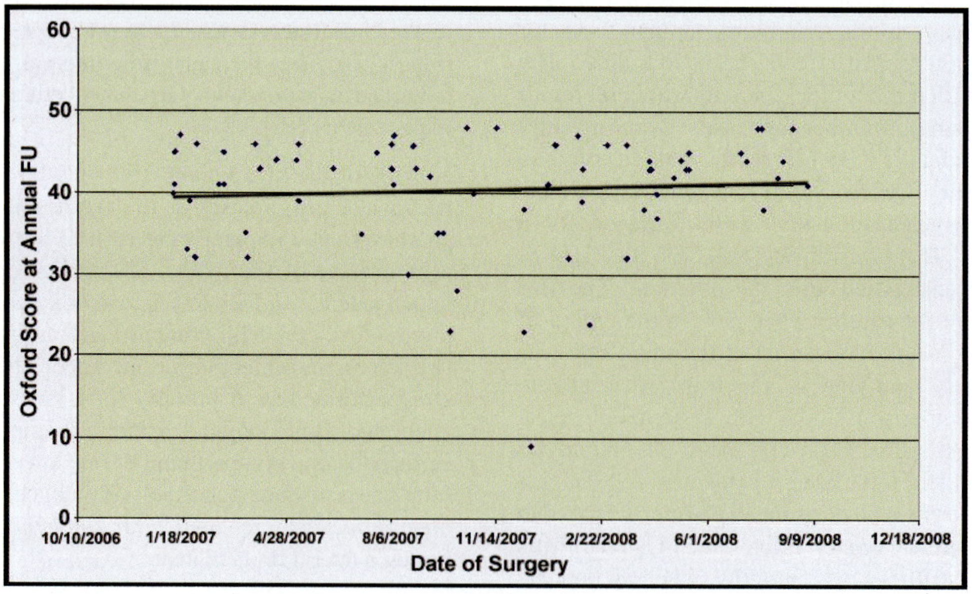

FIGURE 49-7. *Oxford Knee scores at annual follow-up for Genesis II (Smith & Nephew, Memphis, TN) cruciate-retaining total knee replacements performed at the Anderson Orthopaedic Clinic.*

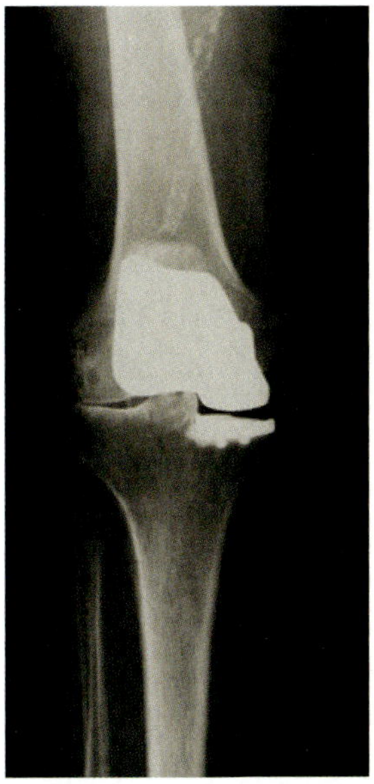

FIGURE 49-8. *A monoblock bicompartmental implant with progressive changes in the lateral tibiofemoral compartment that necessitates further surgery.*

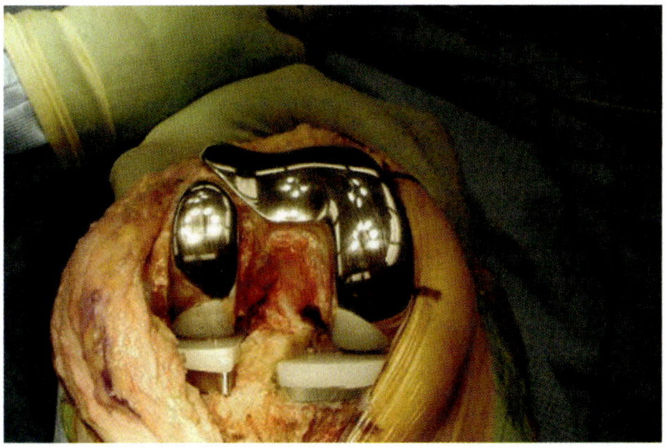

FIGURE 49-9. *The bicompartmental implant was stable and well aligned. The implant was not revised. The lateral compartment arthritis was managed with a unicondylar implant.*

ing total knee replacement. Enrollment of study participants is complete and all subjects have returned for 1-year evaluation. In terms of a more rapid recovery of functional activities, the early results have been better with the less invasive bicompartmental implants. By 1 year after surgery, the patients in both groups had similar Oxford Knee scores and Knee Society scores. Two knees in the total knee arthroplasty group and one knee in the bicompartmental arthroplasty group required manipulation for postoperative stiffness. One patient with a bicompartmental arthroplasty was suspected to have a loose tibial component that was revised at another institution. One patient with a bicompartmental arthroplasty is suspected to have a broken tibial baseplate and is scheduled for revision at our institution.

CONCLUSIONS

Bicompartmental arthroplasty of the medial tibiofemoral and adjacent patellofemoral compartments is a surgical procedure that continues to evolve. Comparison of this surgery will be made with the outcome and survivorship of both unicondylar and total knee arthroplasty. However, direct comparison is fraught with many variables that must be accounted for when making the comparison. First, total knee arthroplasty procedures have the advantage of four decades of implant and instrument upgrades. Bicompartmental arthroplasty is an evolving new technology and results will improve as experience with the procedure grows. As evident from the Anderson Clinic experience, the clinical results will improve as surgeons become more experienced with the surgical technique and as implant manufacturers make upgrades to the implants and instrumentation.

Second, the patient populations are different. The survivorship for all knee arthroplasty procedures is lower in younger, male patients. Unicondylar arthroplasties are more frequently performed in younger and more active male patients[4,15]; bicondylar arthroplasties most likely will be used in a similar patient population. These particular patients are more likely to have an arthroplasty that fails. In the Swedish Registry, the largest age group undergoing unicondylar arthroplasty consists of male patients who are 55 to 64 years old. For total knee arthroplasty, the largest age group consists of patients who are a decade older. Likewise, the gender distribution is different among arthroplasty types. Roughly 50% of patients who undergo unicondylar arthroplasty are male and more than 60% of total knee arthroplasty patients are female.

The threshold for revising a bicondylar arthroplasty with a poor or marginal outcome differs from that with a total knee implant. Surgeons are reluctant to revise a painful total knee arthroplasty without knowing the cause of the pain, but will revise a unicondylar or bicondylar implant more quickly, even without a clearly evident reason for the pain because they have the option to convert to a standard total knee implant. When a failed unicompartmental implant is converted to a primary total knee implant at revision, the outcome is no different than the outcome after primary knee arthroplasty. A failed bicondylar implant converted to a primary total knee implant should also have an outcome similar to primary knee arthroplasty. The result and outcome of surgery for a failed total knee implant is less favorable, because conversion to a revision-style implant has a less predictable outcome.[4]

The early results with bicompartmental arthroplasty are reasonable, although early revisions in the studies available are more frequent than with total knee arthroplasty surgery. Some of the early revisions were primarily for tibial component problems. Similar failures of the tibial compartment have been reported following unicondylar arthroplasty. With a tibial tray that covers only approximately 40% of the tibial plateau, the fixation interface to bone is limited. Overload of the bone may account for some of the early bicompartmental failures, as the tibial component is the same component as used in unicondylar arthroplasty. High stress areas were identified in the medial tibial flare region and are magnified with eccentric loading of the tibial plateau.[16] A unicompartmental tibial tray does not have a stem or keel that extends into the adjacent metaphyseal bone to alleviate the high stresses at the tibial fixation interface.

The ultimate goals for the patient undergoing knee arthroplasty surgery are to alleviate pain and to achieve a high level of functional ability. Retaining both cruciate ligaments and retaining or restoring relatively normal knee kinematics are important means of achieving these goals. The benefit of a knee arthroplasty in which both cruciate ligaments and the lateral tibiofemoral joint are retained was documented by a three-dimensional kinematic analysis of gait in a study that examined eight bicondylar knee arthroplasties with a monoblock femoral component and 10 normal knees. Patients with the bicondylar implants had normal extensor moments and normal gait patterns and knee mechanics.[17]

The techniques for knee arthroplasty will be refined in the next decade. Over the past three decades, little has changed with implants as the focus has shifted to development of technology to optimize knee alignment, soft tissue balance, and customization of the implants to the patient's anatomy. In most studies, progression of arthritis in the unresurfaced compartments is a relatively rare complication with compartmental arthroplasty.[18] As advancements in knee arthroplasty procedures continue, patients will benefit from surgical procedures that are the least disruptive to their normal anatomic structures.

PEARLS AND PITFALLS

When planning a bicompartmental arthroplasty, consider the following:

1. A smooth transition zone between femoral and trochlear implants (in the case of separate components) as well as a smooth transition zone between the trochlear implant and cartilage on the lateral side are essential to pain-free motion. The implant cannot protrude from the articular cartilage or the adjacent component.
2. A monoblock femoral component must be positioned such that the implant does not overhang the tibial component on the medial side and lateral enough to restore the trochlear groove to the correct position.
3. A facetectomy of the lateral facet of the patella may be used to enhance patellar tracking.
4. Independent implants for the trochlea and femoral condyle must be of the correct size, rotation, and translation to assure a smooth transition for the patella as the knee flexes.

REFERENCES

1. Cobb AG, Kozinn SC, Scott RD. Unicondylar or total knee replacement: the patient's preference. *J Bone Joint Surg Br.* 1990;70(1);166.
2. Rougraff BT, Heck DA, Gibson AE. A comparison of tricompartmental and unicompartmental arthroplasty for the treatment of gonarthrosis. *Clin Orthop Relat Res.* 1991;273:157-164.
3. Laurencin CT, Zelicof SB, Scott RD, et al. Unicompartmental versus total knee arthroplasty in the same patient. A comparative study. *Clin Orthop Relat Res.* 1991;273:151-156.
4. The Swedish Arthroplasty Register, Annual Report 2010.
5. Beard DJ, Pandit H, Gill HS, et al. The influence of the presence and severity of pre-existing patellofemoral degenerative changes on the outcome of the Oxford medial unicompartmental knee replacement. *J Bone Joint Surg Br.* 2007;89(12):1597-1601.

6. Hernigou P, Deschamps G. Patellar impingement following unicompartmental arthroplasty. *J Bone Joint Surg Am.* 2002;84(7):1132-1137.
7. Tauro B, Ackroyd CE, Newman JH, et al. The Lubinus patellofemoral arthroplasty. A five- to ten-year prospective study. *J Bone Joint Surg Br.* 2001;83(5):696-701.
8. Kooijman HJ, Driessen AP, van Horn JR. Long-term results of patellofemoral arthroplasty. A report of 56 arthroplasties with 17 years of follow-up. *J Bone Joint Surg Br.* 2003;85(6):836-840.
9. Cartier P, Sanouiller JL, Grelsamer R. Patellofemoral arthroplasty. 2-12-year follow-up study. *J Arthroplasty.* 1990;5(1):49-55.
10. Parratte S, Pauly V, Aubaniac JM, et al. Survival of bicompartmental knee arthroplasty at 5 to 23 years. *Clin Orthop Relat Res.* 2010;468:64-72.
11. Argenson JN, Flecher X, Parratte S, et al. Patellofemoral arthroplasty. An update. *Clin Orthop Relat Res.* 2005;440:50-53.
12. Heyse TJ, Khefacha A, Cartier P. UKA in combination with PFR at average 12-year follow-up. *Arch Orthop Trauma Surg.* 2010;130(10):1227-1230.
13. Palumbo BT, Henderson ER, Edwards PK, et al. Initial experience of the Journey Deuce bicompartmental knee prosthesis – a review of 36 cases. *J Arthroplasty.* 2011;26(6 suppl):40-45.
14. Morrison TA, Nyce JD, Macaulay WB, et al. Early adverse results with bicompartmental knee arthroplasty. A prospective cohort comparison to total knee arthroplasty. *J Arthroplasty.* 2011;26(6 suppl):35-39.
15. Australian National Joint Replacement Registry 2010.
16. Small SR, Berend ME, Ritter MA, et al. Metal backing significantly decreases tibial strains in a medial unicompartmental knee arthroplasty model. *J Arthroplasty.* 2011;26(5):777-782.
17. Wang H, Dugan E, Frame J, et al. Gait analysis after bi-compartmental knee replacement. *Clin Biomech.* 2009;24(9):751-754.
18. Collier MB, Eickmann TH, Anbari KK, et al. Lateral tibiofemoral compartment narrowing after medial unicondylar arthroplasty. *Clin Orthop Relat Res.* 2007;464:43-52.

50 Gap Balancing Versus Measured Resection Techniques for Total Knee Arthroplasty

Yona Kosashvili and Yaron Bar Ziv

There are two distinct classical philosophies for performing total knee replacement: gap balancing and measured resection techniques. The gap balancing technique was developed with the design of cruciate-sacrificing implants, while the measured resection was developed for surgeons who favor cruciate-retaining implants.[1] Modern knee arthroplasties are performed with instrumentation systems that allow surgeons to use features from both techniques. Thus, the distinctions between these philosophies are less evident in everyday practice.

Data indicate that coronal alignment of implants is important for patient satisfaction and implant survivorship after total knee arthroplasty (TKA). The recommended coronal alignment is within 0° to 3° of varus-valgus.[2-6] This principle is based on Insall's opinion that the artificial joint should be parallel to the ground forces. The reason for this neutral alignment is that the stress contact forces will be distributed evenly, avoiding overloading of the medial or lateral compartments. Although the natural native joint line is in 3° of varus, one cannot expect the polyethylene to withstand excessive forces as hyaline cartilage does. Coronal malalignment was found to be associated with an 8-fold increase in early loosening and wear compared to well-aligned components.[3,4] However, a recent study questions the value of coronal alignment. Parratte et al found similar survivorship and patient satisfaction between TKAs with more than 3° of coronal malalignment compared to TKAs within 3° of varus-valgus.[7] Aiming for neutral coronal alignment is also important from a practical point. For most surgeons it is easier to reproducibly perform right-angled bone cuts than an oblique one. A 3° varus cut by itself may be harmless, yet given the human factor, accumulative errors in tibial posterior slope and rotation may result in unfavorable outliers.[1,8]

An additional cause for patient dissatisfaction due to pain and stiffness is rotational malalignment and patellofemoral discomfort (Fig. 50-1). This concept was introduced by Berger et al,[9] who compared computed tomography (CT) scans of 30 patients with isolated patellofemoral complica-

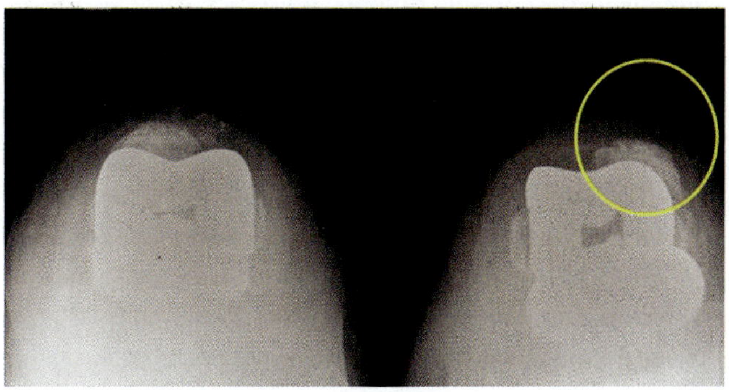

FIGURE 50-1. *Patellar subluxation.*

tions (study group) to CT scans of 20 satisfied patients (control group) post-TKA. The study group was found to have various degrees of combined (femoral and tibial) internal rotation, while the control group was in 0° to 10° of combined external rotation. In that study, the rotation of the femoral component was determined in its relation to the epicondylar axis. The tibial rotation was determined by the angle between two lines. The first line connected the geometrical center of the tibia to the tip of the tibial tubercle, and the second line was perpendicular to the posterior margins of the tibial component. Up to 3° of combined internal rotation resulted in lateral tracking and patellar tilting, 3° to 7° of internal rotation resulted in patellar subluxation, and more than 7° of internal rotation resulted in patellar dislocation.

CLASSIC MEASURED RESECTION TECHNIQUE

Hungerford developed the method of measured resection for cruciate-retaining TKA. The technique is based on a neutral tibial cut, along with femoral cuts based on anatomical landmarks.[10] A key to the measured resection theory is strict adherence to the joint line position, because it is imperative for the function of the retained posterior cruciate ligament (PCL).

The PCL needs to be accurately tensioned in order to function properly. If the PCL is too tight, then excessive tibiofemoral rollback will be induced. Consequently, posterior stress may be increased, risking posterior polyethylene overload. Clinically, PCL tightness may be witnessed by anterior "liftoff" with trial components.[11] The PCL should be routinely released from the Humphrey and Wrisberg ligaments to optimize its function.[11,12] If the PCL is still tight in flexion, additional release can be performed by release from the posterior part of its tibial margin as well as release of its anterior fibers from their femoral origin. In contrast, if the PCL is too loose, then anterior translation of the femoral component may occur, limiting the range of knee flexion due to posterior impingement.[12] This can be addressed by either using a larger femoral component in order to better fill the flexion gap or upsizing the thickness of the polyethylene together with a more extensive release of the posterior capsule.

Distal Femoral Cut

Restoring the native joint line is also important for avoiding patella baja, which may occur after excessive resection of the distal femur in cases of flexion contracture. Figgie et al found that the patella should be within 10 to 30 mm above the joint line in order to avoid patella baja.[13] Because the thickness of the distal femur is 9 mm in most instrumentation systems, the femoral cut should be 9 mm as well, according to the measured resection technique. In cases of flexion contracture, restoring the patient's extension gap is achieved via posterior capsular release rather than additional femoral cuts.

Tibial Cut

Since the minimal polyethylene in most instrumentation systems is 10 mm, the tibial cut should be aimed at a maximum of 10 mm below the less affected side, as this would allow appropriate replacement by the tibial component. However, one should take into account that in severely varus or valgus knees, especially with coronal translation of the femur and flexion contracture, the soft tissues on the less affected side are stretched out. Thus, after ligament balancing, the resulting extension gap may be greater then expected due to the extensive soft tissue release on the affected side. In these cases a more conservative tibial cut of 8 mm, for instance, may be advocated. When there is a substantial tibial defect in such conditions, it is important to refrain from cutting the tibia at its deepest portion of the affected side, as it will result in excessive tibial bone loss.[14,15] Instead, the resulting defect at the affected side that remains after cutting the tibia at 8 to 10 mm below the less affected side can be filled with bone graft[14] or by cement with screw augmentation.[15]

Rotational Alignment of the Femur

Femoral rotation is essential for patellar tracking and restoration of the flexion gap.[16-18] Several anatomical landmarks have been identified as a possible reference:

1. Posterior femoral condyles,
2. Medial and lateral epicondyles,
3. Anterior posterior femoral axis (Whiteside's line), and
4. Proximal tibial cut.

Each landmark has potential limitations. The posterior condylar axis is in relative internal rotation to the femoral rotation due to the larger posteromedial femoral condyle. This tendency to internal rotation is even worse in valgus knees that tend to have hypoplastic lateral femoral condyle.[19] Since various degrees of cartilage wear are present in many arthritic knees, the femoral cut should be in various degrees of external rotation to this landmark.[20] Mantas et al demonstrated that the posterior condylar axis can be in 1° to 9° of internal rotation to the transepicondylar axis, with only 80% within a 3° rotational error margin.[21] Olcott and Scott compared four intraoperative methods to determine femoral component rotation during total knee arthroplasty and found that the transepicondylar axis most consistently recreated a balanced flexion space, whereas 3° of external rotation off the posterior condyles was least consistent, especially in valgus knees.[22] In 100 knees that had TKA, the anteroposterior (Whiteside's) line was found less reliable than the transepicondylar axis, especially in valgus knees and knees with trochlear dysplasia.[23]

However, a navigation study demonstrated that the epicondylar axis, in the worst-case scenario, may lead to a possible external as well as internal rotation of the femoral component of up to 8°.[24] Moreover, there is an average error of 3° of internal rotation when comparing the intraoperative epicondylar axis to the CT-guided epicondylar axis.[25]

Since each landmark for femoral rotational alignment has a potential for error, we suggest cross-checking at least two landmarks [eg, the posterior condylar axis and Whiteside's line (Fig. 50-2) or the transepicondylar axis and the posterior condylar axis (Fig. 50-3)] before completing the femoral cuts. If the marked rotational femoral alignment is confirmed by two landmarks, then it is more reasonable to assume that the correct femoral alignment can be reached with these cuts.

It is possible that with the advancement of technology combining CT or magnetic resonance imaging into preoperative planning, patient-specific instruments may provide more accurate measured resection.[25,26] Despite the potential merits entailed in these implants, more follow-up is required to determine the cost–benefit ratio of these technologies.[27]

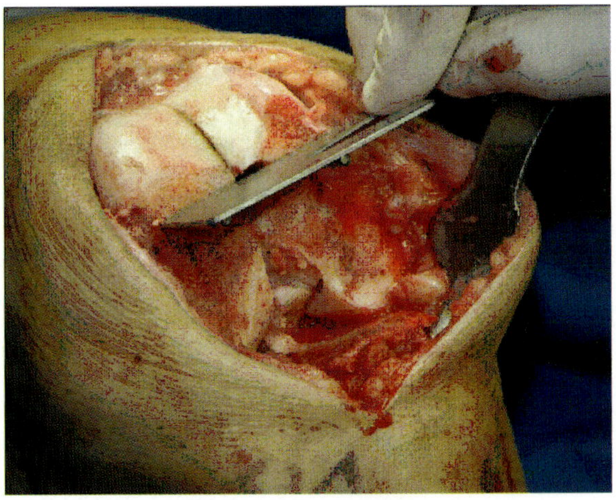

FIGURE 50-2. *Cross-checking anatomical landmarks: a 90° angle between the Whiteside's line and pins placed in 3° of external rotation to the posterior condylar axis.*

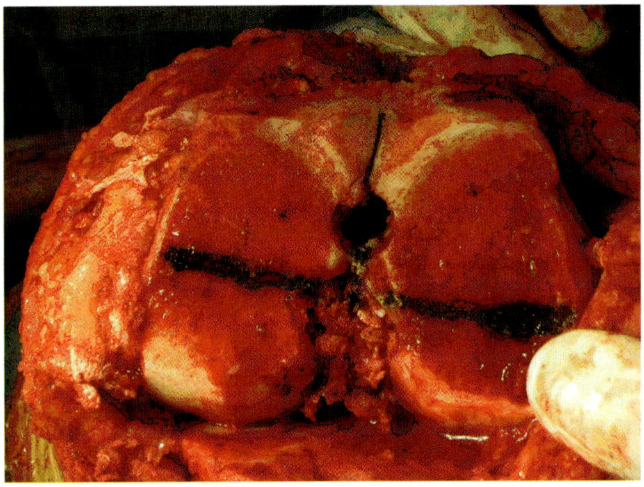

FIGURE 50-3. *Cross-checking anatomical landmarks: a 90° angle between the Whiteside's line and the transepicondylar axis.*

GAP BALANCING

Gap balancing is a technique that focuses on the rectangularity of the flexion gap to determine the femoral component rotation as opposed to bony landmarks in the measured resection technique. This technique favors the use of a cruciate-substituting prosthesis and allows a larger tolerance of the joint line position.[1]

The classic technique of gap balancing was developed by John Insall.[1] The technique used flexion gap balancing first together with ligament releases. According to this technique, the tibial cut is made first. To determine the posterior femoral cut appropriately, the medial or lateral ligamentous structures are released depending on the preoperative deformity to reach an even mediolateral balance.

Ligament balancing is usually performed first in extension. There are several options to achieve ligament balancing in extension with only the proximal tibia cut. The first is to use an intramedullary rod with a plate that allows for a rectangular block to be seated upon. The angle between the plate and rod should match the planned distal femoral cut, usually between 5° and 7° (Fig. 50-4). The plate provides a virtual distal cut, without cutting the distal femur. Spacer blocks are assembled onto the plate and ligament tension, as well as their balance, is examined (Fig. 50-5).

Additional releases are performed as necessary, until reaching an adequate balance in extension. A second option is to use computer navigation to achieve ligament balancing in extension without performing a distal cut.[28] The most popular way to achieve ligament balancing in extension is to establish the extension gap first, which is done by performing the distal femoral cut using an intramedullary rod. This technique is actually a modification of the original gap balancing technique as it is based on extension gap first as opposed to flexion gap first.

Once the ligaments are balanced, the knee is flexed to 90°, and the posterior femoral cut, which establishes the flexion gap, is determined based on the tibial cut and the balanced ligament tension. The femur is distracted anteriorly using a tensioning device or spacer blocks. Tensioning the medial and lateral ligaments in 90° of flexion rotates the distal femur. The axis of rotation of the femur varies according to the tensioning devices used, which could be placed posteriorly at the posterior femoral condyles (Fig. 50-6) or more anteriorly, rotating the femur along the axis of the intramedullary canal via the intramedullary rod (Fig. 50-7).

Since the lateral structures are usually somewhat weaker compared to the medial structures, the distal femur is inter-

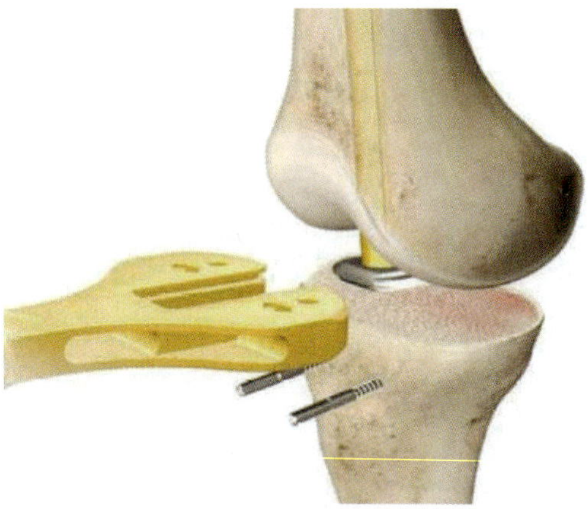

FIGURE 50-4. *A baseplate connected to an intramedullary rod in 5° to 7° of valgus. (© DePuy Orthopaedics, Inc. 2010.)*

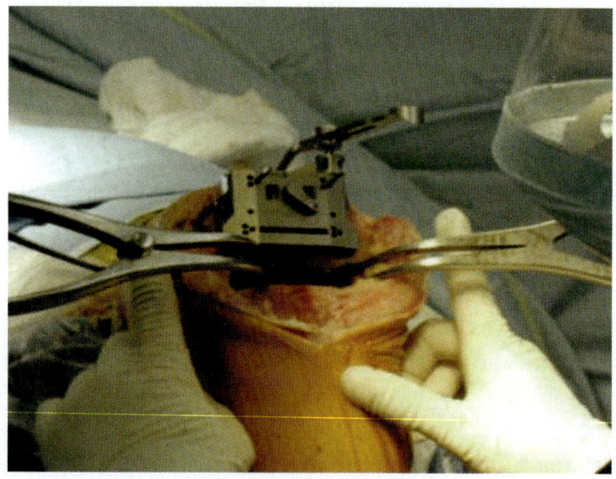

FIGURE 50-6. *Flexion gap tensioning via laminar spreaders placed posteriorly.*

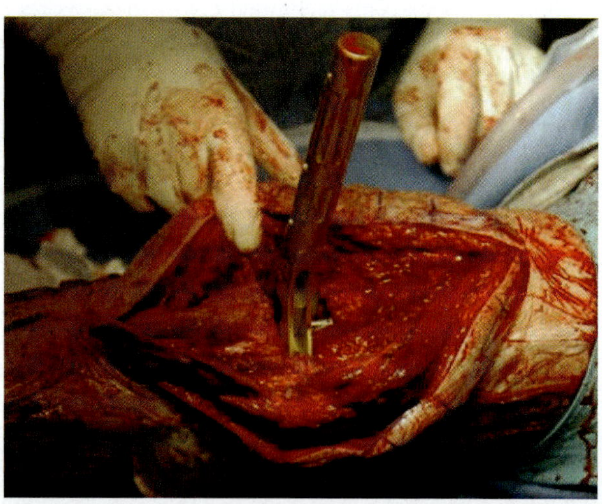

FIGURE 50-5. *Extension gap balance check with spacer blocks assembled onto the baseplate.*

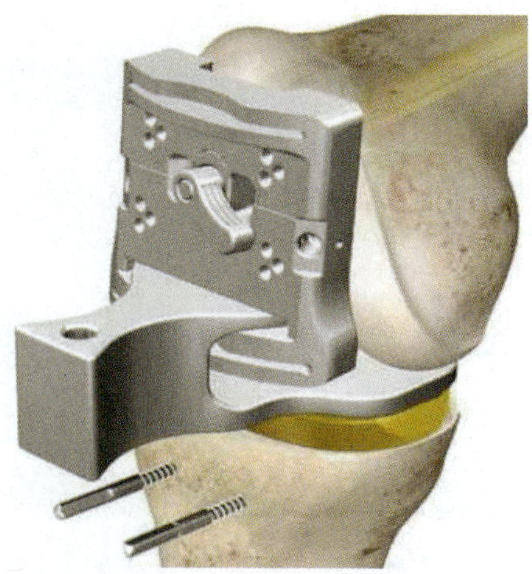

FIGURE 50-7. *Flexion gap tensioning via intramedullary rod. (© DePuy Orthopaedics, Inc. 2010.)*

nally rotated by tensioning the ligaments. Thus, the resulting cut that is made parallel to the proximal tibial surface with the femoral anteroposterior cutting block is actually in external rotation relative to the axis of the posterior femoral condyles.[29]

The advantages of the gap balancing technique over the measured resection technique stem from the variability of the anatomical landmarks as discussed previously in the measured resection section. The gap balancing philosophy is based on achieving balanced rectangular gaps. This principle is important both for both PCL-substituting and PCL-retaining TKAs, because it may reduce the lateral liftoff in flexion and subsequently improve patient satisfaction.[30]

However, the gap balancing technique has several limitations. One of its original advantages was the limited availability of implant sizes, which would usually result in a small femoral size that would cause a large flexion gap that created flexion–extension mismatch. This problem was substantially reduced by the new designs of TKA systems, which provide a much larger variety of implants.[1] The gap balancing relies on the tibial cut, according to which the knee is balanced. However, the tibial cut may not be correct in all three planes (coronal, sagittal, and axial) and an additive error may ensue.[1,27] This possible downside can be addressed by navigation.[27] Since the tibial cut is the cornerstone of the gap balancing technique, verification of the tibial cut alignment cannot be underemphasized. As gap balancing relies on a subjective assessment of soft tissue tension, it is more of an acquired art, which may entail a longer and steeper learning curve. An additional possible limitation of this method is that mediolateral ligament balancing requires soft tissue releases that are done with the knee in extension. However, they potentially influence the flexion gap to a larger extent then expected.[31,32] In order to avoid this pitfall, the soft tissue release from the affected side should be as conservative as possible to achieve gap balancing in extension. Structures such as the superficial medial collateral ligament (MCL) that influence both the flexion and extension gaps should not be overreleased. Thus, most of the release is around the periphery of the proximal tibia and distal femur.

Several techniques are available to achieve mediolateral balance in extension without affecting the flexion gap and femoral component rotation. To facilitate the reading, we refer to varus osteoarthritic knees, although these techniques can be applied for valgus knees as well. The techniques are as follows:

- Tibial plateau reduction,[33,34]
- Removal of the posterior tibial osteophytes,[34,35]
- Removal of the posterior femoral osteophytes before cutting the posterior femoral condyles, and
- Release of the posterior capsule.[1,36,37]

Tibial Plateau Reduction

This technique is practically an extension of the osteophyte removal step (Fig. 50-8). First, the femoral size is measured and then the surface of the proximal tibia is sized to the smallest possible matching size for the respective femur. For example, if the femoral component size is 4 and the minimal matching tibial size is 3, then the tibial surface is reduced to size 3. The reduction has several positive effects[33-35]:

- Decompression of the medial capsular ligamentous sleeve (like osteophytectomy),
- Lateralization of the component,
- Medialization of the tibial tubercle and reducing the Q angle, and
- Tightening the lateral capsular ligamentous sleeve.

Removal of Posterior Tibial Osteophytes

After reduction of the medial border of the tibial proximal surface, one can also release the posterior tibial margins. This will release the medial tension in extension. This

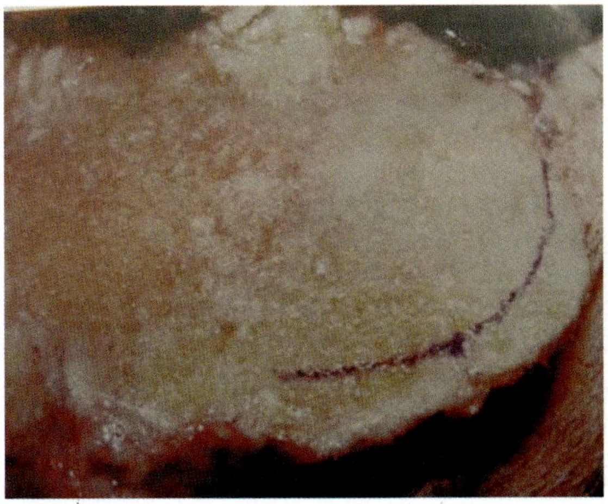

FIGURE 50-8. *Medial tibial plateau reduction osteotomy. The tibial reduction is to the marked line, which represents the medial aspect of the tibial implant.*

step should be performed with good visualization, away from the insertion of the PCL toward the more medial aspect of the tibia. In addition, further release can be achieved via release of the semimembranous and its attachment on the posteromedial corner.

Removal of Posterior Medial Osteophytes Before Resection of Posterior Femoral Condyles

The posterior medial femoral osteophytes tent the posterior capsule and may create a mediolateral imbalance, especially in the presence of flexion contracture. Approaching the posterior femur before cutting the posterior femoral cuts is technically demanding. One way is to use a preliminary cut of the more posterior part of the posteromedial femoral condyle. This cut spares the posterior femoral footing required for the femoral size measurement and creates a window through which access to the posterior aspect of the knee is feasible, making it easier to remove the osteophytes with the knee in flexion (Figs. 50-9 and 50-10).

Release of Posterior Capsule

Contracted adherent capsule to the posterior aspect of the knee may create a mediolateral imbalance in extension. The same posteromedial "window" that was used for removal of posterior osetophytes can also be used to release the adherent capsule with a curved osteotome. This step should be performed with the knee in maximal flexion, and the resected proximal tibia should not be pressed by the osteotome because it may easily be indented. The osteotome should be placed on the surface of the posterior femur and pointed away from the center of the posterior femur to avoid possible vascular injury.

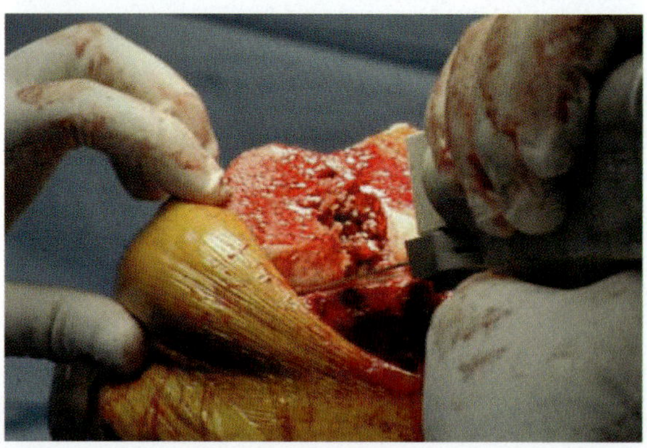

FIGURE 50-9. *Preliminary cut of the more posterior aspect of the posteromedial femoral condyle, opening a posteromedial "window."*

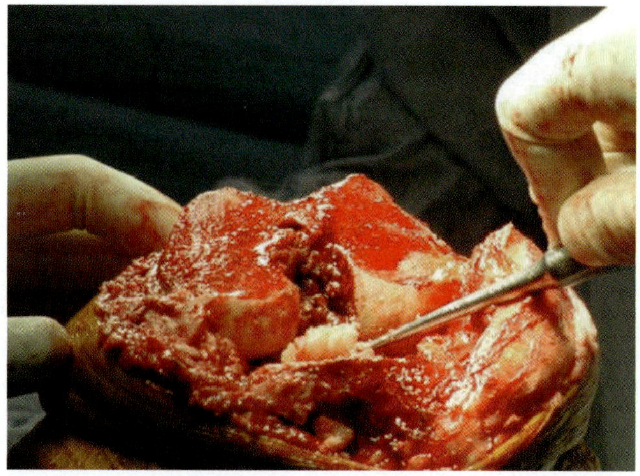

FIGURE 50-10. *Removal of a posteromedial osteophyte from the femur through the "window."*

Mediolateral Ligament Balancing in Extreme Varus Knees

For extreme varus knees, when all of the above are not sufficient, several additional steps are possible:

- Horizontal cut of the posteromedial capsule,[1]
- Pie-crust release of the posterior superficial MCL,[38]
- Release and reattachment of the pes anserinus,[34]
- Vertical release of the superficial MCL from the tibial insertion,[1,32] and
- Medial epicondyle osteotomy and distal advancement.[39,40]

Since each philosophy has its advantages and limitations, many surgeons use principles from both philosophies when performing a TKA. This chapter presents the authors' preferred sequence of steps. For the sake of clarity, the technique for varus osteoarthritic knees is presented (Table 50-1).

CONCLUSION

TKA is a successful surgery that provides the patients long-lasting pain relief and improved function as well as quality of life. Since the collateral ligaments as well as the posterior cruciate ligament (when retained) need to be balanced within a narrow error of margin, the tibial and femoral components need to be well aligned in the coronal, sagittal, and rotational planes. The surgeon can use either the gap balancing or the measured resection techniques in order to achieve this goal. However, modern TKA systems allow using interchangeable motifs during the knee arthroplasty. Combining the techniques may enable the surgeon to cross-check his or her intraoperative decisions and reduce the chances of an accumulative error that may lead to unfavorable outcomes.

TABLE 50-1. Authors' Preferred Approach for Gap Balancing Technique

Technical Step	Surgical Rationale
Medial parapatellar approach.	Facilitated exposure.
Release of medial tibial osteophytes including the posteromedial corner.	Release of the contracted side.
Distal femoral cut using an intramedullary guide.	Preoperative planning with long-standing radiographs for the entry point.
Resection of the proximal tibia using an extramedullary guide.	Avoids errors related to tibial bowing or inappropriate entry point that may occur when using intramedullary guides.
Check the tibial cut on its own, relative to the tibial plafond.	An accurate tibial cut is the cornerstone of the technique.
Establish a balanced extension gap. Use all necessary steps mentioned above for that purpose.	See text for the special steps for achieving a balanced extension gap without affecting the flexion gap.
Check the balance of the extension gap in full extension and 10° of flexion.	Avoid mediolateral imbalance masked by the function of the posterior capsule in full extension.
Mark either the anteroposterior (Whiteside's) axis or epicondylar axis.	Provides an anatomical landmark to cross-check the femoral rotation.
Bring the knee to 90° of flexion and equally stretch laminar spreaders placed onto the medial and lateral posterior femoral condyles.	Establishes the proximal tibia as a reference for the flexion gap and femoral rotation.
Check the balance of the flexion gap in 90° of flexion with the respective measurement block.	Verifying the rectangularity of the flexion gap.
If the flexion gap is balanced, then mark the femoral rotation.	Allows cross-checking the rotational alignment with the previously marked anatomical landmark.
Anteriorize or posteriorize the femoral cuts to match the flexion and extension gaps.	Matching the flexion and extension gaps. Take care to avoid notching of the anterior femoral cortex.
Complete the TKA.	

SURGICAL PEARLS AND PITFALLS

The following are some surgical pearls:

- When using PCL-retaining designs, maintain the original joint line.
- Use long-standing radiographs to determine the entry point to the femoral canal.
- In severe varus cases with deficient tibia, refrain from cutting the medial tibia at its deepest portion. The ensuing defect can reliably be filled with cement with or without screws.
- Use at least two anatomical landmarks for cross-checking the femoral rotation.
- Note that the posterior condylar axis and the anteroposterior axis (Whiteside's) are least reliable in valgus knees.
- When balancing the extension gap, try to limit the tibial release to the proximal margins, in order to avoid releasing soft tissue that also affects the flexion gap.
- Posterior capsule and posterior femoral osteophytectomy via a preliminary cut allow extension gap balancing without affecting the flexion gap.
- While removing the posteromedial osteophyte, place the knee in varus to relax the MCL. Remove the osteophyte using a curette moving from medially to laterally.

The following are some surgical pitfalls:

- Excessive distal femoral cut in knees with flexion contracture for PCL-retaining TKA,
- Determining the femoral entry point in osteoporotic patients,
- Cutting the medial tibia at its deepest portion in severe varus cases with deficient tibia,
- Determining the femoral rotation only on the posterior condylar axis,
- Relying on the posterior condylar axis or anteroposterior axis (Whiteside's) in severe valgus with hypoplastic lateral condyle and trochlear hypoplasia,
- Balancing the extension gap by releasing the hamstrings or superficial MCL from its tibial insertion, and
- Injuring the MCL while removing the posteromedial osteophyte.

REFERENCES

1. Scott WN, ed. *Surgery of the Knee*. 4th ed. Philadelphia, PA: Churchill-Livingstone; 2005.
2. Fang DM, Ritter MA, Davis KE. Coronal alignment in total knee arthroplasty: just how important is it?. *J Arthroplasty.* 2009;24:39-43.
3. Naudie DD, Rorabeck CH. Sources of osteolysis around total knee arthroplasty: wear of the bearing surface. *Instr Course Lect.* 2004;53:251-259.
4. Jeffery RS, Morris RW, Denham RA. Coronal alignment after total knee replacement. *J Bone Joint Surg Br.* 1991;73:709-714.
5. Meding JB, Berend ME, Ritter MA, et al. Intramedullary vs extramedullary femoral alignment guides: a 15-year follow-up of survivorship. *J Arthroplasty.* 2011;26:591-595.
6. Magnussen RA, Weppe F, Demey G, et al. Residual varus alignment does not compromise results of TKAs in patients with preoperative varus. *Clin Orthop Relat Res.* July 26, 2011 [Epub ahead of print].
7. Parratte S, Pagnano MW, Trousdale RT, et al. Effect of postoperative mechanical axis alignment on the fifteen-year survival of modern, cemented total knee replacements. *J Bone Joint Surg Am.* 2010;92:2143-2149.
8. Koyonos L, Stulberg SD, Moen TC, et al. Sources of error in total knee arthroplasty. *Orthopedics.* 2009;32:317.
9. Berger RA, Crossett LS, Jacobs JJ, et al. Malrotation causing patellofemoral complications after total knee arthroplasty. *Clin Orthop Relat Res.* 1998;356:144-153.
10. Hungerford DS, Krackow KA. Total joint arthroplasty of the knee. *Clin Orthop Relat. Res.* 1985; 192:23-33.
11. Lombardi AV Jr, Berend KR. Posterior cruciate ligament-retaining, posterior stabilized, and varus/valgus posterior stabilized constrained articulations in total knee arthroplasty. *Instr Course Lect.* 2006;55:419-427.
12. Scott RD, Chmell MJ. Balancing the posterior cruciate ligament during cruciate-retaining fixed and mobile-bearing total knee arthroplasty: description of the pull-out lift-off and slide-back tests. *J Arthroplasty.* 2008;23:605-608.
13. Figgie HE III, Goldberg VM, Heiple KG, et al. The influence of tibial-patellofemoral location on function of the knee in patients with the posterior stabi-

lized condylar knee prosthesis. *J Bone Joint Surg Am.* 1986;68:1035-1040.

14. Watanabe W, Sato K, Itoi E. Autologous bone grafting without screw fixation for tibial defects in total knee arthroplasty. *J Orthop Sci.* 2001;6(6):481-486.
15. Ritter MA, Harty LD. Medial screws and cement: a possible mechanical augmentation in total knee arthroplasty. *J Arthroplasty.* 2004;195:587-589.
16. Anouchi YS, Whiteside LA, Kaiser AD, et al. The effects of axial rotational alignment of the femoral component on knee stability and patellar tracking in total knee arthroplasty demonstrated on autopsy specimens. *Clin Orthop Relat Res.* 1993;287:170-177.
17. Berger RA, Rubash HE. Rotational instability and malrotation after total knee arthroplasty. *Orthop Clin North Am.* 2001;32:639-647.
18. Rhoads DD, Noble PC, Reuben JD, et al. The effect of femoral component position on the kinematics of total knee arthroplasty. *Clin Orthop Relat Res.* 1993;286: 122-129.
19. Whiteside LA, Arima J. The anteroposterior axis for femoral rotational alignment in valgus total knee arthroplasty. *Clin Orthop Relat Res.* 1995;321:168-172.
20. Asada S, Akagi M, Matsushita T, et al. Effects of cartilage remnants of the posterior femoral condyles on femoral component rotation in varus knee osteoarthritis. *Knee.* March 11, 2011 [Epub ahead of print].
21. Mantas JP, Bloebaum RD, Skedros JG, et al. Implications of reference axes used for rotational alignment of the femoral component in primary and revision knee arthroplasty. *J Arthroplasty.* 1992;7:531-535.
22. Olcott CW, Scott RD. A comparison of 4 intraoperative methods to determine femoral component rotation during total knee arthroplasty. *J Arthroplasty.* 2000;15;22-26.
23. Poilvache PL, Insall JN, Scuderi GR, et al. Rotational landmarks and sizing of the distal femur in total knee arthroplasty. *Clin Orthop Relat Res.* 1996;331:35-46.
24. Stoeckl B, Nogler M, Krismer M, et al. Reliability of the transepicondylar axis as an anatomical landmark in total knee arthroplasty. *J Arthroplasty.* 2006;21:878-882.
25. Van der Linden-van der Zwaag HM, Valstar ER, van der Molen AJ, et al. Transepicondylar axis accuracy in computer assisted knee surgery: a comparison of the CT-based measured axis versus the CAS-determined axis. *Comput Aided Surg.* 2008; 13:200-206.
26. Ng VY, Declaire JH, Berend KR, et al. Improved accuracy of alignment with patient-specific positioning guides compared with manual instrumentation in TKA. *Clin Orthop Relat Res.* August 2, 2011 [Epub ahead of print].
27. Lehnen K, Giesinger K, Warschkow R, et al. Clinical outcome using a ligament referencing technique in CAS versus conventional technique. *Knee Surg Sports Traumatol Arthrosc.* 2011;19:887-892.
28. Pang HN, Yeo SJ, Chong HC, et al. Computer-assisted gap balancing technique improves outcome in total knee arthroplasty, compared with conventional measured resection technique. *Knee Surg Sports Traumatol Arthrosc.* 2011;19:1496-1503.
29. Stiehl JB, Cherveny PM. Femoral rotational alignment using the tibial shaft axis in total knee arthroplasty. *Clin Orthop Relat Res.* 1996;331:47-55.
30. Dennis DA, Komistek RD, Kim RH, et al. Gap balancing versus measured resection technique for total knee arthroplasty. *Clin Orthop Relat Res.* 2010;468: 102-107.
31. Krakow KA, Michalko WM. The effect of medial release on flexion and extension gaps in cadaveric knees: implications for soft tissue balancing in TKA. *Am J Knee Surg.* 1999;12:222-228.
32. Michalco WM, Saleh KJ, Krakow KA, et al. Soft tissue balancing during TKA in a varus knee. *J Am Acad Orthop Surg.* 2009;17:767-774.
33. Dixon MC, Parsch D, Brown RR, et al. The correction of severe varus deformity in total knee arthroplasty by tibial component downsizing and resection of uncapped proximal medial bone. *J Arthroplasty.* 2004;19:19-22.
34. Mullaji AB, Padmanabhan V, Jindal G. Total knee arthroplasty for profound varus deformity: technique and radiological results in 173 knees with varus of more than 20 degrees. *J Arthroplasty.* 2005;20;550-561.
35. Mullaji A, Sharma A, Marawar S, et al. Quantification of effect of sequential posteromedial release on flexion and extension gaps: a computer-assisted study in cadaveric knees. *J Arthroplasty.* 2009;24:795-805.
36. Massin P, Petit A, Odri G, et al. Total knee arthroplasty in patients with greater than 20 degrees flexion contracture. *Orthop Traumatol Surg Res.* 2009;95:7-12.
37. Hanratty B, Bennett D, Thompson NW, et al. A randomised controlled trial investigating the effect of posterior capsular stripping on knee flexion and range of motion in patients undergoing primary knee

arthroplasty. *Knee.* October 29, 2010 [Epub ahead of print].

38. Verdonk PC, Pernin J, Pinaroli A, et al. Soft tissue balancing in varus total knee arthroplasty: an algorithmic approach. *Knee Surg Sports Traumatol Arthrosc.* 2009;17:660-666.

39. Engh GA, Ammeen D. Results of total knee arthroplasty with medial epicondylar osteotomy to correct varus deformity. *Clin Orthop Relat Res.* 1999;367: 141-148.

40. Engh GA. Medial epicondylar osteotomy: a technique used with primary and revision total knee arthroplasty to improve surgical exposure and correct varus deformity. *Instr Course Lect.* 1999;48: 153-156.

51 Principles of Ligament Balancing and Alignment in Total Knee Arthroplasty

Leo A. Whiteside

Alignment and ligament balance in total knee arthroplasty (TKA) continues to be one of the most intellectually challenging aspects of orthopaedic surgery. At the outset, it should be understood that ligament balancing in TKA is effective only when the knee is well aligned. Furthermore, alignment and ligament balancing must be done in both flexion and extension so that flexibility and stability of the knee are maintained throughout the entire functional range of motion of the joint. The three-dimensional mental imaging and dynamic conceptualization necessary to achieve this task are far beyond the realms of mental activity that most surgeons use in normal daily activities.

Although the knee has been studied intensively for decades, it continues to confound investigators and to frustrate surgeons. The intricate ligaments and complex joint surfaces interact in ways that defy description. Nevertheless, the surgeon must repair and reconstruct the damaged and arthritic knee so that its performance is near normal. This requires decisions and adjustments made with reasonable accuracy under the pressure and time constraints of the operating room. Therefore, the subject must be simplified adequately for the surgeon to perform excellent alignment, precise bone cuts, and correct ligament balance every time. This task requires simple instrumentation that is easy to handle and understand and also requires basic rules of resection and alignment that position the joint surfaces so that the ligaments can be balanced through the normal flexion arc. The function of the ligaments must be defined clearly in flexion and extension, and simple techniques must be established to release and balance the ligaments. It is important to emphasize that joint surface position must be established throughout the entire flexion and extension arc so that the ligaments will function with appropriate stability and flexibility characteristics in a fully functional arc of motion.

The lower extremity often is depicted in two dimensions with the hip, knee, and ankle lying in a straight line, the epicondylar axis perpendicular to this line, and the joint line sloped downward medially. When depicted in three dimensions, the lower extremity functions in a plane throughout the flexion-extension arc and the femoral head, the mechanical axis of the femur, the patellar groove, the intercondylar notch, the patellar tendon, the patellar articular crest, and the entire tibia including the ankle remain within this plane as the knee flexes and extends (Fig. 51-1). The axis through which the tibia rotates as the knee flexes and extends is perpendicular to this median anteroposterior (AP) plane and is approximated by the transepicondylar line or epicondylar axis.[1,2] As the knee flexes and extends, the patella is drawn through the patellar groove, which also lies in the AP plane. In the normal knee, the epicondylar axis of the femur remains perpendicular to the AP plane of the lower extremity throughout the flexion and extension arc. This places the tibia nearly perpendicular to the ground and also places the hip in its most favorable position for function (Figs. 51-2 and 51-3).[1,3,4]

The AP axis is the most reliable landmark for resection of the bone surfaces in the flexed position.[3,5] This AP axis is easily constructed by marking the center of the intercondylar notch far posteriorly and the deepest part of the patellar groove just anterior to the intercondylar notch.

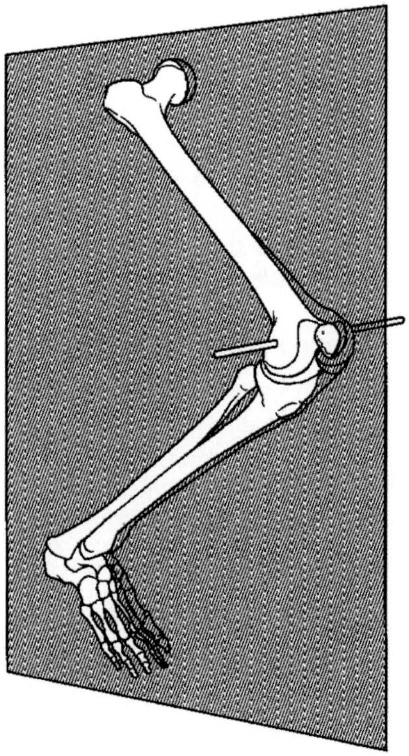

FIGURE 51-1. *The mechanical axis of the lower extremity becomes a plane when flexion and extension in three dimensions are considered. The centers of the hip, knee, and ankle remain within this plane through the flexion-extension arc. The patellar groove (AP axis of the femur) is co-planar with this plane so that the patella is drawn smoothly through the groove as a rope is pulled smoothly through a well-aligned pulley. The epicondylar axis is perpendicular to the AP plane, and the tibia swings through the axis, staying in the AP plane throughout the flexion-extension arc. (Reprinted with permission.[14])*

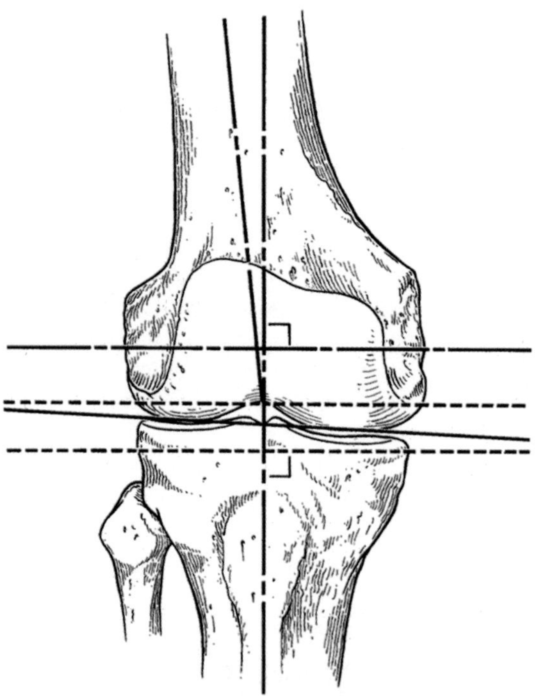

FIGURE 51-2. *In the extended position, the joint surfaces slope medially approximately 3°. Tibial resection is perpendicular to the long axis of the tibia and mechanical axis of the lower extremity. The resection surface is 3° valgus to the articular surface. Femoral resection is perpendicular to the mechanical axis, and 5° valgus to the long axis of the femur. The resection surface is approximately 3° varus to the articular surface. These 3° "errors" in the femoral and tibial surface resections compensate for one another and result in surface resections that are parallel to one another and perpendicular to the mechanical axis. The long axis of the femur serves as the anatomical reference for alignment of the distal femoral cuts, which will be made perpendicular to the mechanical axis and AP plane with the knee in full extension. Cutting the distal femoral surfaces at a 5° valgus angle to the long axis of the femur places the joint surface perpendicular to the AP plane in the extended position. Likewise cutting the upper surface of the tibia perpendicular to the long axis of the tibia places the tibial joint surface perpendicular to the AP plane in full extension. (Reprinted with permission.[12])*

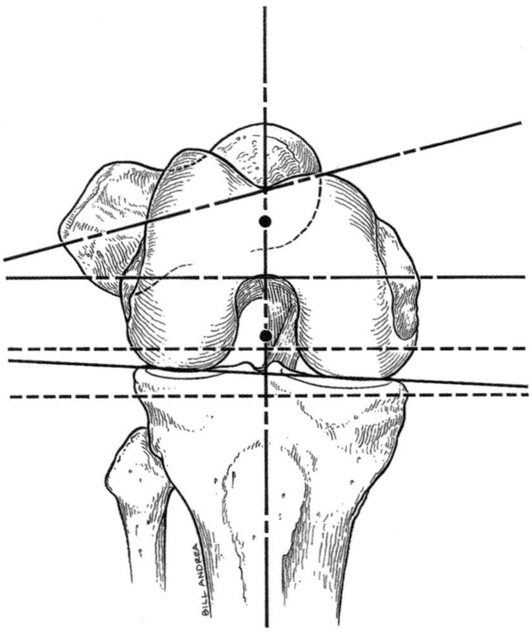

FIGURE 51-3. *With the knee flexed 90°, the joint surface resections are parallel to the epicondylar axis and perpendicular to the AP axis of the femur. The femoral neck is anteverted approximately 15° to the epicondylar axis. When the knee is in functional position in flexion (walking up stairs or standing from a seated position), the positions of the femoral neck and epicondylar axis remain unchanged, and in the normal knee the tibia is vertical. (Reprinted with permission.[12])*

This line then is extended along the deepest part of the patellar groove.[3,5] For convenience of visualization with standard knee alignment and cutting instruments, the AP line is extended onto the tibia so that it can be seen easily with the femoral cutting guide in place. In the face of anterior femoral surface deformity and deficiency in the patellar groove, the two essential landmarks (the center of the intercondylar notch posteriorly and the deepest part of the patellar groove just anterior to the intercondylar notch) always are present and the line constructed by connecting these two points also passes where the normal patellar groove should lie. In the normal knee, the epicondylar axis is very close to perpendicular to the AP axis, but much more difficult to find.[3] In many cases, especially in knees with valgus deformity, the lateral epicondyle is not present, and so the epicondylar axis must be constructed as a line perpendicular to the AP axis (Fig. 51-3).[6]

An important feature of this AP axis is that it lies within the AP plane of the lower extremity, so that when the anterior and posterior surfaces of the femur are resected perpendicular to this line, the knee will align in flexion with the femoral component correctly positioned in the AP plane. The articular surfaces of the knee often are part of the deformity and cannot be used as alignment landmarks; even in the normal knee, the angle made by the articular surface line is highly variable[7] and cannot be used as a reliable landmark for alignment of the knee in flexion. Just as the articular surfaces of the distal femur and upper tibia are not reliable landmarks for resection in extension, they likewise are not reliable landmarks for resection with the knee in flexion.

Ligaments perform throughout the range of flexion and extension, providing stability while maintaining flexibility at all positions of the knee. The anatomic positions of attachment of the ligaments determine their function in flexion and extension. Those attached near the center of rotation of the femur are effective in flexion and extension. Furthermore, those that are attached to the femur anteriorly are more effective in flexion, and those attached posteriorly are more effective in extension (Figs. 51-4 and 51-5).[5,8-15]

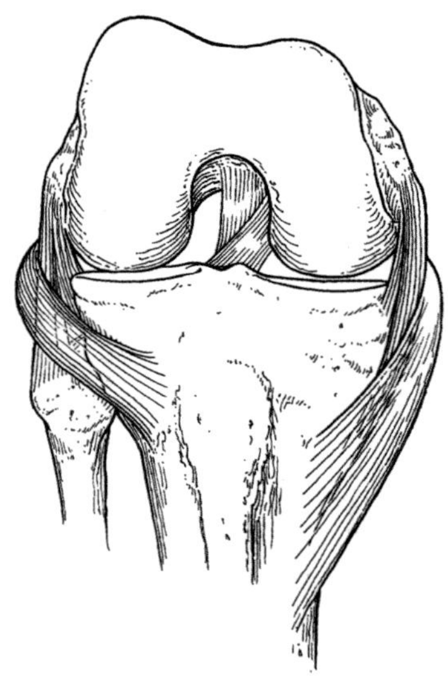

FIGURE 51-4. *With the knee flexed and viewed anteriorly, the deep and superficial medial collateral ligament fibers stabilize the medial side. The lateral collateral ligament and popliteus tendon stabilize the lateral side, and the posterior cruciate ligament is a secondary varus and valgus stabilizing structure. The posterior structures such as the posterior capsule and the posterolateral corner are especially effective in full extension. This also is true of the posterior portion of the iliotibial band. The anterior structures, which in this case are the anterior portion of the iliotibial band and to a certain extent the popliteus tendon, are less effective in the fully extended position because of their position of anatomic attachment. (Reprinted with permission.[28])*

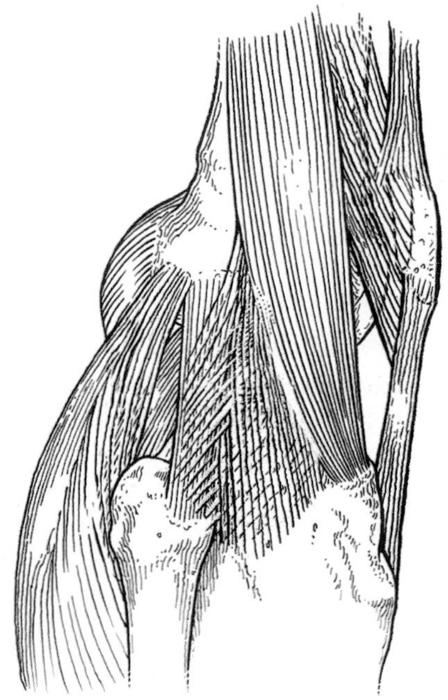

FIGURE 51-5. *Lateral view of the knee showing the major lateral static stabilizing structures with the knee extended. The lateral gastrocnemius tendon (and posterolateral corner capsule), lateral collateral ligament, lateral posterior capsule, popliteus tendon, and posterior portion of the iliotibial band all cross the joint perpendicular (or nearly so) to its surface and are capable of stabilizing the knee in the extended position. The iliotibial band is attached anteriorly to the patella and Gerdy's tubercle and posteriorly to the fibular head, tibial surface, and posterior portion of Gerdy's tubercle. (Reprinted with permission.[13])*

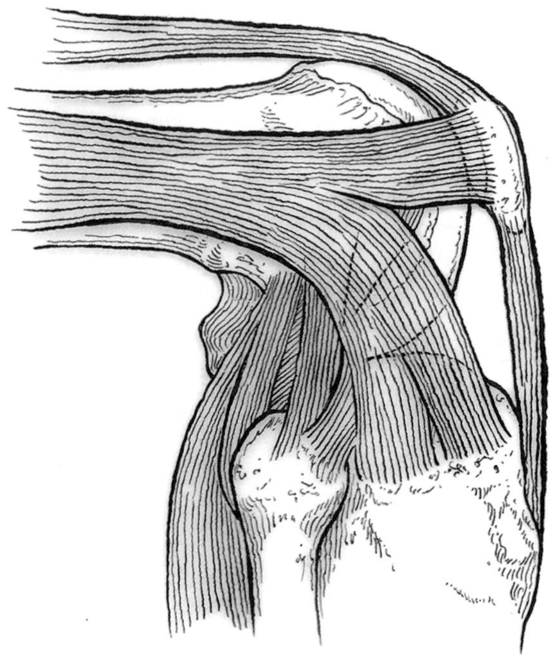

FIGURE 51-6. *Lateral view of the knee showing the major lateral static stabilizing structures with the knee flexed 90°. The lateral gastrocnemius tendon, posterolateral corner capsule, lateral collateral ligament, and popliteus tendon are the only effective lateral stabilizing structures with the knee flexed to this position. The iliotibial band is held anteriorly by its attachment to the patella. Its anterior fibers are effective in flexion. (Reprinted with permission.[13])*

The lateral gastrocnemius tendon and capsule of the posterolateral corner, lateral collateral ligament, and popliteus tendon complex attach near the lateral epicondyle and are stabilizers of the lateral side throughout the flexion arc, but these structures have a differential effect in extension. The structures that attach to the epicondylar area of the femur farther anteriorly, such as the popliteus tendon, are more effective as the knee is flexed, and those attached more posteriorly in the epicondylar area, such as the posterolateral corner, are more effective in extension.[8,10] The iliotibial band, which has broad attachment across the lateral aspect of the knee, has elements that are effective both in flexion and extension (Figs. 51-6 and 51-7).[16]

On the medial side, the medial collateral ligament (anterior and posterior) is attached to the epicondyle and is effective throughout the arc of flexion. The epicondylar attachment is broad enough that there is a difference in function of the anterior and posterior portions of the ligament in flexion and extension. The posterior portion attaches near the epicondylar axis on the femur, but far posteriorly on the tibia, and is tight only in extension (Figs. 51-8 and 51-9).[9,15] The deep medial collateral ligament follows a similar pattern, with its posterior structures tightening in extension and its anterior structures tightening in flexion. Of course the posterior capsule is an extreme posterior structure and slackens in flexion and tightens only in extension.

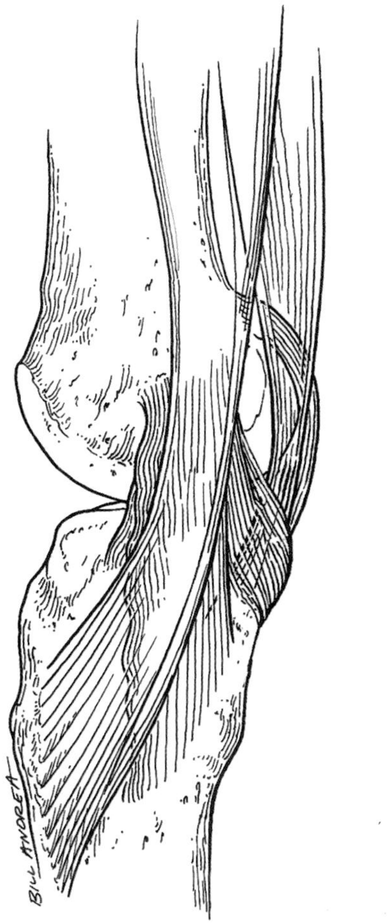

FIGURE 51-7. *On the medial view, the medial collateral ligament (deep and superficial) is the primary medial stabilizer that is tight in extension. The anterior fibers are slackened in full extension and the posterior fibers (posteromedial oblique ligament) are differentially tightened in extension because of their position in the medial femoral condyle and posterior aspect of the tibia. The posterior capsule also is tight. Active medial stability is added by the medial hamstrings through the pes anserinus and semimembranosus. The posteromedial oblique portion of the superficial medial collateral ligament wraps around the tendon of the semimembranosus. (Reprinted with permission.[28])*

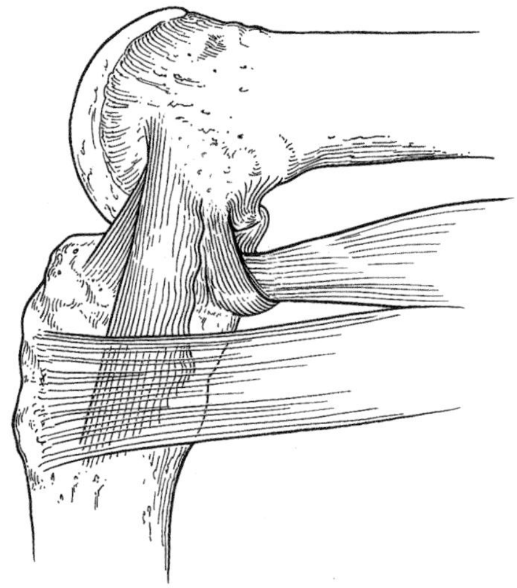

FIGURE 51-8. *Viewed from the medial side with the knee flexed, the medial stabilizing structures are the deep and superficial fibers of the medial collateral ligament. The anterior fibers of the medial collateral ligament are taut and the posterior fibers are relatively lax because of their attachment more posteriorly on the femur. The posterior capsule is slack and is not effective in flexion. The semimembranosus and pes anserina are parallel with the joint and are not capable of supplying active stability in flexion. (Reprinted with permission.[14])*

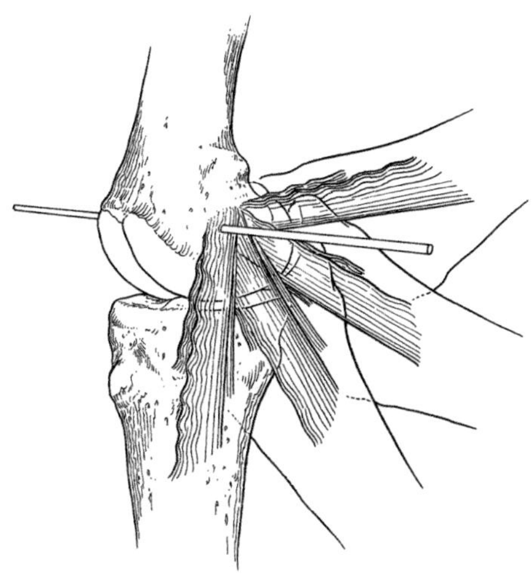

FIGURE 51-9. *Ligaments that attach to the femur near the epicondyles guide the tibia through its arc of flexion and maintain stability throughout the full range of motion. Because the ligaments attach across a broad surface of the femoral epicondyle, the anterior and posterior portions behave differently in flexion and extension. As illustrated in this drawing, the anterior portion of the medial collateral ligament tightens in flexion, and the posterior portion tightens in extension. (Reprinted with permission.[28])*

Knowing this information, the surgeon, after positioning the implants properly with the joint surfaces and axes of the knee, can assess knee stability in flexion and extension and release the structures that are tight. This release can be done by a variety of techniques, including subperiosteal release and direct release of tight structures within the ligament substance (pie-crusting). The surgeon also can adjust the tightness of intact ligaments by changing the position and size of the femoral component, altering the slope of the tibial surfaces, and adjusting the thickness of the polyethylene spacers. AP stability can be altered by changing the configuration of the polyethylene component. The arthritic process often affects the articular surfaces of the joint to cause deformity, placing the tibia in a varus or valgus malposition in all or part of the normal flexion arc. In other words, the tibia and its long axis are displaced outside the normal functional AP plane of the lower extremity. To achieve optimal function of the knee in flexion and extension, the joint surfaces must be returned to their proper positions, the mechanical axes of the long bones brought back into the AP plane, and the ligaments adjusted to their proper tension throughout the functional arc of the knee.

Several factors in the arthritic process affect the functions of ligaments. Osteophytes deform them, causing them to be excessively tight or to restrict their sliding, causing flexion contracture and restriction of flexion. As the joint surfaces collapse, their attachment points come closer together and the ligaments shorten irreversibly. When the joint surfaces separate on the convex side of the deformity, the ligaments usually are elongated permanently (Fig. 51-10). All these abnormalities can be addressed by correct positioning and sizing of the implants, complete debridement of the joint, and finally release of contracted ligaments.

In the knee that is free of deformity in which there is no ligament contracture or stretching of the ligaments, resection of the thickness of the implants from all surfaces and replacement of the thickness of bone with the implant thickness results in restoration of ligament balance throughout the full arc of flexion.[17] This statement is intuitively obvious and also has been demonstrated to be true by experimentation.[17] When no deformity exists, the articular surfaces can be used as landmarks for resection and restoration of joint surface position. However, when deformity does exist, or when normal variations of anatomy are present, anatomical landmarks and axes of reference that are not distorted by the arthritic process must be used to dictate the correct position and alignment for resection of the bone surfaces. In almost all knees with deformity, the unworn surfaces on the convex side of the deformity are in the correct anatomic position and can be used as landmarks for sizing and positioning of the new implant (Fig. 51-11).[5,8-15]

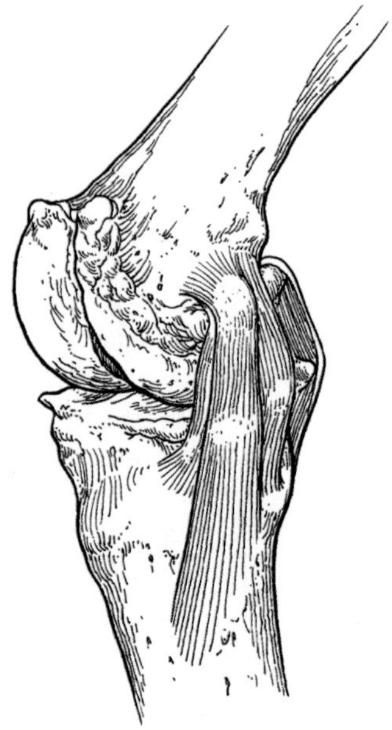

FIGURE 51-10. *Osteophytes are an important factor in ligament balancing. They constrain the deep and superficial fibers of the medial collateral ligament and medial posterior capsule. (Reprinted with permission.[25])*

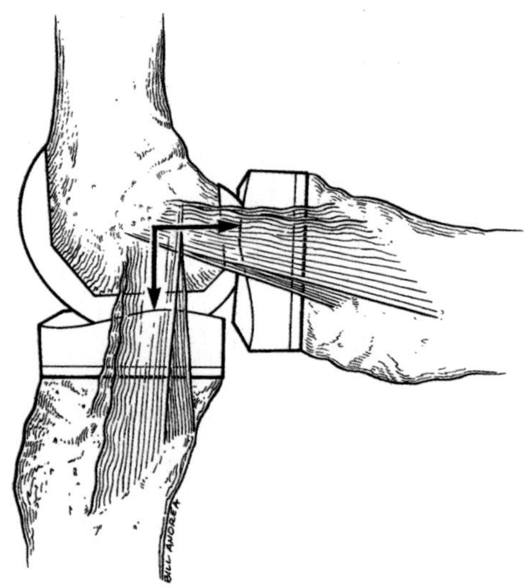

FIGURE 51-11. *In most cases the intact (convex) side of the knee should serve as the landmark for resection both distally and posteriorly. Even when the collateral ligaments are stretched, the distal and posterior surfaces will be positioned correctly to accept a thicker tibial component to achieve stability in flexion and extension, and the ligaments on the contracted (concave) side can be released to achieve correct balance to accommodate this position. (Reprinted with permission.[28])*

PATELLA

The patella maintains a delicate balance in total knee arthroplasty and is dependent on position and configuration of the patellar and femoral articular surfaces, angle of the quadriceps and patellar tendons, and tension of the medial and lateral retinacula. As the knee flexes, the patella engages the patellar groove and then follows this groove through the flexion-extension arc. The apex of the patella stays within the median AP plane in the normal knee and the patellar groove must lie in this plane to accommodate this patellar position.[18] One of the most important aspects of patellar balance and correct tracking is use of the AP axis for femoral component alignment and positioning (Fig. 51-12).[3] The patella, patellar tendon, quadriceps mechanism, tibial tubercle, and intercondylar notch all must be aligned in flexion in the AP plane, which is dictated by the AP axis.[5] Likewise the articular surface of the patella must lie in the same position in both the coronal and sagittal planes.[17] With this correct anatomic relationship established, the complex soft tissue structures that stabilize the patella can be adjusted and adapted to maintain the patella securely in the patellar groove throughout flexion and extension. The patella in this illustration is correctly aligned in the patellar groove, and the implants are correctly aligned in the AP plane of the lower extremity with the long axis of the tibia, the medial third of the tibial tubercle, and the patellar groove, forming a line that forms a plane that crosses the hip just lateral to the center of the femoral head in flexion.[18] The implant articular surfaces are perpendicular to this AP axis. In this illustration all the soft tissue constraints are normally balanced so that the patella tracks smoothly from full extension to deep flexion.

POSTERIOR CRUCIATE LIGAMENT

The posterior cruciate ligament serves a complex purpose throughout the flexion arc, acting primarily to prevent posterior travel of the tibia on the femur, but also performing secondary varus-valgus and rotational stabilizing roles when the collateral ligaments are deficient. It also provides resistance to hyperextension when the posterior capsule is deficient. The posterior cruciate ligament is attached slightly distal and posterior to the epicondylar axis so it slackens in full extension and tightens in flexion. Of course the posterior cruciate ligament is a complex structure and has elements within itself that are differentially effective in flexion and extension.[19,20]

Because the posterior cruciate ligament is a medial structure attached to the medial femoral condyle, it often contracts in the varus knee and stretches in the valgus knee. When it is contracted, it often can be released partially and much of its function can be preserved.[21] Even when it is insufficient to provide adequate posterior stability, it can provide rotational and varus-valgus stabilization.[5,8,9,15,21] If ligaments are to be adjusted, especially the medial collateral ligament, the posterior cruciate ligament often becomes involved as part of the medial stabilizing complex. When the posterior cruciate ligament is sacrificed to accommodate a posterior stabilized total knee system, the collateral ligament structures must be especially carefully maintained because the plastic post that is used to substitute for its posterior stabilizing function is ineffective as a varus-valgus stabilizing structure, and major medial or lateral laxity may occur if the collateral ligaments are insufficient (Figs. 51-13 to 51-15).[5,8,9,15,21]

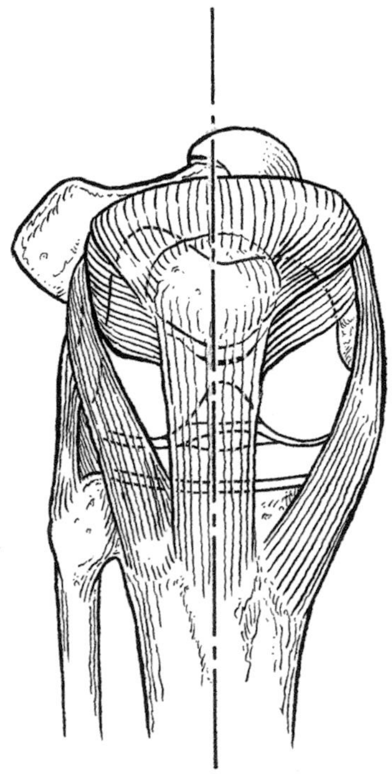

FIGURE 51-12. *The femoral and tibial components are correctly aligned so that the long axis of the tibia, the patellar groove, and the femoral head all lie in the AP plane. Patellar constraints include the vastus medialis, vastus lateralis, and medial and lateral capsular structures including the patellar extension of the iliotibial band. The patellar groove is correctly positioned in the sagittal and coronal planes so that all these constraining structures function at correct tension throughout the arc of flexion, and the tibial component is aligned in rotation so that the patellar tendon and quadriceps hold the patella in the patellar groove.*

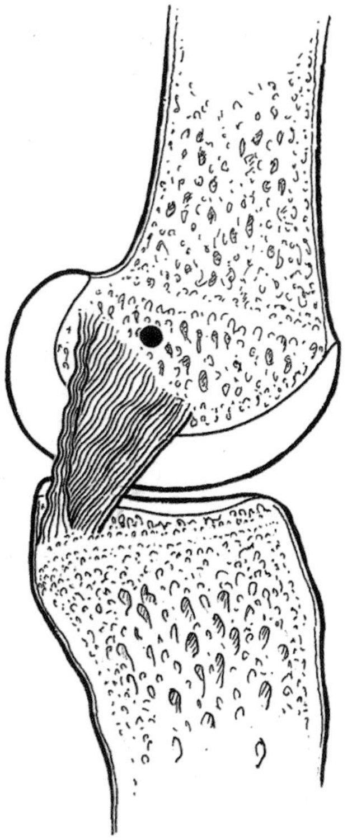

FIGURE 51-13. *The posterior cruciate ligament, like the medial collateral ligament, is attached over a broad band, so its anterior and posterior portions behave differently in flexion and extension. The anterior portion of the posterior cruciate ligament is attached to the femur distal to the epicondylar axis so it tends to loosen in full extension. The posterior portion, being behind the center of rotation, tends to tighten in hyperextension. Both bands are relatively loose at 0° knee flexion. (Reprinted with permission.[28])*

VARUS KNEE—BASIC PRINCIPLES

The contracture and stretching that occur due to articular surface deformity and osteophytes affect medial ligaments unequally and often cause different degrees of tightness or laxity in flexion and extension after the bone surfaces are resected correctly for varus-valgus alignment. The cornerstone of correct ligament balancing is correct varus-valgus alignment in flexion and extension. For alignment in the extended position, the fixed anatomic landmarks such as the intramedullary canal of the femur and the long axis of the tibia are generally well accepted.[22,23] When the joint surfaces are resected at an angle of 5° valgus to the medullary canal of the femur and perpendicular to the long axis of the tibia, the joint surfaces are perpendicular to the mechanical

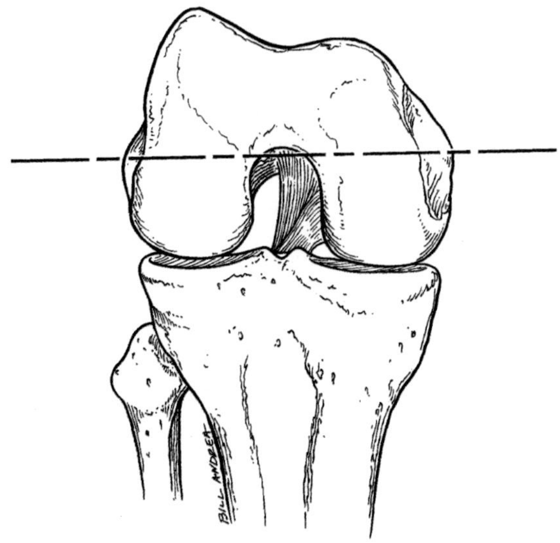

FIGURE 51-14. *In the flexed position, the anterolateral fibers are brought to tension and the posteromedial fibers loosen. (Reprinted with permission.[28])*

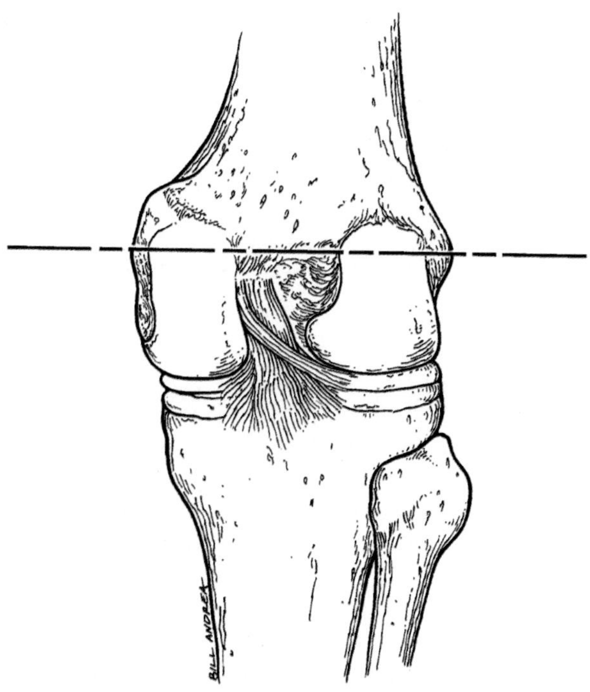

FIGURE 51-15. *Because the posterior cruciate ligament is attached to the medial femoral condyle, it tends to shorten in the varus knee and loosen in the valgus knee. The posterior cruciate ligament has auxillary attachments to the menisci and joint capsule. (Reprinted with permission.[28])*

axis of the lower extremity in the extended position and roughly parallel to the epicondylar axis.[24] In the flexed position, anatomic landmarks are equally important for varus-valgus alignment. Incorrect varus-valgus alignment in flexion not only malaligns the long axis of the femur and tibia, but also incorrectly positions the patellar groove both in flexion and extension.[4,18]

Finding suitable landmarks for varus and valgus alignment has led to efforts to use the posterior femoral condyles, the epicondylar axis, and the AP axis of the femur for varus-valgus alignment of the femoral component in flexion. The posterior femoral condyles and epicondylar axis both are unreliable, and the articular surfaces themselves often are part of the arthritic process and are deformed along with the ligaments.[3,5,9] The AP axis, defined as the center of the intercondylar notch posteriorly and the deepest part of the patellar groove anteriorly, is highly consistent and always lies within the median sagittal plane that bisects the lower extremity in the normal knee.[3,5] If the instrumentation system dictates use of the epicondylar axis or the posterior femoral condylar axis, the AP axis should be drawn first and then the instruments aligned relative to the AP axis, assuming that the other structures are part of the articular deformity (Figs. 51-16 and 51-17).

Once the joint surface has been resected correctly to establish normal varus-valgus alignment in flexion and extension, the trial components are inserted and ligament function is assessed in flexion and extension. Although tensioners and spacers can be used at this point, they do not give a full three-dimensional picture of the knee to the surgeon and furnish no information about flexion contracture, rollback, and rotational laxity abnormalities. The trial components do provide this information, and use of the trial components at this stage of the procedure saves time and effort and also provides better information that allows better ligament balancing. The ligaments then can be released according to their function at each position. The medial collateral ligament (deep and superficial layers) attaches to the medial epicondylar area through a broad band. The posterior oblique portion, which spreads posteriorly over the medial tibial flare and incorporates the sheaths of the semimembranosus tendon, tightens in extension. The anterior portion of the ligament complex, which extends anteriorly along the medial tibial flare, tightens in flexion and loosens in extension. The posterior capsule is loose in flexion and tightens only in full extension.[9,15] With this information, the medial ligament structures of the knee can be released individually according to the position in which excessive tightness is found.

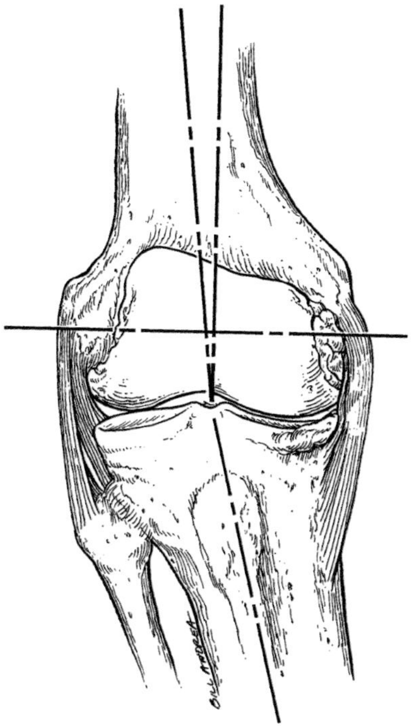

FIGURE 51-16. *The varus knee has a group of bone and ligament abnormalities that must be addressed to correct the deformity. The mechanical axis of the femur is tilted medially relative to the long axis of the tibia. The distal femoral surface usually remains in valgus alignment to the long axis of the femur. Most of the varus deformity is caused by deficiency in the medial tibial plateau. The deep and superficial medial collateral ligaments are contracted and deformed by osteophytes. (Reprinted with permission.[12])*

The sequence in which the procedures are performed is important in total knee replacement. Resection of the femoral surfaces makes the tibial surface accessible. Resection of the tibial surface clears the way to remove the osteophytes. Removal of the osteophytes frees the ligaments so that they may be assessed and released as needed. No ligament should be released until all the osteophytes are removed, otherwise excessive laxity may occur. Extra bone should not be removed to correct a flexion contracture until all ligament balancing has been finished, otherwise inappropriate laxity in extension may occur once ligament release has been done (Figs. 51-18 to 51-22).[25,26]

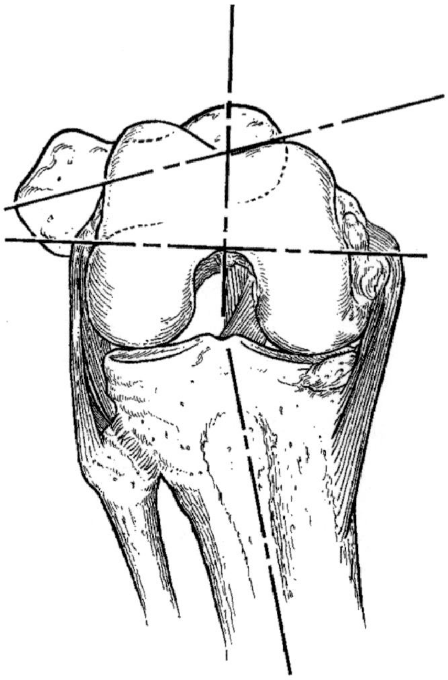

FIGURE 51-17. *In the flexed position, the mechanical abnormalities are similar. The deficiency in the medial tibial plateau causes the tibia to tilt toward varus, and the AP axis of the femur tilts medially relative to the long axis of the tibia. Here the hip is in neutral position with the AP axis passing through the center of the femoral head, and the femoral neck anteverted 15° to the epicondylar axis. The deep and superficial portions of the medial collateral ligament are contracted, and the posterior cruciate ligament, being a medial structure, often is contracted as well. (Reprinted with permission.[28])*

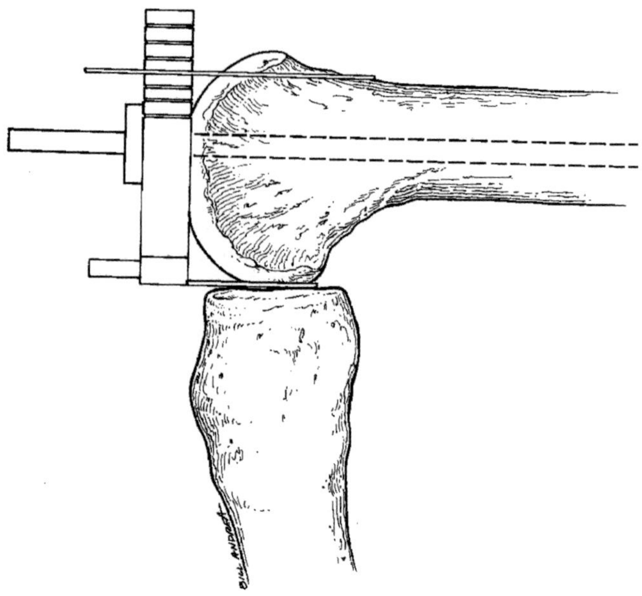

FIGURE 51-18. *The femur is sized from the anterior cortex (just proximal to the joint surface) to the posterior femoral joint surface. Resection guides are used to measure and remove the thickness of the implant from all intact surfaces of the femur. An anterior stylus is used to position the resection guide so that the anterior surface cut aligns flush with the anterior cortex of the femur. Posterior paddles are used to engage the posterior femoral condyles. These posterior paddles are used to confirm the AP size of the femur and not to serve as a guide for rotational alignment (varus-valgus alignment in flexion) of the femoral component. (Reprinted with permission.[28])*

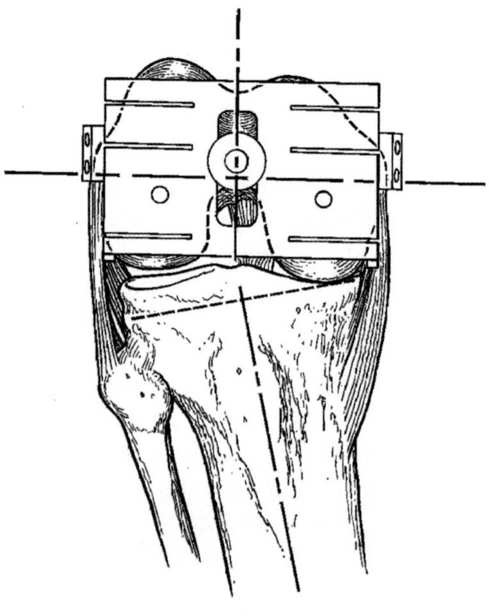

FIGURE 51-19. *Varus-valgus alignment of the femoral component in flexion (rotational alignment) is determined by the AP axis. Here the cutting guide is aligned with the AP axis of the femur. The AP plane of the femur is defined by the center of the intercondylar notch and the deepest point in the patellar groove. This also aligns the femoral surface cuts parallel to the epicondylar axis. (Reprinted with permission.[28])*

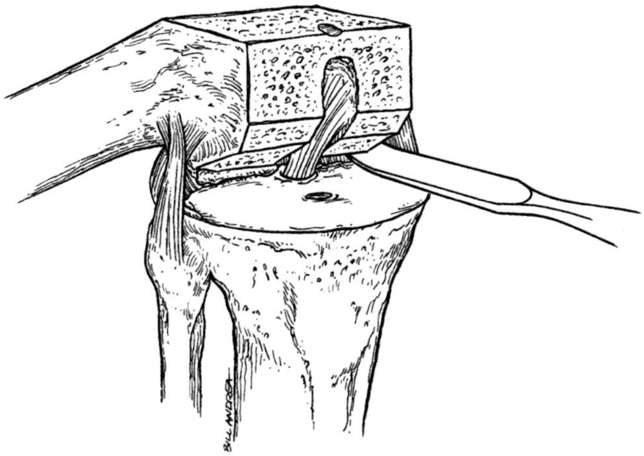

FIGURE 51-20. *After the medial tibial osteophyte has been removed, the knee will be freed enough to allow access to the posterior femoral osteophytes. They are cut free with a curved half-inch osteotome and the same osteotome is used to free the osteophyte in the popliteus recess laterally. (Reprinted with permission.[28])*

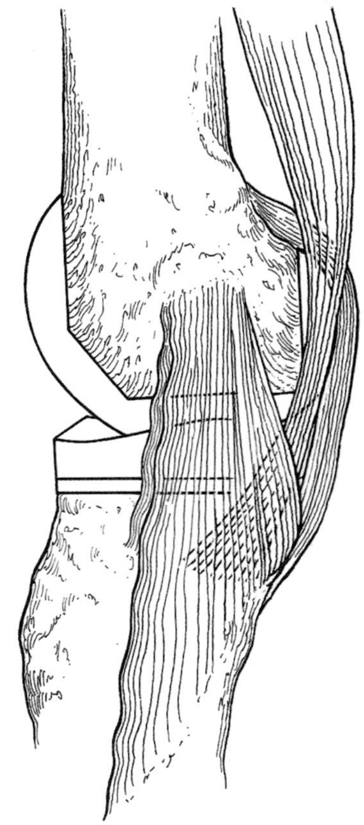

FIGURE 51-21. *The medial collateral ligament attaches to the medial femoral condyle over a fairly broad area, and this affects the function of the ligament in flexion and extension. With the knee fully extended, the posterior capsule and the posteromedial oblique portion of the medial collateral ligament are tight. The posteromedial oblique portion of the medial collateral ligament attaches both to bone and soft tissue, wrapping around the tendon of the semimembranosus where it attaches to the tibia. The anterior portion of the medial collateral ligament loosens in full extension, but being close to the center of rotation, it acts as a stabilizing structure throughout the flexion-extension arc. (Reprinted with permission.[15])*

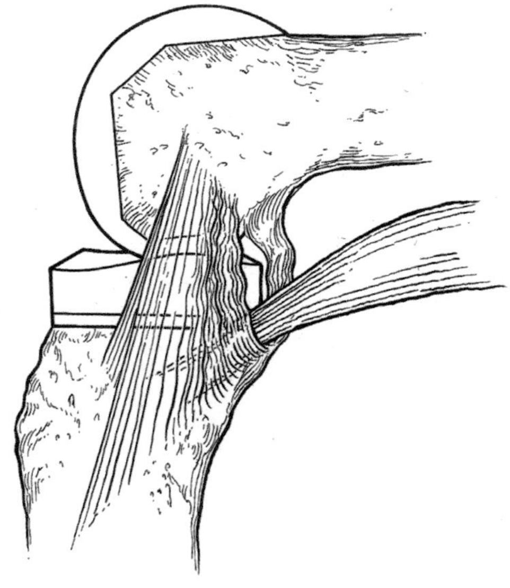

FIGURE 51-22. *When the knee flexes, the posterior capsule and the posteromedial oblique portion of the medial collateral ligament loosen. The anterior portion of the medial collateral ligament tightens. (Reprinted with permission.[28])*

Tight Medially in Flexion Only

In some cases the medial structures are not contracted uniformly, and the knee may be tight medially only in flexion but not in extension (Figs. 51-23 to 51-26). This type of ligament imbalance is corrected best by releasing just the tight anterior structures. The anterior portion of the deep medial collateral ligament can be released easily under direct vision with a sharp osteotome. If this is not enough, subperiosteal release of the anterior fibers of the superficial medial collateral ligament can be done with the same instrument. The anterior structures, which are tight in flexion, are especially amenable to release by multiple puncture (pie-crusting). Because the knee can be flexed to expose the tight structures, gradual release, palpation, and repeated stability testing are done easily. Release of structures in this manner releases only the tight structure and leaves the rest of the ligaments intact to be called into service secondarily, providing stability as the released ligament heals.

Tight Medially in Extension Only

Occasionally the knee is tight medially in extension only, but well balanced in flexion. This leads the surgeon to consider the posterior structures, which normally tighten in extension (Fig. 51-27). The posterior structures are not accessible for multiple puncture and must be released with the knee flexed using an osteotome or similar instrument.[9]

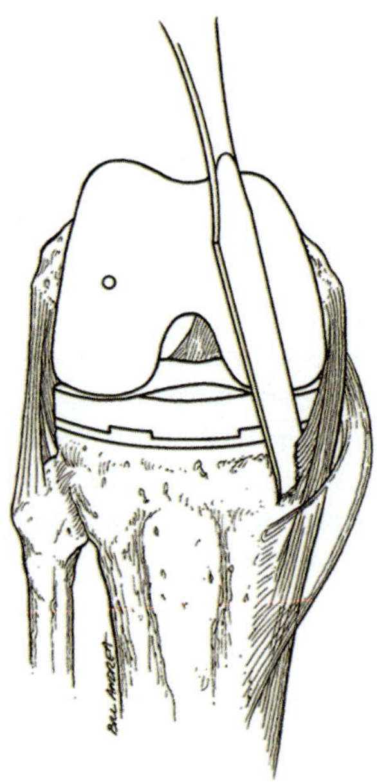

FIGURE 51-23. *Tightness in flexion is corrected by releasing the anterior portion of the medial collateral ligament. The knee is flexed to 90° and a curved ½-inch osteotome is used to elevate the anterior ligament as needed. In some cases release of only the anterior deep medial collateral ligament is sufficient. (Reprinted with permission.[12])*

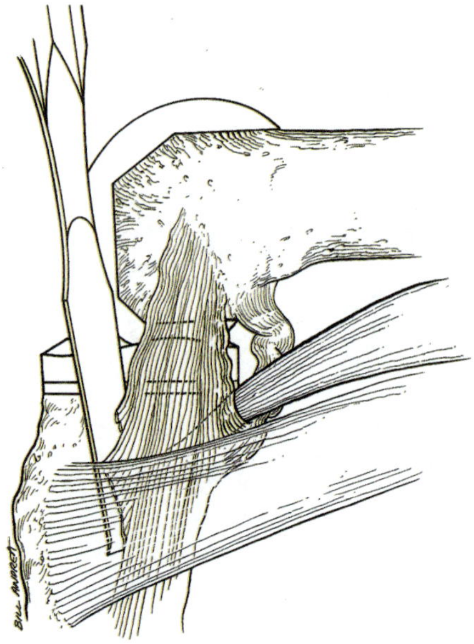

FIGURE 51-24. *If deep medial collateral ligament release is insufficient, the anterior superficial medial collateral ligament is released. The taut anterior fibers are released subperiosteally. These fibers attach fairly far distally (8–10 cm), and the osteotome is passed far enough to completely release the anterior fibers. These fibers also are seen easily and palpated, so they may be released with puncture (pie-crust) technique. The attachment of the pes anserinus and posterior oblique fibers of the medial collateral ligament are left intact. (Reprinted with permission.[15])*

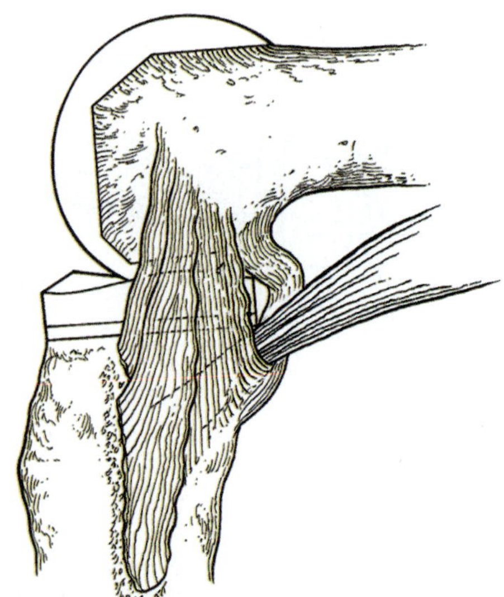

FIGURE 51-25. *In flexion the anterior medial collateral ligament is no longer tight. The posteromedial oblique portion of the medial collateral ligament now acts as a secondary medial stabilizer in flexion. (Reprinted with permission.[28])*

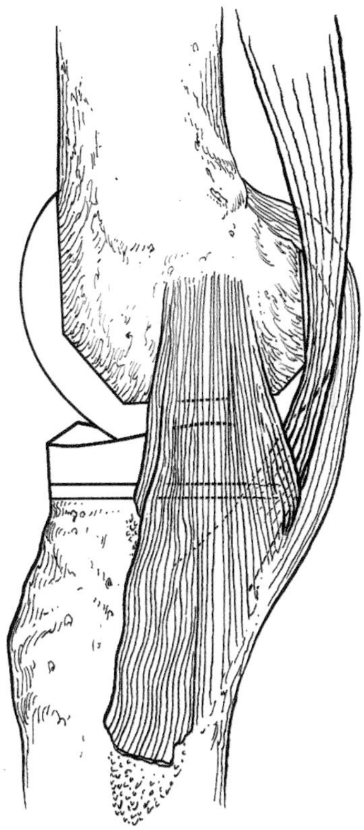

FIGURE 51-26. *The anterior fibers of the medial collateral ligament have been released. Medial stability in extension is near normal because the posterior portion of the medial collateral ligament and the posterior medial capsule function normally. (Reprinted with permission.[28])*

Tight Medially in Flexion and Extension

In many cases with long-standing varus deformity and medial ligament contracture, the knee is tight medially both in flexion and extension. This indicates that the entire medial collateral ligament is contracted. The posterior capsule and posterior cruciate ligament also may be contracted, but the primary contracture is the medial collateral ligament in these cases. The posterior cruciate ligament and posterior capsule cannot be evaluated until the medial collateral ligament contracture has been corrected.

Medial collateral ligament release should begin with the deep fibers of the medial collateral ligament, then proceed to the anterior and posterior structures stepwise as medial stability is tested repeatedly. Release of the entire deep and superficial medial collateral ligament anteriorly and posteriorly still leaves periosteal attachments for these ligaments and also the attachments of these structures to the semimembranosus tendon (Fig. 51-28). The posterior capsule remains also as a secondary stabilizing structure in extension. If the posterior cruciate ligament has been sacrificed in the process of preparing for a posterior stabilized knee, the medial collateral ligament release should be done even more carefully and gradually to avoid overrelease that cannot be compensated by the posterior cruciate ligament.[9,15,21,27]

VALGUS KNEE—BASIC PRINCIPLES

Ligament balancing in the valgus knee continues to challenge arthroplasty surgeons despite advances in instrumentation for bone resection and alignment. However, the application of basic principles of alignment allows the surgeon to correct the deformity and eliminate articular surface deficiency while using reliable anatomic landmarks and axes of the femur and tibia to position the components. The lateral condylar deficiency that is present in most valgus knees and the valgus curvature of the femoral and tibial shafts make total knee replacement in these knees a special

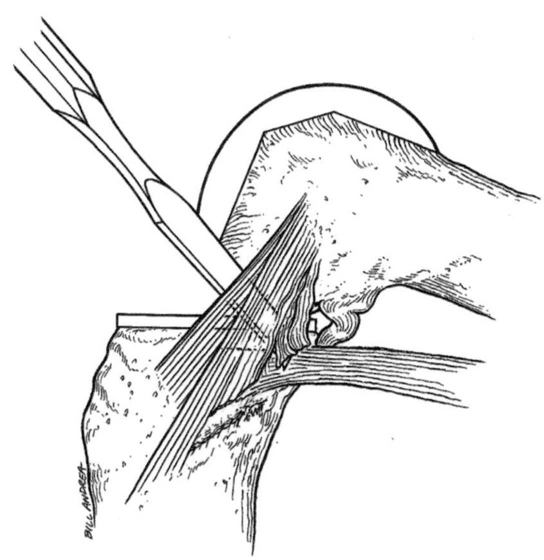

FIGURE 51-27. *In knees that are too tight in extension only, only the posterior portion of the medial collateral ligament should be released first. A curved ½-inch osteotome is used to elevate all but the anterior portion of the medial collateral ligament. The osteotome is directed approximately 45° downward and tapped gently to release the posteromedial oblique fibers from the tibia and from the tendon of the semimembranosus. (Reprinted with permission.[15])*

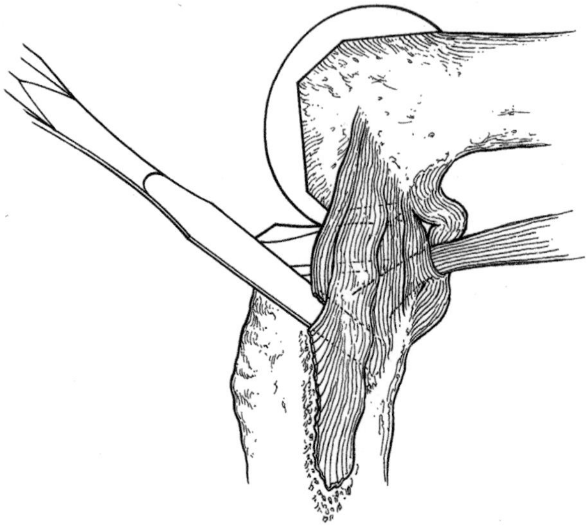

FIGURE 51-28. *If the knee remains tight medially in extension after release of the anterior medial collateral ligament fibers, then the posterior fibers are released. Here the curved ½-inch osteotomy is passed under the released anterior fibers and angled downward 45° to release the posterior oblique fibers of the medial collateral ligament. The fibers attached to the bone and those that wrap around the semimembranosus are released. The medial collateral ligament maintains loose attachment to the pes anserinus, and the distal periosteal attachments to the ligament remain intact as well, so the knee does not become grossly lax as a result of this procedure. The secondary medial stabilizers (the medial posterior capsule in extension and the posterior cruciate ligament in flexion) also are called into play and prevent destabilization of the knee. (Reprinted with permission.[28])*

challenge in anatomic alignment. In these cases the AP axis and the long axes of the femur and tibia will guide the surgeon to a well-aligned knee in virtually every case.[8,10,13] Relying on the articular surface of the intact medial side allows correct placement of the femoral component, and the medial side also gives reliable information for sizing the implant (Figs. 51-29 and 51-30).[22,28]

Ligaments that attach to the femur near the epicondyles (ie, near the axis of rotation of the femur) function through the entire range of flexion of the knee. Those that attach to the femur at a point distant to the epicondylar axis function effectively only in full extension or in positions of fairly deep flexion. On the lateral side of the knee, the structures attaching to the femur near the epicondyles are the lateral collateral ligament, the popliteus tendon, and the posterolateral corner capsule. These three structures are appropriate to release for a knee that is excessively tight laterally both in flexion and extension.[16] The iliotibial band is a complex structure that is attached to the patella, tibia, and fibula. Its posterior fibers tighten in extension and its anterior portion tightens in flexion. It translates posteriorly in flexion, but this posterior positioning is limited by its attachment to the patella. Although the iliotibial band is primarily engaged in lateral stability in extension, it also stabilizes the lateral side of the knee in flexion through its attachments to the patella and to the tibia. The lateral posterior capsular structures are tight only in full extension and are slack when the knee is flexed. Release of either the lateral posterior capsule or the posterior portion of the iliotibial band is appropriate only for a knee that is tight laterally in extension and would have little effect on lateral stability in the flexed position.[8,10,13,28]

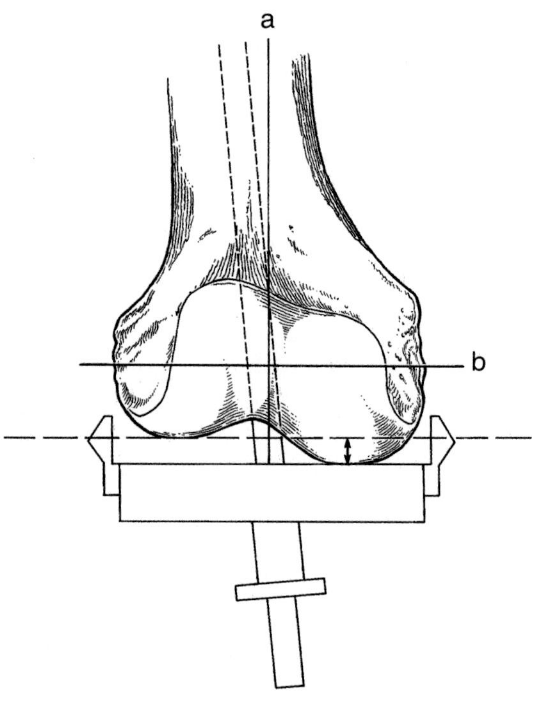

FIGURE 51-29. *The intramedullary alignment rod lies slightly medial to the center of the patellar groove, and the cutting guide is set at a 5° valgus angle. This will align the joint surface perpendicular to the mechanical axis of the femur (**a**), and parallel to the epicondylar axis (**b**). The cutting guide seats against the high (medial) side, which is the reference for resection of the joint surfaces. The thickness of the implant is resected distally from the medial side. In some cases, resection of the thickness of the implant from the medial side results in minimal or no resection from the lateral side of the distal femur. Regardless of the lateral bone deficit, the medial should be used as the reference surface, and augmentation of the lateral surface should be done to make up for the deficit. (Reprinted with permission.[13])*

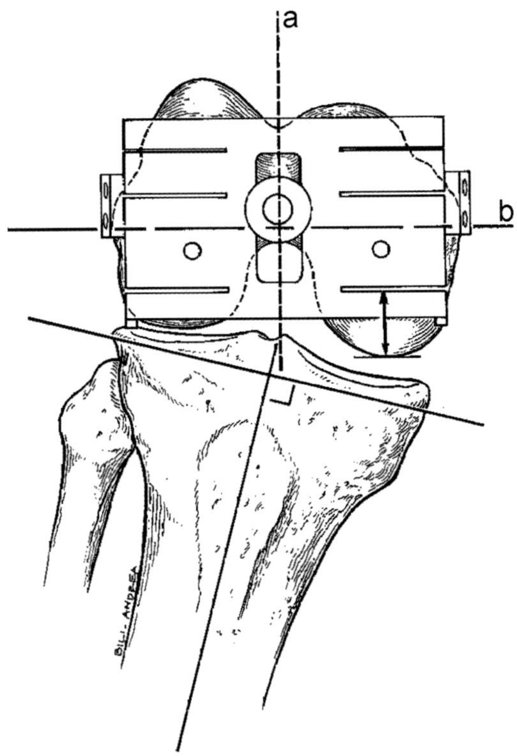

FIGURE 51-30. *The cutting guide for femoral resection is aligned so the surfaces are resected perpendicular to the AP axis of the femur (**a**) and parallel with the epicondylar axis (**b**), resecting the thickness of the implant from the intact medial femoral condylar (**arrow**), and much less from the deficient lateral side. This places the joint surfaces in anatomic position to correct the valgus position in flexion, and places the patellar groove correctly with the mechanical axis of the lower extremity. The tibial surface is resected perpendicular to the long axis of the tibia. The lateral ligaments are still tight, and the tibia is held in valgus malalignment by the ligament contractures. (Reprinted with permission.[13])*

Just as with the varus knee, the distal femoral surfaces are resected at approximately 5° valgus angle to the long axis of the femur, and the anterior and posterior surfaces are resected perpendicular to the AP axis. When the tibial surfaces are resected and the osteophytes are removed, it usually is apparent that the lateral structures are tight and the medial structures are loose. This leaves the joint space in flexion and extension far from rectangular. The ligament balancing procedures will correct this (Fig. 51-31).

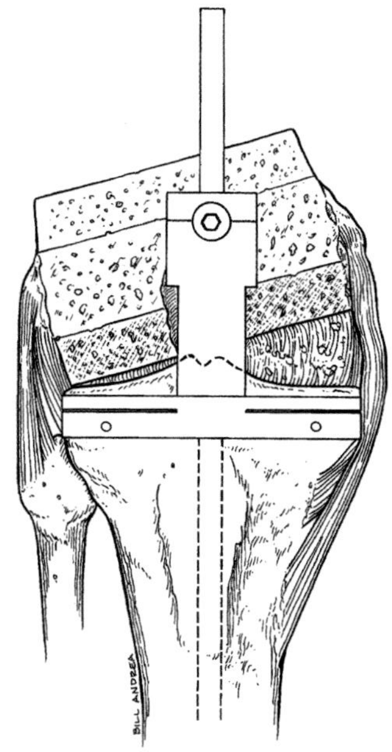

FIGURE 51-31. *After the femoral surfaces are resected and the resected pieces are removed, the tibial surface is resected perpendicular to the long axis of the tibia in the coronal plane, and sloped 4° to 7° posteriorly in the sagittal plane. As is done for the femur, the thickness of the implant is resected from the intact side. Usually there is minimal bone deficiency on the surface of the tibia. (Reprinted with permission.[28])*

Tensioners, spacer blocks, or trial components can be used to assess lateral ligament contractures and medial ligament laxity. (Tensioners should not be used to guide the posterior and anterior resection of the femur. Because the lateral ligaments are tight, the femur would be externally rotated by the tensioner and the cuts made in internal rotation, positioning the knee in marked valgus in flexion while medializing the patellar groove.) As with the varus knee, the valgus knee is tested deliberately in flexion and extension and throughout the entire arc of motion both for valgus laxity and varus tightness as well as for rotational abnormalities.

Tight Laterally Both in Flexion and Extension

When the knee is tight laterally both in flexion and extension, contracted structures attached to the femoral epicondyles should be evaluated and managed first, because the extension-only structures may not be significant deforming forces and cannot be tested adequately until the contracture laterally in the flexed position is addressed (Fig. 51-32). With the trials in place, the lateral ligament structures attached to the epicondyle can be clearly exposed by firmly retracting the patella and patellar tendon laterally. The popliteus tendon is primarily a flexion structure and its release often partially corrects the lateral ligament contracture in flexion.[8,10,13,28] It can be released directly from the bone and retracts only a short distance since it is bound by fibrous tissue to the surrounding soft tissue structures. If this is not enough release to slacken the lateral structures adequately, then the lateral collateral ligament and posterolateral corner should be addressed. Both of these structures can be released by a pie-crusting technique using a No. 11 knife blade to make multiple punctures in the midportion of the ligament and surrounding dense fibrous synovial membrane. Lateral stability should be tested multiple times as the ligaments are released to be sure that the lateral ligaments are not excessively released (Fig. 51-33).

When the lateral ligament contracture has been corrected for the flexed position, the knee is extended and evaluated for ligament contracture in the extended position. If the knee remains tight in the extended position, then the posterior structures should be addressed.[8,10,13,28] The posterior portion of the iliotibial band can be exposed with the knee in full extension by retracting the subcutaneous tissue and deep fascia, dissecting over the anterior surface of the patella and lateral retinacular structures down to the posterior tight portion of the iliotibial band.[16] This structure can be released safely under direct vision down to the biceps femoris muscle and tendon, which are clearly visible from this anterior approach (Fig. 51-34).

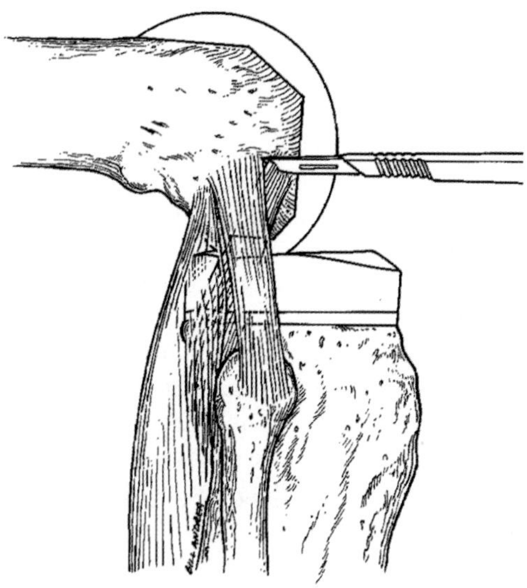

FIGURE 51-32. *To release the lateral epicondylar structures, the knee is flexed to 90°. The popliteus tendon is released directly from the femur and allowed to retract. This tendon is attached to surrounding structures and retracts only partially. (Reprinted with permission.[28])*

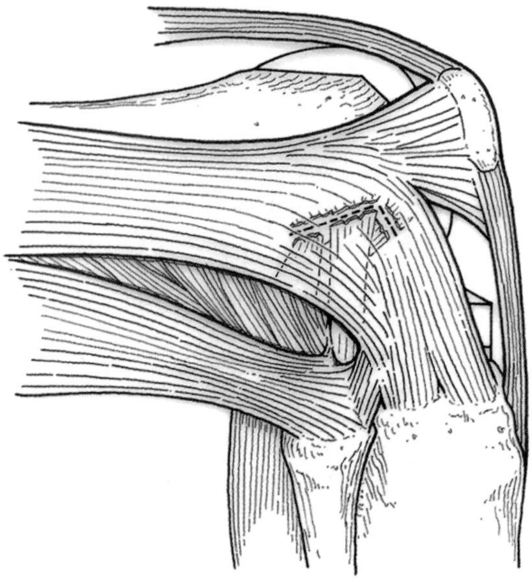

FIGURE 51-33. *Now that the lateral collateral ligament, popliteus tendon, and posterolateral corner have been released, they retract partially, but remain attached to the surrounding capsule and dense overlying synovial membrane, and so continue to function as lateral stabilizers. Release of the popliteus tendon, lateral collateral ligament, and rarely the posterolateral corner capsule always corrects lateral ligament tension in flexion because these are the only major structures that stabilize the lateral side of the knee in flexion. The iliotibial band can still act as a secondary lateral stabilizer in flexion through its attachment to the patella and tibia. The iliotibial band and posterior capsule remain as stabilizers in extension and may still apply deforming forces, but only in the extended knee. (Reprinted with permission.[13])*

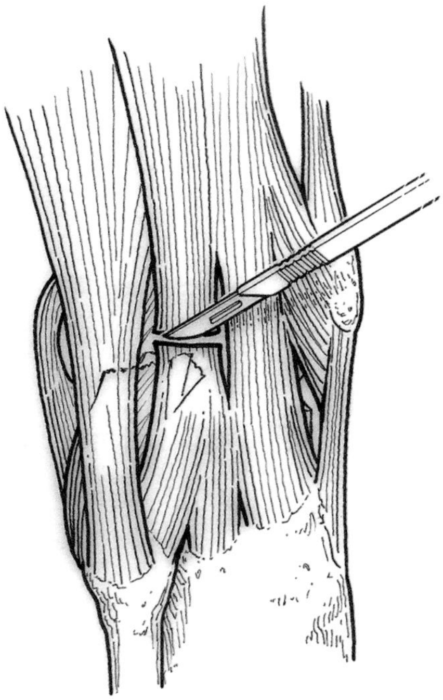

FIGURE 51-34. *If the knee remains tight laterally in extension, the iliotibial band should be released. In this case the release is done just above the joint line, extrasynovially so that the iliotibial band elongates, but remains attached to the synovial membrane and can continue to support the lateral side of the knee in extension. The posterior cruciate ligament, posterior capsule, and biceps femoris remain as lateral stabilizers in extension. (Reprinted with permission.[14])*

Tight Laterally in Extension Only

If the knee is tight laterally in extension only, then the epicondylar structures may be left intact, and the posterior portion of the iliotibial band may be released. If this lateral contracture is accompanied by a flexion contracture, then the lateral posterior capsule likely will need to be released as well (Fig. 51-35).[8,10,13,25,26,28] This release can be done from inside the knee with the tibial polyethylene trial component removed, using a curved osteotome or another sharp instrument applied directly against the bone and releasing the capsule 1 to 1.5 cm proximally.

Tight Laterally in Flexion Only

In rare conditions in which the knee is tight on the lateral side in flexion only, but has normal stability in extension, the epicondylar structures can be partially released until contracture of the lateral ligaments in flexion is corrected. It is not

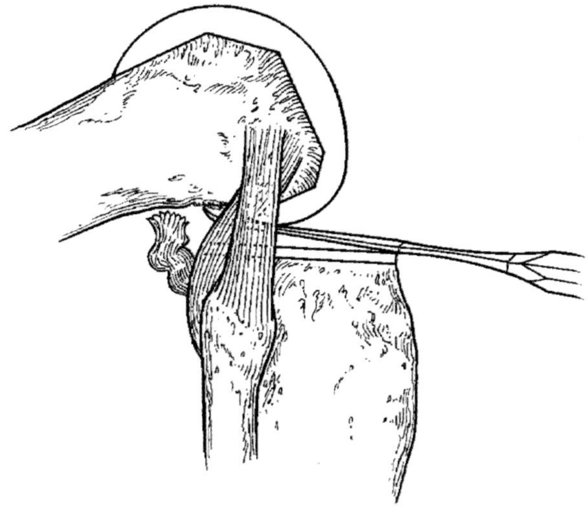

FIGURE 51-35. *The lateral posterior capsule is released by removing the polyethylene spacer and inserting the curved osteotome behind the knee against the femoral attachment of the posterior capsule, then gently tapping the end of the osteotome. This release does not affect stability of the lateral side of the knee in flexion. (Reprinted with permission.[28])*

necessary to take the lateral epicondylar structures completely loose from the femur. Limited release using the pie-crusting technique is sufficient to balance these epicondylar structures.

FLEXION CONTRACTURE

Management of flexion contractures almost always is accomplished by soft tissue release. Most flexion contractures involving either tight medial or lateral structures are corrected by appropriate graduated release of the collateral ligaments and their surrounding soft tissue attachments.[25,26] Occasionally posterior capsular release is necessary, and this release can be done under direct vision using tensioners or with a sharp, curved osteotome elevating the posterior capsule directly from its attachment just proximal to the femoral component of a total knee (Figs. 51-36 and 51-37).

Release of the posterior capsule from the medial side can be done from both the femur and the tibia, but lateral capsular release cannot be done safely from the tibia because of the proximity to the peroneal nerve (Figs. 51-36 and 51-37). Rarely extra resection of the distal femoral bone structure must be done to deal with flexion contracture. Usually resecting approximately half the thickness of the distal femoral component corrects as much as 20° of flexion contracture (Fig. 51-38).[25,26,28]

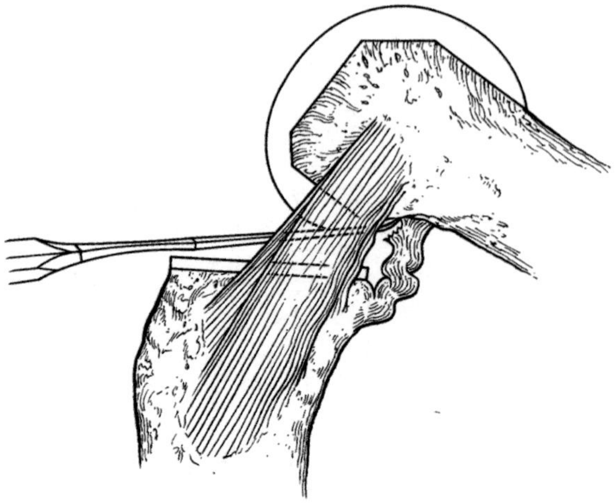

FIGURE 51-36. *The tibial trial polyethylene components have been removed, and a curved ½-inch osteotome is used to elevate the posterior capsule from its femoral attachment. (Reprinted with permission.[26])*

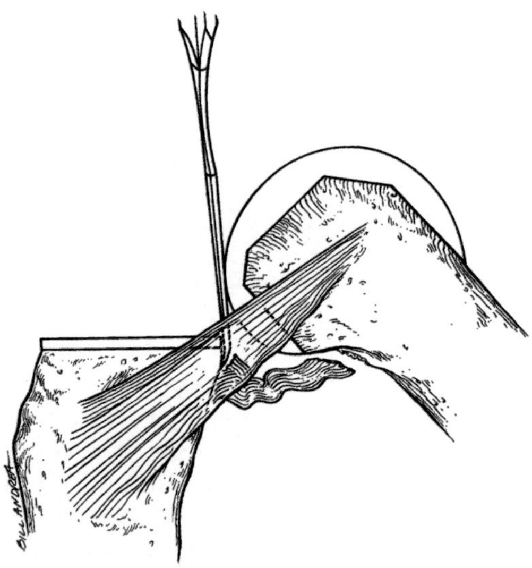

FIGURE 51-37. *With the knee in hyperflexion, the posterior-medial capsule also is elevated from its tibial attachment. It is unsafe to detach the posterior capsule from the lateral tibial surface because the peroneal nerve is easily damaged with this procedure. (Reprinted with permission.[28])*

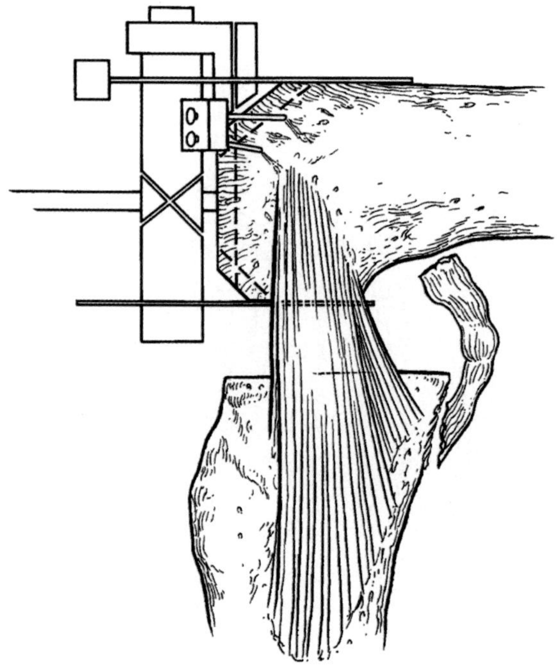

FIGURE 51-38. *Distal resection is done to decrease the cam effect of the femur in extension. Shims are used to position the resection guide, and the guide is placed to resect about 5 mm from the distal surface of the femur and both bevel surfaces. (Reprinted with permission.[25])*

Balancing the Posterior Cruciate Ligament

Posterior cruciate ligament contracture generally is apparent fairly early in the ligament balancing procedure. The femur rolls excessively posteriorly at 90° flexion, and palpation of the ligament reveals that it is very tight, especially in its anterolateral band. This ligament contracture is a common cause of tightening medially in flexion only and is the first thing to look for in these conditions (Fig. 51-39).

With the trial polyethylene component removed, the bone attachment of the posterior cruciate ligament can be accessed with a straight ¼-inch osteotome and this bone segment can be cut loose and elevated, allowing it to ride proximally, thus lengthening the ligament and leaving it attached to surrounding soft tissue structures (Figs. 51-40 and 51-41).

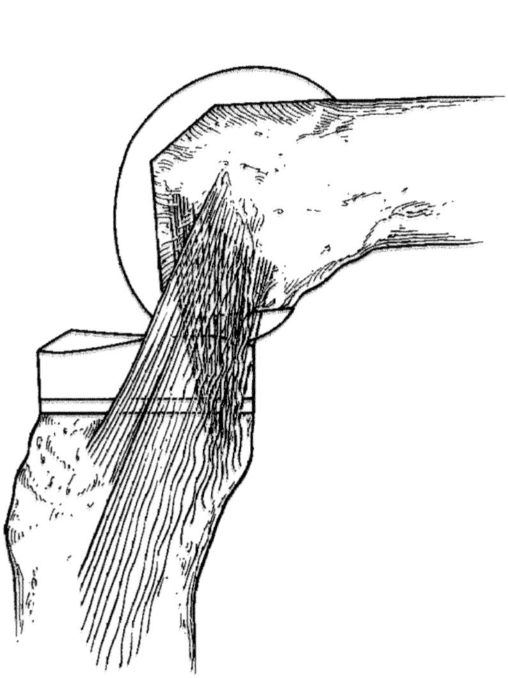

FIGURE 51-39. *On the side view, the femoral component is rolled excessively posteriorly, and is perched on the posterior edge of the tibial component. The anterior band of the medial collateral ligament also may be affected by this posterior position and may seem to be excessively tight. The anterolateral portion of the posterior cruciate ligament is primarily responsible for the excessive posterior rollback. (Reprinted with permission.[28])*

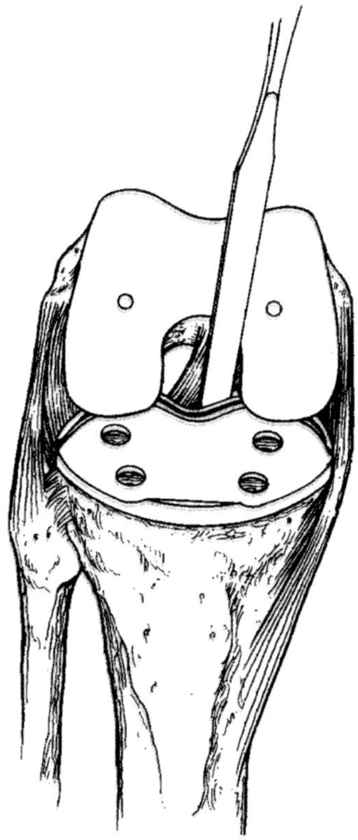

FIGURE 51-40. *The posterior cruciate ligament is released with a small segment of bone from its posterior tibial attachment. A ¼-inch osteotome is used to make several small cuts around the posterior cortical margin, and then the bone piece is levered loose. (Reprinted with permission.[28])*

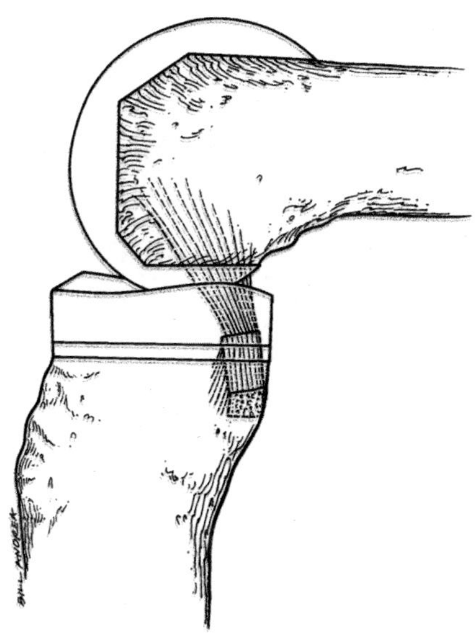

FIGURE 51-41. *The posterior cruciate ligament, in its new position, allows the tibia to slide posteriorly so that the femoral surfaces sit farther forward on the tibia. (Reprinted with permission.[28])*

When the posterior cruciate ligament is released, it is helpful to have a deep-dish or highly conforming polyethylene component available to prevent excessive posterior laxity, especially in flexion. This deep-dish polyethylene component improves anteroposterior stability and rotational stability throughout the flexion arc (Figs. 51-42 and 51-43).

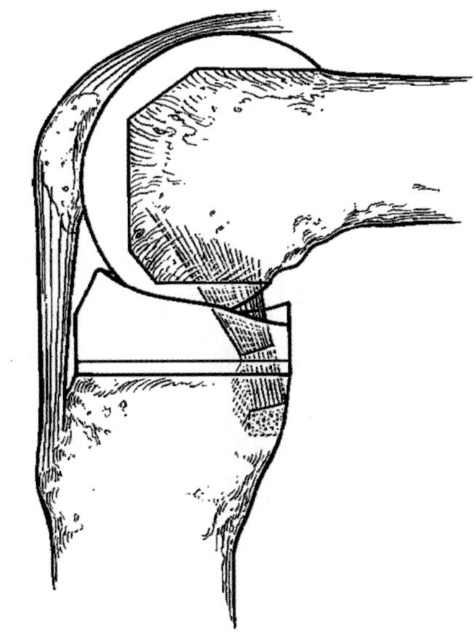

FIGURE 51-42. *When the deep-dish polyethylene insert is applied, posterior sag is controlled, and the tibia is held forward, improving the mechanical advantage of the quadriceps. The barrier to anterior dislocation of the femur (femoral jumping distance) is large both vertically and horizontally. (Reprinted with permission.[28])*

Patellar Ligament Balancing

Patellar ligament balancing is much more commonly necessary than is generally appreciated. If the patella does not track evenly in the patellar groove from 20° to past 120° flexion, the lateral ligamentous structures of the patella are likely to be too tight, and closure of the medial capsular structures will cause undue pressure on the patellar articular surface. Lateral patellar release can be done safely and effectively from outside the joint, approaching the lateral retinaculum directly and leaving the synovial membrane intact. With the knee held in 20° flexion, the lateral patellar retinaculum is exposed under the deep fascia and the connection between the iliotibial band and the lateral patellar edge clearly identified. The fibers from the iliotibial band to the patella can be released approximately 1 cm from the edge of the patella. This release can be extended farther proximally and farther distally, maintaining the lateral blood supply of the patella, which enters superficially over the top of the restraining lateral ligaments (Fig. 51-44).

Rarely the patella continues to tilt and sublux laterally after extensive lateral patellar release, and this is usually caused by abnormal Q angle. Transferring the lateral one-half of the patellar tendon medially over the top of the medial half corrects this with a soft tissue procedure, but in circumstances where the Q-angle abnormality is greater than 30°, the tibial tubercle itself must be transferred medially (Figs. 51-45 and 51-46).[27]

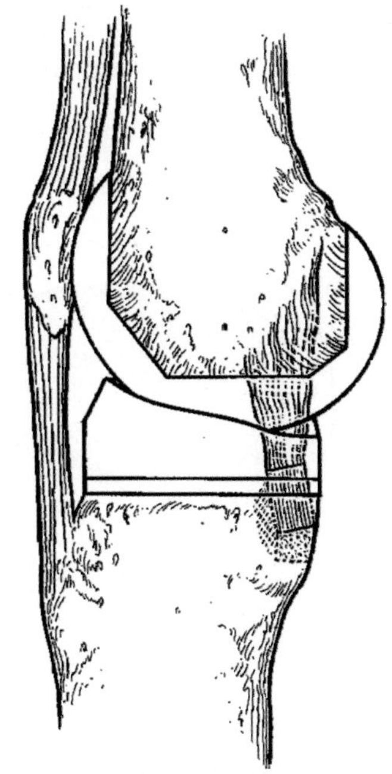

FIGURE 51-43. *In full extension the vertical and horizontal distance of travel required for subluxation also is large, and the tibia is held anteriorly by the anterior wall of the deep-dish prosthesis. (Reprinted with permission.[28])*

SUMMARY

The structure of the knee is complex and its behavior can be unpredictable even in the most experienced surgeon's hands. This is especially true in conditions involving arthritis, joint surface destruction, and deformity. However, the task of replacing the bone surfaces and balancing the ligaments can be made manageable by following a logical plan based on correct alignment throughout the arc of flexion and ligament release based on function of each ligament. Optimal knee function requires correct varus-valgus alignment in all positions of flexion. This requires reliable anatomic landmarks for alignment in flexion and extension.

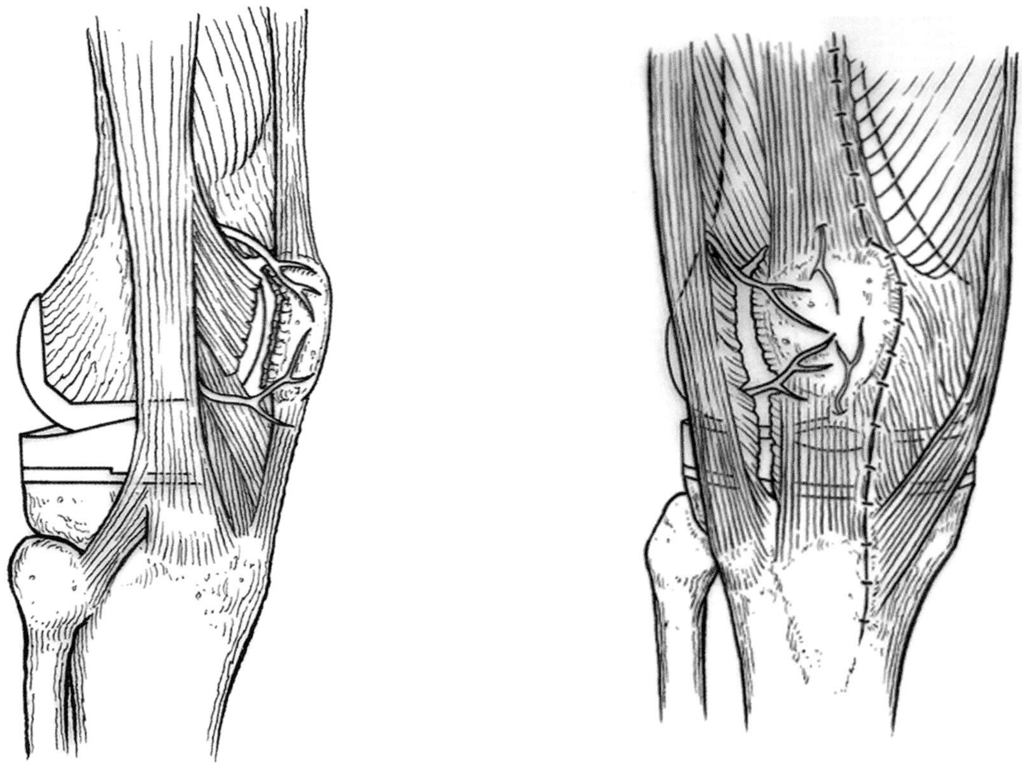

FIGURE 51-44. *Extended lateral patellar release includes the attachment of the oblique fibers of the vastus lateralis and the extension of the iliotibial band to the patellar tendon. This usually can be done extrasynovially without sacrificing the lateral vessels that enter the outer surface of the patella. Because these vessels are in the superficial layers of the lateral retinacular ligaments, the fibrous retinaculum can be released by passing a sharp knife blade under the vessels and transecting the deep fibers.*

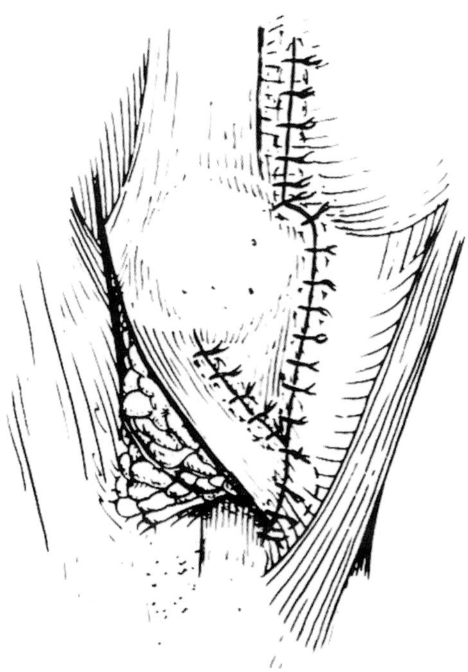

FIGURE 51-45. *The lateral half of the patellar tendon is crossed over the medial half, leaving the fat pad attachments intact, and the distal end is sutured under the medial capsular flap. Other sutures are added to secure its attachment. (Reprinted with permission.[29])*

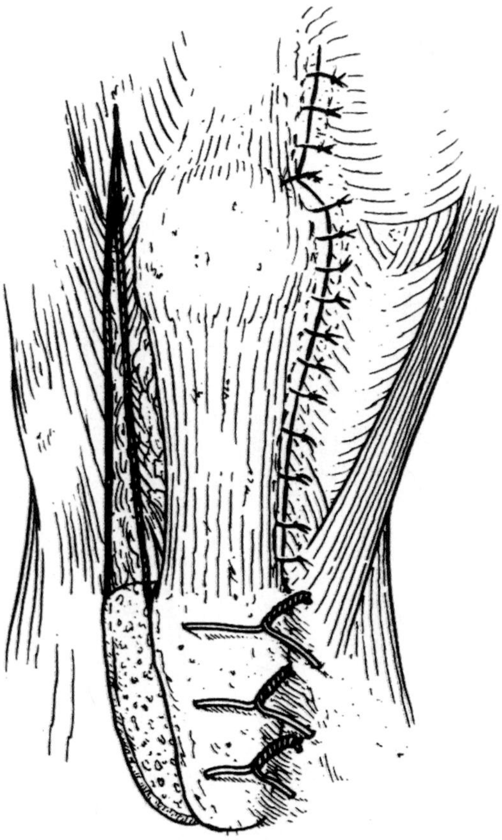

FIGURE 51-46. *The tibial tubercle has been shifted medially, and the medial capsular structures have been sutured. The lateral release has opened slightly to accommodate the medial shift of the quadriceps mechanism. (Reprinted with permission.[29])*

The long axes of the femur and tibia and the AP axis of the femur are highly reliable and provide the guidelines for establishing stable alignment of the joint surfaces by placing the tibia and patellar groove correctly in the median AP plane through the entire arc of flexion. Ligaments perform specific functions and these functions differ in different positions of knee flexion. Knowing their function and testing their tension provides the information necessary to release only the ligaments that are excessively tight, leaving those that are performing normally. Fractional release does not destabilize the knee because other ligaments are retained and because peripheral attachments of the ligament to other soft tissue structures such as the periosteum or synovial capsular tissue allow the released ligament to continue to function. Ligament release does not cause instability. Failure to align the knee and release tight ligaments does cause instability, unreliable function, and excessive wear. This chapter provides an outline of how knee kinematics should be assessed and ligaments balanced in total knee arthroplasty. Although it provides specific examples of common situations encountered by the surgeon, there are thousands of scenarios that can occur during this operation, so this chapter should be viewed as a guide that provides the basic knowledge of how the knee functions. With this knowledge, good instruments, and sound implants, the surgeon can align, balance, and stabilize the knee even in cases with severe bone destruction and ligament contracture.

ACKNOWLEDGMENTS

The author thanks William C. Andrea, MA, CMI, for preparation of the illustrations, and Diane J. Morton, MS, for preparation of the manuscript.

REFERENCES

1. Berger RA, Rubash HE, Seel MJ, et al. Determining the rotational alignment of the femoral component in total knee arthroplasty using the epicondylar axis. *Clin Orthop Relat Res.* 1993;286:40-49.
2. Yoshioka Y, Siu D, Cooke TDV. The anatomy and functional axes of the femur. *J Bone Joint Surg Am.* 1987;69:873-880.
3. Arima J, Whiteside LA. Femoral rotational alignment, based on the anteroposterior axis, in total knee arthroplasty in a valgus knee. *J Bone Joint Surg Am.* 1995;77:1331-1334.
4. Whiteside LA, McCarthy DS. Laboratory evaluation of alignment and kinematics in a unicompartmental knee arthroplasty inserted with intramedullary instrumentation. *Clin Orthop Relat Res.* 1992;274:238-247.
5. Whiteside LA, Arima J. The anteroposterior axis for femoral rotational alignment in valgus total knee arthroplasty. *Clin Orthop Relat Res.* 1995;321:168-172.
6. Akagi M, Yamashita E, Nakagawa T, et al. Relationship between frontal knee alignment and reference axes in the distal femur. *Clin Orthop Relat Res.* 2001;388:147-156.
7. Cooke TD, Pichora D, Siu D, et al. Surgical implications of varus deformity of the knee with obliquity of joint surfaces. *J Bone Joint Surg Br.* 1989;71:560-565.

8. Kanamiya T, Whiteside LA, Nakamura T, et al. Ranawat Award Paper. Effect of selective lateral ligament release on stability in knee arthroplasty. *Clin Orthop Relat Res.* 2002;404:24-31.
9. Saeki K, Mihalko WM, Patel V, et al. Stability after medial collateral ligament release in total knee arthroplasty. *Clin Orthop Relat Res.* 2001;392:184-189.
10. Whiteside LA. Correction of ligament and bone defects in total arthroplasty of the severely valgus knee. *Clin Orthop Relat Res.* 1993;288:234-245.
11. Whiteside LA. Ligament release and bone grafting in total arthroplasty of the varus knee. *Orthopedics.* 1995;18:117-122.
12. Whiteside LA. Positioning the femoral component: the effect of proper ligament balance. *Am J Knee Surg.* 2000;13:173-180.
13. Whiteside LA. Selective ligament release in total knee arthroplasty of the knee in valgus. *Clin Orthop Relat. Res.* 1999;367:130-140.
14. Whiteside LA. Soft tissue balancing. *J Arthroplasty.* 2002;17(4 Suppl 1):23-27.
15. Whiteside LA, Saeki K, Mihalko MW. Functional medial ligament balancing in total knee arthroplasty. *Clin Orthop Relat Res.* 2000;380:45-57.
16. Whiteside LA, Roy ME. Anatomy, function, and surgical access of the iliotibial band in total knee arthroplasty. *J Bone Joint Surg Am.* 2009;91(suppl 6):101-106.
17. Yoshii I, Whiteside LA, White SE, et al. Influence of prosthetic joint line position on knee kinematics and patellar position. *J Arthroplasty.* 1991;6:169-177.
18. Anouchi YS, Whiteside LA, Kaiser AD, et al. The effect of axial rotational alignment of the femoral component on knee stability and patellar tracking in total knee arthroplasty. *Clin Orthop Relat Res.* 1991; 287:170-177.
19. Hagena FW, Hofmann GO, Mittelmeier T, et al. The cruciate ligament in knee replacement. *Int Orthop.* 1989;13:13-16.
20. Hughston JC. The posterior cruciate ligament in knee-joint stability. Proceedings of the American Academy of Orthopaedic Surgeons. *J Bone Joint Surg Am.* 1969;51:1045.
21. Arima J, Whiteside LA, Martin JW, et al. Effect of partial release of the posterior cruciate ligament in total knee arthroplasty. *Clin Orthop Relat Res.* 1998; 353:194-202.
22. Whiteside LA, Kasselt MR, Haynes DW. Varus-valgus and rotational stability in rotationally unconstrained total knee arthroplasty. *Clin Orthop Relat Res.* 1987;219:147-157.
23. Whiteside LA, Summers RG. The effect of the level of distal femoral resection on ligament balance in total knee replacement. In: Dorr LD, ed. *The Knee: Papers of the First Scientific Meeting of the Knee Society.* Baltimore, MD: University Park Press; 1984:59-73.
24. Moreland JR, Bassett LW, Hanker GJ. Radiographic analysis of the axial alignment of the lower extremity. *J Bone Joint Surg Am.* 1987;69:745-749.
25. Mihalko WM, Whiteside LA. Bone resection and ligament treatment for flexion contracture in knee arthroplasty. *Clin Orthop Relat Res.* 2003;406:141-147.
26. Whiteside LA, Mihalko WM. Surgical procedure for flexion contracture and recurvatum in total knee arthroplasty. *Clin Orthop Relat Res.* 2002;404:189-195.
27. Matsuda S, Whiteside LA, White SE, et al. Knee kinematics of posterior cruciate ligament sacrificed total knee arthroplasty. *Clin Orthop Relat Res.* 1997; 341:257-266.
28. Whiteside LA, ed. *Ligament Balancing in Total Knee Arthroplasty. An Instructional Manual.* Berlin: Springer; 2004.
29. Whiteside LA. Distal realignment of the patellar tendon to correct abnormal patellar tracking. *Clin Orthop Relat Res.* 1997;344:284-289.

52 Constraint in Primary Total Knee Arthroplasty

Torrance Walker, Tyler Cannon, and William M. Mihalko

The goals for total knee arthroplasty (TKA) are to relieve pain, restore function, and provide a stable joint that will last for many years. Constraint, as it pertains to TKA, is an important concept to grasp, because it enables the surgeon to obtain excellent long-term survivorship and successful outcomes for his or her patients who undergo a TKA. Instability accounts for up to 25% of all revisions after TKA. Therefore, obtaining appropriate soft tissue balance and component alignment in the coronal and sagittal planes is paramount. When soft tissue is tenuous, the surgeon must have avenues to obtain a stable knee before leaving the operating room. Many times it is the use of implant constraint that allows the surgeon to obtain optimal stability.

Constraint is defined as the resistance to rotation or displacement in the coronal, transverse, and sagittal planes. Constraint is dictated by component design such as the shape and conformity of bearing surfaces and other mechanical design features of the implant that can resist movement in the three anatomic planes. Constraint comes with a price, since increased constraint in the prosthetic design causes increased forces to be transmitted to the component fixation interfaces, which may cause the implant to fail via aseptic loosening. With competent bony and ligamentous architecture, using the least amount of constraint should therefore be the aim for every surgeon, especially when it comes to constraint in the coronal plane. Some surgeons use a stepwise approach during the procedure in which a decision is made at the time of trial implant insertion to retain or sacrifice the posterior cruciate ligament (PCL) based on its pathology or support of the knee in flexion.[1] As the degree of deformity, bone loss, osteopenia, contracture, ligamentous instability, and poor neuromuscular control increases, so might the demand for prosthetic constraint. When ligaments and muscle forces are less reliabile, then the resistance to displacement is then placed on the conformity of the tibial bearing surfaces and friction of the metal–polyethylene interface.

The PCL serves primarily to resist posterior translation of the tibia relative to the femur, but it also has secondary roles in varus-valgus stability of the knee and in limiting internal rotation of the tibia.[2] The origin of the PCL is along the medial aspect of the medial femoral intercondylar notch or along the lateral border of the femoral condyle, while its insertion is on the posterior aspect of the tibial plateau between the two condyles (Fig. 52-1). The PCL elongates during flexion and tightens at 90° and above. This characteristic facilitates femoral rollback during knee flexion. Femoral rollback improves quadriceps efficiency by moving the femoral condyle posteriorly and placing the tibia forward for a better mechanical advantage of the extensor mechanism.[3] Femoral rollback has been shown to be important in knee kinematics and improvement in knee flexion.[4-8] Thus, some advocate preservation of the PCL in TKA in order to reproduce normal knee kinematics via preservation of anatomic femoral rollback, preservation of femoral bone stock, and increased knee range of motion. Several studies have confirmed that normal knee kinematics are not restored after a cruciate-retaining (CR) TKA. Yue et al used dual fluoroscopic imaging to evaluate the in vivo kinematics of the knee with medial compartment osteoarthritis before and after CR TKA.[7] There was no restoration of the normal internal/external tibial rotation or femoral rollback

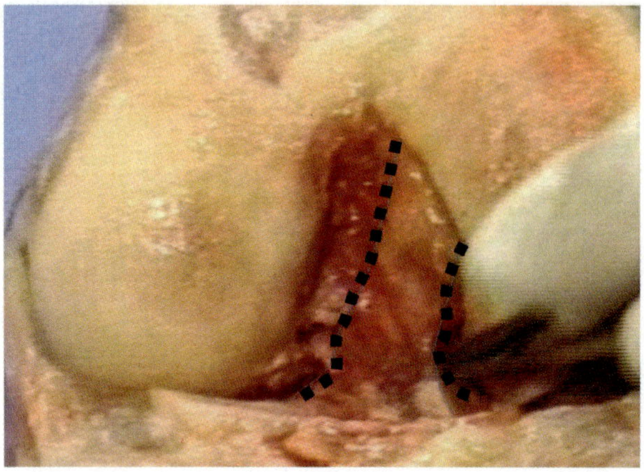

FIGURE 52-1. *A PCL shown from a CR TKA at the time of necropsy. This PCL appeared to remain functioning and intact.*

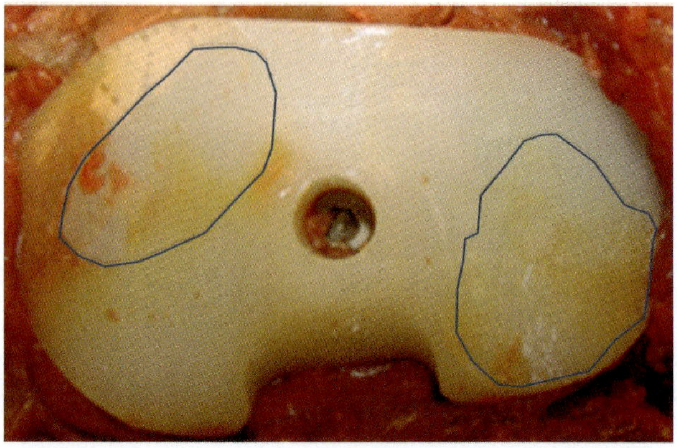

FIGURE 52-2. *A polyethylene tibial insert retrieved at time of necropsy. This insert functioned for over 10 years and the roll-forward wear pattern is evident on the medial side of the insert with no evidence of wear on the posterior medial aspect of the insert.*

after CR TKA. Instead, there was an abnormal anterior femoral translation during early knee flexion. In another study by Dennis and associates, in vivo fluoroscopic analysis showed a "paradoxical motion" in which there was absence of the normal posterior femoral rollback during knee flexion in posterior cruciate-retaining TKA (Fig. 52-2).[8] Instead, there was unpredictable anterior translation of the femoral condyle during deep knee flexion. This is similar to the pattern of cartilage deformation and altered kinematics associated with PCL-deficient knees in which there is a resultant anterior and medial shift of the tibiofemoral contact location and an increase in cartilage deformation in the medial compartment beyond 75° of knee flexion.[9] Zelle et al noticed that femoral rollback patterns during deep knee flexion were only marginally affected when extra posterior tibial slope is added, whereas additional PCL release resulted in paradoxical anterior movement of the femur.[10]

Several factors have been shown to reduce femoral rollback, including increasing tibial polyethylene conformity.[11] Increasing conformity causes increased stresses to be transferred to the bone–cement interface, potentially leading to loosening. Mobile-bearing designs were developed to reduce this potential increased stress at the bone–cement interface and lessen the resulting polyethylene wear to improve TKA survivorship. A recent meta-analysis comparing fixed bearing and mobile-bearing total knee arthroplasty showed a statistically significant improvement in the incidence of tibial radiolucent lines with mobile-bearing devices, but no differences in outcomes such as instability, persistent pain, loosening, Knee Society pain and function scores, and clinical range of motion were found.[12]

There is a continuum of constraint now available in most total knee arthroplasty systems. These implant systems allow seamless transition from a relatively unconstrained, cruciate-retaining articulation to a posterior-stabilized and varus-valgus constrained articulation. The types can be described as (1) cruciate-retaining, (2) posterior-stabilized (PS), and (3) constrained condylar (or one that limits varus-valgus deflection at the knee) unlinked implants.

CRUCIATE-RETAINING TOTAL KNEE ARTHROPLASTY

CR designs have a degree of constraint that is moderate and depend on an intact PCL for posterior stability. The minimized constraint conveys less shear forces at the tibial component–host interface. Another advantage of CR is the preservation of the femoral bone stock for future surgery. Additional benefits of using a CR implant that have been discussed in the literature include fewer patellar complications and the potential for improved proprioception via retained mechanoreceptors.[13] A recent histologic analysis of the PCL retrieved from a well-functioning TKA confirmed the presence of pacini and lamellar-type mechanoreceptors (Fig. 52-3).[13] In addition, a randomized controlled study by Swanik et al[14] revealed mild improvement in proprioception, kinesthesia, and balance after TKA, but retention of the PCL did not appear to show a significant improvement in proprioception and balance when compared with those functions in patients with a PS total knee design.

The decision to use a cruciate-retaining versus a posterior-stabilized implant is still a controversial topic in total knee arthroplasty. CR TKA has shown consistently good long-term results. Some surgeons are devoted to using CR implants for primary TKA because of their training or personal philosophy. These surgeons always retain and "balance" the PCL essentially for any mild, moderate, or severe deformity. Others consistently use a PS device. Still other surgeons preserve the option to retain or substitute the PCL and decide at the time of surgery depending on several factors such as PCL integrity, severe deformity or malalignment, contracture, weight, and age of the patient.

There are no firm disadvantages to using a CR implant. However, there is a rare but potential risk for late rupture of the PCL from a traumatic event, such as a direct blow to the flexed knee in a fall or motor vehicle accident. Also, the PCL could possibly become attenuated over time and provide less stability than was initially obtained at the time of surgery. These patients would report weakness and instability with descending stairs.[15] Due to the possibility of late laxity, some surgeons recommend against PCL retention in patients with rheumatoid arthritis in whom the disease process could lead to attenuation of the ligament and result in flexion instability. But CR advocates point out that the PCL is an extracapsular structure and should not be exposed to rheumatoid arthritis synovitis. Moreover, use of a CR implant may be contraindicated in patients with prior patellectomy. This is because inconsistent rollback kinematics will decrease the moment arm afforded to the extensor mechanism and may significantly decrease the extensor strength of the knee while ascending or descending stairs.

In many knee systems, the CR implant will come with choices for a high-lip or deep-dish polyethylene option (Fig. 52-4). These inserts are utilized during CR TKA in cases in which the PCL support may be tenuous and will limit the amount of anterior translation of the femoral implant condyles on the tibial polyethylene insert.

POSTERIOR-STABILIZED TOTAL KNEE ARTHROPLASTY

PS implants have a somewhat higher constraint of the tibial inserts to increase stability to posterior translation of the femoral condyles on the tibial polyethylene and offset the loss of the PCL. The cam and post in PS implants have been shown to allow more femoral rollback than CR designs, which is also more consistent in nature. The cam-post mechanism provides anteroposterior translational stability, but does not constrain varus-valgus or internal and external rotations. In flexion, however, the design does not inhibit the amount of distraction that may occur if there is a flexion gap mismatch, which may allow the jump height of the polyethylene peg to be overcome and dislocate the post-cam mechanism (Figs. 52-5 and 52-6). Ligament balancing in a varus knee often involves less balancing of the medial structures since the PCL is a secondary varus stabilizer. The surgeon should be cautious not to overrelease structures medially in a varus knee because excessive release of anatomic structures off of the proximal tibia may "overshoot" the targeted medial gap and necessitate a constrained condylar implant, since a PS implant will not constrain the varus and valgus deflection of the knee.

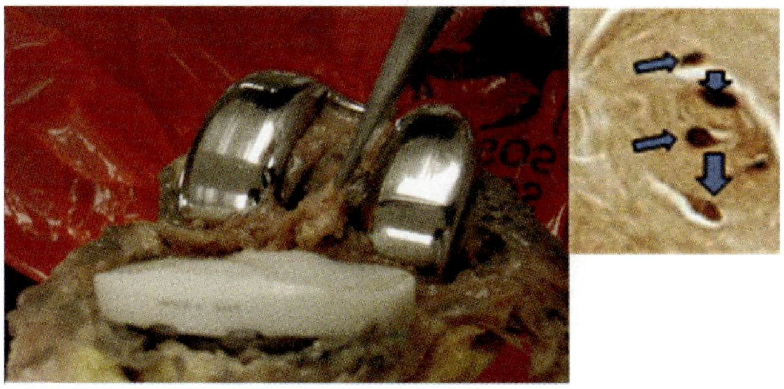

FIGURE 52-3. *A PCL retrieved from a well-functioning TKA at the time of necropsy underwent immunohistochemical staining with neurofilament protein. Examination under ×40 light microscopy revealed the presence of different mechanoreceptors in the ligament.*

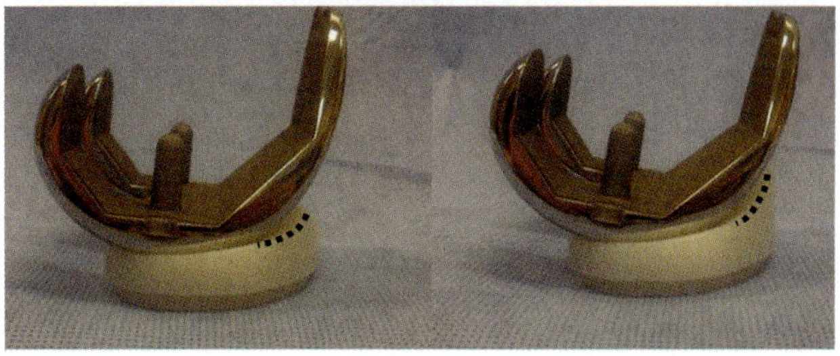

FIGURE 52-4. *Many CR knee systems will include a standard insert (left) and a deep-dished or anterior-lipped insert (right). The deep-dished insert increases anterior support and resists anterior translation or posterior sag in flexion. (Columbus Knee System Aesculap Inc.)*

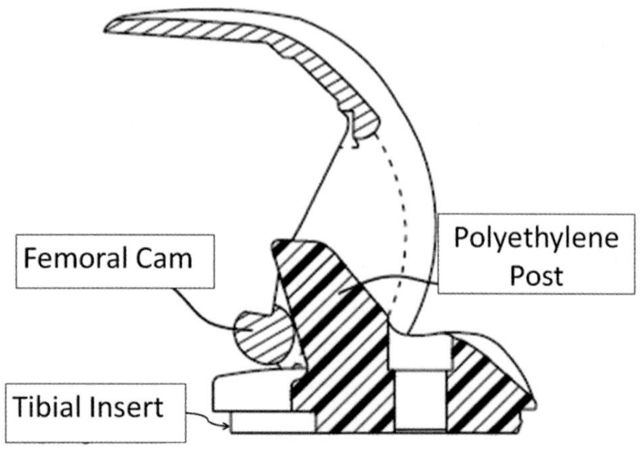

FIGURE 52-5. *Sagittal cross section of a PS knee design. When the cam is located more posterior and superior along the posterior femoral condyles, then the cam will engage later in flexion but will stay low in flexion. This will increase the jump height and decrease the likelihood of the cam jumping the post.*

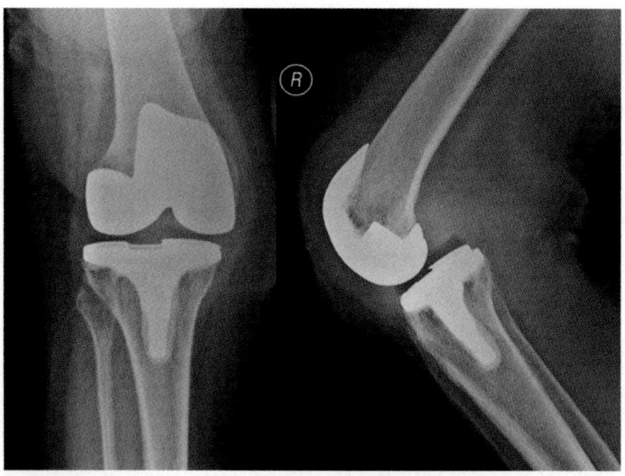

FIGURE 52-6. *An anteroposterior and lateral radiograph of a patient who had a patellectomy at a younger age and then succumbed to a PS TKA for posttraumatic arthritis. After 10 years the patient dislocated the post cam mechanism from post wear and posterior tissue laxity and muscle atrophy.*

The effect of PCL release on the flexion-extension gap ratio has been studied. A cadaveric study by Mihalko and Krackow[16] concluded that PCL sacrifice creates a larger flexion gap at 90° in a range of 3.2 to 9.1 mm but no difference in the joint space in full extension. A study by Schnurr et al[17] using data from computer navigation also revealed that PCL sacrifice had no effect on the extension gap, but it increased the flexion gap >3 mm in 36% of patients, >5 mm in 12%, and had no clinically relevant effect (<2 mm) in 44% of patients. The authors concluded that PCL release had an unpredictable increase on the flexion-extension gap ratio and recommended PCL release before femoral resections are performed.

Several studies have noted that PS TKAs performed better and provided more rollback than did CR designs. Arbuthnot et al[18] concluded that the use of the PS prosthesis for TKA provided a more predictable outcome with regard to posterior sag and a better maximum flexion than a CR implant. The study by Mahoney et al[19] revealed a better extensor mechanism efficiency in PS designs than did CR TKA. It was subsequently suggested that PS designs more closely replicate normal knee kinematics than do CR designs but neither fully restores normal posterior femoral rollback. Thus, the kinematics of the PS knee is more predictable and is dictated by the conforming geometry of the tibiofemoral articulation and the interaction of the tibial post-and-cam mechanism.[3]

Indications for a PS implant include patients who have undergone a previous patellectomy, patients with increased risk for late PCL rupture, and patients with rheumatoid arthritis. The PS knee is considered by many to be an absolute indication for patients with prior patellectomy because of the consistent nature of guided rollback in flexion, which optimizes the quadriceps mechanism moment arm after loss of the patella. These patients have an altered four-bar linkage between the quadriceps and patella tendon and the anterior and posterior cruciate ligaments. The PCL in patellectomy patients sustains a great amount of strain and is prone to developing instability. Also, the use of PS implants have been shown in some studies to be more beneficial in patients at increased risk for late PCL rupture, such as patients with poor neuromuscular control or patients with inflammatory arthropathy. PS TKA should be considered for patients with rheumatoid arthritis, since previous studies have reported on the increased risk of late instability in these patients. Tang et al reported on a series of young patients with rheumatoid arthritis treated with PCL-substituting devices.[20] The mean age at surgery was 41.9 years. Using revision of any component as the end point, the mean 10-year survival rate was 94%.

Disadvantages of PS designs include polyethylene wear from the cam-post mechanism, which can lead to osteolysis, and increased implant bone interface stresses, which may lead to aseptic loosening and failure of the TKA. Patellar clunk syndrome is a well-known soft tissue impingement associated with PS knees. However, its incidence has been reduced with today's design features with longer trochlear groove support. The need for additional bone resection to accommodate the femoral box may predispose to fracture of the femoral condyle as well. Due to the widened flexion space and lack of a PCL in PS knees, there is an increased risk of dislocation or instability in flexion due to flexion-extension gap imbalance. To offset this increase in the flexion gap, some surgeons will increase the distal femoral resection by 1 or 2 mm to allow a larger polyethylene insert to be utilized, which will fill the flexion gap and decrease the risk of flexion instability.

MOBILE-BEARING TOTAL KNEE ARTHROPLASTY

Mobile-bearing (MB) implants for TKA have emerged as a newer design in an attempt to improve polyethylene wear resistance and reduce mechanical loosening in the treatment of disabling knee pain. MB implants are available in multiple forms: rotating platform (allows rotation about an axis without translation, Fig. 52-7), mobile platform (translates a certain amount and rotates with built-in stops), and meniscal-bearing designs, which have independent medial and lateral polyethylene bearings that translate in the anteroposterior direction. The rotating and mobile platforms

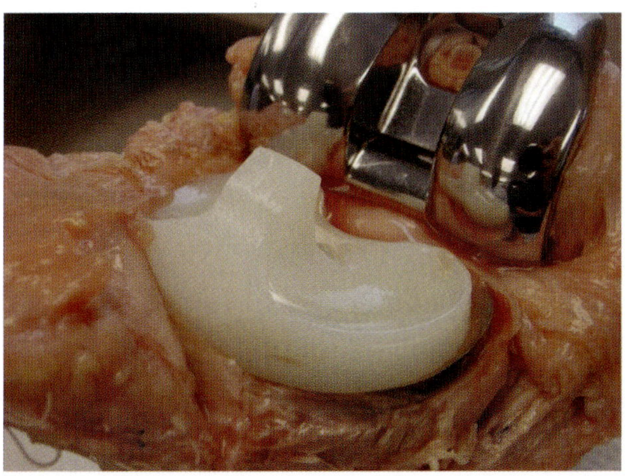

FIGURE 52-7. *A mobile design on a rotating platform retrieved at the time of necropsy. Although well functioning, this implant had significant wear along the anterior aspect of the tibial post from impingement of the anterior aspect of the femoral box and the inferior aspect of the patellar button in flexion.*

are also available in CR and PS designs. Theoretically, this construct ultimately increases contact area for less contact stress and reduction of polyethylene wear. There have been many arguments for and against the decreased wear claim with MB TKA designs. Adding the backside polyethylene bearing also makes it difficult to track how much wear results in these designs and where the particles originate. The decrease in the rotational constraint does decrease the stress that is transferred to the tibial implant–bone interface and is an advantage for both primary and revision TKA. Mobile-bearing implants provide less constraint for greater potential range of motion. However, both CR and PS mobile-bearing constructs seem to have similar ranges of motion.[21,22]

Polyethylene wear may be minimized in MB designs by imparting greater contact area with lower contact stress in the polyethylene. Mobile-bearing TKAs may be more tolerant of small amounts of tibial component malrotation in the transverse plane because the design offers an inherent ability for self-alignment of the tibial component. An additional benefit of mobile-bearing TKAs is enhanced extensor mechanism alignment for potential improvement of patellar tracking and patellofemoral contact stress.[23] Therefore, mobile-bearing knees may provide optimal kinematics secondary to less constraint and improved patellar tracking for ultimately greater potential range of motion and less polyethylene wear.

Disadvantages to mobile-bearing TKAs include spinout (a rotating poly is subluxed where the femoral implant is no longer in contact with the polyethylene) or spitout (a mobile platform is subluxed anteriorly where neither of the femoral condylar articulating surfaces is in contact with polyethylene) and an additional extra bearing surface.[24,25] Most commonly, lateral spinout occurs in meniscal-bearing TKA as a result of surgical technique from a flexion gap imbalance or a tight PCL. Cruciate-retaining components are more frequently associated with spinout due to the presence of the PCL as well as lack of a post for intercondylar restraint. Partial or complete release of the PCL is an initial option, followed possibly by release of the popliteus tendon and addition of a larger insert. Fisher et al[26] reveal that risks for spinout should include female gender, obesity, and preoperative valgus-positioned knees. Medial spinout may be caused by a tight popliteus tendon in flexion which rotates the bearing out medially.

Paradoxical rotation is also a possibility in mobile-bearing TKA as the polyethylene bearing may slip anterior instead of rotating posterior as the knee flexes, thus causing impingement on the posterior edge of the metal tray against the posterior structures of the knee.[27] There have been reports of abnormal rotation in the transverse plane with fluoroscopic kinematic analysis. Paradoxical rotation of the femoral component in flexion to 90° may be a feature more common in CR than PS mobile-bearing knees, and the cam-and-post mechanism is important for posterior femoral roll-back with increasing knee flexion.[28] Similar to fixed-bearing constructs, tibiofemoral dislocation and polyethylene tray dissociation may also develop secondary to flexion gap instability.

Because of the need for optimal flexion and extension gap balancing to prevent spinout, many surgeons advocate preparing the tibia side of the joint first when utilizing MB implants. From here the flexion gap is squared by rotating the femoral component to optimize the rectangular nature of the flexion gap and allow it to be matched to the extension gap with the distal femoral resection depth. Care should be taken, however, if significant soft tissue releases are necessary to balance the extension gap, that a medial soft tissue release does not open the flexion gap to the point that it results in an internally rotated femoral component to equalize the flexion gap. This may occur since a significant release of medial structures off of the proximal tibia has been shown to create more release in flexion than extension.[29]

MB TKA has less constraint in the transverse plane and therefore may have a relative indication for use in patients with an ipsilateral hip fusion to decrease the stresses imparted onto the tibial baseplate fixation interface.

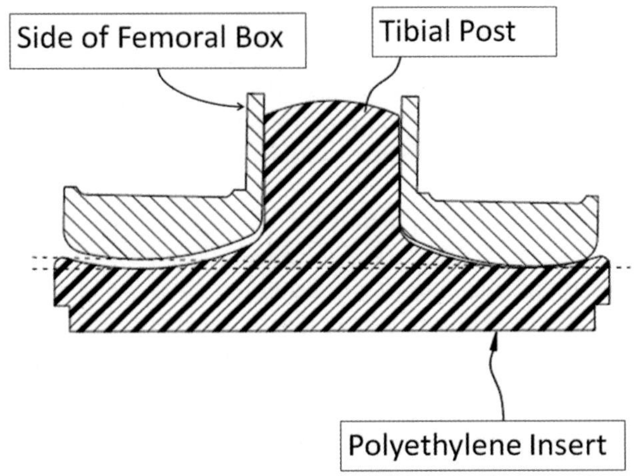

FIGURE 52-8. *A design schematic for a constrained condylar type of peg. In this case 1° to 2° of varus or valgus deflection is allowed before the post is supported against the sides of the box. This gives support to an attenuated medial or lateral soft tissue sleeve.*

CONSTRAINED CONDYLAR TOTAL KNEE ARTHROPLASTY

Constrained condylar implants have more varus-valgus and rotational constraint than do PS implants. This is accomplished by an unlinked, tall tibial post that has a tighter coronal fill in the deep femoral box on the femoral component (Fig. 52-8). Constrained condylar implants are used when the soft tissues are not supportive, especially when one of the collateral ligaments is incompetent. These implants are used more commonly in primary TKA when the medial or lateral collateral ligament is attenuated, such as in patients with severe valgus or varus deformities or in the revision setting with loss of epicondylar support of a collateral ligament. Another instance when these components are utilized is when there is residual instability or irreconcilable flexion-extension imbalances, which may occur after release of the PCL or loss of collateral support.[29] One disadvantage includes the need for removal of more femoral bone stock with some implant systems. Also, with significant soft tissue and ligament compromise, the femoral and tibial components will often require stem extensions to transmit stresses generated by the constrained articulation away from the bone–cement interface to the diaphyseal bone for uncemented stems or dissipate the increased stresses along a broader surface area for cemented extensions. These increased stresses may still lead to aseptic implant loosening and a higher failure rate. Also, excessive stresses at the tibial cam mechanism could result in failure or fracture of the tibial intercondylar eminence. Additionally, these implants are contraindicated when there is loss of epicondylar support from bone loss or complete loss of the collaterals because the flexion space will exceed the jump height for the implant resulting in posterior dislocation.[16]

CLINICAL OUTCOMES

Although there are many differences between PS and CR designs, most studies have found no significant differences in Knee Society scores, patient satisfaction, loosening, and survivorship (Table 52-1).

Whiteside[30] reported on 265 Ortholoc-1 CR TKAs in 202 patients at a minimum of 15 years of follow-up. One knee was revised for loosening and five knees were revised for infection. The survival rate at 18 years was 98.6%. At 15 years after surgery, 79.9% of patients did not have pain, 10.1% had mild pain, 8% had moderate pain, and 2% had severe pain. At 18 years after surgery, 77.6% did not have

TABLE 52-1. Results of Primary Total Knee Arthroplasty

Author(s) (Year)	Number of Knees	Constraint	Mean Follow-up (Range)	Survivorship
Whiteside (2001)	265	PCL-retained	(15-18 years)	98.6% without infection 96.1% without revision
Sextro et al (2001)	66	PCL-retained	15 years	88.7% without infection 85.1% without revision
Dixon et al (2005)	139	PCL-retained	15 years	92.6% at 15 years
Gill and Joshi (2001)	254	PCL-retained	16.8 years	96% at 15 years 82% at 23 years
Schwartz et al (2010)	126	PCL-retained	10 years	97.7% without revision
Rasquinha et al (2006)	150	Posterior-stabilized	12 years	94.6% survivorship
Tang et al (2004)	86	Posterior-stabilized	7.8 years	94% at 10 years
Lee et al (2011)	168	Posterior-stabilized	7 years	98% survivorship
Pavone et al (2001)	34	Posterior-stabilized	23 years	91% survivorship
Smith et al (2011)	Meta-analysis	Mobile-bearing	14 studies	No difference in KSS No difference in ROM
Sykes et al (2011)	Meta-analysis	Mobile-bearing	27 studies	No difference in KSS No difference in ROM
Anderson et al (2006)	70	Constrained condylar	44.5 months (2-6 years)	No loosening No revisions
Anderson et al (2007)	148	Constrained condylar	47 months (24-72 months)	2.5% failure rate

PCL, posterior cruciate ligament; KSS, Knee Society score; ROM, range of motion.

pain, 7.2% had mild pain, 5.2% had moderate pain, and 1% had severe pain. Sextro et al[31] reported on 66 posterior cruciate-retaining total knees in 50 patients at a mean follow-up of 15 years and noted an implant survival rate of 88.7% excluding infection. The 15-year survivorship free of radiographic loosening and/or revision of any component was 85.1%. Dixon et al[32] reported on 139 cruciate-retaining TKAs in 109 patients at a minimum follow-up of 15 years. There were five reoperations, four of which were performed because of wear of the polyethylene insert. There was one revision at 15 years for a loose cemented femoral component. The survival rate without revision or a need for any reoperation was 92.6% at 15 years. Gill and Joshi[33] reported the results of 254 CR TKAs in 223 patients at an average follow-up of 16.8 years. No patient was lost to follow-up. Revision was performed in 10 knees with an implant survival of 96% at 15 years and 82% at 23 years. Schwartz et al[34] reviewed 126 CR TKAs in 113 patients at a minimum follow-up of 10 years. Three knees were revised: one for infection, one for periprosthetic fracture, and one for postoperative arthrofibrosis. Using revision for any reason and revision for aseptic loosening, the authors reported a 97.7% and 100% survivorship, respectively.

Rasquinha et al[35] reported the results of 150 consecutive primary PS modular TKAs in 118 patients. At a mean follow-up of 12 years, there were two revisions for polyethylene wear with femoral osteolysis, one revision for dislocation, and two revisions for infection, for an overall prosthesis survival rate of 94.6%. Tang et al[20] reviewed 86 PCL-substituting TKAs in 52 rheumatoid patients at a mean age of 41.9 years. Revision was performed for one knee because of aseptic loosening of the tibial component, and for three knees because of deep infection. The 10-year survival rate was 94%. The average follow-up period in this study was 7.8 years. Lee et al[36] compared the results of 82 PS TKAs with preoperative severe varus deformity (varus angles ≥ 15°) with those in 86 PS TKAs with mild varus deformity (varus angle ≤ 5°). Both groups showed the same survival rate of 98% at 7 years with no significant differences in terms of perioperative complications. Pavone et al[37] reported the results of 34 total condylar replacements in the 26 patients who were available for clinical follow-up from the overall 80 patients (120 knees). Three revisions occurred in this group of 26 patients available for follow-up, for an implant survivorship of 91% at 23 years follow-up.

Mobile-bearing constructs in TKA appear to have equivalent survivorship to fixed-bearing implants. However, long-term studies are needed for further comparison.[24,25] Smith and colleagues[25] performed a meta-analysis concerning MB TKA outcomes and combined data from 14 studies and found no difference in Knee Society scores, Hospital for Special Surgery scores, and range of motion. Sykes et al[12] performed a meta-analysis comparing MB and fixed-bearing TKA and found similar results. They analyzed 27 studies in the literature and found no clinical difference in range of motion or in Knee Society scores. There was a lower incidence of tibial radiolucent lines in the MB TKA group.

Anderson et al[38] has reported on the use of constrained condylar total knee arthroplasty for valgus deformed knees without the use of stems. This report was a retrospective analysis of 70 consecutive valgus TKA where constrained condylar implants were utilized. At an average of 44.5 months of follow-up, there were no failures and no knees had signs of medial instability or radiographic signs of loosening. Knee Society score and functional scores improved from 34 points and 40 points to 93 and 74 points, respectively. Their conclusions were that avoiding stem extensions in these cases may decrease operative time, prosthetic cost, and canal invasion at surgery. Another larger study by Anderson and colleagues[39] retrospectively reviewed 180 patients with 248 constrained condylar TKAs for severe varus or valgus deformity. There were 192 TKAs in 148 patients available for follow-up at a mean of 47 months. Failure rate in this series was 2.5% with two infections, one aseptic failure, one periprosthetic fracture, and one post failure. The authors questioned the need for stem extensions in these primary TKA cases. However, these studies are both short-term to midterm follow-up studies that may not exhibit the full nature of risk of failures from aseptic loosening at 10 or more years.

It seems that the literature points to the fact that, if performed appropriately, the ranges of constraint used in TKA can result in comparable outcomes. It must be the surgeon who decides when use of the higher constraint is necessary and which primary type of implant (CR, PS, or MB) works best in his or her hands.

SUMMARY

Many TKA systems offer a continuum of constraint that gives the surgeon the flexibility to modify the degree of constraint required based on the soft tissue support and deformity. Knowing when to utilize more constraint is paramount to assure optimal stability before leaving the operating room. When the soft tissue and bony support about the knee allow for anything less than a constrained condylar implant to be utilized and result in a stable knee, then the surgeon should follow through with this rule.

SURGICAL PEARLS AND PITFALLS

When performing a CR TKA, the surgeon should remember that most CR surgeons believe that matched bone resection technique is preferable. The surgeon must make certain that the PCL is not tight in flexion. This will be evident with the trial components in place and liftoff of the trial tibial insert in flexion. The PCL is a medial structure and this happens in varus deformed knees. In this case, the PCL must be recessed or partially released. The anterior fibers are released off of the tibial insertion until the liftoff of the tibial insert no longer occurs. One should be careful that the PCL still is supportive of posterior tibial translation and that the femoral condyles are articulating in the posterior half of the tibial insert. If the PCL is no longer supportive, then use of a high-lipped anterior insert or conversion to a PS TKA should be performed.

During a PS TKA, the surgeon must make certain the PCL is released first before any soft tissue balancing, especially in the varus knee. The surgeon should also be careful not to create an anterior notch when sizing and performing the anterior femoral resection. With the added bone loss from the box preparation, this can increase the possibility of a periprosthetic fracture after surgery. Care should also be taken not to have excessive posterior slope to the tibia because this can increase the chances of cam jumping the peg in flexion.

A mobile-bearing TKA must have proper flexion and extension gap balancing. Proper patient selection is key, since those with large coronal or sagittal plane deformity may not have adequate soft tissue support once release is performed to adequately equalize the flexion and extension gaps. A tight PCL or popliteus can be the source of spinout after surgery. A gap balancing technique with preparation of the tibia first can aid in the gap balancing during MB TKA.

A constrained condylar TKA must have proper rotation of components due to lower tolerance of the cam and peg. A transverse plane malrotation may create a scenario where the peg does not properly engage the sides of the femoral box as the knee flexes. The surgeon must make certain when using a constrained condylar type of knee implant that the flexion space is not too large or loss of collateral support is present. This can result in the cam jumping the peg.

REFERENCES

1. Lombardi AV Jr, Berend KR. Posterior cruciate ligament-retaining, posterior stabilized, and varus/valgus posterior stabilized constrained articulations in total knee arthroplasty. *Instr Course Lect.* 2006;55:419-427.
2. Kazuhiko S, Mihalko WM, Patel V, et al. Stability after medical collateral ligament release in total knee arthroplasty. *Clin Orthop Relat Res.* 2001;392:184-189.
3. Pagnano MW, Cushner FD, Scott WN. Role of the posterior cruciate ligament in total knee arthroplasty. *J Am Acad Orthop Surg.* 1998;6:176-187.
4. Banks SA, Bellemans J, Nozaki H, et al. Knee motions during maximum flexion in fixed and mobile-bearing arthroplasties. *Clin Orthop Relat Res.* 2003;410:131-138.
5. Banks SA, Markovich GD, Hodge WA. In vivo kinematics of cruciate-retaining and -substituting knee arthroplasties. *J Arthroplasty.* 1997;12:297-304.
6. Dennis DA, Komistek RD, Mahfouz MR. In vivo fluoroscopic analysis of fixed-bearing total knee replacements. *Clin Orthop Relat Res.* 2003;410:114-130.
7. Yue B, Varadarajan KM, Moynihan AL, et al. Kinematics of medial osteoarthritic knees before and after posterior cruciate ligament retaining total knee arthroplasty. *J Orthop Res.* 2011;29(1):40-46.
8. Dennis DA, Komistek RD, Mahfouz MR, et al. Multicenter determination of in vivo kinematics after total knee arthroplasty. *Clin Orthop Relat Res.* 2003;416:37-57.
9. Van de Velde SK, Bingham JT, Gill TJ, et al. Analysis of tibiofemoral cartilage deformation in the posterior cruciate ligament-deficient knee. *J Bone Joint Surg Am.* 2009;91:167-175.
10. Zelle J, Heesterbeek PJ, De Waal Malefijt M, et al. Numerical analysis of variations in posterior cruciate ligament properties and balancing techniques on total knee arthroplasty loading. *Med Eng Phys.* 2010;32(7):700-707.
11. D'Lima DD, Chen PC, Colwell CW Jr. Polyethylene contact stresses, articular congruity, and knee alignment. *Clin Orthop Relat Res.* 2001;392:232-238.
12. Sykes J, Snearly C, Benner R, et al. Comparison of mobile bearing and fixed bearing total knee arthroplasty outcomes: a review of the literature. *J ASTM Int.* Feb 11, 2011;8(2) [Epub].
13. Mihalko WM, Creek AT, Mary MN, et al. Mechanoreceptors found in a posteror cruciate ligament from a well-functioning total knee arthroplasty retrieval. *J Arthroplasty.* 2011;26(3):504.e9-504.e12.
14. Swanik CB, Lephart SM, Rubash HE. Proprioception, kinesthesia, and balance after total knee arthroplasty with cruciate-retaining and posterior stabilized prostheses. *J Bone Joint Surg Am.* 2004;86(2):328-334.
15. Wasleiski GL, Marson BM, Benjamin JB. Early, incapacitating instability of posterior cruciate ligament-retaining total knee arthroplasty. *J Arthroplasty.* 1998; 13(7):763-767.
16. Mihalko WM, Krackow KA. Posterior cruciate ligament effects on the flexion space in total knee arthroplasty. *Clin Orthop Relat Res.* 1999;360:243-250.
17. Schnurr C, Eysel P, König DP. Is the effect of a posterior cruciate ligament resection in total knee arthroplasty predictable? *Int Orthop.* June 25, 2011 [Epub ahead of print].
18. Arbuthnot JE, Wainwright O, Stables G, et al. Dysfunction of the posterior cruciate ligament in total

knee arthroplasty. *Knee Surg Sports Traumatol Arthrosc.* 2011;19(6):893-898.

19. Mahoney OM, Noble PC, Rhoads DD, et al. Posterior cruciate function following total knee arthroplasty: a biomechanical study. *J Arthroplasty.* 1994;9:569-578.
20. Tang WM, Chiu KY, Ng TP, et al. Posterior cruciate ligament-substituting total knee arthroplasty in young rheumatoid patients with advanced knee involvement. *J Arthroplasty.* 2004;19(1):49-55.
21. Stiehl JB, Voorhorst PE. Total knee arthroplasty with a mobile-bearing prosthesis: comparison of retention and sacrifice of the posterior cruciate ligament in cementless implants. *Am J Orthop.* 1999;28(4):223-228.
22. Stiehl JB, Dennis DA, Komistek RD, et al. In vivo kinematic comparison of posterior cruciate ligament retention or sacrifice with a mobile bearing total knee arthroplasty. *Am J Knee Surg.* 2000;13(1):13-18.
23. Sawaguchi N, Majima T, Ishigaki T, et al. Mobile-bearing total knee arthroplasty improves patellar tracking and patellofemoral contact stress. *J Arthroplasty.* 2010;25(6):920-925.
24. Carothers JT, Kim RH, Dennis DA, et al. Mobile bearing total knee arthroplasty: a meta-analysis. *J Arthroplasty.* 2011;26(4):537-542.
25. Smith H, Jan M, Mohomed NN, et al. Meta-analysis and systematic review of clinical outcomes comparing mobile bearing and fixed bearing total knee arthroplasty. *J Arthroplasty.* 2011;26(8):1205-1213.
26. Fisher DA, Bernasek TL, Puri RD, et al. Rotating platform spinouts with cruciate-retaining mobile-bearing knees. *J Arthroplasty.* 2011;26(6):877-882.
27. Matsuda S, Whiteside LA, White SE, et al. Knee stability in meniscal bearing total knee arthroplasty. *J Arthroplasty.* 1999;14(1):82-90.
28. Haas BD, Kornistek RD, Stiehl JB, et al. Kinematic comparison of posterior cruciate sacrifice versus substitution in a mobile bearing total knee arthroplasty. *J Arthroplasty.* 2002;17(2):685-692.
29. Mihalko WM, Whiteside LA. Bone resection and ligament treatment for flexion contracture in knee arthroplasty. *Clin Orthop Relat Res.* 2003;406:141-147.
30. Whiteside LA. Long-term followup of the bone-ingrowth Ortholoc knee system without a metal-backed patella. *Clin Orthop Relat Res.* 2001;388:77-84.
31. Sextro GS, Berry DJ, Rand JA. Total knee arthroplasty using cruciate-retaining kinematic condylar prosthesis. *Clin Orthop Relat Res.* 2001;388:33-40.
32. Dixon MC, Brown RR, Parsch D, et al. Modular fixed-bearing total knee arthroplasty with retention of the posterior cruciate ligament. A study of patients followed for a minimum of fifteen years. *J Bone Joint Surg Am.* 2005;87(3):598-603.
33. Gill GS, Joshi AB. Long-term results of cemented, posterior cruciate ligament-retaining total knee arthroplasty in osteoarthritis. *Am J Knee Surg.* 2001;14(4):209-214.
34. Schwartz AJ, Della Valle CJ, Rosenberg AG, et al. Cruciate-retaining TKA using a third-generation system with a four-pegged tibial component: a minimum 10-year follow-up note. *Clin Orthop Relat Res.* 2010;468(8):2160-2167.
35. Rasquinha VJ, Ranawat CS, Cervieri CL, et al. The press-fit condylar modular total knee system with a posterior cruciate-substituting design: a concise follow-up of a previous report. *J Bone Joint Surg Am.* 2006;88(5):1006-1010.
36. Lee BS, Lee SJ, Kim JM, et al. No impact of severe varus deformity on clinical outcome after posterior stabilized total knee arthroplasty. *Knee Surg Sports Traumatol Arthrosc.* 2011;19(6):960-966.
37. Pavone V, Boettner F, Fickert S, et al. Total condylar knee arthroplasty: a long-term followup. *Clin Orthop Relat Res.* 2001;388:18-25.
38. Anderson JA, Baldini A, MacDonald JH, et al. Primary constrained condylar knee arthroplasty without stem extensions for the valgus knee. *Clin Orthop Relat Res.* 2006;442:199-203.
39. Anderson JA, Baldini A, MacDonald JH, et al. Constrained condylar knee without stem extensions for difficult primary total knee arthroplasty. *J Knee Surg.* 2007;20(3):195-198.

53 Minimally Invasive Total Knee Arthroplasty

Alfred Tria, Jr.

Minimally invasive surgery (MIS) for total knee arthroplasty (TKA) began with the work of Repicci in the early 1990s when he was performing unicondylar knee arthroplasty (UKA) with a limited incision.[1,2] The results for UKA were acceptable and were validated by several different centers using different prosthetic designs.[3,4] A few years later, designing surgeons began to look at the possibility of applying the limited incision to TKA.[5-8]

There was considerable early interest in MIS TKA with both positive and negative support. Initially, it was difficult to define the MIS approaches. This led to the concept that any abbreviated skin incision or arthrotomy was MIS. Some surgeons advocated limiting the length of the standard approach and suggested that this would lead to improved results without any compromise of the surgical implant alignment.[9,10] While there was some support for these efforts, the results were not different from the standard TKA.

As the procedures became more common, the definitions became more precise. The anatomy of the approach defines whether it is MIS or not. This does not correlate directly with either the length of the skin incision or the arthrotomy length. When appropriately applied, the MIS approaches have led to faster recoveries, improved range of motion, decreased blood loss, and decreased pain.[11-13] When incorrectly applied, they have led to malalignment and early revision.[14,15]

There are three main MIS approaches: the mini-midvastus, the mini-subvastus, and the quadriceps sparing (Fig. 53-1). The level of difficulty and the incidence of each procedure follow that same order. The approaches are based on the anatomy of the knee and should be applied in well-selected cases if they are to be successful.

PREOPERATIVE EVALUATION

The evaluation of the patient should include an appropriate history, physical examination, and X-ray analysis. There should be no history of a previous arthrotomy or infection. It is always good to know if the other knee was previously replaced and what the patient's impression is of that result. If the first TKA was very successful with an exceptional result, it will be difficult to surpass that; the surgeon should

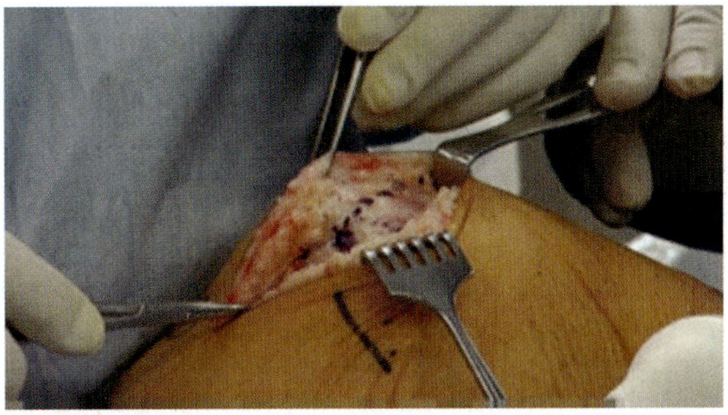

FIGURE 53-1. *The medial aspect of a right knee showing the three MIS incisions drawn with methylene blue.*

take note and, perhaps, follow the approach that was used on the first side. If the opposite knee has not been replaced or has a less than satisfactory result, the surgeon does have a greater freedom of choice with the knee. It is helpful to know what the level of activity of the patient has been and whether the patient was formally very active or sedentary. Patients who are less active are not likely to challenge the total knee after surgery and have limited goals; in these patients, an MIS approach may not be appropriate or necessary.

The physical examination must look for the specific findings that will be favorable to an MIS approach. While obesity is not a direct contraindication to the approaches, it does make the exposure more difficult. If the patient weighs more than 225 pounds or has a body mass index (BMI) greater than 33, the MIS technique will be compromised but not impossible. The girth of the leg is more important than the actual weight of the patient. This can be standardized by measuring the length of the thigh from the anterior superior iliac spine of the pelvis to the middle of the patella with the patient lying supine. Then, the circumference of the knee should be recorded at the level of the patella. Dividing the latter measurement into the thigh length gives a ratio that is ideal for the MIS approaches if it is greater than 3.

The knee should have a good range of motion with no more than a 15° flexion contracture and at least 115° of flexion. The deformity in the coronal plane should not exceed 10° of varus or 15° of valgus. It is ideal if the deformity corrects to neutral with either valgus or varus stress, although this is not an absolute requirement. It is not necessary for either the anterior cruciate or the posterior cruciate ligament to be intact. The MIS approaches can be used both for cruciate-substituting and cruciate-retaining TKA designs. The hip and ankle examinations should be normal in order to support the increased level of activity that the MIS knee should allow the patient. If either of the latter joints has significant limitations in terms of range of motion or associated deformity, it may not be appropriate to attempt an MIS approach that will be severely limited by the associated other joints of the lower limb.

The X-ray evaluation should include a standing anteroposterior view along with a lateral and a skyline patellar view. The standard requirements for the TKA still apply with joint space narrowing and associated sclerosis in all three compartments of the knee. Signs of osteoporosis and associated inflammatory disease are contraindications to the MIS approaches. The limited incisions require some increased retraction for the soft tissues and, if the bone is significantly soft, the retractors may lead to bone injury and loss of substance. Previous osteotomies or other bony procedures are contraindications and make the approach difficult with decreased visualization and possible prosthetic malalignment. The degree of deformity should confirm the findings from the physical examination with no more than 10° of varus, 15° of valgus, and 10° of flexion contracture. The posteroanterior view of the knee can also be helpful and will sometimes show joint space narrowing that is not evident on the standard standing X-ray. While magnetic resonance imaging has become extremely common in the evaluation of the knee, it is not necessary in all cases and should be called for if there is question about the status of the underlying bone, such as in avascular necrosis of the medial femoral condyle not evident on the plain X-ray. Technetium, gallium, and indium scans are also tests that need only be used in specialized cases.

SURGICAL APPROACHES

Mini-arthrotomy Approach

When the MIS approaches started to become popular, there was no doubt that the exposures were quite challenging for most surgeons. Many attempts were made to modify the limited approaches to make them easier. The perioperative pain management programs were improved and the postoperative management was streamlined in an effort to improve the results without requiring the more difficult surgical technique. The mini-arthrotomy was a modification of the standard median parapatellar incision and suggested limiting the quadriceps incision to 4 cm above the superior pole of the patella (Fig. 53-2).[9] This allowed the surgeon to

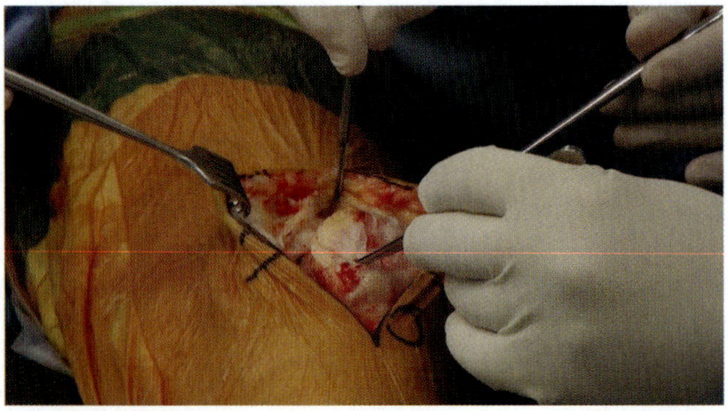

FIGURE 53-2. *The mini-arthrotomy incises the quadriceps tendon for a length of 4 cm from the superior pole of the patella proximally (the knife blade is at the superior extent of the arthrotomy).*

use a smaller skin incision that made the approach look similar to the MIS incision for the patients. However, the clinical result was more like the standard TKA and some surgeons had increased incidence of malalignment even with this technique.[10] The exposure certainly has a place in TKA but should not be equated with the MIS approaches. The perioperative modifications made good sense but they could not produce the same result as the MIS techniques.

Mini-midvastus Approach

The mini-midvastus approach is the most versatile of the techniques and the most popular at the present time.[7,8] The skin incision is limited to 1 or 2 cm above the superior pole of the patella and extends to 2 cm below the tibiofemoral joint line. The incision may be midline or more median parapatellar. The latter approach is more direct and lies immediately over the actual arthrotomy, making the retraction much less difficult. The incision into the vastus medialis is taken from the superior medial pole of the patella proximally in the line of the muscle fibers for a length of 2 cm (Fig. 53-3). It is also helpful to divide the fascia that lies underneath the muscle extending from the joint capsule so that the proximal portion has greater mobility. The arthrotomy is continued distally along the medial side of the patella across the tibiofemoral joint line and extended 2 cm distal to that. The deep portion of the medial collateral ligament is released from the medial side of the tibia.

The quadriceps mechanism is retracted to the lateral side of the knee and the patella is subluxed laterally over the lateral femoral condyle, but it is not everted. Eversion is difficult to perform with the limited incision into the extensor mechanism and is also less desirable because it injures the fibers of the tendon and can lead to patella baja after the surgery. The exposure for the femoral cuts can be completed with minimal retraction of the soft tissues once the incision has been made into the muscle belly of the vastus medialis. The arthrotomy and the skin incision should be retracted medial or lateral and superior and inferior as necessary as a "mobile window." The coordination of the retractors enables the surgeon to use the smaller incision without significantly limiting the visualization of the knee.

The most difficult portion of the surgery is the exposure of the tibial surface and the lateral side of the plateau (Fig. 53-4). This can be expedited with proper use of retractors and balancing of the mobile window to move it more laterally when necessary. Once the femoral and tibial cuts have been completed, there is considerable space in extension and flexion and the patella can be everted without difficulty for resurfacing purposes without placing significant tension on the tendon itself. With the elimination of the tension, the possible patella baja is avoided.

The approach can be compromised if the incision into the vastus medialis is extended beyond the 2 cm. The extension can lead to division of the innervation of the distal portion of the vastus medialis muscle with subsequent weakening of the muscle complex. The lateral muscles of the quadriceps mechanism can become more dominant and can lead to lateral patellar tracking and subsequent patellofemoral pain. In some cases, it may be difficult to obtain proper exposure of the joint because the remaining portion of the vastus medialis is still a bulky muscle that does not allow lateral subluxation of the patella for proper exposure of the entire joint. If

A

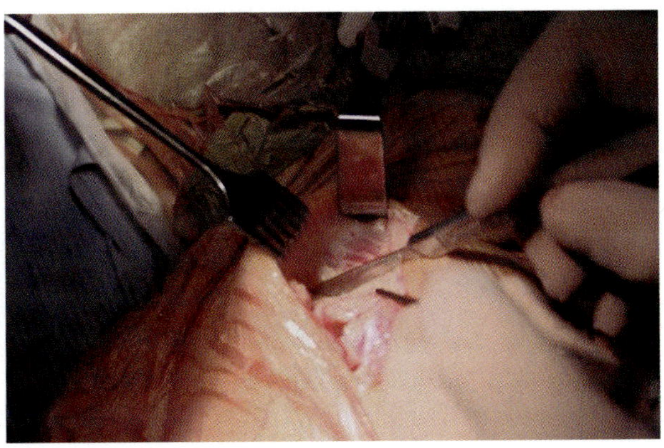

B

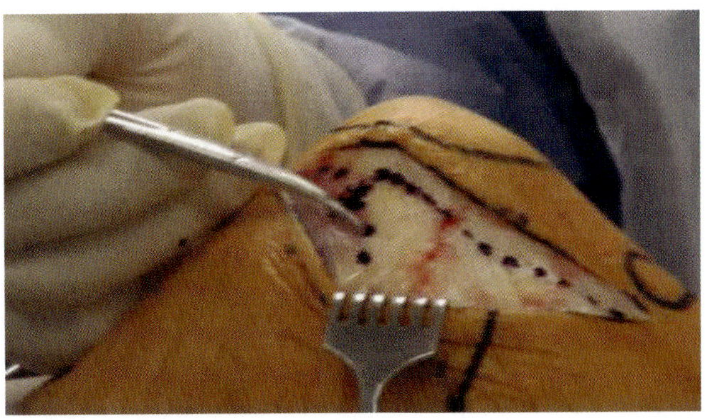

FIGURE 53-3. *(**A**) The knife blade is located at the junction of the distal one-third and the proximal two-thirds of the vastus medialis muscle belly. (**B**) The midvastus arthrotomy incision seen on the medial aspect of a left knee.*

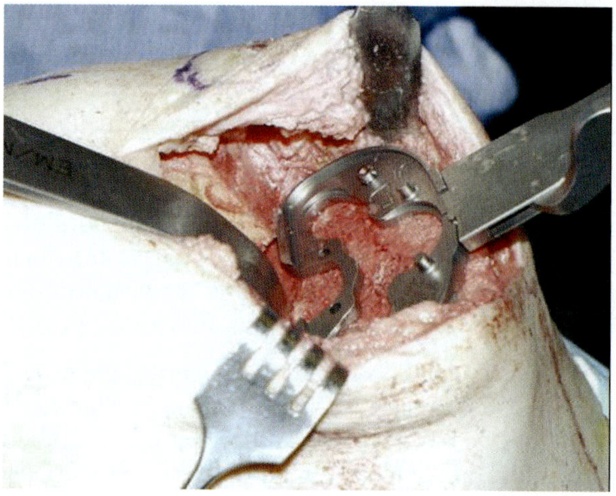

FIGURE 53-4. *The retractor is positioned on the lateral aspect of the tibial cut surface to allow visualization for the placement of the tibial tray.*

the exposure becomes difficult, it is best to continue the medial portion of the arthrotomy proximally into the quadriceps tendon as opposed to extending the muscle incision, which can lead to denervation. It is important to monitor the incision into the vastus medialis throughout the entire operation to be sure that additional retraction of the extensor mechanism does not lead to the superior extension into the muscle.

The medial arthrotomy is closed in the standard fashion. The vastus medialis muscle fibers are not sewn together, but the incised fascia underneath can be reapproximated with sutures.

Subvastus Approach

The subvastus approach is the only approach that preserves the anatomy of the quadriceps mechanism without any invasion of the extensor muscle group.[16-18] The incision is the same as with any of the MIS approaches with either a midline or median parapatellar skin approach. The arthrotomy is performed with the incision just beneath the inferior margin of the vastus medialis muscle belly and is taken distally along the medial side of the patella to 2 cm below the tibiofemoral joint line (Fig. 53-5). The subvastus incision releases the quadriceps mechanism from the medial side of the knee and permits retraction across the anterior aspect of the femur to the lateral side. It is often difficult to retract the entire quadriceps group, especially if the patient is obese or muscular. When the exposure limits the visualization, the natural response of the assistants is to increase the degree of retraction. The increased tension may cause the subvastus incision to extend proximally into the perforating vessels from the femoral artery. If the vessels are avulsed, this can lead to excessive bleeding into the medial aspect of the thigh, which will cause a type of compartment syndrome and lead to a loss of range of motion after the surgery because of the swelling and associated pain.

The patella is subluxed over the side of the femur with the retraction of the entire quadriceps mechanism. Patellar eversion is not possible with this approach but is also less desirable in general. The femur can be exposed and the traditional cuts completed with either standard instruments or instruments that are modified for the limited exposure. The lateral exposure of the tibia can be difficult with the quad mechanism subluxed over the lateral side and it is best to complete the femoral cuts first to give the knee joint more space and laxity for the tibial plateau visualization. Once the femoral and tibial cuts are completed, resurfacing of the patella can be accomplished with gentle eversion, which does not place the patellar tendon under tension when the bone surfaces have been resected.

After relocating the quadriceps mechanism, the medial arthrotomy is closed in the standard fashion. The incision beneath the vastus medialis falls back into anatomic position without any requirement for sutures.

Quadriceps-Sparing Approach

The quadriceps-sparing approach is the most difficult approach of the three MIS procedures.[6,19] The skin incision is similar to the two previous techniques, but the arthrotomy

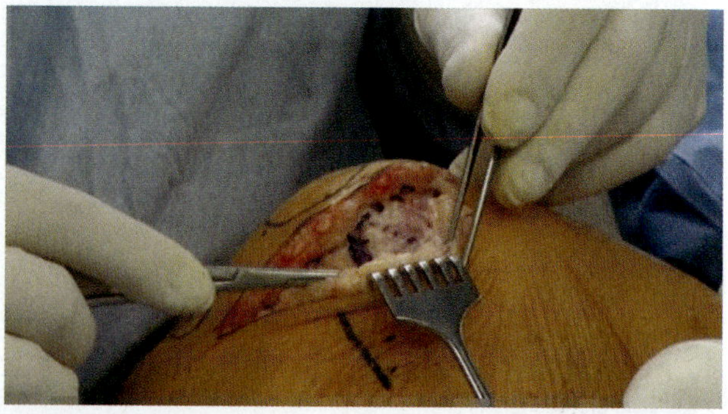

FIGURE 53-5. *The hemostat points to the thick methylene blue line that marks the inferior margin of the vastus medialis where the subvastus incision is made.*

is extremely limited, with the margins from the superior pole of the patella to 2 cm distal to the tibiofemoral joint line (Fig. 53-6). The name of the approach is somewhat misleading because the incision does divide the insertion of the vastus medialis from the medial side of the patella. However, the name was applied early in the development of the approach, and it has become the identifier for the technique.

The exposure is difficult and demands both experience and patience. It depends on the ability to move the arthrotomy and skin incision together as the mobile window for the exposure (Fig. 53-7). The patellar fat pad should be removed and retractors need to be positioned around the lateral side of the tibial cortex without avulsing the insertion of the patellar tendon into the tibial tubercle. It is also difficult to insert the larger implants through the limited incision (Fig. 53-8). This led to some implant modifications with a shortened intramedullary stem on the tibial side or a stem that could be inserted through the tray after it was positioned on the tibial surface while the cement was setting up (Fig. 53-9). There were plans to insert a two- or three-piece femur, but these never came to completion as the technique evolved and proper patient selection made this unnecessary (Fig. 53-10).

As with the other approaches, it is best to start with femoral resection and proceed to the tibia and the patella. During the development of the procedure, newer, unique instruments were designed specifically for the approach. These instruments did fit into the smaller incisions but were not intuitive for the surgeon and did not receive strong support. Most surgeons preferred to use more traditional instruments that were decreased in their overall size (Fig. 53-11). The closure is straightforward with the limited arthrotomy; it is not difficult or time consuming to close the knee.

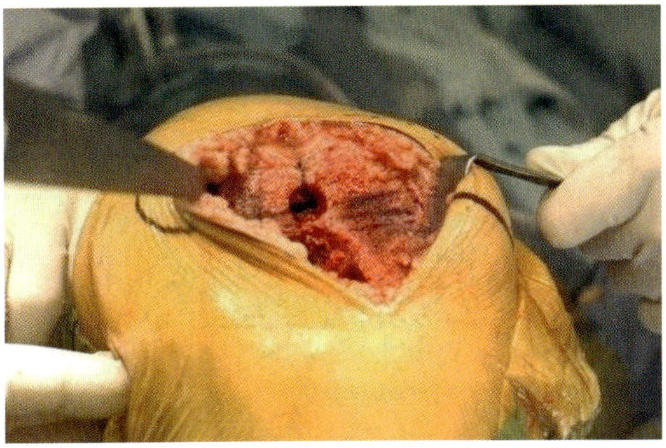

FIGURE 53-7. *The mobile window must be moved medial to lateral and inferior to superior with the coordination of the two retractors.*

Extended Quadriceps-Sparing Approach

The quadriceps-sparing approach can be modified slightly with a 2-cm extension into the quadriceps tendon.[11] The extension improves the visualization with less tension on the incision from the retractors and allows greater accuracy. This technique produces clinical results that are the same as with the MIS quadriceps-sparing approach with much less difficulty for the surgeon who does not perform a high volume of TKAs each year. However, if the incision is extended more than the 2 cm, it becomes a mini-arthrotomy with more standard postoperative results.

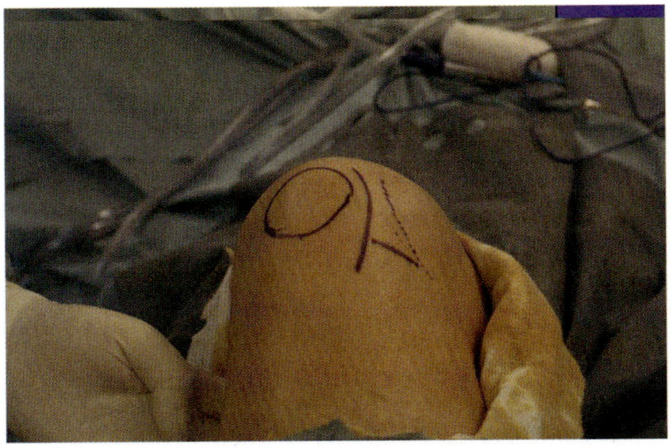

FIGURE 53-6. *The solid line is the skin incision for the quadriceps-sparing approach. The transverse line marks the tibiofemoral joint line and the dotted line marks the medial femoral condyle margin.*

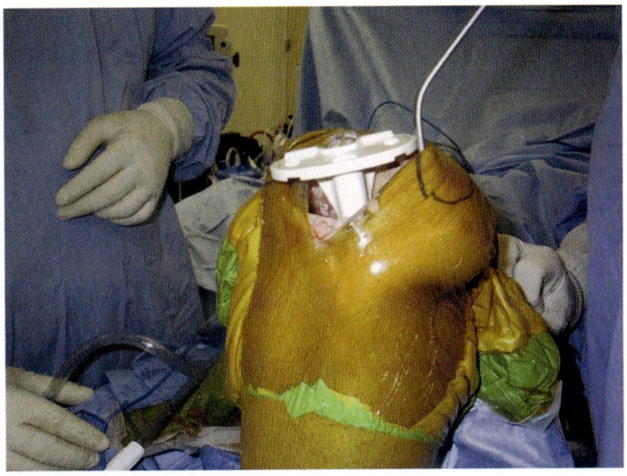

FIGURE 53-8. *The larger size components are difficult to insert in the limited incision.*

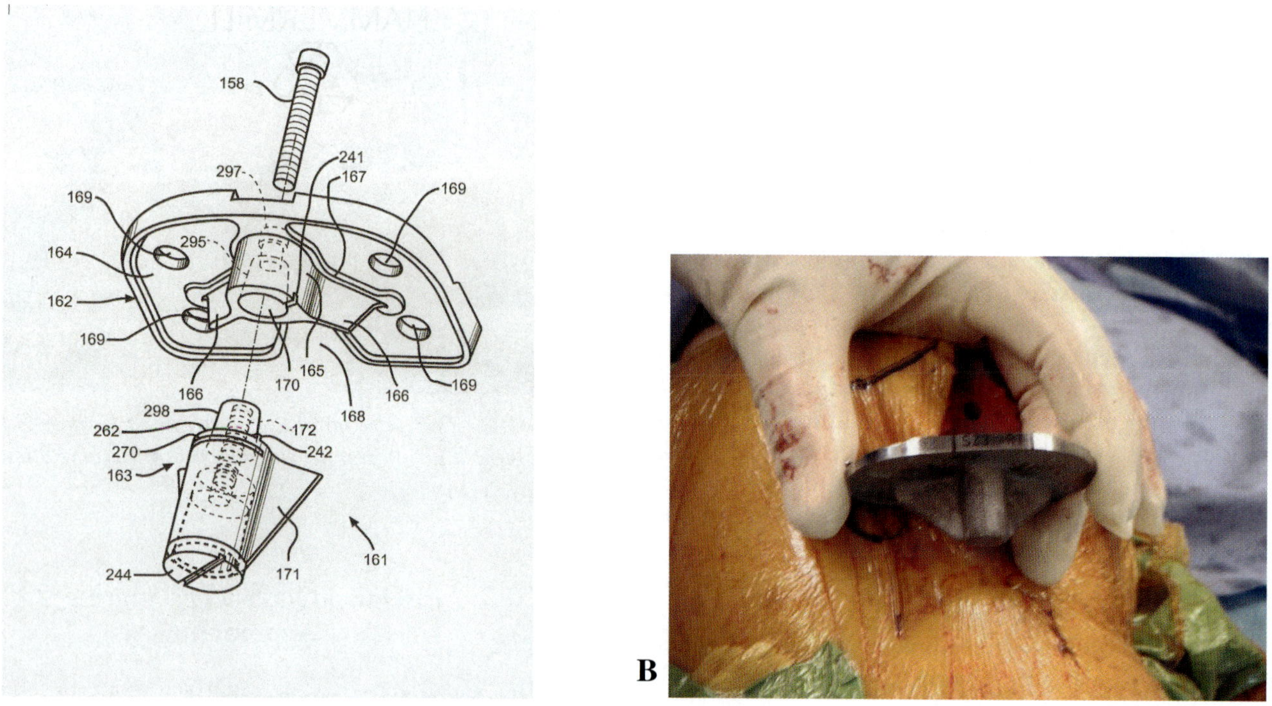

FIGURE 53-9. *(**A**) A diagram of the two-piece tibial component. (**B**) An MIS tibia with a shortened intramedullary stem.*

POSTOPERATIVE MANAGEMENT

As noted above, the MIS approaches invited a more rapid recovery and blended well with improved pain management protocols and more aggressive physical therapy. Patients began to ambulate on the day of surgery and departed from the hospitals in a shorter period of time. The pain associated with the surgery was addressed preoperatively with preemptive narcotics that were given long before the actual pain started. Peripheral nerve blocks that included epidurals, spinals, femoral nerve, and sciatic nerve blocks were introduced, perfected, and oftentimes continued after the surgical procedure for 1 or 2 days while the patient ambulated in the hospital setting. The knee was immobilized for a much shorter period of time after the operation, and physical therapy was more aggressive with more than one scheduled period for exercise each day and with no modifications of the schedule for patients who were in the hospital over weekend days, which were previously considered days of rest.

All of the changes that were introduced with the new approaches helped to improve the final result and helped to shorten the time for recovery and return to full activities of daily living. During the development of the techniques,

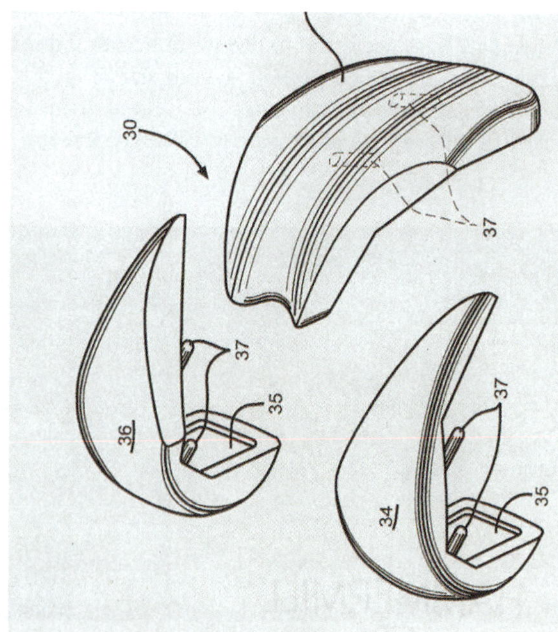

FIGURE 53-10. *A diagram of a proposed three-piece femoral component.*

A 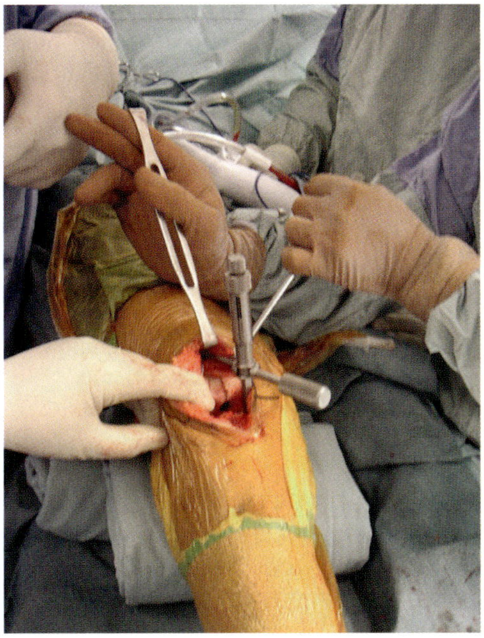

B 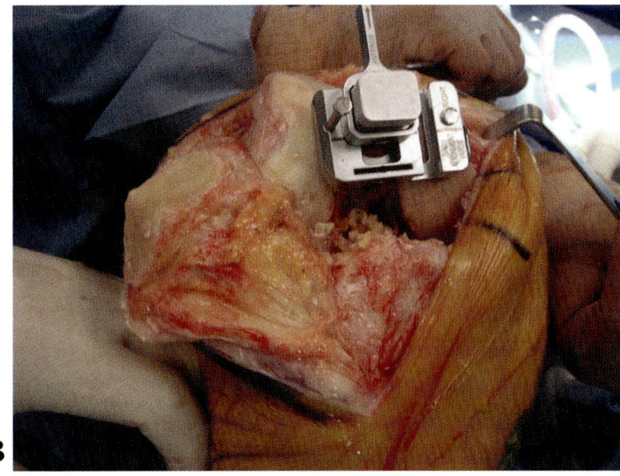

FIGURE 53-11. *(**A**) A unique MIS instrument for anterior femoral resection. (**B**) A modified intramedullary femoral guide that is used here in a standard arthrotomy but can also be used in any MIS approach.*

there was considerable confusion as to which element of the new surgeries contributed most to the final result. There is no doubt that the surgery, the pain management, and the rehabilitation worked together; however, it was the surgical approaches that caused everyone to reconsider the entire management of the total knee patient.

OUTCOMES

The reported clinical results of each of the three MIS techniques are equal to or better than the results reported from the standard TKAs. In the hands of experienced surgeons who have either designed the approaches or who have performed the procedures with some regularity, the results show decreased perioperative pain, less blood loss, faster gain in range of motion, decreased length of stay in the hospital, and faster return to activities of daily living.[5-8,11,13,18,19] Each of the three techniques are equally successful when appropriately applied and implemented.

In the hands of the less experienced surgeon or when the indications for the surgery are expanded, the results become compromised. Malalignment, flexion-extension instability, and even infection can become more common when the indications for each approach are ignored or modified.

CASE EXAMPLE

A patient with a normal BMI (30 or less), a thigh-to-knee ratio of 3 or greater, with deformity that does not exceed 10° to 15° in all planes is ideal for an MIS TKA. The age of the patient is not critical as long as there is an understanding of the purpose of the approach and as long as the patient has the ability to rehabilitate the knee rapidly without significant distractions secondary to health or psychological issues.

It is ideal if the varus or valgus deformity corrects to neutral with stress in the opposite direction. Anterior cruciate or posterior cruciate ligament laxity or absence is not a critical factor. It is best if the ratio of thigh length to knee circumference is 3 or greater in order to avoid the obese or muscular thigh. The knee range of motion should be greater than a total of 115°. The X-ray should agree with the deformity found on physical examination and should be consistent with osteoarthritis and not an inflammatory picture (Fig. 53-12). The patient should understand the goals of the MIS surgery and be able to comply with a more aggressive rehabilitation program to benefit from the surgical approach.

The operating surgeon should be familiar with the surgical technique and have proper instrumentation to support

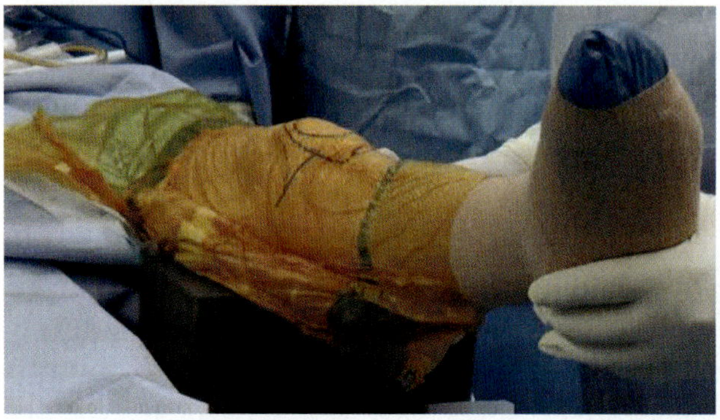

FIGURE 53-12. *An ideal knee for an MIS TKA procedure with limited, supple varus deformity, no obesity, and a good range of motion.*

the operation. The procedure should be completed in a timely fashion and should certainly not require more than 90 minutes of total operating time. Longer operations lead to more medical complications and to a higher infection rate.

The length of stay in the hospital is not critical to the result but is typically shortened if all goes well. The rehabilitation is shortened, and the longevity of the well-performed implant is equal to or better than that of the standard approach.

TIPS AND PEARLS

The curvilinear medial incision gives the best exposure to the knee and it is easiest to extend. The extended quadriceps-sparing approach is the easiest technique for most of the applicable knees. It will not extend with forceful retraction further into the quadriceps tendon and is the most familiar for all surgeons. If there is some difficulty with visualization, the medial capsule can be incised with a "T" extension transversely at the level of the joint line extending to but not across the medial collateral ligament. The midvastus and the subvastus arthrotomies may easily extend proximally, resulting in possible nerve injury with the former and possible hematoma with the latter.

All of the approaches require special attention to the insertion of the patellar tendon into the tibial tubercle. The easiest way to protect the insertion is to release the insertion slightly with a sharp knife from distal to proximal in an oblique fashion coming slightly more lateral at the proximal site. This allows the tendon to peel off slightly with overzealous retraction and does not result in a sudden avulsion. Placing a pin through a portion of the tendon both weakens the tendon and may contribute to tearing by itself.

The prosthetic design is not critical for the MIS surgery, but the cruciate-retaining designs require less exposure and can often be performed without formal dislocation of the tibia beneath the femur. The tibial components usually have short pegs for fixation and require less exposure than the stems for the posterior-stabilized designs. The approaches do not favor cemented or cementless techniques and either one can be used without additional difficulty.

SUGGESTED READING

Scuderi GR, Tria AJ Jr, eds. *MIS of the Hip and the Knee: A Clinical Perspective*. New York: Springer-Verlag; 2004.

Scuderi GR, Tria AJ Jr, Berger RA, eds. *MIS Techniques in Orthopedics*. New York: Springer; 2006.

Scuderi GR, Tria AJ, eds. *Minimally Invasive Surgery in Orthopedics*. New York: Springer; 2010.

REFERENCES

1. Repicci JA, Eberle RW. Minimally invasive surgical technique for unicondylar knee arthroplasty. *J South Orthop Assoc*. 1999;8(1):20-27.
2. Romanowski MR, Repicci JA. Minimally invasive unicondylar arthroplasty: eight year follow-up. *Am J Knee Surg*. 2002;15(1):17-22.
3. Price AJ, Webb J, Topf H, et al. Rapid recovery after Oxford unicompartmental arthroplasty through a short incision. *J Arthroplasty*. 2001;16(8): 970-976.
4. Gesell MW, Tria AJ Jr. MIS unicondylar knee arthroplasty: surgical approach and early results. *Clin Orthop Relat Res*. 2004;428:53-60.
5. Bonutti PM, Mont MA, McMahon M, et al. Minimally invasive total knee arthroplasty. *J Bone Joint Surg Am*. 2004;86(suppl 2):26-32.
6. Tria AJ, Coon TM. Minimal incision total knee arthroplasty: early experience. *Clin Orthop Relat Res*. 2003;416:185-190.

7. Haas SB, Manitta MA, Burdick P. Minimally invasive total knee arthroplasty: the mini midvastus approach. *Clin Orthop Relat Res.* 2006;452:112-116.
8. Laskin RS. Minimally invasive total knee arthroplasty: the results justify its use. *Clin Orthop Relat Res.* 2005;440:54-59.
9. Tenholder M, Clarke HD, Scuderi GR. Minimal incision total knee arthroplasty: the early clinical experience. *Clin Orthop Relat Res.* 2005;440:67-76.
10. Dalury DF, Dennis DA. Mini-incision total knee arthroplasty can increase risk of component malalignment. *Clin Orthop Relat Res.* 2005;440:77-81.
11. Tanavalee A, Thiengwittayaporn S, Itiravivong P. Progressive quadriceps incision during minimally invasive surgery for total knee arthroplasty: the effect on early postoperative ambulation. *J Arthroplasty.* 2007;22(7):1013-1018.
12. Huang HT, Su JY, Chang JK, et al. The early outcome of minimally invasive quadriceps-sparing total knee arthroplasty: report of a 2-year follow-up. *J Arthroplasty.* 2007;22(7):1007-1012.
13. Karpman RR, Smith HL. Comparison of the early results of minimally invasive vs. standard approaches to total knee arthroplasty: a prospective randomized study. *J Arthroplasty.* 2009;24:681-688.
14. Boerger TO, Aglietti P, Mondanelli N, et al. Mini-subvastus versus medial parapatellar approach in total knee arthroplasty. *Clin Orthop Relat Res.* 2005;440:82-87.
15. Kim YH, Kim JS, Kim DY. Clinical outcome and rate of complications after primary total knee replacement performed with quadriceps-sparing or standard arthrotomy. *J Bone Joint Surg Br.* 2007;89(4):467-470.
16. Roysam GS, Oakley MJ. Subvastus approach for total knee arthroplasty: a prospective, randomized, and observer-blinded trial. *J Arthroplasty.* 2001;16(4):454-457.
17. Hofmann AA, Plaster RL, Murdock LE. Subvastus (Southern) approach for primary total knee arthroplasty. *Clin Orthop Relat Res.* 1991;269:70-77.
18. Pagnano MW, Meneghini RM. Minimally invasive total knee arthroplasty with an optimized subvastus approach. *J Arthroplasty.* 2006;21(4 suppl 1):22-26.
19. Chen AF, Alan RK, Redziniak DE, et al. Quadriceps sparing total knee arthroplasty: initial experience with two to four year results. *J Bone Joint Surg Br.* 2006;88(11):1448-1453.

54 Navigation-Assisted Total Knee Arthroplasty

David N. Vegari, Florian F. Dibra, and William J. Hozack

New technologies have the potential to allow for great improvements in the clinical results of total knee arthroplasty (TKA). Computer-assisted TKA is one of those new technologies, but, recently, questions have arisen regarding its overall benefit, its cost-effectiveness, and the ease of its use. The focus of this chapter is to systematically review the literature to explore the proper role for navigation in TKA and what benefits navigation might bring to patients. Also, the chapter discusses how navigation allows the surgeon to accurately and consistently replicate proper mechanical alignment in patients. The system also has a number of other benefits, including decreased blood loss, ease of use with extreme deformities, and potential cost savings. Ultimately, the aim is to provide the surgeon with an evidence-based approach to the benefits of computer-assisted surgery and a detailed outline on how to perform the procedure in a succinct and accurate fashion.

MECHANICAL AXIS

Historically, poor mechanical alignment, particularly in the coronal plane, has been associated with early failure. In a series in the 1970s, Lotke et al found that tibial components positioned in varus had a higher predisposition for mechanical failure of the prosthesis.[1] In 1972, Maquet discovered on long-leg radiographs that a line drawn from the center of the femoral head to the center of the talus passes through the middle one-third of the knee.[2] This has since been referred to as the mechanical axis of the lower extremity. It has been revealed that if, after a TKA, the mechanical axis varied by as a little as ±3° (in either direction) from the medial one-third of the knee, there was an associated higher rate of mechanical failure or loosening of the prosthesis.[3] Also, a postoperative tibiofemoral angle of 4° to 10° correlated strongly with a line passing through the middle third of the knee (Fig. 54-1).[3]

Bargren's data confirm the need to maintain a mechanical axis close to neutral. Bargren found that, both clinically and in cadaver models, TKAs that were loaded eccentrically had a much higher predisposition to failure. Of note, 86% of those knees placed within 1° to 8° of varus failed 86% of the time, when compared to a failure rate of 11% for TKAs placed in 1° to 13° of valgus.[4]

A number of recent studies also profess the importance of the mechanical axis in total knee replacement. One study found that patients within ±3° of coronal alignment had statistically improved International Knee Society scores and Short-Form 12 scores at 6 weeks, 3 months, 6 months, and 1 year postoperatively compared to their outlier counterparts.[5] In another study, patients with ±3° of coronal mechanical alignment had better functional outcomes as measured by the Knee Society scores.[6] Sikorski discusses in detail the importance of the mechanical axis and how it plays a pivotal role in ensuring proper soft tissue balancing.[7]

Berry et al recently questioned the need to restore the mechanical axis so accurately. Their retrospective study found that there was no correlation to improved survivorship when this criterion was followed.[8] However, they acknowledge that their study is not without limitation. Of note, in a commentary by Mont and Mahoney, it is noted

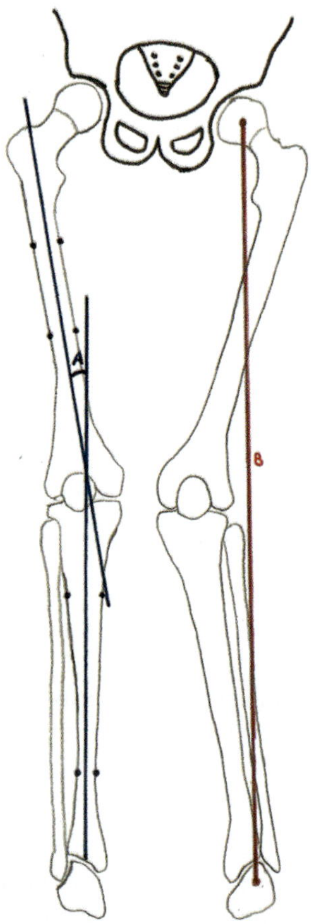

FIGURE 54-1. *Illustration of tibiofemoral angle (**A**) created by the intersection of the anatomic axes of the femur and the tibia. Maquet's line (**B**) passes from the center of the femoral head to the center of the body of the talus.*

that the failure rate within the subgroups was never delineated by those in varus versus valgus deformity. It is quite possible that the varus group is at a much higher predisposition, as historical teaching goes, to failure but this may be masked by the valgus group.[9] Clearly, this would compromise the overall premise of the paper. Perhaps this led the authors to conclude that the current goal of being within ±3° of the mechanical axis continues to be the postoperative goal in total knee arthroplasty.[8]

Despite the marked improvement in both surgical technique and mechanical alignment guides, it has been estimated that over 10% of total knee arthroplasties performed by experienced surgeons result in variations of tibial and femoral alignment of greater than 3°.[10] This problem can be attributed to many factors. Despite the creation of standardized radiographs, there can nevertheless be tremendous variability in these films.[10] Furthermore, these systems manifest an inherent problem: the anatomical variation from one patient to another. Computer-assisted TKA affords the surgeon the opportunity to overcome these obstacles by providing real-time information intraoperatively that is specific to each patient's bony and soft tissue anatomy.

LITERATURE REVIEW

Currently, three types of computer-assisted technologies exist. One uses preoperative templating with magnetic resonance imaging or computer tomography scans with subsequent customized jigs. Another involves robotic technology. This chapter, however, focuses on the third type: image-free intraoperative navigation (Fig. 54-2).

The use of computer-assisted navigation systems has been the topic of a number of original scientific articles. These articles have shown that the routine use of navigation results in better overall coronal alignment than results from the use of standard instrumentation. A meta-analysis of the literature from 1990 to 2007 identified 29 studies of computer-assisted surgery (CAS) that compare it to conventional TKA. The results of the study were profound: mechanical axis malalignment, defined as alignment falling outside of the aforementioned ±3° range, was found to be 9% in the CAS group, while 31.8% in the conventional TKA group.[11]

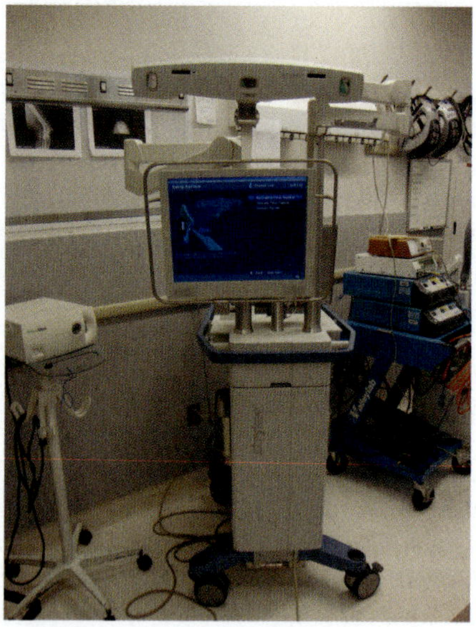

FIGURE 54-2. *The main components of an image-free navigation system for total knee replacement include system equipment trolley and isolation transformer, infrared camera, a computer workstation, and the infrared transmitters (not shown).*

The same meta-analysis also found significant differences when looking at both femoral component alignment and tibial component alignment in the frontal plane. In the CAS group, malalignment of the femoral component, defined as deviation from 90°, was found to be 4.9° and 9.6° at ±3° and ±2°, respectively. However, the conventional TKA patients differed by 16% and 34.1%, respectively. Clearly, there is an improvement in femoral component positioning with the use of CAS. Concomitantly, a statistically significant difference also exists when looking at the tibial component orientation in the frontal plane. Deviation from 90° at ±3° and ±2° for the CAS group was 4% and 4.8%, respectively. The conventional TKA group varied greatly, at 11.1% and 20.3%, respectively. The CAS group shows a benefit over conventional TKA in the frontal planes for both femoral and tibial component alignment.

The case for CAS also has strong level-one evidence in support of its use as well. A study by Matziolis randomized patients to either a CAS group or a conventional TKA group. Postoperatively, measurements were calculated with the use of computer tomography to determine more accurately the mechanical axis variance. The authors found that when comparing mechanical axis alignment in CAS with a conventional cohort, the CAS group consistently had better alignment. Specifically, they found that the CAS mechanical axis ranged from 2.9° of valgus to 3.1° of varus, compared to the conventional group of 4.8° to 6.6°, respectively.[12] The study did not find a statistically significant difference in rotational alignment of femoral and tibial components between the randomized groups.

Yet another prospective, randomized study found significant differences in radiographic alignment in favor of CAS over conventional TKA. Dutton et al found that, in the postoperative radiographic measurements of the randomized CAS group, 92% of patients had a coronal tibiofemoral angle within ±3° of the ideal, as compared to 68% of those patients in the conventional TKA group.[13] This study also shows a statistically significant difference in sagittal alignment of the tibia or posterior tibial slope when looking at a range of 0° to 7° of posterior slope as the ideal. In the CAS group, 90% of patients had tibial slopes in this range, as opposed to 61% of patients in the conventional group.

The substantial difference that CAS makes in patient alignment can be observed in those patients with significant preoperative deformities. Patients with significant deviations from the standard can present real technical challenges even for the most experienced surgeon. These deformities can stem from a multitude of reasons including, but not limited to, trauma, congenital defects, and previous surgery.

In particular, a previous fracture with malunion can make the use of intramedullary and extramedullary guides extremely technically challenging. The CAS system obviates the need to use such guides. In a case series, Hozack et al found that the use of CAS allowed the surgeon to maintain proper mechanical alignment while maintaining appropriate sagittal and rotational alignment (Fig. 54-3).[14]

Furthermore, the study found that when previous trauma resulted in open reduction and internal fixation of either the femur or tibia it necessitated the staging of the TKA. Specifically, the first procedure resulted in the removal of hardware and a period of protective weight bearing—possibly

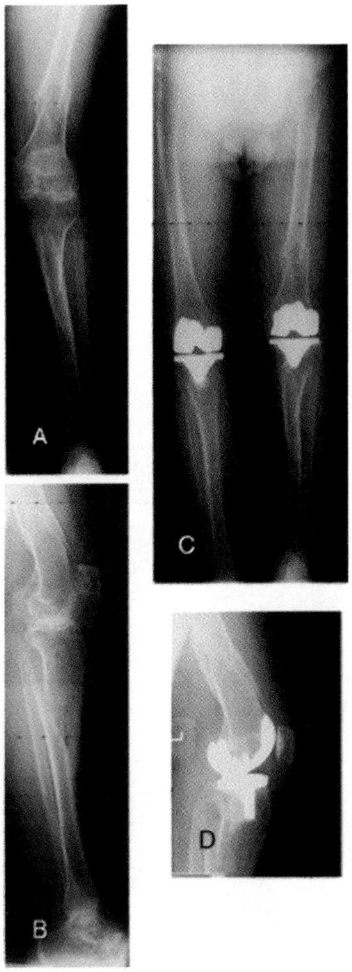

FIGURE 54-3. *Preoperative anteroposterior (AP) (**A**) and lateral (**B**) radiographs of the patient demonstrating both femoral and tibial fracture malunions. Postoperative AP (**C**) and lateral (**D**) radiographs after TKA using navigation. (Reprinted from Klein G, Austin M, Hozack W, et al. Total knee arthroplasty using computer-assisted navigation in patients with deformities of the femur and tibia. J Arthroplasty 2006;21(2):284-288, with permission from Elsevier.)*

up to 6 weeks—to prevent any fracture from the creation of stress risers from the hardware or screw holes. This could delay the TKA for 6 weeks if not longer. However, with the use of CAS, the removal of hardware is not necessary, because there are no guides that need to be passed; anatomic landmarks suffice for appropriate orientation of the cutting guides. This saves the patient the morbidity associated with an additional surgery as well as the loss of patient satisfaction and productivity secondary to a prolonged perioperative course (Fig. 54-4).

In another series, the authors studied 40 patients with significant preoperative deformities, defined as deviation of greater than 10° in the frontal plane. The groups were randomly assigned to CAS and conventional TKA. This series clearly shows a significant improvement in coronal alignment in the CAS group. Specifically, 90% of the patients in the surgical navigation group had a femoral tibial angle within the ±3° range. By contrast, only 50% of patients from the conventional group displayed deviation within this range.[15]

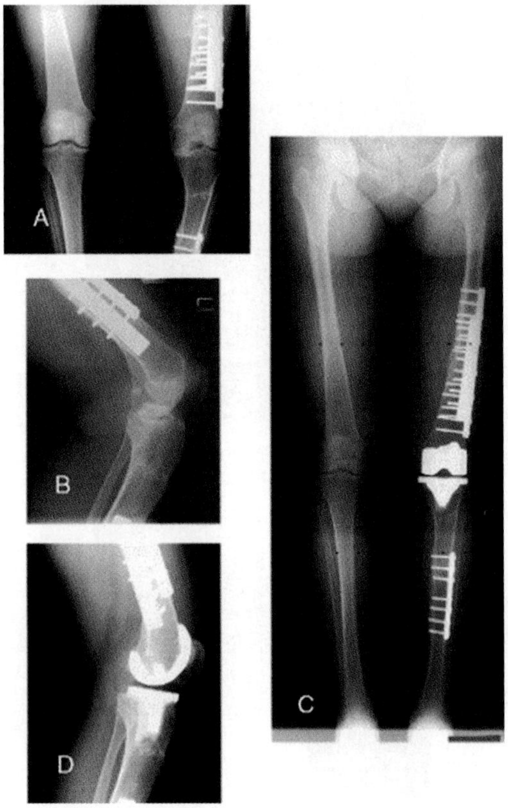

FIGURE 54-4. *Preoperative AP (**A**) and lateral (**B**) radiographs of the patient after open reduction and internal fixation of both the femur and tibia with plates and screws. Postoperative AP (**C**) and lateral (**D**) radiographs of the lower extremity after TKA with navigation. (Reprinted from Klein G, Austin M, Hozack W, et al. Total knee arthroplasty using computer-assisted navigation in patients with deformities of the femur and tibia. J Arthroplasty 2006;21(2):284-288, with permission from Elsevier.)*

The data clearly favor the use of CAS, particularly in the setting of significant preoperative deformity. The surgeon's standard armamentarium of extramedullary and intramedullary jigs does not suffice in these complicated patients. It is necessary that the appropriate landmarks be identified via navigation to better ensure a proper postoperative mechanical axis.

PREOPERATIVE PLANNING

The advantages in preoperative planning with CAS include the accurate determination of the mechanical axis in a patient, which eliminates the need for a long-leg film and for templating. Sizing can be performed in real time by digitization of the anatomic points in the operating room. Preoperative range of motion can be more accurately determined intraoperatively as well by the navigation system. This will better showcase subtleties of the surgery, including tibial slope.

OPERATIVE TECHNIQUE

Positioning

The navigation system is placed opposite the surgeon and generally should be placed at the level of the joint line to ensure proper communication between the instruments during surgery. All setup should take place before surgery and trackers and pointers should be initialized, validated, and calibrated to prevent troubleshooting during the case.

Approach

The surgeon's preferred exposure to the knee need not change with the use of computer-assisted navigation.

Placement of tracker pins

All tracker pins are placed within the incision for simplicity as well as for the prevention of potential stress risers for fracture. This is discussed later in this chapter. The tibia anchoring pin is inserted on the medial tibial plateau in a parallel fashion to the joint line and angled 30° away from the mid-sagittal plane. It also allows for minimization of risk of vascular injury to the posterior structures, particularly when inserted in a knee-flexed position. Drill from the anterior to posterior tibial cortex.

The pins have a self-tapping screw design with antirotation properties that should both be driven bicortically to ensure proper support. The femoral anchoring pin is positioned medially on the anterior surface, just at the proximal aspect of the metaphysic (Fig. 54-5). Care must be taken to ensure that the tracker pin is placed far enough proximally to prevent interference with the femoral cutting jigs and ultimately the trial components. Situating the placement on the medial side allows for a smaller incision, as the medial aspect of the femoral component extends proximally less so than the lateral flange of the femoral component.

Registration

Arguably the most important aspect of navigation is the accurate anatomic registration of various landmarks on the patient. If this is done in error, all readouts and subsequent recommended cuts will not correspond to the patient's own anatomy. Clearly, this must be prevented from occurring. The navigation program is sufficiently sophisticated to prevent a gross error from being registered and will not allow for progression. However, the onus continues to be on the surgeon to ensure proper digitization. The Stryker Navigation System supplies two trackers that can be distinguished by color: blue and green. Green always corresponds to the femur and blue to the tibial anchoring pin. Failure to adhere to this basic color-coding premise will result in inaccurate representation of both the femoral and tibial landmarks.

Femoral head center

The center of the femoral head is identified by rotating the hip while maintaining flexion in the hip and knee joints. This allows the software to accurately identify the center of the femoral head within 1 mm of accuracy vis-à-vis the trackers. Stabilization of the pelvis is critical to the determination, because movement could potentially result in an inaccurate representation of the center of the femoral head (Fig. 54-6).

Distal femur

The distal femur is accurately mapped by identifying the medial and lateral epicondyles and knee center with the pointer. The femoral anteroposterior (AP) axis, or Whiteside's line, is properly identified by aligning the pointer's axis with the most anterior aspect of the intercondylar groove (Fig. 54-7). The computer can also use the epicondylar points to create the transepicondylar axis, which the computer may also use to set the femoral component's rotation. Next, the distal femur is mapped by placing the probe on the anterior cortex and the distal and posterior aspects of the medial and lateral condyles, respectively. When registering each point with the pointer, care should be taken to use the pointer in a "paint-like" fashion to ensure registration. The lateral aspect of the anterior portion of the femur, which is often less prominent, must be included to prevent oversizing of the femoral component.

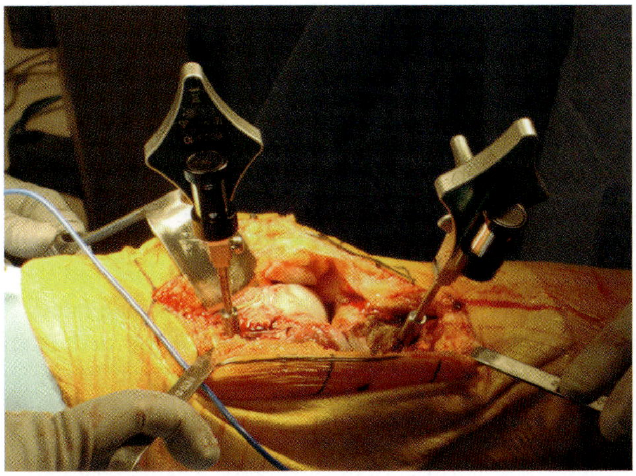

FIGURE 54-5. *Femoral anchoring pin (left) positioned medially on the anterior surface, just at the proximal aspect of the metaphysis. Tibial anchoring pin (right) inserted on the medial tibial plateau.*

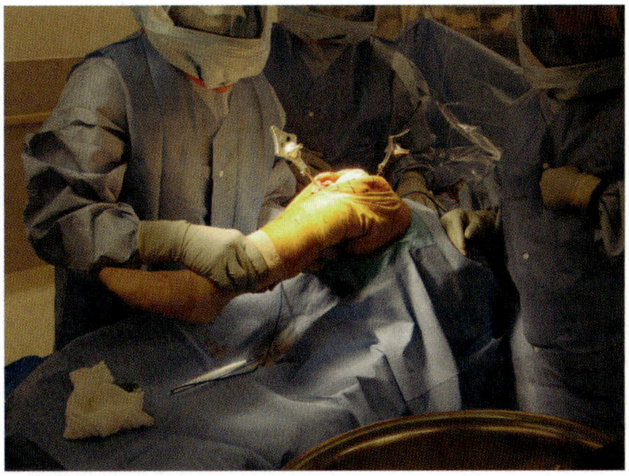

FIGURE 54-6. *The center of the femoral head identified by rotating the hip while maintaining flexion in the hip and knee joints. This allows the software to accurately identify the center of the femoral head within 1 mm.*

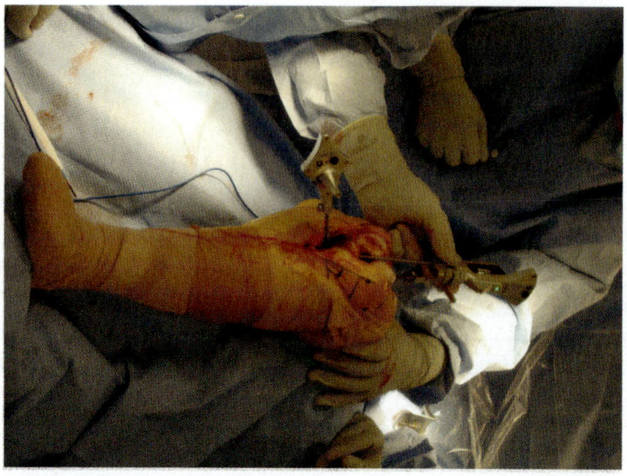

FIGURE 54-7. *Femoral (AP) axis, or Whiteside's line, properly identified by aligning the pointer's axis with the most anterior aspect of the intercondylar groove.*

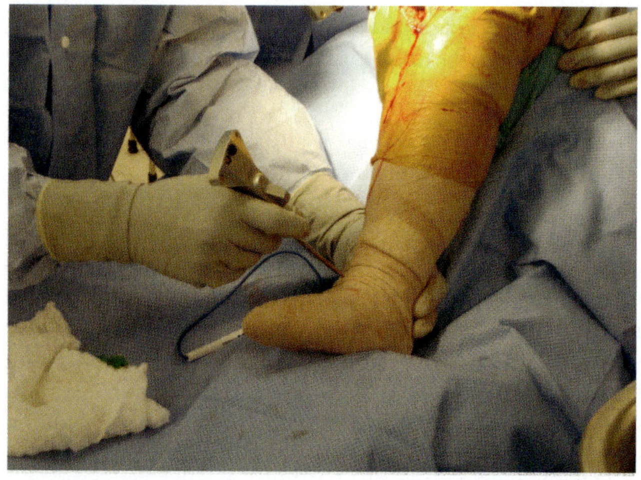

FIGURE 54-8. *The medial and lateral (shown) malleoli digitized with the infrared transmitter in order for the computer to determine the center of the ankle.*

Proximal tibia

The pointer is again used to identify the medial and lateral compartments of the tibia. The lowest point on each condyle must be digitized. The center of the tibial plateau and the AP axis of the tibia are also digitized.

Ankle center

The medial and lateral malleoli are digitized and, based on these two reference points, the computer can now determine the center of the ankle. This will be pivotal in the ultimate determination of the anatomic axis of the tibia and overall anatomic axis of the operative limb (Fig. 54-8).

Preoperative alignment

The initial varus/valgus alignment and range of motion are determined by attaching the trackers after all points have been registered and ranging the knee to the maximums of flexion and extension. This helps determine postoperative range of motion. It also offers necessary information regarding the bone cuts and reveals any potential for soft tissue releases. Should the knee be in excessive varus/valgus, the medial collateral ligament would potentially need to be released further in the former and should be checked for attenuation in the latter scenario. The presence of a flexion contracture might lead the physician to be more aggressive with a posterior capsular release as well as diligently checking for the presence of posterior osteophytes. Alternatively, more distal femur may need to be resected.

Bone Cuts

CAS techniques are amenable to the surgeon's preferences. Either anterior or posterior referencing techniques are supported. The software can also accommodate for a tibia-first approach. However, our preference is to start with the femur. Regardless of surgeon preference, it should be noted that, during femoral cuts, the green tracker is located on the femoral anchoring pin and the blue tracker on the cutting jig. On the tibia this positioning arrangement is reversed.

Distal femoral cut

The computer references the distal femoral cut based on the most distal point of the previously digitized condyles. The computer is able to calculate the length of the perpendicular distance from this digitized point to the point of resection. Next, the horseshoe guide is fixed with two pins on the distal femur. The cutting guide is then attached on the horseshoe with the tracker attached to the tracking interface. This allows the surgeon to adjust the distal and lateral screws on the cutting device until the surgeon has determined that an appropriate cut has been made (Fig. 54-9). Once the appropriate cut is determined and registered, the surgeon can proceed with the resection. The cut can now be verified by placing the tracker and probe on the resected surface.

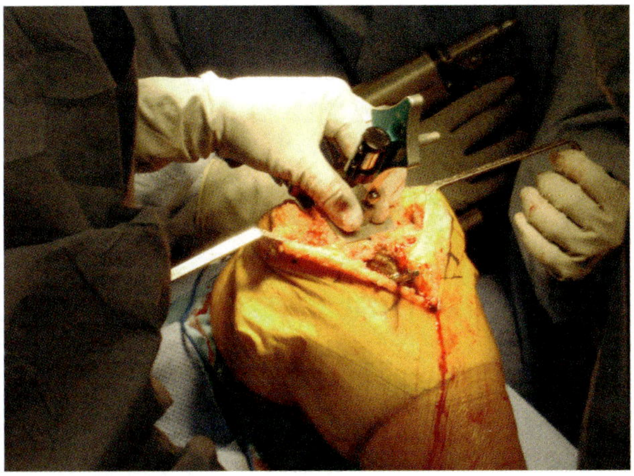

FIGURE 54-9. *Resection plane probe checking the distal femoral cut.*

Femoral rotational cut

The blue tracker is attached to the rotation guide and placed on the distal femoral cut. The surgeon must now choose which rotational reference to use. A stylus is applied to ensure that anterior femoral notching is prevented. The surgeon may now proceed with the cut and the probe may again be applied to check the accuracy of the cut. As the rotational landmarks are less clearly identified than all other landmarks, the surgeon must continue to verify the accuracy of the landmarks documented in the registration process before finalizing the rotational cut.

Finishing cuts: Femur

The 4:1 cutting block is placed and made flush to the anterior cut surface and the final cuts are now made. The computer aids in selecting the appropriate guide, according to sizing. However, the surgeon will make the ultimate decision in determining whether the sizing is accurate. As always, it is safer to err on a larger size.

Proximal tibial cut

The horseshoe guide is again fixed but this time on the tibial surface with two pins. The tibial cutting guide is attached to the horseshoe. The screws on the cutting guide can now be adjusted to determine the depth of the resection and the posterior tibial slope, all while allowing the surgeon to determine in real time via computer logistics the varus/valgus alignment throughout the process. Once the appropriate parameters are selected, the surgeon may proceed with the tibial cut, verified with the resection plane probe (Fig. 54-10).

Tibial rotation

The tibial template can be aligned and pinned in the appropriate position based on the surgeon's determination. The software allows the surgeon to ascertain the positions at which the external rotation increases or decreases, and it can be set accordingly.

Patella and box cut

The patella is resected according to standard principles and is not assessed with the use of navigation. It is noteworthy that the intercondylar box is resected to accommodate for the post and cam mechanism, should a posterior stabilizing knee be selected.

Trialing

Trial components can now be placed with the trackers placed on the pin. This allows for overall alignment to be determined and final range of motion to be assessed. Should there continue to be a residual deformity present, select soft tissue releases may be performed in line with conventional TKA. Once such releases are made, the knee can again be assessed to ensure satisfactory alignment and motion.

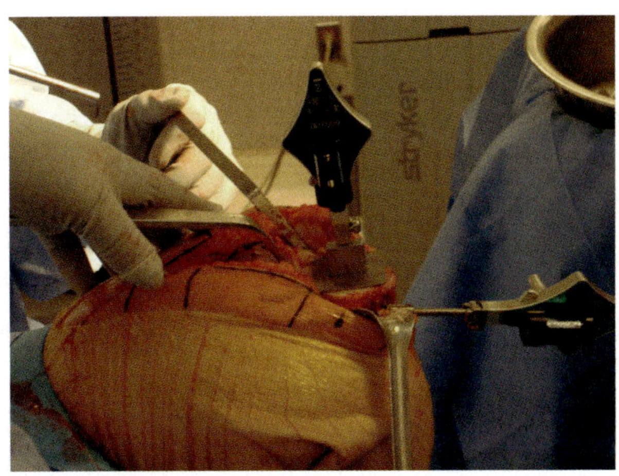

FIGURE 54-10. *Resection plane probe checking the proximal tibial cut.*

Final Components

Final components are cemented in based on standard principles. This can be done with or without the anchoring pins being left in place, should the surgeon prefer to check final alignment and range of motion of the true implant. This is left to the discretion of the surgeon.

COMPLICATIONS

As with any surgical procedure, computer navigation is not without its deficits. However, these complications are commonly seen in conventional total knee arthroplasty as well. Those poor outcomes associated only with navigation knees can be corrected with increased attention to detail and, more important, with experience.

Landmark Variability

As previously mentioned, the key to computer navigation is the accurate identification and digitization of the patient's own anatomic landmarks. Robinson et al found that interobserver reliability for determining patient landmarks can be variable. Specifically, that study asked surgeons to identify four anatomic landmarks on the distal femur of a virtual bone: medial and lateral epicondyles as well as two equidistant points from the articular surface of the posterior femoral condyles. Robinson et al found that no two observers identified the same location for any of the four landmarks.[16] They concluded that perhaps the navigation-assisted implants were placed and "malaligned more precisely." However, the authors did not explain the clinical significance of these differences. Brin et al answered this question when they found that inaccuracies as small as 5 mm can result in a significant detrimental effect to the mechanical axis in a saw bones model.[17] Thus these studies clearly indicate that navigation cannot offset poor surgical technique or lack of attention to detail.

Femoral Fracture

The use of trackers with pin sites has also been associated with fractures. The screw hole may act as a stress riser that subsequently results in potential for fracture.[18] A case report exists which identifies two patients with a periprosthetic fracture through a pin site postoperatively. The authors of the report conclude that, by placing the pins in metaphyseal bone and not diaphyseal bone, there is less of a stress riser phenomenon and subsequent risk of fracture. While the diaphyseal cortical placement of pins may be less intrusive to the surgical field and offers better temporary fixation, the potential catastrophic complication of periprosthetic fracture far outweighs these benefits. They also advocate the use of medial to lateral pins to prevent breeching of the anterior cortex, which represents the tension side of the femur and may be more prone to fracture with pin placement.

OTHER BENEFITS

Decreased Blood Transfusions

A number of studies have found that perioperative blood loss is significantly reduced with navigation, as compared to conventional techniques. Spriggins et al found a significantly decreased rate of transfusion and higher mean hemoglobin levels in the immediate postoperative period of the CAS group when compared to the conventional group, as well as decreased blood loss in obese patients. They found that this decreased the risks associated with blood transfusion, including but not limited to infection and disease transmission. The authors hypothesized that this benefit is secondary to avoiding breach of the intramedullary cavities.[19]

Decreased Embolic Phenomenon

The embolic load seen by the patient secondary to CAS is also significantly decreased. A prospective, double-blind, randomized study compared cardiac embolic load sustained during CAS and conventional TKA as measured by transesophageal echocardiography. The results were startling. The conventional group had a mean embolic score of 6.15, as compared to 4.89 in the CAS group. The authors conclude that CAS can significantly reduce the rates of perioperative cardiovascular dysfunction and postoperative neurologic sequelae.[20]

Soft Tissue Balancing

Soft tissue balancing in TKA can also be improved with CAS when compared with the conventional method. The reason for this is the more accurate measurements of flexion-extension mismatches and the ability to quantify how much has been improved with a soft tissue release. Han et al looked at 60 knees in the CAS group and 56 knees in the conventional group that had a gap difference of greater than 3 mm between the medial and lateral sides in both 90° of flexion and extension. There was a greater outlier group with the conventional method—25% versus 12%.[21] The navigation group ensures a more accurate flexion-extension match that goes beyond intraoperative "feel" by quantifying gap balancing.

Economic Impact

The economic impact of navigation cannot be overlooked either. Specifically, if the rate of revision significantly decreases secondary to improved kinematics and mechanical alignment, then the cost of navigation is more than offset by these savings. A cost-effectiveness study out of Massachusetts General Hospital determined that computer navigation was cost-effective at high-volume institutions ("high volume" refers to institutions seeing more than 250 navigation knees per year). The authors found that an annual revision rate reduction of 2% would make the investment cost-effective when using a Markov Decision Model.[22]

CONCLUSION

In summary, the use of computer navigation for TKA has many benefits. Of upmost importance in TKA is the maintenance of the mechanical axis, which has been shown to correlate with implant longevity. This, combined with additional benefits of diminished blood loss, improved gap balancing, decreased embolic phenomenon, and even economic savings, brings the value of computer navigation into sharp relief. While the initial start-up may be expensive and presents a learning curve that may dissuade its use by experienced surgeons, we strongly advocate the use of computer navigation for more precise and quantitative assessments of total knee arthroplasty.

REFERENCES

1. Lotke PA, Ecker ML. Influence of positioning in total knee replacement. *J Bone Joint Surg Am.* 1977;59:77-79.
2. Maquet P. Biomecanique de la gonarthrose. *Acta Orthop Belg.* 1972;38(suppl. I):S33-S54.
3. Jeffery R, Morris R, Denham R. Coronal alignment after total knee replacement. *J Bone Joint Surg Br.* 1991;73:709-714.
4. Bargren JH, Blaha JD, Freeman MA. Alignment in total knee arthroplasty. Correlated biomechanical and clinical observations. *Clin Orthop Relat Res.* 1983;173:178-183.
5. Choong PF, Dowsey MM, Stoney JD. *J Arthroplasty.* 2009;24(4):560-569.
6. Longstaff LM, Sloan K, Stamp N, et al. Good alignment after total knee arthroplasty leads to faster rehabilitation and better function. *J Arthroplasty.* 2009;24(4):570-578.
7. Sikorski JM. Alignment in total knee replacement. *J Bone Joint Surg Br.* 2008;90:1121-1127.
8. Berry DJ, Parratte S, Pagnano MW, et al. Effect of postoperative mechanical axis alignment on the fifteen-year survival of modern, cemented total knee replacements. *J Bone Joint Surg Am.* 2010;92:2143-2149.
9. Mont MA, Mahoney MO. Commentary on: Parratte S, et al. Effect of postoperative mechanical axis alignment on the fifteen-year survival of modern, cemented total knee replacements. *J Bone Joint Surg Am.* 2010;92:e16 1-2.
10. Stulberg DS, Loan P, Sarin V, et al. Computer-assisted navigation in total knee replacement: results of an initial experience in thirty-five patients. *J Bone Joint Surg Am.* 2001;84:90-98.
11. Mason JB, Fehring T, Fahrbach K et al. Meta-analysis of alignment outcomes in computer-assisted total knee arthroplasty surgery. *J Arthroplasty.* 2007;22(8): 1097-1106.
12. Matziolis G, Krocker D, Perka C, et al. A prospective, randomized study of computer-assisted and conventional total knee arthroplasty: three-dimensional evaluation of implant alignment and rotation. *J Bone Joint Surg Am.* 2007;89:236-243.
13. Dutton AQ, Yeo S, Chong H, et al. Computer-assisted minimally invasive total knee arthroplasty compared with standard total knee arthroplasty: a prospective, randomized study. *J Bone Joint Surg Am.* 2008;90:2-9.
14. Klein G, Austin M, Hozack W, et al. Total knee arthroplasty using computer-assisted navigation in patients with deformities of the femur and tibia. *J Arthroplasty.* 2006;21(2):284-288.
15. Hernandez-Vaquero D, Noriega-Fernandez A, et al. Computer assistance increases precision of component placement in total knee arthroplasty with articular deformity. *Clin Orthop Rel Res.* 2010;468:1237-1241.
16. Robinson M, Eckhoff D, Bach J, et al. Variability of landmark identification in total knee arthroplasty. *Clin Orthop Rel Res.* 2006;442:57-62.
17. Brin Y, Livshetz I, Zukor D, et al. Precise landmarking in computer assisted total knee arthroplasty is critical to final alignment. *J Orthop Res.* 2010;28:1355-1359.
18. Wysocki R, Sheinkop M, Della Valle C, et al. Femoral fracture through a previous pin site after com-

puter-assisted total knee arthroplasty. *J Arthroplasty.* 2008;23:462-465.

19. Kalairajah Y, Simpson D, Cossey AJ, et al. Blood loss after total knee arthroplasty: effects of computer-assisted surgery. *J Bone Joint Surg Br.* 2005;87:1480-1482.
20. Church J, Scadden J, Janes G, et al. Embolic phenomena during computer-assisted and conventional total knee replacement. *J Bone Joint Surg Br.* 2007;89:481-485.
21. Lee D-H, Park J-H, Song D-I, et al. Accuracy of soft tissue balancing in TKA: comparison between navigation-assisted gap balancing and conventional measured resection. *Knee Surg Sports Traumatol Arthrosc.* 2010;18:381-387.
22. Slover J, Bozic K, Malchau H, et al. Impact of hospital volume on the economic value of computer navigation for total knee replacement. *J Bone Joint Surg Am.* 2008;90:1492-1500.

55

Robotically Assisted Unicompartmental Knee Arthroplasty

Jess H. Lonner

Currently approximately 10% of patients who undergo knee arthroplasty for arthritis receive unicompartmental knee arthroplasty (UKA).[1] That number may increase to 20% or more, as patients continue to present for treatment of their arthritis at an earlier stage than patients typically did in the past, particularly if combined with patellofemoral arthroplasty.[2] UKA is becoming more germane, given the interest of both patients and surgeons in early intervention strategies, which tend to be more conservative and leave a more "normal" feeling knee than total knee arthroplasty. UKA is also a particularly relevant option, considering that knee replacement patients today tend to be more active, younger, and often present with an earlier stage of arthritis than in years past.

The results and durability of unicompartmental arthroplasty are affected by a variety of factors, including the pattern of arthritis, deformity and pain location, prosthesis design, polyethylene quality, and implant alignment and fixation. Excessive posterior tibial slope or varus of the tibial component and/or mechanical axis of the limb may predispose the prosthesis to early failure.[3-5] Achieving consistently accurate alignment of the tibial component in UKA using conventional approaches is difficult.[3,6-8] Outliers beyond 2° of the desired alignment may occur in as many as 40% to 60% of cases using conventional methods,[8,9] and the range of component alignment varies considerably, even in the hands of skilled knee surgeons.[3] The problem is compounded when using minimally invasive surgical approaches, which is how most contemporary UKAs are likely performed.[6,7,10] One study analyzing the results of 221 consecutive UKAs performed through a minimally invasive approach found a large range of tibial component alignment, with a mean of 6° (SD = ±4) and a range from 18° varus to 6° valgus.[7]

Computer navigation was introduced in an effort to reduce the number of outliers and improve the accuracy of UKA. However, even with computer navigation, the number of outliers (beyond 2° of the preoperatively planned implant position) may approach 15%, since there remains an element of imprecision with the use of standard cutting guides and conventional methods of bone preparation, even when positioning of the guides is guided by computer navigation.[8] Robotic guidance was therefore introduced to capitalize on the improvements seen with computer navigation but also to further refine and enhance the accuracy of bone preparation, even with minimally invasive techniques, by better interfacing and integrating the planning and performance of bone preparation.[9,11,12]

INDICATIONS AND CONTRAINDICATIONS OF ROBOTICALLY ASSISTED UKA

The indications and contraindications for robotically assisted UKA are identical to those used for conventional approaches, with typical variations depending on surgeon philosophy and tolerances. These are outlined in Chapter 56.[2,5,12-18] There are no specific contraindications to the use of robotic assistance for unicompartmental arthroplasty, although the added duration of surgery early in the learning curve may make it undesirable for some patients in whom a briefer anesthetic time is warranted. Anesthetic times may be as long as 2 hours during the initial few cases with robotic assistance but quickly decrease soon thereafter to approximately 1 hour, as the surgical team becomes more proficient with the setup, preparation, and nuances of the surgical procedure.

ROBOTIC SYSTEM DESCRIPTION

The currently available robotic system in the United States is the Robotic Arm Interactive Orthopaedic System (RIO) (MAKO Surgical Inc., Ft. Lauderdale, FL), a surgeon-interactive robotic arm that uses preoperative computed tomography images of the patient's lower extremity to allow accurate preoperative planning, intraoperative navigation, and robotic assistance to prepare bone for implantation of UKA components (Fig. 55-1). Other systems, such as autonomous Robodoc (Curexo Technology Corp, Fremont, CA) and semiautonomous Acrobot (Acrobot Ltd, London, UK) are not currently approved for use in knee surgery by the United States Food and Drug Administration.

The RIO system provides a stereotactic interface, which constrains the surgeon in the preparation of the femur and the tibia. Stereotactic boundaries are virtual walls created by the software and implemented through the robotic arm hardware to restrict the cutting tip to within a predefined resection volume.

The RIO technology is an alternative to standard UKA instrumentation with their intra- and extramedullary guides, pinned cutting blocks and jigs, and saws. In their place are burrs of varying sizes, which have reduced inventory and further optimized the application of minimally invasive approaches to UKA without having to squeeze miniaturized, but still bulky, instruments into a small wound. The RIO robotic arm is enabling technology that has improved the accuracy and the performance of unicompartmental arthroplasty through a minimally invasive approach.

PREOPERATIVE PLANNING

Once the patient is considered a candidate for unicompartmental or bicompartmental knee arthroplasty, the preoperative planning becomes focused on the robotic arm and RIO software and technology. A preoperative computer tomography (CT) scan is performed of the patient's hip, knee, and ankle to gather the patient-specific data on limb alignment (mechanical axis) and anatomic features so that the operative plan for resection can be developed. The RIO software converts the CT scan data into segmented slices, which create the patient-specific bone model from which the operative plan can be determined by the surgeon before surgery. The RIO software allows manipulation and coordination of the collected data to model the limb and accurately plan the implant size, alignment, and corresponding volume and orientation of bone resection (Figs. 55-2 and 55-3). The system can also accommodate the performance of patellofemoral arthroplasty (PFA) for isolated patellofemoral arthritis or when there is bicompartmental arthritis for the performance of bicompartmental knee arthroplasty with a modular combination of UKA and PFA.[12]

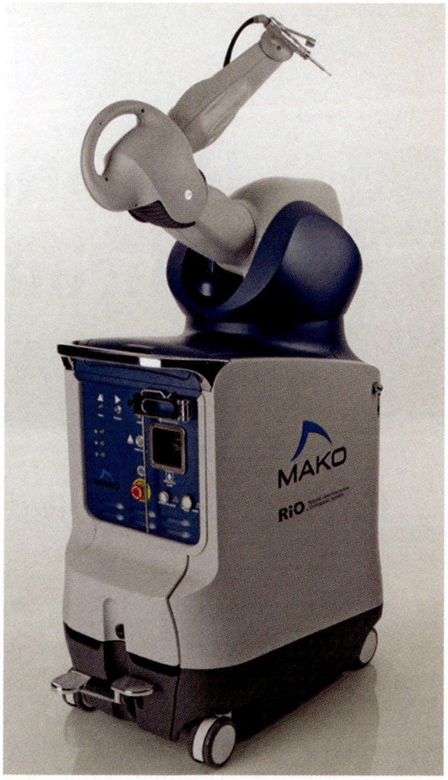

FIGURE 55-1. *RIO Robotic Arm (MAKO Surgical Inc, Ft. Lauderdale, FL).*

TECHNIQUE FOR UKA

The patient is positioned supine on the operating table and the surgical limb is positioned in a table-mounted leg holder. The robotic arm is sterilely draped and brought into the surgical field (Fig. 55-4). A 6-mm burr is attached to the "hand" of the robotic arm, also called the end effector. Bicortical partially threaded pins are drilled percutaneously into the proximal tibia and distal femur and optical tracking arrays are clamped to the respective pins, approximately 1 cm above the skin surface.

Standard arthrotomies are made, depending on surgeon preference. Minimally invasive incisions are effective for unicompartmental knee arthroplasty, with slightly larger incisions for bicompartmental or modular total knee arthroplasties. Next, surface landmarks, including the medial and lateral malleoli, medial and lateral epicondyles, and numerous points along the articular cartilage of the knee and periarticular surfaces of the distal femur and proximal tibia, are identified and registered using optical probes. The RIO integrates the registration points and preoperative CT data.

Once the registration has been completed, osteophytes are excised on the surgical side of the knee (medial or lateral) and a dynamic soft tissue balancing algorithm is initiated. The virtual modeling of the patient's knee and intraoperative tracking allows real-time adjustments of component position to balance the flexion and extension spaces. With an applied valgus stress to tension the medial collateral ligament (for medial UKA) or a varus stress to tension the lateral structures (for lateral UKA), the three-dimensional position of the femur and the tibia are captured throughout a passive range of knee motion. By providing a virtual representation of flexion and extension gap spacing, an assessment can be made of whether the planned position of the femoral and tibial components is appropriate through a full range of motion (Fig. 55-5). With each planned position of

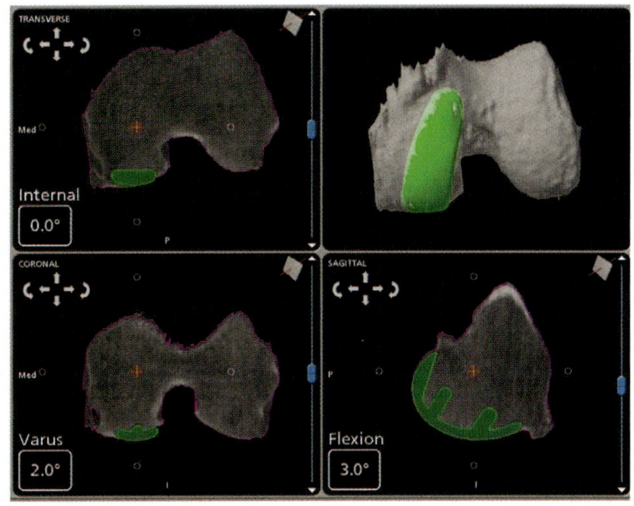

FIGURE 55-3. *The femoral component is similarly templated.*

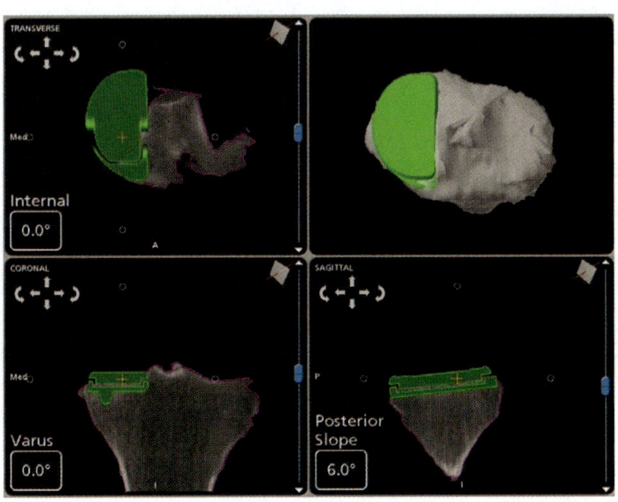

FIGURE 55-2. *The tibial component is virtually templated preoperatively, including selection of size, alignment, and position within the proximal tibia.*

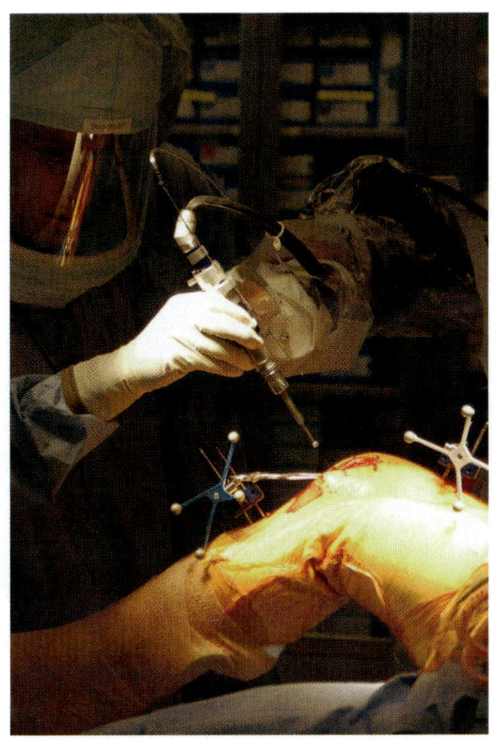

FIGURE 55-4. *The robotic arm is sterilely draped and moved next to the operating table and patient.*

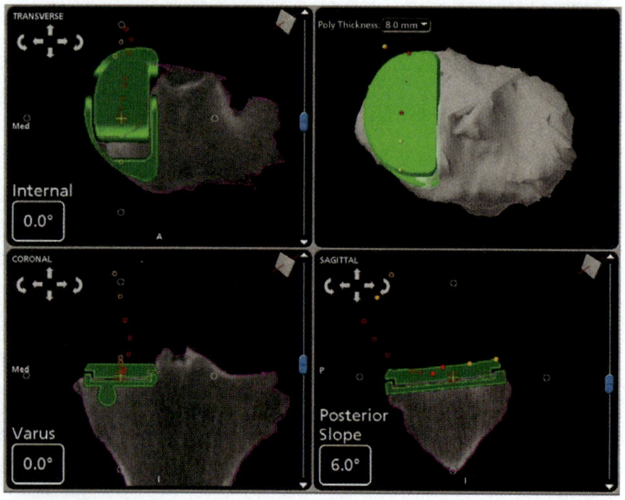

FIGURE 55-5. *During the preoperative planning, three-dimensional positions of the femur and tibia are captured through a passive range of motion and an assessment of tracking of one component on the other is made. In this case, the red dots on the tibial component illustrate the central tracking of the midportion of the femur through an arc of motion.*

the implants, a visual representation of the "tightness" or "looseness" of the knee is displayed at every captured flexion angle. The distance between planned components is displayed on a bar graph at the corresponding flexion angles captured (Fig. 55-6). Each "bar" represents relative knee tightness or laxity between the femoral and tibial components at a particular degree of knee flexion. By adjusting the implant position, the flexion and extension gaps can be planned a priori to achieve the desired postsurgical values.

Bone resection is then performed with the robotic arm, which applies stereotactic boundaries to a cutting burr positioned on its end. The surgeon moves the cutting burr within the predefined volume in burring mode to resect bone, without resistance. If, however, the burr tip is moved to the boundaries of the haptic zone, the arm applies a force simulating contact with a rigid wall, thereby confining the tip to the correct region in space and safeguarding against inadvertent bone removal. Thus the robotic arm effectively acts as a three-dimensional virtual instrument that precisely executes the preoperative plan.

The femur is addressed first and resected at varying degrees of flexion and extension to gain access to different parts of the condyle. More extension helps access the ante-

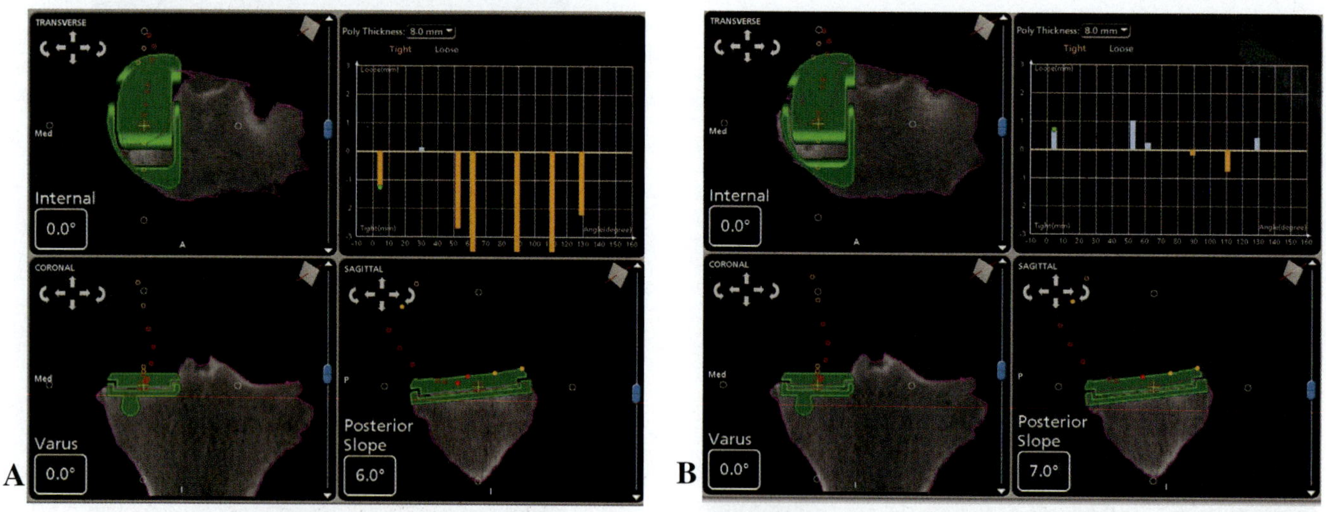

FIGURE 55-6. *A bar graph showing relative tightness or laxity of the knee in different degrees of flexion based on where the femoral and tibial components are preoperatively templated. Adjustments can be made to tighten or loosen the knee in different areas by adjusting the virtual position of the components. (**A**) Demonstrates relative tightness of the joint through an entire range of motion (orange bars). (**B**) Shows that a slight increase in posterior slope and removal of 1.4 mm of additional tibial bone improves the balance and tissue tension in the joint.*

rior aspect of the femur and allows retraction of the anterior soft tissue; deeper flexion helps gain exposure for preparation of the posterior femoral condyle. Preparation of the proximal tibia is performed in a similar fashion (Fig. 55-7).

The trial femoral and tibial components are provisionally implanted and optical probes are used to trace the surfaces of the prostheses to confirm that the implant position matches the preoperative virtual plan (Fig. 55-8). An assessment of range of motion and stability is made. If necessary, additional bone can be removed by making adjustments to slope or depth of resection in the surgical plan on the computer and then resculpting the bone surfaces. Once satisfactory alignment and stability are achieved and if no additional adjustments are needed, the bony surfaces are irrigated with pulsatile lavage and dried, and the components are cemented into place.

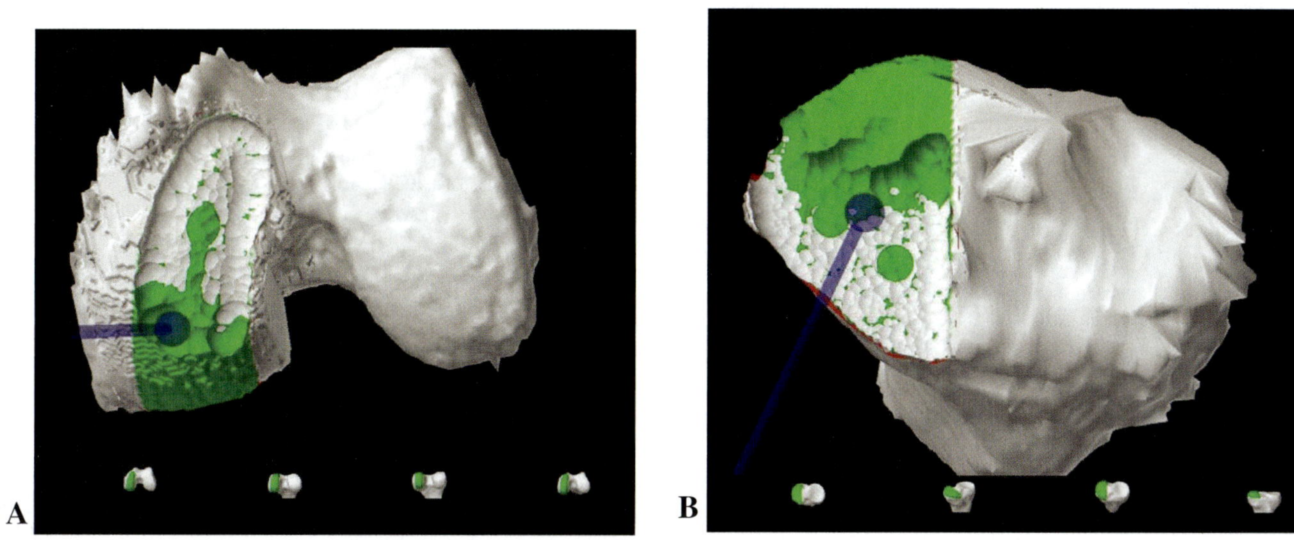

FIGURE 55-7. *Femoral (**A**) and tibial (**B**) preparation as seen in real-time virtual imaging.*

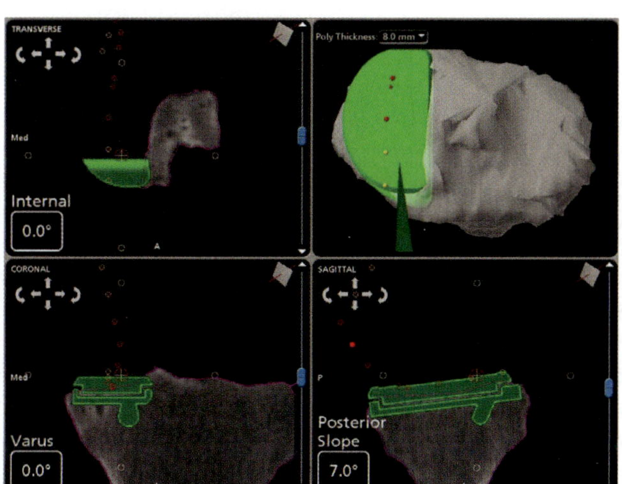

FIGURE 55-8. *Trialing of the components is performed and an optical probe is used to trace the articulating surfaces of the femoral and tibial components to ensure that their positions match the preoperative plan. In this image, the tip of the probe is on the articulating surface of the tibial component (represented by the crosshairs) and is perfectly aligned with the preoperative plan.*

RESULTS

Lonner et al reviewed their experience with their initial 31 cases of robotic arm-assisted UKA. In that series, the radiographic alignment of the tibial component was compared to the preoperatively planned position in 31 consecutive knees in 31 patients undergoing UKA using robotic arm-assisted bone preparation and in 27 consecutive patients who underwent unilateral UKA using conventional manual instrumentation to determine the error of bone preparation and variance with each technique (Fig. 55-9). The root-mean-square (RMS) error of the tibial slope was 3.1° with the conventional manual technique compared with 1.9° robotically. In addition, the variance using manual instruments was 2.6 times greater ($p = .02$) than the robotic arm-guided bone preparation method. In the coronal plane, the average error of tibial alignment was 2.7° ± 2.1° more varus using manual instruments compared with 0.2° ± 1.8° when bone preparation was performed with robotic arm assistance ($p < .0001$), and the varus-valgus RMS error was 3.4° manually compared with 1.8° robotically.[19] Roche et al evaluated their first 43 patients who underwent UKA using robotic assistance. Of the 344 X-ray measurements that were analyzed, less than 1% were considered outliers.[11] These studies, which reviewed the authors' early experiences with a robotic arm technique show that the accuracy of bone preparation is significantly improved compared to conventional minimally invasive surgery techniques, even early after technology adoption.

A series by Roche et al reported on the results of robotically assisted UKA in 84 patients with a minimum 1-year follow-up from a multicenter registry. At a minimum of 1 year after UKA, there were statistically significant improvements in range of motion ($p < .02$), Knee Society scores ($p < .0001$), and Western Ontario and McMaster Universities Osteoarthritis Index (WOMAC) scores ($p < .01$), particularly pain ($p < .01$) and stiffness ($p < .01$), compared to preoperative values.[11]

The application of this robotic system for modular bicompartmental knee arthroplasty has been equally successful (Fig. 55-10). John et al reviewed the initial 30 consecutive modular unlinked bicompartmental UKAs and PFAs performed by this author and found that at a minimum 1-year follow-up (range, 1 year to 2.5 years), WOMAC pain score decreased from 11.0 to 2.8 ($p = .0001$); WOMAC function score decreased from 13.6 to 3.2 ($p = .0008$); WOMAC total score decreased from 24.6 to 6.0 ($p = .0001$); range of motion increased from 122° to 138° ($p = .0001$); and Knee Society function and knee scores increased from 56 to 92 and 40 to 88, respectively ($p = .0001$). There were no perioperative complications and no radiographic evidence of loosening, polyethylene wear, or progressive arthritis of the lateral tibiofemoral compartment.[20]

COMPLICATIONS

Typical complications after unicompartmental arthroplasty, in general, can also occur with robotic arm assistance, including loosening of the prostheses, polyethylene wear, progressive osteoarthritis of the unresurfaced compartments of the knee, infection, stiffness, instability, thromboembolic complications, and others.

Surgical complications resulting from robotic arm-assisted UKA are identical to those encountered with surgical navigation in general. The pin sites create a stress riser in the cortical bone, which poses a risk for fracture. Inadvertent pin placement could theoretically cause neurovascular laceration. While some have found surgical time to be excessive with the use of autonomous robotic systems applied to total knee arthroplasty, the surgical times with this semiautonomous system are well within an acceptable range. In this author's experience, for instance, the surgical time from insertion of tracking pins to implantation was reduced from approximately 2 hours to less than 1 hour before 10 cases had been completed.

A study by Chun et al reported the need to abandon 22% of cases using an autonomous robotic-assisted technology (Robodoc, Curexo Technology Corp, Fremont, CA). Conversely, the need to abandon the procedure with the semiautonomous, surgeon-driven technology used by this author has been less than 0.5%.[21]

POSTOPERATIVE MANAGEMENT

Physical therapy is typically commenced on the day of surgery, once the spinal anesthetic has worn off, unless the procedure is performed later in the day, in which case it begins on the first postoperative day. Patients are encouraged to ambulate immediately with a cane, crutches, or a walker. Range-of-motion exercises begin immediately. Patients are most often discharged 1 day after surgery. Use of a cane can be terminated once the patient recovers adequate balance and strength. Most patients have been able to ambulate without a cane as soon as 1 to 2 weeks after surgery. For thromboembolic disease (TED) prophylaxis, this author prefers the use of enteric coated aspirin in a dosage of 325 mg used twice daily for 4 to 6 weeks, depending on activity level and tolerance. Alternatively, low-dose warfarin is used in patients who are at higher risk for TED or unable to take aspirin.

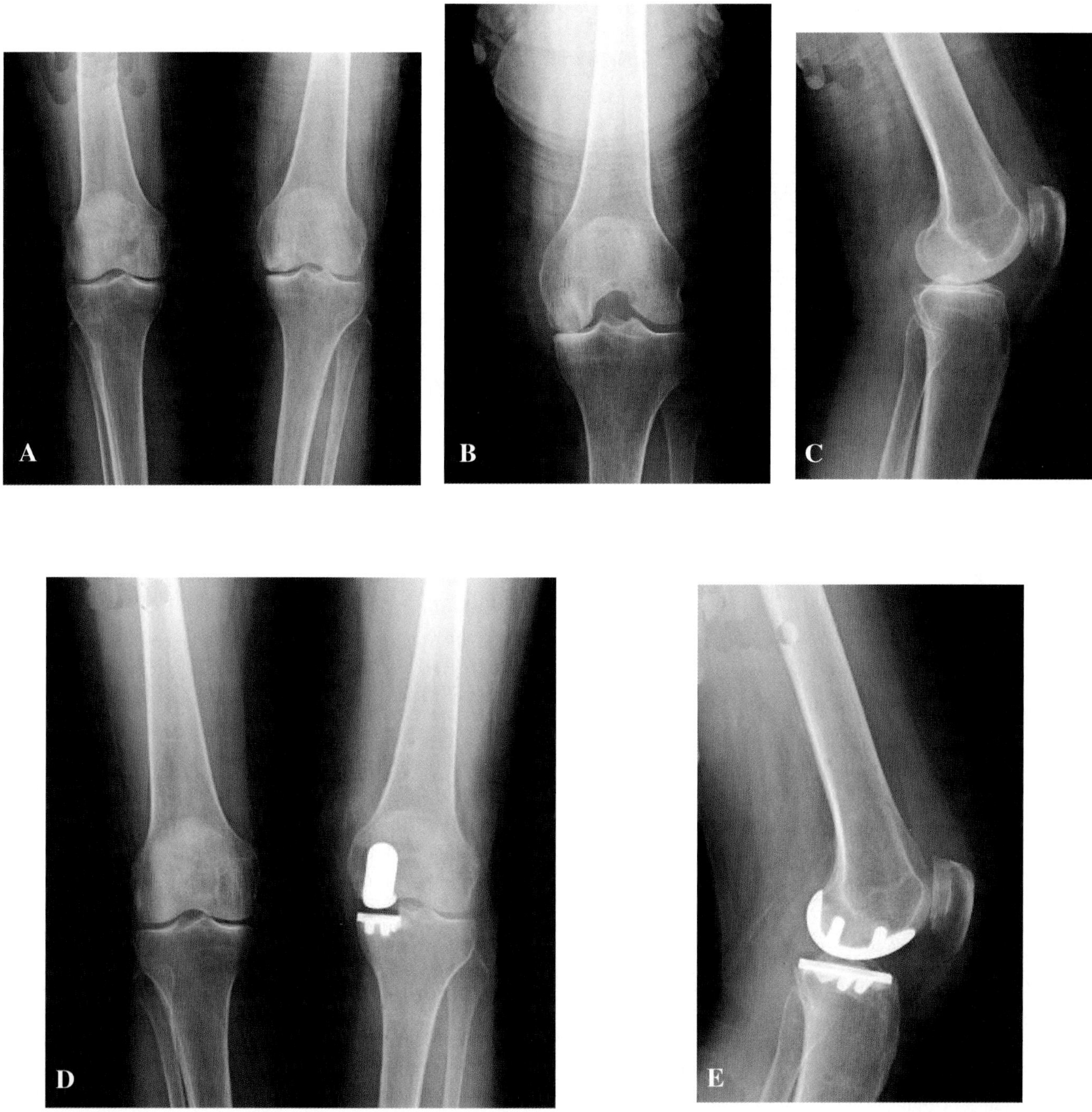

FIGURE 55-9. *Preoperative standing anteroposterior (**A**), midflexion posteroanterior (**B**), and lateral (**C**) radiographs showing advanced medial compartment arthritis and spontaneous osteonecrosis of the knee. Postoperative anteroposterior (**D**) and lateral (**E**) radiographs show a well-aligned implant that corresponds to the preoperative plan.*

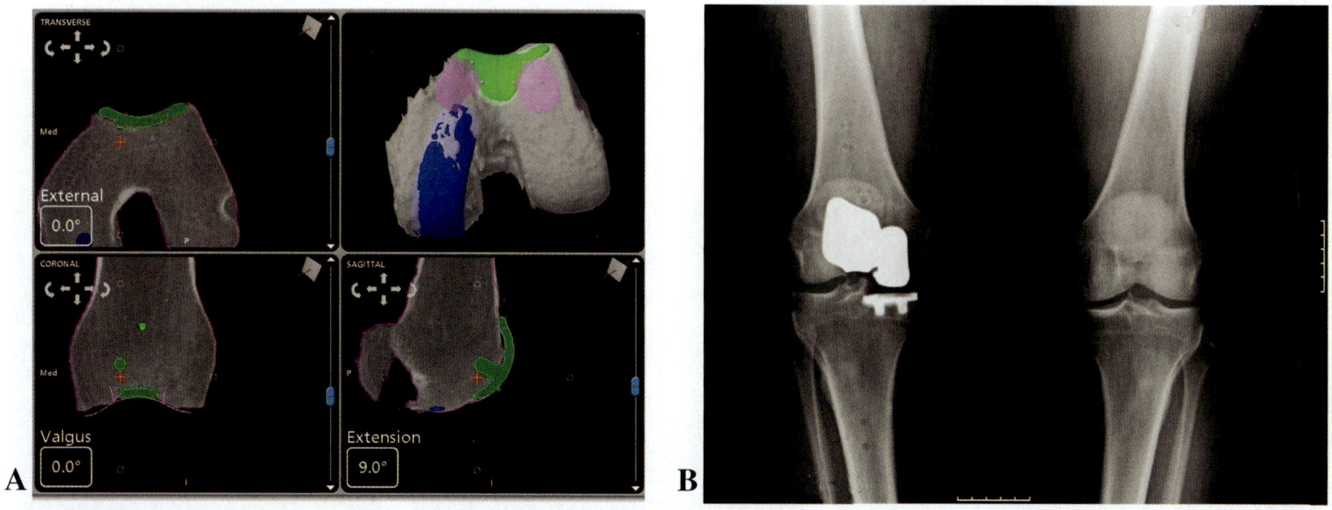

FIGURE 55-10. *Preoperative plan for robotically assisted modular bicompartmental knee arthroplasty (**A**) and postoperative anteroposterior radiographs (**B**).*

PEARLS AND PITFALLS

The following are some pearls and pitfalls of robotically assisted UKA:

- Preoperative "templating" is important; follow sound principles of implant positioning.
- Plan conservative bone resection. Adjustments can be made intraoperatively to volume of resected bone and slopes. Overresection cannot be corrected; underresection can.
- Like all navigated cases, conventional or robotic, the need for accurate intraoperative landmarking and registration is important.
- Whether or not image-guided or imageless systems are superior is not established; however, the fact that this system is image guided does seem to provide a safeguard.
- Adequate surgical exposure remains critical, even though the procedure is amenable to minimally invasive techniques.
- At all times make sure the bone being resected corresponds to the plan and "makes sense" before starting the bone resection process. This can be done by "tracing the field."
- Be sure to protect the soft tissues during bone preparation.
- As with standard techniques, careful cementing is important. Try not to leave cement behind.
- If there is a need to abandon use of the robot either because the preparation does not seem to correspond to the plan or if there is an electromechanical problem with the system, be sure to have manual (conventional) instruments available.

REFERENCES

1. Riddle DL, Jiranek WA, McGlynn FJ. Yearly incidence of unicompartmental arthroplasty in the United States. *J Arthroplasty.* 2008;23:408-412.
2. Lonner JH. Modular bicompartmental knee arthroplasty with robotic arm assistance. *Am J Orthop.* 2009;38(2 suppl):28-31.
3. Collier MB, Eickmann TH, Sukezaki F, et al. Patient, implant, and alignment factors associated with revision of medial compartment unicondylar arthroplasty. *J Arthroplasty.* 2006;21(suppl):108-115.
4. Hernigou P, Deschamps G. Alignment influences wear in the knee after medial unicompartmental arthroplasty. *Clin Orthop Relat Res.* 2004;423:161-165.
5. Hernigou P, Deschamps G. Posterior slope of the tibial implant and the outcome of unicompartmental

knee arthroplasty. *J Bone Joint Surg Am.* 2004;86: 506-511.

6. Fisher DA, Watts M, Davis KE. Implant position in knee surgery: a comparison of minimally invasive, open unicompartmental, and total knee arthroplasty. *J Arthroplasty.* 2003;18(suppl):2-8.
7. Hamilton WG, Collier MB, Tarabee E, et al. Incidence and reasons for reoperation after minimally invasive unicompartmental knee arthroplasty. *J Arthroplasty.* 2006;21(suppl):98-107.
8. Keene G, Simpson D, Kalairajah Y. Limb alignment in computer-assisted minimally-invasive unicompartmental knee replacement. *J Bone Joint Surg Br.* 2006; 88:44-48.
9. Cobb J, Henckel J, Gomes P, et al. Hands-on robotic unicompartmental knee replacement. *J Bone Joint Surg Br.* 2006;88:188-197.
10. Romanowski MR, Repicci JA. Minimally invasive unicondylar arthroplasty: eight-year follow-up. *J Knee Surg.* 2002;15:17-22.
11. Sinha RK. Outcomes of robotic arm assisted unicompartmental arthroplasty. *Am J Orthop.* 2009;38 (suppl):20-22.
12. Lonner JH. Indications for unicompartmental knee arthroplasty and rationale for robotic arm-assisted technology. *Am J Orthop.* 2009;38(2 suppl):3-6.
13. Berend KR, Lombardi AV Jr, Adams JB. Obesity, young age, patellofemoral disease, and anterior knee pain: identifying the unicondylar arthroplasty patient in the United States. *Orthopedics.* 2007;30(5 suppl): 19-23.
14. Berend KR, Lombardi AV Jr, Mallory TH, et al. Early failure of minimally invasive unicompartmental knee arthroplasty is associated with obesity. *Clin Orthop Relat Res.* 2005;435:171-180.
15. Borus T, Thornhill T. Unicompartmental knee arthroplasty. *J Am Acad Orthop Surg.* 2007;15:9-18.
16. Kozinn SC, Scott RD. Unicondylar knee arthroplasty. *J Bone Joint Surg Am.* 1989;71:145-150.
17. Pennington DW, Swienckowski JJ, Lutes WB, et al. Unicompartmental knee arthroplasty in patients sixty years of age or younger. *J Bone Joint Surg Am.* 2003; 85:1968-1973.
18. Schai PA, Suh JT, Thornhill TS, et al. Unicompartmental knee arthroplasty in middle aged patients: a two to six year follow-up evaluation. *J Arthroplasty.* 1998;13:365-372.
19. Lonner JH, John TK, Conditt MA. Robotic arm-assisted UKA improves tibial component alignment: a pilot study. *Clin Orthop Relat Res.* 2010;468:141-146.
20. John T, Sheth N, Lonner JH. Modular bicompartmental arthroplasty of the knee. Proc., Knee Society, September 2010.
21. Chun YS, Kim KI, Cho YJ, et al. Causes and patterns of aborting a robot-assisted arthroplasty. *J Arthroplasty.* 2011;26:621-625.

56 Computer-Assisted Imageless Unicompartmental Knee Replacement Surgery

Dinesh K. Nathwani and Gareth G. Jones

In an attempt to improve the reliability of implant positioning and soft tissue balancing, computer-assisted surgery (CAS) in knee arthroplasty is gaining popularity. Currently its role can be broadly divided into two groups: image-based navigation, in which data are primarily obtained from preoperative and intraoperative computerized tomography (CT) scans, and imageless navigation, in which key landmarks are identified and registered intraoperatively. Robotic-assisted surgery most commonly works in conjunction with image-based navigation systems to guide or replace the surgeon during bone resection.

The use of unicompartmental knee arthroplasty (UKA) to treat isolated medial or lateral osteoarthritis is widely accepted; it is less invasive and bone conserving when compared with total knee arthroplasty (TKA), has a shorter recovery period,[1] and results in improved physiological knee kinematics[2] with increased flexion.[3,4]

Unicompartmental knee replacement (UKR) was initially performed through the same open approach employed for a total knee arthroplasty. The move to a minimally invasive approach with a smaller skin incision and no eversion or dislocation of the patella was popularized by the introduction of the phase 3 Oxford knee instrumentation in 1998.[5]

Published survival rates of UKA performed through an open approach in clinical follow-up studies are good, with a 10-year survival rate of 94% to 100%.[6,7] The Oxford group has published a 10-year survival rate of 96% for minimally invasive phase 3 arthroplasties. And a recent systematic review of worldwide joint register data sets found the revision rate to be 15.3% at 10 years. No doubt the difference is multifactorial but inaccurate implant positioning is a likely contributory factor.

Implant position and soft tissue balancing in TKA are understandably thought to have a role in implant survival.[8,9] Postoperative radiographic analysis has suggested that unicondylar prosthesis positioning is less accurate than total knee prosthesis positioning, and minimally invasive unicondylar knee replacement is less accurate again compared with an open procedure.[10] Meta-analysis of studies comparing CAS TKA with conventional surgery concluded that there was a significant improvement in component orientation and mechanical axis when CAS was used.[11] Hence it is somewhat surprising that a questionnaire survey of the British Association for Surgery of the Knee found that only 8.5% of UKR surgeons occasionally used navigation for unicondylar knee arthroplasty, especially because the majority of operations are now performed via a minimally invasive approach.[12] The identification of intraoperative landmarks presents a real challenge.

PREOPERATIVE EVALUATION

Classically, patients give a history of predominant medial or lateral knee pain. Anterior knee pain may also be present but has been demonstrated by the Oxford group not to affect clinical outcome.[13] A full past medical and social history is obtained to identify patients suitable for an arthroplasty procedure. All patients are asked to complete an Oxford knee score.[14]

Preoperative assessment includes weight-bearing anteroposterior full extension, lateral, and skyline radiographs. The authors also routinely obtain 45° posteroanterior flexion radiographs as described by Rosenberg et al.[15]

PREPARATION OF PATIENT FOR SURGERY

Patients undergo a routine anesthetic-led preoperative assessment, with appropriate investigations as prescribed by the NHS National Institute for Health and Clinical Excellence preoperative tests guidelines[16]; a blood type and screen is performed during this assessment. Before admission, it is mandatory for patients to attend Joint School, which aims to educate them and forms part of an enhanced recovery program designed to improve patient experience and reduce length of stay.

INDICATIONS AND CONTRAINDICATIONS FOR SURGERY

The authors' patient inclusion criteria include predominantly unicompartmental osteoarthritis (radiological grade 3–4 using Ahlbäck's classification[17]), a functionally intact anterior cruciate ligament, fully correctable varus-valgus deformity of 10° to 15° of flexion, and a fixed flexion deformity of less than 15°.

Some patellofemoral osteoarthritis is accepted, provided there is no severe lateral osteoarthritis with bone loss and subluxation. This is supported by the findings of Beard et al,[18] who prospectively found no difference in the functional outcome scores of patients undergoing Oxford UKAs with intraoperative full-thickness patellofemoral cartilage loss. One has to exercise caution in those found intraoperatively to have "substantial bone loss with eburnation and grooving in the lateral part of the patellofemoral joint." In the authors' own series, many of these underwent a TKA, a decision supported by the poorer outcomes in patients with radiological obliteration of the lateral patellar facet joint space.[13]

Large reviews such as that of the Norwegian Arthroplasty Register[4] demonstrating that resurfacing of the patella has no clinical effect on pain and function after TKA also add credence to the decision not to exclude patients with patellofemoral osteoarthritis.

The intraoperative finding of a nonfunctioning anterior cruciate ligament (ACL) or grade 3/4 osteoarthritis (Outerbridge classification[19]) affecting the other tibiofemoral compartment is grounds for abandoning the procedure and performing either a combined ACL reconstruction and UKA, or a TKA.

SURGICAL APPROACH AND TECHNIQUE

Approach

The authors' experience involves the Accuris fixed-bearing unicompartmental knee replacement (Smith & Nephew UK Ltd), together with the BrainLAB Vector Vision (BrainLAB, Helmstetten, Germany) image-free navigation system. As detailed in the operative technique below, the Vector Vision software utilizes two reference arrays (tibia and femur) plus registration of intraoperative anatomical landmarks with a blunt pointer, to morph a generic three-dimensional (3D) model of a knee joint. Leg alignment and flexion-extension gap can then be assessed visually in real time and bone resection parameters are planned (mechanical axis set at 0°, posterior slope 3°), guided, and checked by the navigation system at each stage.

Technique

The procedure begins with the patient supine, tourniquet applied, and a side support and foot stop to support the limb. The tourniquet is routinely released before closure and hemostasis are achieved, thus avoiding the necessity of drains postoperatively. A minimally invasive approach can be utilized and the patellar subluxed rather than everted. At this stage all three compartments are assessed for ongoing wear and this assessment is recorded. Reference arrays are then inserted into the femur (two 4-mm threaded pins) and the authors' preference is to use the surgical incision for these pins. The tibial pins (two 3-mm threaded pins) are inserted away from the incision site. The reflective reference arrays are attached to the pins according to the required orientation. The markers on the arrays reflect the infrared beam that is emitted from the BrainLAB hardware module and camera (Fig. 56-1). The hardware picks up these *x,y,z* axes reflections and identifies the fixed bony landmarks of the femur and tibia, respectively.

A process of "registration" takes place and the software guides the surgeon through all the necessary steps to allow the computer system to build up a 3D model of the affected

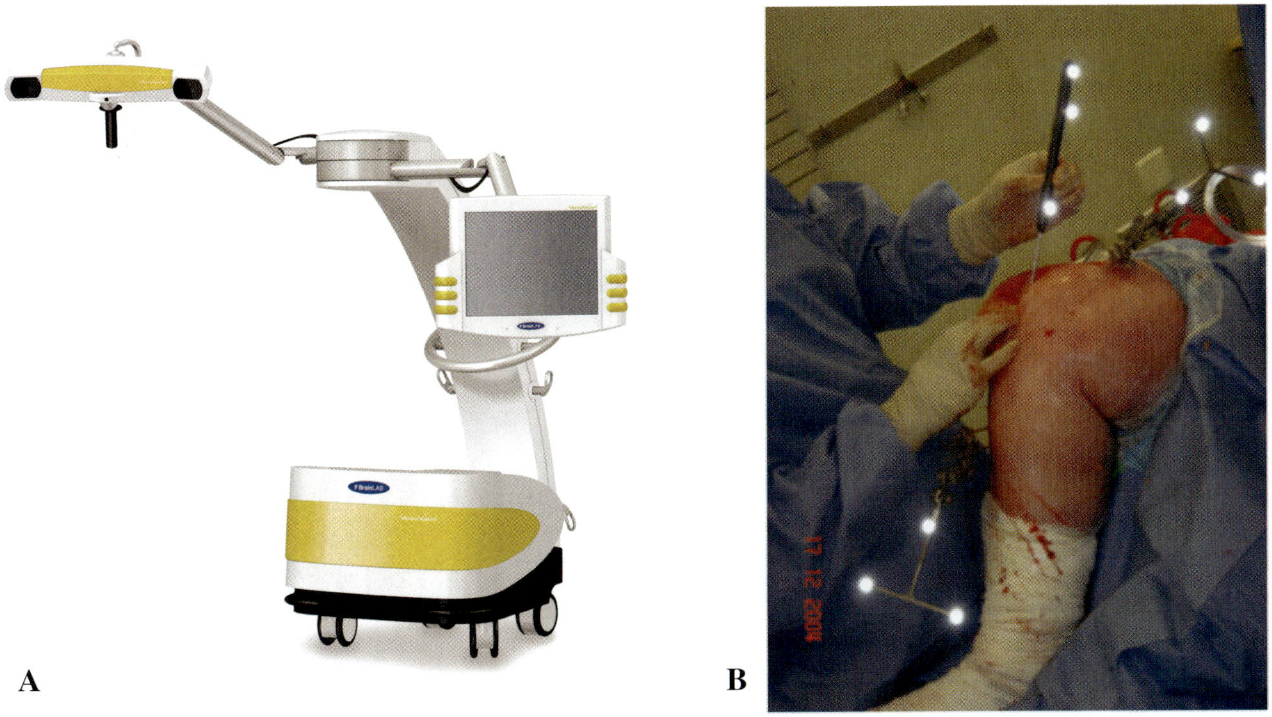

FIGURE 56-1. *BrainLAB machine showing camera setup (**A**) and intraoperative image of navigation process (**B**).*

knee in current time and space and matches these data to the nearest CT scan data stored within the system. Clearly this process is critical in defining the outcome and accuracy of the final product and meticulous care should be taken when identifying the bony landmarks. These include the medial and lateral malleolus of the tibia, the mechanical axis points of the tibia and femur, the femoral rotational axis points, and an evaluation of the center of the hip joint to establish the center point of hip rotation, thus helping to identify the mechanical axis. Once this mechanical axis is identified, all subsequent plans for cuts can be referenced to this axis. This is a major deviation from conventional surgery, where the anatomical axis is invariably used and there is wide variation of this axis from one patient to the next, hence potential inaccurate alignment. The registration process also maps out the wear within the joint, especially the lowest point from which cuts can be planned.

Following registration the surgeon can evaluate the exact amount of fixed flexion deformity, varus-valgus alignment, and range of motion preoperatively and assess whether these can be easily corrected from the minimal releases already performed as part of the approach. Using the shims supplied with the Accuris system, it is then straightforward to visualize which shim would be required both in flexion and extension to obtain the optimal position (Fig. 56-2).

The cutting block is then navigated freehand into position and secured with pins. A planning screen then helps the surgeon identify what would happen to the alignment, gaps, and residual deformities if he or she were to execute this planned position. If the surgeon is happy with the plan, the guiding array is removed from the block and cuts are performed. Following these cuts, the guiding array can be reapplied to the cut surface and real-time assessment is displayed on the screen to assess the alignment and level of cut achieved in all three planes of measurement and, if necessary, this will then allow the surgeon to modify the cut. Again this is a unique step not performed routinely in conventional, nonnavigated surgery (Fig. 56-3).

The finishing blocks can then be attached to complete the bone surface preparation and the components are cemented into position. A layered closure is then performed in the routine manner and dressings are applied. The patient is mobilized from day 1 and most are usually discharged by the 2nd or 3rd postoperative day.

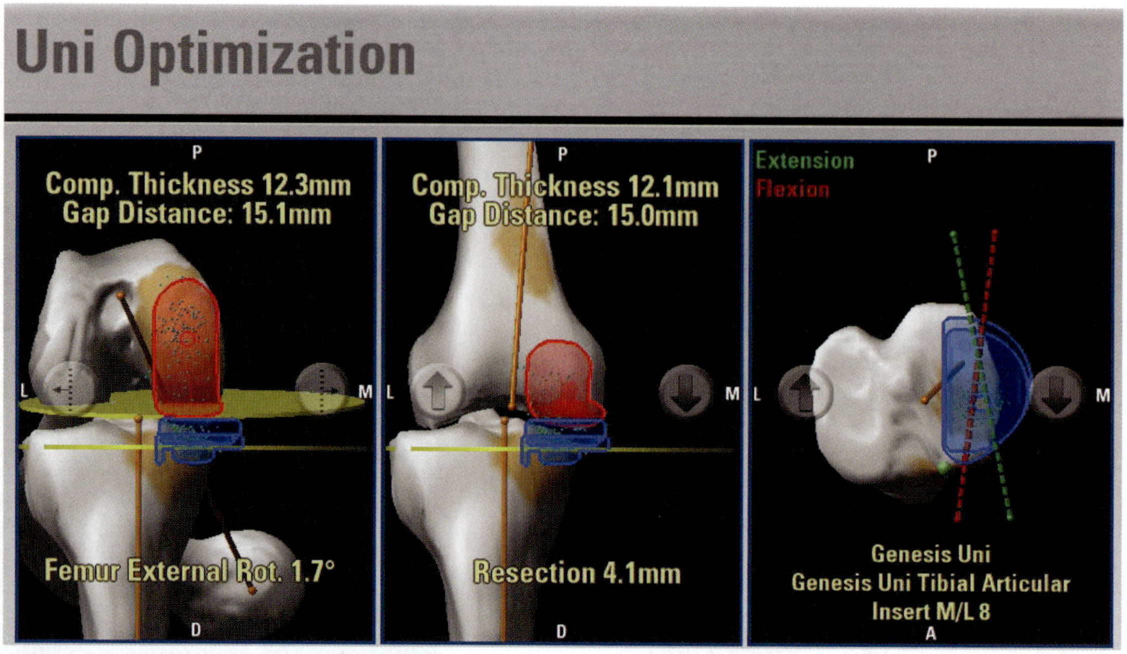

FIGURE 56-2. *Uni planning screen.*

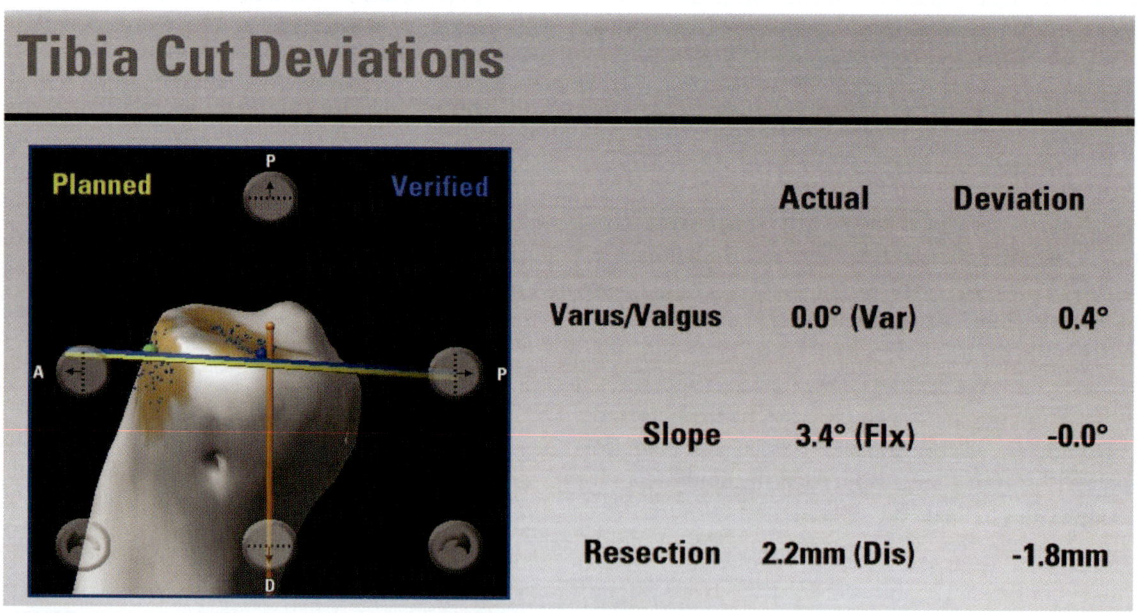

FIGURE 56-3. *Verification of cuts.*

POSTOPERATIVE MANAGEMENT

Postoperative anteroposterior and lateral radiographs are obtained, together with an Oxford knee score,[14] and Knee Society function score[20] at follow-up. Length of stay, postoperative hemoglobin levels, transfusion requirement, and any complications are recorded.

COMPLICATIONS

There are some disadvantages associated with CAS. Investigation of the learning curve in a large Pan-European study comprising 368 TKA cases showed no difference in accuracy of implant positioning between experienced and inexperienced centers.[21] However, the inexperienced centers took approximately 20 minutes longer per case for the first 30 cases. Indeed, even in experienced hands, operative time is approximately 10 minutes longer than conventional surgery.[22]

In addition to the potential operative risks associated with traditional UKA, there are possible complications related to pin placement, including case reports of stress fractures,[23,24] although these are not thought to occur to any significant level[25] with the advent of newer pin stabilization configurations.

OUTCOME

The authors' current series includes 100 consecutive UKAs performed in 92 patients (50 male, 42 female), with an average age of 66 years. Follow-up varies from 7 to 45 months.

Tibial component alignment is measured on digital postoperative radiographs: the mean coronal alignment variation being –0.75° (range –3° to +2°) from a planned 90° angle between the horizontal axis of the tibial component and the mechanical axis of the tibia (Fig. 56-4), and a mean sagittal variation of –2.32° (range 0° to –6°) from a planned 3° posterior slope (ie, the angle between the perpendicular to the middle part of the diaphysis of the tibia and the posterior inclination of the tibial component). A negative value indicates amount of posterior slope and varus alignment (Fig. 56-4).

The average Oxford knee score[14] is 7.75 (range 0–24). Mean length of stay is 3.7 days (range 2–7 days), which compares favorably with the National Joint Registry (NJR) for England and Wales' reported average 4.2 days length of stay.[26] Complications include one superficial infection and two arthroscopies to treat meniscal tears in the remaining compartment. Only one knee has required revision to another UKR arthroplasty, which compares favorably with NJR data, suggesting an up to 12% revision rate at 3 years.

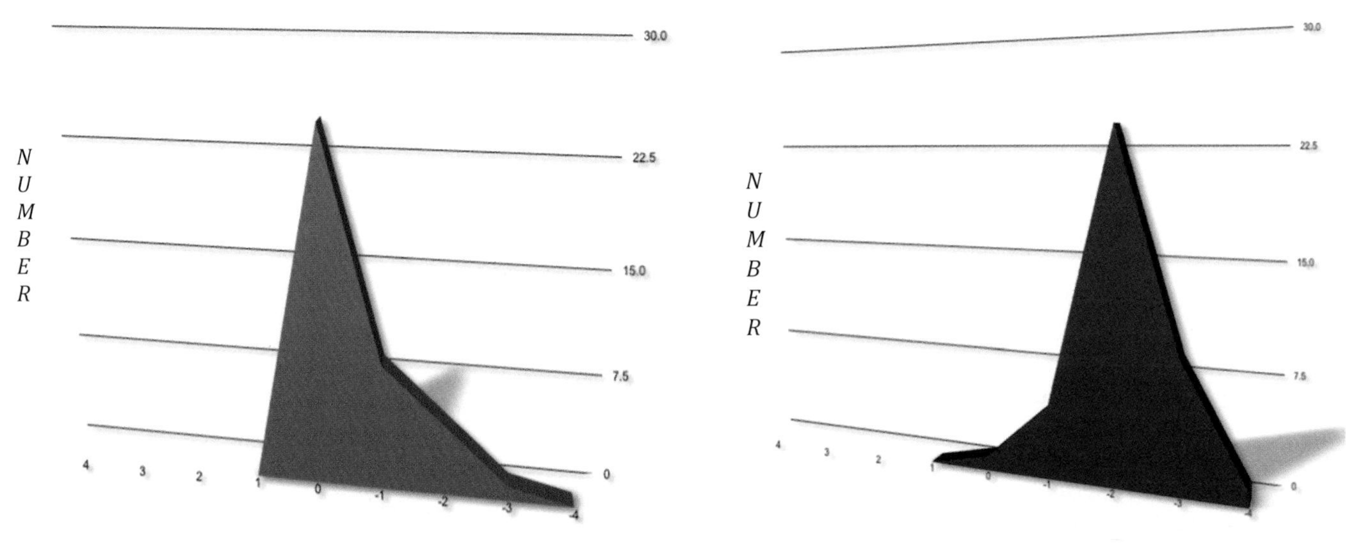

A *VARUS (-)/ VALGUS (+)* **B** Slope: Anterior (+)/ Posterior (-)

FIGURE 56-4. *Tibial component alignment in the authors' series of 100 consecutive navigated UKRs: (**A**) coronal alignment; (**B**) sagittal alignment.*

Postoperative hemoglobin drop (mean 1.6 g/dL) and length of inpatient stay (mean 3.7 days) are both significantly lower than our total knee arthroplasty cohort.

Elsewhere, two studies have also demonstrated a lower frequency of nonoptimal implantation UKR using imageless navigation techniques with an open surgical technique.[27,28] The same improvement in postoperative alignment has been found more recently with imageless minimally invasive CAS.[22,29,30]

Attempts to correlate an improved unicondylar implant alignment with short-term functional outcome are ongoing. A recent longer-term follow-up (mean 6.9 years) also found no functional difference between navigated and nonnavigated groups, albeit the study is compromised by a modest cohort (21 patients) and implant inconsistency between the two groups.[31]

More recent studies looking at functional outcomes and alignment in TKA indicate promise: a randomized control study (115 patients) found that accurately aligned total knee implants defined as a mechanical axis within 3° of neutral have superior International Knee Society and Short-Form 12 physical scores at 1.5, 3, 6, and 12 months postoperatively.[32] A CT analysis of femoral and tibial components in TKAs found significant improvements in the Knee Society scores at 1 year in those well-aligned prostheses, significant for overall alignment and femoral coronal alignment. These same patients also had a shorter length of hospital stay.[33]

Should the body of evidence eventually find no significant functional difference or longevity between poorly and well-aligned UKAs, which is unlikely, the outcome will merely raise questions as to current theories of alignment and implant design. It has been highlighted by others that CAS will play an important role in limiting the potential confounding error of implant positioning when assessing optimum implant design and alignment.[34]

In addition to improving accuracy of mechanical alignment, image-based CAS also provides an objective measure of flexion and extension gaps and ligament balancing. As detailed in the operative technique (above), the Accuris fixed-bearing unicompartmental knee replacement (Smith & Nephew UK Ltd) requires the insertion of increasingly thick shims at the beginning of the procedure until ligamentous balance is achieved; this is used as a reference to guide the subsequent osteotomies. Indeed, a study comparing flexion-extension gap distance between traditional and CAS surgery found that navigation-assisted soft tissue balancing in TKA reduced not only the postoperative alignment outliers but also the medial gap difference and achieved a more rectangular flexion and extension gap compared with conventional TKA.[35]

Other advantages of CAS knee surgery include reduced blood loss[36] and a reduction in systemic embolic events as measured by transesophageal and transcranial Doppler ultrasonography.[37,38]

CT-BASED COMPUTER NAVIGATION AND ROBOTICS

CT-based computer navigation requires an intraoperative probe to register anatomical features, which are then mapped onto the previously acquired CT model. This allows for the guidance of preplanned bony resections, usually in conjunction with robotic assistance, and theoretically removes the error of inaccurate anatomical landmark selection present in imageless surgery.[39]

The use of robotics initially centered on a robot autonomously carrying out the bone cuts, with the surgeon purely acting as an emergency stop.[34] But more recently, robotic systems have tended to be semiactive or hands-on, whereby the surgeon controls the robot (ie, as an intelligent tool).

Some robot-assisted devices require either the robot to be rigidly fixed to the patient or the limb to be rigidly fixed via bony pins. However, a recent report on the first 10 clinical cases using a combination of semiactive robot CT-guided planning, together with an intraoperative optical tracking device, appears to allow for more movement.[40]

Arguably, although imageless CAS provides a powerful intraoperative visual aid, bone resection remains dependent on the potentially inaccurate surgeon/oscillating saw/jig combination. This is supported by a study comparing BrainLAB planned bony resection parameters with physical measurement (Vernier callipers) of the excised bone, where there were found to be a number of outliers. The use of robotic high-speed cutting devices that prevent the surgeon from removing bone outside of a predetermined area (planned using preoperative CT scanning) has proved more successful. Indeed, a prospective randomized controlled trial of 28 unicondylar knee replacements demonstrated that the Acrobot (Stanmore Implants) achieved coronal tibiofemoral alignment angles within 2° of the CT planned resection, which was significantly more accurate than the conventional group.[41]

Drawbacks of CT-based computer navigation include the increased cost, operative time (average of 16 minutes longer than conventional surgery in one study[41]), challenging theater setup, and increased patient exposure to radiation.

CASE EXAMPLE

An active 75-year-old woman presented with significant knee pain (Oxford score 38/48). The patient had returned to normal household chores at 12 weeks postoperatively, with a range of movement from full extension to 120° of flexion. The postoperative Oxford knee score at 6 months was 2/48 (Fig. 56-5).

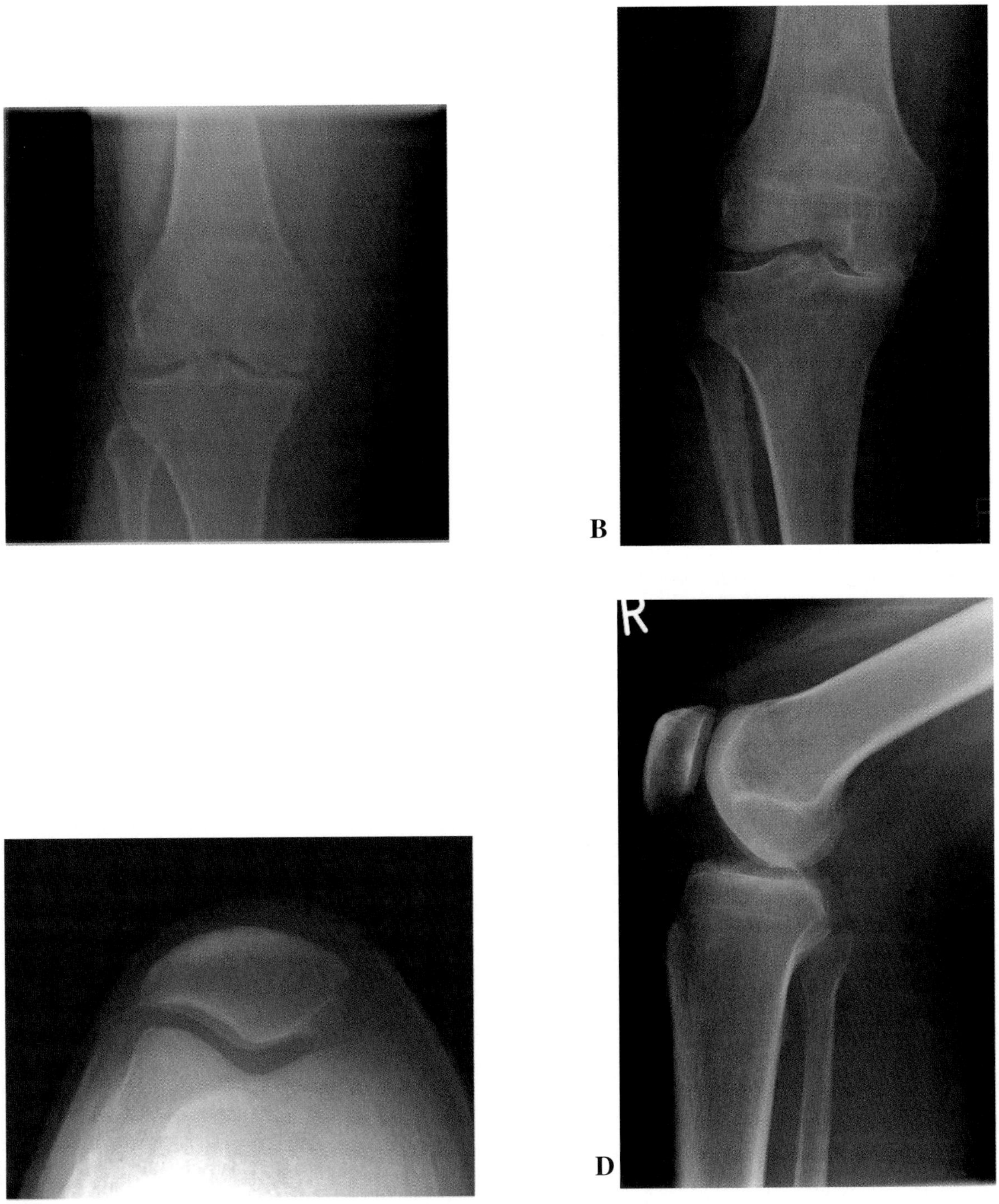

FIGURE 56-5. *Case example: an active 75-year-old woman with significant knee pain.* *(**A**) Weight-bearing anteroposterior full extension; (**B**) Rosenberg view; (**C**) skyline; (**D**) lateral;* **Continued**

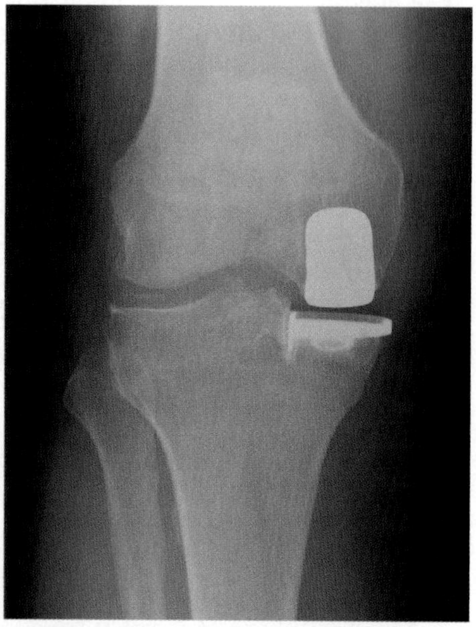

E

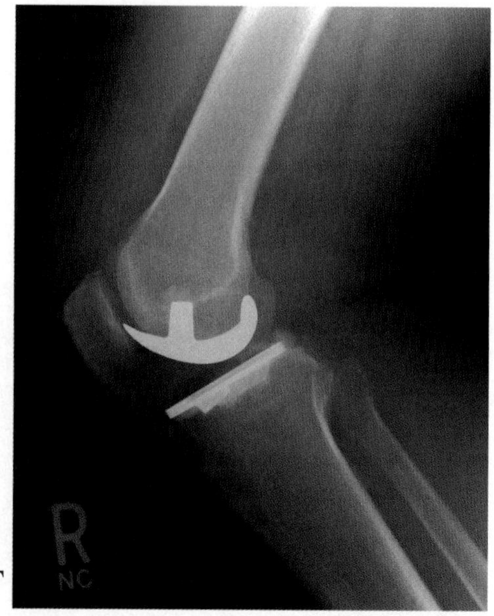

F

FIGURE 56-5 Continued. *(E, F) postoperative X-rays.*

ECONOMICS

After an initial investment, CAS could become an economic as well as a clinical choice. Although more expensive than conventional surgery due to the cost of computer hardware and software and ongoing maintenance costs, potentially this could be offset by reduced revision costs (as a consequence of poorly aligned implants). A recent paper employed a Markov decision model to examine the cost-effectiveness of CAS compared with the volume of TKAs performed.[42] The results hold promise. Using current values, it is estimated that CAS would be cost-effective given a 2% annual reduction in revision rate in a 250 arthroplasties per year center; pro-rata, a 25 arthroplasties per year center would require a 13% annual reduction in revision rate.

CONCLUSION

Computer-assisted surgery improves accuracy of unicondylar implant positioning and allows operations to be safely carried out through smaller incisions, which ipso facto assist postoperative recovery. While the evidential base for improved component positioning on revision rate is still being established, arguably consistent alignment should allow for more accurate assessment of implant design and positioning. Costs are likely to be reduced as the technology advances and the practice becomes more commonplace.

PEARLS AND PITFALLS

The following are some pearls and pitfalls:

- Use of smaller-diameter pins (3 and 4 mm) has significantly reduced the incidence of periprosthetic fractures from pin placement to zero. Two 4-mm threaded pins are used within the incision in the femur and two 3-mm threaded pins are inserted into the anteromedial border of the tibia using the guide. These are inserted from anteromedial to posterolateral in both bones to allow line of sight with the hardware. A stop-start drilling technique is used to minimize bone necrosis and subsequent weakening.
- Preoperative planning is important to ensure that only minimal bone resection is performed especially on the tibial side. The usual amount is 4 mm from the lowest tibial point registered. This ensures that should the UKR need revising at a later stage to a total knee replacement (TKR) for progression of arthritis, then a cleanup cut should suffice in allowing a normal primary TKR inser-

tion rather than needing stems and wedge augments. This fits with the bone-conserving philosophy of partial joint replacement.

- The uniqueness of the cutting block ensures an 8-mm flexion gap at all times and so the need for recutting is minimized and an 8-mm poly insert should fit every time with balanced gaps providing that the intraoperative plan has been executed precisely.
- The ligament balance screen during trialing of the prostheses allows accurate final alignment assessment and, rather than relying on the surgeon's "feel" of balance, one can objectively assess the impact of increasing polyethylene thickness on final alignment, thus ensuring the joint is not pushed into overall valgus, which will progress wear in the unaffected compartment if doing a medial UKR. Gap measurements and dynamic kinematic assessments are also seen on the screen before final implantation.

REFERENCES

1. Newman J, Pydisetty RV, Ackroyd C. Unicompartmental or total knee replacement: the 15-year results of a prospective randomised controlled trial. *J Bone Joint Surg Br.* 2009;91(1):52-57.
2. Patil S, Colwell CW Jr, Ezzet KA, et al. Can normal knee kinematics be restored with unicompartmental knee replacement? *J Bone Joint Surg Am.* 2005;87: 332–338.
3. Amin AK, Patton JT, Cook RE, et al. Unicompartmental or total knee arthroplasty?: results from a matched study. *Clin Orthop Relat Res.* 2006;451:101-106.
4. Lygre SH, Espehaug B, Havelin et al. Pain and function in patients after primary unicompartmental and total knee arthroplasty. *J Bone Joint Surg Am.* 2010; 92(18):2890-2897.
5. Pandit H, Jenkins C, Gill HS, et al. Minimally invasive Oxford phase 3. Results of 1000 cases. *J Bone Joint Surg Br.* 2011;93(2):198-204.
6. Svärd UC, Price AJ. Oxford medial unicompartmental knee arthroplasty: a survival analysis of an independent series. *J Bone Joint Surg Br.* 2001;83:191-194.
7. Keys GW, Ul-Abiddin Z, Toh EM. Analysis of first forty Oxford medial unicompartmental knee replacement from a small district hospital in UK. *Knee* 2004;11(5):375-377.
8. Bejek Z, Sólyom L, Szendrõi M. Experiences with computer navigated total knee arthroplasty. *Int Orthop.* 2007;31(5):617-622.
9. Ritter MA, Faris PM, Keating EM, et al. Postoperative alignment of total knee replacement: its effect on survival. *Clin Orthop Relat Res.* 1994;299:153-156.
10. Fisher DA, Watts M, Davis KE. Implant position in knee surgery: a comparison of minimally invasive, open unicompartmental, and total knee arthroplasty. *J Arthroplasty.* 2003;18(7 suppl 1):2-8.
11. Mason JB, Fehring TK, Estok R, et al. Meta-analysis of alignment outcomes in computer-assisted total knee arthroplasty surgery. *J Arthroplasty.* 2007;22(8): 1097-1106.
12. Schindler OS, Scott WN, Scuderi GR. The practice of unicompartmental knee arthroplasty in the United Kingdom. *J Orthop Surg. (Hong Kong)* 2010;18(3): 312-319.
13. Beard DJ, Pandit H, Ostlere S, et al. Pre-operative clinical and radiological assessment of the patellofemoral joint in unicompartmental knee replacement and its influence on outcome. *J Bone Joint Surg Br.* 2007;89(12):1602-1607.
14. Dawson J, Fitzpatrick R, Murray D, et al. Questionnaire on the perceptions of patients about total knee replacement. *J Bone Joint Surg Br.* 1998;80(1):63-69.
15. Rosenberg TD, Paulos LE, Parker RD, et al. The forty-five-degree posteroanterior flexion weight-bearing radiograph of the knee. *J Bone Joint Surg Am.* 1988;70(10):1479-1483.
16. National Institute for Health and Clinical Excellence. Preoperative tests: the use of routine preoperative tests for elective surgery. *Clinical Guideline 3*; 2003.
17. Ahlbäck S, Rydberg J. X-ray classification and examination technics in gonarthrosis [in Swedish]. *Lakartidningen* 1980;77(22):2091-2093.
18. Beard DJ, Pandit H, Gill HS, et al. The influence of the presence and severity of pre-existing patellofemoral degenerative changes on the outcome of the Oxford medial unicompartmental knee replacement. *J Bone Joint Surg Br.* 2007;89(12):1597-1601.
19. Outerbridge RE, Outerbridge HK. The etiology of chondromalacia patellae. *Clin Orthop Relat Res.* 2001;389:5-8.
20. Insall JN, Dorr LD, Scott RD, et al. Rationale of the Knee Society clinical rating system. *Clin Orthop Relat Res.* 1989;248:13-14.
21. Jenny JY, Miehlke RK, Giurea A. Learning curve in navigated total knee replacement. A multi-centre

study comparing experienced and beginner centres. *Knee* 2008;15(2):80-84.

22. Rosenberger RE, Fink C, Quirbach S, et al. The immediate effect of navigation on implant accuracy in primary mini-invasive unicompartmental knee arthroplasty. *Knee Surg Sports Traumatol Arthrosc.* 2008; 16(12):1133-1140.
23. Massai F, Conteduca F, Vadalà A, et al. Tibial stress fracture after computer-navigated total knee arthroplasty. *J Orthop Traumatol.* 2010;11(2):123-127.
24. Ossendorf C, Fuchs B, Koch P. Femoral stress fracture after computer navigated total knee arthroplasty. *Knee.* 2006;13(5):397-399.
25. Owens RF Jr, Swank ML. Low incidence of postoperative complications due to pin placement in computer-navigated total knee arthroplasty. *J Arthroplasty.* 2010;25(7):1096-1098.
26. *National Joint Registry for England and Wales: 7th Annual Report.* COMOC; 2010:119-120.
27. Jenny JY, Boeri C. Unicompartmental knee prosthesis implantation with a non-image-based navigation system: rationale, technique, case-control comparative study with a conventional instrumented implantation. *Knee Surg Sports Traumatol Arthrosc.* 2003;11(1):40-45.
28. Perlick L, Bäthis H, Tingart M, et al. Minimally invasive unicompartmental knee replacement with a non-image-based navigation system. *Int Orthop.* 2004;28 (4):193-197.
29. Keene G, Simpson D, Kalairajah Y. Limb alignment in computer-assisted minimally-invasive unicompartmental knee replacement. *J Bone Joint Surg Br.* 2006; 88(1):44-48.
30. Jung KA, Kim SJ, Lee SC, et al. Accuracy of implantation during computer-assisted minimally invasive Oxford unicompartmental knee arthroplasty: a comparison with a conventional instrumented technique. *Knee.* 2010;17(6):387-391.
31. Konyves A, Willis-Owen CA, Spriggins AJ. The long-term benefit of computer-assisted surgical navigation in unicompartmental knee arthroplasty. *J Orthop Surg Res.* 2010;31(5):94.
32. Choong PF, Dowsey MM, Stoney JD. Does accurate anatomical alignment result in better function and quality of life? Comparing conventional and computer-assisted total knee arthroplasty. *J Arthroplasty.* 2009;24(4):560-569.
33. Longstaff LM, Sloan K, Stamp N, et al. Good alignment after total knee arthroplasty leads to faster rehabilitation and better function. *J Arthroplasty.* 2009;24 (4):570-578.
34. Davies BL, Rodriguez y Baena FM, Barrett AR, et al. Robotic control in knee joint replacement surgery. *Proc Inst Mech Eng H.* 2007;221(1):71-80.
35. Lee DH, Park JH, Song DI, et al. Accuracy of soft tissue balancing in TKA: comparison between navigation-assisted gap balancing and conventional measured resection. *Knee Surg Sports Traumatol Arthrosc.* 2010;18(3):381-387.
36. Kalairajah Y, Simpson D, Cossey AJ, et al. Blood loss after total knee replacement: effects of computer-assisted surgery. *J Bone Joint Surg Br.* 2005;87(11): 1480-1482.
37. Kalairajah Y, Cossey AJ, Verrall GM, et al. Are systemic emboli reduced in computer-assisted knee surgery?: a prospective, randomised, clinical trial. *J Bone Joint Surg Br.* 2006;88(2):198-202.
38. Church JS, Scadden JE, Gupta RR, et al. Embolic phenomena during computer-assisted and conventional total knee replacement. *J Bone Joint Surg Br.* 2007;89(4):481-485.
39. Yau WP, Leung A, Liu KG, et al. Interobserver and intra-observer errors in obtaining visually selected anatomical landmarks during registration process in non-image-based navigation-assisted total knee arthroplasty. *J Arthroplasty.* 2007;22(8):1150-1161.
40. Pearle AD, O'Loughlin PF, Kendoff DO. Robot-assisted unicompartmental knee arthroplasty. *J Arthroplasty.* 2010;25(2):230-237.
41. Cobb J, Henckel J, Gomes P, et al. Hands-on robotic unicompartmental knee replacement: a prospective, randomised controlled study of the acrobot system. *J Bone Joint Surg Br.* 2006;88(2):188-197.
42. Slover JD, Tosteson AN, Bozic KJ, et al. Impact of hospital volume on the economic value of computer navigation for total knee replacement. *J Bone Joint Surg Am.* 2008;90(7):1492-1500.

57

Kinematically Aligned Total Knee Arthroplasty with Patient-Specific Cutting Guides

Joseph V. Vernace and Stephen M. Howell

Kinematically aligned total knee arthroplasty (TKA) is an evolving concept that challenges the commonly accepted principles of traditional TKA that uses lower limb mechanical alignment. Mechanically aligned TKA aligns the femoral and tibial components perpendicular to their respective mechanical axes, adjusts internal and external femoral component position to equalize the flexion and extension gaps, and then balances the knee with appropriate collateral ligament and capsular releases. Kinematically aligned TKA, in contrast, positions the components to restore the more recently understood parallel and perpendicular relationship of the femoral, patellar, and tibial kinematic axes of the knee. Co-aligning the transverse axis of a best fitting, single-radius femoral implant with the flexion-extension axis (FE axis) of the femur simultaneously aligns the implant parallel to the FE axis of the patella. Aligning the tibial implant perpendicular to the longitudinal axis of the tibia simultaneously aligns the implant parallel to both the flexion-extension axes of the femur and patella. After aligning the implants to the three kinematic axes, the removal of osteophytes restores ligament length, motion, and stability and nearly eliminates the need for collateral and retinacular ligament releases.

Patient-specific custom cutting guides (OtisKnee, OtisMed, Inc, Alameda, CA) are preoperative navigation tools that enable the surgeon to kinematically align the femoral and tibial implants accurately. The cutting guides are created from three-dimensional (3D) models made from a magnetic resonance image (MRI) of the knee and are machined to fit each patient. The use of the cutting guides shortens the operative time, reduces instrumentation in part because the sizes of the implants are known, shortens turnover time, and has improved the clinical outcome when compared to our prior 20-year experience with mechanically aligned TKA.[1-4]

This chapter reviews the history of mechanical alignment, the concepts of knee kinematics, the rationale and technique of using custom cutting guides for TKA, and early clinical results.

HISTORY OF MECHANICALLY ALIGNED TKA: KNOWN LIMITATIONS

There is universal agreement that mechanically aligned TKA improves the quality of life of patients with end-stage knee arthritis. However, international arthroplasty registries in the United Kingdom, Canada, and New Zealand have shown that 20% to 25% of patients with mechanically aligned TKA are dissatisfied.[5-7]

Mechanically aligned TKA has evolved over the years, including many changes in implant designs, materials, surgical approaches, and techniques. Although early implants and instrumentation were primitive, the failures that occurred were attributed to implant alignment. The concept of the three kinematic axes of the knee was unknown at that time, so the principle of mechanical alignment evolved in which the implants were aligned perpendicular to a straight line running from the center of the femoral head through the center of the knee to the center of the ankle. However, studies have shown that the normal mechanical axis varies widely from patient to patient and is not a straight line.[8-10] Although mechanical alignment has been the accepted principle for aligning TKA, this methodology changes the alignment of the limb and knee from normal in the majority of patients and may not be desirable and would be unnatural for most patients.[9,10] The change in limb and knee alignment from normal often causes uncorrectable ligament imbalances, instability, and limited motion, which might be one of the primary causes of the dissatisfaction of patients with mechanically aligned TKA.

The literature is often quoted as supporting the theory that malalignment off this neutral mechanical axis results in early failures; however, most of this repeatedly cited literature has major pitfalls.[11,12] Most papers examined short-leg X-rays (that cannot properly evaluate the mechanical axis) and reviewed surgical results from the 1970s and early 1980s at a time when instrument systems were poor or nonexistent and implant designs were biomechanically inferior to modern arthroplasty components.[13-19] Only one of these papers examined long-leg standing X-rays for alignment; however, that implant (Denham Knee) was a roller and trough design that was positioned with primitive instrumentation and has no similarities to more modern implant designs.[20] One has to question the possibility of poorly designed components implanted with little or no instrumentation and coincidentally positioned in varus failing for other reasons, such as gross instability, implant choices, and overload.[21]

As this questionable evidence regarding malalignment causing failure mounted, an arbitrarily acceptable range of hip-knee-ankle (HKA) alignment from 3° of varus to 3° of valgus off the 0° HKA axis was adopted as the goal of TKA. Better instrument systems and eventually computerized intraoperative navigation became available and have been in use for many years. Although many studies have shown a decrease in outliers from this "acceptable" limb alignment, these studies have failed to produce better clinical results, even though the target goal of limb alignment has been achieved much more readily.[12,22-25]

Accepting the premise that the optimal goal of lower limb alignment is within the parameters of ±3° from the 0° mechanical axis and recognizing that this goal is now more readily achievable, yet clinical results have not improved, leaves only one of two conclusions to be reached: either TKA is as good as it is ever going to be or an incorrect alignment goal has been chosen.

To accept the idea that the best possible TKA results have been attained with mechanically aligned TKA is disturbing, considering most studies show patient satisfaction at approximately 80%.[5-7] In other words, one of five patients who have undergone TKA is dissatisfied with the results. Even if all the knees implanted never failed under those ideal mechanical alignment conditions, a clinical failure rate of 20% would still exist, even if implant survival is 100%. While it is difficult to accurately evaluate the 3D spatial relationships of a postoperative TKA, reducing its overall potential for clinical success and long-term survival to a single-view, nonstanding, short-leg X-ray film seems suspect at best.

OtisMed technology was born out of a desire to kinematically align the femoral and tibial components in three dimensions to restore a more normal functioning TKA than mechanically aligned TKA. The use of patient-specific cutting guides mimics the normal alignment of the knee, recommended by Hungerford, who favored "... anatomic orientation in the coronal plane wherein the joint line forms approximately a 2-3 degree varus angle relative to the mechanical axis."[26] Although rarely referenced in the TKA literature or in presentations, there are many studies showing that varus alignment of the tibial component has no effect on outcomes.[11,20,27-31] Even with one study showing that as much as 7° of tibial component varus has no effect on survivorship up to 10 years, the bias toward mechanical alignment remains.[32]

Traditional teaching recommends aligning the femoral component in 5° to 6° of valgus and the tibial component perpendicular to the long axis of the tibia, both of which are nonanatomic. External rotation of the femoral component is therefore necessary to change the trapezoidal shape of the flexion gap into a rectangular configuration (not because it helps patellar tracking, which it may). Once all these nonanatomic bone cuts have been made, balancing the ligament structures about the knee is performed as necessary in both flexion and extension. Many knees, even if balanced in this manner, will continue to have midflexion instability for reasons discussed in the kinematic section of this chapter.

The completed TKA needs to function as a complex unit of musculature, ligamentous complexes, and femoral and tibial component articulation in flexion-extension and rotation. Curiously, during mechanically aligned TKA surgery, the femoral and tibial components are approached independently and then expected to function as a unit when they are brought together. In other words, the knee is exposed, the tibia is cut perpendicular to its long axis and then ignored, while the femur is then prepared for the femoral component in whatever position the surgeon desires based on conventional or navigation parameters. When that has been done, the trials are placed and the two independently positioned implants are brought together and are expected to be balanced and properly aligned. When they are not, conventional teaching says that the soft tissues have contracted or stretched, and therefore balancing the knee is necessary in order to restore normal ligament tension, because TKA is a "soft tissue procedure."

A carpenter would never make a door in one room and the door frame in another room, cut in the hinge slots, bring them together, and expect the hinges to match up perfectly. They might be close and the door may still swing open or closed, but it may rub the floor or the door frame or not open or close all the way easily. He would not blame the surrounding wall for the problem and adjust the drywall; he would fix the mismatch of the door and frame and assume he made an error in the fitting of the two.

When we do nonanatomic bone resection and nonkinematic TKA and do not match the tibial component to the properly placed kinematically aligned femoral component, we cannot reproduce the proper mechanics of the knee. Although we might get close, we have not re-created normal anatomy and therefore have altered the surrounding soft tissues into abnormal tensions. The need for soft tissue balancing in mechanically aligned TKA is compensatory and is brought about by nonanatomic bone cuts and outdated multiradius designed implants.

With proper kinematic alignment and properly placed anatomic bone cuts, the authors have noted almost no need for ligament balancing, including medial and lateral ligament releases, posterior capsular release, and an extremely low number of lateral retinacular releases. Kinematic alignment changes the concept of TKA from being a soft tissue balancing procedure to a true bony resurfacing procedure.

HISTORY OF THE THREE AXES THAT DESCRIBE NORMAL KNEE KINEMATICS

In the 1980s, the rotation of the tibia on the femur was thought to take place on variable or multiple axes and the femur was thought to have multiple radii or an oval shape. The oval shape was represented as "J" shaped and is the biomechanical basis for the design of some femoral components still in use today. Although the concept that the knee has a variable axis is still taught, Hollister et al showed for the first time in 1993 that there is a single transverse axis in the femur about which the tibia flexes and extends. This single axis, which passes through the center of the medial and lateral femoral condyles that are circular in shape, has since been verified by others.[9,33-35] This is the primary axis that controls knee kinematics

There are three axes that describe the kinematics of the knee. The primary axis is the transverse axis in the femur about which the tibia flexes and extends, which is substantially different from the transepicondylar axis (TEA), which is a line connecting the medial and lateral epicondyles.[34] These two axis have an average difference of 5° (range, 2°–11°), which means that rotationally aligning the femoral component to the TEA causes malalignment (Fig. 57-1).[9,30,34-36]

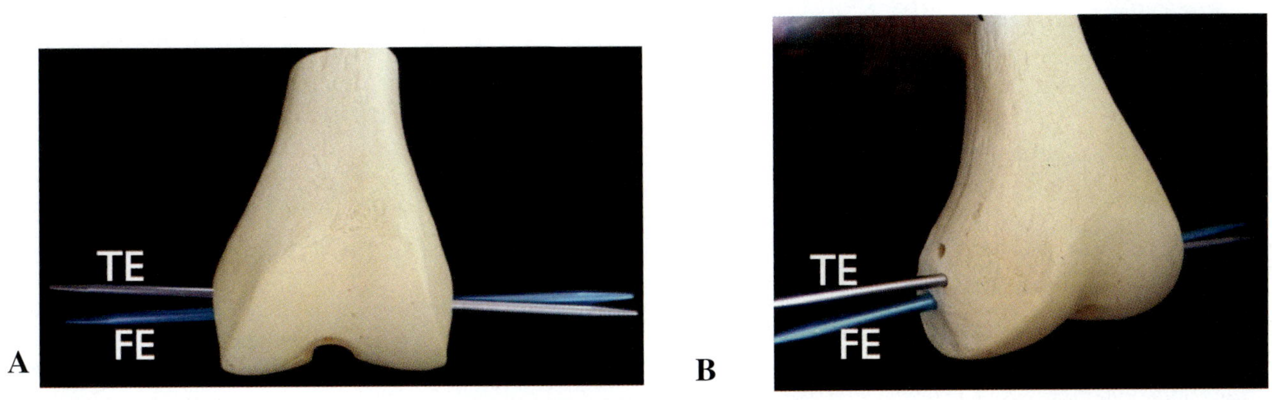

FIGURE 57-1. *(**A**) AP view of a 3D model of a left knee made from an MRI of an actual patient. Shown is the average 3D difference between the transepicondylar (TE) axis and the flexion and extension (FE) axis of the femur, about which the tibia flexes and extends, which is 5° (range, 2°–11°). Aligning the femoral component to the TE axis results in kinematic malalignment of the femoral component. (**B**) Oblique view demonstrates the typical difference between the TE axis and the FE axis of the distal femur on the medial femoral condyle.*

It is disturbing that current literature continues to perpetuate the notion that the TEA is the functional axis of flexion.[37,38] Another axis is the transverse axis in the distal femur about which the patella flexes and extends and this patellar axis is parallel to the primary axis.[35] The third axis is the longitudinal axis of the tibia about which the tibia internally and externally rotates on the femur and is perpendicular to the two transverse axes (Fig. 57-2). The orientation of these three axes is not related to the center of the femoral head or the location of the ankle, which means that mechanical alignment of the knee disregards the kinematics of the knee.[9,33-35,39,40]

A single-radius implant is ideal for kinematic reconstruction because there is no significant clinical difference in the medial or lateral femoral condyles of a varus or valgus knee with end-stage osteoarthritis.[36] The critical step in aligning the femoral component is co-aligning the transverse axis of the component with the primary transverse axis in the femur, which restores the kinematics of the knee without releasing collateral or retinacular ligaments.[41-43]

The inability of mechanical alignment to consistently improve clinical outcomes might be related to a subset of these knees being kinematically malaligned. In contrast, kinematically aligned TKA strives to restore the natural alignment of the limb by removing osteophytes, preserving ligament integrity without the need for ligament balancing.[41-43] In other words, resurfacing the distal femur and proximal tibia within the undisturbed soft tissue envelope should allow a more normal feeling for the patient, with a more rapid recovery of range of motion, independent ambulation, and functionality because the soft tissues have not only not been altered, but are returned to their previous normal lengths and alignment.[1] This "natural alignment" approach has been extremely successful with mobile-bearing unicompartmental knee arthroplasty.[44-46]

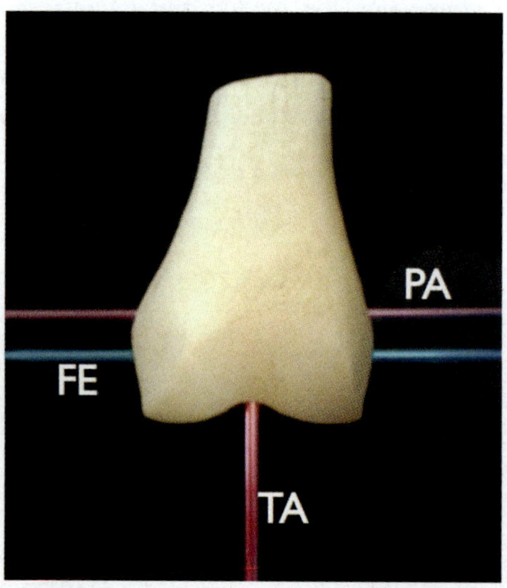

FIGURE 57-2. *AP view shows the parallel relationship between the flexion extension (FE) axis of the distal femur, about which the tibia flexes and extends, and the patella axis (PA) in the femur, about which the patella flexes and extends. Also shown is the perpendicular relationship between the tibial axis (TA), about which the tibia internally and externally rotates on the femur, and the two, parallel transverse axes in the femur. These three axes determine the kinematics of the knee.*

PREOPERATIVE EVALUATION

The general history and physical examination should include a history of the patient's overall medical condition and consider general health and potential risks for undergoing a major surgical procedure. Consultations with other specialists should be considered when appropriate for preoperative clearance. A specific history of the patient's prior treatments to the knee, including both nonoperative and operative, should ensure that they are candidates for TKA. Any previous complications should be noted, especially prior infection, deep venous thrombosis, or pulmonary embolism.

The physical examinations should include a thorough hip and knee exam with assessments of range of motion, angular alignment, ligament integrity, effusion, and tenderness. Lower extremity vascular or neurologic abnormalities should be noted. In general, the preoperative history and physical exam are no different than for a mechanically aligned TKA.

IMAGING

Standard radiographs including a standing posteroanterior flexion view, a lateral view, and a Merchant view are essential to determine the extent of arthritic changes of the three compartments. The location of osteophytes should be noted, especially posterior osteophytes, because these will need to be removed and are not as readily noticeable as medial and lateral osteophytes at the time of surgery. An MRI of the knee is obtained for manufacturing the patient-specific guides, the details of which are discussed later in the chapter.

INDICATIONS AND CONTRAINDICATIONS

Kinematic alignment can be performed in almost every patient requiring TKA. The authors have not found a varus or valgus deformity or flexion contracture that was so extensive that kinematic alignment could not be used. If a patient is unable to have a preoperative MRI because of a pacemaker, defibrillator, metal near the knee joint, is unable to remain still during the scan, or has a thigh too thick to fit in a dedicated knee coil, then a computed tomography (CT) arthrogram can be performed. The only contraindication to a CT arthrogram is an allergy to contrast agents.

Patients with multiple deformities in the limb due to a malunion of a femoral or tibial shaft fracture or an osteotomy need special consideration. Correcting angular deformity at the knee does not correct an angular deformity of the long bones and may leave the limb malaligned. Kinematic alignment is designed to retain the posterior cruciate ligament (PCL), so a patient with a torn PCL may require 2 mm of extra bone removal from the distal femur to compensate for the 2 mm of extra flexion space and balance the flexion-extension gap when using a PCL-substituting femoral component.

PREPARATION FOR SURGERY: MRI SCANNING AND MANUFACTURING PATIENT-SPECIFIC CUTTING GUIDES

The process of manufacturing patient-specific cutting guides begins once the patient schedules surgery. Patients should be screened for the ability to undergo MRI scanning or CT arthrogram of the knee.

A sagittal magnetic resonance imaging scan of the arthritic knee is obtained with a dedicated knee coil with use of a 1.5- to 3.0-T scanner. Axial and coronal localizers are used to customize the sagittal imaging plane perpendicular to the transverse axes in the femur about which the tibia and patella flex and extend (Fig. 57-3).[39] General scanning parameters included a 16-cm field-of-view centered at the joint line of the knee, 256 matrix, 2-m slice thickness, and 2 excitations. Specific parameters such as echo time (TE), repetition time (TR), and bandwidth are unique for the brand of the MRI scanner and are provided by OtisMed, Inc.

Proprietary software segments each image, retaining the femur, tibia, articular cartilage, and osteophytes. The segmented images are meshed together to form a 3D model of the arthritic knee (OtisMed Corp.). In a similar process a 3D model of the prearthritic or normal knee is formed by filling in articular cartilage and bone defects, removing osteophytes, and correcting the varus-valgus alignment by adjusting the tibial position until the medial and lateral joint spaces are equal (Fig. 57-4).

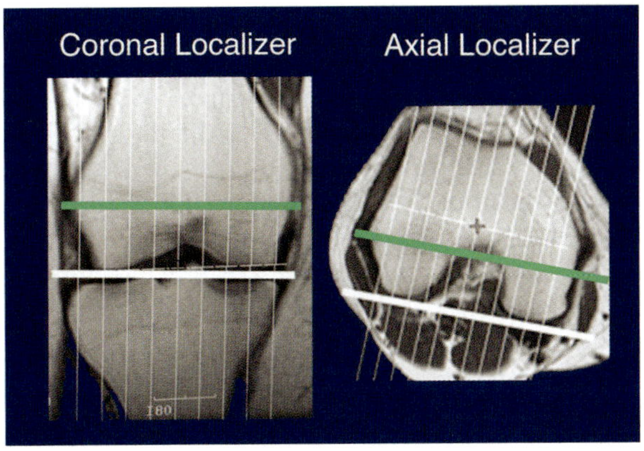

FIGURE 57-3. *A schematic diagram shows the coronal (left) and axial (right) localizer, the femoral joint line (thick white line), the transverse axis in the femur about which the tibia flexes and extends (green line), and the plane for the nonorthogonal, oblique, sagittal scan (parallel, thin lines). Aligning the nonorthogonal, oblique, sagittal scan perpendicular to both the distal femoral joint line (thick white line) in the coronal localizer and the posterior femoral joint line (thick white line) in the axial localizer aligns the nonorthogonal, oblique, sagittal scan perpendicular to the transverse axis in the femur about which the tibia flexes and extends (green line), which projects the femoral condyles as a circle in the same plane that the tibia flexes and extends about the femur.*

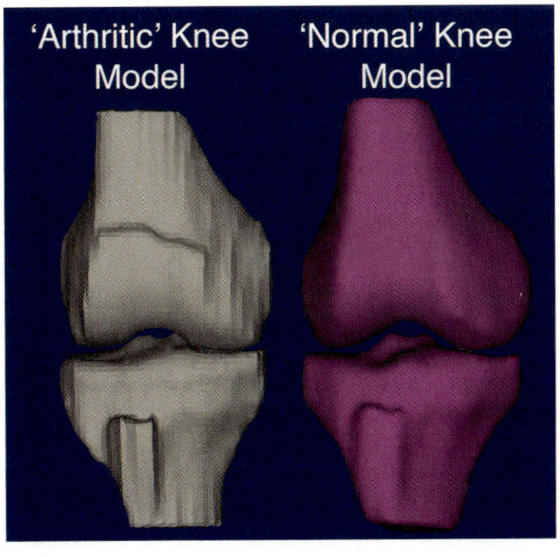

FIGURE 57-4. *3D models of the arthritic knee (left) and the virtually realigned "normal" knee (right) are created using proprietary software. Prearthritic alignment is restored by filling in bone and cartilage defects, removing osteophytes and positioning the tibia to equalize the medial and lateral joint spaces.*

The position and optimal size of each component is determined by shape-matching the best fitting femoral and tibial components to the 3D normal knee model. Shape-matching the tibial articulating surface of the femoral condyles of the femoral component to the femur co-aligns the transverse axes of the femoral component and the FE axis of the femur about which the tibia and patella flex and extend. The anteroposterior axis of the tibial component is set perpendicular to the transverse axis of the femoral component, which kinematically aligns the tibial component to the femoral component. Finally, the tibia is centered under the tibial component, which kinematically aligns the tibia with the tibial component (Fig. 57-5).

The distal and posterior cut planes of the femur and proximal cut plane of the tibia are then transferred from the 3D normal knee model to the 3D arthritic knee model. Custom femoral and tibial cutting guides are machined to match the arthritic knee model from biocompatible plastic (Delran). A saw slot is placed in each guide, which sets varus-valgus, proximal-distal, and flexion-extension positioning of the femoral and tibial component. Two articular pin holes are placed in each guide, which sets internal-external rotation, anterior-posterior, and medial-lateral positioning of the femoral and tibial component. The articular pin fixation holes in each guide correspond to the rotational alignment of the four-in-one cutting guide for the femur and the base plate fixation holes on the tibia. Therefore, each guide provides the surgeon with the size and 6 degrees of freedom of placement for the femoral and tibial components.

SURGICAL APPROACH AND TECHNIQUE

Instrumentation and Surgical Exposure

Before the start of the procedure, during the time out, the surgeon and operating room staff should confirm that the patient information etched on each patient-specific guide matches the patient and surgeon. The etching records the initials and birth date of the patient, the name of the surgeon, the size of each component, and an "R" or "L" to signify the side being operated upon.

The instruments can be limited to one tray by opening only those conventional instruments and trial components that match the size of the implants predicted by the preoperative plan. Only the patellar instruments, four-in-one femoral cutting block, tibial punch, and trial components for the sized femoral and tibial components are needed. A full set of sterilized backup instruments should be available for the uncommon event that they are needed. The number of trays necessary is reduced from the usual 8 to 1, which allows more rapid setup and turnover time and reduction in costs for sterilization and instrument inventory (Fig. 57-6).

Both a medial parapatellar and midvastus exposure have been routinely used with kinematically aligned TKA with patient-specific cutting guides. The key step in the exposure

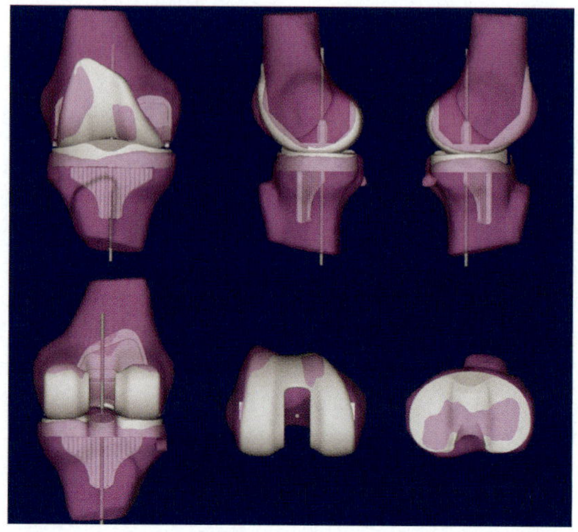

FIGURE 57-5. *Schematic shows the shape-matching of the best fit femoral and tibial components to the restored 3D normal knee model, which kinematically aligns the TKA (see text for details).*

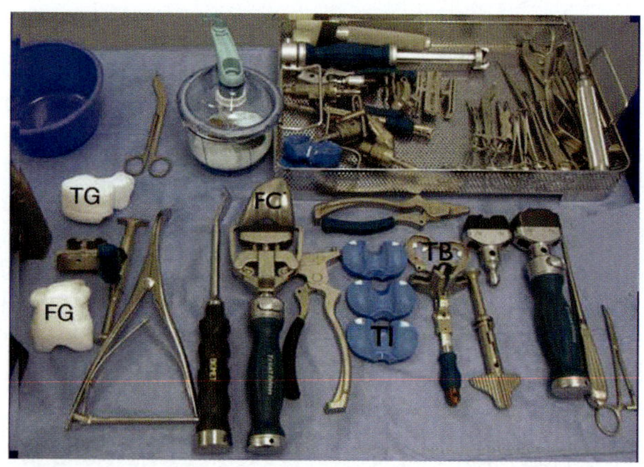

FIGURE 57-6. *Operating room table shows all the necessary instruments for performing a kinematically aligned TKA with use of custom cutting guides. Specificallly, the tibial guide (TG), femoral guide (FG), and the trial femoral component (FC) and trial tibial baseplate (TB) with three tibial inserts (TI) corresponding to the planned size of the components.*

is clear visualization of the anterior femoral cortex, femoral condyles, and proximal tibia. The patient-specific guides are not designed for use with very small incisions or a lateral approach.

Begin exposing the femur by removing the synovial tissue and fat proximal to the trochlear grove on the anterior femur and the lateral fat pad. Release the lateral synovial fold above the patellar tendon and elevate the medial soft tissue envelope off the tibia to expose the anterolateral and posteromedial tibial plateau, respectively. Displace the patella lateral with a retractor and flex the knee to 90°.

Femoral Preparation

Bring the anterior flange of the femoral guide into contact with the anterior cortex of the distal femur and then gently compress the guide proximally and posteriorly at a 45° angle on the distal femoral articular surface (Fig. 57-7A). The guide should be centered medially and laterally and fit snuggly with no medial and lateral or rotational play. If there is slight flexion-extension instability, then reposition the guide until the flat portion of the anterior flange is seated on the anterior cortex and the two feet of the guide are on the medial and lateral condyles (Fig. 57-7B). The femoral guide does not use an intramedullary rod because the use of a rod kinematically malaligns some knees due to the varying longitudinal shape of the femoral shaft.[40,47]

Pin the femoral guide in place by drilling the two articular pins and then the two anterior pins. Insert the saw in the slot, remove the medial pin, and make the distal cut on the medial condyle. Replace the medial pin, remove the lateral pin, and complete the distal cut by sawing the lateral condyle. Remove the femoral guide and measure the thickness of the distal resections with a caliper. The distal resection should be 7 to 8 mm thick on the unworn side and 1 to 2 mm thinner on the worn side. When a condyle is underresected, shave off more bone until the desired resection is met. When a condyle is overresected, then lift the chamfer block off the overresected side until the desired resection is met and fill the gap during cementation.

Select the four-in-one cutting guide that matches the planned size of the femoral component and insert it in the two articular pin holes. Make the posterior cuts and measure the thickness of each bone resection with the caliper. Each posterior resection should equal the thickness of the distal resections after correcting for cartilage and bone wear.[41-43] When a condyle is underresected, rotate the guide anteriorly until the desired resection is met. When a condyle is overresected, rotate the chamfer block posteriorly on the overresected side until the desired resection is met and fill the gap with cement during cementation.

Tibial Preparation

Expose the tibia by removing osteophytes from the intercondyler notch overlying the anterior and posterior cruciate ligament. Excise the anterior cruciate ligament, insert a posterior retractor preserving the insertion of the posterior cruciate ligament, and dislocate the tibia anteriorly. Remove the menisci, anterior, medial and lateral osteophytes, and

A

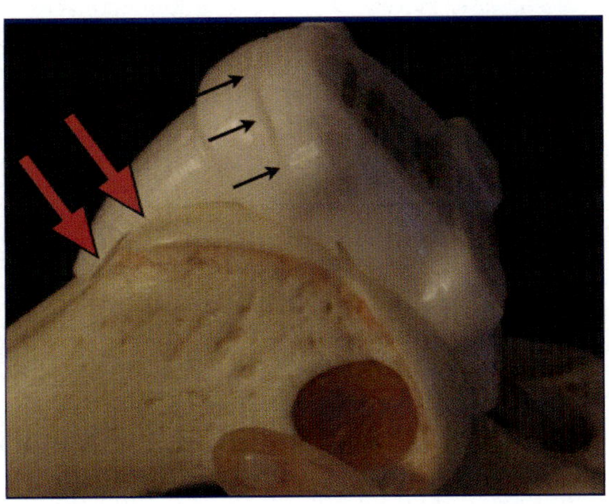

B

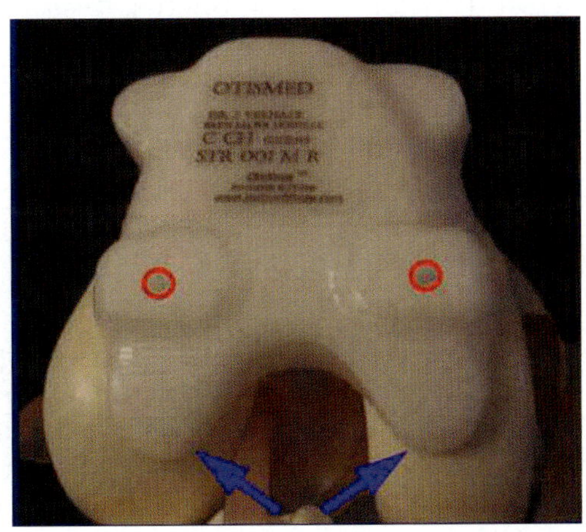

FIGURE 57-7. *(**A**) Lateral view of the femoral cutting guide shows the anterior flange (pink arrows) fitted against the anterior femoral cortex and the distal femoral cutting slot (black arrows). (**B**) Axial view of the femoral cutting guide shows the "feet" of the guide (blue arrows) abutting the medial and lateral femoral condyles and the articular pinholes (red circles).*

any fat pad. Flex the knee to 70° to increase the space between the anterior tibia and patella tendon. Insert the tibial cutting guide and place the anterolateral flange against the tibia, centering the feet of the guide on the tibial articular surface (Fig. 57-8A). Removal of any anterior osteophytes on the anterior tibia is necessary, because these may prevent proper seating of the guide. The medial and lateral feet should fit tightly against the tibial articular surface (Fig. 57-8B).

Pin the tibial guide in place by drilling the two articular pins and then the two anterior pins. Insert the saw in the slot, remove the medial pin, and cut the medial tibia. Replace the medial pin, remove the lateral pin, and complete the tibial cut. Remove the tibial guide and assess the thickness of the tibial resection. The worn side should be thinner than the unworn side by the amount of wear and the anterior resection should be slightly thicker than the posterior resection, which preserves the PCL and neutralizes the posterior slope. The tibial guide does not use an intramedullary or extramedullary rod because the use of these rods kinematically maligns some knees due to the varying longitudinal shape of the tibial shaft.[40,48]

Select the tibia baseplate that matches the planned size of the tibial component and set the internal-external rotation by aligning the holes in the baseplate with the two articular pin holes. Make slight anteroposterior and medialateral adjustments to center the baseplate as needed without changing the rotation. The articular pin holes are more reliable than the tibial tubercle and "floating trial" method, as these techniques have been shown to be unreliable and not repeatable.[49,50] Use the tibial punch to complete the tibial preparation.

Resurface the patella. A personal follow-up study at 1 year of patients with bilateral TKA with a resurfaced patella in one knee and not in the other showed that the resurfaced kinematically aligned knee was preferred over the unresurfaced kinematically aligned knee and that the unresurfaced kinematically aligned knee was preferred over a resurfaced mechanically aligned knee (authors' experience, unpublished data).

Trial Reduction

Perform a trial reduction and adjust the thickness of the tibial liner until the knee is stable to varus-valgus testing at 30° intervals. If the tibial trial lifts off or anterior translates with the knee in 90° of flexion, then increase the posterior slope 1° to 2°. If the knee does not fully extend, remove any posterior femoral and tibial osteophytes, perform a gentle manual manipulation, or, if necessary, release the posterior capsule on either side of the PCL. Removal of bone from the distal femur is rarely needed to balance the knee unless the PCL is inadvertently damaged.[51] When the PCL is nonfunctional, an additional 2 mm of distal femoral resection often balances the knee and a cruciate-retaining component can still be used. If the knee is tight medially, remove medial osteophytes from the femur and tibia and, if necessary, recut the tibia in 1° to 2° of more varus. If the knee is tight laterally, then remove lateral osteophytes from the femur and tibia and, if necessary, recut the tibia in 1° to 2° of

A

B

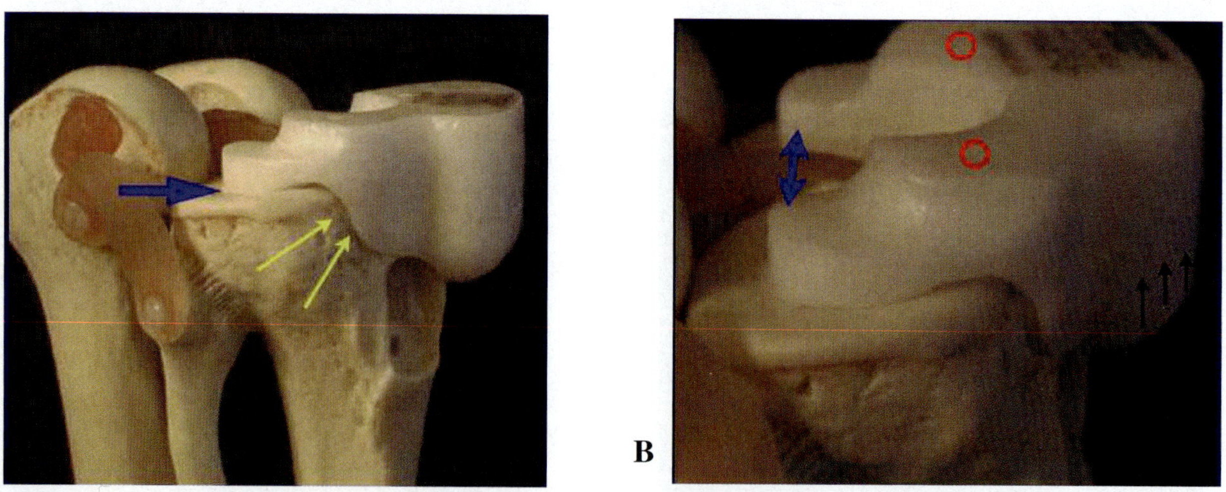

FIGURE 57-8. *(**A**) Lateral view of the tibial cutting guide shows the fit of the lateral foot of the guide (yellow arrow) on the lateral tibal plateau and the fit of the anterolateral flange (blue arrows) against the anterolateral tibia (behind the patellar tendon which has been removed). (**B**) An axial view close-up shows the medial and lateral feet (blue arrows), the articular pin holes (red circles), and the tibial saw slot (thin black arrows).*

more valgus.[41-43] Check patella tracking. A lateral release is rarely needed in the kinematically aligned knee because the three rotational axes are restored to normal.[37] The final step is implantation of the components and closure, which are performed the same as in the mechanically aligned TKA.

COMPLICATIONS

Complications following kinematically aligned TKA are similar to those for mechanically aligned TKA and include postoperative infection, deep venous thrombosis, pulmonary embolism, nerve injury, persistent swelling, anemia, postoperative medical complications such as cardiac and pulmonary issues, and long-term dissatisfaction with the results. Complications such as fracture from pinning the guides or osteolysis from plastic debris caused by drilling and sawing through the plastic guides have not been observed (personal experience of the authors).

RESULTS

Several early studies have looked not only at the alignment issues with kinematic TKA, but also at the early benefits of the procedure. Data were gathered on hand-held computer devices (OrthoSight, Conshohocken, PA) in order to eliminate interviewer bias as patients were surveyed utilizing the Oxford score, Knee Society score SF-12, and several custom questions. This device was also used to input operative time, implant sizes, the need for ligament releases, bone recuts, and guide fit.

In general, operative times are shorter and patient satisfaction, Oxford scores, and Knee Society scores are higher than noted in conventional or computer-navigated studies.[1-3,22,23] One study noted a decrease in surgical time of 14%.[3] There was a low incidence of transfusion in unilateral knee patients of 5.3%, which is attributed to not releasing soft tissues and not violating the femoral canal with an intramedullary rod.[1,2] The manipulation rate was low at 0.7%.[2] Eighty percent of patients walked without a cane by the end of the 4th postoperative week and by 6 months to 1 year postoperatively, 96% judged their knee as normal or nearly normal with 50% rating their knee as "normal."[1,2] Knee Society scores and Oxford scores were higher (179–181) than comparative studies of mechanically aligned conventional and navigated TKA (144–149).[1-3,22,23,52] A level I study found the average Western Ontario and McMaster Universities Osteoarthritis Index (WOMAC), Oxford, and Knee Society scores at 6 months postoperatively to be significantly better in the kinematically aligned group than in the mechanically aligned group[53] (Fig. 57-9).

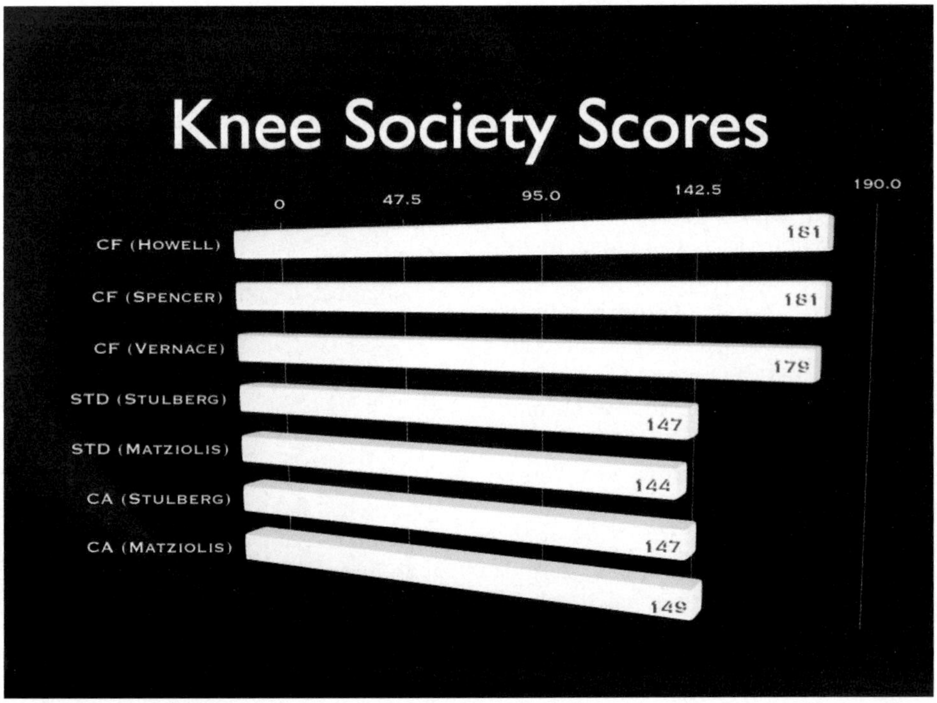

FIGURE 57-9. *The 6-month Knee Society scores are shown highlighting that the scores of the kinematically aligned TKA (Howell, Spencer, Vernace, Dossett) are better than mechanically aligned TKA with standard instrumentation (STD Stulberg, STD Matziolis, STD Dossett) and computer navigational instrumentation (CA Stulberg, CA Matziolis).*

A study of contact kinematics of kinematically aligned TKA performed with patient-specific guides performed by three surgeons with their preferred cruciate-retaining implant showed negligible adduction or medial separation of the components with standing and kneeling. The low prevalence of adduction in the kinematically aligned TKA is in contrast to the high prevalence in mechanically aligned TKA.[54] Limiting adduction is important for preventing medial overload and loosening and may be related to key principles of the kinematically aligned TKA, which are restoration of the normal joint line and not releasing collateral ligaments.[52,55]

The risk of placing the tibial component in varus for long-term wear is controversial. Berend et al noted that mechanically aligned tibial components may fail, whereas tibial components aligned in varus may not. The 10-year survivorship of tibial components implanted in an average of 3° of varus was 96%.[32] The underlying cause of failure is adduction or medial lift-off, which amplifies dynamic forces by up to four times body weight and was a more significant factor than a tibial component placed in more than 4° of varus.[21] Berend concluded that "...components in greater than four degrees varus that had lower stress estimates had lower failure rates *despite* the malalignment." Kinematically aligned TKA unloads the medial side by reducing or eliminating adduction and might reduce the prevalence of short- and long-term implant failure even when the tibia is positioned in a few degrees of varus.

Another benefit of kinematically aligned TKA performed with patient-specific guides is that internal tibial rotation with kneeling is more normal than in the mechanically aligned TKA. Internal tibial rotation, which is normally approximately 16°, was noted to be better in the our contact kinematic group than in comparable previous studies. Internal tibial rotation has been shown to be significantly reduced (average 4°) in both posterior-stabilized and cruciate-retaining TKA done with mechanical alignment and reversal of the normal tibial internal rotation occurred in 21% to 60% of the knees studied.[54] Our contact kinematic group as a whole had reversal of rotation of 15% and had an average internal tibial rotation ranging from 9° to 11°.[52,55] Therefore, minimization of adduction and medial overload should decrease tibial baseplate and polyethylene wear, while re-establishment of more normal rotation provides for a more normal feeling knee.

CONCERNS OVER NONMECHANICAL AXIS ALIGNMENT

A concern over the use of kinematic alignment with custom cutting guides has arisen from a published pilot study conducted in 2006 at the request of an implant company to evaluate the first-time use of these custom guides before release for general use. The study was based on only four knees and was conducted in the earliest phases of the development of the guides. The currently in-use rotational alignment protocol for the MRI had not been developed. Review of the MRIs from two of the four knees showed malrotation of the knee, and by today's standards they would have been rescanned. The authors claimed that malalignment in the coronal plane occurred with the use of the guides.[56] However, the determination of malalignment was based on intraoperative navigation and not the more customary use of long-leg CT scanograms or radiographs.

Although the primary goal of kinematically aligned TKA is to restore the normal limb and joint line alignment before the onset of arthritis, the alignment of the limb is nearly identical to mechanically aligned TKA. Two level III studies have shown that the average variation from the 0° HKA axis is less than 1.5°. One study of 21 subjects found an average HKA axis of 1.2° of varus with fewer outliers than many previously reported studies utilizing conventional or computer-assisted techniques.[3] The second study with 48 subjects found an average HKA axis of 1.4° of valgus.[1] The most common finding on long-leg X-rays with kinematic alignment with respect to the HKA axis is that the overall alignment is within the 0° ± 3°; however, the femoral component is in more valgus and the tibial component is in more varus than the mechanically aligned TKA. This would be expected when trying to recreate normal anatomy rather than a conceptually based mechanical alignment.

CASE EXAMPLES

Kinematically aligned TKA with patient-specific guides has been successfully performed on severe varus and valgus deformities (Fig. 57-10), as well as in patients with malunions above or below the knee joint (Fig. 57-11) or in patients with prior trauma and retained hardware that would limit the use of conventional instrumentation (Fig. 57-12).

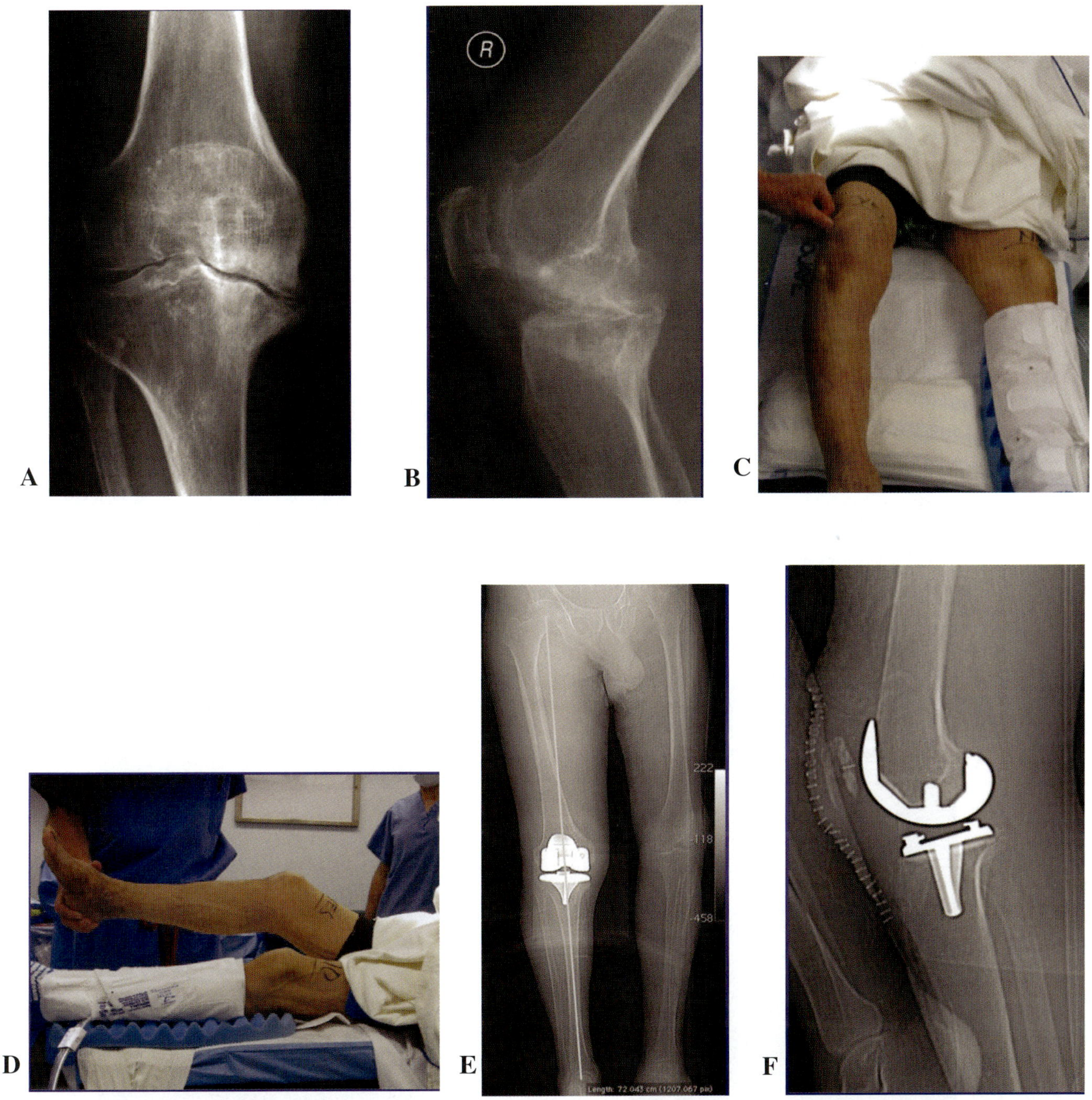

FIGURE 57-10. *Case example. AP (**A**) and lateral (**B**) preoperative radiographs of a 57-year-old male with a malunion of a tibial plateau initially treated with percutaneous pins 20 years ago with subsequent development of severe medial posttraumatic osteoarthritis. Intraoperative photographs (**C**, **D**) show the severe flexion contracture and varus deformity. AP (**E**) and lateral (**F**) postoperative CT scanograms show restoration of a neutral hip-knee-ankle angle without the need for medial augments following kinematically aligned TKA. The tibial joint line is anatomic and in slight varus.*

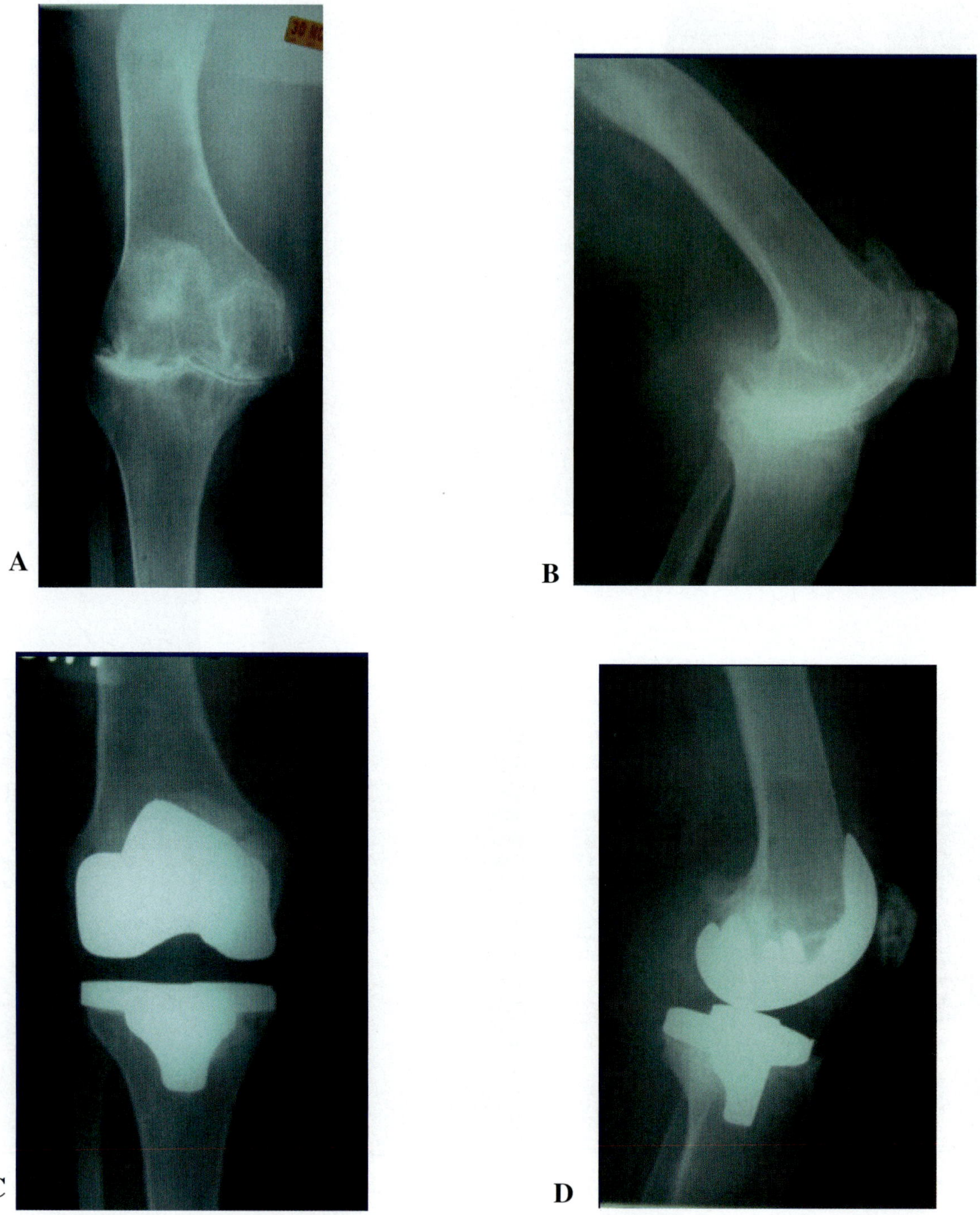

FIGURE 57-11. *Case example. AP (**A**) and lateral (**B**) radiographs of a 64-year-old female with a 30-year-old malunion of a femoral shaft fracture with severe tricompartmental osteoarthritis. (**C**, **D**) Kinematically aligned TKA with custom cutting guides was performed without intramedullary instrumentation or computer navigation. This patient was ambulating without assistive devices 2 weeks postoperatively.*

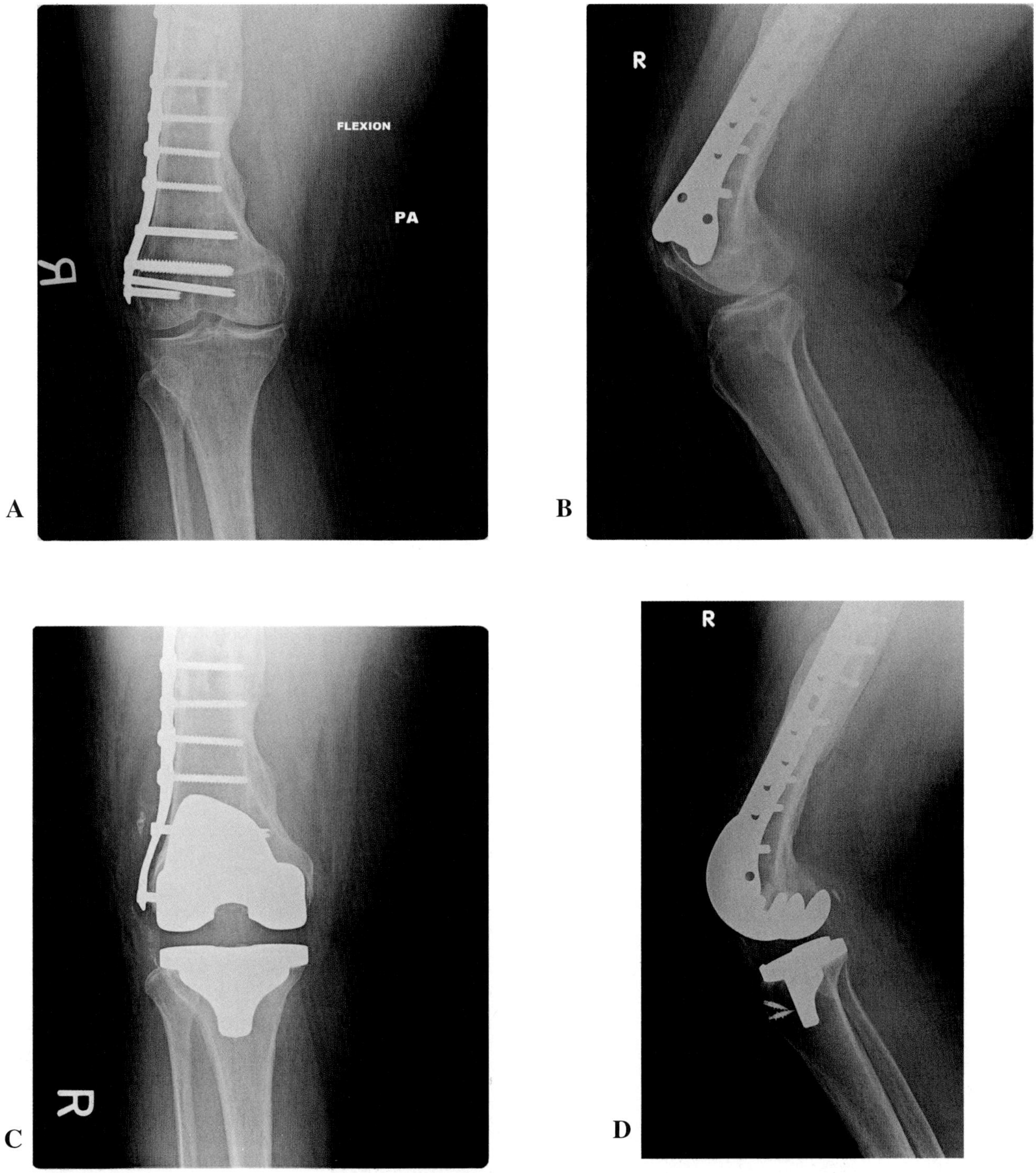

FIGURE 57-12. *Case example. AP (**A**) and lateral (**B**) radiographs of a 52-year-old female with a distal femoral shaft fracture treated with plate and screw fixation with resultant malunion and secondary posttraumatic osteoarthritis. Postoperative AP (**C**) and lateral (**D**) radiographs show a kinematically aligned TKA performed with patient-specific guides without an intramedullary rod and without hardware removal. The distal anterior flange of the plate was resected intraoperatively to avoid prominence and skin irritation.*

SUMMARY

The aim of kinematically aligned TKA is to restore normal knee anatomy, knee function, and patient satisfaction to the highest level without disrupting the normal soft tissue envelope, essentially performing a total knee resurfacing procedure. Early studies have indicated that concerns over gross lower limb malalignment with this technique are unsubstantiated and the average HKA axis is similar to that in mechanically aligned TKA. Concern over tibial varus and early failure has been based on old literature that reported on surgical techniques and implant designs that are now considered inferior with respect to modern-day TKA. Newer studies have questioned the advisability of restoring the limb to a neutral mechanical axis since this procedure changes the alignment of most limbs from normal. Kinematic studies have conclusively established that there are three axes that govern knee kinematics and that these axes are not related to the location of the femoral head and center of the ankle. The principle of kinematically aligned TKA is to position the implants to restore these axes. Most major implant companies have or are developing patient-specific cutting guides for use in TKA; however, they all strive to align the limb mechanically, and not kinematically, which might still result in the undesirable prevalence of 20% patient dissatisfaction shown in international registry studies of mechanically alignned TKA. Further level I studies are needed to confirm the benefits and limitations of kinematically aligned TKA and its ability to reduce the unacceptable patient satisfaction currently seen in mechanically aligned TKA using conventional and computer-navigated instrumentation.

PEARLS AND PITFALLS

Reliable guide placement is the key to successfully performing a kinematically aligned TKA. Care must be taken, as in any instrument system, to ensure proper seating of the guides, including removal of any anterior femoral or tibial osteophytes, which might prevent proper seating. Adequate exposure can be achieved through a small incision, but is paramount in guide placement. Removal of all osteophytes, including those on the posterior femur, is key to restoring normal ligament lengths and motion.

REFERENCES

1. Howell SM, Kuznik K, Hull ML, et al. Results of an initial experience with custom-fit positioning total knee arthroplasty in a series of 48 patients. *Orthopedics*. 2008;31(9):857-863.
2. Vernace JV. Custom fit total knee replacement: early clinical reuslts of 200 knees in 175 consectutive patients. Presented at Pennsylvania Orthopaedic Society Meeting, Philadelphia, PA , Nov. 22, 2008.
3. Spencer BA, Mont MA, McGrath MS, et al. Initial experience with custom-fit total knee replacement: intra-operative events and long-leg coronal alignment. *Int Orthop.* 2009;33(6):1571-1575.
4. Siegel H. MRI guided custom fit total knee replacement: the first six weeks. Presented at the Alabama/ Mississippi Joint Orthopaedic Meeting, Sandestin, FL, May 3, 2008.
5. *The New Zealand Joint Registry 10 Year Report: January 1999 to December 2008;* 2009.
6. Baker PN, van der Meulen JH, Lewsey J, et al. The role of pain and function in determining patient satisfaction after total knee replacement. Data from the National Joint Registry for England and Wales. *J Bone Joint Surg Br.* 2007;89(7):893-900.
7. Bourne RB, Chesworth BM, Davis AM, et al. Patient satisfaction after total knee arthroplasty: who is satisfied and who is not? *Clin Orthop Relat Res.* 2010; 468(1):57-63.
8. Moreland JR, Bassett LW, Hanker GJ. Radiographic analysis of the axial alignment of the lower extremity. *J Bone Joint Surg Am.* 1987;69(5):745-749.
9. Eckhoff DG, Bach JM, Spitzer VM, et al. Three-dimensional mechanics, kinematics, and morphology of the knee viewed in virtual reality. *J Bone Joint Surg Am.* 2005;87(suppl 2):71-80.
10. Bellemans J, Colyn W, Vandenneucker H, et al. The Chitranjan Ranawat award: Is neutral alignment normal for all patients? The concept of constitutional varus. *Clin Orthop Relat Res.* 2012;470(1):45-53.
11. Paratte S, Pagnano MW, Trousdale RT, et al. Effect of mechanical axis alignment on fifteen-year survival of modern, cemented total knee replacement. *J Bone Joint Surg Am.* 2010;92:2143-2149.
12. Alden KJ, Pagnano MW. Computer-assisted surgery: a wine before its time. *Orthopedics.* 2008;31(9):936, 939.
13. Moreland JR. Mechanisms of failure in total knee arthroplasty. *Clin Orthop Rel Res.*1988;226:49-64.
14. Lotke PA, Ecker, ML. Influence of positioning of prosthesis in total knee replacement. *J Bone Joint Surg Am.* 1977;59(1):77-79.

15. Bargren JH, Blaha JD, Freeman MA. Alignment in TKA: correlated biomechanical and clinical observations. *Clin Orthop Relat Res.* 1983;173:178-183.

16. Hvid I, Nielsen S. Total condylar knee arthroplasty: prosthetic component positioning and radiolucent lines. *Acta Ortho Scand.* 1984;55:160-165.

17. Ritter MA, Faris PM, Keating EM, et al. Postopertive alignment of TKR, its effect on survival. *Clin Orthop Relat Res.* 1994;299:740-746.

18. Berend ME, Ritter MA, Meding JB, et al. Tibial component failure mechanisms in TKA. *Clin Orthop Relat Res.* 2004;428:26-34.

19. Rand JA, Coventry MB. Ten year evaluation of geometric total knee arthroplasty. *Clin Ortho Rel Res.* 1988;232:168-173.

20. Jeffery RS, Morris RW, Denham RA. Coronal alignment after total knee replacement. *J Bone Joint Surg Br.* 1991;73(5):709-714.

21. Berend ME, Ritter MR, Hydahl HC, et al. Implant migration and failure in total knee arthroplasty is related to body mass index and tibial component size. *J Arthroplasty.* 2008;23(6 suppl 1):104-109.

22. Stulberg SD, Yaffe MA, Koo SS**.** Computer-assisted surgery versus manual total knee arthroplasty: a case-controlled study. *J Bone Joint Surg Am.* 2006;88 (suppl 4):47-54.

23. Matziolis G, Krocker D, Weiss U, et al**.** A prospective, randomized study of computer-assisted and conventional total knee arthroplasty. Three-dimensional evaluation of implant alignment and rotation. *J Bone Joint Surg Am.* 2007;89(2):236-243.

24. Dutton AQ, Yeo SJ, Yang KY, et al. Computer-assisted minimally invasive total knee arthroplasty compared with standard total knee arthroplasty. A prospective, randomized study. *J Bone Joint Surg Am.* 2008;90(1):2-9.

25. Bauwens K, Matthes G, Wich M, et al. Navigated total knee replacement: a meta-analysis. *J Bone Joint Surg Am.* 2007;89:261-269.

26. Hungerford DS, Krackow KA. Total joint arthroplasty of the knee. *Clin Ortho Relat Res.* 1985;192: 23-33.

27. Aglietti P, Buzzi R. Posterior stabilized total-condylar knee replacement: three to eight years follow-up of 85 knees. *J Bone Joint Surg Br.* 1988;70: 211-216.

28. Collier MB, Engh CA, McAuley JP, et al. Factors associated with loss of thickness of polyethylene tibial bearings after knee arthroplasty. *J Bone Joint Surg Am.* 2007;89:1306-1314.

29. Callaghan J, Liu, S, Warth C. Computer-assited surgery: a wine before its time. In the affirmative. *J Arthroplasty.* 2006;4:27-28.

30. Morgan SS, Bonshahi A, Pradhan N, et al. The influence of postoperative coronal alignment on revision surgery in total knee arthroplasty. *Int Orthop.* 2008;32 (5):639-642.

31. Tew M, Waugh W. Tibiofemoral alignment and the results of knee replacement. *J Bone Joint Surg Br.* 1985;67:551-556.

32. Malkani AL, Rand JA, Bryan RS, et al. Total knee arthroplasty with the kinematic condylar prosthesis. A ten year follow-up study. *J Bone Joint Surg.* 1995;77: 423-431.

33. Hollister, AM, Jatana S, Singh AK, et al. The axes of rotation of the knee. *Clin Orthop Relat Res.* 1993; 290:259-268.

34. Eckhoff D, Hogan C, DiMatteo L, et al. Difference between the epicondylar and cylindrical axis of the knee. *Clin Orthop Relat Res.* 2007;461:238-244.

35. Coughlin KM, Incavo SJ, Churchill DL, et al. Tibial axis and patellar position relative to the femoral epicondylar axis during squatting. *J Arthroplasty.* 2003; 18(8):1048-1055.

36. Lustig S, Lavoie F, Si Selmi TA, et al. Relationship between the surgical epicondylar axis and the articular surface of the distal femur: an anatomic study. *Knee Surg Sports Traaumatol Arthrosc.* 2008;16:674-682.

37. Sikorski JM. Alignment in total knee replacement. *J Bone Joint Surgery Br.* 2008;90:1121-1127.

38. Benjamin J. Component alignment in total knee arthroplasty. *AAOS Instruct Course Lect.* 2006;55: 405-412.

39. Howell SM, Howell SJ, Hull ML. Assessment of the radii of the medial and lateral femoral condyles in varus and valgus knees with osteoarthritis. *J Bone Joint Surg Am.* 2010;92(1):98-104.

40. Howell SM, Kuznik K, Hull ML, et al. Longitudinal shapes of the tibia and femur are unrelated and variable. *Clin Orthop Relat Res.* 2010;468:1142-1148.

41. Howell SM, Hull ML. Kinematic alignment in total knee arthroplasty: definition, surgical technique, and challenging cases. *Orthopedic Knowledge Online.* American Academy of Orthopaedic Surgeons; 2011: 1255-1268.

42. Howell SM, Hull ML. Kinematically aligned TKA with use of MRI based cutting guides in improving accuracy in knee arthroplasty. In: Thienpont E, ed.

Improving Accuracy in Knee Arthroplasty. New Delhi, India: Jaypee Brothers Medical Publishers (P) Ltd.; 2012;207-232.

43. Howell SM. Principles of kinematic alignment in total knee arthroplasty with and without patient specific cutting blocks (OtisKnee). In: Scott WN, Scuderi G, eds. *Insall and Scott Surgery of the Knee*. 5th ed. Philadelphia, PA: Elsevier; 2012;121:1-14.
44. Goodfellow JW, Kershaw CJ, Benson MK, et al. The Oxford Knee for unicompartmental osteoarthritis. The first 103 cases. *J Bone Joint Surg Br.* 1988;70(5):692-701.
45. Pandit H, Jenkins C, Barker K, et al. The Oxford medial unicompartmental knee replacement using a minimally-invasive approach. *J Bone Joint Surg Br.* 2006;88(1):54-60.
46. Price AJ, Webb J, Topf H, et al. Rapid recovery after oxford unicompartmental arthroplasty through a short incision. *J Arthroplasty.* 2001;16(8):970-976.
47. Jiang CC, Insall JN. Effect of rotation on the axial alignment of the femur. Pitfalls in the use of femoral intramedullary guides in total knee arthroplasty. *Clin Orthop Relat Res.* 1989;248:50-56.
48. Matsuda S, Mizu-uchi H, Miura H, et al. Tibial shaft axis does not always serve as a correct coronal landmark in total knee arthroplasty for varus knees. *J Arthroplasty.* 2003;18(1):56-62.
49. Ikeuchi M, Yamanaka N, Okanoue Y, et al. Determining the rotational alignment of the tibial component at total knee replacement: a comparison of two techniques. *J Bone Joint Surg Br.* 2007;89(1):45-49.
50. Siston RA, Goodman SB, Patel JJ, et al. The high variability of tibial rotational alignment in total knee arthroplasty. *Clin Orthop Relat Res.* 2006;452:65-69.
51. Smith CK, Chen JA, Howell SM, et al. An in vivo study of the effect of distal femoral resection on passive knee extension. *J Arthroplasty.* 2010;25:1137-1142.
52. Howell SM, Hodapp EE, Vernace JV, et al. Kneeling is safe for patients with kinematically aligned, cruciate-retaining total knee arthroplasty: an intersurgeon analysis of consecutive series. Submitted for publication.
53. Dossett GH, Swartz GJ, Estrada NA, et al. Kinematically versus mechanically aligned total knee arthroplasty. *Orthopaedics*. 2012;35(2):97.
54. Dennis DA, Komistek RD, Walker SA, et al. Femoral condylar lift-off in vivo in total knee arthroplasty. *J Bone Joint Surg Br.* 2001;83:33-39.
55. Hodapp EE, Howell SM, Vernace JV, et al. Different surgeons minimize undesirable contact kinematics: a study of kinematically aligned total knee arthroplasty. Poster exhibit presented at 2010 National Predoctoral Clinical Research Training Program Meeting, St. Louis, MO, May 3-4, 2010.
56. Klatt BA, Goyal N, Austin MS, et al. Custom-fit total knee arthroplasty (OtisKnee) results in malalignment. *J Arthroplasty.* 2008;23(1):26-29.

58

Patient-Matched Instruments

David J. Mayman, Denis Nam, Michael B. Cross, and Steven B. Haas

This chapter reviews the history of instrumentation used for total knee replacement, the evolution of these instruments over time, and how we have arrived at patient-specific instruments. A discussion is presented on the development of the technology, the process that is used to create the patient-matched instruments, the potential advantages and disadvantages, and literature that has been published on the topic. The potential for improvement in intraoperative efficiency with these instruments is analyzed and, finally, potential future directions based on this technology are discussed.

HISTORY

Knee replacements have been performed using evolving mechanical instruments for close to 50 years. Instruments have evolved over time in order to improve ease of use, accuracy of implantation, and minimization of soft tissue trauma.

The current mechanical instruments have advantages and disadvantages. These instruments are familiar to knee surgeons and relatively straightforward to use. These instruments are, however, quite inaccurate. Literature shows that overall lower extremity mechanical malalignment occurs in 20% to 30% of cases using conventional techniques.[1-3] On the tibial side, this persists with the use of both intramedullary and extramedullary guides.[4-12] Reed et al noted extramedullary tibial alignment guides to be only 65% accurate, versus 85% for intramedullary guides, in obtaining a coronal alignment within 2° of neutral to the mechanical axis in the coronal plane.[6] In addition, varus tibial component positioning has been associated with an increased risk of aseptic component failure.[13] On the femoral side, malalignment is also common, likely due to several factors. The cutting guides are based on the anatomic axis of the femur and not the mechanical axis. The guide is dependent on a rigid fit of the intramedullary (IM) rod in the femoral canal, which is rarely obtained. The guide is also dependent on the position of the entrance hole through the distal femur into the IM canal. A combination of these issues leads to errors of greater than 3° in up to 20% of cases.[14-17] Invasion of the IM canal has also been implicated in fat embolism[18] as well as increased blood loss in knee replacement surgery.[19-21]

In an attempt to alleviate these issues of malalignment and invasion of the IM canal, companies began developing computer-navigated instruments over a decade ago. Although these computerized guides have improved accuracy, they have not become the standard of care for a number of reasons. Computerized systems can be expensive, with capital equipment costs of $100,000 or greater. Computerized systems have also been criticized for the need for extra incisions and pins in the tibia and femur.[22] Likely the largest impediment to implementation of computerized guides is the large learning curve for the surgeon and increased operating time required for the procedure. This increased time converts into frustration for the surgeon and increased expenses for the hospital. Modern navigation systems have attempted to address these issues and are improving, but have not been able to penetrate a large volume of knee replacement surgery. The goal of patient-matched instruments has been to obtain accuracy of implant alignment, including tibial and femoral rotation, while improving operating room efficiency.

DEVELOPMENT

Patient-matched cutting blocks were first introduced by OtisMed Corporation (Alameda, CA). Although these blocks were eventually removed from the market, the idea was felt to be of sound principle. Since that time, multiple companies have developed or are currently developing patient-matched cutting blocks. Several technological hurdles have needed to be crossed in the development process.

In order to create these instruments, planning of the surgical procedure needed to be moved well into the preoperative time period. Preoperative imaging needs to be done in order to determine appropriate alignment of the leg and the cutting blocks as well as to create a three-dimensional model of the knee to manufacture blocks that fit appropriately in the operating room. After the imaging is performed and the three-dimensional (3D) re-creation of the knee is achieved, a surgical plan needs to be created. This involves the virtual implantation of implants to match the patient's anatomy and to create appropriate flexion and extension gaps. Once the surgical plan is created and approved by the surgeon, the blocks need to be manufactured and shipped to the hospital for the appropriate surgery. The blocks are opened for the surgical procedure, allowing for fewer instruments to be used intraoperatively and the procedure to be carried out in a more accurate and efficient manner.

Each of these steps has been a very large change from the standard technique of knee replacement surgery and has created hurdles that have needed to be overcome. Some of these hurdles are still being dealt with today.

The first question was how to obtain mechanical axis alignment of the leg. Some companies have gone with a full leg magnetic resonance imaging (MRI), some use a full leg computed tomography (CT) scan, and one uses a combination of a full-length standing X-ray of the leg. X-rays have been the classic technique that we have used to measure long leg alignment, but X-rays are limited by technique and rotation of the leg (Fig. 58-1). Alignment in patients who have large flexion contractures can be difficult with X-rays. Concerns over radiation dosages remain with CT scan, and MRI has never previously been used to measure alignment. Issues with MRI distortion in measuring alignment have been discovered and are still being worked on.

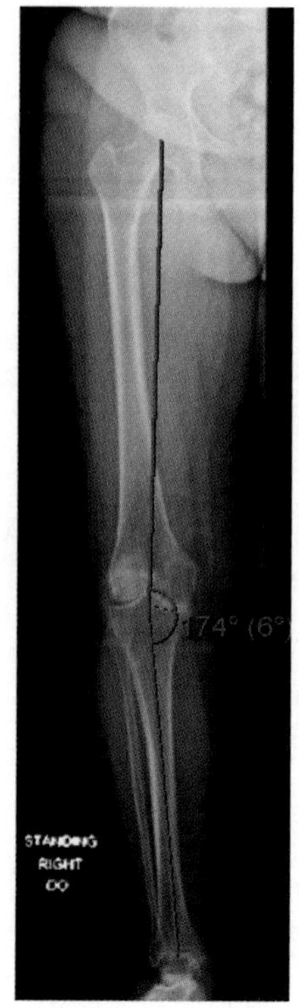

FIGURE 58-1. *Preoperative AP hip to ankle X-ray.*

The next hurdle was creating a 3D model of the distal femur and proximal tibia. Currently either CT or MRI is used. MRI has the advantage of being able to build cartilage into the model and does not expose patients to additional radiation. CT allows for easier bone modeling and is cheaper but does not show cartilage and exposes patients to ionizing radiation. Imaging centers have been creating 3D models from CT scans for years, but before this endeavor 3D bone images had never been created from MRI scans. Early on it was discovered that the MRI scanners needed to be appropriately calibrated or errors could be introduced from the scan. The 3D models from MRIs are still being done manually, adding time and cost to the procedure. Software engineers continue to work on the automation process to allow digitization and automatic creation of 3D models from MRI. Other imaging techniques such as 3D ultrasound have been discussed, but are not currently being used clinically (Figs. 58-2 and 58-3).

Although surgeons have talked about common techniques for measuring bone resection in total knee arthroplasty for many years, it was discovered early on that the same words can mean different things for different surgeons. Since the surgical plan is initially being created by an engineer and not the surgeon, it has been critical that the

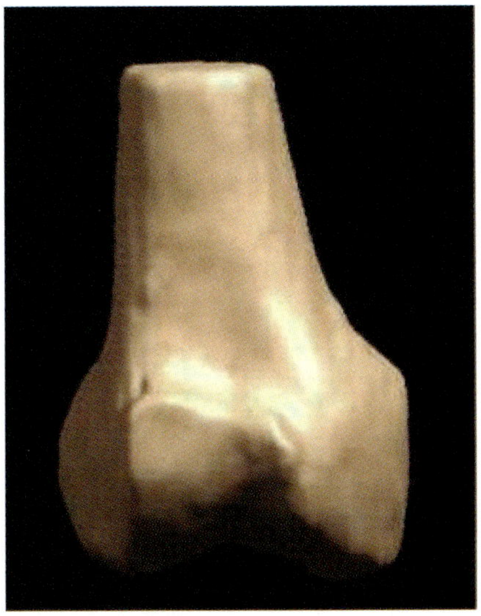

FIGURE 58-2. *Three-dimensional model femur.*

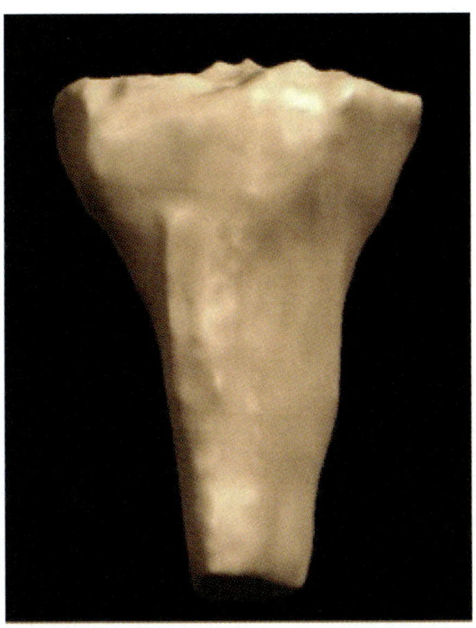

FIGURE 58-3. *Three-dimensional model tibia.*

surgeon and the engineer can communicate effectively to create these surgical plans. Definitions such as aggressive cut versus conservative cut and maximum coverage versus overhang are often seen differently between surgeons. Current systems use Web-based systems to communicate surgeon preferences to the engineers. These preferences often change over time after several surgical plans have been created and this actually ends up being a large part of the learning curve involved in this process.

Once the provisional surgical plan has been created, this is available for the surgeon to view and fine-tune. The initial plan sizes the femur and tibia as well as sets cut depths for the proximal tibia and distal femur. Rotation of the implants is set based on surgeon preferences. Typically the surgeon will view this provisional plan and either approve it as is or can make changes such as asking for extra bone to be removed because of a preoperative flexion contracture or upsizing or downsizing of the femur to optimize bony coverage, flexion gap, and amount of anterior bone cut (Figs. 58-4 to 58-7).

Once the plan is approved by the surgeon, the blocks are engineered and manufactured. The engineering and manufacturing of these blocks is a process that is entirely new to orthopaedic implant manufacturers. Some companies have chosen to outsource this process, while others have purchased equipment and facilities to do this in house.

Because of the disposable nature of these blocks and the rapid manufacturing required, there has been much debate about materials of the blocks, whether the blocks should be actual cut blocks or just pin guides for standard blocks. Typically blocks made from CT scans have been pin guides only and blocks made from MRIs that better fit the articular surface including cartilage can be manufactured as cut blocks or pin guides. These blocks can be shipped sterile or nonsterile (Figs. 58-8 to 58-11).

SURGICAL TECHNIQUE

All preoperative planning has been moved to the surgeon's office, giving this technique the nickname "preoperative navigation." The knowledge of implant sizes preoperatively has allowed for optimization of surgical trays, minimizing the total number of instruments and trays required for the surgical procedure.

Standard exposures are used for these instruments. Tibial or femoral cuts can be made. It is critically important that soft tissue be removed from bone at any contact point with the instruments but that osteophytes not be removed.

The femoral block fits onto the distal femur and is pinned in place. Depending on the block, it can be used as the distal femoral cutting block or can be used as a pin guide for the company's standard distal femoral cutting block. The blocks that are created as cutting blocks put the pins in the same location as the pins for standard cut blocks, allowing

Patient-Matched Instrumentation **TKA CUTTING BLOCK SURGICAL ALIGNMENT PLAN**	
PATIENT	
ANATOMY	**RIGHT**
SURGEON	
IMPLANT	
SURGERY DATE	
X-RAY MEASUREMENTS	
PRE-OP FULL LEG DEFORMITY	4 VARUS°
MECHANICAL AXIS FEMUR VALGUS ANGLE	4.6°
TIBIA DEFORMITY	1.7°
FEMUR PART NO.	
VARUS/VALGUS ALIGNMENT	MECHANICAL AXIS OFF PATIENT X-RAY
MECHANICAL VARUS PREFERENCE	.0°
EXTERNAL ROTATION	A/P AXIS
FLEXION	4°
DISTAL FEMORAL RESECTION	IMPLANT THICKNESS (9.5MM)
SIZE	7
DISTAL MEDIAL RESECTION	9.5 mm
DISTAL LATERAL RESECTION	8.0 mm
DISTAL SULCUS RESECTION	.0 mm
POSTERIOR MEDIAL RESECTION	10.5 mm
POSTERIOR LATERAL RESECTION	8.0 mm
TIBIA PART NO.	
VARUS/VALGUS ALIGNMENT	MECHANICAL AXIS OFF PATIENT X-RAY
EXTERNAL ROTATION	ALIGN W/MEDIAL 1.3 TIB TUBERCLE
POSTERIOR SLOPE	3 DEGREE
PLANNED INSERT THICKNESS	9 mm (Standard resection +1)
SIZE	6
PROXIMAL MEDIAL RESECTION	5.0 mm
PROXIMAL LATERAL RESECTION	10.0 mm
RESECTION TO EMMINENCE	22.0 mm

FIGURE 58-4. *Written surgical plan.*

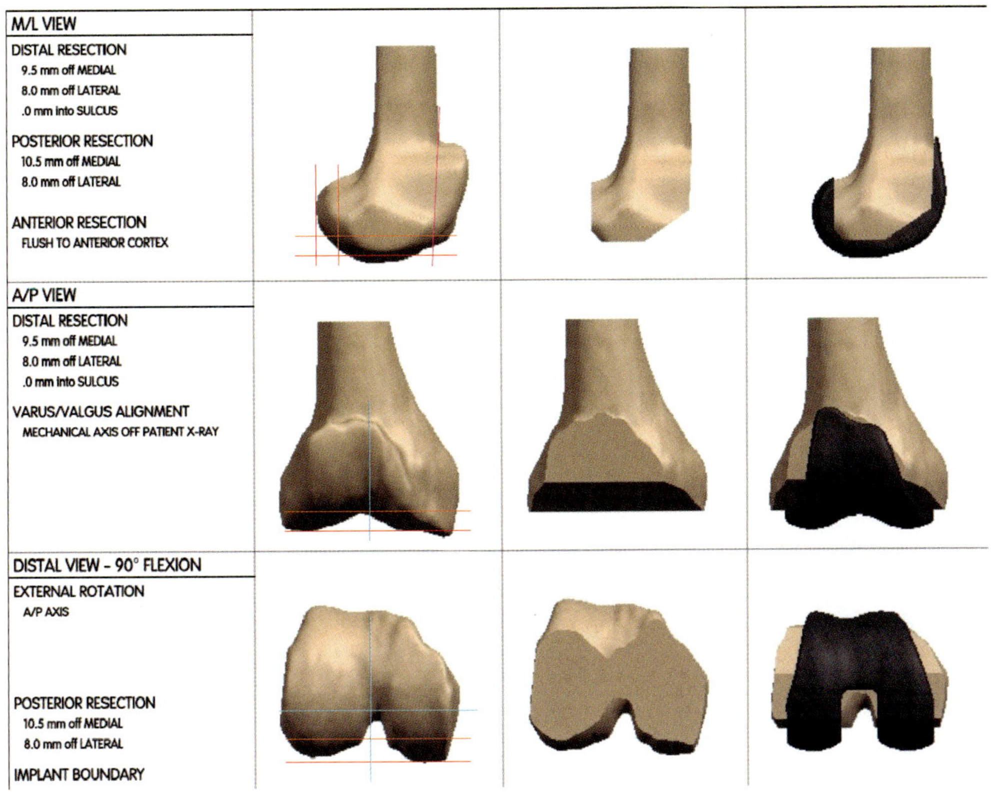

FIGURE 58-5. *Femoral plan.*

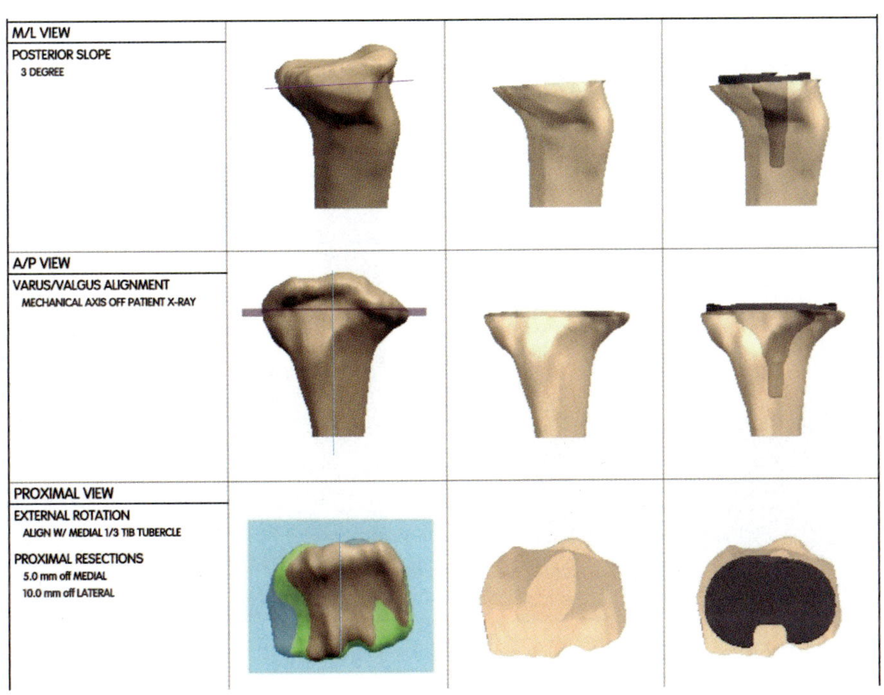

FIGURE 58-6. *Tibial plan.*

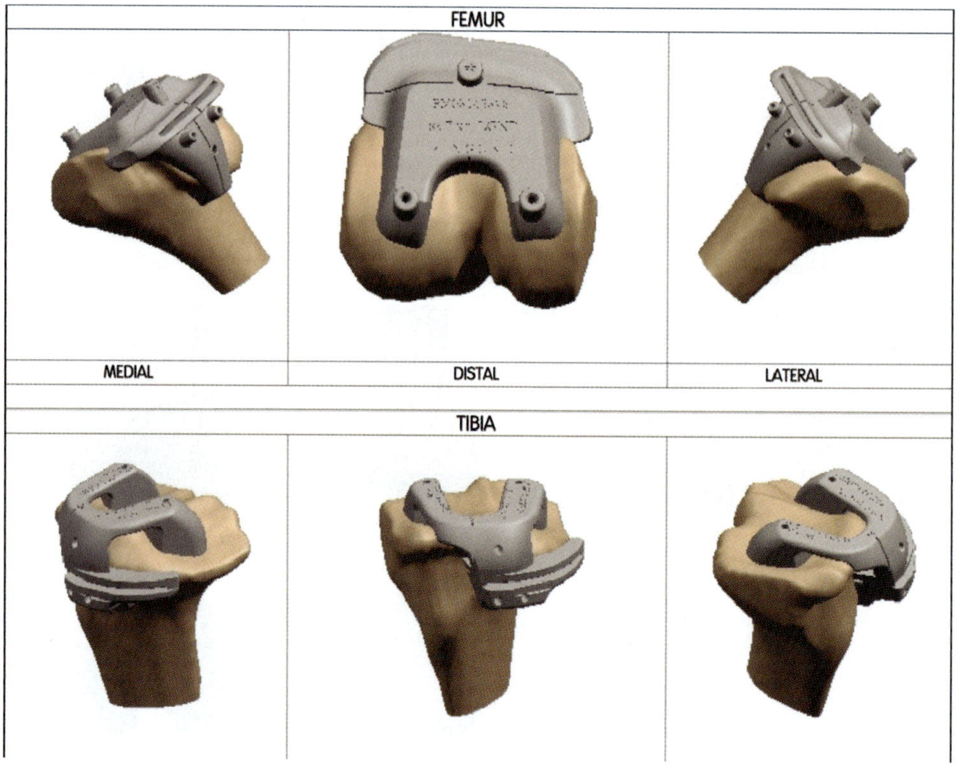

FIGURE 58-7. *Surgical plan with cutting blocks.*

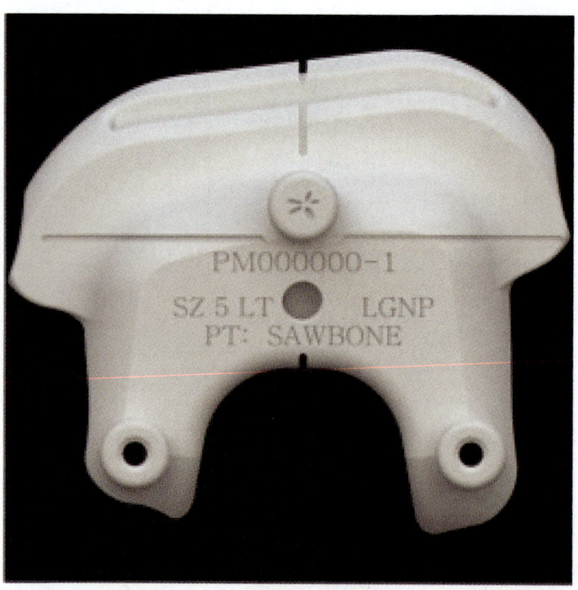

FIGURE 58-8. *Femoral cut block.*

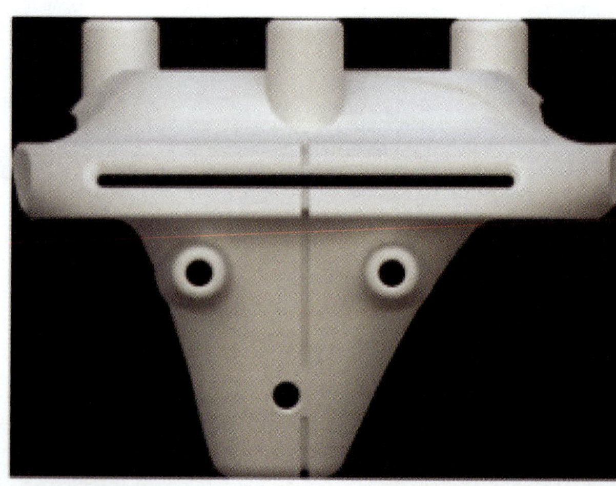

FIGURE 58-9. *Femoral cut block.*

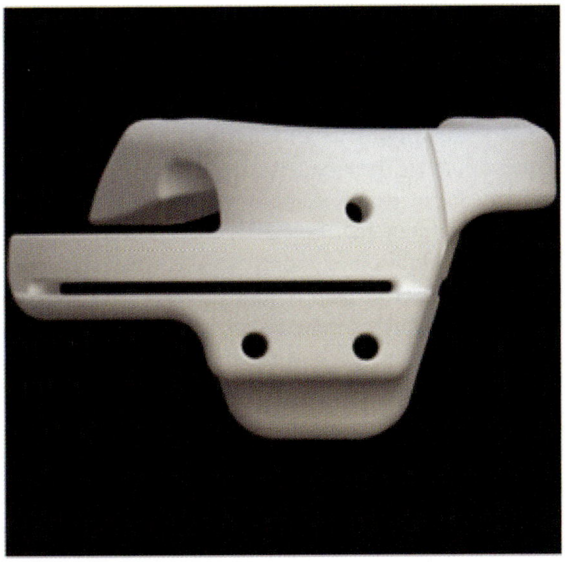

FIGURE 58-10. *Tibial cut block.*

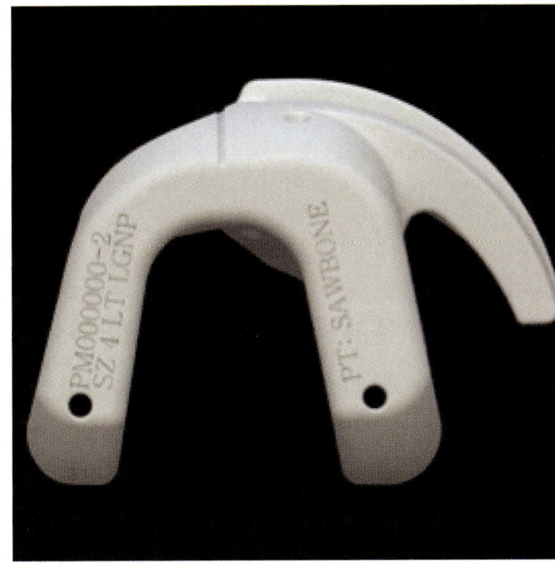

FIGURE 58-11. *Tibial cut block.*

the surgeon to convert to standard cutting blocks if the surgeon chooses to cut more or less bone. The cut blocks also have pin holes to set rotation of the standard anteroposterior (AP) cut blocks. The distal femoral cut is made and the custom cutting block is removed. The femoral block typically fits well due to the complex geometry of the distal femur. Moderate-sized osteophytes allow for an easier fit to the bone. Depending on surgeon preference, the standard AP cutting block can be put on and the AP cuts can be made as determined by the preoperative plan, or the surgeon can move to the tibia and make the tibial cut before the AP cuts on the femur (Figs. 58-12 and 58-13).

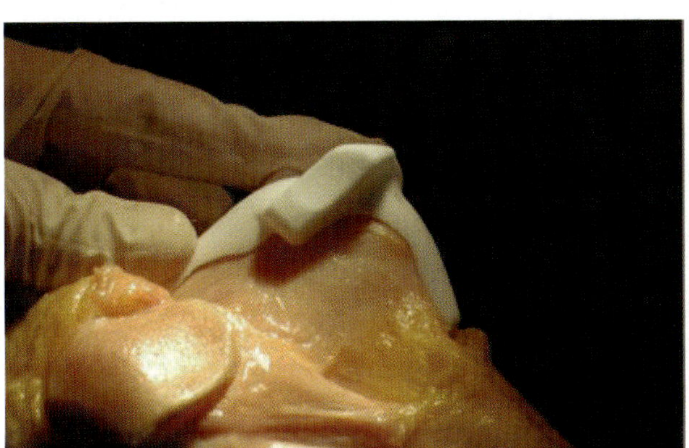

FIGURE 58-12. *Intraoperative femoral cut block placement.*

The tibial blocks have been more difficult to use than the femoral blocks. Again, it is critically important to remove all soft tissue that comes into contact with the block because any soft tissue can malalign the block. Depending on the system, the tibial custom block can be used simply to put pins in for standard cut blocks or can be used directly as the

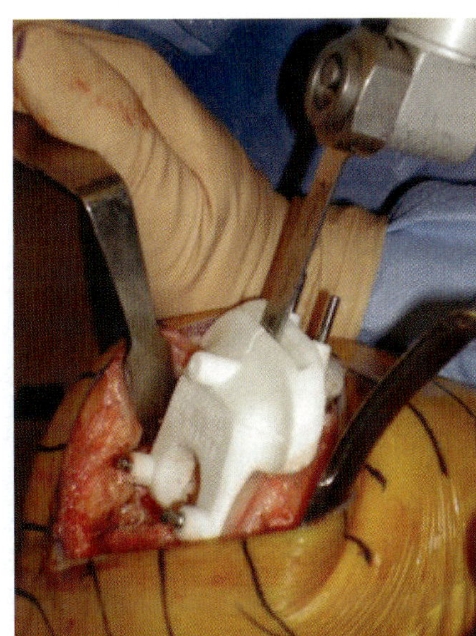

FIGURE 58-13. *Intraoperative femoral cut.*

cutting block. Pin holes in the blocks on the surface of the plateau correspond with the holes in the tibial trial in order to set tibial component position and rotation on correlation to the preoperative plan. Most systems have the ability to insert a drop rod into the tibial block in order to get a second check of alignment (Fig. 58-14). Once the tibial cut is made, the extension gap can be assessed and any ligament balancing can be performed, just as with standard instrumentation.

Potential Advantages of Custom Cut Blocks

The following are potential advantages of custom cut blocks:

1. Preoperative planning,
2. Improved alignment over standard cut blocks,
3. Better rotational alignment than even standard navigation,
4. More efficient surgery with less instrumentation, and
5. No invasion of the femoral canal.

Preoperative planning of knee replacement surgery with knowledge of amounts of bone that should be cut from each area of the knee as well as sizing and rotation information allow the surgeon to go into the procedure with a better understanding of the individual procedure and the intricacies of each procedure.

Abundant literature shows that standard mechanical guides are not very accurate in regard to mechanical axis alignment of the leg after knee replacement surgery. Computer navigation techniques have greatly improved these mechanical axis results but have added large capital equipment costs, long learning curves, complexity to the surgery, and increased surgical times.[22,23]

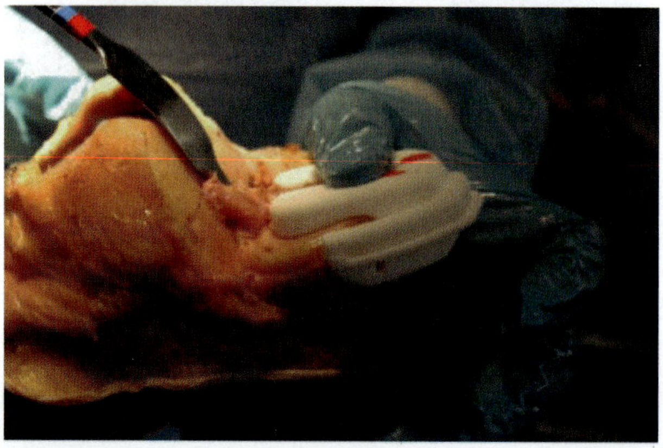

FIGURE 58-14. *Intraoperative tibial block placement.*

Although computer navigation has improved mechanical axis alignment, rotational alignment of the femur has still been questionable because of the difficulty in obtaining high-quality input data for the navigation system.[24] Tibial rotational alignment has been largely ignored in standard navigation techniques and attempts to set tibial rotation with navigation have not proven reliable.[25] Preoperative MRI or CT scan used in patient-matched cut blocks has allowed for accurate assessment of the epicondylar axis, posterior condyles, and trochlear sulcus for assessment of rotation. This has been incorporated into the building of these cut blocks. On the tibial side, the CT or MRI clearly defines the tibial tubercle and tibial crest, allowing for accurate matching of rotation with the cut blocks.

The custom cut blocks have allowed for removal of many instruments for the surgery. The only instruments required on the tibial side are the trials and keel punch. On the femoral side, AP and chamfer cut blocks as well as trials are still needed. This potentially allows for less surgical setup time, less instrument trays to be opened, and theoretically a savings for the hospital due to decreased sterilization costs. However, at this time, no studies have been reported in the literature to support this notion.[26,27] Slover et al performed a cost-effectiveness analysis of custom total knee cutting blocks using a Markov decision model and concluded that the routine use of custom cutting blocks would not be cost-effective unless it results in a significantly reduced revision rate.[27] Therefore, further studies are required to determine if custom cut blocks are truly cost-effective.

The distal femoral cut block is put on without an intramedullary rod. This avoids opening and reaming of the femoral canal. This potentially could lead to less fat emboli and a decreased blood loss if we assume that this is similar to computer navigation techniques.[18-21,28] These advantages are all potentially significant improvements over current mechanical instrument technique, but because this technology is new, there is still very little supporting literature.

Potential Disadvantages of Custom Cutting Blocks

The potential disadvantages of custom cutting blocks include the following:

1. Errors in imaging can cause errors in the final product.
2. Lead time required for imaging, planning, and creation of the blocks can delay surgery.

3. Cost of imaging and blocks can add to the overall cost of surgery.
4. Current systems set rotation on a bony resection model only and do not set rotation for ligament balancing techniques.

As discussed previously, different companies use different imaging modalities (MRI, CT, or X-ray) to define mechanical axis alignment of the leg for these cut blocks. MRI has not been previously used to measure mechanical axis alignment and there have been issues with some MRI systems in measuring these values. X-ray has classically been used to measure mechanical axis alignment but has been shown to be variable depending on rotation of the leg. Large flexion contractures can also compromise accuracy of alignment measurements using X-ray. The current systems require engineers who manually digitize points on the MRI in order to create the 3D model. Rotational axis points such as trochlear sulcus, epicondyles, and posterior condyles are also manually picked.

Additional time is required for the planning and creation of these custom cut blocks. Imaging studies need to be done, the imaging studies need to be analyzed, and a surgical plan must be created. The plan needs to be approved and then the blocks need to be manufactured. The blocks then need to be labeled and shipped for the appropriate patient. Typically this process can be completed in approximately 3 weeks. It is rare that a patient would be having surgery in less than 3 weeks after being seen by the surgeon; however, at this time with current technology, this could potentially be a delay in surgery.

The cost of imaging, engineering support, and manufacturing of the blocks is at the center of the debate of overall cost-effectiveness of the use of these custom cutting blocks. The cost of the MRI or CT scan is clearly an additional cost to the system over standard X-rays required for the use of mechanical instruments. The amount of money being spent by industry on engineers developing and manufacturing the blocks are additional costs when compared to standard. Financial models argue that hospitals can save money on the efficiency of the procedure and decreased costs of sterilization. There are also potential savings to the company in not having to manufacture expensive mechanical instrument trays or maintain expensive inventory on hospital shelves because the sizes are determined preoperatively. These financial models are currently being tested at many sites, but there is still very little literature looking at the overall cost to the company and the health care system.

Current custom cut blocks set rotational alignment of the femur on a bony resection model, using surgeon preference of trochlear sulcus, epicondylar axis, or posterior condylar axis. They do not include a ligament balancing technique. There has been criticism of these systems based on their lack of intraoperative flexibility and allowance for the surgeon to make intraoperative changes based on intraoperative conditions. Most surgeons can agree that we are aiming for neutral mechanical axis of the leg with a perpendicular joint line. Most literature has suggested that alignment within 3° of neutral mechanical axis is ideal. The custom blocks allow the surgeon to plan mechanical axis alignment and are typically set to remove bone equal to the thickness of the implant in order to create appropriate gaps. The blocks put pins in a position that is compatible with the standard cut blocks to allow the surgeon to take more or less bone, still in the appropriate alignment, in order to compensate for any intraoperative findings that require more or less bone to be taken. The systems do set rotational alignment based on bony resection; however, if the surgeon believes that a ligament balancing technique should be used, then after the distal femoral cut and proximal tibial cut are made, standard ligament tensioning devices can be used to set femoral rotation. Sizing of the implants can also be changed if the surgeon feels that this is necessary. Significant effort has been made to build in as much preoperative planning as possible while still allowing for the surgeon to make intraoperative assessments and changes as necessary to deal with the intraoperative environment.

RESULTS

Although the concepts behind patient-matched cutting blocks seem sound, the technology is new and there is very little scientific literature looking at outcomes. The first publication on the topic was a review of four patients undergoing OtisKnee, custom-fit total knee. An image-free navigation system was used to measure the recommended cuts and showed recommended cuts outside of 3° of neutral mechanical with wide variations of recommended cut angles.[29]

Other studies, including a larger study by Howell et al, using the OtisKnee blocks showed acceptable alignment with excellent short-term results and shorter operative times than a similar cohort of patients whose knees were operated on with mechanical instruments.[30]

FUTURE DIRECTIONS

The development of these custom blocks is really still in its infancy. Although there seems to be potential for improvements in alignment and efficiency with these systems, rigorous scientific evaluation needs to be performed to evaluate these systems. A recently published paper by Mont et al looking at surgeon perceptions reported that 10 of 50 surveyed surgeons had used patient-matched instruments. Twenty-nine of the remaining 40 said that they were interested in trying the technology.[31]

The technology has the potential to evolve into the development of fully disposable instruments for custom procedures. This has the potential to improve efficiency and accuracy of the procedure, eliminating large, expensive instrument trays and removing millions of dollars of inventory from hospital shelves, but each step of this procedure will also add potential costs and errors that need to be thoroughly investigated throughout the development and implementation process. In today's health care environment, any new technique or instrumentation development technique needs to be guided by the principles of improving patient outcomes while also improving efficiency within the system.

REFERENCES

1. Mason JB, Fehring TK, Estok R, et al. Meta-analysis of alignment outcomes in computer-assisted total knee arthroplasty surgery. *J Arthroplasty.* 2007;22(8): 1097-1106.
2. Mulhall KJ, Ghomrawi HM, Scully S, et al. Current etiologies and modes of failure in total knee arthroplasty revision. *Clin Orthop Relat Res.* 2006;446:45-50.
3. Sikorski JM. Alignment in total knee replacement. *J Bone Joint Surg Br.* 2008;90(9):1121-1127.
4. Dennis DA, Channer M, Susman MH, et al. Intramedullary versus extramedullary tibial alignment systems in total knee arthroplasty. *J Arthroplasty.* 1993;8(1):43-47.
5. Brys DA, Lombardi AV Jr, Mallory TH, et al. A comparison of intramedullary and extramedullary alignment systems for tibial component placement in total knee arthroplasty. *Clin Orthop Relat Res.* 1991;263:175-179.
6. Reed MR, Bliss W, Sher JL, et al. Extramedullary or intramedullary tibial alignment guides: a randomised, prospective trial of radiological alignment. *J Bone Joint Surg Br.* 2002;84(6):858-860.
7. Simmons ED Jr, Sullivan JA, Rackemann S, et al. The accuracy of tibial intramedullary alignment devices in total knee arthroplasty. *J Arthroplasty.* 1991;6(1):45-50.
8. Teter KE, Bregman D, Colwell CW Jr. Accuracy of intramedullary versus extramedullary tibial alignment cutting systems in total knee arthroplasty. *Clin Orthop Relat Res.* 1995;321:106-110.
9. Thienpont E. Extramedullary or intramedullary tibial alignment guides: a randomised, prospective trial of radiological alignment. *J Bone Joint Surg Br.* 2003;85(6):932; author reply, 932.
10. Yang SH, Liu TK. Intramedullary versus extramedullary tibial alignment guides in total knee arthroplasty. *J Formos Med Assoc.* 1998;97(8):564-568.
11. Maestro A, Harwin SF, Sandoval MG, et al. Influence of intramedullary versus extramedullary alignment guides on final total knee arthroplasty component position: a radiographic analysis. *J Arthroplasty.* 1998;13(5):552-528.
12. Mihalko WM, Krackow KA. Differences between extramedullary, intramedullary, and computer-aided surgery tibial alignment techniques for total knee arthroplasty. *J Knee Surg.* 2006;19(1):33-36.
13. Berend ME, Ritter MA, Meding JB, et al. Tibial component failure mechanisms in total knee arthroplasty. *Clin Orthop Relat Res.* 2004;428:26-34.
14. Deakin AH, Basanagoudar PL, Nunag P, et al. Natural distribution of the femoral mechanical-anatomical angle in an osteoarthritic population and its relevance to total knee arthroplasty. *Knee.* 2012;19(2):120-123.
15. Cates HE, Ritter MA, Keating EM, et al. Intramedullary versus extramedullary femoral alignment systems in total knee replacement. *Clin Orthop Relat Res.* 1993;286:32-39.
16. Kinzel V, Scaddan M, Bradley B, et al. Varus/valgus alignment of the femur in total knee arthroplasty. Can accuracy be improved by preoperative CT scanning? *Knee.* 2004;11(3):197-201.
17. Bardakos N, Cil A, Thompson B, et al. Mechanical axis cannot be restored in total knee arthroplasty with a fixed valgus resection angle: a radiographic study. *J Arthroplasty.* 2007;22(6 suppl 2):85-89.
18. Church JS, Scadden JE, Gupta RR, et al. Embolic phenomena during computer-assisted and conventional total knee replacement. *J Bone Joint Surg Br.* 2007;89(4):481-485.
19. Hinarejos P, Corrales M, Matamalas A, et al. Computer-assisted surgery can reduce blood loss after total knee arthroplasty. *Knee Surg Sports Traumatol Arthrosc.* 2009;17(4):356-360.

20. Schnurr C, Csécsei G, Eysel P, et al. The effect of computer navigation on blood loss and transfusion rate in TKA. *Orthopedics.* 2010;33(7):474.
21. Millar NL, Deakin AH, Millar LL, et al. Blood loss following total knee replacement in the morbidly obese: the effect of computer navigation. *Knee.* 2011;18(2):108-112.
22. Canale ST, Beaty JH. *Campbell's Operative Orthopaedics.* 11th ed. Philadelphia, PA: Elsevier Inc.; 2008.
23. Confalonieri N, Manzotti A, Pullen C, et al. Computer-assisted technique versus intramedullary and extramedullary alignment systems in total knee replacement: a radiological comparison. *Acta Orthop Belg.* 2005;71(6):703-709.
24. Siston RA, Patel JJ, Goodman SB, et al. The variability of femoral rotational alignment in total knee arthroplasty. *J Bone Joint Surg Am.* 2005;87(10): 2276-2280.
25. Siston RA, Goodman SB, Patel JJ, et al. The high variability of tibial rotational alignment in total knee arthroplasty. *Clin Orthop Relat Res.* 2006;452:65-69.
26. Watters TS, Mather RC III, Browne JA, et al. Analysis of procedure-related costs and proposed benefits of using patient-specific approach in total knee arthroplasty. *J Surg Orthop Adv.* 2011;20(2):112-116.
27. Slover J, Rubash H, Malchau H, et al. Cost-effectiveness analysis of custom total knee cutting blocks. *J Arthroplasty.* 2011 Jun 13 [Epub ahead of print].
28. Kalairajah Y, Simpson D, Cossey AJ, et al. Blood loss after total knee replacement: effects of computer-assisted surgery. *J Bone Joint Surg Br.* 2005;87(11): 1480-1482.
29. Klatt BA, Goyal N, Austin MS, et al. Custom-fit total knee arthroplasty (OtisKnee) results in malalignment. *J Arthroplasty.* 2008;23(1):26-29.
30. Howell SM, Kuznik K, Hull ML, et al. Results of an initial experience with custom-fit positioning total knee arthroplasty in a series of 48 patients. *Orthopedics.* 2008;31(9):857-863.
31. Mont MA, Johnson AJ, Zywiel MG, et al. Surgeon perceptions regarding custom-fit positioning for total knee arthroplasty. *Surg Technol Int.* 2010;20:348-351.

59 Total Knee Arthroplasty Using Mobile Bearing

Douglas A. Dennis and Raymond H. Kim

Initial condylar total knee arthroplasty (TKA) designs were primarily used in elderly, low-demand patients with advanced arthritic degeneration. The excellent 10- to 15-year clinical outcomes in this patient cohort[1-5] have resulted in performance of TKA on younger patients who have higher functional demands and the need for increased implant longevity. Quantitative assessments of walking activity have demonstrated that joint replacement subjects walk between 1 and 2 million cycles per year, with some subjects walking more than 6 million cycles annually.[6,7] Typically, younger subjects have increased activity requirements and longevity expectations approaching three decades or more. To meet the demands of these younger patients, future TKA designs must improve functional performance and reduce articular bearing surface wear while maintaining the excellent long-term fixation typically obtained in properly aligned and balanced TKAs currently in use today. One successful design concept that has evolved over the past three decades to meet these increased demands is the development of the mobile-bearing TKA. The purpose of this chapter is to review the design rationale, surgical implantation issues, and clinical outcomes of use of mobile-bearing TKA.

DESIGN RATIONALE OF MOBILE-BEARING TKA

Early TKAs were performed before comprehensive understanding of the importance of alignment and soft tissue balancing and often resulted in early failures due to malalignment, instability, and the use of implants with excessive prosthetic constraint. While increased prosthetic constraint provided by hinged or extremely conforming unlinked TKA systems enhance the stability of TKA, the torsional, coronal, and sagittal stresses normally shared by the surrounding soft tissue stabilizing structures are transferred through the implant to the fixation interface,[8] resulting in premature TKA failure secondary to aseptic component loosening.[9-12] Biomechanical studies have demonstrated that highly conforming fixed-bearing TKA designs are intolerant of higher rotational and anterior-posterior translational kinematic motion patterns that are commonly encountered after TKA, with accelerated polyethylene wear frequently observed.[11,13-17] Implant malalignment worsens the elevated subsurface polyethylene stresses already present in highly conforming fixed-bearing TKA systems greater than in less conforming fixed or highly conforming mobile-bearing TKA designs.[13,16,17]

The premature failure of first-generation TKA implants resulted in the development of an implant that relied more on the load-sharing and stabilizing roles of the native capsular and ligamentous structures. This was accomplished by reducing articular conformity and typically incorporated the use of round-on-flat or flat-on-flat articular geometries. These designs allowed rotation and multiplane translation to occur at the articulating interface and relied more on the surrounding soft tissue structures than conformity of the articular surfaces for stability and dispersion of the applied loads.

While these low-conformity TKA designs significantly reduced stresses transmitted to the fixation interface, they created a detrimental decrease in contact area between the femoral component and the polyethylene bearing surface and a subsequent increase in cross-shear forces. Since the contact stress experienced at the polyethylene surface is inversely proportional to the degree of conformity between the femoral condyles and the tibial polyethylene insert, reduction of contact area with low-conformity designs led to accelerated polyethylene wear and subsequent premature TKA failure.[18,19]

Fluoroscopic kinematic evaluations of low-conformity, posterior cruciate ligament-retaining (PCL-retaining) TKA articulations have also demonstrated an increased incidence of both paradoxical anterior femoral translation during deep flexion (instead of controlled posterior femoral rollback) and reverse axial rotation patterns. These abnormal kinematic patterns are likely secondary to a reduction in articular conformity with resulting instability.[10,11,20-23] This paradoxical motion produces detrimental cyclical tensile shear stresses at the articulating surface, further increasing the risk of accelerated polyethylene wear.[8,24]

Strategies employed to reduce polyethylene wear have included use of thicker polyethylene bearings,[8,25] enhancements in polyethylene locking mechanisms of modular tibial components to reduce backside wear,[26-28] improved sterilization techniques,[29-34] returning to the use of TKA implants with increased articular surface conformity,[1-3,35-37] and the use of mobile-bearing TKA systems.[1-3,35-37] Analysis of contact area versus contact stress demonstrates a dramatic reduction of contact stress as contact area is increased. Due to the logarithmic relationship between contact area and stress, increasing the contact area beyond 350 to 400 mm² does reduce contact stresses further but to a substantially lesser degree[38] (Fig. 59-1). In contrast to total hip arthroplasty, where conformity may be achieved in all planes, the focus in TKA is primarily on achieving sagittal and coronal plane conformity. Increasing coronal plane conformity has been shown to be the most critical in reduction of peak polyethylene stresses,[8,15] particularly in the presence of femoral condylar liftoff.[8,14,15,39] Increasing sagittal plane conformity provides the opportunity of improved control of anterior-posterior translation with reduced paradoxical anterior femoral translation, particularly when tested during gait.[22,40]

Advantages of Mobile-Bearing TKA

Mobile-bearing TKA designs offer the advantage of allowing increased implant conformity and contact area in both the sagittal and coronal planes without dramatically increasing stresses transmitted to the polyethylene bearing or the fixation interface. The incorporation of polyethylene bearing mobility, such as in a rotating platform TKA design, allows smooth rotation through the tibial tray–polyethylene bearing articulation and effectively minimizes the transfer of torsional stresses to the fixation interface that are typically present with fixed-bearing TKA implants.[41] While

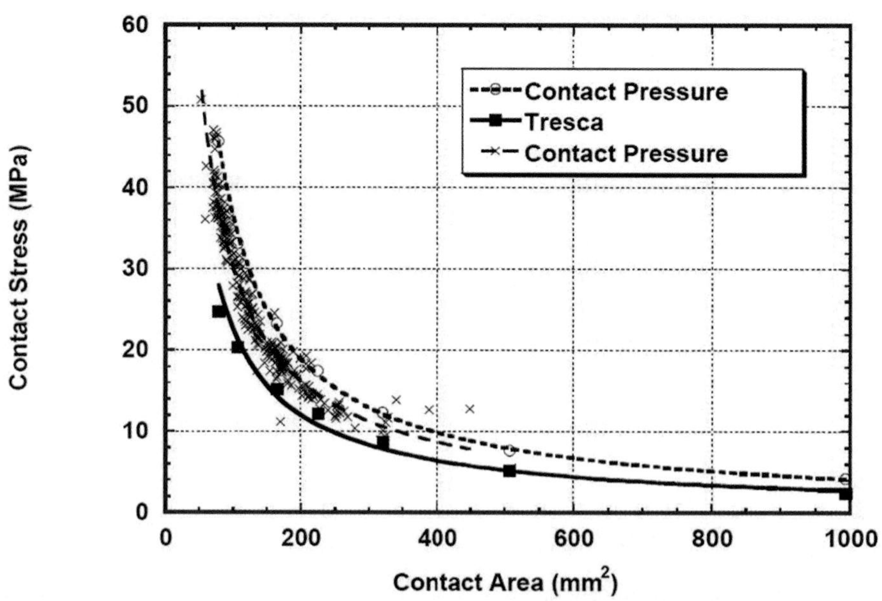

FIGURE 59-1. *Graph demonstrating experimental and finite element analyses of polyethylene contact area (mm²) and resultant contact stresses (MPa).[38] (Reprinted with permission.)*

ultracongruent fixed-bearing TKA implants have been developed, they typically exhibit increased conformity in only the sagittal plane. If increased congruence was present in both the sagittal and coronal planes, excessive stresses within the polyethylene and at the fixation interface would be incurred, resulting in premature failure.[9-12]

The importance of coronal plane conformity and its effect on polyethylene stresses has been demonstrated using TekScan analysis.[42] When a flat-on-flat design is tested in good alignment with equal loading of each condyle, peak polyethylene stresses reach approximately 16 MPa. When the same design is loaded in 3° of varus malalignment, shifting load to one condyle as occurs with femoral condylar lift-off, the peak stresses dramatically increase to 38 MPa, which far exceeds the yield strength of polyethylene (20–22 MPa). When similar testing was performed with a TKA design with increased coronal conformity, peak polyethylene stresses increased to only 16 MPa when tested under varus loading conditions (Fig. 59-2).

The increased conformity of mobile-bearing TKA designs has been shown to substantially increase contact area, reduce contact stresses, and lower polyethylene wear in numerous other scientific evaluations.[8,14,17,24,43-46] Greenwald and Heim[43] demonstrated that contact areas of mobile-bearing TKA during gait range from approximately 400 to 800 mm², which equates to contact stresses at 14 MPa or less (Fig. 59-3). This magnitude of contact area is significantly greater than is typically seen in most fixed-bearing TKA designs (200–250 mm²) (Fig. 59-4). Finite element evaluations also demonstrate reduced polyethylene contact stresses as a direct result of increased contact area.[46-49] These findings are supported by results of knee simulator wear studies of fixed-bearing versus mobile-bearing TKA, which have demonstrated significantly reduced polyethylene wear rates with highly conforming rotating platform designs when compared with fixed-bearing systems.[44,45] McEwen et al[44] noted over a 4-fold reduction in wear with testing of a rotating-platform TKA design (Fig. 59-5). Reduced polyethylene wear has similarly been observed in retrieval studies. Atwood et al reported results from their retrieval studies on the long-term volumetric wear rate of 54 mm^3 annually for a rotating-platform mobile-bearing knee design versus 120 mm^3 per year secondary to backside wear in fixed-bearing TKAs.[50]

For the benefits of increased conformity and lower contact and cross-shear stresses to be recognized, the mobile polyethylene bearing must remain congruent with the femoral component throughout knee motion. Rotating-platform

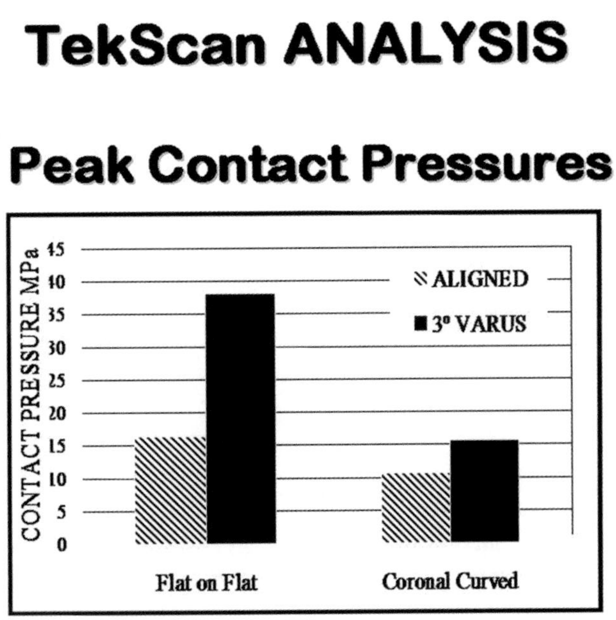

FIGURE 59-2. *Histogram demonstrating peak polyethylene contact stresses (MPa) of high-versus low-conformity TKA designs in neutral and 3° varus alignment. (Reprinted with permission from Medscape. Available at: http://www.medscape.com/viewprogram/3133. © 2004 Medscape.)*

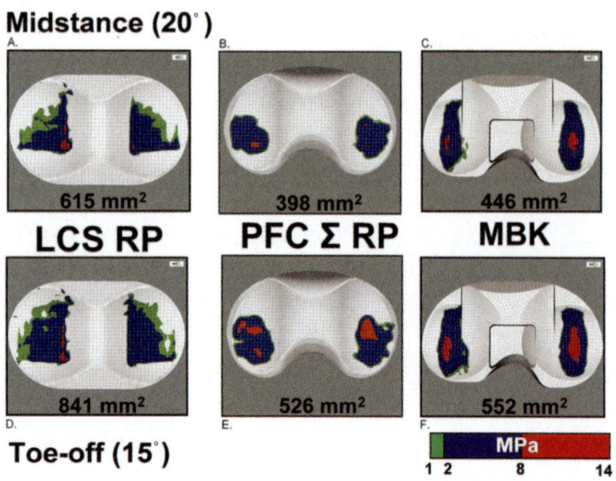

FIGURE 59-3. *Contact area and stress analysis demonstrating high polyethylene contact areas (mm^2) and low peak stresses (MPa) of three mobile-bearing TKA designs. (Reprinted with permission from Greenwald AS, Heim CS: Mobile-bearing systems: ultra-high molecular weight polyethylene wear and design issues. In Pellegrini VD (ed): Instructional Course Lectures 54. Rosemont, IL: American Academy of Orthopaedic Surgeons, 2005, pp. 195-206.)*

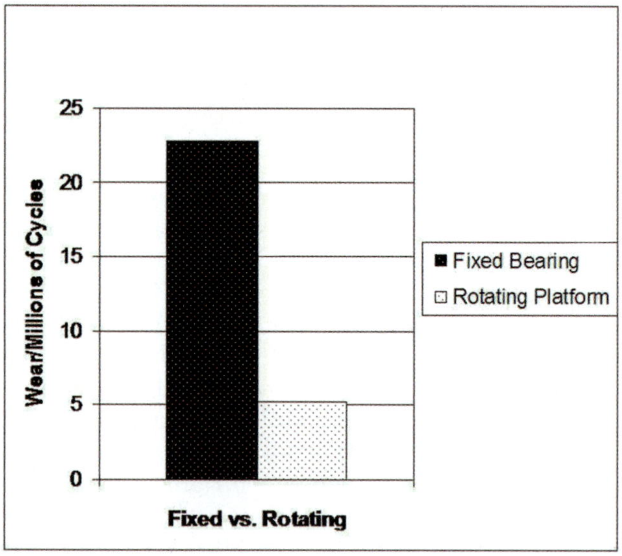

FIGURE 59-5. *Histogram of a high kinematic knee simulator analysis comparing polyethylene wear (mg) per million cycles in a rotating-platform versus a fixed-bearing TKA. (Reprinted with permission from Medscape. Available at: http://www.medscape.com/viewprogram/3133. © 2004 Medscape.)*

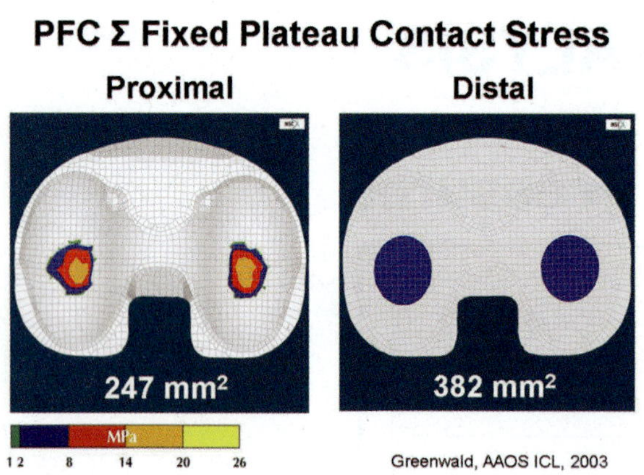

FIGURE 59-4. *Contact area and stress analysis demonstrating a lower polyethylene contact area (mm^2) and higher peak stress (MPa) in a fixed-bearing TKA design. (Reprinted with permission from Greenwald AS, Heim CS: Mobile-bearing systems: ultra-high molecular weight polyethylene wear and design issues. In Pellegrini VD (ed): Instructional Course Lectures 54. Rosemont, IL: American Academy of Orthopaedic Surgeons, 2005, pp. 195-206.)*

systems utilize a flat tibial tray–polyethylene counter surface that allows unimpeded freedom of the polyethylene insert to rotate around a central post on a highly polished, cobalt-chrome surface with a very low surface roughness. In vivo fluoroscopic kinematic studies in which tantalum beads are implanted within the transparent polyethylene bearing have confirmed that rotation in rotating-platform TKA systems predictably occurs in all subjects tested at time intervals out to 5 years following implantation.[51,52] These analyses have demonstrated that the majority of axial rotation in these rotating-platform designs occurs at the polyethylene bearing–tibial tray interface as the polyethylene bearing "follows" the rotation of the femoral component, maintaining congruency of the bearing with the femoral component.[11,51,52]

Rotation of the rotating-platform polyethylene insert with the femoral component, independent of the rotation of the firmly fixed tibial tray, creates the potential for self-alignment of the polyethylene bearing with the femoral component. Self-alignment of the bearing with the femoral component optimizes prosthesis kinematics, reduces cross-shear stresses experienced by the polyethylene bearing surface, and avoids excessive load transfer to PCL-substituting tibial posts, which can occur when rotational malalignment exists between fixed-bearing femoral and tibial components. This self-aligning behavior with a highly conforming design has been shown to maintain large, centrally located surface contact areas at the femorotibial articulation during both flexion-extension and axial rotation of the knee,[17] which is much more difficult to achieve in fixed-bearing TKA designs.

An additional advantage of bearing self-alignment of rotating-platform TKA systems is facilitation of central patellar tracking.[53] In a fixed-bearing TKA, if substantial internal rotation of the tibial component relative to the femoral component is present, the tibial tubercle becomes lateralized, enhancing the risk of patellar subluxation. A rotating-platform design, through bearing rotation, typically provides for greater self-correction of the component malalignment, allowing better centralization of the extensor mechanism. The authors reviewed 1318 consecutive primary TKAs performed by the senior author (D.A.D.) over a 6-year period.[53] All subjects were implanted using a single posterior-stabilized knee design (Sigma Press-Fit Condylar; Depuy, Warsaw, IN). The femoral and patellar components were identical and the tibial component type was either a mobile-bearing rotating-platform design or a fixed-bearing tibial design (all-polyethylene or modular metal-backed tibial component). The selection of a fixed- versus mobile-bearing TKA was primarily based on patient age with subjects less than 70 years of age receiving a mobile-bearing TKA. Mobile-bearing TKA devices were implanted in 940 cases (71.3%; 940 of 1318) and fixed-bearing knees were implanted in 378 cases (28.7%; 378 of 1318). A lateral release was performed in any case in which perfect patellar tracking (patella centered in the trochlear groove with bicondylar contact through 90° of flexion with no subluxation or separation of a patellar facet from the trochlear groove) was not obtained. The overall prevalence of lateral release was 7.9% (104 of 1318 knees). The incidence of lateral release in the fixed-bearing group (14.3%; 54 of 378) was found to be significantly higher ($p < .0001$) than in the mobile-bearing group (5.3%; 50 of 940).

Kinematic patterns of differing rotating-platform knee designs, however, can vary. Garling et al[54] performed a fluoroscopic kinematic evaluation of 10 rheumatoid patients implanted with a different rotating-platform TKA (NexGen LPS mobile; Zimmer, Warsaw, IN) and found that the femoral component underwent greater axial rotation than the mobile polyethylene bearing insert, suggesting that the femoral component was sliding on the top of the insert. They attributed this to the limited articular conformity in this design, an anterior (versus central) pivot point for the rotating platform, insert impingement, or fibrous tissue caught between the insert and the tibial tray. Therefore the kinematic finding of polyethylene bearing rotation in conjunction with the femoral component is a design-specific condition.

Last, use of mobile-bearing TKA implants may prove advantageous in cases of revision TKA. In revision TKA, significant bone loss secondary to osteolysis or iatrogenic resection is commonly encountered. As a result, obtaining rigid fixation becomes increasingly difficult in the context of diminished bone stock. Disrupted or unbalanced soft tissue supporting structures may also be encountered, which necessitate use of revision components with increased constraint. While increased prosthetic constraint can solve problems with ligamentous instability, it results in increased stress transmission to the fixation interface, which may lead to premature component loosening as well as increased polyethylene post wear secondary to increased torque on the constraining mechanism. Potential advantages of mobile-bearing use in revision TKA include reduction in polyethylene wear, decreasing fixation stresses, and protection of the constraining mechanisms.

In summary, the rotational freedom provided in mobile-bearing TKA designs assists in maintaining alignment of both the patellofemoral and femorotibial articulations throughout knee flexion in addition to lessening fixation stresses. Self-alignment via polyethylene bearing rotation improves postoperative TKA kinematics, lessens polyethylene surface stresses, and minimizes posterior-stabilized post impingement, increasing the potential for enhanced polyethylene longevity.

Fears Associated With Mobile-Bearing TKA

Despite the many demonstrated advantages of use of a mobile-bearing TKA, several concerns have been expressed with their use, including the need for a more exacting surgical technique, the occurrence of bearing instability,[2,36,55,56] the risk of enhanced polyethylene wear resulting from creation of a second articulating surface, and the question of whether the polyethylene particles generated from the inferior aspect of the bearing will be smaller with greater osteolytic potential.

Dislocation ("spin-out") of the polyethylene bearing in rotating-platform TKA most commonly occurs during deep knee flexion when the bearing rotates 90° around its central axis in the tibial tray and the posterolateral polyethylene lip slips posteriorly underneath the lateral femoral condyle and the anteromedial polyethylene lip slips anteriorly underneath the medial femoral condyle (Fig. 59-6). This may be irreducible by closed attempts and require operative reduction. The highest incidence of bearing spin-out [3.3% (5/149)

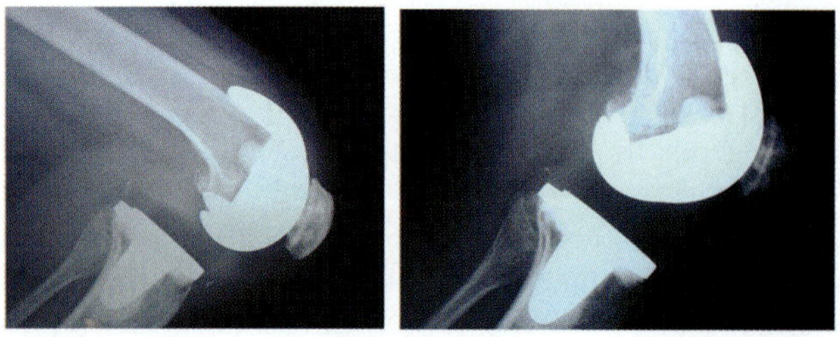

FIGURE 59-6. *Lateral radiographs of a rotating-platform TKA demonstrating a dislocated polyethylene bearing (left) and following closed reduction of the dislocated bearing (right).*

to 12% (2/17)][11,14] has been associated with early outcome evaluations of rotating-platform TKA, when attention to flexion gap tension and balance was less emphasized. Improvements in surgical implantation instrumentation, a better understanding of the importance of flexion and extension gap tension and balance, and more precise femoral component rotation have decreased the incidence of bearing instability following mobile-bearing TKA. Several recent outcome evaluations have reported a 0% to 2.2% incidence of bearing spin-out in primary TKA at up to 20 years following the operative procedure.[1-3,56] A meta-analysis of clinical results of mobile-bearing TKAs performed at the authors' institution determined the incidence of bearing instability in reports after 1995 to be 0.1%.[57]

The additional polyethylene–metal interface at the undersurface of the polyethylene bearing has raised concerns about the generation of additional polyethylene particles and accelerated wear. With fixed-bearing TKA systems, "backside" polyethylene motion against a rough tibial tray that is not designed to accommodate motion has shown significant polyethylene wear and subsequent periprosthetic osteolysis.[26-28] In rotating-platform systems, a rotating, polyethylene bearing is matched against a flat, highly polished, cobalt-chromium surface with extremely low surface roughness. To date, backside polyethylene wear has not emerged as a clinically significant issue in rotating-platform designs. Studies examining the backside bearing surface of retrieved rotating-platform polyethylene inserts have reported only limited evidence of significant undersurface wear.[12,56] Currier et al[58] recently analyzed in vivo backside wear of rotating-platform retrievals using three-dimensional surface profilometry and observed that surface damage represented plastic deformation rather than material removal in contrast to evaluation of fixed-bearing retrievals, which demonstrated material loss due to multidirectional wear.

An explanation for the lack of clinically significant backside polyethylene wear is the decoupling of multidirectional motions occurring at the articular interfaces with rotating-platform TKA designs.[33,44] In fixed-bearing systems, all rotational, translational, and flexion-extension motion patterns are experienced on the superior aspect of the polyethylene articular surface, thereby resulting in multidirectional motion pathways. In a rotating-platform design that allows no anterior-posterior translation, the inferior or tibial tray–polyethylene counter surface is designed to experience purely rotational (reciprocal/unidirectional) motion patterns. If the polyethylene bearing tracts with the femoral component,[51,52] the superior articular surface (femoral component–polyethylene interface) primarily experiences flexion-extension (reciprocal/unidirectional) motion, since rotation is occurring on the inferior aspect of the bearing. Pooley and Tabor[59] reported that when high-density polyethylene is subjected to unidirectional sliding, the molecules tend to align along the direction of sliding, lowering the coefficient of friction and reducing wear of the material. Conversely, when the material is exposed to multidirectional wear pathways, increased cross-shear stresses are created that enhance polyethylene wear. Additional laboratory studies have shown that the multidirectional shear stresses experienced at the single articulating polyethylene interface in fixed-bearing systems can result in the generation of 4 to 10 times the amount of polyethylene wear experienced at the unidirectional interfaces in rotating-platform designs.[36,41,44] Therefore, use of rotating-platform TKA designs can reduce polyethylene wear by decoupling multidirectional motions to unidirectional motion patterns at two differing interfaces, thus reducing cross-shear stresses and wear occurring at both interfaces.[36,41,44]

Another explanation for minimal undersurface polyethylene wear is the presence of high contact area (typically >700 mm²) at the inferior mobile articulation[49] (Fig. 59-7), which generates peak subsurface stresses of less than 17 MPa and mean subsurface stresses of less than 8 MPa at this articulation when subjected to forces up to five times body weight.[16] These low subsurface stresses result in minimized polyethylene wear.[3]

In contrast to a purely rotating-platform TKA design, additional mobile-bearing TKA systems exist that permit both rotation and anterior-posterior translation to occur on the inferior aspect of the polyethylene bearing, which creates multidirectional motion patterns. Jennings et al[60] compared wear of a rotating-platform TKA (LCS RP; Depuy, Warsaw, IN) with a design that allowed both rotation and anterior-posterior translation (LCS AP Glide; Depuy, Warsaw, IN) in a knee simulator wear analysis. At 5 million

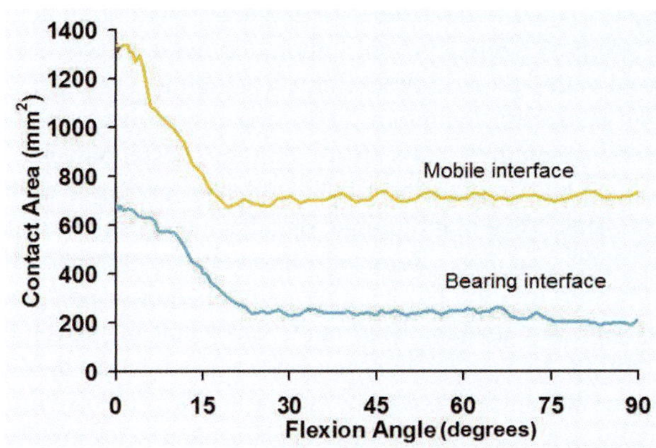

FIGURE 59-7. *Contact area analysis of the superior and inferior aspects of a rotating-platform TKA demonstrating the high contact areas (mm^2) present at the articular (superior) and mobile (undersurface) interfaces throughout knee flexion. (Reprinted with permission from Otto JK, Callaghan JJ, Brown TD. Mobility and contact mechanics of a rotating platform total knee replacement. Clin Orthop Relat Res. 2001;392:24-37.)*

cycles, they observed over twice the amount of polyethylene wear in the LCS AP Glide TKA (Fig. 59-8). Therefore, close follow-up evaluation of this type of mobile-bearing TKA is merited to see if premature failure due to backside wear occurs secondary to the multidirectional motion on the inferior aspect of the mobile polyethylene bearing.

Last, the fear that polyethylene wear microparticulate debris created in mobile-bearing designs will result in increased osteolysis has yet to be clinically relevant. Fisher et al[61] analyzed wear debris created in both fixed-bearing and rotating-platform TKA designs in a knee simulator analysis under high kinematic conditions, attempting to simulate the activity patterns of the younger patient. They observed no differences in microparticulate size but felt the osteolytic potential was much higher in fixed-bearing designs since substantially more debris particles were generated in the fixed-bearing TKA cohort.

SURGICAL TECHNIQUE ISSUES

Meticulous attention to symmetric ligament balancing, reproduction of neutral mechanical alignment, and creation of balanced flexion and extension gaps are critical for the long-term success of both fixed-bearing and mobile-bearing TKA. Proper attention to these fundamental concepts result in more uniform loading of the articular bearing surface rather than placing excessive eccentric loads on either the

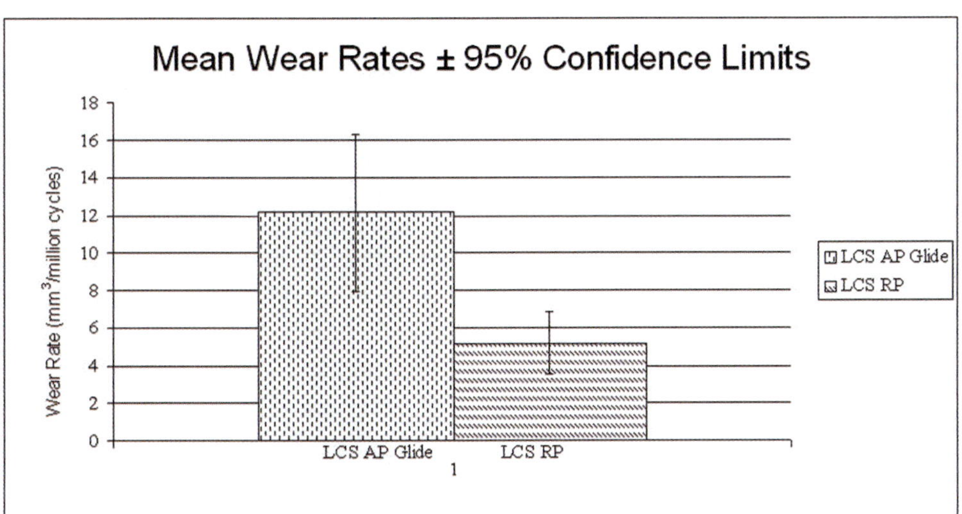

FIGURE 59-8. *Histogram of a knee simulator analysis comparing polyethylene wear (mg) per million cycles of a rotating-platform (LCS RP) versus a mobile-bearing TKA which allows both rotation and anteroposterior translation (LCS AP Glide).[60] (Reprinted with permission.)*

medial or lateral aspects of the polyethylene surface. As previously discussed, failure to obtain flexion-extension gap balance is of particular importance in a mobile-bearing TKA because of the risk of bearing dislocation. The authors favor the use of a gap-balancing methodology rather than measured resection techniques when using a mobile-bearing TKA implant because coronal plane stability is more reproducibly obtained.[62]

Flexion-extension gap balance can be achieved by several methods. The authors initially resect the distal femur and proximal tibia to establish the extension gap before addressing the flexion gap and determining femoral component rotation. After the extension gap has been created, it is assessed for gap height and symmetry medially and laterally using spacer blocks, laminar spreaders, or other tensioning devices. If the extension gap is asymmetric, soft tissue releases are to be performed to obtain a balanced, symmetric extension gap. When using a mobile-bearing TKA implant, symmetric laxity of 1 to 2 mm medially and laterally with varus and valgus stress testing is desired.

Obtaining a balanced flexion gap requires proper rotation of the femoral component and can be achieved by multiple methods[63-70] (Fig. 59-9), including (1) use of cutting jigs that rotate the femoral component a predetermined amount (typically 3° to 5°) externally relative to the posterior condylar axis,[63] (2) femoral component placement either parallel to the trans-epicondylar axis[64-66] or perpendicular to the anterior-posterior axis (Whiteside's line),[67] or (3) by utilizing the gap-balancing method in which the femoral component is placed parallel to the tibial cut with the medial and lateral collateral ligaments equally tensioned.[68-70] All methods have been shown to have potential shortcomings and combined use of all rotational landmarks is wise. The critical step in use of gap balancing involves placement of the anterior-posterior cutting block to ensure the flexion gap height is equal to the extension gap height without notching the femur. A decision about femoral component size is confirmed at this point in time. Since tensioning is utilized with a gap-balancing technique, it is imperative that all osteophytes, including posterior femoral osteophtyes, be removed before placement of the anterior-posterior cutting block, since they may impinge on adjacent capsular and ligamentous structures. Removal of osteophytes after femoral component rotation has been set and the anterior and posterior femoral cuts have been made can result in flexion gap instability. Using a tensioning device placed within the flexion gap the anterior-posterior cutting block is adjusted rotationally to ensure that the flexion gap is symmetric medially and laterally and parallel to the tibial cut with each collateral ligament equally tensioned. Secondary checks are then performed to ensure a reasonable rotational position relative to the transepicondylar and anterior-posterior axes (Fig. 59-10). Use of this technique facilitates obtaining balanced flexion and extension gap heights and a rectangular flexion gap that is symmetric medially and laterally. If a flexion-extension gap balance cannot be obtained or substantial incompetence of the collateral ligamentous structures exists, it is wise to consider use of a fixed-bearing TKA to reduce the risk of polyethylene bearing spin-out.

The coronal plane stability of knee arthroplasties implanted using either measured resection or gap-balancing techniques has been studied in our research laboratory using video fluoroscopy. The incidence of femoral condylar liftoff

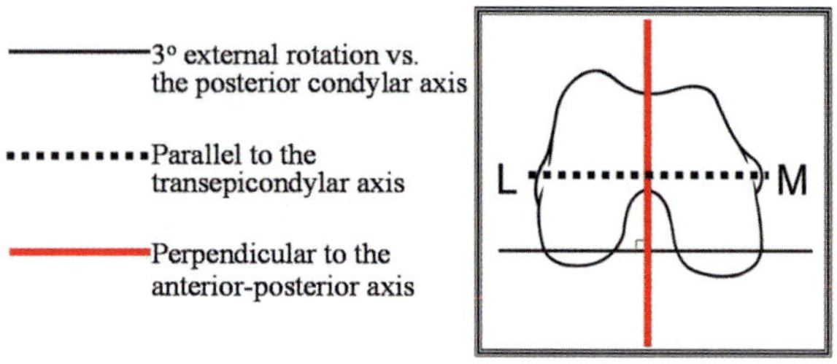

FIGURE 59-9. *Diagram demonstrating the three measured resection methods available to assist in obtaining correct femoral component rotation. (Reprinted with permission from Kim RH, Dennis DA. Mobile bearing total knee arthroplasty: technique and results. In: The Knee–A Comprehensive Review, Chapter 20, World Scientific Publishing, Singapore and New Jersey, 2010, pp 467-486.)*

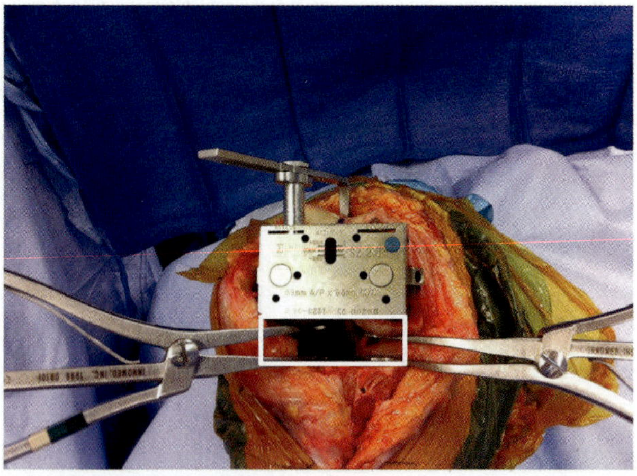

FIGURE 59-10. *Intraoperative photograph demonstrating a gap-balancing technique in which the anterior-posterior cutting block is placed parallel to the resected tibia with each collateral ligament equally tensioned.*

greater than 0.75 mm was 80% (maximum 2.9 mm) and 70% (maximum 2.5 mm) for PCL-retaining and -substituting TKA cohorts performed using measured resection in contrast to 35% (maximum 0.88 mm) for gap-balanced TKAs (p =.003). Liftoff greater than 1.0 mm occurred in 60% and 45% of the PCL-retaining and -substituting TKAs using measured resection versus none in the gap-balanced group ($p < .0001$).[62]

CLINICAL RESULTS OF MOBILE-BEARING TKA

Reports of fixed-bearing TKA have demonstrated survivorship rates greater than 90% at 10 to 15 years.[26,71-75] Most of these reports focus on patients with advanced age (>60–65 years) and, subsequently, lesser activity levels. With current trends to use TKA implants in younger, more active patients, there is greater interest in minimizing polyethylene wear in order to reduce osteolysis, aseptic loosening, and the need for revision TKA. Prospectively randomized studies comparing results of fixed- versus mobile-bearing TKA are limited,[76-82] have demonstrated similar clinical results, and have inadequate follow-up duration to provide valuable information regarding the high-demand, younger TKA patient who may require multiple decades of implant survival. Future long-term, prospectively randomized controlled trials are required to see if the basic science analyses showing reduced polyethylene wear and fixation stresses in mobile-bearing TKA design are confirmed by long-term clinical outcomes.

Long-term clinical reports of mobile-bearing TKA show satisfactory results with limited loosening and osteolysis. In the initial experience with the LCS meniscal bearing and rotating-platform systems, Buechel and Pappas[2] reported 95.1% and 98.2% (cemented and cementless) good to excellent results at a follow-up period of up to 10 years. When evaluating only the rotating-platform LCS system, Buechel et al[35]reported survivorship rates of 97.7% at both 10 and 20 years with end points defined as revision for any mechanical reason or a poor clinical knee score. Survivorship of the cementless LCS rotating-platform system with loosening as the end point was determined to be 99.4% at 20 years.[1] Callaghan et al[3] evaluated the 15-year results of the LCS rotating-platform design and reported no failures secondary to loosening, osteolysis, wear, or bearing instability. Sorrels and Stiehl[83] reported a survivorship of 90.3% with this design 13 years following the operative procedure. Various studies evaluating primary TKA implanted with a rotating-platform system reported no evidence of radiographic loosening, even at 20-year radiographic follow-up[1-3,35] and reported that revision TKA was required in 0% to 0.2% due to aseptic loosening.[1-3,35]

A meta-analysis of clinical results of mobile-bearing TKA was performed at the authors' institution, which involved a review of 19 manuscripts that met criteria for analysis.[57] A total of 3506 knees using a mobile-bearing TKA implant design were analyzed, including rotating-platform (RP group), meniscal bearing, and mobile-bearing designs that allowed bearing rotation as well as anterior-posterior translation (APGR group). Survivorship at 15 years was superior in the RP cohort (96.4%) versus the meniscal bearing group (86.5%; Table 59-1). Radiographic component loosening rates for the entire study group was 0.33%. Bearing complication (polyethylene bearing fracture or dislocation) rates of implants placed before 1995 were greater (1.6%) than in those placed after 1995 (0.1%; Table 59-2). The authors hypothesize that the significant reduction in bearing complications is related to improvements in surgical technique, particularly recognition of the importance of flexion-extension gap balancing, which was less emphasized in the early years of TKA.

TABLE 59-1. Implant Survivorship

Implant Design	5-Year	10-Year	15-Year
MeBe	97.7%	93.3%	86.5%
RP	98.4%	96.5%	96.4%*
APGR	97.8%	96.7%	NA

* p = .0032 compared to the 15-year MeBe TKA subgroup.

TABLE 59-2. Bearing Complication Occurrence Based on Date of Surgery (Entire Cohort)

Date of Surgery	TKA Number	Bearing Complications
Pre-1995	2037	33 (1.6%)
Post-1995	838	1 (0.1%)*

* p = .00019 compared to entire cohort pre-1995.

Between January 2000 and November 2006, a total of 341 revision TKA procedures were performed by three surgeons at our institution. Of the 341 revisions, 143 revisions (137 patients) were performed using a mobile-bearing TKA system (PFC Sigma and LCS posterior-stabilized rotating-platform implants; Depuy, Warsaw, IN). Factors used to determine use of a mobile-bearing implant design were patient age, activity requirements, longevity expectations, and the ability to achieve both a symmetrical extension and flexion gap balance. A posterior-stabilized rotating-platform insert was used in 88 knees, while a constrained condylar rotating-platform prosthesis was implanted in 55 knees. At a mean follow-up duration of 3.6 years (range, 2–8 years), the mean Knee Society clinical scores improved from 48.4 preoperatively to 89 points postoperatively, while the Knee Society functional scores improved from 49.3 points preoperatively to a mean of 79.2 points. There were no cases of bearing instability and no revision procedures were required for prosthetic loosening. Longer follow-up is necessary to see if the theoretical benefits of mobile-bearing use in revision TKA are clinically observed.

PEARLS AND PITFALLS

Mobile-bearing TKA implants were introduced with the goal of increasing implant survivorship by reducing polyethylene wear and aseptic component loosening. The basic scientific data which demonstrate reduced polyethylene contact forces, reduced cross-shear, and lessened fixation stresses are supported by clinical results after three decades of use with these devices. Fears of accelerated wear from the mobile articulating polyethylene interface and substantial bearing instability have yet to be recognized. Additional advantages of mobile-bearing use are reduced load transmission to stabilizing posts and facilitation of patellar tracking. The main pitfall with the use of mobile-bearing devices has been bearing instability. Precise surgical technique to assure satisfactory flexion-extension balance is imperative. If adequate gap balance cannot be obtained, one should consider use of a rotating-platform constrained condylar design or select a fixed-bearing implant. Ten to 15-year analyses of fixed- and mobile-bearing devices have shown similar clinical results, although these reports have typically involved elderly subjects with lesser activity levels. Longer follow-up is required to see if results remain comparative in the 50-year-old subject who will demand 30 years or more of function at activity levels of greater than 2 million cycles annually.

REFERENCES

1. Buechel FF Sr. Long-term follow-up after mobile-bearing total knee replacement. *Clin Orthop Relat Res.* 2002;404:40-50.
2. Buechel FF, Pappas MJ. New Jersey low contact stress knee replacement system: ten-year evaluation of meniscal bearings. *Orthop Clin North Am.* 1989; 20:147-177.
3. Callaghan JJ, O'Rourke MR, Iossi MF, et al. Cemented rotating-platform total knee replacement. A concise follow-up, at a minimum of fifteen years, of a previous report. *J Bone Joint Surg Am.* 2005;87(9): 1995-1998.
4. Ranawat CS, Boachie-Adjei O. Survivorship analysis and results of total condylar knee arthroplasty: eight- to 11-year follow-up period. *Clin Orthop Relat Res.* 1988;226:6-13.
5. Schai PA, Thornhill TS, Scott RD. Total knee arthroplasty with the PFC system: results at a minimum of ten years and survivorship analysis. *J Bone Joint Surg Br.* 1998;80:850-858.
6. Schmalzried TP, Szuszczewicz ES, Northfield MR, et al. Quantitative assessment of walking activity after total hip or knee replacement. *J Bone Joint Surg Am.* 1998;80(1):54-59.
7. Silva M, Shepherd EF, Jackson WO, et al. Average patient walking activity approaches 2 million cycles per year: pedometers under-record walking activity. *J Arthroplasty.* 2002;17(6):693-697.
8. Bartel DL, Bicknell VL, Ithaca MS, et al.The effect of conformity, thickness and material on stresses in ultra-high molecular weight components for total joint replacement. *J Bone Joint Surg Am.* 1986;68: 1041-1051.
9. Bert JM. Dislocation/subluxation of meniscal bearing elements after New Jersey low-contact stress total knee arthroplasty. *Clin Orthop Relat Res.* 1990;254: 211-215.
10. Dennis DA, Komistek RD, Mahfouz MR. In vivo fluoroscopic analysis of fixed-bearing total knee replacements. *Clin Orthop Relat Res.* 2003;410:114-130.
11. D'Lima DD, Trice M, Urquhart AG, et al. Tibiofemoral conformity and kinematics of rotating-bearing knee prostheses. *Clin Orthop Relat Res.* 2001;386:235-242.
12. Huang CH, Ma HM, Liau JJ, et al. Osteolysis in failed total knee arthroplasty: a comparison of mobile-bearing and fixed-bearing knees. *J Bone Joint Surg Am.* 2002;84:2224-2229.

13. Cheng CK, Huang CH, Liau JJ, et al. The influence of surgical malalignment on the contact pressures of fixed and mobile bearing knee prostheses–a biomechanical study. *Clin Biomech*. 2003;18:231-236.

14. D'Lima DD, Chen PC, Colwell Jr CW. Polyethylene contact stress, articular congruity, and knee alignment. *Clin Orthop Relat Res*. 2001;392:232-238.

15. Liau JJ, Cheng CK, Huang CH, et al. The effect of malalignment on stresses in polyethylene component of total knee prostheses–a finite element analysis. *Clin Biomech*. 2002;17:140-146.

16. Matsuda S, White SE, Williams II VG, et al. Contact stress analysis in mobile bearing total knee arthroplasty. *J Arthroplasty*. 1998;13:699-706.

17. Stukenborg-Coleman C, Ostermeier S, Hurschler C, et al. Tibiofemoral contact stress after total knee arthroplasty: comparison of fixed and mobile-bearing inlay designs. *Acta Orthop Scand*. 2002;73:638-646.

18. Lonner JH, Siliski JM, Scott RD. Prodromes of failure in total knee arthroplasty. *J Arthroplasty*. 1999;14:488-492.

19. Sharkey PF, Hozack WJ, Rothman RH, et al. Why are total knee arthroplasties failing today? *Clin Orthop Relat Res*. 2002;404:7-13.

20. Banks S, Bellemans J, Nozaki H, et al. Knee motion during maximum flexion in fixed and mobile-bearing arthroplasties. *Clin Orthop Relat Res*. 2003;410:131-138.

21. Dennis DA, Komistek RD, Colwell CE, et al. In vivo anteroposterior femorotibial translation of total knee arthroplasty: a multicenter analysis. *Clin Orthop Relat Res*. 1998;356:47-57.

22. Dennis DA, Komistek RD, Mahfouz MR, et al. Multicenter determination of in vivo kinematics after total knee arthroplasty. *Clin Orthop Relat Res*. 2003;416:37-57.

23. Dennis DA, Komistek RD, Mahfouz MR, et al. A multicenter analysis of axial femorotibial rotation following total knee arthroplasty. *Clin Orthop Relat Res*. 2004;428:180-189.

24. Blunn GW, Walker PS, Joshi A, et al. The dominance of cyclic sliding in producing wear in total knee replacements. *Clin Orthop Relat Res*. 1991;273:253-260.

25. Bartel DL, Burstien AH, Toda MD, et al.The effect of conformity and plastic thickness on contact stress in metal backed plastic implants. *J Biomech Eng*. 1985; 107:193-199.

26. Engh GA, Lounici S, Rao AR, et al. In vivo deterioration of tibial baseplate locking mechanisms in modular total knee components. *J Bone Joint Surg Am*. 2001;83:1660-1665.

27. Rao AR, Engh GA, Collier MB, et al. Tibial interface wear in retrieved total knee components and correlation with modular insert motion. *J Bone Joint Surg Am*. 2002;84:1849-1855.

28. Wasielewski RC, Parks N, Williams I, et al. Tibial insert undersurface as a contributing source of polyethylene wear debris. *Clin Orthop Relat Res*. 1997;345:53-59.

29. Bargmann LS, Bargmann BC, Collier JP, et al. Current sterilization and packaging methods for polyethylene. *Clin Orthop Relat Res*. 1999;369:49-58.

30. Bell CJ, Walker PS, Abeysundera MR, et al. Effect of oxidation on delamination of ultrahigh-molecular-weight polyethylene tibial components. *J Arthroplasty*. 1998;13:280-290.

31. Blunn G, Brach delPreva EM, Costa L, et al. Ultra high molecular-weight polyethylene (UHMWPE) in total knee replacement: fabrication, sterilization and wear. *J Bone Joint Surg Br*. 2002;84:946-949.

32. Collier JP, Satula LH, Currier BH, et al. Overview of polyethylene as a bearing material. *Clin Orthop Relat Res*. 1996;333:76-86.

33. McNulty DE, Liau YS, Haas BD. The influence of sterilization method on wear performance of the low contact stress total knee system. *Orthopaedics*. 2002;25(S):243-246.

34. Williams IR, Mayor MB, Collier JP. The impact of sterilization method on wear in knee arthroplasty. *Clin Orthop Relat Res*. 1998;356:170-180.

35. Buechel FF Sr, Buechel FF Jr, Pappas MJ, et al.Twenty-year evaluation of the New Jersey LCS rotating platform knee replacement. *J Knee Surg*. 2002;15:84-89.

36. Murray DW, Goodfellow JW, O'Connor JJ. The Oxford unicompartmental arthroplasty: a ten-year survival study. *J Bone Joint Surg Br*. 1998;80:983-989.

37. Psychoyios V, Crawford RW, O'Connor JJ, et al. Wear of congruent meniscal bearings in unicompartmental knee arthroplasty: a retrieval study of 16 specimens. *J Bone Joint Surg Br*. 1998;80:976-982.

38. Rullkoetter PJ, Gabriel SM, Colleran DP, et al.The relationship between contact stress and contact area with implications for TKR evaluation and design. Transactions 45th Annual Meeting of Orthopaedic Research Society, Anaheim, CA; 1999.

39. Scuderi GR, Komistek RD, Dennis DA, et al. The impact of femoral component rotational alignment

on condylar lift-off. *Clin Orthop Relat Res*. 2003; 410:148-154.

40. Stiehl JB, Dennis DA, Komistek RD, et al. In vivo kinematic analysis of mobile bearing total knee prosthesis. *Clin Orthop Relat Res*. 1997;345:60-66.

41. Jones VC, Barton DC, Fitzpatrick DP, et al. An experimental model of tibial counterface polyethylene wear in mobile bearing knees: the influence of design and kinematics. *Biomed Mater Eng*. 1999;9:189-196.

42. Sharma A, Komistek RD, Ranawat CS, et al. In vivo contact pressures in total knee arthroplasty. *J Arthroplasty*. 2007;22(3):404-416.

43. Greenwald AS, Heim CS. Mobile-bearing knee systems: ultra-high molecular weight polyethylene wear and design issues. *Instr Course Lect*. 2005;54:195-205.

44. McEwen HM, Barnett PI, Bell CJ, et al. The influence of design, materials and kinematics on the in vitro wear of total knee replacements. *J Biomech*. 2005;38 (2):357-365.

45. McNulty DE, Swope SW, Auger DD, et al. The effect of crosslinking UHMWPE on in-vitro wear rates of fixed and mobile bearing knees. Presented at ASTM Symposium on Crosslinked and Thermally Treated UHMWPE for TJR; Nov 2002.

46. Otto JK, Callaghan JJ, Brown TD. Gait cycle finite element comparison of rotating-platform total knee designs. *Clin Orthop Relat Res*. 2003;410:181-188.

47. Bartel DL, Rawlinson JJ, Burstein AH, et al. Stresses in polyethylene components of contemporary total knee replacements. *Clin Orthop Relat Res*. 1995;317:76-82.

48. Miller GJ, Petty W, Goll C. Congruency and varus/valgus loading effect on prosthetic knee contact stress. Combined Orthopaedic Research Society (English Speaking World), San Diego, CA; Nov 6-8, 1995.

49. Otto JK, Callaghan JJ, Brown TD. Mobility and contact mechanics of a rotating platform total knee replacement. *Clin Orthop Relat Res*. 2001;392:24-37.

50. Atwood SA, Currier JH, Mayor MB, et al. Clinical wear measurement on low contact stress rotating platform knee bearings. *J Arthroplasty*. 2008;23(3):431-440.

51. Dennis DA, Komistek RD, Mahfouz MR, et al. Mobile-bearing total knee arthroplasty: do the polyethylene bearings rotate? *Clin Orthop Relat Res*. 2005;440:88-95.

52. Komistek RD, Dennis DA, Mahfouz MR, et al. In vivo polyethylene bearing mobility is maintained in posterior stabilized total knee arthroplasty. *Clin Orthop Relat Res*. 2004;428:207-213.

53. Yang CC, McFadden LA, Dennis DA, et al. Lateral retinacular release rates in mobile-versus fixed-bearing TKA. *Clin Orthop Relat Res*. 2008;466(11):2656-2661.

54. Garling EH, Kaptein BL, Nelissen RG, et al. Limited rotation of the mobile-bearing in a rotating platform total knee prosthesis. *J Biomech*. 2007;40(suppl 1): S25-S30.

55. Dendrinos GK, Mavropoulou A, Polyzoides AJ. Late failure and revisions of old-type total knee replacements. *Acta Orthop Belg*. 1991;57:274-284.

56. Huang CH, Ma HM, Liau JJ, et al. Late dislocation of rotating platform in New Jersey low-contact stress knee prosthesis. *Clin Orthop Relat Res*. 2002;405:189-194.

57. Carothers JT, Kim RH, Dennis DA, et al. Mobile-bearing total knee arthroplasty: a meta-analysis. *J Arthroplasty*. 2011;26(4):537-542.

58. Currier J, Porter E, Carlson E, et al. 3D surface profilometry of wear in rotating platforms. Orthopedic Research Society #2248 Transactions Vol. 35, New Orleans, LA; 2010.

59. Pooley C, Tabor D. Friction and molecular structure: the behavior of some thermoplastics. *Proc R Soc Lond*. 1972;329A:251.

60. Jennings LM, Galvin AL, McEwen HM, et al. The influence of design on the wear of mobile bearing total knee replacements. ORS poster #2002, 54th Annual Meeting of the Orthopaedic Research Society; 2008.

61. Fisher J, McEwen H, Tipper J, et al. Wear-simulation analysis of rotating-platform mobile-bearing knees. *Orthopedics*. 2006;29(9 Suppl):S36-S41.

62. Dennis DA, Komistek RD, Kim RH, et al. Gap balancing versus measured resection technique for total knee arthroplasty. *Clin Orthop Relat Res*. 2010;468(1):102-107.

63. Nagamine R, Miura H, Inoue Y, et al. Reliability of the anteroposterior axis and the posterior condylar axis for determining rotational alignment of the femoral component in total knee arthroplasty. *J Orthop Sci*. 1998;3(4):194-198.

64. Berger RA, Rubash HE, Seel MJ, et al. Determining the rotational alignment of the femoral component in total knee arthroplasty using the epicondylar axis. *Clin Orthop Relat Res*. 1993;(286):40-47.

65. Griffin FM, Math K, Scuderi GR, et al. Anatomy of the epicondyles of the distal femur: MRI analysis of normal knees. *J Arthroplasty*. 2000;15(3):354-359.

66. Poilvache PL, Insall JN, Scuderi GR, et al. Rotational landmarks and sizing of the distal femur in total knee arthroplasty. *Clin Orthop Relat Res*. 1996; 331:35-46.
67. Whiteside LA, Arima J. The anteroposterior axis for femoral rotational alignment in valgus total knee arthroplasty. *Clin Orthop Relat Res*. 1995;321:168-172.
68. Dennis, DA. Measured resection: an outdated technique in total knee arthroplasty. *Orthopedics*. 2008; 31(9):940, 943-944.
69. Fehring TK. Rotational malalignment of the femoral component in total knee arthroplasty. *Clin Orthop Relat Res*. 2000;380:72-79.
70. Katz MA, Beck TD, Silber JS, et al. Determining femoral rotational alignment in total knee arthroplasty: reliability of techniques. *J Arthroplasty*. 2001; 16(3):301-305.
71. Berger RA, Rosenberg AG, Barden RM, et al. Long-term followup of the Miller-Galante total knee replacement. *Clin Orthop Relat Res*. 2001;388:58-67.
72. Brassard MF, Insall JN, Scuderi GR, et al. Does modularity affect clinical success? A comparison with a minimum 10-year followup. *Clin Orthop Relat Res*. 2001;388:26-32.
73. Laskin RS. The Genesis total knee prosthesis: a 10-year followup study. *Clin Orthop Relat Res*. 2001; 388:95-102.
74. Ritter MA, Berend ME, Meding JB, et al. Long-term followup of anatomic graduated components posterior cruciate-retaining total knee replacement. *Clin Orthop Relat Res*. 2001;388:51-57.
75. Sextro GS, Berry DJ, Rand JA. Total knee arthroplasty using cruciate-retaining kinematic condylar prosthesis. *Clin Orthop Relat Res*. 2001;388:33-40.
76. Aglietti P, Baldini A, Buzzi R, et al. Comparison of mobile-bearing and fixed-bearing total knee arthroplasty: a prospective randomized study. *J Arthroplasty*. 2005;20:145-153.
77. Beard DJ, Pandit H, Price AJ, et al. Introduction of a new mobile-bearing total knee prosthesis: minimum three year follow-up of an RCT comparing it with a fixed-bearing device. *Knee*. 2007;14:448-451.
78. Bhan S, Malhotra R, Kiran EK, et al. A comparison of fixed-bearing and mobile-bearing total knee arthroplasty at a minimum follow-up of 4.5 years. *J Bone Joint Surg Am*. 2005;87:2290-2296.
79. Kim YH, Kook HK, Kim JS. Comparison of fixed-bearing and mobile-bearing total knee arthroplasties. *Clin Orthop Relat Res*. 2001;392:101-115.
80. Kim YH, Yoon SH, Kim JS. The long-term results of simultaneous fixed-bearing and mobile-bearing total knee replacements performed in the same patient. *J Bone Joint Surg Br*. 2007;89:1317-1323.
81. Kim YH, Kim DY, Kim JS. Simultaneous mobile- and fixed-bearing total knee replacement in the same patients: a prospective comparison of mid-term outcomes. *J Bone Joint Surg Br*. 2007;89:904-910.
82. Price AJ, Rees JL, Beard D, et al. A mobile-bearing total knee prosthesis compared with a fixed-bearing prosthesis: a multicentre single-blind randomized controlled trial. *J Bone Joint Surg Br*. 2003;85:62-67.
83. Sorrels RB, Stiehl JB. Long-term outcomes of a rotating platform mobile bearing prosthesis after TKA. *J Arthroplasty*. 2004;19:255.

60

Current Trends and Indications for All-Polyethylene Tibial Components

Morteza Meftah, Anthony C. Wong, Amar S. Ranawat, and Chitranjan S. Ranawat

The place of all-polyethylene tibial (APT) components in total knee arthroplasty (TKA) continues to be an area of debate. Early APT designs had problems with fatigue failure of the polyethylene and loosening. This led to the introduction of metal-backed tibial (MBT) components. Currently, MBT components in TKA dominate the orthopaedic market. The *Annual Report of the National Joint Registry for England and Wales* in 2007 showed that only 3.9% of primary TKAs utilized APT components.[1] Proponents of MBT components cite greater intra-operative flexibility due to modularity and the ability to apply a porous coating among the reasons to utilize MBT components.[2,3] Despite these advantages, many studies comparing APT to MBT have not been able to demonstrate a significant difference in terms of implant survivorship.[1,4-6] This has renewed the interest in APT components.

ALL-POLYETHYLENE TIBIAL VERSUS METAL-BACKED TIBIAL COMPONENTS

When TKAs were first introduced, only APT components were available. High rates of loosening, instability, and deformation were observed. These findings were initially associated with the inability of the polyethylene to accommodate and distribute stresses appropriately.[7] Metal-backing was first introduced to improve load distributions over the tibial plateau at the interface between the prosthesis and bone.[2] In vitro biomechanical studies have shown that this is possible, but in vivo radiostereometric analysis (RSA) studies have not been able to confirm these results.[4]

MBT components can be either modular or nonmodular. Modular designs with a metal baseplate and a modular polyethylene insert, either fixed or rotating, are the most common. This design offers several advantages. The surgeon has the option of matching the bearing surface with the femoral component, independent of the choice of tibial baseplate.[8] MBT components also offer various options of stems and augments that cannot be used with APT designs. It must be noted that cases requiring stems and augments represent only a minority of primary TKAs.[4] Several authors have also indicated the advantage of MBT components at revision surgery where worn polyethylene components can be exchanged without disrupting the bone–prosthesis or cement–prosthesis interfaces.[8] It must be stressed that there are very specific situations in which it is appropriate to replace only the polyethylene component: acute infection, polyethylene spinout, or late wear with well-fixed components.

The major drawback to the use of MBT designs is that modular tibial components introduce an additional site of relative motion between the baseplate and the insert. This leads to additional production of polyethylene wear particles. These particles can lead to an inflammatory response, which has been shown to result in osteolysis and failure of the prosthesis. A study investigating the backside wear of polyethylene tibial inserts in TKAs determined that the average volumetric wear rate was 138 ± 95 mm^3/year.[8] The authors determined that this was not due to creep or cold flow of the polyethylene through the screw holes on the baseplate, but due primarily to the wear of the inserts. This type of wear is accelerated in thin (< 8 mm) polyethylene components that were commonly used with MBT implants.[1]

APT components also have their advantages. From a technical viewpoint, the tibial resection can be more conservative to accommodate the minimum satisfactory thickness of polyethylene. The lack of modularity eliminates the issue of backside wear. The absence of a metal baseplate allows the use of thicker polyethylene inserts, thus reducing the amount of wear and reducing shear stresses occurring at the cement–prosthesis and cement–bone interfaces. Of relevance to the current economic climate, the potential for cost-savings is huge. This has been highlighted by other authors, with Apel et al recognizing the cost differential between APT and MBT components as early as 1991.[9] The prerequisites for using APT components include minimal deformity in the coronal plane, good tibial bone stock, and normal proximal tibial anatomy. It follows then that they are not as versatile as MBT components.

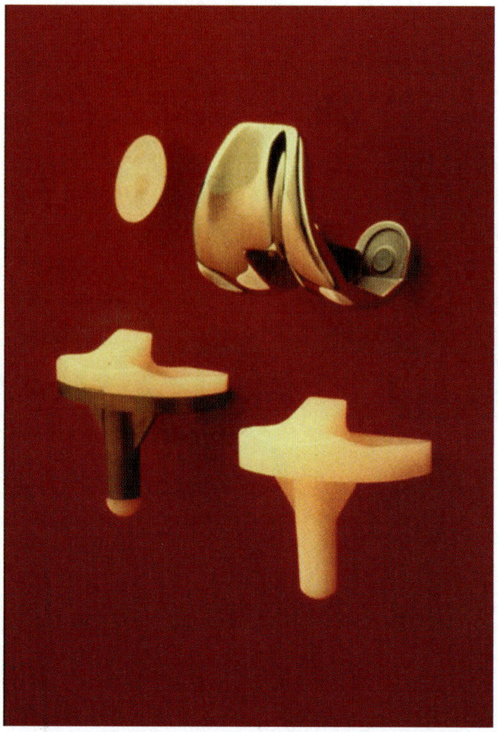

FIGURE 60-1. *A photograph of Sigma all-polyethylene tibial (right) and metal-backed (left) designs (DePuy Orthopaedics) with identical femoral component.*

SURVIVORSHIP AND FUNCTION

A study conducted at our institution investigated the 10- to 18-year follow-up for 44 APT TKAs (Fig. 60-1) in 32 patients (12 bilaterals) who were 60 years and younger.[10] Good to excellent clinical outcomes were obtained in 96% of the patients. The implants were either posterior-stabilized press-fit condylar (PFC) modular or Sigma designs (DePuy Orthopaedics, Inc, Warsaw, IN). Clinical analysis included pre- and postoperative Knee Society Score (KSS), Knee Society Function Score (KSFS), Western Ontario and McMaster Universities Osteoarthritis Index (WOMAC), UCLA activity score, and a detailed patient administered questionnaire (ROC-PAQ) containing separate sections for pain, daily living activities, sport participation, and satisfaction that has been used in several prior publications.[11-13] Anteroposterior and lateral weight-bearing radiographs of the patients were also evaluated for loosening, wear, and osteolysis using digital imaging software. The KSS improved from 38.3 ± 9.7 to 94 ± 7 and KSFS improved from 51.5 ± 14.1 to 89 ± 20 at an average of 12.4 ± 2.7 years of follow-up. Implant survivorship looking at failure for all causes was 95.5%. None of the patients in the study indicated that they were dissatisfied (satisfaction score less than 5 on the ROC-PAQ) and the mean satisfaction score was 9.2 ± 1.4. All patients, except for one with severe hip and spine osteoarthritis, were able to perform activities of daily living without significant difficulty. Sixty-two percent of patients were participating in sporting activities such as running, gym exercises, and playing tennis or golf (Table 60-1). The radiographic analysis indicated satisfactory alignment of the components without evidence of loosening, wear, or osteolysis (Fig. 60-2).

Kaplan-Meyer survivorship in this study for mechanical failure and failure for all causes was 97.7% and 95.5%, respectively (Fig. 60-3). The survivorship observed in our study is consistent with several other studies[1,3,14-18] at a follow-up of 8 to 20 years (Table 60-2). Our reported scores for performance of daily living and sporting activities are promising. Our results indicate that APT components can have favorable results in a group of young active patients and their continued use should be considered.

TABLE 60-1. Sport Activities at 5 Years and 12 Years Postoperatively

Activity	5 Years[a] 38 pts[a]	12 Years 36 pts[a]
Walking > 1 mile	16	14
Running	1	0
Swimming	9	4
Gym	13	10
Tennis/Squash	3	3
Golf	8	8
Biking	-	1
Yoga/Dance	-	2

[a]Some patients were participating in more than one activity.

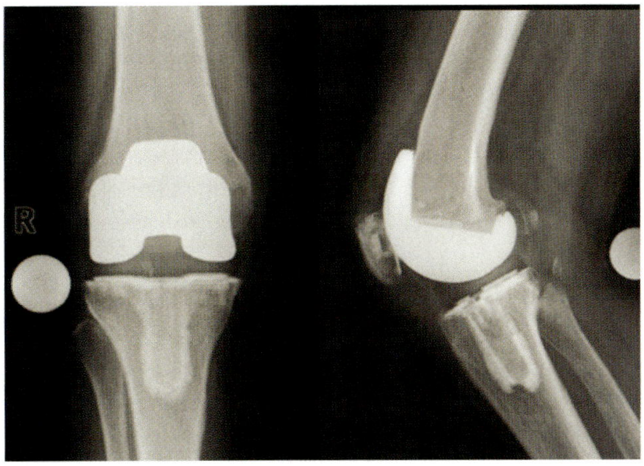

FIGURE 60-2. *Anteroposterior (left) and lateral (right) radiographs of a patient, 16 years post APT with UCLA score of 6, who participates in biking and golf.*

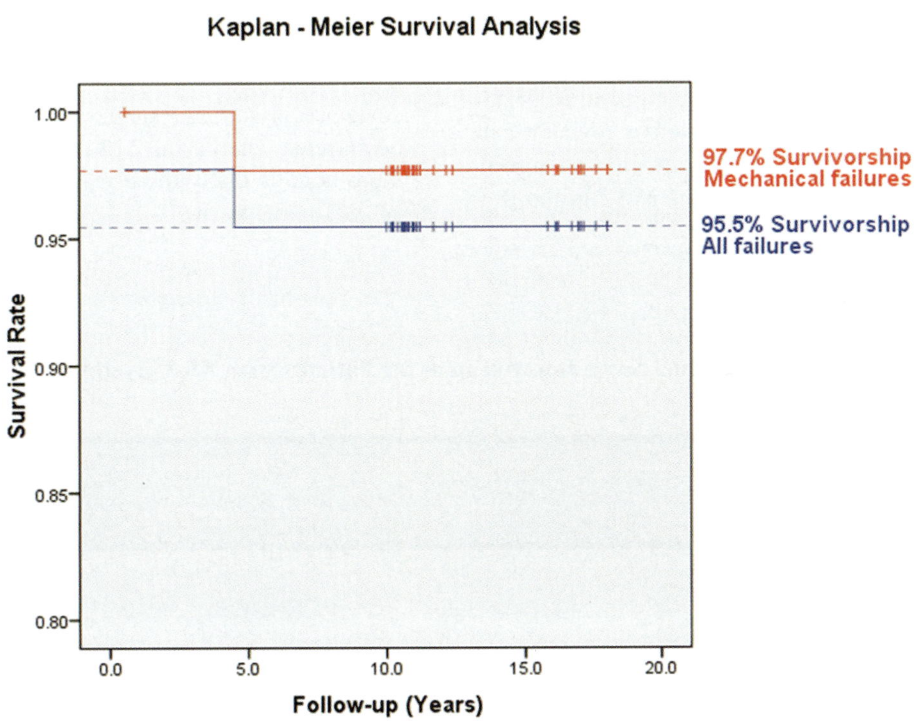

FIGURE 60-3. *Kaplan-Meyer survivorship for mechanical failure and failure for all causes.*

TABLE 60-2. Comparison of Overall Survivorship of All-Polyethylene Tibial Components from Various Studies

Investigators	Overall Survivorship	Average Length of Follow-up (years)
Meftah et al[10]	95.5%	12.4
Bettinson et al[1]	94.5%	10
Campbell et al [17]	89%	7.4
Gioe et al[3]	99.4%	14.3
Pagnano et al [15]	98%	14
Rodriguez et al[14]	96%	7

The survivorship of MBT TKAs is widely reported in the literature and ranges from 88.9% to 97.2% at 8 to 13 years.[4,19-22] A number of good-quality studies have also compared survivorship and function of APT and MBT TKAs (Table 60-3).[1,4] The general conclusion has been that the results are similar at 10 years with regard to function, survivorship, patient satisfaction, and radiological parameters. One study has even shown APT TKAs to perform better.[3] This was a prospective study that followed patients with APT TKAs over a 14-year period. The cumulative survival was 99% as compared to 95.1% for the MBT population. The cumulative revision rate (CRR) for the APT group was 1%, which was significantly lower than the 4.9% CRR in the MBT group ($p = .02$).

COMPARISON OF SURGICAL TECHNIQUES

The general principles of TKA are to be followed whether one is doing an APT or an MBT TKA. There are some key differences in the surgical steps which are worth highlighting to the surgeon inexperienced in using APT components.

When using an APT component, the femoral component must be cemented before the tibial component. Since the APT comprises a one-piece tibial component, cementing the tibia first is likely to obscure visualization and not allow for proper removal of excess cement from the posterior portion of the femoral component (Fig. 60-4). When using a posterior-stabilized APT with a post, it may be impossible to place the femoral component on the distal femur if the tibia is inadvertently cemented first.

The implantation of an MBT component utilizes a separate polyethylene insert, which is inserted last. This allows the surgeon proper visualization for cement removal even after both the femoral component and the tibial baseplate are cemented in place. It also gives the option of performing a further trial reduction of the knee joint with polyethylene inserts of varying thickness before the definitive insert is attached to the baseplate. This opportunity to perform a final trial reduction after cementing the femoral component is not available to the surgeon when using an APT component and is one of the main reasons why surgeons prefer MBT.

The MBT design's metal tibial baseplate also allows for the utilization of intramedullary stems, wedges, and augments. The clear benefits of this modularity do, however, come at a price to the surgeon and patient; more bone must be resected when using MBT components and, in revision, more bone is likely to be resected compared with revising an APT component.

TABLE 60-3. Comparison of Functional Score Improvement for Patients with All-Polyethylene Tibial Components from Various Studies

Investigators	Preoperative KSS	Postoperative KSS	Preoperative KSFS	Postoperative KSFS
Meftah et al [10]	38.3	94	51.5	89
Adalberth et al [16]	43	93	45	90
Campbell et al [17]	37	84	-	-
Najibi et al [18]	51.3	89.0	44.3	64.1

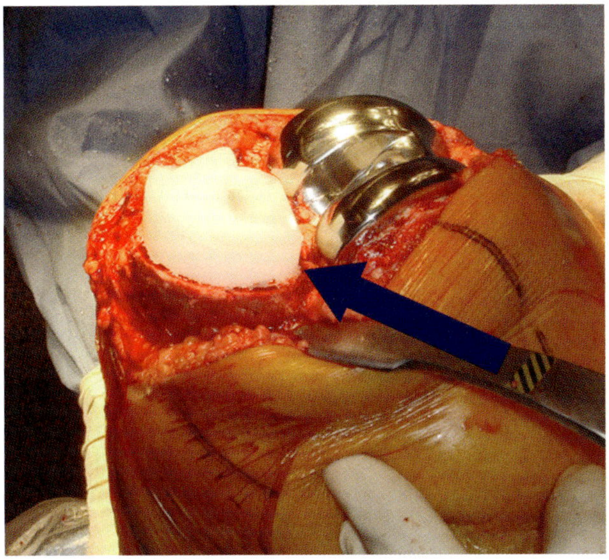

FIGURE 60-4. *Cementation of the femur before that of the tibia allows adequate visualization for proper removal of excess cement from the posterior portion of the femoral component (blue arrow), especially when using a posterior-stabilized implant.*

COST COMPARISON

The cost differential between APT and MBT components presents a significant advantage for the APT group and has been reported by numerous studies. One such study quoted the inflation-adjusted implant cost of a TKA with an APT component as $841 (range, $292–$1,535) less than a TKA with an MBT component.[3] Because the survivorship between the two groups is very similar, the cost advantage may represent a major determining factor in performing an APT TKA.

CONCLUSION

The utilization of APT components in TKA clearly has its place. As indicated by the study conducted at our institution, the survivorship of APT TKAs in young and active patients is comparable to that of MBT TKAs and excellent clinical results were observed after 10 to 18 years. The cost advantage of APT components is several hundred dollars per implant and represents a significant advantage over MBT components. Although APT components lack modularity and do not allow for the usage of stems and augments in more complicated primary TKAs, they completely eliminate the concerns surrounding the issue of backside wear. We believe that APT components still have a major role to play in contemporary TKA surgery and should be considered as an excellent option for uncomplicated primary TKAs.

REFERENCES

1. Bettinson KA, Pinder IM, Moran CG, et al. All polyethylene compared with metal backed tibial components in total knee arthroplasty at ten years: a prospective, randomized controlled trial. *J Bone Joint Surg Am*. 2009;91:1589-1594.
2. Small SR, Berend ME, Ritter MA, et al. A comparison in proximal tibial strain between metal-backed and all-polyethylene anatomic graduated component total knee arthroplasty tibial components. *J Arthroplasty*. 2010;25(5):820-825.
3. Gioe TJ, Sinner P, Mehle S, et al. Excellent survival of all-polyethylene tibial components in a community joint registry. *Clin Orthop Relat Res*. 2007;464:88-92.
4. Gioe TJ, Stroemer ES, Santos ER. All polyethylene and metal-backed tibias have similar outcomes at 10 years. *Clin Orthop Relat Res*. 2006;455:212-218.
5. Blumenfeld RJ, Scott RD. The role of the cemented all-polyethylene tibial componenet in total knee replacement: a 30-year patient follow-up and review of the literature. *Knee*. 2010;17:412-416.
6. Robinson RP, Green TM. Eleven-year implant survival rates of the all-polyethylene and metal backed modular Optetrak posterior stabilized knee in bilateral simultaneous cases. *J Arthroplasty*. Epub 2011 Mar 15.
7. Adalberth G, Nilsson KG, Byström S, et al. Low-conforming all-polyethylene tibial component non infe-

rior to metal-backed component in cemented total knee arthroplasty. *J Arthroplasty.* 2000;15(6):783-792.

8. Conditt MA, Thompson MT, Usrey MM, et al. Backside wear of polyethylene tibial inserts: mechanism and magnitude of material loss. *J Bone Joint Surg Am.* 2005;87(2):326-331.
9. Apel DM, Tozzi JM, Dorr LD. Clinical comparison of all-polyethylene and metal-backed tibial components in total knee arthroplasty. *Clin Orthop Relat Res.* 1991;273:243-252.
10. Meftah M, Ranawat AS, Sood AB, et al. All-polyethylene tibial implant in young, active patients: a concise follow-up, 10 to 18 years. *J Arthroplasty.* Epub 2011 Jul 19.
11. Rasquina VJ, Ranawat CS, Cervieri CL, et al. The press-fit modular total knee system with a posterior-cruciate substituting design: a concise followup of a previous report. *J Bone Joint Surg Am.* 2006;88:1006–1010.
12. Cooper JH, Ranawat AS, Potter HG, et al. Early reactive synovitis and osteolysis after total hip arthroplasty. *Clin Orthop Relat Res.* 2010;468:3278-3285.
13. Ranawat AS, Rossi R, Loreti I, et al. Comparison of the PFC Sigma fixed-bearing and rotating-platform total knee arthroplasty in the same patient: short-term results. *J Arthroplasty.* 2004;19:35-39.
14. Rodriguez JA, Baez N, Rasquinha V, et al. Metal-backed and all-polyethylene tibial components in total knee replacement. *Clin Orthop Relat Res.* 2001;392:174-183.
15. Pagnano MW, Levy BA, Berry DJ. Cemented all-polyethylene tibial components in patients age 75 years and older. *Clin Orthop Relat Res.* 1999;367:73.
16. Adalberth G, Nilsson KG, Bystrom S, et al. All-polyethylene versus metal-backed and stemmed tibial components in cemented total knee arthroplasty. A prospective, randomised RSA study. *J Bone Joint Surg Br.* 2000;83:825.
17. Campbell MD, Duffy GP, Trousdale RT. Femoral component failure in hybrid total knee arthroplasty. *Clin Orthop Relat Res.* 1998;356:58-65.
18. Najibi S, Iorio R, Surdam JW, et al. All-polyethylene and metal-backed tibial components in total knee arthroplasty: a matched pair analysis of functional outcome. *J Arthroplasty.* 2003;18(7 suppl 1):9.
19. Bozic KJ, Kinder J, Menegini M, et al. Implant survivorship and complication rates after total knee arthroplasty with a third-generation cemented system: 5 to 8 years followup. *Clin Orthop Relat Res.* 2005;430:117-124.
20. Ehrhard J, Gadinsky N, Lyman S, et al. Average 7-year survivorship and clinical results of a newer primary posterior stabilized total knee arthroplasty. *HSS J.* 2011;7(2):120-124.
21. Parsch D, Krüger, Moser MT, et al. Follow-up of 11-16 years after modular fixed-bearing TKA. *Int Orthop.* 2009;33:431-435.
22. Stern SH, Insall JH. Posterior stabilized prosthesis. *J Bone Joint Surg Am.* 1992;74(7):980-986.

61 Uncemented Total Knee Arthroplasty Using Tantalum

Michael J. Dunbar, Christopher Jones, Shane Guerin, and Glen Richardson

Uncemented total knee arthroplasty implants have been used since the early 1980s in an attempt to improve durability by creating a biological bond between the implant and bone. Several surface coatings and early porous metals were developed, such as cobalt chrome sintered beads, titanium plasma spray, and diffusion-bonded fiber metal mesh.[1] These techniques provided for a three-dimensional surface applied to the substrate of the implant in an effort to encourage osteointegration. The volume of space afforded was limited by the thickness of the applied material and substrate to which it was applied. These materials were further limited by relatively high moduli of elasticity and low frictional characteristics. The Swedish Knee Arthroplasty Register reported specifically on survivorship of uncemented and cemented tibial components from this period of uncemented proliferation, 1985–1994 (Fig. 61-1).[2] The risk ratio for revision for any reason was 1.5 times higher in the uncemented tibial group compared to the cemented group during this period. Perhaps as a result of these reported outcomes, the use of uncemented fixation in Sweden has fallen since the mid-1980s, such that now the vast majority of all total knee arthroplasties (TKAs) in Sweden are cemented. Cemented fixation in TKA, especially of the tibial component, remains the gold standard. Despite this, TKA has limited survivorship.

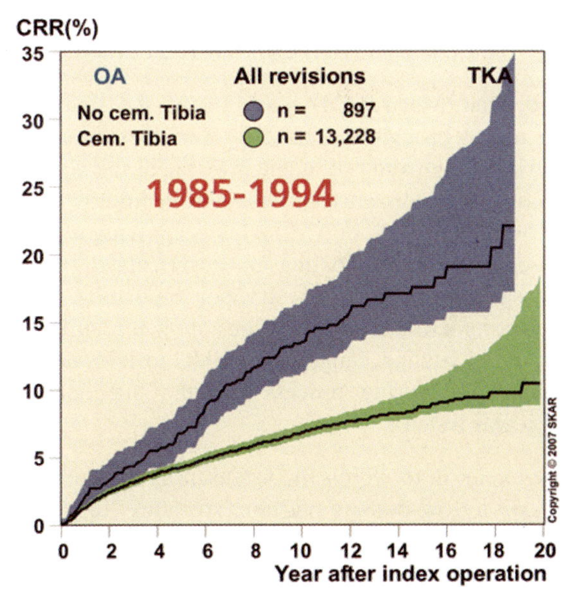

FIGURE 61-1. *The cumulative revision rate (CRR) for TKA inserted 1985–1994 in which the tibial component was fixed with or without cement. Uncemented TKA was more common in Sweden during this period. The risk ratio for revision of an uncemented tibial component during this period was 1.5 (1.2–2.8). (From the Swedish Knee Arthroplasty Register 2009 Annual Report.)*

Aseptic loosening and osteolysis are the leading causes of failure in TKA.[2-4] Failure rates for these reasons are significantly higher in younger age groups receiving TKA. This is of concern given that the average age is decreasing and body mass index is increasing in the average TKA patient.[4] In Canada, over a recent 10-year period, the demand for TKA in the 45- to 54-year age group increased more than 300%, and 87% of all patients receiving TKA were obese or overweight.[4] The numbers are likely similar in the United States. Clearly, the biomechanical demand on modern TKA has increased and prolonged survivorship is of particular importance in young patients. In young patients in which a TKA is expected to last for multiple decades, not only is the mechanical interface of concern, but so too is the quality of the periprosthetic bone stock. Modern porous metal materials have been adapted to current TKA designs, partly to address these concerns.

Modern porous metal uncemented fixation may offer an advantage in younger, higher demand patients if new materials and manufacturing techniques could provide an uncemented implant with (1) greater inherent stability, (2) larger volumes for osteointegration, and (3) reduced stress shielding. Modern porous metals have addressed these issues to various degrees, depending on the manufacturer, by providing materials with (1) high coefficients of friction, (2) large volumes of interconnected porosity, and (3) low moduli of elasticity.

TANTALUM MATERIAL PROPERTIES

Trabecular Metal (TM) was one of the first modern porous metals brought to market by Zimmer (Warsaw, Indiana), originating from a strategic investment in and eventual acquisition of Hedrocel technology from Implex Corporation. The manufacture of TM involves applying a commercially pure tantalum coating to a reticulated pyrolized carbon skeleton by a chemical vapor deposition process.[5] The resulting surface characteristics show a relatively high coefficient of friction, ranging from 0.82 to 1.75, depending on the manufacturing process and the material against which it was tested.[5]

The skeleton to which the tantalum is applied is composed of a low-density carbon structure of repeating dodecahedrons. The resulting structure is not dissimilar to cancelous bone (Fig. 61-2). The ability to determine the shape of the skeleton allows considerable scope in terms of implant design, particularly with respect to porosity. Porosity of TM varies between 75% and 85%, compared to 30% to 35% for cobalt chrome sintered beads and 40% to 50% for fiber metal.[5] The interconnected pores promote bone ingrowth and provide three-dimensional fixation.[6,7]

Tantalum has high bioaffinity. It forms a stable oxide layer, Ta_2O_5, which then interacts with surrounding bodily

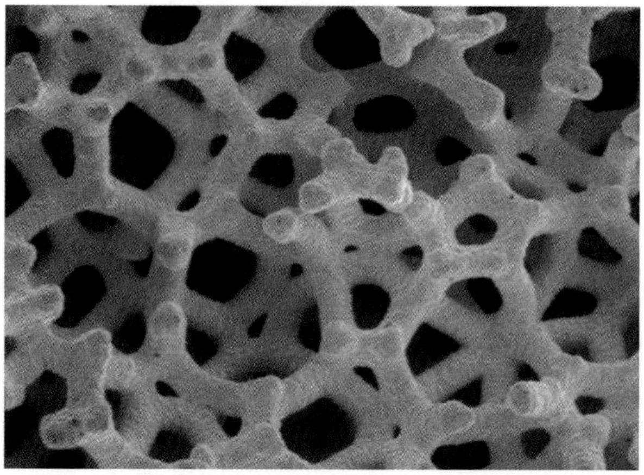

FIGURE 61-2. *Dodecahedral microstructure of porous tantalum (Trabecular Metal) with large area of interconnected porosity, somewhat resembling cancellous bone.*

fluids to develop a bone-like apatite layer.[5] As such, tantalum may have osteoinductive properties.

The porosity of tantalum results in a significant reduction in the stiffness of the construct, with TM having a modulus of elasticity of approximately 3 GPa, which is similar to that of subchondral bone.[5] This optimal elasticity may create a more physiological transfer of stresses to the periprosthetic bone, theoretically decreasing detrimental stress shielding and possibly preventing tibial component lift-off from asymmetrically applied loads.[8]

CLINICAL APPLICATIONS OF TANTALUM IN PRIMARY TKA

TM is available as part of the Zimmer NexGen TKA system on the tibial and patellar component. The tibial component is available in monoblock or modular version. The monoblock has two hexagonal pegs and no central keel (Fig. 61-3A). The polyethylene is direct compression molded into the porosity of the TM (Fig. 61-3B). The advantages of such an approach are elimination of backside wear and a low modulus, relatively flexible component that may avoid stress shielding. Disadvantages include greater difficulty in implanting, inability to balance soft tissue with polyethylene thickness after tibial component implantation, and perhaps inability to use cross-linked polyethylene. The TM tibial component is also available in a modular version,

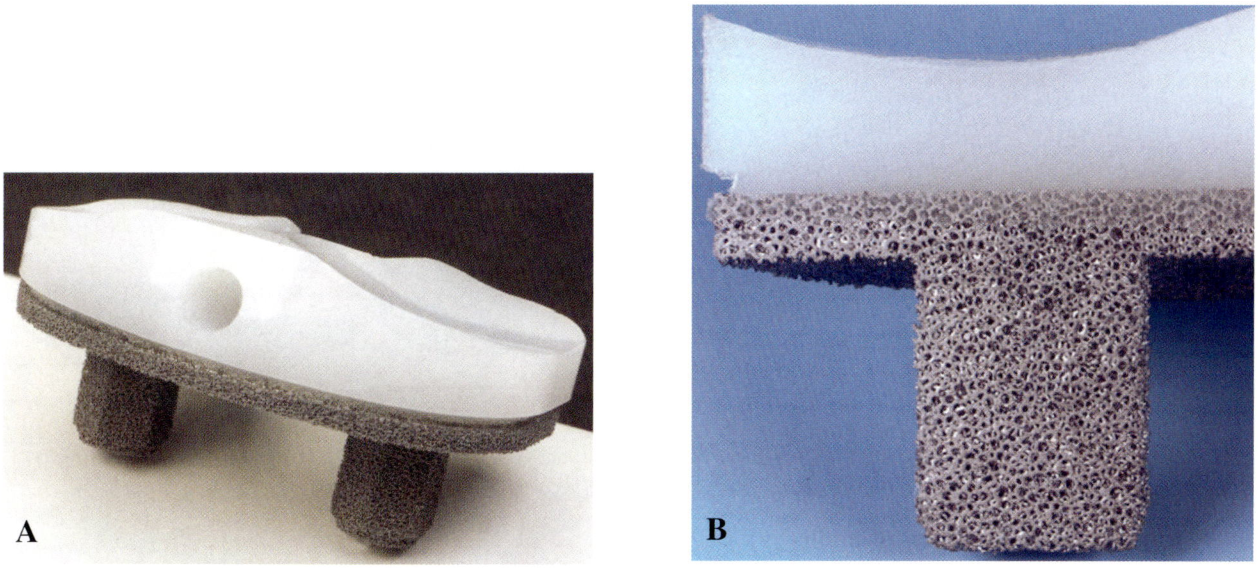

FIGURE 61-3. *(**A**) The Zimmer NexGen monoblock TM tibial component. Note the hexagonal pegs. (**B**) Cross section of a monoblock TM tibial component demonstrating the porosity of the TM and the extent of the interdigitation of the polyethylene.*

again with two hexagonal pegs but with the addition of a smaller central boss, required to accommodate enhanced fixation of thicker polyethylene inserts (Fig. 61-4). The TM is applied to a substrate of titanium, which makes up the locking mechanism as well. The advantages include greater ease of implantation, ability to exchange the polyethylene, and perhaps the ability to use cross-linked polyethylene.

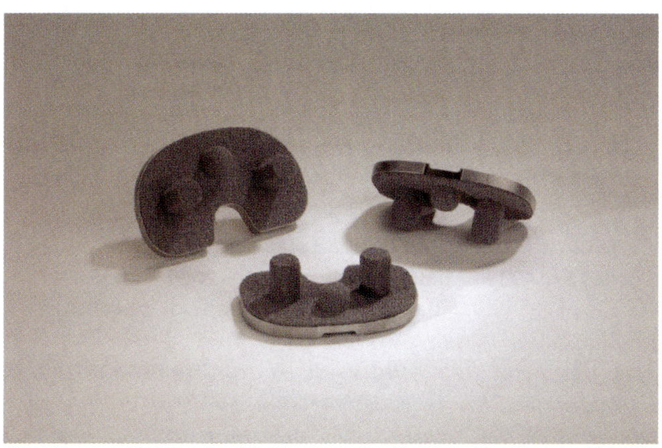

FIGURE 61-4. *The Zimmer NexGen modular TM tibial component. Note the anterior boss and modular tray.*

The primary disadvantage is the increased stiffness and higher modulus associated with bonding the TM to the titanium baseplate.

The TM patellar component is also available in a monoblock and modular form. The monoblock TM patellar component has a central hexagonal peg (Fig. 61-5A). The modular TM patellar component has a dome-shaped TM surface with a peripheral ring used for suture augmentation (Fig. 61-5B). The polyethylene component is cemented onto the TM base. The modular TM patellar component is used primarily in situations with bony insufficiency of the patella, such as in revisions. Augments, wedges, and cones, although useful in the complex primary situation, are more commonly used in the revision setting and are outside the scope of this chapter.

INCIDENCE OF TANTALUM USE IN TKA

It is difficult to ascertain the incidence or even numbers of tantalum prostheses implanted. More generally, there is variability between countries regarding the overall incidence of cementless fixation in TKA. In Sweden, either cementless or hybrid fixation accounted for approximately

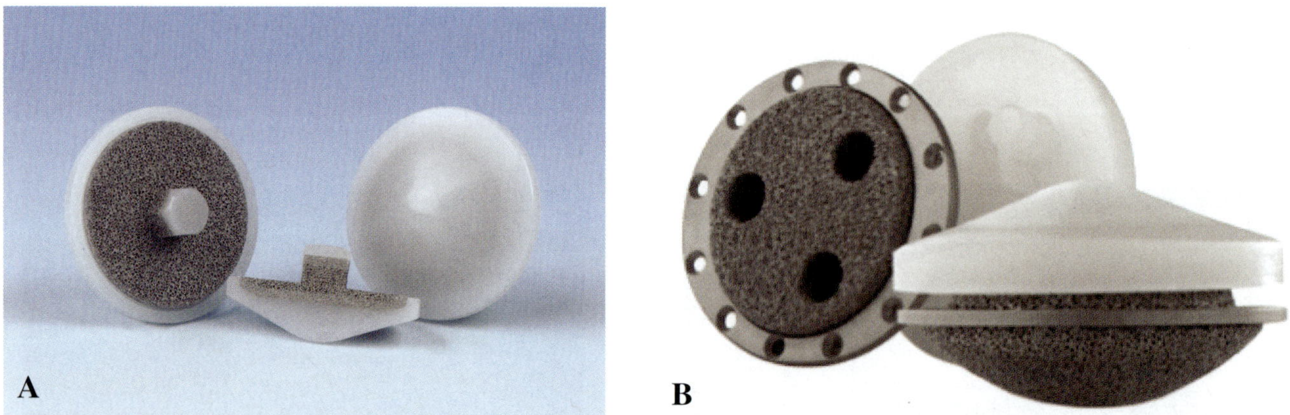

FIGURE 61-5. *(**A**) TM monoblock patellar component with central hexagonal peg. (**B**) TM modular patellar component with dome-shaped metal surface and peripheral fixation augmentation ring.*

25% of all cases in 1985 (Fig. 61-6).[2] This has decreased since to less than 2% of all cases in 2009. In Canada, only 16% of cases in 2007 used either cementless (6%) or hybrid (10%) fixation.[4] The rates of cemented fixation have remained relatively constant since 2003. In Australia, the number of cemented cases has risen slightly since 2003 to slightly over 50% of all cases. In 2009 approximately 25% of cases used cementless fixation and 25% used hybrid fixation.[3]

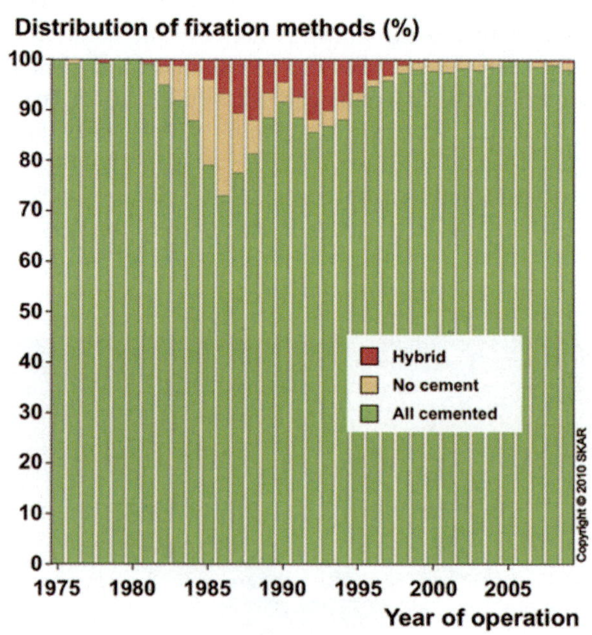

FIGURE 61-6. *The relative yearly distribution of the use of cement in TKA in Sweden from 1975 to 2009. Uncemented fixation peaked in the mid 1980s and has decreased since to less than 5% of all cases in 2009. (From the Swedish Knee Arthroplasty Register 2009 Annual Report.)*

PREOPERATIVE EVALUATION

History and Examination

Generally, the history and physical examination is the same as for routine primary TKA. Specifically, patient height, weight, and body mass index should be assessed. Visual assessment of gait to identify significant varus thrust should be considered because gait has been shown to have an effect on roentgen stereophotogrammetric analysis (RSA) migration patterns of monoblock TM tibial components. A history of inflammatory arthropathy should be elicited. As inflammatory joint disease is in general a contraindication to uncemented TKA, and given there is little published outcomes on TM in this patient population, inflammatory disease should be of concern.

Imaging

As for routine primary total knee replacement, plain radiographs include weight-bearing anteroposterior (AP), lateral, and 30° flexed posteroanterior (PA) radiographs, as well as skyline patellar views. In some complex primary situations, computed tomography is important to outline the available bone stock and help to define the need for cones or augments.

Preparation of Patient for Surgery

In addition to the routine preoperative preparation for total knee arthroplasty, the informed consent process should include the fact that although TM implants have promising features and good midterm results, their long-term success has yet to be determined.

SURGERY

Indications for TM

Modern cementless fixation is potentially advantageous in young, active patients where a high-friction, high-porosity, and low-modulus implant may be desirable to enhance fixation and reduce long-term stress shielding. Uncemented monoblock TM tibial implants have performed better in RSA studies than both cemented and low-porosity uncemented tibial implants.[8-11] Uncemented monoblock TM tibial implants have also shown less percentage bone loss on dual X-ray absorptiometry (DEXA).[12,13]

Patients with a high varus adduction moment and with certain electromyographic (EMG) muscle firing patterns across the knee, both preoperatively, have been shown to have high migration patterns or deformation of the tibial component.[8,11,14,15] This may prove to be a beneficial behavior, but long-term follow-up is required.[8,10,13,16]

The use of the TM modular patellar component in patients with patellar deficiency after trauma or partial patellectomy has documented success in the literature.[17,18] Note, however, that >50% host bone contact is required, and patellar replacement with a porous metal component is not indicated following total patellectomy.[17,18] TM may be considered in cases were metal sensitivity is a concern because of its high biocompatibility.[5,19,20]

Contraindications Specific to Tantalum

There are no specific contraindications. Caution is potentially advised with the use of the uncemented TM monoblock tibia in tall, heavy males. Meneghini and de Beaubien reported an early failure rate of 7.5% using a posterior cruciate-substituting monoblock TM tibial component in this patient demographic.[21]

Anatomy, Surgical Approach, and Technique

As for any joint replacement surgery, the surgeon must be familiar with the manufacturer's surgical technique specific to the implant being used before undertaking the operation. The approach, anatomy, and implantation technique for porous metal implants are the same as for routine primary total knee arthroplasty, with specific attention to the following details.

Tibia

The porous metal tibial components are typically implanted without cement. However, in the event of unexpectedly poor proximal tibial bone quality, cement may be used. Cement should be only applied to the tibial baseplate and proximal tibia and not to the fixation pegs.[22] A conventional cemented tibial option is advisable in case adequate initial fixation cannot be achieved.

The exposed peripheral edge of the TM tibial components is rough. Care should be taken in particular not to overhang a porous metal tibial component. Conversely, high migration has been seen in some patients in whom the component is undersized within the cortical mantle.[8] Care should be taken not to undersize the tibial component in the face of significantly osteoporotic subchondral bone.

Cruciate-retaining and cruciate-substituting designs are both available. If a monoblock cruciate-substituting design is used, it is usually recommended that the tibial component be implanted after the femoral component so that the post on the tibial component does not interfere with femoral component implantation. In this situation the polished articulating surface of the femoral component must be meticulously protected during the retraction required to facilitate implantation of the tibial component.

Uncemented components in general have an intuitive appeal for more minimally invasive surgery (MIS) by negating the need to clear posteriorly extruded cement. Results of MIS have been mixed, with some authors reporting improved short-term outcomes, while others caution against increased tourniquet time and increased incidence of malalignment.[23,24] Based on recent meta-analysis data, the results are equivocal given conventional outcome metrics.[25] Given this, in general, a standard incision and surgical approach is recommended by the authors for use with TM tibial components.

Patella

Like the tibial components, the monoblock TM patella component is typically inserted without cement. If cement is required, it is recommended that it only be applied to the undersurface of the implant and not to the peg itself.

During implantation of the monoblock TM patella component, care must be taken to ensure correct alignment of the peg with the predrilled peg hole before clamping the implant in place. The implantation of the component should be able to be started with the thumb and forefinger across the patella and implant. If the component is implanted and the peg is malaligned with the drill hole, the patella may be at increased risk of fracture during implantation. Sufficient patella thickness (at least 12 mm) must remain to safely accommodate the peg of the component. If the residual patella is insufficiently thick, a primary cemented all-polyethylene component should be used instead. The TM monoblock patella component may be implanted using either an inset or an onlay technique. The manufacturer's surgical technique should be reviewed for the specific implant to be used. For further details on the exact technique, see http://www.zimmer.com/content/pdf/en.[26]

The modular TM patella currently available is designed for use in patella deficiency. The patella is reamed and the unpegged porous metal component is sutured in place using nonabsorbable suture material. The polyethylene component is then cemented into the porous metal component. We recommend reviewing the manufacturer's surgical technique for further information.[27] Significant residual patellar bone stock is a requisite for success.[17]

A viable patella is necessary in order to achieve osteointegration. As such, situations in which significant compromise of patellar blood supply arises, such as the need for a lateral release, should be considered a contraindication for use.

POSTOPERATIVE TREATMENT AND COMPLICATIONS

Rehabilitation

Postoperative rehabilitation is similar to that in routine primary total knee arthroplasty, including allowing immediate unrestricted weight bearing and joint range of motion. There is currently no direct evidence to support restricted weight bearing. EMG muscle firing patterns have been shown to correlate to RSA migration patterns, suggesting that in the future there may be a role for a patient-specific rehabilitation program.[15]

Complications

TM has been shown to have similar perioperative complications associated with TKA, as compared to conventional implants with cemented fixation.[8,9,28,29] There have been limited reports of isolated failures of TM tibial components related to fibrous ingrowth.[30]

The excellent fixation of the TM implant may create difficulties if removal is required at revision for reasons such as infection.[31,32] Typically an oscillating saw is required at the bone–implant interface, with the pegs being cut off by the saw and subsequently retrieved from the metaphyseal bone. This creates significant tantalum metal debris, which may be problematic despite meticulous protection of the surrounding tissues.[31] Klein et al described an alternative technique using osteotomes to break the pegs instead of cutting them with a saw, which created no macroscopic metal debris.[32]

Monoblock TM tibial components are at risk of high initial migration and potentially deformation under physiological loads, as defined by RSA.[8,10] Longer follow-up is required to definitively determine if this is a complication or actual benefit.

The two-peg press-fit design of the TM tibial implant intuitively confers improved rotational and coronal plane stability over keeled or stemmed primary implants, but introduces the risk of peg penetration of medial and, more commonly, lateral cortex, particularly in smaller females in which the tibia is overresected. The clinical consequences of this are not clear at present, with reports of implant stability and excellent function despite this complication, likely due to the favorable biomechanical properties of the TM.[33]

Patella fracture following successful implantation of a monoblock TM patellar component has been reported.[34] However, the patient had a fall onto the knee, and at surgery for successful fracture fixation the implant was well fixed. There have been no reports to date of worn patellar polyethylene leading to exposed TM.

The modular TM patellar implant has a high incidence of failure when used with less than 50% host bone contact with the patella.[17,18]

OUTCOMES

Monoblock TM Tibia

Although long-term follow-up is unavailable for the monoblock TM tibial component, the short- to intermediate-term data on component survivorship and clinical outcomes are encouraging. Based on the following, including multiple conventional, DEXA, and RSA studies, the TM monoblock tibia has been extensively studied.

Conventional studies

O'Keefe et al implanted 125 monoblock posterior stabilized TM tibial components with cement.[33] At minimum 5-year prospective follow-up, no components were identified as being at risk of loosening. Two tibial implants were revised: one for arthrofibrosis and one for late infection at 4 years. The survivorship with regard to tibial component loosening was 100%.

Helm et al prospectively reviewed a cohort of 105 consecutive uncemented TM monoblock components for a minimum of 3 years and found results as good as those published for commonly used cemented prostheses.[28] They observed no radiolucent lines under the tibial component and significant improvements in functional knee scores. One patient sustained postoperative trauma necessitating revision of a well-fixed tibial component at 2 months post implantation.

Unger and Duggan performed 108 minimally invasive subvastus total knee arthroplasties using an uncemented cruciate-retaining monoblock TM tibial component, an uncemented fiber-metal femoral component, and a combination of 90 uncemented monoblock and 18 cemented all-polyethelyne patellae.[34] At an average of 4.5 years, they reported no progressive radiolucencies. Mean Knee Society scores improved from 36 (objective) and 46 (functional) preoperatively to 88 and 85, respectively. Three patients had poor results on both knee scores. One reoperation was performed for aseptic loosening of the femoral component. At revision surgery the well-fixed TM tibial component was removed. Although there were no reoperations for TM tibial components, one tibial component had subsided 4 mm at 6 months and 8 mm at 3 years. The knee was painful and rated as poor on Knee Society scores. The patient refused revision surgery.

Tigani et al published a case report in 2009 on a failure of a TM monoblock tibial component at 7 months' follow-up.[30] A reactive fibrous tissue was found on histology at the bone–implant interface.[30] No bone ingrowth was seen. The patient was an 80-year-old osteoarthritic male with multiple comorbidities.

In 2011 Kamath et al reported the prospective results of a minimum 5-year follow-up on 100 monoblock TM components in patients less than 55 years.[29] This group was compared to a control group of 312 cemented controls. There were no differences in complications and operative times were lower in the TM group. Clinical outcomes were the same in both groups. Three monoblock TM components were revised, but none due to failure of fixation. There were 5 failures in the cemented group.

DEXA studies

Harrison et al published in 2010 the results of 41 monoblock TM tibial components in patients 60 years old or under with DEXA reported as the main outcome metric.[12] DEXA of 3 zones of interest around the tibial component were compared to the contralateral tibia and to historic controls for cemented components. DEXA was performed at 2 months, 1 year, and 2 years postoperatively. Bone mineral density (BMD) percentage change was different between the operative and nonoperative tibia in one zone at 2 months only. BMD percentage change was better than historic controls. There were no failures.

In a similar study in 2010, Minoda et al published the results of a DEXA study on 28 uncemented monoblock TM tibial components and 28 cobalt chrome cemented tibial components.[13] Like Harrison, 3 zones of interest were studied at 2 months, 1 year, and 2 years postoperatively[12] Knee Society score, range of motion, and bone mineral density of the lumber spine were the same in both groups. Percent change in BMD in the lateral tibial plateau was significantly less in the TM group, however.

RSA studies

Henricson et al used RSA to compare an uncemented cruciate-retaining monoblock porous tantalum tibial component with a cemented cruciate-retaining tibial component in patients younger than 60 years.[9] After initial migration, all the porous tantalum components stabilized by 3 months with the exception of external rotation, which stabilized by 12 months. Most of the porous tantalum components showed subsidence only, without the contralateral lift-off seen in metal-backed components, and the authors postulate that this is likely due to the elasticity of the porous tantalum implant.[35,36] The cemented components performed similarly to the porous tantalum components in this study, with stabilization of migration after 6 weeks to 3 months. This is in contrast to previous RSA studies of cemented tibial components that demonstrate continuous migration indicating bone resorption at the bone–cement interface.[37,38] One patient continuously complaining of pain and with greater migration of the tibial component than the group average was revised at 19 months. Macroscopically, the tibial component was felt to be well fixed. Microscopically, examination of the retrieved tibial component showed well-organized continuous layer of dense fibrous tissue at the bone–implant interface, with only small areas of bone ingrowth. This was not dissimilar to Tigani's findings.[30] The revision was subsequently complicated by early deep infection. Though infection of the initial implant was not formally diagnosed, it cannot be discounted.

Comparing an uncemented posterior stabilized monoblock porous tantalum tibial component with a conventional cemented posterior stabilized tibial component, Dunbar et al found that the proportion of porous tantalum components considered to be at risk of early aseptic loosening was significantly lower than the group of cemented components (0 of 28 and 4 of 21, respectively).[8] The continued migration of the cemented components considered at risk of aseptic loosening was almost exclusively rotational in the axial plane and the cemented components exhibited significantly more occurrences of lift-off than the porous tantalum components. Subsidence without contralateral lift-off, as reported by Henricson, was also seen by Dunbar et al, and in some cases was reported as actual deformation of the monoblock TM component. Cemented components not considered at risk of aseptic loosening had higher migration from 12 to 24 months than the monoblock TM tibial components as a group. However, although more stable from 12 months, the overall migration of the porous tantalum components was significantly higher than that of the cemented components, with more subsidence, more posterior tilt, and more internal rotation. Despite this behavior, the components remained stable.

Wilson et al, in a follow-up on the same cohort as Dunbar et al, showed significantly less inducible displacement in the TM monoblock group when compared with RSA to a cemented tibial component of the same design.[11] This is in contrast to other RSA studies that have shown uncemented implants to have higher inducible displacement.[39,40] The authors attribute their results to the quality and volume of the bone–implant interface of the porous tantalum implant.

Stilling et al used RSA to compare stability of an uncemented TM monoblock tibial component to that of an uncemented titanium pegged fiber-metal component with additional screw fixation.[10] They found that most of the migration of the porous tantalum components occurred over 3 months, whereas migration of the titanium components continued for 12 months. The porous tantalum components migrated less overall than the titanium components at 12 and 24 months, and at 24 months there was significantly less continued migration of porous tantalum components than titanium components (2 of 24 and 12 of 22, respectively). They concluded that the porous tantalum component had better mechanical fixation and better long-term survival could be expected.

Modular TM Tibial Components

Having been introduced more recently, there is insufficient published data to comment on specific outcomes related to the modular TM tibial component. However, the application of TM to the more rigid substrate of the modular TM tibial component changes some material properties and may result in different deformation and periprosthetic stress loading patterns in vivo, as previously reported in the monoblock TM tibial component.[8,12,13] The implications of this are unclear and long-term follow-up is necessary.

TM Patellar Components

Unger and Duggan performed 90 patellar resurfacings with a monoblock TM implant.[34] Using a minimally invasive midvastus approach, they cut the patella freehand without everting it. Four implants required reoperation. One patient sustained a traumatic transverse patella fracture that was managed with a tension band wire construct. The TM patellar component was well-fixed both radiologically and clinically at operation and the outcome was ultimately good with no extensor lag. Two patients were revised to an all-polyethylene patella because of anterior knee pain. Both implants were found to be loose at revision operation. One patient complained of persistent anterior knee pain and skyline radiographs demonstrated an oblique patellar cut causing symptomatic subluxation. The implant was well-fixed at revision surgery and the patella was recut, a cemented all-polyethylene component implanted, and a lateral release performed with good result.

Ries et al retrospectively reviewed a group of 16 patients (18 knees) with patellar bone deficiency at both primary (2 knees) and revision (16 knees) TKA managed with a modular TM patellar implant.[17] Ten of 11 implants that had at least 50% host bone contact remained stable at 12 months, compared to zero of 7 implants with no host bone contact. The implant that failed despite host bone contact was complicated by deep infection. In the knees with stable implants the average extensor lag was 0.5°. Tigani et al found similar results in their series of 10 knees (3 primary, 7 revision) with patellar bone deficiency managed with a modular TM patellar implant.[18] In the 9 patients with greater than 50% host bone contact, the implant remained stable at a mean follow-up of 45 months (range, 18-65 months). One patient was post patellectomy with no residual bone stock and developed loosening of the patellar implant at 17 months postoperatively.

CASE EXAMPLES

Case 1

A 62-year-old male retiree presents with pain and stiffness associated with osteoarthritis and a valgus deformity 20 years after an open lateral menisectomy (Fig. 61-7A). A posterior stabilized uncemented monoblock TM tibial component with cemented femoral component and cemented inset patellar button was used with satisfactory results and stable fixation, as defined by RSA (Fig. 61-7B).

Case 2

A 52-year-old male laborer presents with pain and stiffness and a varus deformity associated with osteoarthritis (Fig. 61-8A). A posterior stabilized uncemented modular TM tibial component with cemented femoral component and cemented inset patellar button was used with satisfactory results and stable fixation, as defined by RSA (Fig. 61-8B).

PEARLS AND PITFALLS

Some pearls and pitfalls with the use of TM tibial components are as follows:

1. Early to midterm results of monoblock TM tibial components show promising outcomes, as defined by favorable RSA migration patterns and conventional studies.[8-10,29,34]
2. The low-modulus monoblock TM tibial components can demonstrate significant subsidence and deformation

A

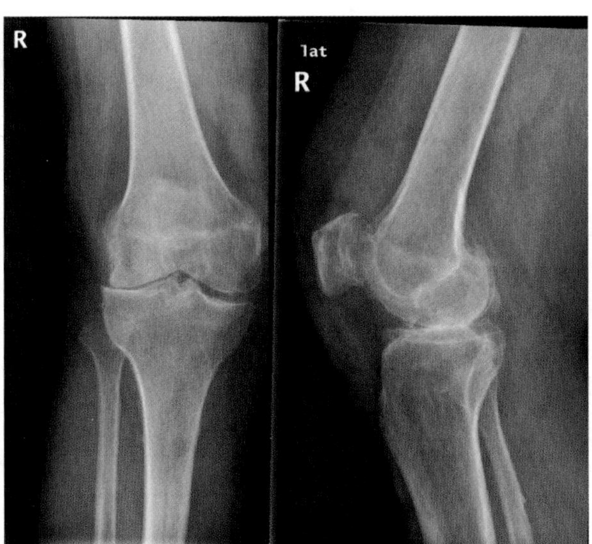

B

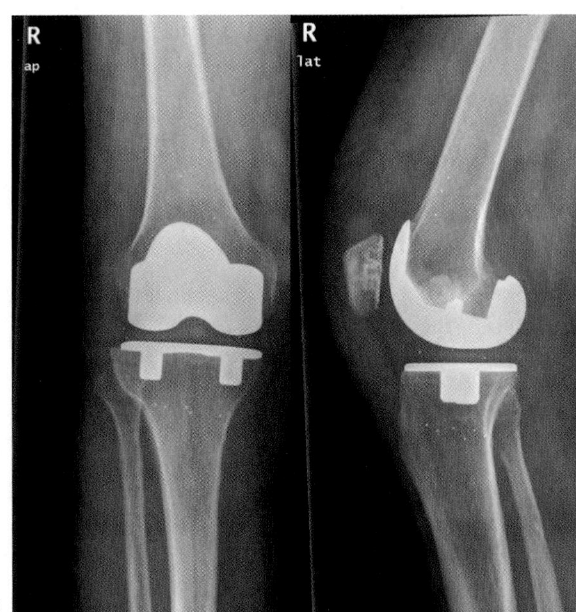

FIGURE 61-7. *(**A**) Preoperative AP and lateral radiographs of a right knee. (**B**) Postoperative AP and lateral radiographs demonstrating a well-fixed uncemented monoblock TM tibial component, cemented NexGen femur, and cemented inset patellar button. Note the RSA beads.*

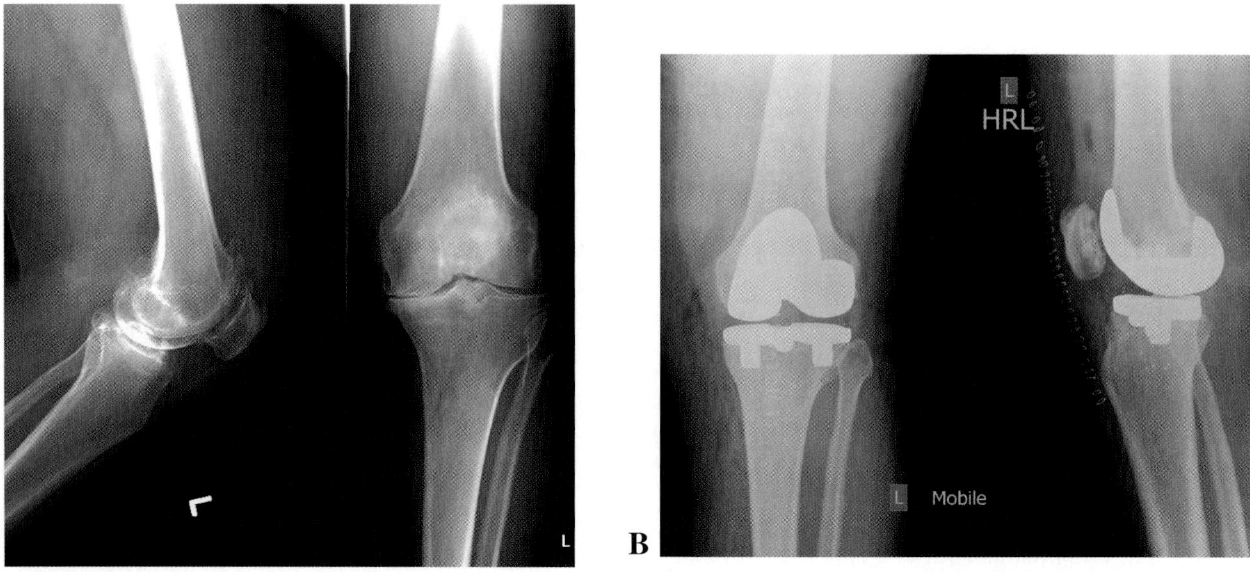

FIGURE 61-8. *(**A**) Preoperative lateral and AP radiographs of a left knee. (**B**) Postoperative AP and lateral radiographs demonstrating an uncemented modular TM tibial component, cemented NexGen femur, and cemented inset patellar button. Note the RSA beads.*

under biomechanical loads.[8-11,14,15] To date, these patterns of motion have not been detrimental to survivorship, and some have speculated that these behaviors may in fact be beneficial, particularly with respect to maintenance of periprosthetic bone stock.[8-12] Long-term follow-up is required.

3. Initial stable fixation is necessary when using uncemented TKA components. The surgeon must be prepared to change technique if this cannot be obtained in the operating room.
4. The exposed edge of TM tibial implants is rough. As such, avoid significant overhang, especially medially.
5. Undersizing the tibial component in osteoporotic subchondral bone may lead to significant subsidence.[8] Try to obtain cortical contact in such cases.
6. Tantalum patellar augmentation is only successful in the setting of at least 50% host bone contact.[17]

SUGGESTED READING

Fukuoka S, Yoshida K, Yamano Y. Estimation of the migration of tibial components in total knee arthroplasty. A roentgen stereophotogrammetric analysis. *J Bone Joint Surg Br.* 2000;82:222-227.

Meneghini RM, Hanssen AD. Cementless fixation in total knee arthroplasty: past, present, and future. *J Knee Surg*. 2008;21:307-314.

Ryd L, Albrektsson BE, Carlsson L, et al. Roentgen stereophotogrammetric analysis as a predictor of mechanical loosening of knee prostheses. *J Bone Joint Surg Br.* 1995;77:377-383.

REFERENCES

1. Ranawat CS. History of total knee replacement. *J South Orthop Assoc.* 2002;11(4):218-226.
2. Robertsson O. *Annual Report 2009: The Swedish Knee Arthroplasty Register.* Lund, Sweden: Department of Orthopaedics, Lund University Hospital; 2009.
3. *Hip and Knee Arthroplasty Annual Report 2010.* Adelaide, South Australia: Australian Orthopaedic Association National Joint Replacement Registry; 2010.

4. Information CIfH. *Hip and Knee Replacements in Canada.* Ottawa, Canada: Canadian Institution for Health Information; 2008.
5. Levine BR, Sporer S, Poggie RA, et al. Experimental and clinical performance of porous tantalum in orthopedic surgery. *Biomaterials.* 2006;27(27):4671-4681.
6. Bobyn JD, Stackpool GJ, Hacking SA, et al. Characteristics of bone ingrowth and interface mechanics of a new porous tantalum biomaterial. *J Bone Joint Surg Br.* 1999;81(5):907-914.
7. Bobyn JD, Toh KK, Hacking SA, et al. Tissue response to porous tantalum acetabular cups: a canine model. *J Arthroplasty.* 1999;14(3):347-354.
8. Dunbar MJ, Wilson DA, Hennigar AW, et al. Fixation of a trabecular metal knee arthroplasty component. A prospective randomized study. *J Bone Joint Surg Am.* 2009;91(7):1578-1586.
9. Henricson A, Linder L, Nilsson KG. A trabecular metal tibial component in total knee replacement in patients younger than 60 years: a two-year radiostereophotogrammetric analysis. *J Bone Joint Surg Br.* 2008;90(12):1585-1593.
10. Stilling M, Madsen F, Odgaard A, et al. Superior fixation of pegged trabecular metal over screw-fixed pegged porous titanium fiber mesh: a randomized clinical RSA study on cementless tibial components. *Acta Orthop.* 2011;82(2):177-186.
11. Wilson DA, Astephen JL, Hennigar AW, et al. Inducible displacement of a trabecular metal tibial monoblock component. *J Arthroplasty.* 2010;25(6):893-900.
12. Harrison AK, Gioe TJ, Simonelli C, et al. Do porous tantalum implants help preserve bone?: evaluation of tibial bone density surrounding tantalum tibial implants in TKA. *Clin Orthop Relat Res.* 2010;468(10):2739-2745.
13. Minoda Y, Kobayashi A, Iwaki H, et al. Comparison of bone mineral density between porous tantalum and cemented tibial total knee arthroplasty components. *J Bone Joint Surg Am.* 2010;92(3):700-706.
14. Astephen Wilson JL, Wilson DA, Dunbar MJ, et al. Preoperative gait patterns and BMI are associated with tibial component migration. *Acta Orthop.* 2010; 81(4):478-486.
15. Hubley-Kozey CL, Hatfield GL, Wilson JL, et al. Alterations in neuromuscular patterns between pre- and one-year post-total knee arthroplasty. *Clin Biomech (Bristol, Avon).* 2010;25(10):995-1002.
16. Hansson U, Ryd L, Toksvig-Larsen S. A randomised RSA study of peri-apatite HA coating of a total knee prosthesis. *Knee.* 2008;15(3):211-216.
17. Ries MD, Cabalo A, Bozic KJ, et al. Porous tantalum patellar augmentation: the importance of residual bone stock. *Clin Orthop Relat Res.* 2006;452:166-170.
18. Tigani D, Trentani P, Trentani F, et al. Trabecular metal patella in total knee arthroplasty with patella bone deficiency. *Knee.* 2009;16(1):46-49.
19. Patil N, Lee K, Goodman SB. Porous tantalum in hip and knee reconstructive surgery. *J Biomed Mater Res B Appl Biomater.* 2009;89(1):242-251.
20. Sheth NP, Lonner JH. Clinical use of porous tantalum in complex primary total knee arthroplasty. *Am J Orthop (Belle Mead NJ).* 2009;38(10):526-530.
21. Meneghini MR, de Beaubien, BC. Early failure of cementless porous tantalum monoblock tibial components is likely related to patient height, weight and gender. *J Arthroplasty.* 2010;25(3):e66.
22. US/NexGen Trabecular Metal Monoblock Tibial Components Surgical Technique Addendum (97-7255-134-00) (04 2007). Available at: http://www.zimmer.com/content/pdf/en. Accessed July 18, 2011.
23. Bonutti PM, Zywiel MG, Ulrich SD, et al. A comparison of subvastus and midvastus approaches in minimally invasive total knee arthroplasty. *J Bone Joint Surg Am.* 2010;92(3):575-582.
24. Khanna A, Gougoulias N, Longo UG, et al. Minimally invasive total knee arthroplasty: a systematic review. *Orthop Clin North Am.* 2009; 40(4):479-489, viii.
25. Smith TO, King JJ, Hing CB. A meta-analysis of randomised controlled trials comparing the clinical and radiological outcomes following minimally invasive to conventional exposure for total knee arthroplasty. *Knee.* 2012;19(1):1-7.
26. US/NexGen Trabecular Metal Primary Patella Surgical Technique (97-7255-112-00) (08 2005). Available at: http://www.zimmer.com/content/pdf/en. Accessed July 18, 2011, 2011.
27. US/NexGen Trabecular Metal Augmentation Patella Surgical Technique (97-7255-004-00 Rev 2)(4 2008). Available at: http://www.zimmer.com/content/pdf/en Accessed July 18, 2011, 2011.
28. Helm AT, Kerin C, Ghalayini SR, et al. Preliminary results of an uncemented trabecular metal tibial component in total knee arthroplasty. *J Arthroplasty.* 2009;24(6):941-944.

29. Kamath AF, Lee GC, Sheth NP, et al. Prospective results of uncemented tantalum monoblock tibia in total knee arthroplasty minimum 5-year follow-up in patients younger than 55 years. *J Arthroplasty.* 2011; 26(8):1390-1395.

30. Tigani D, Sabbioni G, Raimondi A. Early aseptic loosening of a porous tantalum knee prosthesis. *Chir Organi Mov.* 2009;93(3):187-191.

31. Sanchez Marquez JM, Del Sel N, Leali A, et al. Case reports: tantalum debris dispersion during revision of a tibial component for TKA. *Clin Orthop Relat Res.* 2009;467(4):1107-1110.

32. Klein GR, Levine HB, Hartzband MA. Removal of a well-fixed trabecular metal monoblock tibial component. *J Arthroplasty.* 2008;23(4):619-622.

33. O'Keefe TJ, Winter S, Lewallen DG, et al. Clinical and radiographic evaluation of a monoblock tibial component. *J Arthroplasty.* 2010;25(5):785-792.

34. Unger AS, Duggan JP. Midterm results of a porous tantalum monoblock tibia component clinical and radiographic results of 108 knees. *J Arthroplasty.* 2011;26(6):855-860.

35. Hyldahl H, Regner L, Carlsson L, et al. All-polyethylene vs. metal-backed tibial component in total knee arthroplasty—a randomized RSA study comparing early fixation of horizontally and completely cemented tibial components: part 2. Completely cemented components: MB not superior to AP components. *Acta Orthop.* 2005;76(6):778-784.

36. Hyldahl H, Regner L, Carlsson L, et al. All-polyethylene vs. metal-backed tibial component in total knee arthroplasty—a randomized RSA study comparing early fixation of horizontally and completely cemented tibial components: part 1. Horizontally cemented components: AP better fixated than MB. *Acta Orthop.* 2005;76(6):769-777.

37. Nilsson KG, Karrholm J. Increased varus-valgus tilting of screw-fixated knee prostheses. Stereo-radiographic study of uncemented versus cemented tibial components. *J Arthroplasty.* 1993;8(5):529-540.

38. Nilsson KG, Karrholm J, Ekelund L, et al. Evaluation of micromotion in cemented vs uncemented knee arthroplasty in osteoarthrosis and rheumatoid arthritis. Randomized study using roentgen stereophotogrammetric analysis. *J Arthroplasty.* 1991;6(3):265.

39. Toksvig-Larsen S, Ryd L, Lindstrand A. Early inducible displacement of tibial components in total knee prostheses inserted with and without cement: a randomized study with roentgen stereophotogrammetric analysis. *J Bone Joint Surg Am.* 1998;80(1):83-89.

40. Uvehammer J, Karrholm J. Inducible displacements of cemented tibial components during weight-bearing and knee extension observations during dynamic radiostereometry related to joint positions and 2 years history of migration in 16 TKR. *J Orthop Res.* 2001; 19(6):1168.

62 Uncemented Total Knee Arthroplasty Using Porous Titanium

Aidin Eslam Pour, Peter F. Sharkey, and James B. Hept

The goal of total knee arthroplasty (TKA) is to provide pain relief and improve function in patients with osteoarthritis. Cemented TKA has been evaluated in many studies and has demonstrated good functional improvement and reasonable longevity. The usual mechanisms of failure of TKA implants include polyethylene wear, osteolysis, and loosening. TKA that has failed due to loosening may be difficult to revise because of the severity of osteolysis and poor remaining bone. The functional level after revision arthroplasty is typically not as great as after the primary procedure. For these reasons, knee replacement has been often considered a procedure for the older population with lower activity levels in order to increase the longevity of the implants. However, younger patients with degenerative or inflammatory knee arthritis who experience significant knee pain resulting in substantial decrease in functional level are not uncommon. Surgeons may be reluctant to carry out TKA in these patients, even if the only alternatives are nonoperative treatment, osteotomy, or knee fusion. Nevertheless, this young patient population often demands TKA because of the good pain relief and potential return to their normal life and work (Fig. 62-1).

A

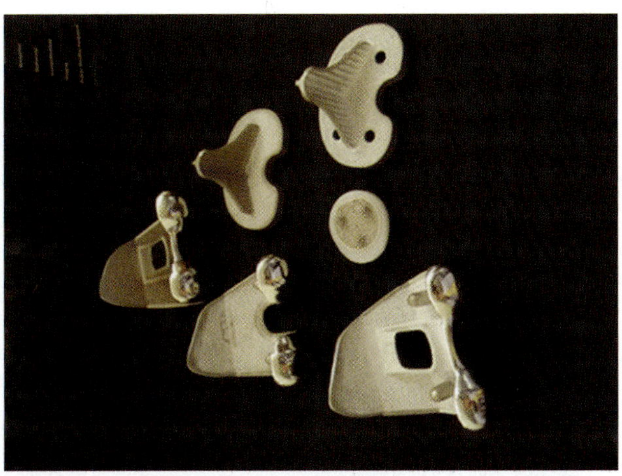

B

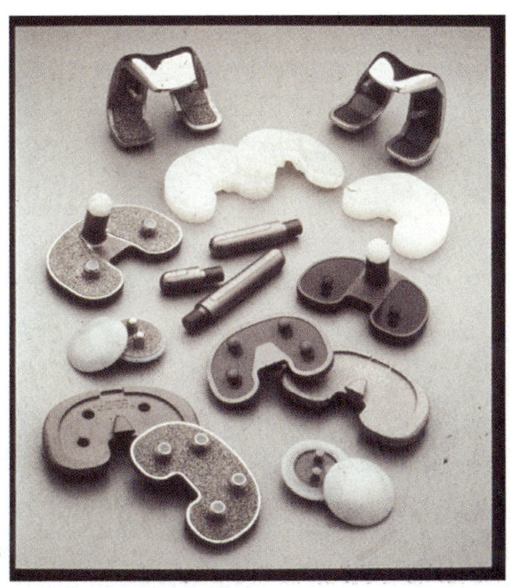

FIGURE 62-1. *(**A**) The Triathlon PS cementless knee system, beaded with Peri-Apatite. Screw fixation and non-screw fixation options available. (Compliments of Stryker Orthopaedics, Mahwah, NJ.) (**B**) The Miller-Galante cementless total knee system. (Compliments of Zimmer Orthopaedics, Warsaw, IN.)*

Prosthetic loosening is a complex phenomenon. Important factors are implant design, the polyethylene material used in production, alignment of components, the position of the implants, and cementing technique. One of the important considerations is the bone–cement interface. Methylmethacrylate is toxic to osteoblasts and osteoclasts. The exothermic reaction caused by cement causes thermal necrosis in the bone. Even in the arthroplasty with optimal cementing technique, there is a layer of fibrous tissue separating the bone and cement junction. The rate of failure due to loosening will be likely higher in a younger patient population with more activity-induced stress on the implant–cement–bone interface.

Considering the excellent results of noncemented total hip arthroplasty in long-term follow-up studies, TKA implant designers have developed and are developing cementless TKA implants as an alternative to cemented TKA implants. Many early uncemented designs were unsuccessful and there are few implants with demonstrated long-term follow-up (Table 62-1).

The most important factors in determining the longevity of an implant are quality of fixation and component durability. The major forces on a TKA implant are eccentric compression, rotational torque, and transitional shear. For long-term success, an implant must minimize stress shielding, be resistant to osteolysis, and be reproducibly implanted with sufficient initial stability to consistently achieve bone ingrowth.

The other proposed advantage of the cementless fixation is easier revision in case of loosening and infection. By removing the implant, the interface will be removed and there will be no need to remove the cement fragments. Especially, with loosening, the fibrous fixation around the implant will make extraction of the implant easier with less bone loss.

The shorter operative time might be considered another possible advantage. There is no need to wait for operation room personnel to mix the cement or cement polymerization after implantation. Also, there is less concern regarding the cement fragments around the implant needing debridement.

BIOMECHANICS AND IMPLANT DESIGN

Femoral Implant

The biomechanics and fixation of the femoral total knee implant have been studied. The survivorship of uncemented femoral implant components has been reported to be better compared with cementless tibial and patellar implants (Fig. 62-2). Studies by Walker et al[1] and Whiteside and Pafford[2] have shown that in extension the implant–bone interface around the anterior and posterior flange will undergo shear stress while weight bearing when there is strong bone–implant interface. In flexion, the bone–implant interface on the distal femur will experience high shear stress. This finding suggests that diffuse bone ingrowth, in all component regions, is critical to ensure long-term success.

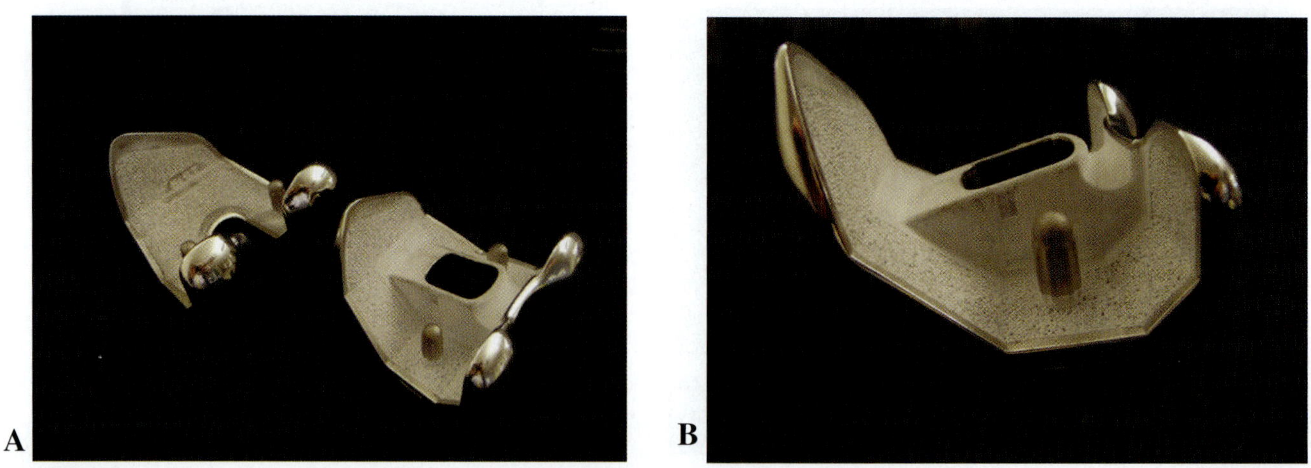

FIGURE 62-2. *The Triathlon PS femoral component, beaded with Peri-Apatite. (Compliments of Stryker Orthopaedics, Mahwah, NJ.)*

TABLE 62-1. Published Studies Reporting High Failure Rate in Cementless TKA

Author	Publication Year	Failed Implant	Implant Manufacturer
Femoral implant			
Duffy et al[42]	2007	7% failure of ingrowth of femoral implant; 6% femoral loosening with osteolysis; 3% femoral implant fracture	Hybrid fixation; press-fit condylar; Johnson and Johnson
Goldberg and Kraay[14]	2004	Osteolysis around 17% of the femoral implants	Miller-Galante I; Zimmer
Chockalingam and Scott[51]	2000	9.8% failure of femoral implant due to loosening	Freeman-Samuelson modular (Suzzer orthopaedics)
Tibial implant			
Barrack et al[38]	2004	8.2% failure of tibial implant due to loosening	Low-contact-stress mobile bearing, DePuy
Goldberg and Kraay[14]	2004	Osteolysis around 21% of the tibial implants	Miller-Galante I; Zimmer
Berger et al[24]	2001	8% failure of tibial implant due to loosening; 12% osteolysis around the tibial implant	Miller-Galante I; Zimmer
Duffy et al[52]	1998	28% failure of tibial implant due to loosening	Hybrid fixation; press fit condylar; Johnson and Johnson
Regner et al[53]	1997	11.8% failure of the tibial implant due to loosening; 22% progressive varus tilting of the tibial implants	Freeman-Samuelson modular (Suzzer orthopaedics)
Patellar implant			
Ritter and Meneghini[28]	2010	16.5% failure of metal-backed patella	AGC; Biomet
Tarkin et al[54]	2005	7% failure of metal-backed patella	Low-contact-stress mobile bearing, DePuy
Goldberg and Kraay[14]	2004	10.5% failure of metal-backed patella	Miller-Galante I; Zimmer
Kraay et al[25]	2001	21.5% failure of metal-backed patella	Miller-Galante I; Zimmer
Parker et al[40]	2001	37.4% failure of metal-backed patella	Miller-Galante I; Zimmer
Berger et al[24]	2001	48% failure of metal-backed patella; 12% femoral implant failure due to abrasion from the patellar implant	Miller-Galante I; Zimmer
Duffy et al[52]	1998	36.9% failure of metal-backed patella	Hybrid fixation; Press fit condylar; Johnson and Johnson
Lombardi et al[55]	1988	5.4% failure of metal-backed patella	Porocoat Synatomic knee system; DePuy
Stulberg et al[22]	1988	11% failure of metal-backed patella	Miller-Galante I; Zimmer

Radiolucencies around the femoral implant were studied by Kobs and Lachiewicz.[3] They evaluated 41 TKAs using hybrid Miller-Galante total knee prostheses with uncemented porous-coated femoral implants. Their study showed that only 15% of the implants had radiolucent lines. They found bone hypertrophy in 83% of the implants, which was mostly noted around the anterior flange. They concluded that extensive contact between the cancellous bone and porous-coated femoral implant surface is achieved more readily compared to the tibial implant. Compression of the implant during weight bearing consistently provided immediate stability in the early postoperative period satisfactory for bone ingrowth. Other studies have shown that a press-fit femur might also be sufficient for consistent bone ingrowth for most patients.[4,5]

Tibial Implant

The literature demonstrates that many of the failures of cementless TKA designs are secondary to the tibial implant (Fig. 62-3).[6-8] Initial fixation of the tibial implant can be

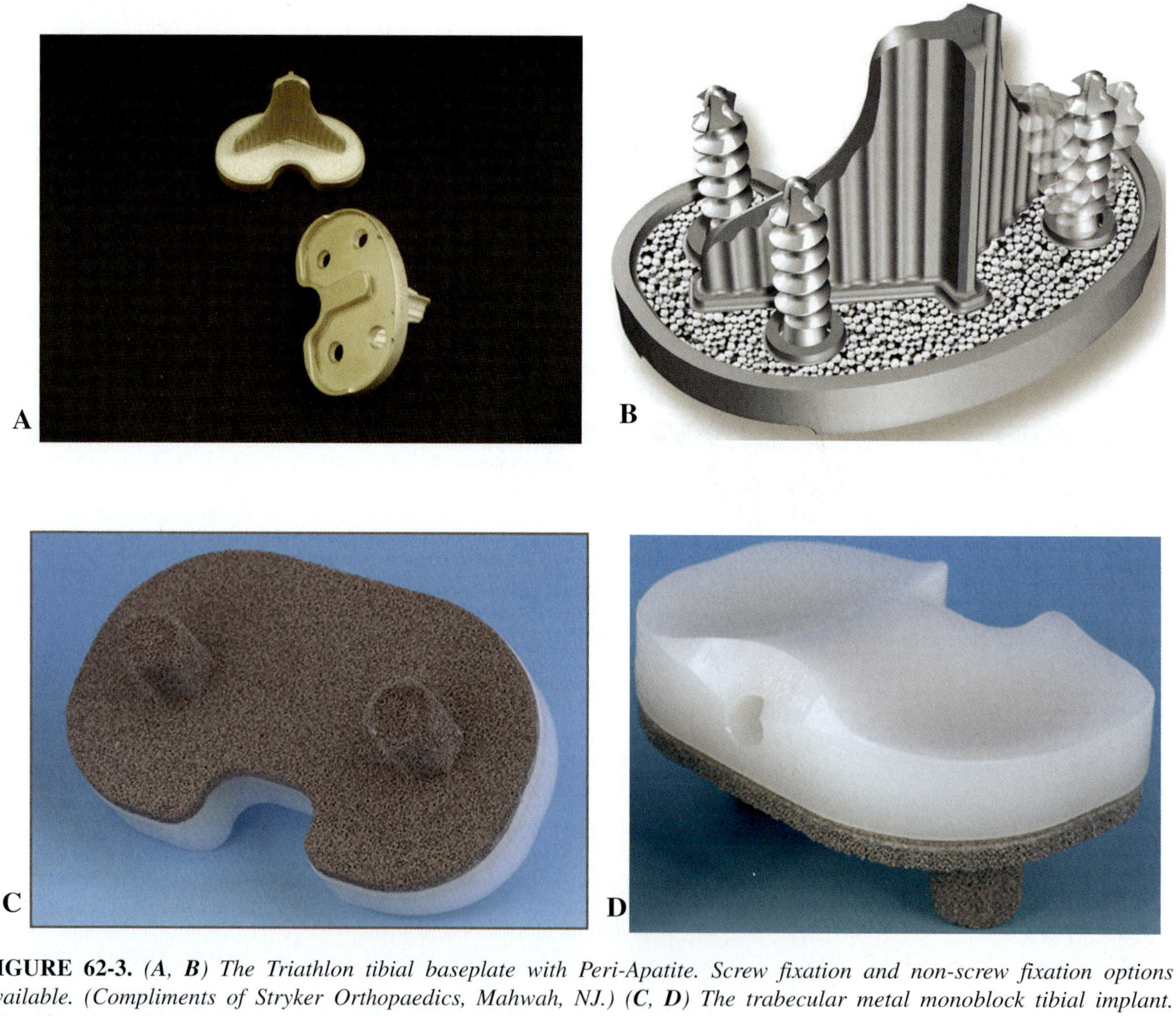

FIGURE 62-3. *(**A**, **B**) The Triathlon tibial baseplate with Peri-Apatite. Screw fixation and non-screw fixation options available. (Compliments of Stryker Orthopaedics, Mahwah, NJ.) (**C**, **D**) The trabecular metal monoblock tibial implant. (Compliments of Zimmer Orthopaedics, Warsaw, IN.)*

achieved through press fitting the stem and pegs or with screws. Hydroxyapatite coating may increase the speed of bone ingrowth into the implant surface. The surgical goal is to achieve implant initial stability leading to consistent bone ingrowth. Early full weight bearing after TKA is critical. The forces generated in the knee during weight bearing can reach as high as 3 to 4 times body weight. Any varus or valgus malalignment of the tibia coupled with sliding and rollback of the femoral implant on the tibia can cause micromotion at the bone–implant interface Excessive micromotion at the bone–implant interface can lead to failure of bone ingrowth. It has been shown that motion of more than 150 μm will compromise the bone ingrowth process.[6]

The proximal tibia surface provides little rotational stability for the tibial implant. Further, the cancellous bone of the proximal tibia inconsistently offers resistance to compressive forces.[9] The peripheral cortical bone of the tibia is of variable thickness and may not provide adequate stability either.[10-12]

Volz et al[6] studied four different designs of uncemented TKA components. They found that tibial implants fixed with four screws placed peripherally in the four quadrants of the tibial plateau had the highest stability, and the least stability was found with a 2-peg design. Miura et al also showed the benefits of screws for enhancing in the initial fixation of the tibia implant. They compared implants with and without supplemental screw fixation and found that addition of screws reduced liftoff by more than 90%.[13] Other authors reported better implant–bone contact with use of screws.[14] Implants with central stems decrease side-to-side toggle of the implant while weight bearing, but using a stem may result in stress shielding of the proximal tibia.[8] For this reason, a shorter stem is often used. Depending on the tibial cut, the forces applied to the implant with or without a central stem may result in liftoff contralateral to compressive forces, resulting in bone ingrowth failure and implant subsidence. Despite these biomechanical findings, other authors have shown good and consistent medium-term survival of uncemented tibial implants with pegs with or without supplemental screw fixation.[15-18]

An important consideration is the variable bone quality of the proximal tibia. It has been shown that the strength of bone in a surgically prepared proximal tibia is lowest in the anterolateral and intercondylar regions of the tibia.[19] This inconsistent bone quality provides emphasis on the importance of achieving rim fit and using implants with supplemental fixation (stem, pegs, and/or screws) when performing TKA with uncemented tibial components.

The material used for implant production is another important issue. Implants with lower modulus of elasticity may bend and thus increase micromotion of the implant.[13] Bending can be reduced by using materials with higher modulus of elasticity or different implant design in the form of a thicker tibial tray; however, these changes likely would increase stress shielding. The optimal design, which balances these competing considerations, has not been clinically determined.

Patellar Implant

To perform uncemented patellar resurfacing, a component of metal–polyethylene composite has been designed (Fig. 62-4). Historically, the hostile biomechanical requirements of the patellofemoral articulation have proven challenging to implant designers. Theoretically, a metal-backed patellar component provides uniform load distribution to the underlying patellar bone. However, metal backing results in reduced polyethylene thickness, which causes increased wear, particulate debris, and finally, after wear, metal-on-metal articulation and metal-induced synovitis.[20,21] Another problem with uncemented patella fixation is that high shear stresses on bone–implant interface can lead to peg fracture.[22,23] The failure rate of metal-backed patellar implants has been reported to be up to 50%.[24] A newer generation of metal-backed patellar implants has been reported to have better outcome.[25] One design is composed of an anatomically shaped polyethylene that can rotate freely on a polished baseplate. The implantation technique for an uncemented patella is more demanding and requires accurate bone preparation. Also, greater patellar bone loss or patellar fracture may be encountered when revising an uncemented patella.[14,26]

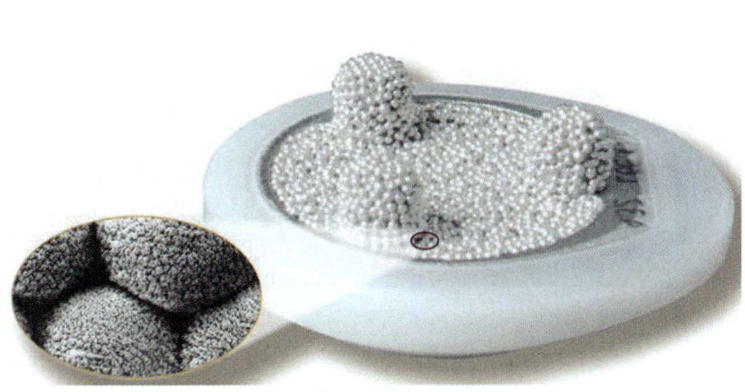

FIGURE 62-4. *The Triathlon metal-backed patella along with Peri-Apatite. (Compliments of Stryker Orthopaedics, Mahwah, NJ.)*

DESIGNING A CEMENTLESS TOTAL KNEE IMPLANT: AN ENGINEERING VIEW

When designing a cementless knee, it is important to address both long-term fixation and initial implant stability. Initial fixation is affected by several factors, including the geometry and fixation features that are in direct apposition to the bone, as well as the articulation and kinematics of the knee system itself (Fig. 62-5).

In the case of cementless femurs, a press fit onto the resected distal femur along with ancillary fixation pegs has proven successful in limiting micromotion, allowing for bone ingrowth and reliable long-term fixation. Unfortunately, cementless tibial components have not enjoyed the same clinical success.

Since the tibial component is placed on a single, planar cut, it is more susceptible to micromotion due to the load transferred through the bone–implant interface. In order to minimize this motion, the implant needs to have sufficient load-carrying capabilities. Optimally, the underside of the tibial baseplate would feature a keel shape, which resists torsional loads. Additionally, peripherally placed, supplemental fixation pegs underneath the tibial baseplate would minimize rocking. Equally as important is optimal kinematics to limit the torsional and anteroposterior loading of the tibial component. An implant system that allows the soft tissues to guide the motion of the knee inherently limits the torsional stresses being transferred to the implants. Moreover, an implant geometry that limits instability throughout the range of motion will prevent excessive anteroposterior shifting of the femoral-tibial contact point and subsequently the axial load.

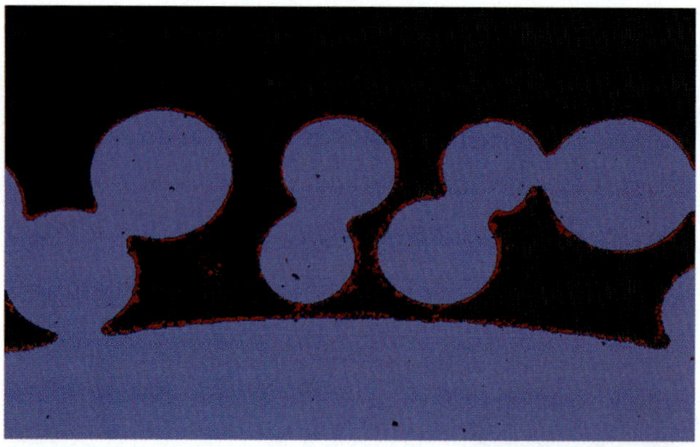

FIGURE 62-5. *A 360° coverage with Peri-Apatite (PA) hydroxyapatite (HA). The attached image depicts the distinct advantage of the PA technique. PA uniformly wraps itself around the circumference of the porous surface, increasing the HA surface available for potential fixation.*[1] *(Compliments of Stryker Orthopaedics, Mahwah, NJ.)*

Another important consideration when designing a cementless knee is the performance of the polyethylene in the metal-backed patellar component. Although metal-backed patellar components have historically demonstrated reliable ingrowth, the performance of the bearing surface has not been as successful. The most common mechanisms of failure for metal-backed patellar components were disassociation of the polyethylene from the metal backing and excessive polyethylene wear. These failures were driven by high stresses in the patella articulation due to poor patellofemoral track designs, relatively thin polyethylene that results from the use of a metal backing, and the shortcomings of early polyethylenes. These failure modes can be addressed through the advent of high-performance polyethylenes, as well as through the design of the patellofemoral articulation. Ideally, a laterally flared, anatomic patella track that is relatively open in extension will guide the patella into a deepened trochlear groove through flexion. This would minimize the shear forces on the patella, thereby limiting the shear stresses between the polyethylene and metal backing. Also, the use of a polyethylene material that demonstrates excellent mechanical properties, increased wear resistance, and high oxidation resistance is a crucial consideration for a successful metal-backed patellar component design.

An additional consideration when designing a cementless knee is the ingrowth architecture itself. Specific aspects to consider when developing the osseointegration architecture include the percent porosity, pore size, and coefficient of friction of the ingrowth material itself. Biologic fixation will be improved through the use of newly developed biomaterials, such as highly porous metals, specifically titanium and tantalum.

In summary, the design of a successful cementless knee relies not only on the geometry of the implants that are implanted into the resected bone, but also on the kinematics of the knee system. Therefore, to maximize long-term biologic fixation and clinical success, an ideal cementless knee platform should

- Optimize the load-carrying geometry of the tibial component through the use of a keel and fixation pegs;
- Provide freedom of internal and external rotation and consistent ligamentous stability throughout the range of motion to minimize torsional loads and anteroposterior load shifting;

- Incorporate a laterally flared, anatomic patellofemoral track that minimizes shear stresses in the patellar component;
- Incorporate a highly porous, biofriendly material to maximize biologic fixation; and
- Utilize a highly cross-linked polyethylene to minimize polyethylene wear.

The incorporation of these key tenants should lead to more successful cementless total knee replacements.

CLINICAL RESULTS

Since the introduction of cementless TKA, many implants have been designed and studied (Figs. 62-6 and 62-7). There has been substantial improvement in implant design and survival rates. Eriksen et al[27] published a 20-year follow-up with results for 102 patients who underwent TKA with a cementless AGC 2000 prosthesis (Biomet, Warsaw, IN). They reported an 84.4% survival rate for all components, and the revision in their patient population

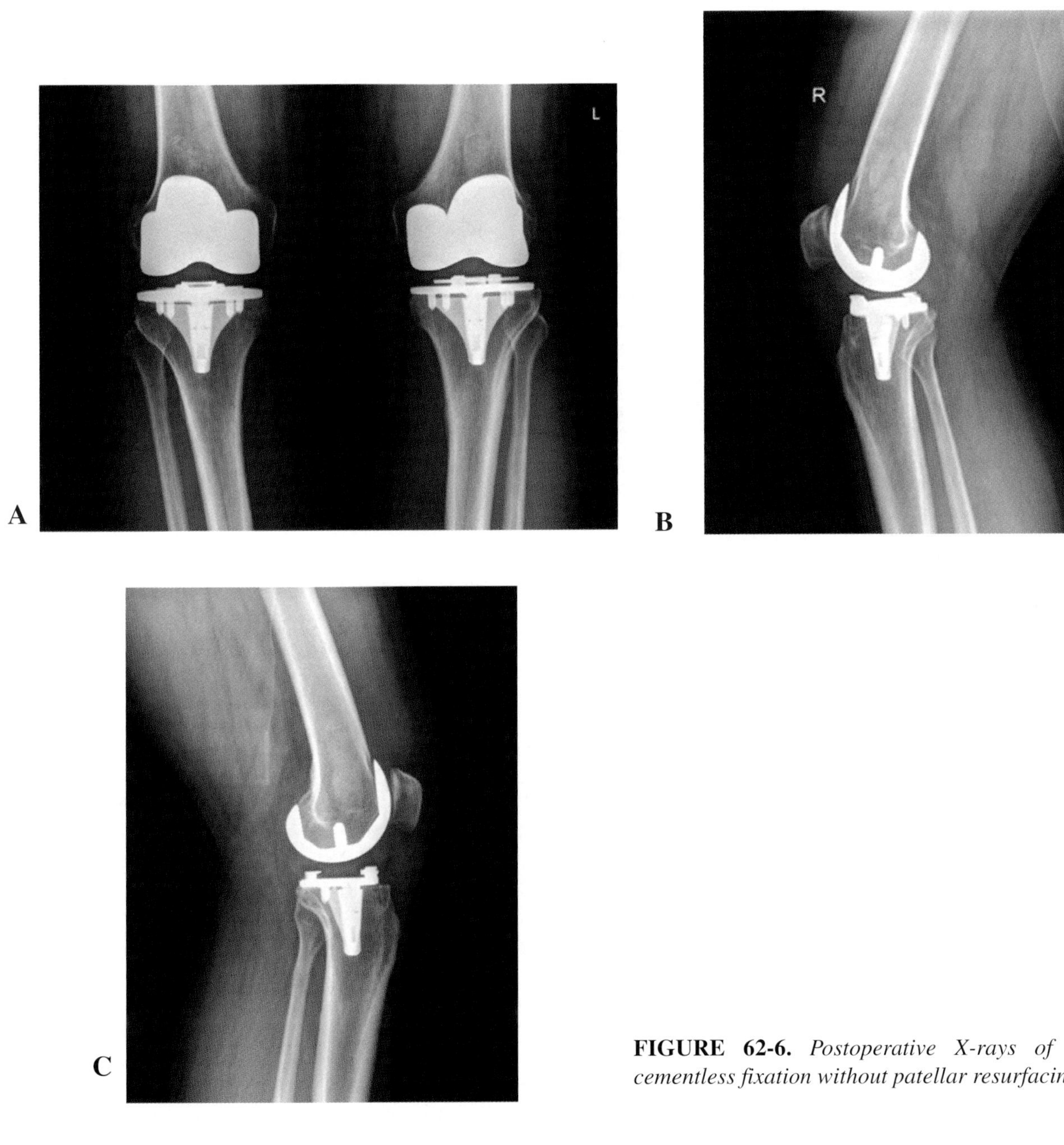

FIGURE 62-6. *Postoperative X-rays of TKA with cementless fixation without patellar resurfacing.*

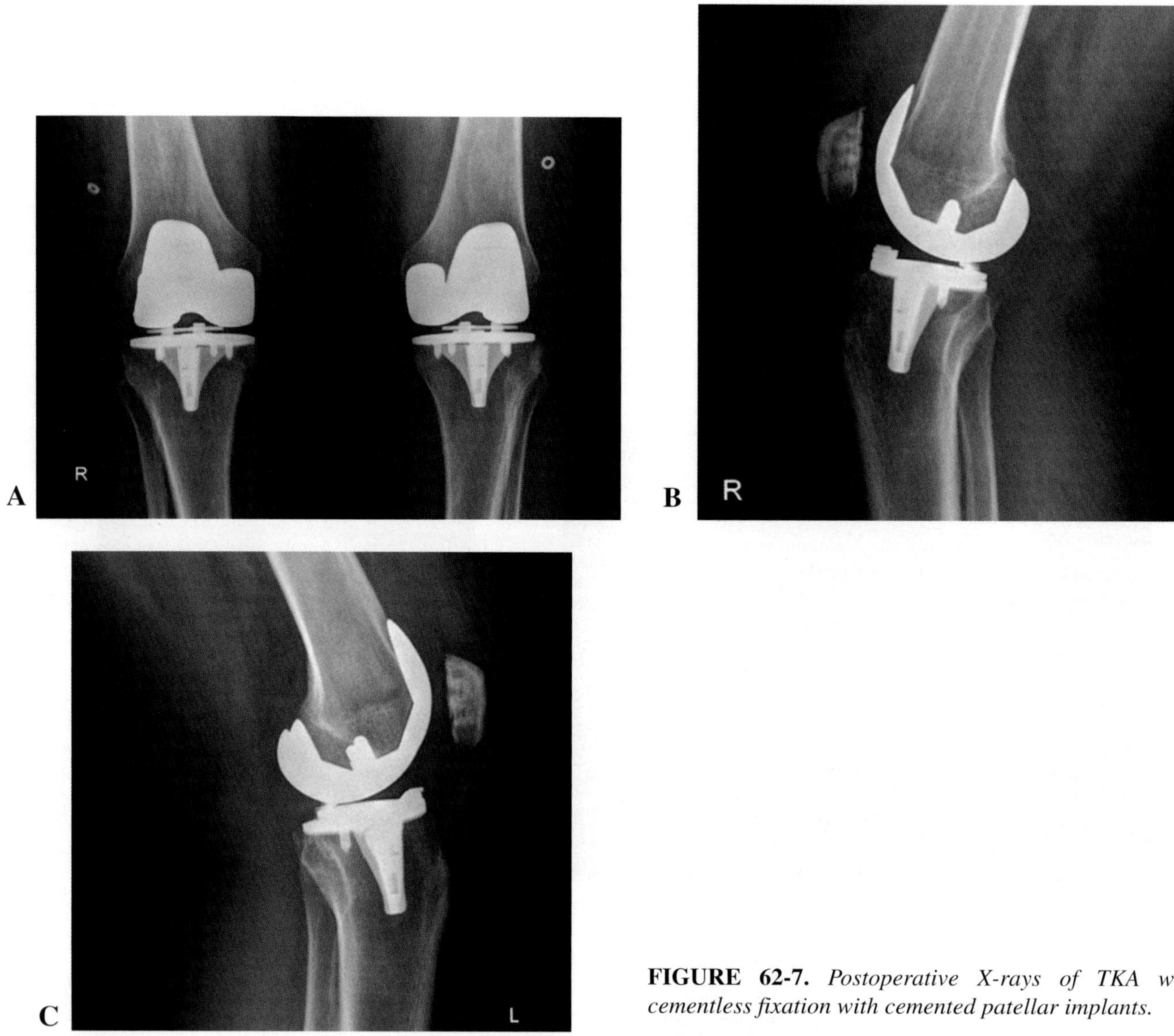

FIGURE 62-7. *Postoperative X-rays of TKA with cementless fixation with cemented patellar implants.*

was predominantly secondary to early tibial and late patellar implant failure. The survival rates for the femoral and tibial implants were 100% and 97.2%, respectively. Similar results have been reported by Ritter and Meneghini.[28] Most of the failures in Ritters's study were reported to be secondary to the metal-backed patellar implant and the survivorship, including and excluding the patellar implant, was 76.4% and 96.8%, respectively, at 20-year follow-up. Chana et al[29] reported 98.6% survival for a cementless hydroxyapatite-coated Duracon implant (Stryker, Mahwah, NJ) and reported tibial plate subsidence in 1 of 219 knees. They also found that all radiographic gaps visible at the bone–implant interface on initial postoperative radiographic evaluation resolved substantially over the first year following surgery. In a recent study, Baker et al[30] randomized 501 primary TKAs for comparison of cemented and cementless knee replacement. The 15-year survival rate for cemented and cementless fixation was 80.7% and 75.3%, respectively, which was not significantly different. Interestingly, they reported a higher failure rate for male patients using cementless fixation. In another randomized study, Beaupre et al[31] compared a hydroxyapatite-coated tibial implant (Scorpio, Stryker, Mahawah, NJ) with a cemented component in 81 patients and found no difference in functional outcome or failure rate of the implant at 5-year follow-up. Cross and Parish[32] published the outcome of cementless fixation in 1000 consecutive hydroxyapatite-coated cementless TKAs. They reported a 0.5% failure rate primarily due to periprosthetic infection. The survival rate, with revision as the end point at 10-year follow-up, was reported to be 99%.

Rotating Platform TKA with Cementless Fixation

The outcome of cementless rotating platform TKA designs has also been studied. This tibial design theoretically decreases the stress on the bone–implant interface. Efstathopoulos et al[33] reported 98% survival of cementless low-contact-stress rotating platform total knee implant in 423 TKAs in 10-year follow-up. In this series, patella resurfacing with a metal-backed patellar implant was not performed. Sansone et al[34] reported a 93.7% survival rate for cementless fixation of a mobile-bearing total knee inplant in 110 TKAs in an average 6-year follow-up. The main causes of failure in their study were aseptic loosening of the tibial implant and dislocation of the rotating polyethylene. Similar results have been reported by other investigators.[35-37] Conversely, Barrack et al[38] compared a cemented and cementless mobile-bearing total knee implant and found substantially higher subsidence and loosening rates in the cementless fixation group (8% vs. 0%) at a minimum 2-year follow-up.

Hybrid Fixation

Hybrid fixation (uncemented femur and cemented tibia) of TKA implants has also been studied. Wright et al[39] reported good to excellent outcomes with midterm follow-up using a hybrid fixation technique. The only mechanical failure in their study was secondary to loosening of a metal-backed patellar implant. Kobs and Lachiewicz[3] reported 88% good to excellent results in their patients who underwent hybrid TKA with midterm follow-up. The main cause of failure in their study was patellar component fracture requiring revision. In a randomized study, Parker et al[40] compared the cemented and hybrid cementless implants and found equivalent results if a metal-backed patellar implant was excluded. Similar results have been reported in other studies.[41] However, Duffy et al[42] followed 65 consecutive patients who underwent hybrid TKA with 15-year follow-up. They reported a 27% revision rate for the femoral implant. The main cause of failure was loosening. Also, they reported two femoral implant fractures.

Younger Patient Population

The outcome of cementless fixation has also been studied in a younger patient population. In this patient population the stress on the implant–bone interface is likely higher when compared to an older and more sedentary population. Nilsson et al[43] published the results of 97 TKAs in patients younger than 65. They randomized the patients into three groups to include cemented fixation, cementless fixation with screws, and cementless fixation without screws. They found more implant migration in the uncemented group during the first 3 months after surgery and there was no difference between the screw fixation and screwless implant design. One uncemented tibial tray migrated enough to require revision. Tai and Cross[44] reported 97.5% survival of cementless components, excluding infection, at 12-year follow-up for patients who were younger than 55 at the index procedure. The main causes of failure in their series was infection, tibial baseplate loosening, and polyethylene wear. Both studies concluded that uncemented knee arthroplasty is an acceptable option for a younger patient population. In another study, Hofmann et al[45] studied the outcomes of cementless TKA in 57 patients younger than 50 years old. They found no implant loosening and failure and the main reason for reoperation was infection. Lyback et al[46] reported good to excellent outcome in 77 cementless TKAs in patoents with an average age of 33 (range 16-64) with survival rate of 99% at 5 years.

Rheumatoid Arthritis Patients

The medium- and long-term survival of uncemented total knee implants has been studied in rheumatoid arthritis patients. Woo et al[47] reported successful results at 10-year follow-up with uncemented TKA in this population. Schroder et al[48] investigated the outcome of 51 cementless TKAs in rheumatoid patients. The medium follow-up time was 54 months. They reported one tibial component had loosened and a 97% implant survival rate in this population. Similar results have been reported in other studies.[49,50]

CONCLUSION

Cementless TKA was introduced to the orthopaedic society about 3 decades ago (Figs. 62-8 and 62-9). The proposed advantages of this type of fixation are improved longevity of the implant, especially in younger patients, shorter operation time, and possibly easier revision arthroplasty. The clinical outcome of cementless TKA is a combination of success and failure. As the understanding of the knee biomechanics, biomaterials, bone ingrowth, and implant design improves, engineers can produce better implants with less failure and better longevity. The newer designs of the cementless TKA implants have successful medium- to long-term results that are nearly equal to cemented TKA as the current gold standard. Orthopaedic surgeons should choose the implants they use in surgery based on the evidence in the literature supporting their use.

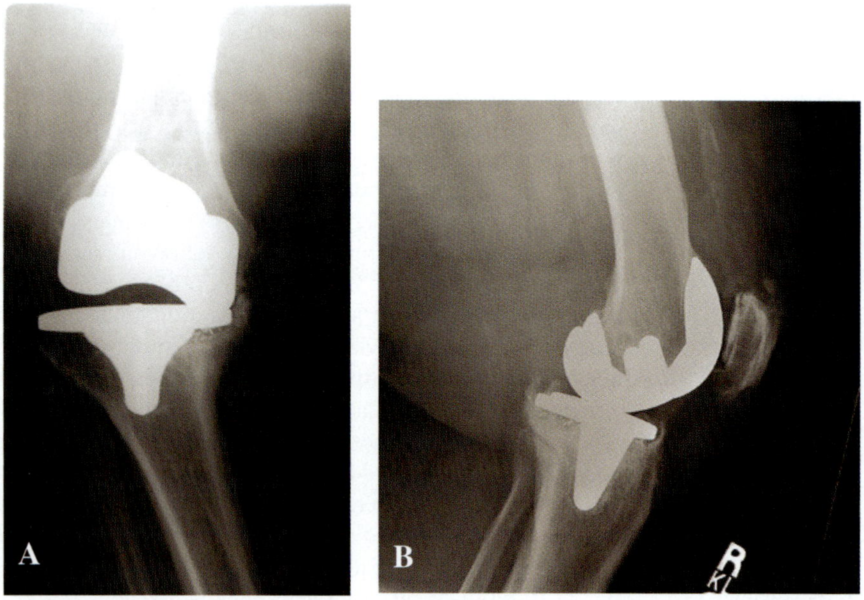

FIGURE 62-8. *Postoperative X-rays of TKA with cementless fixation. Patient was found to have loosening and subsidence of the tibial implant with significant osteolysis 6 years after surgery, requiring revision TKA. (Courtesy of Greg A. Erens, MD.)*

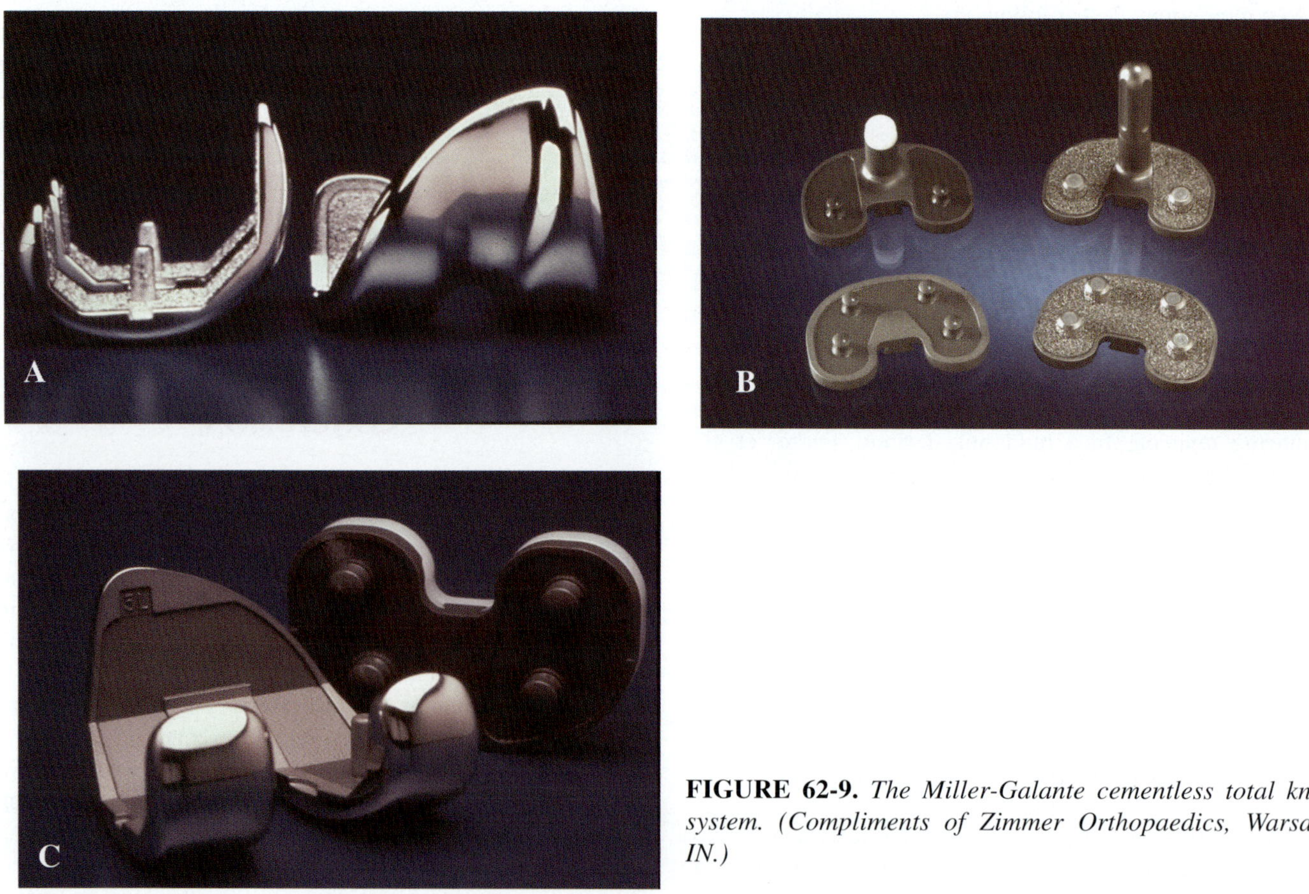

FIGURE 62-9. *The Miller-Galante cementless total knee system. (Compliments of Zimmer Orthopaedics, Warsaw, IN.)*

SUGGESTED READING

Lombardi AV, Berasi CC, Berend KR. Evolution of tibial fixation in total knee arthroplasty. *J Arthroplasty.* 2007;22(4 suppl 1):25-29.

Rand RJ, Trousdale RT. Factors affecting the durability of total knee arthroplasty. *J Bone Joint Surg Am.* 2003; 85:259-265.

Stiehl JB. Clinical results and complications in mobile bearing total knee arthroplasty. *Instr Course Lect.* 2005; 54:233-240.

REFERENCES

1. Walker PS, Granholm J, Lowrey R. The fixation of femoral components of condylar knee prostheses. *Eng Med.* 1982;11:135-140.
2. Whiteside LA, Pafford J. Load transfer characteristics of a noncemented total knee arthroplasty. *Clin Orthop Relat Res.* 1989;239:168-177.
3. Kobs JK, Lachiewicz PF. Hybrid total knee arthroplasty. Two- to five-year results using the Miller-Galante prosthesis. *Clin Orthop Relat Res.* 1993;286:78-87.
4. Freeman MA, McLeod HC, Levai JP. Cementless fixation of prosthetic components in total arthroplasty of the knee and hip. *Clin Orthop Relat Res.* 1983;176: 88-94.
5. Freeman MA, Samuelson KM, Bertin KC. Freeman-Samuelson total arthroplasty of the knee. *Clin Orthop Relat Res.* 1985;192:46-58.
6. Volz RG, Nisbet JK, Lee RW, et al. The mechanical stability of various noncemented tibial components. *Clin Orthop Relat Res.* 1988;226:38-42.
7. Reilly D, Walker PS, Ben-Dov M, et al. Effects of tibial components on load transfer in the upper tibia. *Clin Orthop Relat Res.* 1982;165:273-82.
8. Murase K, Crowninshield RD, Pedersen DR, et al. An analysis of tibial component design in total knee arthroplasty. *J Biomech.* 1983;16:13-22.
9. Johnson JA. An evaluation of the load bearing capibility of the cancellous proximal tibia with special interest in the design of the knee implants. *Trans Orthop Res Soc.* 1983;8:403.
10. Walker PS, Greene D, Reilly D, et al. Fixation of tibial components of knee prostheses. *J Bone Joint Surg Am.* 1981;63:258-267.
11. Walker PS, Hajek JV. The load-bearing area in the knee joint. *J Biomech.* 1972;5:581-589.
12. Walker PS, Soudry M, Ewald FC, et al. Control of cement penetration in total knee arthroplasty. *Clin Orthop Relat Res.* 1984;184:155-164.
13. Miura H, Whiteside LA, Easley JC, et al. Effects of screws and a sleeve on initial fixation in uncemented total knee tibial components. *Clin Orthop Relat Res.* 1990;259:160-168.
14. Goldberg VM, Kraay M. The outcome of the cementless tibial component: a minimum 14-year clinical evaluation. *Clin Orthop Relat Res.* 2004;428:214-20.
15. Schepers A, Cullingworth L, van der Jagt DR. A prospective randomized clinical trial comparing tibial baseplate fixation with or without screws in total knee arthroplasty a radiographic evaluation. *J Arthroplasty.* May 27, 2011 [Epub ahead of print].
16. Stilling M, Madsen F, Odgaard A, et al. Superior fixation of pegged trabecular metal over screw-fixed pegged porous titanium fiber mesh: a randomized clinical RSA study on cementless tibial components. *Acta Orthop.* 2011;82:177-186.
17. Ferguson RP, Friederichs MG, Hofmann AA. Comparison of screw and screwless fixation in cementless total knee arthroplasty. *Orthopedics.* 2008;31:127.
18. Cooke C, Walter WK, Zicat B. Tibial fixation without screws in cementless total knee arthroplasty. *J Arthroplasty.* 2006;21:237-241.
19. Hvid I, Hansen SL. Trabecular bone strength patterns at the proximal tibial epiphysis. *J Orthop Res.* 1985; 3:464-472.
20. Buechel FF, Pappas MJ, Makris G. Evaluation of contact stress in metal-backed patellar replacements. A predictor of survivorship. *Clin Orthop Relat Res.* 1991;273:190-197.
21. Bartel DL, Bicknell VL, Wright TM. The effect of conformity, thickness, and material on stresses in ultra-high molecular weight components for total joint replacement. *J Bone Joint Surg Am.* 1986;68: 1041-1051.
22. Stulberg SD, Stulberg BN, Hamati Y, et al. Failure mechanisms of metal-backed patellar components. *Clin Orthop Relat Res.* 1988;236:88-105.
23. Rosenberg AG, Andriacchi TP, Barden R, et al. Patellar component failure in cementless total knee arthroplasty. *Clin Orthop Relat Res.* 1988;236:106-114.
24. Berger RA, Lyon JH, Jacobs JJ, et al. Problems with cementless total knee arthroplasty at 11 years followup. *Clin Orthop Relat Res.* 2001;392:196-207.

25. Kraay MJ, Darr OJ, Salata MJ, et al. Outcome of metal-backed cementless patellar components: the effect of implant design. *Clin Orthop Relat Res*. 2001; 392:239-244.
26. Sundfeldt M, Johansson CB, Regner L, et al. Long-term results of a cementless knee prosthesis with a metal-backed patellar component: clinical and radiological follow-up with histology from retrieved components. *J Long-Term Effects Med Implants*. 2003;13:341-354.
27. Eriksen J, Christensen J, Solgaard S, et al. The cementless AGC 2000 knee prosthesis: 20-year results in a consecutive series. *Acta Orthop Belg*. 2009;75:225-233.
28. Ritter MA, Meneghini RM. Twenty-year survivorship of cementless anatomic graduated component total knee arthroplasty. *J Arthroplasty*. 2010;25:507-513.
29. Chana R, Shenava Y, Nicholl AP, et al. Five- to 8-year results of the uncemented Duracon total knee arthroplasty system. *J Arthroplasty*. 2008;23:677-682.
30. Baker PN, Khaw FM, Kirk LM, et al. A randomised controlled trial of cemented versus cementless press-fit condylar total knee replacement: 15-year survival analysis. *J Bone Joint Surg Br*. 2007;89:1608-1614.
31. Beaupre LA, al-Yamani M, Huckell JR, et al. Hydroxyapatite-coated tibial implants compared with cemented tibial fixation in primary total knee arthroplasty. A randomized trial of outcomes at five years. *J Bone Joint Surg Am*. 2007;89:2204-2211.
32. Cross MJ, Parish EN. A hydroxyapatite-coated total knee replacement: prospective analysis of 1000 patients. *J Bone Joint Surg Br*. 2005;87:1073-1076.
33. Efstathopoulos N, Mavrogenis AF, Lallos S, et al. 10-year evaluation of the cementless low-contact-stress rotating-platform total knee arthroplasty. *J Long-Term Effects Med Implants*. 2009;19:255-263.
34. Sansone V, da Gama MM. Mobile-bearing total knee prosthesis: a 5- to 9-year follow-up of the first 110 consecutive arthroplasties. *J Arthroplasty*. 2004;19: 678-685.
35. Buechel FF Sr, Buechel FF Jr, Pappas MJ, et al. Twenty-year evaluation of meniscal bearing and rotating platform knee replacements. *Clin Orthop Relat Res*. 2001;388:41-50.
36. Buechel FF Sr, Buechel FF Jr, Pappas MJ, et al. Twenty-year evaluation of the New Jersey LCS rotating platform knee replacement. *J Knee Surg*. 2002;15:84-89.
37. Jordan LR, Olivo JL, Voorhorst PE. Survivorship analysis of cementless meniscal bearing total knee arthroplasty. *Clin Orthop Relat Res*. 1997;338:119-123.
38. Barrack RL, Nakamura SJ, Hopkins SG, et al. Early failure of cementless mobile-bearing total knee arthroplasty. *J Arthroplasty*. 2004;19:101-106.
39. Wright RJ, Lima J, Scott RD, et al. Two- to four-year results of posterior cruciate-sparing condylar total knee arthroplasty with an uncemented femoral component. *Clin Orthop Relat Res*. 1990;260:80-86.
40. Parker DA, Rorabeck CH, Bourne RB. Long-term followup of cementless versus hybrid fixation for total knee arthroplasty. *Clin Orthop Relat Res*. 2001;388:68-76.
41. Illgen R, Tueting J, Enright T, et al. Hybrid total knee arthroplasty: a retrospective analysis of clinical and radiographic outcomes at average 10 years follow-up. *J Arthroplasty*. 2004;19:95-100.
42. Duffy GP, Murray BE, Trousdale RR. Hybrid total knee arthroplasty analysis of component failures at an average of 15 years. *J Arthroplasty*. 2007;22:1112-1115.
43. Nilsson KG, Henricson A, Norgren B, et al. Uncemented HA-coated implant is the optimum fixation for TKA in the young patient. *Clin Orthop Relat Res*. 2006;448:129-139.
44. Tai CC, Cross MJ. Five- to 12-year follow-up of a hydroxyapatite-coated, cementless total knee replacement in young, active patients. *J Bone Joint Surg Br*. 2006;88:1158-1163.
45. Hofmann AA, Heithoff SM, Camargo M. Cementless total knee arthroplasty in patients 50 years or younger. *Clin Orthop Relat Res*. 2002;404:102-107.
46. Lyback CO, Belt EA, Hamalainen MM, et al. Survivorship of AGC knee replacement in juvenile chronic arthritis: 13-year follow-up of 77 knees. *J Arthroplasty*. 2000;15:166-170.
47. Woo YK, Kim KW, Chung JW, et al. Average 10.1-year follow-up of cementless total knee arthroplasty in patients with rheumatoid arthritis. *Can J Surg*. 2011;54:179-184.
48. Schroder HM, Aaen K, Hansen EB, et al. Cementless total knee arthroplasty in rheumatoid arthritis. A report on 51 AGC knees followed for 54 months. *J Arthroplasty*. 1996;11:18-23.
49. Armstrong RA, Whiteside LA. Results of cementless total knee arthroplasty in an older rheumatoid arthritis population. *J Arthroplasty*. 1991;6:357-362.
50. Stuchin SA, Ruoff M, Matarese W. Cementless total knee arthroplasty in patients with inflammatory

arthritis and compromised bone. *Clin Orthop Relat Res*. 1991;273:42-51.

51. Chockalingam S, Scott G. The outcome of cemented vs. cementless fixation of a femoral component in total knee replacement (TKR) with the identification of radiological signs for the prediction of failure. *Knee*. 2000;7:233-238.

52. Duffy GP, Berry DJ, Rand JA. Cement versus cementless fixation in total knee arthroplasty. *Clin Orthop Relat Res*. 1998;356:66-72.

53. Regner L, Carlsson L, Karrholm J, et al. Clinical and radiologic survivorship of cementless tibial components fixed with finned polyethylene pegs. *J Arthroplasty*. 1997;12:751-758.

54. Tarkin IS, Bridgeman JT, Jardon OM, et al. Successful biologic fixation with mobile-bearing total knee arthroplasty. *J Arthroplasty*. 2005;20:481-486.

55. Lombardi AV Jr, Engh GA, Volz RG, et al. Fracture/dissociation of the polyethylene in metal-backed patellar components in total knee arthroplasty. *J Bone Joint Surg Am*. 1988;70:675-679.

63 Total Knee Arthroplasty for Varus Knee

Jiying Chen and Yan Wang

Varus deformity of the knee, by definition, means inversion of the tibia relative to the femur. The mechanical axis migrates medially from the center of the knee and the medial compartment is overloaded (Fig. 63-1A). Varus deformity is much more prevalent among patients with knee osteoarthritis who undergo total knee arthroplasty (TKA) than valgus deformity. Varus knee is usually classified according to the severity of the deformity, but there are no unanimously accepted criteria. Extra-articular deformity, either developmental or traumatic, as a special form of varus knee, usually can be corrected through proper intra-articular bone resection and soft tissue balance. Navigation is helpful for some of these cases. The goal of TKA for varus knee is to replace the damaged joint (surface), but to maintain acceptable soft tissue balance and correct the malalignment. A constrained prosthesis may be indicated when balance or stability is in doubt.

PREOPERATIVE EVALUATION

History and Examination

Most varus deformities of the knee are caused by osteoarthritis (OA). With the wear and loss of the medial meniscus, articular cartilage, and bone, the varus deformity occurs. The deformity usually steadily deteriorates and long-standing malalignment usually causes medial soft tissue contracture with or without laxity of the lateral soft tissue envelope.[1,2] Extra-articular deformity caused by dysplasia, rickets, or fracture malunion constitutes special forms of varus knees, which are discussed more extensively in other chapters.

Before operation, a careful physical examination of the knee should be made. Routine items such as lower limb alignment, gait, tenderness, range of motion, and stability must be assessed. The overall leg alignment is assessed in the weight-bearing position; the degree of the varus deformity is also noted. Furthermore, flexion contracture may coexist with varus deformity, which can be reflected by the range of motion. Apart from these examinations of the knee, particular attention should be paid to the special test for varus knee.[3]

Tilting of knee with single-leg stance

Medial compartment OA may cause a varus tilt when the knee is close to full extension. This is best appreciated from behind the patient in contrast to lateral compartment OA, which may cause a valgus tilt and is best appreciated from in front of the patient.

Valgus stress test (for medial collateral ligament)

This examination should be performed at 30° of flexion. If the deformity can be corrected by the valgus stress test, it suggests that the varus deformity is mainly caused by erosion of cartilage and bone, and there is little adaptive ligamentous change. If the deformity cannot be corrected, it usually means that the medial structure is contracted. This type of deformity is also called fixed varus knee.

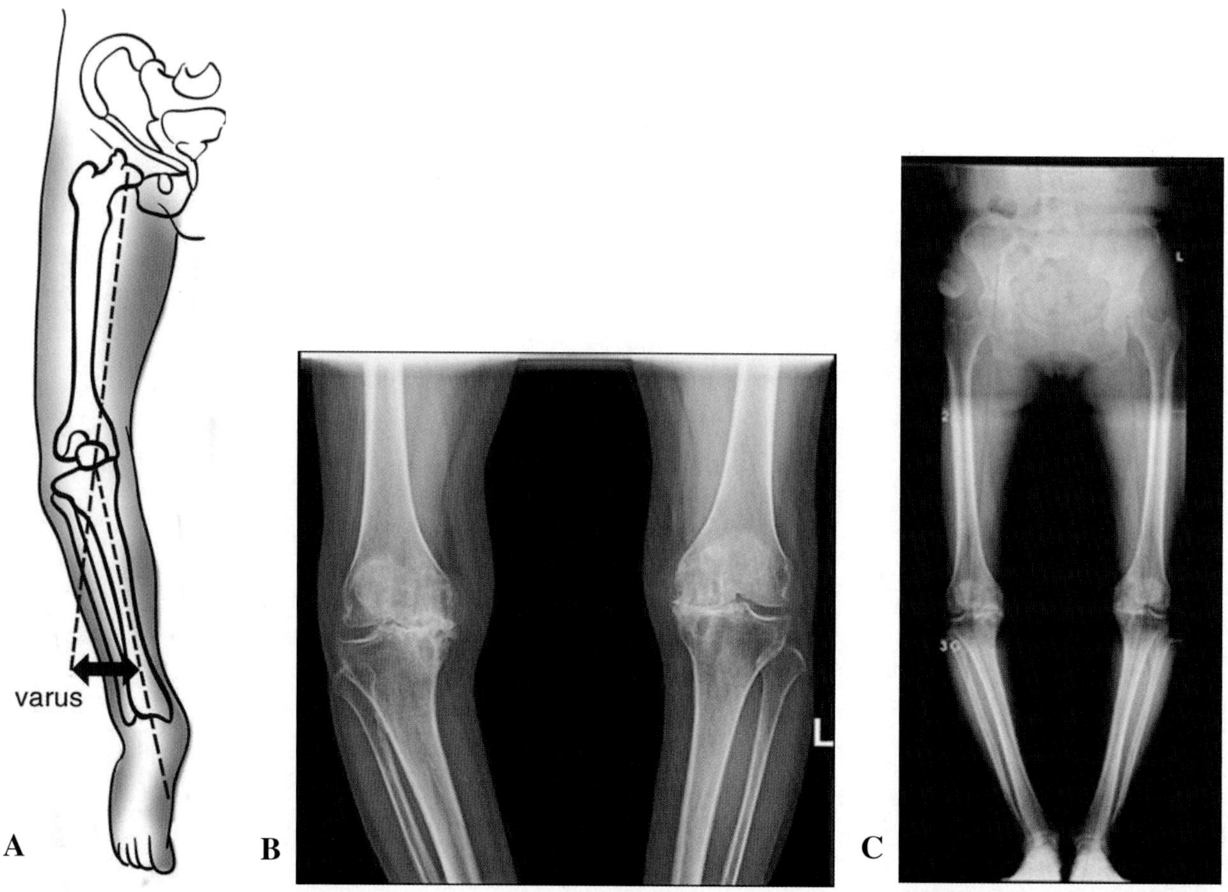

FIGURE 63-1. *(**A**) Illustration of the deformity of varus knee. (**B**) Weight-bearing anteroposterior view of the varus knee on plain radiographs. (**C**) A full-length standing hip-to-ankle view showing the overall alignment of lower extremity.*

Varus stress test (for lateral collateral ligament)

This test, also performed at 30° of flexion, is useful to assess the laxity of lateral collateral ligament (LCL).

Imaging

Much information can be acquired from plain radiographs. Detailed preoperative radiographs, including weight-bearing anteroposterior (AP), lateral, a full-length standing hip-to-ankle view, and some other special positional radiographs, should be made for accurate preoperative assessment.[3]

Weight-bearing radiographs are helpful in the assessment of the degrees of varus deformity, erosion of cartilage, bone defect, and the laxity of the LCL (Fig. 63-1B). The lateral radiographs could help to show the position of the patella, the medial laxity relative to the notch, the position and depth of the tibial defects, and the magnitude of the posterior osteophytes.

The full-length standing hip-to-ankle view shows the overall alignment and mechanical axis of the lower extremity, revealing any bowing of the tibia or femur (Fig. 63-1C). The centers of the hip, the femoral notch, and the ankle can be identified and the hip-knee-ankle (HKA) angle can be measured. Additionally, the mechanical tibial angle (MTA), the mechanical femoral angle (MFA), and the hip-knee-shaft (HKS) angle can also be recorded. MTA is the medial angle between the mechanical axis of the tibia and a line tangential to the tibial plateau. MFA is the medial angle between the mechanical axis of the femur and a line tangential to the distal femoral condyles. HKS is the angle between the mechanical axis and the femoral medullary axis, which is helpful in setting the valgus angle of the distal femoral cut.

Coronal stress radiographs may be helpful in determining ligament integrity and predicting the difficulty in correcting deformity and balancing soft tissue intra-operatively.

PREPARATION OF PATIENT FOR SURGERY

There is no special need for preoperative preparation for patients with mild to moderate varus knee deformity. But for severe deformity with major bony defect, augmentation metal blocks or wedges, allograft, or modular stems may be needed intraoperatively. And preparation of constrained prosthesis or modular inserts is advised for inadvertent overrelease or instability.

SURGICAL CONSIDERATIONS

Indications

Careful preoperative evaluation should be made to determine the indication for TKA surgery. Generally, the prime indications for TKA in patients with varus knee are still severe pain and functional disability, deformity, instability, and loss of motion.[4] However, before TKA surgery is selected, the patient should undergo conservative treatment for at least half a year without obvious effect.

Contraindications

Recent or active infection of the knee or its adjacent metaphysis of the femur or tibia remains an absolute contraindication to TKA. If any possibility of infection exists, two-stage arthroplasty should be considered. Other absolute contraindications include inadequate soft tissue coverage of the knee with or without associated poor vascularity. Those patients with severe peripheral vascular disease are also not candidates for joint arthroplasty. In addition, these patients who have cardiopulmonary insufficiency and cannot stand the anesthesia should not immediately undergo surgery; those situations should be considered as relative contraindications.

Anatomy of Varus Knee

Before performing soft tissue release, essential anatomy and function of the medial structures of the knee should be well acknowledged. These structures include superficial and deep medial collateral ligament (SMCL and DMCL), semimembranosus (SM), pes anserinus, posterior oblique ligament (POL), joint capsule, and posterior cruciate ligament (PCL).[5]

Superficial medial collateral ligament and posterior oblique ligament

The SMCL has its tibial insertion on the medial aspect of the upper tibia and femoral insertion on the medial epicondyle. The POL is a part of the MCL and its fibers run in an oblique fashion from the upper aspect of the SMCL fibers to the posteromedial aspect of the proximal tibial flare.

The SMCL functions as the primary restraint against valgus stress and a restraint to external rotation of the tibia. The anterior portion of the SMCL is under tension from full extension to 90° of flexion, but becomes maximally taut at 90° of flexion. The posterior oblique portion of the SMCL has the maximal tension at full extension.

Semimembranosus

The SM has five insertions to the posteromedial aspect of the tibia and blends with the POL and the posterior capsule. The SM affects mainly the extension space. Release of this structure is usually only necessary in cases of significant varus deformity with flexion deformity.

Pes anserine tendons

The insertions of the sartorius, gracilis, and semitendinosus lie in order from superior to inferior just medial to the proximal portion of the anterior crest of the tibia and constitute the pes anserinus. These tendons also affect mainly the extension gap. In general, this structure does not need to be released unless a significant varus deformity is still present after other structures have been released.

Posterior cruciate ligament

The PCL is a posterior and medial structure of the knee and functions as a secondary stabilizer of medial side of the knee. It has the maximal taut at full flexion. In a varus knee, the PCL is often contracted.

SURGICAL TECHNIQUE

Approach

A standard surgical approach of midline incision followed by medial parapatellar arthrotomy is most commonly used to obtain adequate exposure in most cases of varus knee. The approach can also be extended proximally or distally to achieve greater exposure with excellent visualization of both medial and lateral structures and minimal neurovascular injury.[6,7] A bent Hohman retractor should be placed in the lateral aspect of the tibial plateau to retract the extensor mechanism laterally and aid in exposure. Care should be taken to minimize tension on the extensor mechanism to prevent avulsion of the insertion on the tuberosity.

Subvastus arthrotomy and midvastus muscle-splitting approach can also be used in the varus knee if the leg is not too fat or too muscular.[8] These two approaches could benefit the postoperative rehabilitation by preserving a larger portion of the extensor mechanism. However, difficulty in retraction or eversion of the patella may cause inadequate exposure.[9]

Procedure

For patients with mild varus deformity, a standard surgical technique can be used to obtain a stable and balanced knee. However, for a moderate or severe fixed varus case, further medial soft tissue release may be necessary. In addition, some special techniques may be needed for some retractable severe deformity.[4]

Standard Technique

Medial exposure and preliminary release

The standard procedure includes preliminary medial soft tissue release and standard tibial and femoral resection. Preliminary medial soft tissue release is a part of the normal exposure procedure during TKA, which includes releasing the tibial insertion of the capsule, the DMCL, and the posteromedial corner of the knee joint. Generally, the anteromedial tibial soft tissue sleeve is released approximately 1 to 2 cm below the medial joint line by subperiosteal dissection with a scalpel or electrocautery (Fig. 63-2, B and C).[5,10,11]

Removal of osteophytes

The presence of osteophytes on the medial aspect of the tibial plateau and femoral condyle can substantially tighten the medial soft tissue sleeve. Removal of the osteophytes that impede on the medial structures is often enough to provide a balanced flexion and extension gap in the minimal to moderate varus knee (Fig. 63-2A).[12]

Tibial bone cut

The tibial and femoral bone cuts are normally performed by using the measured resection technique in the varus knee. Gap technique may be difficult to use because of medial tissue contracture and gross imbalance. The tibial bone cut should be perpendicular to the mechanical axis of the tibia, and approximately 8 to 10 mm of bone from the normal lateral tibial plateau should be removed.[13] Medial defects of the tibial plateau may remain after bone resection. Any attempt to eliminate any existing medial tibial defects by bone cut should be avoided, especially when severe medial tibial bone loss is present.[13-15] By removing the defect, softer cancellous bone can be exposed, and the bearing surface of the proximal tibia may become smaller. This may impair the matching between tibial and femoral implant and the long-term fixation of tibial tray. Yet, an additional 1 to 2 mm of tibia bone cut is reasonable for reducing the bone defect.[14] The medial defects of the tibial plateau can be addressed with cement, metal augment, or bone graft.[16-18] For the sclerotic surface of the tibia, some holes should be drilled to fix cement. Occasionally, the tibial component can be shifted slightly laterally, away from the medial defect, so that it rests on healthier, intact bone.

Femoral bone cut

The distal femoral cut is generally performed with 5° to 7° valgus relative to the femoral intramedullary canal. But this angle can be adjusted according to the HKS angle measured on the long-standing AP X-ray. At this point, the width and balance of femorotibial gap in extension of the knee should be checked. The cause of any imbalance should be analyzed. The posterior condyle should be checked for major defects, and a decision must be made as to whether the posterior condylar axis could be used as the reference of rotational orientation of femoral resection. The transepicondyle line may be used if a posterior condyle defect is present.[13]

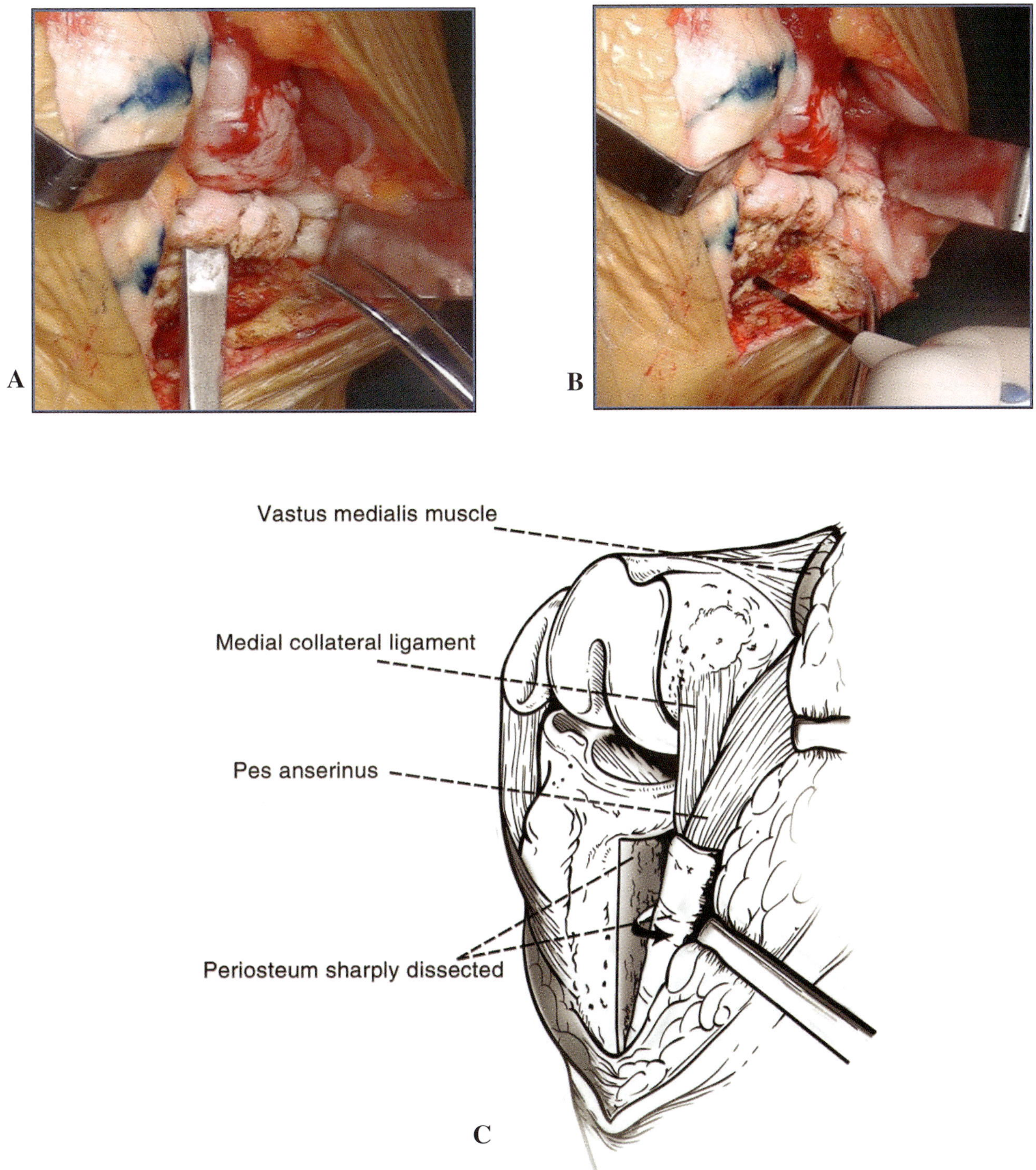

FIGURE 63-2. *Osteophytes on the medial aspect of the tibial plateau are removed by osteotome (**A**), then the anteromedial side of the tibia is released with electrocautery (**B**). (**C**) Illustration of subperiosteal dissection in anteromedial aspect.*

Medial Soft Tissue Release Technique

If the soft tissue balance in flexion and extension cannot be achieved with the standard surgical technique, further medial releasing may be necessary. This is often encountered in moderate to severe fixed varus knee deformities.[4,5,19,20]

Medial soft tissue release may be the most important step in the procedure of arthroplasty of varus knee. The goal of release is to lengthen the medial structure to create a rectangular space between the cut surfaces of the femur and the tibia. This space should be approximately equal in flexion and extension. Inadequate release may cause residual deformity, which may limit the range of motion, accelerate polyethylene wear, or cause premature loosening. Conversely, overrelease may cause instability.

Contractured soft tissue in the fixed varus deformity can often be classified as dynamic and static stabilizers. The dynamic stabilizers are the compliant musculotendinous structures such as pes anserinus and the semimembranosus tendon complex. The static stabilizers include the medial and posteromedial capsule, the SMCL, the DMCL, and the POL.[21] To release these structures effectively and safely, a proper sequence should be taken.[22] Not every surgeon agrees on the details of the procedure; the authors prefer the following order of steps.

Step 1: Release the DMCL and the posteromedial corner of the knee.

Step 2: Remove all osteophytes on the femur and the tibia.

Step 3: Release the POL and the posterior capsule.

Step 4: Release the SM tendons.

Step 5: Further release the SMCL, up to 6 to 8 cm, and release the pes anserinus.

The release of the DMCL and posteromedial corner (step 1) and removal of all osteophytes (step 2) are usually performed during the standard surgical techniques as described previously.

The next step is to release the POL and the posterior medial capsule (step 3). This step is especially indicated when the knee has varus flexion deformity and is tighter in extension than in flexion after bone resection (Fig. 63-3).[5] The posterior medial capsule can be released by periosteal elevator (or curved osteotome) from behind the posterior femoral condyle and/or from the posterior medial tibia, or cut between the femur and the tibia. Care should be taken not to injure the posterior structures, including the blood vessels (Fig. 63-4).

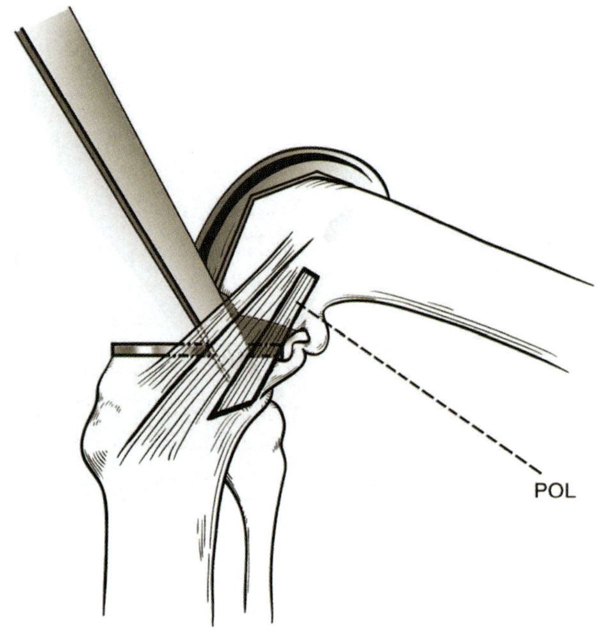

FIGURE 63-3. *Illustration of the release of POL on the posteromedial aspect of the upper tibia.*

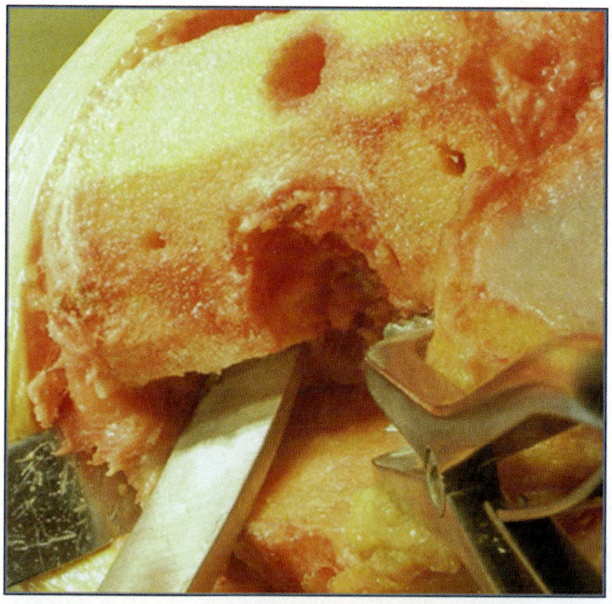

FIGURE 63-4. *The posteromedial capsule is released from behind the posterior femoral condyle using a curved osteotome; osteophytes are also removed.*

If imbalance with medial tightness continues after step 3, releasing of the SM tendons (step 4) may be necessary, especially with severe varus deformity or combined varus with flexion contracture deformity.[5] The release of the SM tendon affects the extension space more than the flexion space. Sharp dissection can proceed posteromedially with the tibia externally rotated and the knee flexed after the osteophytes in this area are removed (Fig. 63-5B).

During the release in Steps 3 and 4, it is difficult to expose these structures since they are located in the posteromedial corner of the knee. A "4" figure position of the knee can facilitate access to these structures (Fig. 63-5A). With the patient supine, the ipsilateral hip is flexed and externally rotated, the knee is flexed, the tibia is externally rotated and shifted anteriorly with a Hohman retractor, and the posteromedial corner is well exposed.

The final step of medial soft tissue release is to release the SMCL, up to 6 to 8 cm if needed, and the pes anserinus (step 5). The SMCL is the most important medial stable structure. It has been demonstrated to affect both the flexion and extension gaps.[21] Release of the anterior portion of this ligament affects the flexion gap more than the extension space. Yet release of the posterior portion can increase the extension more than the flexion gap. With the knee placed in either flexion or extension, the surgeon pulls the leg of the patient or uses a laminar spreader to stretch the soft tissue envelope. Then the tension of the SMCL can be palpated with one finger, and the tightest portion can be identified, and release can be done by passing the osteotome distally and subperiosteally at the tightest part. The release is continued until tension on the laminar spreader is reduced and the imbalance is corrected. Since the release of the SMCL has the potential risk of overlengthening or instability, careful assessment of the cause of the imbalance is necessary before putting an osteotome under this ligament. When a tightened SMCL has undergone release, the elevation should be done gently and slowly and the instrument should be well controlled by two hands. Multiple reassessments of soft tissue balance are necessary to prevent potential overrelease. Normally, the pes anserinus does not need to be released in the varus knee. And some surgeons believe this release could not increase much of the space. However, when evaluation shows this structure to be the culprit for imbalance, it can be released.

In particular, the PCL must be assessed for balance as well when a cruciate-retaining (CR) prosthesis is used. The PCL, which is situated in the intercondylar notch, originates from the medial femoral condyle and inserts at the posterior aspect of the tibia. The PCL can be released at its femoral insertion. The knee is put at 90° flexion with tibial and femoral trial in place; the PCL is touched with the index finger and the tightest part of the ligament is pointed with a cautery until it gets the proper tension. Or it can be released at the tibial insertion by elevation subperiosteally under the PCL downward. Proper tension is not easy to achieve, and a taut PCL can add to medial tension, especially in flexion, causing imbalance, spin-out, and increased polyethylene wear. Conversely, a loose PCL can cause paradox anterior translation of the femur.

A B

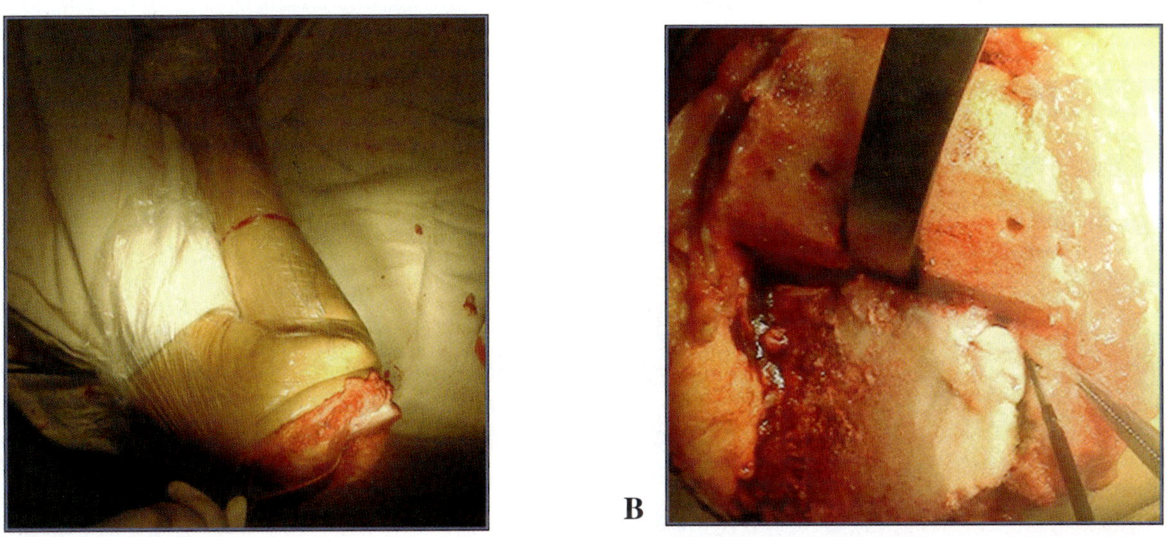

FIGURE 63-5. *With the patient supine, the hip flexed and externally rotated, the knee maximally flexed, and the tibia dislocated anteriorly, the posteromedial side of the knee is well exposed (**A**). The posteromedial corner, posterior oblique ligament, and semimembranosus could be released (**B**).*

Medial Tibial Reduction Osteotomy

This technique is based on the principle that the MCL is indirectly lengthened by downsizing and lateralizing the tibial component and removing the exposed proximal medial tibia around the component. This procedure was first described by Dixon et al and recommended as an adjunct to the medial soft tissue release for moderate to severe varus deformity.[23] After standard tibial bone resection, trial components can be used to assess the coverage and the soft tissue balance (Fig. 63-6A). If balance is unacceptable and the proximal tibia has enough bearing surface, a smaller sized (usually one size smaller) trial component is used (Fig. 63-6B). The downsized tibial component is lateralized to the lateral cortical margin of the tibia and the remaining medial tibial overhang is removed flush with the medial edge of the tibial tray by a vertical saw cut (Fig. 63-6C). This technique could minimize the medial flare of the proximal tibia and help to balance the space without extensive soft tissue release. In addition, releasing the contracted medial soft tissue sleeve along with relative medialization of the tibial tubercle may improve the patellar tracking. This technique, however, may increase the stress on the downsized tibial component. It is best reserved for cases in which the tibial component is found to be between sizes.

A

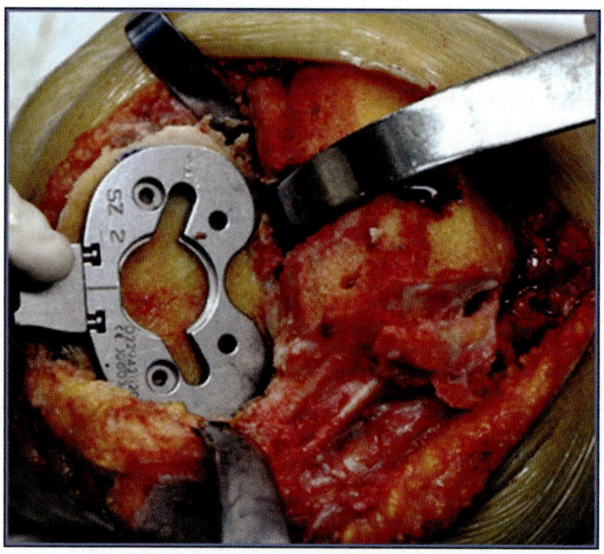

B

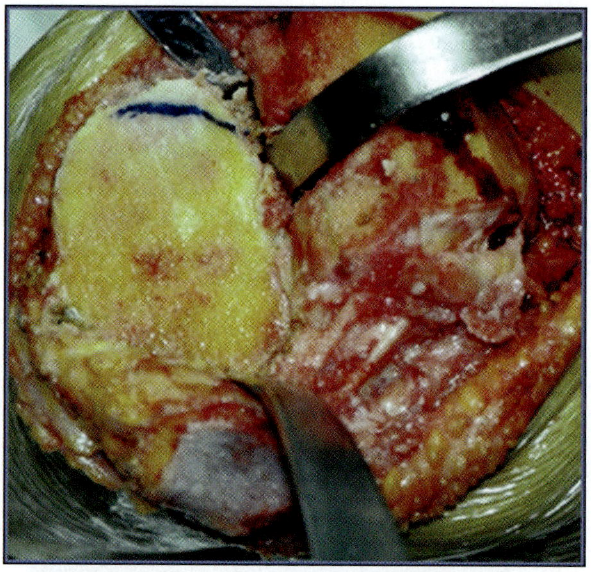

C

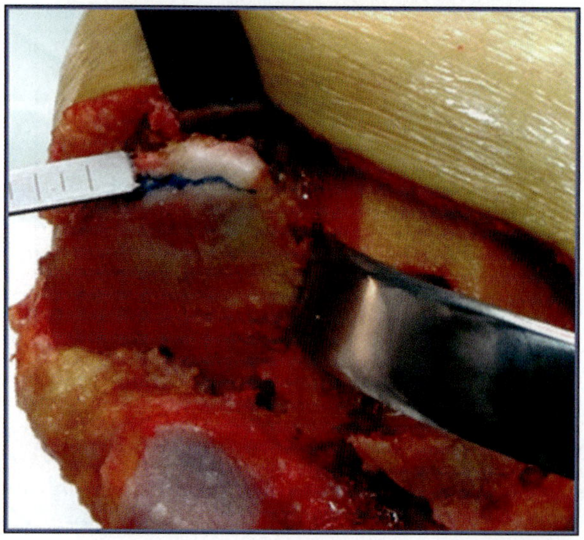

FIGURE 63-6. *Appropriate downsizing and lateralization of the tibial tray on the proximal tibia. (**A**) Templating with the trial. (**B**) The resection area of the medial side of the tibial plateau is marked. (**C**) The medial side of the tibial plateau is cut by saw along the marked line.*

Pie Crust and Needle Puncture Techniques

The pie crust technique was originally used for releasing the iliotibial band in the valgus knee.[24-26] It can effectively lengthen the contracted ligament or tendon via multiple stab incisions in the tightest portion. In varus knee deformity, the pie crust technique is mainly used to address the contracted SMCL by making multiple horizontal perforations in the tight fibers of the SMCL.[27] The procedure can be done from the inside-out at the joint line level using a No. 11 blade (Fig. 63-7A) and can specifically and individually lengthen the contracted SMCL fibers by approximately 6 to 8 mm in both flexion and extension.

An alternative procedure is the needle puncture technique. It is indicated for moderate varus deformity.[28] A standard 19-gauge aspiration needle is used to pierce the tensest fibers by puncturing in a perpendicular or slightly oblique fashion (Fig. 63-7B), whereas the knee is stressed in valgus. Punctures are performed every 3 to 5 mm apart proximodistally and anteroposteriorly through both the tight fibers of the SMCL as well as the DMCL. The punctures are carried out respectively in extension or flexion only, or in both, depending on the tightness observed by palpation; the mediolateral balance of the knee is reassessed every 5 to 10 punctures until the appropriate release is achieved.

Medial Epicondyle Osteotomy

Medial femoral epicondylar osteotomy was developed by Engh and is indicated for the most severe fixed varus deformities, especially for the combined deformity with a fixed flexion contracture.[29,30] The procedure is performed in 90° of knee flexion. All the synovial tissue on the medial femoral condyle should be excised to expose the epicondyle. The osteotomy is performed with an osteotome or an oscillating saw directed in the long axis of the femur. A wafer of bone approximately 1 cm thick and 4 cm in diameter is separated from the condyle. After implantation of total knee components, the wafer of bone needs to be reattached to the medial femoral condyle with No. 2 or heavier nonabsorbable suture or by a screw with washer. The osteotomized wafer of bone should be placed somewhat distal and posterior to the original location. Proper position of this bony fragment could be done by placing the knee in extension and then in 90° of flexion; the attached MCL will pull it to the isometric point. Sutures are placed through the epicondyle and then beneath a bridge of metaphyseal cortical bone that represents the junction between the anterior femoral resection and the adjacent epicondylar osteotomy (Fig. 63-8). A minimum of two to three sutures is recommended to

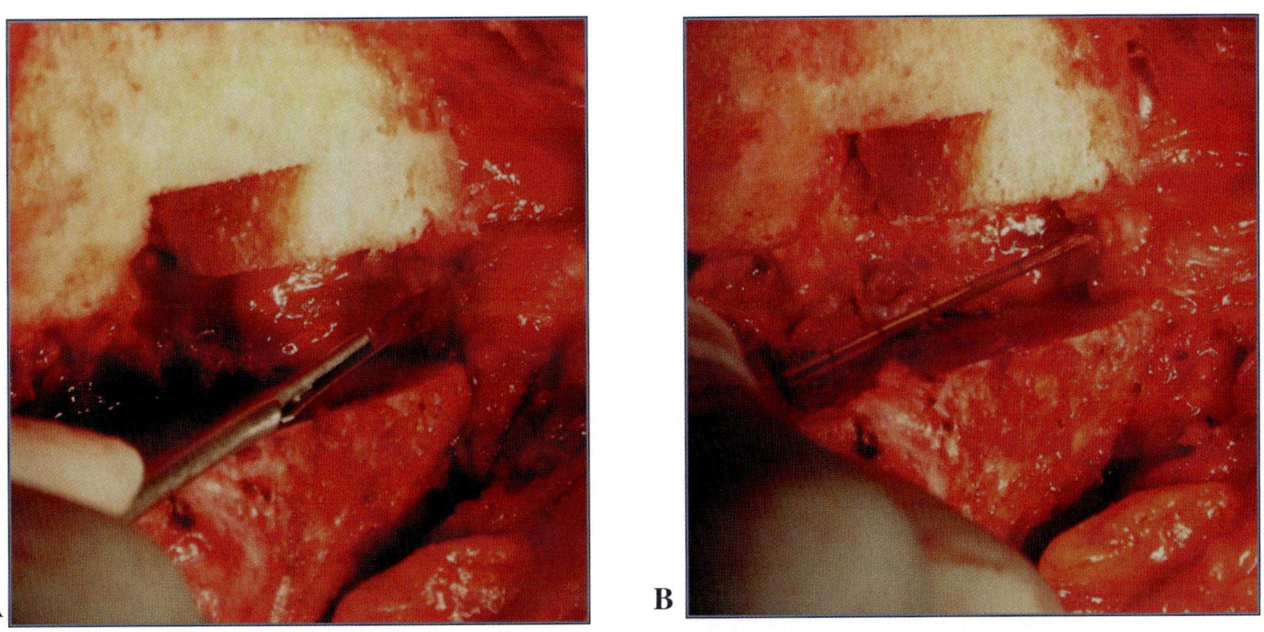

A B

FIGURE 63-7. *The medial collateral ligament is pierced with a No. 11 blade in a "pie crust" fashion (**A**) or a needle in a "needle puncture" fashion (**B**).*

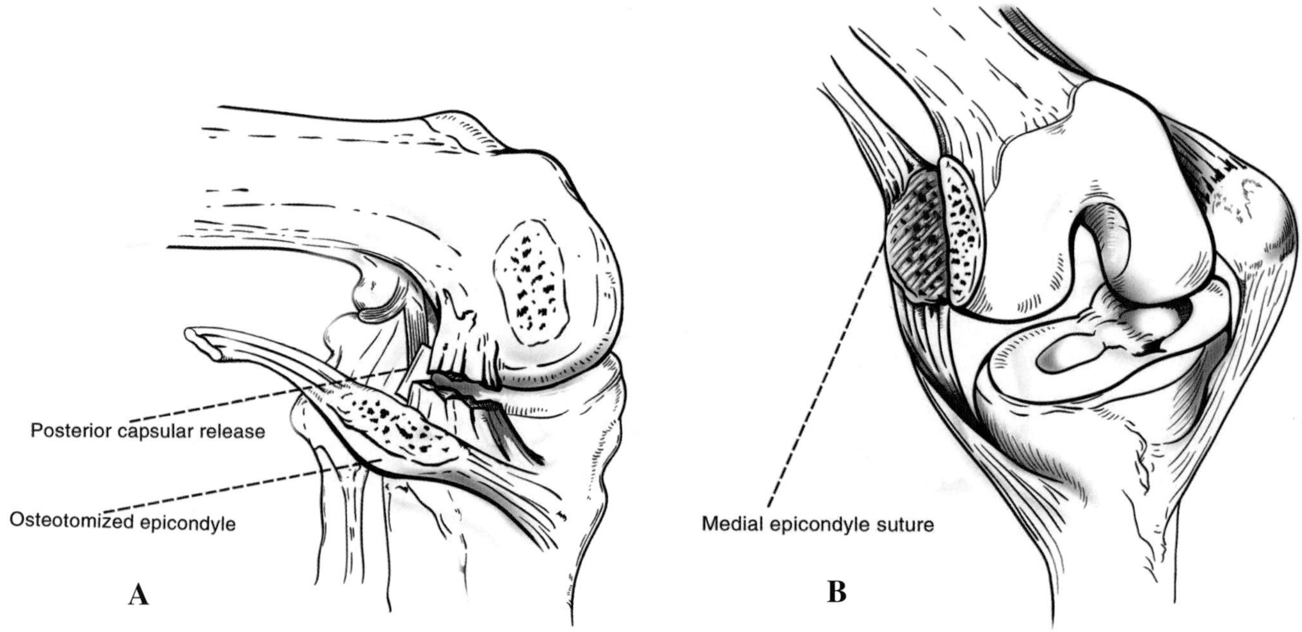

FIGURE 63-8. *(**A**) A wafer of bone is separated from the condyle along the long axis of the femur at 90° of flexion. (**B**) Suture repair of the epicondyle in flexion, maintaining the femoral origin of the MCL.*

restore the knee stability in flexion. While performing this procedure, the knee is stable in extension due to the proximal to distal continuity of the collateral ligaments and the adductor magnus tendon. But it is temporarily unstable in flexion on the medial side, hence a CR prosthesis is recommended to limit the potential increase in flexion space. The epicondylar osteotomy preserves the integrity of the MCL and facilitates the approach to the posterior femoral condyle for additional capsular release.[29]

Lateral Collateral Ligament Advancing Technique

The LCL advancing technique has been described by Krackow[31] and is indicated for severe varus deformities with significant lateral collateral laxity and large lateral thrust during gait. If complete release of the medial structures is performed and there continues to be an imbalance, advancing the LCL to correct the imbalance may be considered.

This procedure can be accomplished by osteotomizing the proximal fibula. The proximal fibular segment is first predrilled along the intramedullary canal for later fixation, and a transverse osteotomy of the proximal fibula is performed. Care is taken to protect the peroneal nerve as it courses around the neck of the fibula. With trial components in place, the proximal portion of the fibula with the LCL insertion is tightened until the ligament is providing adequate support to the lateral joint. The level of overlapping bone is marked, and the excess is removed. The fibular head is then fixed in place with an intramedullary screw and washer (Fig. 63-9). Also, the LCL can be advanced proximally at the femoral attachment and fixed with a washer and screw. The technique prevents overlengthening of the leg after release of the MCL.

POSTOPERATIVE REHABILITATION

Wound closure after TKA with medial release and postoperative rehabilitation are the same as with standard TKA, regardless of the technique used to correct the varus deformity.

COMPLICATIONS

Complications that are relatively common in varus knee arthroplasty are often related to soft tissue balance and

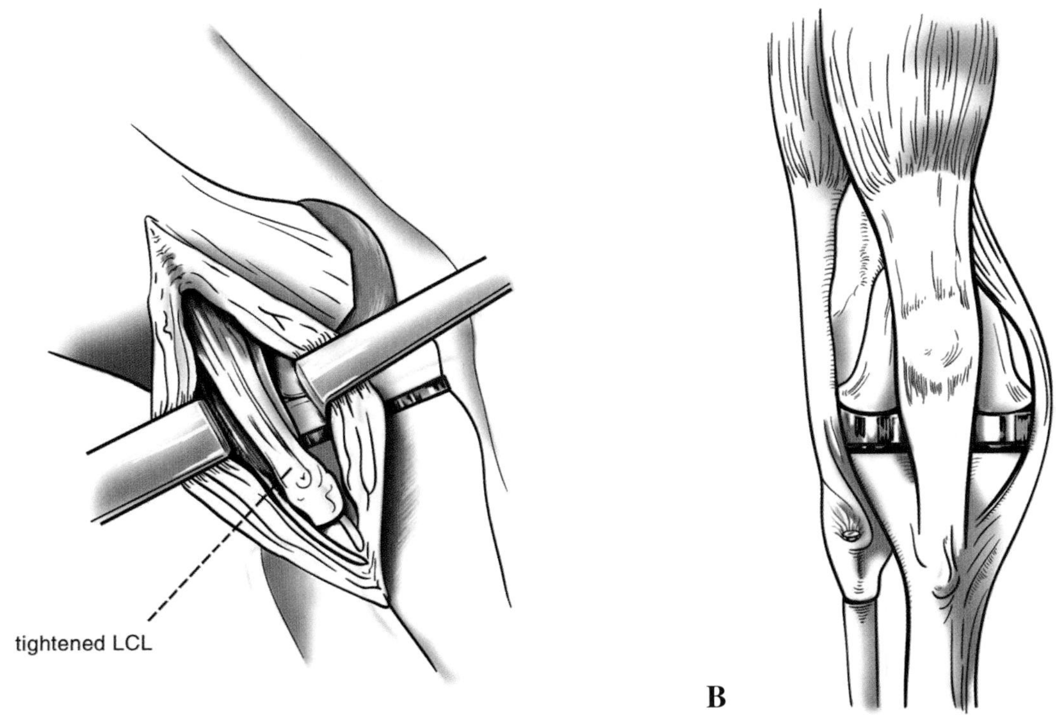

FIGURE 63-9. *Proximal portion of the fibula with the LCL insertion tightened in place with an intramedullary screw and washer.*

alignment. Inadequate release will cause residual imbalance, which may cause knee symptoms and asymmetric wear of the insert leading to premature failure of the TKA. Hence meticulous assessment with tensional device, measuring blocks, or trial components is necessary to make sure the balance is acceptable.

Overrelease of the medial soft structures during subperiosteal dissection is a common intraoperative complication in fixed varus deformity. It can be avoided by intermittently checking the balance while doing the soft tissue release. Once overrelease is committed, varied degrees of instability of the knee will occur. The greatest instability happens when the knee is in flexion. Different techniques of medial soft tissue sleeve or MCL repair or tensioning have been described. Suture anchors can be used to tighten the MCL by screwing one to two anchors into the anteromedial tibial cortex about 1 cm anterior to the MCL insertion and pulling the anterior portion of the MCL anteriorly with the attached wire, with the knee in 30° of flexion. Staples can be used to fix the overreleased MCL in the similar way.

A complete cut of the SMCL in performing the pie crust technique is perhaps the most difficult problem to handle. Repair could be accomplished with a trial tibial insert 2 mm thinner than the final insert to be placed. A full-length knee brace should be used after operation to protect ligament repair. Residual medial laxity or instability is common no matter what technique has been used for amendment of the overrelease. Changing the prosthesis to a constrained one or using a modular high post constrained insert intraoperatively may be the wisest and safest solution for this difficult situation.

Alignment in varus knee arthroplasty is relatively more difficult, especially in cases with massive bone defect or with primary or secondary extra-articular deformity. In the former situation, a stem may be helpful for both keeping the alignment and neutralizing the stress. In the latter situation, careful preoperative planning should be done, extra-articular guiding should be used, and navigation may be helpful in the really serious case.

OUTCOMES

The techniques described in this chapter for releasing the medial structures, balancing the collateral ligaments, and restoring the normal alignment of the knee have been proven to be successful. The survivorship data and results of clinical and radiographic follow-up studies have shown that TKA for treating knee arthroplasty with varus deformity is both predictable and durable.

Recently, Bae et al[32] reported the results of TKA using a CR prosthesis (67 knees) or posterior-stabilized implants (70 knees) in patients with slight deformity of approximately 4.1° varus. The increased Knee Society score (KSS) and function score did not vary significantly between the different prostheses and the postoperative alignment was corrected to varus 5.8°. The clinical outcome of TKA for the slight varus deformity was satisfactory after a follow-up of 3.9 years, no matter whether the PCL was retained or sacrificed.

As for moderate varus deformity of the knee, Laskin[33] reported that the CR prosthesis in knees with a deformity of greater than 15° varus contracture led to statistically inferior results, such as less range of motion, greater pain, and increased loosening, at a mean follow-up of 10 years. All these results suggest that a posterior cruciate release should be performed and a posterior-stabilized type of implant should be used for the patient with a fixed moderate varus contracture. However, another study reported that TKA using a CR prosthesis in patients with varus deformity of at least 15° can present good results with a 93% revision-free survivorship at 10 years and no revisions for instability or loosening.[34]

Implant longevity and improved function after TKA in severe varus deformity have also been reported. Dixon et al[23] presented the correction of a mean varus deformity of up to 24° by using a technique of downsizing and lateralizing the tibial component in 12 knees. The femorotibial angle was corrected to an average of 4° valgus postoperatively, and the KSS increased from 24 preoperatively to 94 at a mean follow-up of 42 months. Another study compared 39 primary TKAs using PCL-retaining prostheses for severe varus deformity of 20° with much less severe deformity at an approximately 6-year follow-up. There was no statistical difference in knee score, alignment, or revision.[35]

In a series of studies, the technique of reduction osteotomy of posteromedial tibial flare was used to treat severe intra- and extra-articular varus deformity of greater than 20° in 173 knees.[36-38] At an average follow-up of 2.6 years, mean KSS improved from 22.8 to 91.1 and function score from 22.8 to 72.1. Mean femorotibial varus of 22.8 preoperatively was corrected to 5.38 valgus postoperatively. Of 30 grafts for posteromedial tibial defects, 28 were successfully incorporated without reported significant instability. Only three knees (1.7%) showed tibial component loosening with recurrence of deformity. These techniques were proven to be reliable in restoring alignment and stability without the need for constrained implants. To conclude, although some studies have been reported with satisfactory clinical outcomes after the short-term or midterm follow-up of TKA in varus knee, the results of long-term follow-up of more than 20 years still need to be known in a large patient cohort.

PEARLS AND PITFALLS

Attention should be paid to adhere to some principles when performing TKA for varus knee. Before operation, the type of deformity should be identified. Correctable varus deformity mainly caused by bone and cartilage defect is relatively easy to address by standard TKA alone and further medial soft tissue release is usually unnecessary. Fixed varus deformity is relatively more complex and needs further medial soft tissue release or special techniques. Some key points for the performance of medial soft tissue release need to be acknowledged.

- The medial structure release should be done with proper sequence. Not every surgeon agrees with the exact steps of the sequential release.
- Release should be done millimeter by millimeter. Carefully titrate the medial release at each stage; palpate the remaining medial soft tissue envelope with a finger and identify particular areas of tightness. Intermittent reassessment of gaps is important to avoid overrelease.
- An intact soft tissue sleeve at the anteromedial part of the tibia must be maintained. Subperiosteal release is necessary during the whole maneuver. An interrupted soft tissue sleeve may cause instability of the medial side or difficulty in wound closure.
- When assessing soft tissue balancing, it should be remembered that the medial structure is naturally tighter than the lateral side. Two to three millimeters of more laxity on the lateral side is acceptable during the toggle test with the trial in place.
- When big osteophytes exist on the X-ray, more care should be paid to the tenuated medial tissue; the deformity is often not as difficult as estimated to correct. The balance is usually achieved dramatically when the osteophytes are removed. So, do not do too much release before performing this step.
- Varus knee caused by extra-articular deformity is usually more fixed. Medial soft tissue releasing usually needs to be more extensive, and balance is more difficult to achieve.

- Puncture release, like the pie crust technique, is not as safe as a lateral release because the medial collateral ligament is a narrower string. It should be used with great caution.

SUGGESTED READING

Whiteside LA. Soft-tissue balancing: the knee. *J Arthroplasty.* 2002;17(4 suppl 1):23-27.

REFERENCES

1. Laskin RS, Schob CJ. Medial capsular recession for severe varus deformities. *J Arthroplasty.* 1987;2:313.
2. Teeny SM, Krackow KA, Hungerford DS. Primary total knee arthroplasty in patients with severe varus deformity. A comparative study. *Clin Orthop Relat Res.* 1991;273:19-31.
3. Robbins GM, Masri BA, Garbuz DS, et al. Preoperative planning to prevent instability in total knee arthroplasty. *Orthop Clin North Am.* 2001; 32(4):611-626.
4. Karachalios T, Sarangi PP, Newman JH. Severe varus deformities treated by total knee arthroplasty. *J Bone Joint Surg Br.* 1994;76(6):938-942.
5. Mihalko WM, Saleh KJ, Krackow KA, et al. Soft-tissue balancing during total knee arthroplasty in the varus knee. *J Am Acad Orthop Surg.* 2009;17(12): 766-774.
6. Insall JN. A mid-line approach to the knee. *J Bone Joint Surg Am.* 1971;53:1584.
7. Insall JN. Total knee replacement. In: Insall JN, ed. *Surgery of the Knee.* New York: Churchill Livingstone; 1984.
8. Keating EM, Faris PM, Meding JB, et al. Comparison of the midvastus muscle-splitting approach with the median parapatellar approach in total knee arthroplasty. *J Arthroplasty.* 1999;14(1): 29-32.
9. Maestro A, Suarez MA, Rodriguez L, et al. The midvastus surgical approach in total knee arthroplasty. *Int Orthop.* 2000;24:104-107.
10. Saeki K, Mihalko WM, Patel V, et al. Stability after medial collateral ligament release in total knee arthroplasty. *Clin Orthop Relat Res.* 2001;392:184-189.
11. Matsueda M, Gengerke TR, Murphy M, et al. Soft tissue release in total knee arthroplasty. Cadaver study using knees without deformities. *Clin Orthop Relat Res.* 1999;366:264-273.
12. Mihalko WM, Whiteside LA, Krackow KA. Comparison of ligament-balancing techiniques during total knee arthroplasty. *J Bone Joint Surg Am.* 2003; 85:132.
13. Brooks P. Seven cuts to the perfect total knee. *Orthopedics.* 2009;32(9):680.
14. Plaskos C, Hodgson AJ, Inkpen K, et al., Bone cutting errors in total knee arthroplasty. *J Arthroplasty.* 2002; 17(6):698-705.
15. Bäthis H, Perlick L, Tingart M, et al. Intraoperative cutting errors in total knee arthroplasty. *Arch Orthop Trauma Surg.* 2005;125(1):16-20.
16. Dorr LD, Ranawat CS, Sculco TA, et al. Bone graft for tibial defects in total knee arthroplasty. *Clin Orthop Relat Res.* 2006;446:4-9.
17. Cuckler JM. Bone loss in total knee arthroplasty: graft augment and options. *J Arthroplasty.* 2004;19(4 suppl 1):56-58.
18. Engh GA, Ammeen DJ. Bone loss with revision total knee arthroplasty: defect classification and alternatives for reconstruction. *Instr Course Lect.* 1999;49:167-175.
19. Engh GA. The difficult knee. Severe varus and valgus. *Clin Orthop Relat Res.* 2003(416):58-63.
20. Whiteside LA, Saeki K, Mihalko WM. Functional ligament balancing in total knee arthroplasty. *Clin Orthop Relat Res.* 2000;380:45.
21. Peters CL. Soft-tissue balancing in primary total knee arthroplasty. *Instr Course Lect.* 2006;55:413-417.
22. Yagishita K, Muneta T, Ikeda H. Step-by-step measurements of soft tissue balancing during total knee arthroplasty for patients with varus knees. *J Arthroplasty.* 2003;18:313.
23. Dixon MC, Parsch D, Brown RR, et al. The correction of severe varus deformity in total knee arthroplasty by tibial component downsizing and resection of uncapped proximal medial bone. *J Arthroplasty.* 2004;19(1):19-22.
24. Mihalko WM, Krackow KA. Anatomic and biomechanical aspects of pie crusting posterolateral structures for valgus deformity correction in total knee arthroplasty: a cadaveric study. *J Arthroplasty.* 2000;15(3):347-353.
25. Clarke HD, Schwartz JB, Math KR, et al. Anatomic risk of peroneal nerve injury with the "pie crust"

technique for valgus release in total knee arthroplasty. *J Arthroplasty.* 2004;19(1):40-44.

26. Clarke HD, Fuchs R, Scuderi GR, et al. Clinical results in valgus total knee arthroplasty with the "pie crust" technique of lateral soft tissue releases. *J Arthroplasty.* 2005;20(8):1010-1014.
27. Verdonk PCM, Pernin J, Pinaroli A, et al. Soft tissue balancing in varus total knee arthroplasty: an algorithmic approach. *Knee Surg Sports Traumatol Arthrosc.* 2009;17:660-666.
28. Bellemans J, Vandenneucker H, Lauwe JV, et al. A new surgical technique for medial collateral ligament balancing: multiple needle puncturing. *J Arthroplasty.* 2010;25(7):1152-1156.
29. Engh GA, Ammeen D. Result of total knee arthroplasty with medial epicondylar osteotomy to correct varus deformity. *Clin Orthop Relat Res.* 1999; 367:141-148.
30. Engh GA. Medial epicondylar osteotomy: a technique used with primary and revision total knee arthroplasty to improve surgical exposure and correct varus deformity. *Instr Course Lect.* 1999;48: 153-156.
31. Krackow KA, Phillips MJ, Mihalko WM. Ligament advancement techniques in primary and revision total knee arthroplasty. *Techn Knee Surg.* 2003;3: 138-143.
32. Bae DK, Song SJ, Cho SD. Clinical outcome of total knee arthroplasty with medial pivot prosthesis: a comparative study between the cruciate retaining and sacrificing. *J Arthroplasty.* 2011;26(5):693-698.
33. Laskin RS. Total knee replacement with posterior cruciate ligament retention in patients with a fixed varus deformity. *Clin Orthop Relat Res.* 2003(331): 29-34.
34. Kubiak P, Archibeck MJ, White RE. Cruciate-retaining total knee arthroplasty in patients with at least fifteen degrees of coronal plane deformity. *J Arthroplasty.* 2008;23(3):366-370.
35. Ritter MA, Faris GW, Faris PM, et al. Total knee arthroplasty in patients with angular varus or valgus deformities of > 20°. *J Arthroplasty.* 2004;19(7):862-865.
36. Mullaji AB, Padmanabhan V, Jindal G. Total knee arthroplasty for profound varus deformity: technique and radiological results in 173 knees with varus of more than 20 degrees. *J Arthroplasty.* 2005;20(5): 550-561.
37. Mullaji A, Marawar S, Sharma A. Correcting varus deformity. *J Arthroplasty.* 2007;22(4 suppl 1):15-19.
38. Lee BS, Lee SJ, Kim JM, et al. No impact of severe varus deformity on clinical outcome after posterior stabilized total knee arthroplasty. *Knee Surg Sports Traumatol Arthrosc.* 2011;19(6):960-966.